a **LANGE** medical book

Dermatology

a LANGE medical book

Dermatology

First Edition

Edited By:

Milton Orkin, MD
Clinical Professor
University of Minnesota School
    of Medicine
Minneapolis, Minnesota

Howard I. Maibach, MD
Professor of Dermatology
University of California School
    of Medicine
San Francisco, California

Mark V. Dahl, MD
Professor of Dermatology
University of Minnesota School
    of Medicine
Minneapolis, Minnesota

APPLETON & LANGE
Norwalk, Connecticut/San Mateo, California

0-8385-1288-7

Notice: Our knowledge in clinical sciences is constantly changing. As new
information becomes available, changes in treatment and in the use of drugs
become necessary. The authors and the publisher of this volume have taken
care to make certain that the doses of drugs and schedules of treatment are
correct and compatible with the standards generally accepted at the time of
publication. The reader is advised to consult carefully the instruction
and information material included in the package insert of each drug or
therapeutic agent before administration. This advice is especially
important when using new or infrequently used drugs.

91 92 93 94 95 / 10 9 8 7 6 5 4 3 2 1

Prentice Hall International (UK) Limited, *London*
Prentice Hall of Australia Pty. Limited, *Sydney*
Prentice Hall Canada, Inc., *Toronto*
Prentice Hall Hispanoamericana, S.A., *Mexico*
Prentice Hall of India Private Limited, *New Delhi*
Prentice Hall of Japan, Inc., *Tokyo*
Simon & Schuster Asia Pte. Ltd., *Singapore*
Editora Prentice Hall do Brasil Ltda., *Rio de Janeiro*
Prentice Hall, *Englewood Cliffs, New Jersey*

ISBN: 0–8385–1288–7
ISSN: 1051–9796

PRINTED IN THE UNITED STATES OF AMERICA

To Our Wives
Etta Fay, Siesel, and Arlene
And to the Patience and Persistence of the Chapter Authors

Table of Contents

SECTION IV: DISORDERS OF STRUCTURE & FUNCTION

Preface

Books in the Lange series are characterized by simplicity in the face of complexity. We have tried to continue this philosophy by including most of the dermatologic diseases that afflict our patients. The discussions are in the "Lange format" used so successfully in other books in the series, which consists—with variations where appropriate—in listing "Essentials of Diagnosis" followed by introductory remarks about causes, pathogenesis, incidence, and so on, and then the conventional descriptions of symptoms and signs, laboratory findings, prevention, treatment, and prognosis.

Editing the first edition of a book of this kind has been a great adventure. We have tried to impose uniformity of style and format on each chapter but we wanted each of our authors to express his or her individual style. We wanted to be comprehensive but not duplicative. If we have succeeded in these endeavors, it has only been with protracted effort on the part of everyone involved and several revision cycles. We cannot begin to express our admiration of and gratitude to the authors who have endured with us the arduous tasks involved in book publication.

Because dermatology is a visual specialty, color photographs should ideally be used to illustrate dermatologic diseases. Even with color, however, the variations that every physician knows characterize all skin diseases, the different presentations in patients with different pigmentary characteristics, and the difficulty even with excellent color photos of showing three dimensions on book paper—and above all the need to keep the book affordable by students and others—have supported our decision to depend on black and white illustrations. We have listed color atlases in our bibliographic recommendations in Chapter 6, and we urge our readers to buy one and consult it frequently while using this book.

We want this book to serve the needs of medical students, primary care physicians, and dermatologists as well as other physicians, nurses, and ancillary medical personnel. *Dermatology* will be useful both as a teaching aid and as a resource manual when difficult cases must be dealt with in daily clinical practice.

Because there is no "cookbook" way to manage dermatologic diseases successfully, we do not offer a cookbook. Once the diagnosis is made, a successful treatment plan must be devised that considers the age of the patient, the region affected, the severity of expression of the disease, and matters to do with patient compliance, for example, a topical drug's cosmetic impact, odor, and cost. For these reasons, specific treatment recommendations must always be tailored to the specific patient's specific needs.

Dosages and treatment methods in this book are for adults unless otherwise specified.

Acknowledgments

In addition to the regular reviewers, Christian G. Schrock, MD reviewed the chapters on infectious diseases. Nancy Evans, our sponsoring editor, shepherded the book through its many drafts. James Ransom, our development editor, perfected grammar, spelling, and tables. Charles Evans, our production editor, put this book into its present form. We wish to thank these special people.

Minneapolis and San Francisco
October 1990

Milton Orkin, MD
Howard I. Maibach, MD
Mark V. Dahl, MD

The Authors

Raza Aly, MPH, PhD
Professor of Dermatology and Microbiology, University of California School of Medicine, San Francisco.

Klaus E. Andersen, MD, PhD
Professor, Department of Dermatology, Odense University Hospital, Odense, Denmark.

Kenneth A. Arndt, MD
Dermatologist-in-Chief, Beth Israel Hospital, Boston; Professor of Dermatology, Harvard Medical School, Boston.

Joseph Beninson, MD
Clinical Associate Professor of Dermatology, Department of Dermatology, University of Michigan, Ann Arbor; Director, Leg Ulcer Clinic; Director, Peripheral Vascular Disease, Dermatology, Henry Ford Hospital, Detroit.

Martin M. Black, MD, FRCP
Consultant Dermatologist, St. Thomas Hospital, London; Senior Lecturer in Histopathology, Institute of Dermatology, UMDS, University of London.

Paul Brooke, MD
Chief Resident, Department of Dermatology, University of Alabama School of Medicine, Birmingham.

Turner M. Caldwell III, MD
Assistant Clinical Professor, Texas Tech University Medical School; Director, Melanoma Clinic, Harrington Regional Cancer Center, Amarillo, Texas.

Jeffrey P. Callen, MD
Professor and Chief, University of Louisville School of Medicine, Louisville.

William A. Caro, MD
Professor of Clinical Dermatology, Northwestern University Medical School, Evanston, Illinois.

Mark V. Dahl, MD
Professor of Dermatology, University of Minnesota School of Medicine, Minneapolis.

D. Joseph Demis, MD, PhD
Clinical Professor of Dermatology, Albany Medical College, Albany, New York.

José M. De Moragas, MD
Professor of Dermatology and Chairman, Department of Dermatology, Hospital, Sant Pau. Barcelona, Autonomous University.

Patricia G. Engasser, MD
Clinical Associate Professor of Dermatology, University of California School of Medicine, San Francisco.

Ervin Epstein, Jr., MD
Clinical Professor of Dermatology, University of California, San Francisco.

Ervin Epstein, Sr., MD
Associate Clinical Professor of Dermatology, University of California School of Medicine, San Francisco.

John H. Epstein, MD
Clinical Professor of Dermatology, University of California School of Medicine, San Francisco.

Nancy B. Esterly, MD
Professor of Pediatrics, Professor of Dermatology, Medical College of Wisconsin, Milwaukee.

David S. Feingold, MD
Professor and Chairman, Department of Dermatology, Tufts University School of Medicine, Boston.

Yehudi M. Felman, MD
Clinical Professor of Dermatology, Downstate Medical School, Brooklyn.

Jo-David Fine, MD
Associate Professor and Director of Dermatologic Research, Department of Dermatology, University of Alabama School of Medicine; Chief, Dermatology Section, Birmingham Veterans Administration Medical Center, Birmingham.

Frederick S. Fish, MD
Director, Department of Dermatology and Cutaneous Surgery, St. Paul Ramsey Medical Center; Assistant Clinical Professor of Dermatology, University of Minnesota, Minneapolis.

Mitchell H. Friedlaender, MD
Division of Ophthalmology, Scripps Clinic and Research Foundation, La Jolla, California.

Lowell A. Goldsmith, MD
Professor and Chair, Department of Dermatology, and James H. Sterner Professor of Dermatology, University of Rochester, Rochester, New York.

Robert W. Goltz, MD
Professor of Medicine/Dermatology, University of California, San Diego School of Medicine, San Diego.

David J. Gross, MD
Dermatology Resident, University of Arkansas for Medical Sciences, Little Rock.

Leonard C. Harber, MD
Rhodebeck Professor and Chairman, Department of Dermatology, Columbia University College of Physicians and Surgeons; Director, Dermatology Service, Presbyterian Hospital, New York.

Harry J. Hurley, MD, DSc (Med)
Clinical Professor of Dermatology, University of Pennsylvania, Philadelphia.

Michael T. Jarratt, MD
Clinical Associate Professor, Baylor College of Medicine, Austin, Texas.

Henry Earl Jones, MD
Clinical Professor of Dermatology, Emory University School of Medicine, Atlanta, Georgia.

Harold B. Kaiser, MD
Clinical Professor of Medicine, University of Minnesota Medical School, Minneapolis.

Edward A. Krull, MD
Chairman, Department of Dermatology, Henry Ford Hospital, Detroit.

Christy A. Lorton, MD
Clinical Instructor, Department of Dermatology, University of Cincinnati Medical Center, Cincinnati.

Alan Lyell, MD, FRCPE
Consultant in Charge of Skin Department, Royal Infirmary, Glasgow, Scotland.

Howard I. Maibach, MD
Professor, Dermatology, University of California School of Medicine, San Francisco.

Sandy Martin, MD
Clinical Assistant Professor, Dermatology and Cutaneous Surgery, University of Miami School of Medicine, Miami; Staff, Delray Community Hospital, Delray Beach, Florida.

Charles Gordon Toby Mathias, MD
Dermatology Consultant, Group Health Associates, Cincinnati, Ohio; Associate Clinical Professor, Department of Dermatology and Environmental Health, University of Cincinnati Medical Center, Cincinnati.

Karen C. McKoy, MD
Clinical Instructor, Department of Dermatology, Harvard Medical School, Boston.

Beno Michel, MD
Clinical Professor of Dermatology, Case Western Reserve University, Cleveland.

Samuel L. Moschella, MD
Clinical Professor, Harvard Medical School, Boston.

Jess Mottaz, BS
Research Fellow in Dermatology, University of Minnesota School of Medicine, Minneapolis.

Sigfrid A. Muller, MD
Professor and Chairman, Department of Dermatology, Mayo Medical School and Mayo Clinic, Rochester, Minnesota.

James J. Nordlund, MD
Professor and Chairman, Department of Dermatology, University of Cincinnati College of Medicine, Cincinnati.

Milton Orkin, MD
Clinical Professor, University of Minnesota School of Medicine, Minneapolis.

Amy S. Paller, MD
Associate Professor of Pediatrics and Dermatology, Northwestern University School of Medicine, Evanston, Illinois; Head, Division of Dermatology, The Children's Memorial Hospital, Chicago.

Frank Parker, MD
Professor and Chairman, Department of Dermatology, Oregon Health Sciences University, Portland.

John M. Pelachyk, MD
Director of Dermatopathology, Department of Dermatology, Henry Ford Hospital, Detroit; Clinical Assistant Professor, Department of Dermatology, University of Michigan Medical School, Ann Arbor.

Paul G. Quie, MD
Professor of Pediatrics, University of Minnesota School of Medicine, Minneapolis.

Harry H. Roenigk, Jr., MD
Walter J. Hamlin Professor of Dermatology; Chairman, Department of Dermatology, Northwestern University Medical School, Evanston, Illinois.

Roy S. Rogers III, MD
Professor of Dermatology, Mayo Medical School, Rochester, Minnesota.

Theodore Rosen, MD
Associate Professor of Dermatology, Baylor College of Medicine; Chief of Dermatology, Veterans Administration Medical Center, Houston, Texas.

Bijan Safai, MD
Memorial Sloan-Kettering Cancer Center, New York.

Peter Derrick Samman, MD, FRCP
Honorary Consultant, St. John's Hospital for Diseases of the Skin; Honorary Consultant, Westminster Hospital, London.

Walter B. Shelley, MD, PhD
Professor of Dermatology, Medical College of Ohio, Toledo.

Robert S. Stern, MD
Associate Professor of Dermatology, Beth Israel Hospital, Harvard Medical School, Boston.

John S. Strauss, MD
Professor and Head, Department of Dermatology, University of Iowa College of Medicine, Iowa City.

Frank Taliercio, MD
Director, Dermatology Division, St. Agnes Hospital; Clinical Instructor in Dermatology, New York Medical College, White Plains, New York.

Gerhard Tappeiner, MD
Associate Professor of Dermatology, Department of Dermatology I, University of Vienna, Austria.

Denny L. Tuffanelli, MD
Clinical Professor, Department of Dermatology, University of California, San Francisco.

C.F.H. Vickers, MD
Professor and Head, University Department of Dermatology, Royal Liverpool Hospital, Liverpool, England.

Robert R. Walther, MD, FACP
Associate Clinical Professor, Columbia University, College of Physicians and Surgeons, New York.

Stephen B. Webster, MD
Associate Clinical Professor, University of Minnesota Medical School, Minneapolis; Associate Clinical Professor, University of Wisconsin Medical School, Madison.

Ronald C. Wester, PhD
Associate Research Dermatologist and Associate Adjunct Professor in Pharmacy, University of California, San Francisco.

Klaus Wolff, MD
Professor and Chairman, Department of Dermatology, University of Vienna.

Herschel S. Zackheim, MD
Clinical Professor, Department of Dermatology, University of California, San Francisco.

Alvin S. Zelickson, MD
Clinical Professor, University of Minnesota School of Medicine, Minneapolis.

Section I:
Normal Skin

Structure & Function of the Skin

1

Frank Parker, MD

The skin is a complex, dynamic organ of many cell types and specialized structures serving multiple functions crucial to health and survival. One of the largest and most versatile of organs, the skin provides a number of unique functions:

(1) It protects deeper cells from the environment (ie, desiccation; chemical and mechanical injury; microbial, fungal, and parasitic invasion; damaging effects of ultraviolet light).

(2) It regulates and helps maintain body temperature.

(3) It serves as a neuroreceptor organ in monitoring diverse environmental stimuli.

(4) It processes antigenic substances presented to it.

(5) It provides cosmetic adornment as an organ with specialized keratinized structures—hair and nails—that serve some protective function as well.

These functions may be correlated with specific structures and properties of the epidermal and dermal regions (Table 1–1 and Fig 1–1). The stratified squamous epithelium (the epidermis) differentiates to form the stratum corneum of anucleate cornified cells. In aggregate, these constitute a relatively impermeable protective barrier to the inward penetration of liquids, irritating chemicals, allergens, and microorganisms. These tightly packed lamellae of cornified surface cells—in conjunction with the brown pigment melanin, produced by specialized cells in the epidermis, the melanocytes—play an important role in protection against the carcinogenic and aging effects of ultraviolet radiation. The skin plays an important role in immunologic defense by virtue of the Langerhans cells, found in the mid epidermis, serving as the most peripheral outpost of the immune system. Langerhans cells present antigens as the first step necessary for delayed hypersensitivity reactions. Cytokine mediators such as interleukin-1 produced by keratinocytes aid these cell-mediated immune reactions in skin.

The connective tissue, which makes up the preponderance of the dermis, is composed of collagen and elastic fibers and ground substance. It provides strength, elasticity, and protection against shearing forces to the skin (Table 1–1 and Fig 1–1). The dermis provides nourishment to the epidermis and interacts with the epidermis during embryogenesis, wound repair, and remodeling. Two components of the dermis—its unique circulatory system and the specialized cutaneous appendages, the eccrine sweat glands—play a vital role in the body's thermoregulatory function. Furthermore, the extensive innervation of the skin and its appendages (the hairs have networks of nerves surrounding the hair bulbs) make the skin an important neuroreceptor sense organ interacting with the environment, registering such sensations as pain, itch, vibration, heat, and cold. The dermis also contains complex tubular structures in the axillas and in the genitocrural and mammary areas, ie, the apocrine sweat glands, which secrete a viscous fluid which, when acted upon by resident bacteria, emits distinctive body odors.

THE EPIDERMIS

Two major zones of epidermis can be distinguished: an inner region of viable, moist cells termed the malpighian layer and the outer layer of anucleate, flattened, nonviable, desiccated cells known as the **stratum corneum,** or horny layer (Fig 1–2). Three substrata of living cells are recognized: the basal, spinous, and granular layers (Fig 1–2). These 3

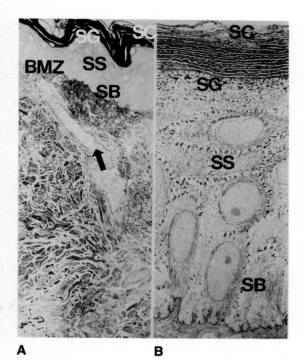

A   **B**

Figure 1–1. Light **(A)** and electron microscopic **(B)** view of the skin. The light microscopic picture on the left shows the stratum corneum (SC), stratum granulosum (SG), 6–7 layers of stratum spinosum (SS) beneath, and the stratum basale (SB) abutting the basement membrane zone (BMZ). Taking up most of the picture is the dermis, in which a portion of a blood vessel is seen (arrow). In **B,** the epidermis and a small area of dermis are pictured under the electron microscope. The epidermis is composed of an outer layer, the stratum corneum (SC), with anucleate, flattened, horny cells; and the underlying layers, the stratum granulosum (SG), stratum spinosum (SS), and stratum basale (SB).

layers represent progressive stages of differentiation and keratinization of the living keratinocyte as they move toward the skin's surface to become stratum corneum. Thus, the columnar basal cells continually divide and give birth to daughter cells that are displaced toward the skin surface. Here in the spinous stratum they are polyhedral, but they flatten as they move into the granular layer (Fig 1–1). The spinous cells adhere to one another mechanically by numerous attachment devices called desmosomes (Fig 1–2), which represent complex modifications of the cell membrane. Large bundles of submicroscopic keratin filaments (formerly called tonofilaments) synthesized in the spinosum cells attach or "loop through" the desmosomes. To early observers, these desmosomal junctions imparted a spinous profile to the cells in the mid portion of the stratum germinativum—hence the designation "stratum spinosum."

As the cells move from the basal to the spinous layer and become more flattened, several additional structural changes occur. **Keratin filaments** form a network within the cytoplasm, and refractile **keratohyaline granules** and submicroscopic **lamellar granules** appear. Bundles of **keratin filaments** fill the cytoplasm and form intracellular networks that extend across cells and loop about the perinuclear space of the cells in the stratum spinosum.

Keratin filaments of the epidermis—hair and wool—are structurally homologous fibrous proteins composed of "building blocks" of chains of fibrous proteins assembled around one another in an α-helix coil.

Keratohyaline granules synthesized in the upper germinative layer account for the distinctive granules in the granular layer (Fig 1–3). Keratohyaline gran-

Table 1–1. Correlations of structure with functions of the skin.

Components of the Skin and the Appendages	Known and Presumed Functions
Stratum corneum	Prevents skin desiccation; protects against external chemical and antigen damage; impedes microbial, fungal, parasitic, and insect injury.
Viable keratinocytes	Produce keratin and stratum corneum.
Basement membrane zone	Attaches epidermis to dermis.
Dermal collagen, elastin, and glycosaminoglycans	Protects against mechanical shearing effects; provides strength and stretchability.
Melanin	Protects against ultraviolet light.
Dermal vasculature and eccrine sweat glands	Thermoregulation; vasculature provides the epidermis with nutrients.
Dermal nerves and neuroreceptor network in upper dermis and around hair follicles	Monitor environment; vasculature provides the epidermis with nutrients.
Langerhans cells	Process antigens and function as macrophages.
Fibroblasts	Produce collagen, elastin, and glycosaminoglycans.
Mast cells	Synthesize substances that mediate inflammatory responses.
Sebaceous glands	Produce sebum, which maintains the soft texture of the skin surface.
Apocrine glands	Secrete sweat, which, when acted on by diphtheroids, create odor.
Hairs over scalp, body, eyelashes, and nasal hair	Provide aesthetic adornment and protect eyes from small particles and filter air breathed into nose.
Fingernails	Assist in grasping objects and in self-defense.

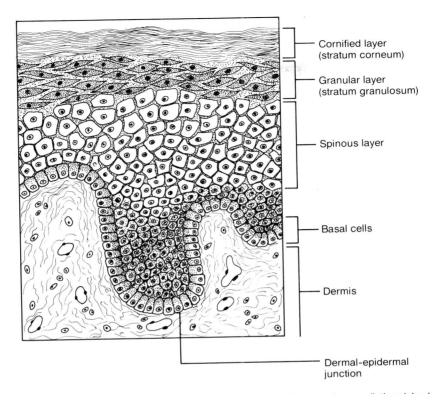

Cornified layer
(stratum corneum)

Granular layer
(stratum granulosum)

Spinous layer

Basal cells

Dermis

Dermal-epidermal
junction

Figure 1–2. Schematic drawing of the epidermis. Three major layers of living cells are distinguished: The columnar cells, comprising the basal layer, nearest the dermis; the spinous layer, composed of polyhedral cells with many desmosomal attachments on the cell surfaces (modification of the cell membranes where cells of the spinous layer attach to one another); and the granular layer, interposed between the spinous layer and the stratum corneum, where cells take on a flattened configuration and contain dense keratohyaline granules.

ules are probably composed of both sulfur-rich proteins (cysteine residues) and phosphorylated histidine-rich proteins. In the stratum granulosum, keratohyalin accrues incrementally among the keratin filaments to form larger and larger masses enclosing the filaments (Fig 1–3). Histidine-rich basic protein has been demonstrated to facilitate the assembly of keratin filaments into macrofibrils. This substance has been termed filagrin because it seems to aggregate and align the keratin filaments into large, insoluble fibrous structures, or macrofibrils. Filagrin is also found in large quantities in the stratum corneum.

Also in the upper layers of the spinous layer are **lamellar granules.** These structures contain lipid lamellae that appear to be extruded from the cells into the intercellular spaces. The function of the lamellar granules is unknown but may have something to do with both accumulating lipid materials between the stratum corneum cells that add to the barrier properties of the corneum as well as adding to the thickening of the corneum cell membranes.

The final stage of keratinization—the abrupt change from the granular layer to the stratum corneum—is attended by a variety of dramatic morphologic and biochemical degenerative alterations,

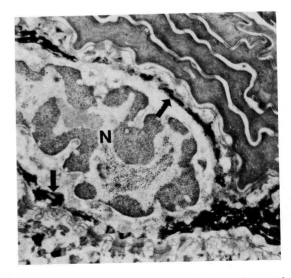

Figure 1–3. A higher magnification electron micrograph of the stratum granulosum just below the flattened, anucleate stratum corneum squames. Note the dense keratohyaline granules (arrows) surrounding the pyknotic degenerating nucleus (N) of the granulosa cell.

including the degradation of cellular organelles and nuclei (Fig 1–3) (carried out by lysosomal hydrolytic enzymes) as well as by the appearance of a thickened cellular envelope of stratum corneum cells that provides them with the useful property of extreme resistance to degradation by various chemicals. The corneum cells are filled with a 2-phased ordered system of low-density filaments (keratin filaments) embedded in a denser continuous matrix (filagrin). The cornified layer consists of up to 25 layers of anucleate dead cells held tightly together by means of desmosomes. Horny cells at the surface of the skin are continuously and imperceptibly shed. Normally, 0.5–1 g of horny cells are lost daily.

The basal layer of the epidermis has a permanent population of germinal cells known as stew cells whose progeny undergo the specific pattern of differentiation (keratinization) just described in a period of 26–42 days (transit time). New epidermal cells continually form to compensate for those that exfoliate. Cells in the germinativum require 12–14 days to move from the basal layer to the stratum corneum and another 14 days for the corneum cells to be shed.

The control of this continuous mitotic activity in the basal layer may be mediated by intracellular concentrations of cAMP/cGMP, prostaglandins, and other compounds derived from arachidonic acid, polyamines, calcium, glucocorticoids, and a variety of additional regulatory proteins such as chalones and epidermal growth factor.

Precise control of proliferation of basal cells and their subsequent orderly differentiation into keratinized stratum corneum cells result in a smooth, pliable skin surface. Alterations in the homeostatic state of basal cell division, defects in epidermal differentiation, or alterations in exfoliation of the stratum corneum cells all may lead to irregularities in the skin surface, characterized clinically as roughening, scaling, and fissuring of the skin. Thus, a variety of skin diseases present with alterations in the skin surface due to defects in these processes, ie, increased cell division and turnover of basal cells (psoriasis), altered keratinization (Darier's disease), and defects in exfoliation (ichthyosis vulgaris).

Organisms must be protected from their environment to survive. In humans, a large measure of this protection is afforded by the epidermis. The major barrier function resides in the stratum corneum. The low permeability of this horny layer not only effectively retards water loss from the inner milieu but also shields against damage from the environment, preventing entrance of toxic substances, allergens, and infectious agents. The barrier properties of the horny layer are of practical importance in the physician's care of patients from several viewpoints. First, excessive drying or inflammatory reactions of the skin lead to roughness and scaling as the normally uniformly packed layers of stratum corneum are disrupted. If extensive areas of the horny layer are disrupted (as is seen in burns of the skin or in toxic epidermal necrolysis), there is impressive transepidermal water loss such that total fluid loss can be appreciable, contributing to life-threatening fluid and electrolyte imbalance. Second, with breaks in the horny layer, external substances gain entrance to the underlying epidermis. Haptens and antigens may induce delayed hypersensitivity and contact dermatitis. Unwanted absorption of toxic chemicals may damage underlying living cells directly. Third, the disruption of the barrier layer increases the chance of colonization by pathogenic bacteria.

The percutaneous absorption of various topical medications used in treating inflammatory skin conditions is regulated by the stratum corneum. Most medications are absorbed by passive diffusion. Although topical steroids do not readily permeate the corneum, they do penetrate enough to exert anti-inflammatory effects on the underlying living epidermis and dermis. In treating extensive inflammatory skin conditions, significant amounts of steroids may be absorbed, leading to suppression of the pituitary-adrenal axis.

MELANOCYTES & LANGERHANS CELLS

Melanocytes are dendritic cells. Their dendrites touch numerous keratinocytes in their vicinity. Melanocytes form a network of cells near the basal layer of the stratum germinativum (Fig 1–4). Melanocytes synthesize the yellow, red, and brown biochromes—melanin—which are large polymers bound to protein. Melanin absorbs light over a broad range of wavelengths (200–2400 nm), thus serving as an excellent screen against the damaging cutaneous effects of solar ultraviolet radiation.

Melanin is synthesized within unique organelles called **melanosomes.** Ultrastructurally, these consist of an orderly helical, filamentous internal structure upon which melanin accumulates (Fig 1–5). Once the melanosome is filled with pigment, it is called a melanin granule. Granules are transferred to adjacent keratinocytes by moving out to the tips of the melanocyte dendrites. The ends of the dendrites that contain melanin granules are phagocytosed and internalized by keratinocytes. In this way, all the keratinocytes acquire protective melanin, accumulating "caps" of melanin over their nuclei.

Melanin synthesis begins with the oxidation of tyrosine by the enzyme tyrosinase to form 3,4-dihydroxyphenylalanine (dopa) within the melanosomes. A second oxidation, also under the control of tyrosinase, forms dopaquinone, and additional nonenzymatically mediated oxidation and polymerization alterations in the resulting quinone molecule then occur to form the final products—either eumelanin (brown or black) or phaeomelanin (red, yellow).

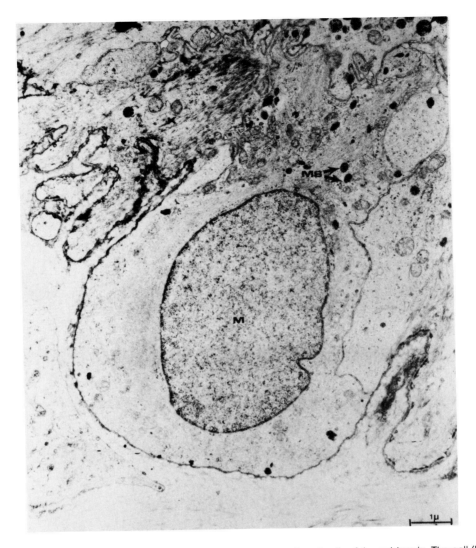

Figure 1–4. An electron microscopic picture of a melanocyte between basal cells of the epidermis. The cell (M) contains many melanosomes (MS) with dark melanin pigment within.

Phaeomelanin is formed by the addition of cysteine to dopaquinone.

Neither sex nor race affects the number of melanocytes. Negroid skin contains the same number of melanocytes as Caucasian skin, but the pigmentation is more intense as a result of genetically determined increased melanin synthesis in Negroid skin as well as the diffuse distribution of melanin granules within the keratinocytes. Individuals of Causasoid or Mongoloid genetic background produce fewer melanin granules, and the granules are packed into cytoplasmic aggregates (melanosome complexes) within the keratinocytes rather than being individually packaged and spread diffusely throughout the cytoplasm, as occurs in Negroid skin.

Two factors profoundly influence melanin synthesis: ultraviolet light and hormones. Exposure to ultraviolet light, both in UVB and UVA wavelengths, increases melanin synthesis and transfer of melanin to keratinocytes, causing the characteristic tanning of the skin. In addition, 2 trophic hormones in the pituitary gland, α-MSH and β-MSH, cause generalized hyperpigmentation. α-MSH and β-MSH are components of a pituitary stem peptide that is cleaved to release the 2 melanocyte-stimulating hormones.

Lack of MSH, as in hypopituitarism, results in a generalized decrease in skin color. Occasionally, pituitary and lung carcinomas secrete MSH to cause hyperpigmentation. In Addison's disease, an increase of the pituitary common stem peptide causes increased MSH release due to lack of adrenal cortico-steroids. A more extensive discussion of pigmentation can be found in Chapter 22.

Langerhans cells constitute a small proportion of epidermal cells located in the mid zone of the stratum spinosum. These cells bear surface receptors for the Fc portion of immunoglobulin molecules and for the C3b complement component. They can take up and present antigen to reactive lymphocytes. They have been implicated as pivotal antigen-presenting cells. Langerhans cells are of mesenchymal origin, probably derived from the bone marrow. Langerhans cells lack desmosomes and keratin filaments and contain unique organelles—trilaminar, racket-shaped granules (Fig 1–5).

Langerhans cells are also found in the dermis, lymph nodes, and thymus, relating to the role of these cells in picking up antigens in skin and circulating to the draining lymph nodes via dermal lymphatics in order to bring about "sensitization" of lymphocytes to the specific antigen or to elicit a cell-mediated immune reaction.

THE DERMAL-EPIDERMAL JUNCTION

The structures situated at the dermal-epidermal junction constitute an anatomic functional unit that serves to weld the epidermis to the underlying dermis. This junction also acts as a barrier to the movement of inflammatory and neoplastic cells between the dermis and epidermis.

The dermal-epidermal junction is undulated, forming dermal papillae (upward projections of the dermis into the epidermis) and rete ridges (downward fingerlike growths of epidermis). A thin, intensely staining PAS-positive basal lamina follows the papillae and ridges. Under the electron microscope (Fig 1–6 and 1–7), the basal lamina appears as an electron-dense (lamina densa), continuous feltwork of proteoglycans and type IV collagen separated from the plasma membrane of the epidermal basal cells by a thin, clear, amorphous space (lamina lucida). Several substructural dermal fibrous elements, including collagen and specialized anchoring fibrils (type VII collagen) and microfibrillar bundles, are found coursing perpendicularly to the basal lamina and help secure the epidermis to the dermis.

THE DERMIS

The dermis lies between the epidermis and the subcutaneous adipose tissue. In humans, the whole mass of the dermis may constitute 15–20% of the total body weight (Fig 1–1). The dermis has many functions. It protects deeper structures from mechanical injury. The dermis provides nourishment to the epidermis and interacts with the epidermis during embryogenesis, morphogenesis, and wound repair and remodeling. It gives the skin its strength, elasticity, and softness.

Grossly, the dermis is a tough, resilient tissue with viscoelastic properties. A 3-dimensional matrix of loose connective tissue is composed of fibrous proteins (collagen and elastin) embedded in an amorphous gel of ground substance (glycosaminoglycans)

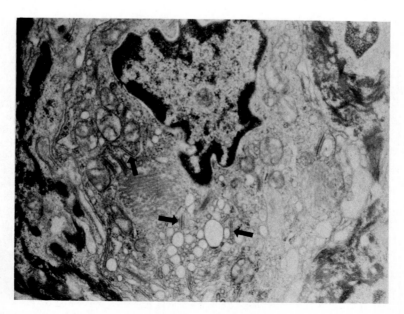

Figure 1–5. An electron microscopic picture of a Langerhans cell in the mid zone of the stratum spinosum. These cells contain unique trilaminar rod-shaped granules (arrow).

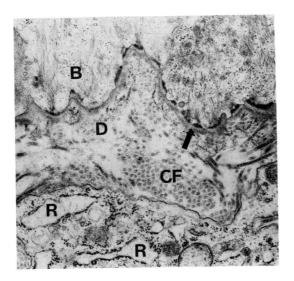

Figure 1–6. An electron microscopic picture of the epidermal-dermal junction, showing a basal epidermal cell (B) above and the dermis (D) below. A portion of a fibroblast is seen in the lower portion of the picture. Note the rough endoplasmic reticulum (R) organelles in the fibroblast, where collagen synthesis is carried out. Collagen fibers (CF) of the dermis are cut in longitudinal and cross section. The thin, dense, continuous fibrillar basal lamina (arrow) is seen just below the plasma membrane of the basal cell, separated from it by a thinner, clear space, the lamina lucida.

(Fig 1–1). The fibrous matrix serves as a scaffolding within which networks of blood vessels, nerves, and lymphatics intertwine. The dermis also contains epidermal appendages such as sweat glands and pilosebaceous units and provides support and protection for these structures.

The dermis can be divided into an upper papillary layer, characterized by interlacing fine collagen fibers and ample interfibrillar spaces, and the deeper reticular dermis, recognized by the thicker, aggregated bundles of collagen with lesser amounts of interfibrous space. Elastic fibers are intertwined within the collagenous network.

COLLAGEN & ELASTIC FIBERS

Collagen, which comprises 77% of the fat-free dry weight of the skin, accounts for the tensile strength of the dermis. Type I collagen is the major collagen, with type III collagen contributing only 15% of the total collagen mass. Collagen is composed of elongated rodlike tropocollagen molecules, each containing 3 polypeptide chains (chains of about 1000 amino acids) aligned in a parallel direction and arranged in a triple helix, much like the strands of a stiff rope. The component polypeptide chains are characteristic for the tissue source. The type I collagen of skin and bone contains 2 tropocollagen chains, α_1 and α_2. Glycine occupies every third position of the amino acid sequence along the entire length of each chain, and copious amounts of proline and hydroxyproline are also present.

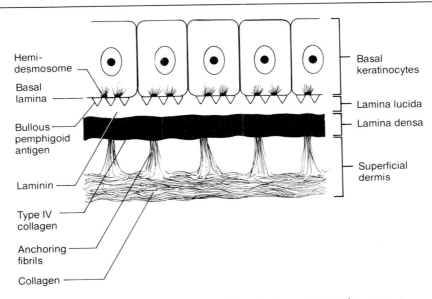

Figure 1–7. Schematic diagram of the skin basement membrane zone.

Hemi-desmosome
Basal lamina
Bullous pemphigoid antigen
Laminin
Type IV collagen
Anchoring fibrils
Collagen

Basal keratinocytes
Lamina lucida
Lamina densa
Superficial dermis

Elastic fibers constitute a small percentage of the remaining fibrillar systems in the dermis. Like rubber, the elastic fibers have a low coefficient of elasticity; ie, they can be deformed by a small force, and they recover their original dimensions. Elastic fibers consist of microfibrils embedded in an amorphous matrix. The central amorphous portion of elastic fibers—elastin—is composed of unique amino acids, desmosine and isodesmosine, derived from lysine. The cross-linking of these desmosine amino acids found in long peptide chains results in a structure similar to that of rubber.

Collagen molecule synthesis begins in the fibroblasts' rough endoplasmic reticulum (Fig 1–6). Proline and lysine residues in the nascent collagen chain are acted on intracellularly by the enzymes prolylhydroxylase and lysylhydroxylase to form hydroxyproline and hydroxylysine. These hydroxylating enzymes require ascorbic acid as a cofactor, which explains why collagen synthesis is impaired in scurvy. The collagen molecule chains are glycosylated and secreted through the fibroblasts' Golgi complexes, and this so-called tropocollagen is then released from the cell in soluble form. Extracellularly, the tropocollagen aggregates to initiate fibrillogenesis, a process that involves intra- and intermolecular cross-linkings. The extent of cross-linking determines the tensile strength that collagen imparts to the skin as well as the solubility and resistance to enzymatic degradation. Recently synthesized collagen is solubilized more readily (less cross-linking) than older collagen that contains more covalent cross-links. Such linking increases with age. Thus, general body collagen in a mature individual is relatively inert and has an estimated half-life of 5 years.

Collagen synthesis and degradation continue throughout life. Degradation processes are under the influence of a collagenolytic enzyme, collagenase, the only known mammalian enzyme that splits the collagen helix.

GROUND SUBSTANCE

The ground substance of the dermis consists largely of the acidic mucopolysaccharides, chondroitin sulfate and hyaluronic acid. These hydrophilic carbohydrate-protein complexes (glycosaminoglycans) account for only 0.1–0.2% of the dry weight of the dermis. In company with other nonfibrous proteins (serum proteins and other mucoproteins), water, and electrolytes, they form an extrafibrillar viscoelastic gel. Glycosaminoglycans act as a barrier to bacterial penetration. Hyaluronic acid avidly binds water and maintains dermal turgor. In fact, the dermis may function as a water storage organ that helps to maintain hydration of other tissues under mild water deprivation. The water-binding properties of the glycosaminoglycans also serve to maintain the internal milieu of the dermis and thereby allow nutrients and salts from the circulation to "percolate" to the actively metabolizing epidermal cells. The glycosaminoglycans are metabolized and degraded by fibroblasts and mast cells.

CELLULAR ELEMENTS OF THE DERMIS

The cellular elements of the dermis consist predominantly of the ubiquitous fibroblasts dispersed through the dermal connective tissue. Fibroblasts are responsible for the synthesis of collagen and elastic fibers and the ground substance.

Mast cells are the other dominant cellular dermal constituent. They commonly are found in close association with small vessels in the papillary dermis. Mast cells are recognized by their distinctive metachromatic granules (granules that impart a different color than the dye applied to them). These granules contain the anticoagulant heparin as well as the vasoactive substance histamine and proteases. Although not stored within the granules, prostaglandins and leukotrienes are also synthesized and released by mast cells during the degranulation process.

Mast cells play an important role in a variety of inflammatory reactions. Histamine is synthesized in the mast cells from histidine by the enzyme histidine decarboxylase. Histamine increases capillary permeability and initiates vasodilatation and can evoke edema and redness. Human mast cells contain chymotrypsin and trypsin-like enzymes, which have a potent biologic action, ie, formation and inactivation of kinins and participation in the clotting sequence. Trypsin-like enzymes can cleave human C3 to generate mediators. Mast cells also synthesize leukotrienes as well as prostaglandin 2, which evoke potent inflammatory reactions characterized by redness, edema, and itching.

IgE complexed with antigen on the cell membrane, physical stimuli such as heat, cold, and pressure, and direct chemical liberators (eg, opioids) all cause mast cell degranulation.

THE VASCULATURE OF THE SKIN

The skin encloses a vast 3-dimensional meshwork of blood vessels whose 2 predominant planes comprise netlike plexuses parallel to the skin surface. Vertically oriented communicating vessels link these superficial and deep vessel networks. Microcirculatory units arise from these interconnecting small arterioles to nourish the epidermis and the metabolically active skin appendages.

The extensive cutaneous vasculature has several functions: It provides nutrition to the entire skin; it helps maintain the body at a constant temperature;

and it participates in the inflammatory response. In comparison to other organs, the metabolic requirements for nutritional blood flow are low. The skin utilizes only 5 mL of oxygen per minute, and only 1 vol% of oxygen is extracted from arterial blood as it passes through the skin.

Blood flow in normal and warm thermal environments is higher in the digits and other acral skin areas. This may relate to the presence of special arteriovenous shunts called glomus bodies found in the mid dermis of acral skin regions.

Dermal blood flow varies over a wide range in response to changes in core body temperature and the temperature of the external environment. Hypothalamic centers in the brain control dermal blood flow through vasoconstriction by the sympathetic nervous system. The total skin blood flow of a 70-kg man at rest in a normal indoor environment is 20–500 mL/min, and the maximum value is calculated to be 2.1–3.5 L/min attained with exercise in a warm environment. Direct heating of the skin over the whole body can increase the cardiac output of a 70-kg man to almost 7 L/min, most of which is distributed to the skin. Skin blood flow is important in regulation of blood pressure. An increase in metabolic rate can increase skin blood flow. This explains the warm, soft texture to the skin observed in hyperthyroidism.

SKIN APPENDAGES

ECCRINE SWEAT GLANDS & THERMOREGULATION (See Chapter 27.)

The eccrine sweat glands are a highly developed and responsive part of the thermoregulatory apparatus (Figs 1–8 and 1–9). Their function is to manufacture and pump a hypotonic solution to the skin surface for evaporative cooling in times of heat stress. With maximal thermal stimulation, sweating rates of 2–3 L/h can be attained for short periods. An increase in body core temperature, acting through temperature-sensitive centers in the hypothalamus, is the most potent stimulus for generalized sweating. The initiation of bodily exercise causes immediate neurogenic stimulation of generalized sweating. With continuation of exercise, rises in temperature of hypothalamic centers contribute to the sweating response. Eccrine glands receive a single set of innervating fibers which are excitatory and cholinergic functionally but are derived anatomically from the sympathetic nervous system.

The primary thermoregulatory function of the skin

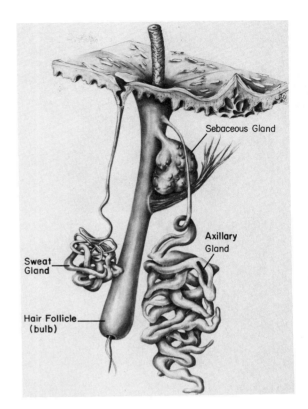

Figure 1–8. A diagrammatic depiction of the "gross" structure and anatomic relationships of the eccrine (sweat gland), apocrine (axillary gland), and sebaceous glands to the hair follicle. Note the highly coiled eccrine gland connected to the skin surface by an elongated duct that is straight until it takes a spiral course within the epidermis. The apocrine gland is much larger but as highly convoluted as the eccrine gland. The apocrine duct usually opens into the hair follicle, but occasionally it may open directly onto the skin surface. The multilobular sebaceous gland is tucked between the hair follicle and the arrector pili muscle (not labeled). The sebaceous gland empties sebum through the sebaceous duct into the hair follicle infundibulum. (Courtesy of W Montagna.)

is to control heat loss. The skin does this by varying skin circulatory and sweat gland function. In order for body temperature to remain relatively constant, heat losses must be balanced against heat gains. Body heat is lost through evaporation of eccrine sweat on the skin surface as well as by radiation, conduction, and convection. The cutaneous circulation acts much as a "radiator" in a hot-water heating system. It can vary rates of blood flow to the skin, much like adjusting the valve on a radiator (ie, the greater the flow, the greater the loss of heat); or it can vary the cutaneous blood volume by changing the capacity of the venous bed (this changes the surface area at the interface between warm blood and tissues), much like varying the number of coils in the radiator. Heat is conducted

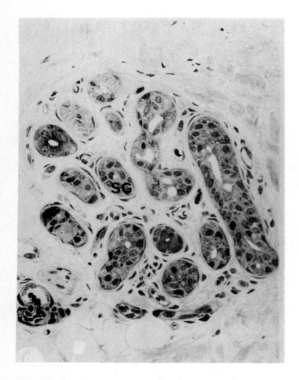

Figure 1–9. Light microscopic sections through the eccrine sweat glands (SG). The hypotonic sweat is produced by these glandular elements, which consist of highly coiled, tubular structures (see Fig 1–8), which discharge the sweat onto the surface of the skin by way of an elongated duct.

to the skin surface. Normally, the distance between the cutaneous circulation and the skin surface is small enough so that the rate of heat conduction is not a limiting factor in heat transfer. However, when the body is cold, it "shuts down" the cutaneous circulation. Most of the blood then flows deeper, so that conduction becomes a limiting factor for heat loss.

APOCRINE SWEAT GLANDS
(See Chapter 27.)

A second type of sweat gland is the apocrine gland. Apocrine glands are complex tubular structures with compound secretory coils. They secrete a viscous material which, when acted upon by surface bacteria, causes musky odors that give us our distinctive human body odors. It may be that apocrine sweat is the human equivalent of pheromones.

Apocrine glands occur in greatest numbers in the axillas, the genitocrural skin, within the mammary areolae, and in the external auditory canal (ceruminous glands) (Figs 1–8 and 1–10). The secretory segment is enclosed by large myoepithelial cells (smooth muscle-like cells arranged helically around secretory tubules) that may serve to contract and push the apocrine secretion onto the skin surface. The cuboidal secretory cells contain vesicles that are released from the tips of the cells into the glandular lumen by apical decapitation of the tips of the secretory cells (apocrine secretion) and exocytosis of the granules (Fig 1–10).

The apocrine glands are enclosed in a meshwork of nerve fibers composed of both sympathetic and parasympathetic fibers. Adrenergic nerves play the major role in the control of apocrine secretion, in part by stimulating the myoepithelial cells' contractions.

SEBACEOUS GLANDS
(See Chapter 3.)

The sebaceous glands are lipid-secreting simple or compound acinar structures which are holocrine glands that empty their fatty secretion into the follicular canal at the level of the infundibulum of hair follicles (Fig 1–8). Over the scalp, forehead, face, and upper chest, they occur with a frequency of 400–900/cm^2, whereas over most of the rest of the body they are found in numbers approximating 100/cm^2.

The germinative undifferentiated sebaceous cells lie at the periphery of the acinus, resting upon a basal lamina. As these cells divide, they move toward the central areas of the acini and synthesize increasing quantities of triglyceride-rich sebum (approximately 60% triglycerides and diglycerides, 25% wax esters, 15% squalene, and lesser amounts of sterol esters). The lipids contained in sebum are synthesized by mitochondria and stored in Golgi vacuoles. The lipid-storing vacuoles increase in size and number until they replace the entire cell cytoplasm. As the fully differentiated sebum-laden cells approach the sebaceous duct, their plasma membranes disintegrate, disgorging fragments of the cells and the lipid droplets into the sebaceous duct (holocrine secretion) and then into the pilary canal and out onto the skin surface.

Androgens control the mitotic rate of the undifferentiated cells at the periphery of the acinus, and these hormones also affect the subsequent growth, differentiation, and synthesis of sebum within the sebaceous cells. Sebaceous glands are extremely sensitive androgen end organs, being stimulated by small quantities of a variety of androgens in the circulation. Sebaceous glands metabolize various androgens to dihydrotestosterone (the most potent androgen yet identified) by way of a 5α-reductase enzyme. Thus, at puberty, when significant levels of androgens are secreted into the circulation in both males and females, the glands convert these to dihydrotestosterone, which initiates the synthesis of specific enzyme systems that induce sebaceous gland growth and differentiation.

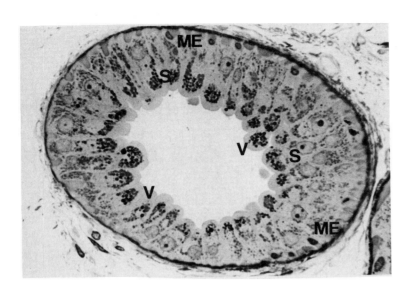

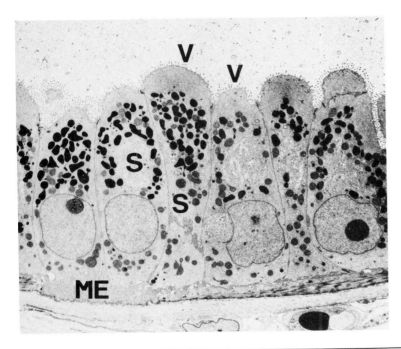

Figure 1–10. Light **(above)** and electron microscopic **(below)** picture of apocrine gland. Myoepithelial cells are seen at the base of the cuboidal secretory cells, which contain electron-dense granules in their apical portions. Microvillous processes can be seen extending from the tips of the secretory cells' luminal surfaces, probably important in the secretion of apocrine sweat.

DERMAL NERVES & INNERVATION; ITCHING

The skin is a mosaic of nerve terminals from axons that ramify in areas 1 cm in diameter with considerable functional overlap. Some free nerve endings are sensitive to cooling and heating, while others mediate pain, pressure, and itch. These nerve endings lie within the papillary and reticular dermis, and some may extend into the lower portion of the epidermis.

Accumulations of sensory nerves also encircle hair follicles and hair bulbs, so that fine body hairs also serve as sensing appendages. Two types of nerves

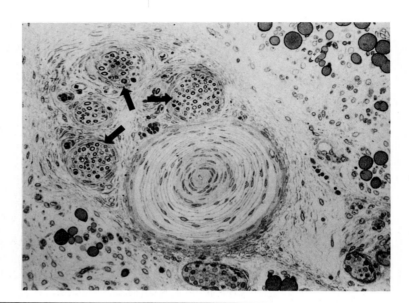

Figure 1–11. Several myelinated nerve fibers (arrow) seen in this light micrograph surrounding the "onion skin"-like, encapsulated specialized Meissner corpuscle.

concentrate around hair follicles: (1) lanceolate nerve fibers lying in close proximity to the external root sheath and hair bulb and (2) Ruffini corpuscles of cylindric encapsulated nerve endings enclosed in a connective tissue compartment encircling hair follicles just below the sebaceous duct.

Three specialized nerve endings are found in the skin: (1) Meissner's touch corpuscles, (2) pacinian corpuscles, and (3) hederiform endings. Meissner's corpuscles are oval structures composed of coils of terminal axons enclosed within a basal lamina and collagen fibers. They are found predominantly in the dermal papillae of the palms and soles and seem to subserve the sensory function of touch (Fig 1–11).

Pacinian corpuscles are ellipsoidal structures composed of an unmyelinated axon core surrounded by a multilaminated capsule, found in the deep portion of the plantar and palmar dermis. Digital pacinian corpuscles are closely associated with the specialized glomerular arteriovenous anastomosis (glomus vascular body). The thick-walled vein draining the corpuscle enters the venous outlet of the adjacent glomus. When the arteriovenous shunt is open, the increased venous pressure is transmitted to the corpuscle receptors, signaling local changes in blood flow. More deeply situated pacinian corpuscles seem to serve as vibratory sensors.

Hederiform ("ivy-shaped") endings involve the Merkel cells. These cells lie singly or in groups in the basal epidermis and are associated with an adjacent flattened axon terminal plate. These Merkel-neuron structures may function as mechanoreceptors for touch, but their exact function is unclear.

PHYSIOLOGY OF ITCH

The physiology of itch (pruritus) is not well understood. Presumably, various chemomediators (histamine, proteases, leukotrienes, prostaglandins) liberated by a wide variety of stimuli and noxious agents act on fine free terminal unmyelinated C nerve fibers near the basal portion of the epidermis to elicit this distinctive sensation. Itch and pain sensations are transmitted along these small, slow-conducting sensory neurons in the spinal nerves to the spinothalamic tract and then to the thalamus and sensory cortex. It is not clear how scratching relieves itching, but scratching may disturb the rhythm of afferent impulses traveling toward the spinal cord.

Pruritus is an important and bothersome feature of many skin diseases as well as some systemic diseases. The motor response of scratching it evokes, if not controlled, leads to further cutaneous damage, often with perpetuation and intensification of the symptom.

REGIONAL DIFFERENCES IN STRUCTURE & FUNCTION OF THE SKIN

The skin varies in its anatomy and physiologic functions from area to area. For example, there are differences in the thickness of the epidermis or dermis in certain regions. The stratum corneum is extremely thick on the palms and soles. Calluses (large masses of stratum corneum) form in areas of increased friction or pressure. In addition, prominent linear ridges (fingerprints) are seen on the volar surfaces of the digits. These, in conjunction with sweat glands, whose orifices are arranged in a regular manner along the apices of the ridges, help increase friction and enhance the function of the digits in grasping and twisting. The overall thickness of the dermis is greatest over the dorsal portions of the body, whereas such regions as the scrotum have a very thin epidermis.

The flexibility and elasticity of the skin varies from region to region. For example, the skin over the large joints (elbows, knees) is somewhat redundant, flexible, and mobile, while that over the digits and scalp tends to be bound down and less mobile.

There is also considerable regional variation in the number and distribution of various appendages, but the functional significance of these differences is not clear. For example, sebaceous glands are found in greatest concentrations over the head and upper chest; the apocrine glands are found in the axillary, genital, and mammary regions and the external ear canal. Special arteriovenous anastomoses—glomus bodies—are found in the acral regions of the body, most likely for thermoregulatory functions.

THE NAIL
(See Chapter 29.)

The hard, durable epidermal appendage, the nail plate, located on the dorsal tip of the distal phalanges of each digit, protects the end of the digit and serves as a grasping tool and weapon.

The nail plate is composed of tightly packed, multiple layers of horny cells firmly cemented together and filled with keratin. The nail plate is formed by rapidly dividing, keratinizing epidermal cells under the proximal nail fold (nail matrix region) as well as on the nail bed. Substances (eg, arsenic or chemotherapeutic agents) or diseases (eg, psoriasis) that alter epidermal mitosis, differentiation, and keratinization cause defects in nail growth such as longitudinal ridging and pitting.

The nail bed has a rich vascular supply that functions to deliver nutrients to support rapid cellular turnover and keratinization. Numerous glomus bodies are found in the nail bed. Nails grow an average of 0.1 mm/d, but more slowly with age. Serious systemic illness temporarily stops or slows nail growth.

Like the keratin in the stratum corneum, that in the nail is also composed of aggregates of filaments 7–10 nm long embedded in an amorphous matrix. The hardness of nails is related to these components. The fibrils made of keratin are rather tightly arranged

within each nail cell perpendicular to the axis of growth and parallel to the nail plate surface. The fibrils are embedded in a matrix protein rich in cystine and held tightly by disulfide bonds.

HAIR
(See Chapter 28.)

These keratinous fibers grow within epithelial follicles found over the entire skin surface except for the palms and soles. Two major types of hairs—terminal and vellus—are recognized. Terminal hairs are thick, pigmented, and long and are seen on the scalp, eyebrows, axillas, and genital areas of men and women and, to a large extent, on the trunk of adult males (Fig 1–12). Vellus hairs are small in diameter, short, and

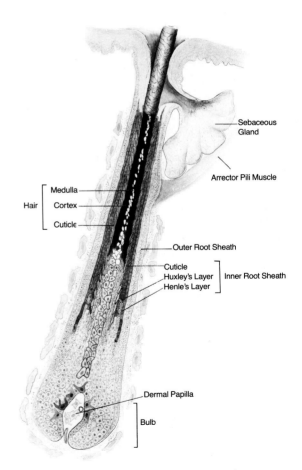

Figure 1–12. A cross-sectional diagrammatic representation of a hair follicle and bulb showing the 3 layers of human terminal hairs (medulla, cortex, and cuticle) as well as the outer and inner root sheaths. The relationship of the sebaceous gland to the hair follicle is also depicted. (Courtesy of W Montagna.)

nonpigmented and therefore are difficult to discern. Even in the apparent "nonhairy" areas of the skin (eg, forehead, eyelids), vellus hairs are found.

Hairs undergo growth cycles, so that the length of terminal and vellus hairs is determined by the specific body region as well as by the genetic makeup of each individual. These recurring cycles consist of active hair growth (anagen), hair follicle regression (catagen), and a rest period (telogen). Each follicle in human skin maintains an independent rhythm of growth cycles. Thus, on the scalp, 80–85% of hairs are in anagen and 15–20% in telogen at any given time. Furthermore, the duration of anagen may be as long as 5–6 years in scalp follicles, followed by only a few months of telogen rest period.

The hair shaft is produced by mitotic activity of the follicular epithelium. This mitotic activity—and, therefore, the length of anagen and the rapidity of hair growth as well as the diameter of the hair fiber—are controlled by androgenic, growth, and thyroid hormones.

Mild androgenic stimulation of hair growth is all that is required to bring on terminal hair growth in some follicles in the male (beard, tip of nose, ears, midline, lower abdomen, and chest). Excessive growth of hair in these areas in females is often indicative of underlying alterations in androgen metabolism (ie, adrenal and ovarian hyperandrogen states). Growth hormone is thought to maintain the growth of hair on the extremities, while hyper- or hypothyroid states result in diffuse loss of scalp and body hair.

The hair shaft is formed in the hair bulb, composed of the dermal papilla and the hair matrix (Fig 1–12). The papilla is an accumulation of dermal connective tissue that invaginates the hair matrix cells. The papilla contains many vascular channels, providing nourishment for the rapidly dividing cells of the matrix (Fig 1–12).

The cells in the matrix are several layers deep and divide every 23–72 hours during anagen, providing cells that stream upward and undergo keratinization, hardening, and orientation into tightly packed layers that form the hair shaft. At the end of the anagen phase of the follicular cycle, continuous cell division slows down and finally ceases temporarily in catagen.

The hair develops and grows within an inner root sheath (consisting of 3 distinct cellular layers from within outward: the cuticle, Huxley's and Henle's layers) which arise from the matrix cells (Fig 1–12). The inner root sheath is in turn surrounded by the outer root sheath, which is a sleeve of cells that is an extension of the surface epidermis (Fig 1–12). The matrix cells surrounding the dermal papilla are thus precursors of the hair fiber, and the more peripheral matrix cells give rise to the various layers of the inner root sheath.

Human terminal hairs consist of several layers of cells. The main portion of the fully keratinized hair is the cortex, which is made up of closely packed, interdigitating spindle-shaped cells whose long axis is parallel to the hair axis. Covering the cortex is the cuticle, composed of 6–8 layers of flattened cells that overlap each other from root to tip. The third component is the central medulla. It consists of specialized cells that contain air spaces (Fig 1–12).

The chemical composition of hair is 65–95% protein by weight. The keratinous protein is found mostly in the cortical cells and is a condensation polymer of amino acids. Other constituents of the hair include water, lipids, pigment, and trace elements. The keratinous protein is insoluble and resistant to proteolytic enzymes and shows the typical electron microscopic configuration of keratin, namely, light staining fibrils embedded in an electron-dense matrix. Large amounts of the sulfur-containing amino acid cystine is found in hair. There are many disulfide bonds in the keratin molecule, which provides strength and rigidity to the hair. Thioglycolates—potent reducers of disulfide bonds—are used to soften hairs in the permanent waving process.

REFERENCES

Clark RAF: Cutaneous tissue repair: Basic biologic considerations. J Am Acad Dermatol 1985;13:701.

Fine JD: The skin basement membrane zone. Adv Dermatol 1987;2:283.

Galvin S et al: The major pathways of keratinocyte differentiation as defined by keratin expression: An overview. Adv Dermatol 1989;4:277.

Goldsmith LA: *Biochemistry and Physiology of the Skin.* Oxford Univ Press, 1983.

Katz SI: The epidermal basement zone-structure ontogeny and role in disease. J Am Acad Dermatol 1984;11:1025.

Kerdel FA, Sotor NA: The mast cell in mastocytosis and pediatric dermatologic disease. Adv Dermatol 1989;4: 159.

Montagna W, Parakkal PF (editors): *The Structure and Function of Skin,* 3rd ed. Academic Press, 1974.

Parker F: The biology of pigmentation. Chap 8, pp 79–91, in: Birth Defects. Original article series, vol XVII, No. 2, March of Dimes Birth Defects Foundation, 1981.

Ryan TJ, Mortimer PS, Jones RL: Lymphatics of the skin: Neglected but important. Int J Dermatol 1986;25:411.

Sato E et al: Biology of sweat glands and their disorders. I. Normal sweat gland function. J Am Acad Dermatol 1989;4:537.

Percutaneous Absorption

2

Ronald C. Wester, PhD

The skin acts as a barrier to absorption of chemicals and invasion by microorganisms. It also acts as a barrier to the loss of water and other substances from the body to the outside. This function usually serves a physiologic purpose; however, in order to treat skin disease effectively, drugs and medications must be able to penetrate the barrier properties of skin. Furthermore, if too much medication is absorbed, systemic toxicity may result.

The factors to be considered in topical treatment of skin disorders include not only the diagnosis and the topical drug of choice but also the concentration of drug, the site of treatment, the age of the patient, and the vehicle into which the drug is incorporated. In topical therapy, the strongest drug is not necessarily the best one.

The skin is the body's main interface with the environment. While it functions as a barrier to absorption, it can also serve as a pathway for drugs or other chemicals to enter the circulation. Percutaneous absorption is the process by which a substance moves from the skin surface to its site of action or to the systemic circulation. The substance may be a drug or chemical administered with therapeutic intent, or it may be some noxious extraneous material that the skin contacted.

Fig 2–1 depicts a schema of percutaneous absorption. If a topical therapeutic agent is to be effective, it must first be absorbed. The drug must penetrate in adequate concentration to its intended site of action to produce the desired pharmacologic response.

The skin acts as a barrier in that it prevents noxious chemicals and other materials from entering the body while at the same time preserving the homeostatic milieu of viable cells just millimeters beneath the skin. The barrier effect is generally beneficial, but it may interfere with treatment because the barrier also inhibits absorption of pharmacologic agents.

In general, absorption follows Fick's law of diffusion:

$$J = \frac{KD\,(\Delta C)}{\gamma} \qquad \text{Penetration} = \frac{\text{Partition coefficient} \times \text{Concentration gradient}}{\text{Thickness of stratum corneum}}$$

where
- J = the penetration flux,
- K = the partition coefficient of the barrier,
- D = the diffusion constant,
- Δ = the difference in concentration across the barrier, and
- γ = the thickness of the stratum corneum.
- C = the permeability constant

As a simplification, the flux at a given skin site is directly proportionate to the concentration of the drug.

Factors in Skin Absorption

Skin absorption is affected by many factors.

(1) Absorption occurs by diffusion around and through the cells that make up the skin. Some absorption takes place along hair follicles or through sweat ducts. Putting a drug on the skin does not automatically mean that the drug will reach the intended site of therapeutic action.

(2) Substances such as organic solvents may damage the stratum corneum and permit easier penetration by such chemicals.

(3) Skin thickness and barrier permeability are different in different areas. For example, hydrocortisone is absorbed through the skin 6 times better on the forehead than on the arm, and 44 times better on the scrotum.

(4) Applying more of a substance increases the amount absorbed. Incrementation stops, however, when the skin is saturated. Systemic absorption is also increased if the concentration of a substance is higher and if more body area is exposed.

(5) The skin of preterm infants is more permeable than the skin of full-term infants and adults.

(6) Diseased skin is not necessarily more permeable than normal skin.

(7) Occluded or well-hydrated skin is more permeable than nonoccluded or dry skin.

(8) The vehicle may affect absorption of the drug. In fact, many drugs have been developed to be optimally absorbed with specific vehicles. Compounding a drug extemporaneously with various creams or lotions may result in decreased percutaneous absorption despite an apparent equal concentration, and generic equivalents may not be really equivalent.

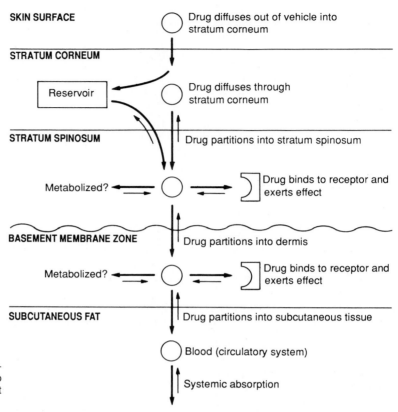

SKIN SURFACE — Drug diffuses out of vehicle into stratum corneum

STRATUM CORNEUM

Reservoir ← Drug diffuses through stratum corneum

STRATUM SPINOSUM — Drug partitions into stratum spinosum

Metabolized? ← ○ → Drug binds to receptor and exerts effect

BASEMENT MEMBRANE ZONE — Drug partitions into dermis

Metabolized? ← ○ → Drug binds to receptor and exerts effect

SUBCUTANEOUS FAT — Drug partitions into subcutaneous tissue

Blood (circulatory system)

Systemic absorption

Figure 2–1. Schema of percutaneous absorption. In order to work, a drug must reach its target cell in adequate amounts.

METHODS OF DETERMINING PERCUTANEOUS ABSORPTION

The 2 basic ways of quantifying percutaneous absorption are the in vitro diffusion cell method and direct in vivo determination. In the in vitro technique, a piece of excised human or animal skin is placed in a diffusion chamber; a chemical (usually with a radioactive label) is applied to one side of the skin, and on the other side an assay is performed to detect the chemical in a collection vessel. The skin sample may be wholly intact or separated into stratum corneum, epidermis, and dermis. The in vitro technique is easy to use and provides results quickly, but results may not be the same as with in vivo absorption.

Percutaneous absorption in vivo is calculated by measuring the levels of drug or a radioactive label on the drug in blood and excreta after topical application of the labeled chemical. Radiolabeled chemicals are often necessary because concentrations of the chemical in blood and excreta following topical applications may be low and otherwise not easily measured. The amount of material detected in blood or excreta following topical application is compared to the amount following parenteral administration, in which

bioavailability is assumed to be 100%. Percutaneous absorption is then expressed as follows:

$$\text{Percentage of dose} = \frac{\text{Total radioactivity following topical administration}}{\text{Total radioactivity following parenteral administration}} \times 100$$

The disadvantage of both methods is that they may require radioactive tracers. In addition, measurement of radioactivity does not distinguish between that of the chemical and that of its metabolites, such as may occur as a result of skin metabolism during absorption.

Other methods of estimating percutaneous absorption—eg, biologic assay (vasoconstriction), autoradiography, and fluorescence studies—are more qualitative than quantitative.

DOSE & DOSING REGIMEN

The concentration of the applied dose, the surface area of the site, and the elapsed time the chemical is on the skin are the main variables affecting percutaneous absorption. As the concentration of a drug is increased, the total amount absorbed into the skin and body also increases. Increasing the surface area of the applied dose also increases absorption. Absorption occurs over time. Thus, the longer the substance is on the skin, the greater the chance for continued absorption. Toxicity following percutaneous and systemic absorption is most likely to occur when high concentrations of a drug are spread over a large area of skin.

The total amount absorbed over a 24-hour period may differ for a single application and for the same amount applied in divided doses; eg, absorption from a single application of a preparation with a high concentration of hydrocortisone has been shown to be greater than when a preparation with the same concentration is applied in several equally divided doses. This finding suggests that the skin becomes saturated with the first topical application, so that absorption from subsequent applications may be altered. In clinical practice, therefore, one daily application of a topical drug may be all that is required if the medication is sufficiently potent and present in sufficient concentration.

VARIATIONS IN ABSORPTION BY INDIVIDUAL & SITE

As with most things individual patients vary in the amount of medication they absorb through the skin. Physicians must consider this when they evaluate the results of topical therapy. For example, the *median* percutaneous absorption of hydrocortisone studied in one group of 18 healthy adult males was 0.9% of the applied dose. Several individuals absorbed only one-third as much, and one subject absorbed 3 times more than the median amount.

The extent of absorption varies also with the site of application of the drug or chemical, and this general pattern of regional variation holds also for different types of chemicals. High total absorption is found on the head, neck, scrotum, and axillas, where exposure to both cosmetics and the environment is greater than that of other body parts (Fig 2–2). The female genitalia show greater absorption than forearm skin but not as much as scrotal skin.

Other physiologic or pathologic factors may also affect percutaneous absorption. More detailed discussion is beyond the scope of this text.

PERCUTANEOUS ABSORPTION IN DISEASED SKIN

The percutaneous absorption of hydrocortisone and certain other dermatologic drugs is usually studied in normal skin, but in clinical practice, drugs are usually applied to diseased skin. It is often assumed that the

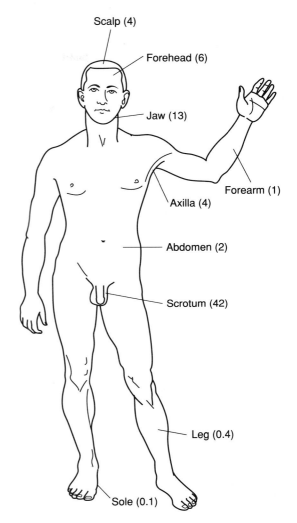

Figure 2–2. Relative percutaneous absorption of hydrocortisone at various anatomic sites.

skin's ability to act as a barrier is compromised when the skin is diseased and that enhanced penetration by topical agents results. In practice, however, absorption differs for different drugs and for different dermatologic disorders. The skin in acute exfoliative erythroderma is more permeable than normal skin. The percutaneous absorption of carmustine (BCNU) in mycosis fungoides in one study was 7.2% for uninvolved skin and 20.6% for diseased skin.

In contrast, the percutaneous absorption of hydrocortisone applied to sharply defined erythematous plaques with silvery scales in 4 patients hospitalized with psoriasis was 2.3%; the absorption of the same dose in 6 normal subjects was 2.4%. The same was true for the absorption of anthralin. Thus, the percutaneous absorption of hydrocortisone and anthralin in skin with presumably stable psoriatic plaques is the same as in normal skin, and a penetrating vehicle and occlusion are needed to enhance delivery of drug to the lesions.

PERCUTANEOUS ABSORPTION IN THE NEONATE

Little is known about percutaneous absorption in children and infants; however, it is in infants that the greatest potential toxicologic response to topical administration can occur.

Infants have a proportionately larger ratio of body surface area to body weight than do adults. An attendant may apply liberal amounts of drug over large areas of skin and then cover the infant with diapers, rubber pants, and other clothing. The combination of large surface area, occlusion produced by clothing, and natural wetness (sweat, urine) tends to enhance absorption of the drug. Other considerations, such as the inherent toxicity of a drug add to the potential for toxic reactions.

Infants are more likely both to develop cushingoid features after applications of topical corticosteroids and to experience seizures from excessive use of lindane cream used as a scabicide. Because of their increased skin permeability, premature infants are probably more susceptible to poisoning owing to topical absorption. In term infants, the skin's capacity to act as a barrier is probably intact, but these infants are still vulnerable to topical poisoning.

REFERENCES

Bronough R, Maibach HI: *Percutaneous Absorption.* Marcel Dekker, 1985.

Feldmann RJ, Maibach HI: Regional variation in percutaneous penetration of ^{14}C cortisol in man. J Invest Dermatol 1967;48:181.

Maibach HI: In vivo percutaneous penetration of corticoids in man and unresolved problems in their efficacy. Dermatologica 1976;152(Suppl 1):11.

Riegelman S: Pharmacokinetic factors affecting epidermal penetration and percutaneous absorption. Clin Pharmacol Ther 1974;16:873.

Wester RC, Bucks DA, Maibach HI: In vivo percutaneous absorption of hydrocortisone in psoriatic patients and normal volunteers. J Am Acad Dermatol 1983;5:645.

Wester RC, Maibach HI: Cutaneous pharmacokinetics: Ten steps to percutaneous absorption. Drug Metab Rev 1983;14:169.

Wester RC, Maibach HI: Percutaneous absorption: Neonate compared to the adult. In: *Neonatal Skin: Structure and Function.* Maibach HI, Boisits E (editors). Marcel Dekker, 1982.

Sebum

3

John S. Strauss, MD

Sebaceous glands are holocrine structures—ie, their discharged secretion contains the entire secreting cells—whose cells synthesize lipids. When a cell completes its life cycle and ruptures, the mixture of lipids, called **sebum,** is discharged into the sebaceous duct and then into the follicular canal to be carried to the skin surface. Since the sebaceous glands are holocrine structures, the production of sebum is roughly proportionate to gland size, and measurements of the rate of sebum production have been used to determine the average size of the glands. Discussion of variations in the rates of secretion in sebaceous glands is therefore almost synonymous with discussion of changes in sebaceous gland size; eg, there are marked changes in sebaceous gland size in relation to age, and these are reflected in changes in the production of sebum.

Sebum has no known function in humans. Before the nature of sebum is discussed, it is necessary to briefly outline how the functional capacity of the glands (sebum production) is measured.

Human sebaceous glands vary greatly in size and shape from one gland to another, in the number of glandular acini per follicular unit, and in their relationship to the follicular unit itself. Unless surface area (planimetric) methods are used, therefore, only major changes in gland size can be appreciated in histologic sections. Because of this limitation—as well as the problems associated with repeated biopsies—measurements of the functional capacity of the glands have been used in most studies to determine the response of the sebaceous glands. The advantage of measuring the functional capacity is that many glandular units are sampled, so that the variations in individual glandular units average out. In addition, since these methods are noninvasive, multiple collections can be made over time to follow any changes in sebaceous gland size and function.

The major technologic drawback to all collection techniques is that the measurements are made at the surface of the skin. Skin surface lipids are composed of a *mixture* of sebum and lipids liberated from epidermal cells during keratinization. Since there are major differences in the composition of lipids from

these 2 sources, it may be difficult to assess the functional capacity of sebaceous glands by assessing the amounts or composition of surface lipids. This drawback can be overcome by making measurements from sebaceous gland-rich areas, such as the face, as described below.

There are many different methods of measuring sebaceous gland activity. Adequate techniques involve collecting the skin surface lipids from a defined area of the skin at a fixed interval of time after suitable baseline conditions have been established. The collected lipid can be analyzed by various methods, including weighing, spectroscopy, photometry, nephelometry, and specific identification of lipid components of sebaceous origin. It should be apparent that when surface measurements are made, the gland output itself is not measured. On areas such as the face, where most of the lipid is of sebaceous origin, the epidermal component is minor and probably does not significantly influence the results. On the extremities, however, where the sebaceous glands are small, there could be a large sampling error because the epidermal lipid component of the skin surface film is proportionately greater. Therefore, on these areas it becomes particularly important to identify lipids that are specifically and uniquely of sebaceous origin.

COMPOSITION OF SEBACEOUS, EPIDERMAL, & SKIN SURFACE LIPIDS

Pure human sebum, as excreted by the sebaceous glands, contains approximately 50–55% triglycerides, 25–30% wax esters, 10–15% squalene, and a small amount of cholesterol and cholesterol esters. Squalene represents the end product of a blocked cholesterol synthesis pathway. Squalene and wax esters are unique to sebum; they are not found in epidermally derived lipid. They are the lipids that should be identified as reference standards to identify sebum. There are no free fatty acids in freshly secreted sebum. The free fatty acids found on the skin surface result from the partial hydrolysis of triglycerides by bacteria in the follicular canal and on the skin surface. Epidermally derived lipids have about the same proportion of triglycerides as sebum, but the rest of the lipid consists of cholesterol and cholesterol esters. Skin surface lipid, then, is a mixture of sebum and epidermal lipids, and the exact composition of the skin surface varies depending on the relative proportions of sebaceous and epidermal lipids in the collection area.

If radiolabeled acetate is injected into human skin, the average time for peak recovery of the label in surface lipids is 8 days. Synthesis takes about $7\frac{1}{2}$ days, and half a day is needed for sebum to pass from the ruptured sebaceous cell to the surface of the skin. The double bonding in the fatty acids of sebum is at the 6–7 position, rather than at the usual 9–10 position found in fatty acids in all other body tissues— evidence that there is de novo synthesis of lipids rather than incorporation of circulating lipids.

FACTORS INFLUENCING SEBUM EXCRETION

There are no known external factors that influence sebaceous gland secretion. Sebum secretion is in fact a continuous process that is not influenced by external forces. In a protected area, sebum will continue to accumulate over extended periods. However, in unprotected sites, the lipid will either flow away or be wiped away, thereby making it appear as though there is a limit to the amount of sebum that is secreted. Although the skin looks oilier in summer than in winter, this is not due to any change in the secretory rate related to temperature. The presence of more surface moisture causes the lipid to spread as a monolayer owing to its content of fatty acids and other polar lipids that become oriented at the oil-water interface. The effect of water can be demonstrated by using an atomizer to spray water onto the forehead of a person who appears to have dry skin; the skin instantly becomes more oily.

The rate of sebum secretion depends on gland size. There are thus regional variations in sebaceous secretion. Sebaceous gland secretion is under hormonal control, as discussed below. Therapeutic agents may also influence sebaceous gland secretion (see Chapter 26).

Regional Variations

The size and number of the sebaceous glands show wide regional variations, with corresponding differences in the lipid film at the surface of the skin. Sebaceous glands are largest and most numerous on the face and scalp and progressively decrease in size and number from the trunk to the extremities. There are no sebaceous glands on the palms and soles. On the chest and back, larger and more numerous glands are found on the midline than laterally.

Hormonal Factors

There is no motor innervation of the sebaceous glands; variation in size and activity of the gland with age is hormonally related.

At birth, the sebaceous glands are well-developed, but shortly thereafter they atrophy and do not enlarge again until puberty. Animal and human studies show that the glands are stimulated by androgens. Development of the sebaceous glands at birth is probably related either to stimulation by the fetal adrenal gland or to transplacental hormonal stimulation.

Stimulation of the glands during puberty is one of the earliest manifestations of the pubertal process. Sebaceous glands are androgen-sensitive, and it is likely that the small increase in androgen production accompanying adrenarche is capable of stimulating the human sebaceous glands.

The changes in sebaceous gland activity that occur shortly after birth and during early puberty can be detected by changes in the composition of skin surface lipid. Sebaceous lipid contains wax esters and squalene but little cholesterol and cholesterol esters, whereas epidermal lipid is rich in cholesterol and cholesterol esters and low in wax esters and squalene. Therefore, if skin surface lipid is composed mainly of epidermal lipid, it will have a high cholesterol content and a low content of squalene and wax esters; if it is rich in sebaceous lipid, the cholesterol level will be low, but there will be significant amounts of wax esters and squalene. In the newborn, the skin surface lipid of the face reflects the greater contribution of lipid from the sebaceous glands. During childhood, however, surface lipid is of the epidermal type. When sebaceous gland function begins to increase at about 8 years of age in most individuals, the composition of the skin surface lipids again shows that sebaceous gland lipid is the major component. The change in composition is a sensitive measurement that is useful only when the sebaceous component is small; once it is more than 10–15%, no further changes can be detected in the composition of the surface lipid film.

Sebum secretion decreases slowly after puberty. Sebum secretion is less in women than in men, probably due to a lesser stimulatory effect of the combined adrenal and ovarian androgens compared to the stimulation in men by testosterone and its derivatives. Circulating estrogen levels are probably insufficient to influence sebaceous gland secretion, though large amounts of exogenous estrogen decrease sebaceous gland activity. (This is the basis for the therapeutic use of estrogens in acne.) Although pharmacologic doses of exogenous progesterone may stimulate the glands, physiologic endogenous progesterone levels are not sufficient to do so.

Animal studies show that sebaceous gland secretion depends on pituitary activity. There are few human data on this point, but sebum secretion is decreased in primary and secondary hypopituitarism. Whether this is a direct effect or mediated through changes in gonadotropin secretion has not been determined, though in gonadotropin deficiency, sebaceous gland activity is restored by administration of gonadotropin.

Secretion of sebum is increased in parkinsonism, but the cause is not known.

Nutritional Factors

Near-total starvation has pronounced effects on sebaceous gland activity. Within 10 days of the onset of a severe fast ($<$ 50 kcal/d), the amount of squalene in surface skin lipids increases. This represents a relative increase in the squalene concentration resulting from a decrease in the synthesis of other components of sebum while squalene synthesis remains constant. Clinical studies in severe pellagra have confirmed these findings, and when patients with pellagra are given nutritional support, the changes in lipid composition are promptly reversed. The mechanisms involved are unknown. It is not known if changes occur with intermediate levels of caloric deprivation.

REFERENCES

Downing DT, Stranieri AM, Strauss JS: The effect of accumulated lipids on measurements of sebum secretion in human skin. J Invest Dermatol 1982;79:226.

Downing DT, Strauss JS: On the mechanism of sebaceous secretion. Arch Dermatol Res 1982;272:343.

Downing DT, Strauss JS: Synthesis and composition of surface lipids of human skin. J Invest Dermatol 1974;62:228.

Greene RS et al: Anatomic variation in the amount and composition of human surface lipid. J Invest Dermatol 1970;54:240.

Greene SC et al: Variation in sebum fatty acid composition among adult humans. J Invest Dermatol 1984;83:114.

Harris HH et al: Sustainable rates of sebum secretion in acne patients and matched normal controls. J Am Acad Dermatol 1983;8:532.

Jacobsen E et al: Age-related changes in sebaceous wax ester secretion rates in men and women. J Invest Dermatol 1985;85:483.

Kligman AM, Shelley WB: An investigation into the biology of the sebaceous gland. J Invest Dermatol 1958; 30:99.

Pochi PE, Strauss JS: Endocrinologic control of the development and activity of the human sebaceous gland. J Invest Dermatol 1974;62:191.

Pochi PE, Strauss JS: Studies on the sebaceous glands in acne and endocrine disorders. Bull NY Acad Med 1977;53:359.

Pochi PE, Strauss JS, Downing DT: Age-related changes in sebaceous gland activity. J Invest Dermatol 1979; 73:108.

Ramasastry P el at: Chemical composition of human skin surface lipids from birth to puberty. J Invest Dermatol 1970;54:139.

Stewart ME et al: Suppression of sebum secretion with 13-cis-retinoic acid: Effect on individual skin surface lipids and implications for their anatomic origin. J Invest Dermatol 1984;82:74.

Stewart ME et al: Measurement of sebum secretion rates in young children. J Invest Dermatol 1985;84:59.

Strauss JS, Pochi PE: The quantitative gravimetric determination of sebum production. J Invest Dermatol 1961;36:293.

Strauss JS, Downing DT, Ebling FJ: Sebaceous glands. Pages 569–595 in: *Biochemistry and Physiology of the Skin.* Goldsmith LA (editor). Oxford Univ Press, 1983.

4

Cutaneous Microbiology

Raza Aly, MPH, PhD

Healthy individuals harbor limited numbers of bacteria at any given skin site; these total numbers are made up of a uniform range of species. At birth, the newborn infant is virtually free of bacteria but quickly acquires typical "normal flora" in a remarkably consistent manner. The neonate is exposed to bacteria from the mother's vaginal and fecal microflora during birth and then from the external environment.

Conventionally, cutaneous bacteria are classified as "residents" or "transients." To qualify as residents, organisms must be able to multiply on the skin, not merely survive there. The transient bacteria are merely present on the skin. They may or may not become residents, depending on several ecologic factors.

The majority of the resident microorganisms live in the most superficial layers of the epidermal stratum corneum and in the upper parts of the hair follicles. The remainder of the resident skin bacteria reside in the deeper areas of the follicular canals, some of which are beyond the reach of ordinary disinfection procedures. These inaccessible bacteria serve as a reservoir of recolonization after surface bacteria are removed by artificial means.

The types of organisms present on the skin change from season to season, with micrococci preponderating during the winter and coryneforms in the summer in temperate climes. The survival of bacteria and the extent to which they become resident probably depends partly upon the exposure of skin to a particular environment and partly on the innate and species-specific bactericidal activity of the skin. In general, there are 3 regions that differ in their bacterial flora: (1) the axillas, the perineum, and the webs of the toes; (2) the hands, face, and abdomen; and (3) the upper arms, legs, and trunk. Anatomic sites where partial occlusion is the rule (axillas, perineum, toe webs) yield greater numbers of microorganisms than normally exposed areas (arms, legs, trunk). The differences may relate to increased amounts of moisture, higher body temperature, and concentrations of skin lipids in the occluded areas. The axillas, perineum, and toe webs are more frequently colonized by gram-negative bacilli than drier areas. Areas of skin with sebaceous gland-rich areas, such as the face, scalp,

and upper trunk, bear large numbers of anaerobic propionibacteria and *Pityrosporum ovale*.

The size of the bacterial population in each region remains relatively constant (Fig 4–1). Certain subjects may be characterized as having consistently high bacterial counts, whereas others show relatively constant low counts.

Colonization Versus Infection

Colonization is the presence on the skin (or a lesion) of bacteria or other pathogens without any significant associated host reaction. A smear for microscopic examination may be helpful in determining whether colonization or infection is occurring. The presence of polymorphonuclear leukocytes in the smear is evidence that host defenses are involved. Leukocytes are usually not present in lesions merely colonized by pathogens. However, many nonbacterial stresses are capable of eliciting polymorphonuclear leukocyte responses. The absence of bacteria in smears from such lesions indicates that the origin of the lesion is nonbacterial. These findings must be correlated with clinical data before firm diagnostic conclusions can be reached.

RESIDENT SKIN FLORA

Staphylococci

At least 10 *Staphylococcus* species living on humans have been characterized: *S aureus, S epidermidis, S hominis,* and *S saprophyticus* are the more common species. *S aureus* is potentially pathogenic and thus has received the most attention; the nose and perineum are the common resident carrier sites. This organism, however, is rarely resident on normal skin, with an incidence of less than 10%. In diseased skin, colonization is common. The incidence of *S aureus* in patients with atopic dermatitis is 93% in lesions and 76% on adjacent normal skin. On eczematous skin, it is the predominant organism, constituting 90% of the total aerobic flora.

S epidermidis and *S hominis* are the most frequently isolated staphylococci from the axillas, head,

22

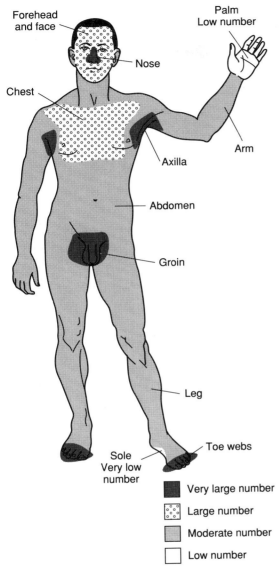

Figure 4–1. Relative numbers of bacteria on the skin surface at various anatomic sites.

Forehead and face
Palm Low number
Nose
Chest
Arm
Axilla
Abdomen
Groin
Leg
Sole Very low number
Toe webs

■ Very large number
▦ Large number
▨ Moderate number
□ Low number

legs, and arms. Micrococci are usually found in much smaller numbers on human skin than on staphylococci. Eight different *Micrococcus* species have been isolated from human skin—*M luteus (Sarcina luteus)* is the major species—but they probably have even lower pathogenicity than *S epidermidis*.

Coryneforms

The aerobic coryneforms of skin are commonly known in the medical literature as the "diphtheroids," a name designed to indicate a close relationship with the diphtheria bacillus. However, except for some morphologic resemblance, they have little in com-

mon; therefore, the better term "coryneform" is used in the current skin microbiology literature.

Skin coryneforms are conveniently categorized on the basis of lipolytic activity. The lipophilic coryneforms are usually found in the axilla and other moist area of the skin; nonlipophilics are common in the glabrous skin.

Brevibacterium species are nonlipophilic coryneforms and prefer to live in humid regions of the skin, particularly the toe webs.

Propionibacterium acnes

This bacterium is the predominant anaerobe in areas rich in sebaceous glands. The major pathogenic process with which *P acnes* has commonly been associated is acne vulgaris. Two other propionibacteria (*P granulosum* and *P avidum*) are also found in the skin.

Streptococci

Streptococci, especially beta-hemolytic streptococci, are not frequently isolated on the skin. Alpha-hemolytic streptococci are predominantly present in the oropharynx and may spread to adjoining skin areas, especially in infants. In some geographic areas with high streptococcal skin infection rates, carriage of beta-hemolytic streptococci on normal skin has been reported.

Gram-Negative Bacteria

The aerobic gram-negative bacteria form a small proportion of the skin flora of healthy individuals. They occur primarily on the perineum and moist intertriginous areas. *Escherichia coli, Klebsiella-Enterobacter,* and *Proteus* species predominate. *Acinetobacter (Mima-Herellea)* is sometimes present in the intertriginous regions. Infrequent, usually transitory carriage of gram-positive *Bacillus* species and mycobacteria has also been reported.

Pityrosporum

Pityrosporum species are the only yeasts found in significant numbers on human skin. The 3 morphologic forms found on the skin—oval, round, and filamentous—gave rise to the delineation of 3 separate species: *P ovale, P orbiculare,* and *Malassezia furfur*. These 3 forms are morphologic variants of the same species.

FACTORS CONTROLLING SKIN BACTERIAL FLORA

Several factors influence survival of bacteria—including pathogens—on human skin. When *S aureus* and group A beta-hemolytic streptococci are experimentally applied on human skin, they do not survive for more than a few hours. Yet on some individuals, these bacteria not only survive but also multiply and initiate disease. Skin itself controls in part the survival of organisms that come in contact with it.

Cutaneous Barrier

The barrier presented by the skin and mucous membranes constitutes a strong defense against invading organisms. The skin not only has a resistant barrier in the outer keratinous layer, but it is also protected against microbial infection by several other host and bacterial factors.

When skin is damaged, cutaneous infection can develop. The organisms most likely to be involved in such infections are those that normally inhabit the hair follicles and sweat glands.

Many transient pathogenic microorganisms are capable of penetrating mucous membranes in the absence of trauma. The toxic products of bacteria may damage the surface epithelial cells, thus facilitating their entry. Once the barrier is breached, the host then relies on the next line of defense: The cellular defense mechanism against bacteria primarily consists of the ingestion and intracellular killing of invading microorganisms. Humoral factors (antibodies and complement) can opsonize or damage bacteria, facilitating their removal by phagocytosis. On repeated contact with bacteria, specifically sensitized lymphocytes elaborate lymphokines that activate macrophages and enhance phagocytosis and intracellular killing.

Other Host Factors

Mechanical factors alone cannot be entirely responsible for skin resistance to bacterial invasion. The **low pH** (3.0–5.0) of the skin discourages growth of many environmental bacteria. Skin surface lipids comprising fatty acids are antimicrobial; these act against *Streptococcus pyogenes* and *Staphylococcus aureus* but not against certain gram-negative bacteria, eg, *E coli* and *Pseudomonas aeruginosa*. For some skin bacteria, cutaneous **surface lipids** may have a stimulatory rather than inhibitory role. Oleic acid promotes growth of *P acnes* and other coryneforms.

A variety of **antimicrobial antibodies** occur in external secretions of the normal host. These antibodies play an important role in the regulation of the resident flora and the survival of pathogenic bacteria. IgA antibodies found in the saliva can inhibit attachment of oral streptococci to epithelial cells without the involvement of phagocytes or the complement system. A deficiency in this mechanism may render the host susceptible to certain infections.

Desquamation, a continuous process, is an important host factor that limits the bacterial population. Epithelial cells colonized with bacteria are always being shed. Bacteria that can recolonize the keratinous surface become part of the resident flora, while those that cannot will eventually be eliminated. Clinicians have used chemicals (eg, salicylic acid) that promote shedding of horny scales with this effect in mind.

Humidity has a profound effect on the total flora and on its composition. The effects of increased hydration have been studied by occluding the skin with plastic film for several days. The pH of the skin, which is acidic (4.5–5.5) before occlusion, becomes neutral (7.0) after 4 days of occlusion. In addition, surface levels of carbon dioxide, which promote microbial growth and alter microbial metabolism, tend to rise. These changes plus the hydration of the skin caused by the occlusion produce exponential rises in microbial counts.

Bacterial adherence to the skin surface is another factor determining colonization. Not all bacteria adhere to skin even when competition from other microorganisms is eliminated. The binding is a specific phenomenon brought about by the molecular interaction of bacterial and host cellular surface components. The pili in gram-negative bacteria and fimbriae in gram-positive bacteria—both proteins—are involved. When bacteria and skin epithelial cells are mixed experimentally, significant adherence occurs with *S aureus*, *S epidermidis*, *S pyogenes*, *P aeruginosa*, and coryneforms but not with *Streptococcus viridans* or alpha-hemolytic streptococci. The feeble adherence of these streptococci may account for their scarcity on normal skin. *P aeruginosa* and *S pyogenes* show good attachment despite the fact that they are infrequently encountered on healthy skin. Since the nose serves as a reservoir of *S aureus*, the ability of this organism to adhere to nasal epithelial cells is also important. The teichoic acid component of the cell wall of *S aureus* seems to mediate adherence of the organism to nasal mucosal cells. Adherence of *S aureus* to fibronectin is another factor to be considered for adherence and colonization.

The host's general health status and regular use of hypodermic needles are important factors as well. Drug addicts, patients with diabetes injecting themselves with insulin, and those receiving allergy shots all have an increased carriage rate of *S aureus* in the nose.

Microbial Factors

Microbial antagonism is a complex regulator of the resident skin flora. This phenomenon can be attributed in part to competition for essential nutrients and in part to the production of inhibitory substances. Bacteriocins produced by bacteria are chemically heterogeneous and include polypeptides, glycoproteins, and lipoproteins. The phenomenon of bacterial interference has been utilized to control recurrent furunculosis and staphylococcal epidemics in the hospital nursery by the prophylactic application of *S aureus* strain 502A (see Chapter 12).

The opposite action—**satellitism or syntrophism**—wherein one organism produces a growth enhancement factor for another, also may be an effective population regulator. It is not known whether the bacteria involved in this phenomenon exert these effects by production of essential factors, by destruction of toxic substances, or by both mechanisms.

In general, intact skin provides a formidable barrier against bacterial invasion. Breaches in mucosal or skin surface defenses often result in the host becoming infected by members of its own resident flora. Periodontal disease, caries, and endocarditis are major examples. Procedures that impair host defenses—eg, immunosuppression, chemotherapy, and irradiation—may also render the host susceptible to the resident flora or especially to transient pathogens, ordinarily suppressed by the normal flora.

Disinfection of Skin

Physicians and others in contact with patients who may or may not harbor infections are required to prevent spread of infection from one patient to the next. Realistically, it is not necessary to remove the entire skin flora to achieve this purpose—the aim should be rather to decrease the transient flora (which may include pathogens) and keep the normal flora to a minimum.

The transient skin flora is not firmly attached to the skin and can usually be removed easily and almost as effectively by handwashing with soap or detergent and water as with an antiseptic agent. Antiseptics may produce excessively dry skin if used frequently, and any regimen of handwashing that leads to dermatitis should be discontinued or modified. Antiseptics should be used when longer periods of antibacterial activity are needed, such as during surgery and other invasive procedures of high risk or in handling newborn infants. Chlorhexidine, iodine, and hexachlorophene are widely used for this purpose.

During venipuncture, reduction of bacterial flora is required only for a short time. In this instance, 70% alcohol is very effective, and its protein-precipitating action makes dispersal of microcolonies unlikely. The antibacterial activity ends with evaporation of the alcohol.

REFERENCES

Aly R, Shinefield HR (editors): *Bacterial Interference.* CRC Press, 1982.

Aly R et al: Survival of pathogenic microorganisms on human skin. J Invest Dermatol 1972;58:205.

Kloos WE, Musselwhite MS: Distribution and persistence of *Staphylococcus* and *Micrococcus* species and other aerobic bacteria on human skin. Appl Microbiol 1975;30:381.

Maibach HI, Aly R (editors): *Skin Microbiology: Relevance to Clinical Infection.* Springer-Verlag, 1981.

Marples RR, Leyden JJ: Bacterial infection: Fundamental cutaneous microbiology. Pages 590–599 in: *Dermatology,* 2nd ed. Moschella SL, Hurley HJ (editors). Saunders, 1985.

Noble WC: *Microbiology of Human Skin,* 2nd ed. Lloyd-Luke, 1981.

Sheagren JN: *Staphylococcus aureus:* The persistent pathogen. N Engl J Med 1984;310:1368.

5

Care of Normal Skin, Hair, & Nails

Patricia G. Engasser, MD

The skin and its appendages constitute a resilient organ that does not require elaborate care for optimal functioning. The misinformation provided the public about skin, hair, and nail care has understandably resulted in confusion. Physicians should therefore serve as a source of reliable information on these matters for their patients and should begin by directing attention to the skin in relation to general health. Special foods or vitamins in excess of normal requirements do not significantly enhance the quality of the skin, hair, or nails; however, fad diets with protein deprivation may have disastrous dermatologic consequences, such as profuse hair loss. Systemic disorders and environmental factors may also profoundly influence the condition of the skin and its appendages.

SKIN CARE

SKIN CLEANSING

Skin cleansing removes dirt, cosmetics, cellular debris, body secretions, sweat, and microorganisms. The frequency and vigor with which the skin should be cleansed depend on the individual's skin, daily activities, and environment. Washing is the most efficient method. Water alone removes many soils; a surface-active agent (soap or detergent) aids removal of lipids. In the USA, soaps account for 90% of the toilet bars sold. Promoters have claimed that detergent bars are milder than soaps, allegedly because they do not create an alkaline pH. The skin's excellent buffering system accurately maintains an acid pH, however, and claims that products are superior because they protect the "acid mantle" cannot be substantiated.

All soaps and detergents are at least mildly irritating, and individuals differ significantly in their ability to tolerate various products. The skin of infants and young children may be irritated by detergents in bubble baths marketed for this age group, for example. As adults age, the need and tolerance for washing with soap and water decreases, and bathing or showering with warm water once or twice a week using a cleansing bar only in intertriginous or odor-producing areas may suffice for the elderly. Bath oils temporarily smooth the skin and decrease dryness caused by bathing, but they have the important disadvantage of causing the tub or floor to become dangerously slippery.

Some people with normal-appearing complexions complain that soap and water cause burning and irritation; such patients can generally use plain water to wash and should be instructed to use a toilet bar sparingly on occasion. Soap-free cleansers or emollients (eg, Cetaphil lotion) may be used by people with sensitive skins. Women who use only cleansing creams and never wash their faces may develop seborrheic dermatitis, acne, or acne rosacea. Abrasive sponges or scrubs are acceptable if they are tolerated, but vigorous scrubbing is not recommended.

Astringents, fresheners, toners, or refining lotions are generally alcohol-in-water solutions used by people with oily complexions to remove sebum or makeup. Facial masks, which cause drying by evaporation, are unnecessary in routine skin care and may be irritating.

REDUCTION OF BODY ODOR & SWEATING

Attention to personal cleanliness is the first step in reducing body odor. Bathing or showering removes dirt, bacteria, sweat, sebum, and cellular debris. Clean clothes are also important to control body odor.

Axillas

People in the USA spend about $800 million annually on antiperspirants and deodorants to reduce axillary sweating and modify its odor. There are 2 types of axillary sweat glands (see also Chapter 27). The output of the numerous eccrine sweat glands is a clear, watery fluid that is secreted in greater amounts in response to thermal or emotional stimuli. The apocrine sweat glands secrete minute amounts of milky, odorless, sterile fluid that produces a distinctive body odor when metabolized by the axillary flora. Because the apocrine glands develop under the control of androgenic hormones, axillary odor does not occur until puberty.

Deodorants contain modestly effective antimicrobial agents and may contain fragrances to disguise axillary odor. **Antiperspirants** contain aluminum or aluminum-zirconium salts, which block the eccrine sweat duct and obstruct delivery of sweat to the skin surface. These metallic salts also exert a deodorant effect because of their antimicrobial properties, and the drier environment they produce reduces the number of odor-causing bacteria.

Commercial antiperspirants cause a 20–40% reduction in axillary sweating. Their effectiveness can be increased by applying them both in the morning and at bedtime. Because these products may be mildly irritating, they should not be applied to moist or inflamed skin, nor should they be used soon after shaving. Shaving axillary hair aids in reducing odor, because hair increases the surface area for the production and release of odor-causing chemicals.

For patients with extreme hyperhidrosis, aluminum chloride hexahydrate, 20% solution in absolute alcohol (Drysol), may be prescribed by a physician for use on the axillas, palms, or soles. The product is applied at bedtime under an occlusive plastic film but may cause irritation, especially if used frequently.

Pubes

Feminine hygiene sprays are deodorants sprayed on the vulva. Many patients have suffered adverse local reactions to these products, and women are best advised to cleanse the vulva gently with toilet soap and water. Until the relationship of talc to ovarian carcinoma has been clarified, cosmetics containing perfumed talc should not be used on the vulva simply to mask body odor. However, obese males or male athletes may find that talcum powder dusted in the groin helps to prevent chafing.

Feet

The synthetic materials used in shoes today do not dissipate sweat as well as leather does. Shoes made of synthetic materials create a damp, warm environment favoring the growth of bacteria and fungi. Removing these shoes at home and wearing open slippers or sandals may be necessary for some people to avoid bromhidrosis or tinea pedis. Dusting the feet with drying powders (eg, Zeasorb powder) is helpful.

MOISTURIZING

Dry Skin

The stratum corneum remains flexible as long as its water content is at least 10%. When the moisture content of air is reduced (eg, in dry weather or in air-conditioned rooms), the stratum corneum may become dry and brittle. The usual desquamation process is deranged, so that the skin flakes and small fissures appear. The skin feels rough and looks scaly. The intercellular lipid bilayer plays a role in barrier function and desquamation. Repeated contact with soaps, detergents, or lipid solvents depletes these lipids and leads to dry skin. Dry skin on the body causes pruritus. If the condition progresses, inflammation develops.

Moisturizers

Cosmetic moisturizers soften and lubricate dry skin and function in the same way as dermatologic emollient creams and lotions. *Moisturizers do not prevent aging of the skin.* Addition of DNA, RNA, placenta extract, or similar materials does not improve their effectiveness.

Most moisturizers are oil-and-water emulsions. Soon after they are applied, the water evaporates to leave an occlusive film of residual oil that inhibits further evaporation of water and allows gradual rehydration of the stratum corneum. In general, thick moisturizers containing petrolatum or lanolin are the most effective even if the least aesthetic. Lighter, thinner lotions or creams are less effective for severely dry skin, and more frequent applications may be required. In addition to adding a layer of oil, most moisturizers affect keratinization so that with regular use the cells of the stratum corneum are more compact. This retards water loss. Humectants such as lactic acid and urea augment this effect.

Moisturizers counteract the taut feeling caused by washing. They also disguise the "ashy" appearance associated with black skin when it flakes. Moisturizers can prevent chapping in persons whose hands are repeatedly immersed in detergents and water or are exposed to cold dry weather. Emollients should be used after bathing by persons with dry or flaking skin, because they can relieve pruritus and discomfort.

In some women, the repeated use of moisturizers may cause an acneiform eruption on the lower face. Although moisturizers are considered bland preparations by the general public, they contain emulsifiers, preservatives, and fragrances that can cause irritant or allergic contact dermatitis.

PREVENTION & REPAIR OF SUN DAMAGE

Aging Skin & Sun-Damaged Skin

Only in the last 2 decades have dermatologic scientists and clinicians separated the changes observed in skin due to intrinsic aging from those of sun-induced aging (photoaging). With aging, there is a flattening of the dermal-epidermal junction, decrease in numbers of pigment-producing melanocytes, thinning of the dermis, and reduction in the number of skin appendages. Often this thinner, more translucent skin becomes rough and dry.

Sun-induced aging occurs predominantly in light-exposed areas on fair-skinned people. Actinic damage causes irregular epidermal cellular proliferation, which can lead to atypia and ultimately to skin cancer. Irregular pigmentation is common. Ultraviolet light (UVL) damages dermal fibroblasts, causing degeneration of elastin and collagen that results in wrinkling.

Sun Protection

Although acute sun damage is easily recognized as a painful sunburn, the delayed injurious effects are cumulative, initially less noticeable, and often disregarded. The incidence of skin cancers, including melanoma, increases as distance from the equator decreases, ie, as the intensity of UVL exposure increases.

The skin normally defends itself against damage from UVL by synthesizing melanin, the pigment responsible for tanning. Fair-skinned people who tan poorly and freckle or those who tan moderately but are subjected to prolonged or intense UVL exposure need protection other than the skin's natural defenses. Clothing is helpful, though a single layer of light clothing does not offer total protection, and as much as 50% of the incidental light may be reflected onto the skin under a wide-brimmed hat.

A. Sunscreens: Sunscreens are topical preparations that absorb or scatter UVL. Their efficacy in shielding skin from UVL damage and their cosmetic acceptability have improved significantly in the last decade. The sun protection factor (SPF) is a numerical value that signifies the degree of protection provided by each product against sunburning wavelengths of ultraviolet radiation. The SPF value is assigned after clinical testing has determined the preparation's ability to prevent sunburn. An amount of UVL that causes a very mild sunburn is called the minimal erythema dose (MED). Using fair-skinned subjects and either natural sunlight or a solar simulator, the SPF is calculated as follows:

$$SPF = \frac{\text{MED of skin protected with test sunscreen}}{\text{MED of unprotected skin}}$$

The resulting number is generally rounded off and stated as 2, 4, 6, 8, 15, or higher. If a person usually sunburns after 30 minutes of exposure, wearing a sunscreen with a rating of SPF 8 *theoretically* would enable that person to be out of doors for up to 4 hours without sunburning; however, protection may be significantly reduced by sweating, swimming, or friction or if the subject applies too thin a layer of sunscreen. Furthermore, the solar simulator may not accurately reproduce natural conditions of exposure of skin to sunlight.

Sun damage is cumulative, so that the use of sunscreens should be started in childhood. Fair-skinned individuals anticipating significant outdoor exposure should apply a sunscreen (preferably with a rating of SPF 15 or higher) each morning from spring through fall and reapply it after swimming or sweating. Although persons who are able to tan and insist on tanning may choose to use sunscreens with a rating of SPF 6 or 8, they should be reminded that tanning itself always signifies that the skin has been injured. Users should experiment to find a sunscreen with the base they prefer. Adolescents with oily skin or acne ordinarily use a clear, alcohol-based sunscreen. Children and mature women usually prefer alcohol-free lotions and creams that do not sting when applied. Sun-screening lip balms are also helpful. Designations of "water-resistant" or "waterproof" indicate that the sunscreen has withstood testing for staying power during water immersion.

There is increasing evidence from animal experiments that UVL (320–400 nm) contributes to acute and chronic actinic damage, and this has prompted a search for screening agents effective against long-wave UVL (ie, UVA). Butyl methoxydibenzoylmethane (Parsol 1789) has been introduced as a chemical that offers significant UVA protection (Photoplex).

Occasionally, a patient develops contact or photo-contact dermatitis after using sunscreens. This may represent an allergic reaction to one of the product's ingredients, eg, aminobenzoic acid (*p*-aminobenzoic acid, PABA). Patch testing can guide recommendations for a suitable alternative product by identifying the allergen.

B. Lotions to Augment Suntan: Despite claims to the contrary, so-called quick-tanning lotions are of little or no medical value. They do not enhance the natural tanning process, ie, increase the production of melanin. Some products may stain the skin, mimicking a tan, but this stain offers little or no protection from sunburn.

C. Tanning Booths and Beds (Solariums): Exposure of skin to long-wavelength ultraviolet radiation in a solarium produces a natural-appearing tan. Although this may confer some degree of protection to the skin from subsequent exposure to sunlight, the solarium exposure itself may damage the skin. Until the true risks are better known, cosmetic tanning in solariums is not recommended.

Repair of Actinic Damage

Tretinoin is a vitamin A derivative that when applied topically can repair actinic damage as detected visually and histologically. The role this agent will ultimately play in skin care is not settled. Although retinoids have been studied for years for their anticarcinogenic properties, under certain specialized conditions in animal experiments, tretinoin can act as a promoter for chemical carcinogenesis.

Despite the foregoing, tretinoin (Retin-A cream 0.025%, 0.05%, and 0.1%) is being prescribed widely to reverse actinic damage. A small amount (pea-sized) is applied to the face or other light-exposed areas at bedtime. To minimize irritation, application should be delayed for 20 minutes after washing. Applications should be initiated gradually every second or third night. Tretinoin may be irritating at first, but tolerance develops with time. Because tretinoin causes desquamation, the skin is more vulnerable to UVL damage during treatment and must be protected with clothing and sunscreens.

HAIR CARE
(See also Chapter 28.)

HAIR WASHING

The hair and scalp are washed with shampoos to remove sebum, cellular debris, microorganisms, cosmetics, and other soils. Shampoos today usually contain anionic detergents rather than soaps. Because they remove oil efficiently, people with oily scalps do not really need to choose specially formulated shampoos. People usually choose a shampoo for aesthetic, not medical, reasons.

Although most North Americans shampoo more frequently than hygiene requires, frequent—even daily—shampooing rarely causes difficulties, and there is no substantial evidence that the practice increases sebum production.

Many different kinds of shampoos have been developed.

Antidandruff Shampoos

Dandruff is characterized by desquamation of corneocytes in visible groups. It is hypothesized that the yeastlike organism *Pityrosporon ovale* plays a causative role. There is no "cure" for dandruff. Frequent shampooing alone is sufficient for mild cases. Se-

lenium sulfide, zinc pyrithione, tar sulfur, and salicylic acid are useful agents found in shampoos specifically designed to treat dandruff. It may be necessary to rotate the use of different antidandruff shampoos for optimal effect. Many people find that it is most practical to apply the shampoo when they first enter the shower or bath and then to leave the lather on for 5 minutes to give the active ingredients time to be deposited. Following these shampoos with a conditioner (cream rinse) does not reduce their efficacy but does increase manageability of the hair—a function antidandruff shampoos often fail to perform. Seborrheic dermatitis and the treatment of stubborn dandruff are discussed in Chapter 40.

Acid-Balanced Shampoos

The claims have been made for acid-balanced shampoos are unjustified. Using a shampoo with an acid pH on normal hair or scalp provides no benefits. Hair damaged by sunlight or alkaline oxidation due to processing with hair dyes, bleaches, or straighteners is slightly soluble in an alkaline medium and will feel slimy if regular shampoos are used. For damaged hair, an acid pH shampoo may impart a more normal texture.

Baby Shampoos

Baby shampoos are useful in young children because they contain amphoteric detergents designed to be minimally irritating, especially to the eyes.

Conditioning Shampoos

Conditioners (see below) are added to shampoos to enhance the manageability and appearance of the hair. However, it is generally more effective to apply a separate conditioner after shampooing.

Conditioning Agents

Scanning electron microscopic studies of scalp hair show overlapping cuticle scales protecting the inner cortical fibers. As it grows out, scalp hair is subject to weathering and chemical and mechanical injury. These injuries are not repaired because the hair shaft is composed of dead cells and biologic repair is thus impossible. Cuticle scales near the scalp are smooth and uniform, but near the ends of hairs cuticle that has been repeatedly traumatized may be partially or totally worn away, exposing the inner cortical fibers and resulting in split ends.

Exposure to intense sun and chlorine in swimming pools may cause perceptible undesirable changes in the texture and feel of hair because of oxidative changes in the keratin. Alkaline oxidation damage also occurs from the use of hair dyes, bleaches, and hair straighteners, which rupture the cross-linking disulfide bonds of hair formed by cystine and permit formation of cysteic acid. Hair can tolerate elective cosmetic processes such as permanent waving or dyeing if they are undertaken carefully and not too often.

Combing and brushing may cause significant mechanical injury to the cuticle scales. Because the frictional coefficient is higher in Caucasian hair when it is wet, grooming of wet or damp hair causes more damage than styling of dry hair. In contrast, the curly hair of blacks is more easily managed when it is wet or heavily lubricated, so hair should be groomed under these conditions and may benefit from a conditioner, which will help prevent damage due to tangles and will impart some sheen.

Conditioning agents (cream rinses) are usually quaternary cationic polymers that form a layer on the hair and thereby lubricate it so that the damage caused by combing or brushing is reduced. They also enable the hair to be combed so that the strands are aligned and light reflects uniformly to give a lustrous appearance. The hair of blacks in particular may benefit, because tightly curled hair does not align uniformly and therefore appears dull. Anionic detergent shampoos remove oil, so that hair develops a static electric charge and "flyaway" appearance. Conditioners help to dissipate this charge and allow the hair to be groomed more easily. Some cream rinses have oils added for lubrication. The addition of partially degraded collagen to conditioners may improve the texture of damaged hair.

Damaged and processed hair benefits from the use of conditioners because they reduce further damage caused by grooming and improve appearance and feel. Fine hair can be overconditioned and will look dull and greasy as a result.

HAIR REMOVAL

Beard Removal
Although improved implements have made shaving easier, the process still results in numerous microscopic cuts and abrasions.

A. Wet Shaving: Shaving with a blade requires wetting the beard thoroughly to soften it. The beard hair can absorb up to 30% of its weight in water, but softening requires at least 2 minutes of contact with warm water. Stretching the skin and shaving against the grain for close shaves may cause ingrown hairs. Cosmetic products used prior to wet shaving are designed to hydrate and soften the beard and to lubricate the skin and thus reduce friction. However, shaving soaps and lathering shaving creams that contain large amounts of soap remove the sebum from the beard and wet the hair most thoroughly.

Styptic pencils made from alum staunch bleeding from small cuts incurred while shaving.

B. Dry Shaving: Shaving with an electric shaver requires a dry beard. Pre-electric shaving lotions are hydroalcoholic solutions (alcohol in water) that may contain a lubricant. Alternatively, powders containing talc may be used to remove sebum and sweat.

These cosmetics may make shaving more pleasant but are not necessary.

C. Aftershave Products: Hydroalcoholic aftershave lotions are primarily fragrance products that impart a "bracing" sensation. Their claimed effectiveness in preventing skin infections is unproved. Emollient lotions are preferable if the skin is dry or chapped. Hydrocortisone cream 1% may help to alleviate occasional irritation caused by shaving but should not be used as a face cream.

D. Pseudofolliculitis Barbae: Not all men can easily look clean-shaven. Some men—especially blacks with heavy, curly beards (see Chapter 52)—may develop pseudofolliculitis barbae from shaving. Tender erythematous papules arise when closely cut hairs grow out and pierce the hair follicle or curl back and reenter the skin to cause a foreign body reaction. Shaving less closely "with the grain" and carefully freeing each of the entrapped hairs with a clean needle or toothpick bring relief. Tretinoin (Retin-A cream 0.05%) applied daily may be helpful but is not uniformly successful. Depilatories, which dissolve hair and leave soft ends, may be a satisfactory alternative to shaving for some men. Powdered depilatories are preferred by patients because they work more quickly, but they are irritating and have an unpleasant odor. Irritation can be minimized by refraining from daily use and by treating irritated skin with hydrocortisone cream 1–2.5%. Many black men find that the most satisfactory treatment is to grow a beard.

Superfluous Hair in Women
The normal amounts of facial and body hair in women vary depending upon genetic background; a sudden increase in facial or body hair warrants a diagnostic endocrine examination. However, women who have no hormonal abnormalities often wish to have superfluous hair removed from the face or body.

A. Bleaching: Some fine dark hairs become inconspicuous when they are bleached; melanin is converted to colorless leucomelanin when it is oxidized. Bleaching can be achieved by mixing 1 oz of hydrogen peroxide (6%) with 20 drops of ammonia and applying it for up to 30 minutes. It may be useful to practice with a small test area first. Commercially prepackaged bleaching materials are available.

B. Shaving: Most women who remove hair from the legs and axillas shave, usually with a razor. Because they shave at the end of a shower or bath, when the hair is wet and soft, they rarely use preshave preparations. Women with warts on their legs should be advised to avoid shaving this area temporarily, because they can easily inoculate the wart virus into the many tiny cuts produced by shaving. As shaved hair grows out, the cut ends feel thick and bristlelike; however, shaving does not cause hair to grow thicker or faster. For women, shaving is a practical but not commonly used means of removing facial hair. The pseudofolliculitis caused by shaving in black men has also been reported in black women who shave their facial hair.

C. Chemical Depilatories: Much of the strength in the keratin of hair is derived from its high cystine content (17%), which forms strong disulfide bonds and cross-links. Chemical depilatories contain an alkaline-reducing agent that cleaves these disulfide bonds, so that the hair swells and partially dissolves. The cuticle of hair within the follicle is more easily penetrated than the cuticle of hair above the follicle, and this allows depilatories to act below the surface of the skin. Because the chemical structure of the keratin of the epidermis resembles that of hair, depilatories left on the skin too long cause skin irritation. Older preparations contained alkaline earth sulfides that are fast-acting but have an unpleasant odor and are irritating. They are still used in powder form for removal of beard hair by black men. Thioglycolates combined with calcium hydroxide are the most popular preparations.

Although chemical depilatories give a smoother feel to the skin for a longer time than shaving, fewer than 1% of women in the USA use them exclusively for hair removal; 8% of women use them along with other methods. Depilatories are costly and slow, may be ineffective or irritating, and have an unpleasant odor.

D. Epilation: Epilation removes hair at the root.

1. Plucking– A few facial or body hairs may be removed by plucking with tweezers every 2–10 weeks. Many women shape their brows in this manner.

2. Waxing– Waxing strips many hairs from their roots at one time. Solid mixtures of wax and rosin are heated until they liquefy and are then applied to the hairy areas. As the wax cools, it solidifies and traps the hairs. When the wax is pulled off, the embedded hairs are extracted at the root. An alternative method uses appropriate tacky materials layered on strips of paper or cloth. These methods are used for hair removal on the face and body. However, the procedure is slightly painful, and a skilled operator can often perform the task with less discomfort. Waxing is most frequently performed in beauty salons. When it is done on the upper lip or legs, it frequently causes folliculitis.

3. Electrolysis– In contrast to electrolysis, all the methods discussed above provide only temporary hair removal. In electrolysis, a fine needle is passed down the hair follicle to the root and electric current is discharged that destroys the root and removes hair permanently. Older machines used direct current, but machines using high-frequency alternating current have become more popular, because the operator can treat more hair per session.

The success of electrolysis depends on the electrologist's skill in locating the hair root with blind probing. A competent operator destroys 50–80% of the hair roots treated. Electrolysis can be helpful, but it is a costly, uncomfortable process that may take years of weekly treatments. Complications include infection, scarring, and hyperpigmentation.

CARE OF NAILS

FINGERNAILS
(See also Chapter 29.)

The nail plate protecting the distal phalanx is composed of hard keratin whose strength is derived from disulfide bonds formed as a result of the high cystine content. Normal nails vary in thickness and flexibility. Fingernails grow more slowly, become thinner, and may develop longitudinal ridges with age. Fingernails may become brittle and split in layers distally as a result of trauma or chemical exposure. Skin diseases (eg, psoriasis, lichen planus, or eczema) or systemic diseases such as endocrinopathies may cause nail dystrophies not amenable to ordinary care.

Little can be done to strengthen a normal fingernail. Ingestion of gelatin or calcium does not help. Gentle care and protection can prevent injuries arising from everyday activities.

Nails should not be used to pry open objects. Small splits should be filed promptly with a "diamond dust" file, which is finer than an emery board. Light cotton gloves for household chores and heavy cotton gloves for gardening help protect fragile nails. Repeated immersion of hands in water and detergents causes nails to become brittle, and cotton-lined rubber or neoprene gloves worn during wet work may prevent this damage. However, rubber gloves should not be worn for so long that the hands sweat.

PRESERVATION OF THE
EPONYCHIUM
(Cuticle)

Cooks, bartenders, homemakers, and others whose occupations require that they frequently have their hands in water often develop chronic paronychia (inflammation of the posterior nail fold), in which the nail fold becomes swollen and the eponychium is lost. Physicians should emphasize to patients that intact eponychium prevents infections of the posterior nail fold and that it performs this important function by acting as a seal between the posterior nail fold and the underlying nail plate. When hands are damp after washing, the eponychium can be gently pushed back, preferably with a soft towel. Hand cream massaged into the eponychium prevents development of a dry and ragged surface. Cuticle removers, which are used to achieve a smooth, neat-appearing eponychium, are creams or lotions containing alkali, frequently potassium hydroxide, that dissolves the disulfide bonds of the keratin and softens it. The potential hazards of these caustic products should be explained, and women with paronychiae should not use them at all. Although many manicurists trim or clip the eponychium, the practice should be discouraged, because it can result in inflammation of the posterior nail fold.

Hangnails

Hangnails, which are partially detached dried pieces of eponychium at the lateral nail fold, should be cut close to the base. Patients should be warned not to pick or tear at loose pieces of skin, because this habit perpetuates the development of hangnails and may encourage secondary infections. Using suitable gloves and emollients when hands are exposed to dry, cold weather, water, or detergents prevents the development of painful hangnails.

Manicures

The nail matrix, which extends from the lunula to 5 mm beneath the posterior nail fold, is the site of manufacture of the nail plate, and trauma to this area may cause not only paronychiae but also deformities of the nail itself. Overzealous removal of dirt from beneath the free edge of the nail can cause distal onycholysis. Women who buff their nails with abrasive powders for a natural look should be cautioned against excessive abrasion, which this may injure the matrix.

Repeated application and removal of nail polish can exert a drying effect on the nail and surrounding skin. Nail polish removers contain ketones, usually acetone. However, if the manicure is carefully preserved and repaired, it is generally beneficial. Patients who become allergic to nail polish usually do not break out on the fingers but rather on the eyelids or neck, where percutaneous absorption is more likely. Some nail enamels, called hardeners, are polishes that form a particularly thick coat or contain nylon

fibers, and they may provide some extra protection or shielding for the nail. In the past, nail hardeners contained formaldehyde, which causes physical change in nail keratin. Because these products caused many adverse reactions, including hemorrhage in the nail bed, they were removed from the market in the USA.

Using cyanoacrylate glues and thin fibrous paper patches to repair or wrap the distal end of nails is a tedious but generally harmless procedure that can help women grow longer fingernails. Repeated application of linen or silk over the entire nail plate should be discouraged. Use of methacrylates as glues for wrapping nails can result in onycholysis, paronychiae, and nail destruction.

Sculptured Nails

Sculptured nails are molded false nails created by polymerizing an acrylic monomer on the nail plate. The process is popular because it creates attractive long nails. However, because nail elongators frequently produce painful separation of the nail plate from the nail bed and inflammation of the surrounding nail folds, the practice should be discouraged.

TOENAILS

Ingrown toenails usually result from improper care. The most common initiating factor is ill-fitting footwear that presses on the lateral nail folds and nail plate. Fashionable shoes often do not allow sufficient room for the toes, and people with foot deformities due to arthritis have a difficult time finding properly fitted shoes.

Toenails should always be clipped straight across. Nails should never be cut down at the corners, because the sharp ends formed will dig into the lateral nail folds and cause pain and swelling; ultimately, a foreign body reaction occurs, and granulation tissue forms. In the initial stages, the patient should be shown how to introduce cotton between the sharp corner of the nail and the skin. The cotton should be replaced daily after a shower or bath, when the nail is soft, until the nail has grown out enough to allow it to be shaped properly.

REFERENCES

Elias PM: Epidermal lipids, barrier function, and desquamation. J Invest Dermatol 1983;80(Suppl):44S.

Frosch PJ: Irritancy of soaps and detergent bars. In: *Principles of Cosmetics for the Dermatologist.* Frost P, Horwitz SN (editors). Mosby, 1982.

Gilchrest BA: *Skin and Aging Processes.* CRC Press, 1984.

Lowe NJ, Weingarten D, Wortzman M: Sunscreens and phototesting. Clin Dermatol (July–Sept) 1988;6:40.

Pathak MA: Sunscreens: Topical and systemic approaches for protection of human skin against harmful effects of solar radiation. J Am Acad Dermatol 1982;7:285.

Proceedings of Emerging Role of Retinoids in the Treatment of Aging and Skin Cancer. J Cutan Aging Cosmet Dermatol 1988;1:1.

Quatrale RP et al: The mechanism of antiperspirant action by aluminum salts. 3. Histological observations of human eccrine sweat glands inhibited by aluminum zirconium chlorhydrate glycine complex. J Soc Cosmet Chem 1981;32:195.

Shuster S: The aetiology of dandruff and the mode of action of therapeutic agents. Br J Dermatol 1984;111:235.

Weiss JS et al: Topical tretinoin improves photoaged skin: A double-blind, vehicle-controlled study. JAMA 1988;259:527.

Wilkinson JB, Moore RJ (editors): *Harry's Cosmeticology,* 7th ed. Chemical Publishing Co, 1982.

Zviak C (editor): *The Science of Hair Care.* Vol 7 of: *Dermatology.* Calnan CD, Maibach HI (editors). Marcel Dekker, 1986.

Section II:
Dermatologic Diagnosis

Principles of Clinical Diagnosis in Dermatologic Practice

6

Walter B. Shelley, MD, PhD

Dermatologic diagnosis is delightfully direct. You look, you recognize, and you name—all in a fraction of a second. Making a clinical diagnosis of a skin disease is a simple act of pattern recognition not different from the pattern recognition that enables you to look, to recognize, and to name birds, cars, or friends.

Dermatologic diagnosis is thus set apart from general medical diagnosis, where the "bird" is never seen but is recognized by its shadow, its call, its droppings, or its nest. In internal medicine, the pattern to be recognized must first be woven by the clinician out of threads called symptoms, laboratory test results, and imaging procedures. This calls for a special skill in spinning and weaving. With skin disease, the pattern is already there in the skin, waiting to be seen and recognized.

What makes for difficulty is that the simple act of seeing a skin disease may prove not to be so simple after all in every case. As outlined in Table 6–1, the lighting must not only be "adequate" but varied in angle and intensity. Too much light masks subtle pigmentary changes. Indeed, the faint glow of Wood's light permits one to see otherwise invisible yet diagnostically essential ash leaf-shaped hypopigmented macules that favor the diagnosis of tuberous sclerosis and thus may explain the origin of convulsive seizures. The ultraviolet rays of Wood's light also bring out the diagnostic fluorescence of fungal *(Microsporon)* and bacterial (erythrasma) infections.

Just as one should vary distance and angle when looking at skin lesions, one should view selected areas under magnification with a 2.7 × power loupe. One should look for the unique or distinctive primary lesion (Table 6–2), since much of what is seen is nonspecific, nondiagnostic secondary change that

Table 6–1. How to look at skin lesions.

Technique	Value
Use good lighting—vary intensity and angle	To perceive otherwise inapparent lesions.
Use special lighting—Wood's light	Tinea capitis-infected hairs fluoresce blue-green. Erythrasma fluoresces a bright coral red color.
Vary distance of inspection	Both distribution and lesions are assessed.
Vary field of study—use magnification loupe (2.7 power), diascopy (firm pressure with overlying glass slide).	Close-up view. Evaluates vascular contribution to color and bulk of lesion.
Examine entire mucocutaneous surface: oral mucosa, retroauricular, inframammary, perianal, feet	Avoids overlooking tumors, candidiasis, tinea, leukoplakia.
Palpate lesion firmly and stroke normal skin	Locates occult scleroderma, deep cysts; elicits dermographism.
Examine patient lying down and standing	Accentuates atrophic areas on abdomen (induces fat herniation, eg, piezogenic pedal papules).
See patient again—after no bath for 1 week, after covering lesion	Lesions may evolve in more recognizable form. Scabies may become more evident. Psoriasis lesions may develop recognizable scales.
Imagine the lesions transposed to another location	Stimulates new diagnostic thoughts.
Look for unique lesion	The burrow of scabies, the black dot of warts; the comedo of acne.

must be ignored temporarily in the search for a recognizable diagnostic pattern.

The diagnostician never focuses only on what the patient points out. The more "global" the inspection, the greater the diagnostic yield. Look in the mouth, behind the ears, in the scalp. These sites may disclose the only recognizable signs of lichen planus, carcinoma, or psoriasis, respectively. The patient may stoutly assert that his feet are unaffected when inspection may reveal a florid tinea pedis that in turn makes the diagnosis of trichophytid for the patient's chief complaint of a rash on his trunk. The more you look, the more you find. "Look" with your fingers too. Scleroderma may be inapparent until you feel its tautness. Look again at the next visit. You may see the pattern of skin changes evolve into one that is easily recognizable. Mentally transposing the lesion to another site can be helpful. A scaly lesion of the back may rapidly be recognized as psoriasis when transposed to the elbow.

But what if you have looked and looked and have not recognized? In that case, asking someone who knows—a clinician with more years of experience examining more thousands of patients—is the easiest way to add to your memory bank of recognizable visual images of disease. If there is no one to ask, search the color atlases looking for a "match." The du Vivier atlas (1986) is the most comprehensive one now available, but there are many smaller, highly valuable atlases that provide self-instruction not possible with black and white photographs. As you continue to use your atlases as "bird guides," you will gradually build your visual memory to where you can recognize 75 portraits of skin disease. Although there are several thousand other rare diseases, Lynch (1987) has pointed out that a memory bank of 75 diseases allows you to immediately recognize 95% of all the skin lesions you will ever see.

Table 6–2. What to look for in skin lesions.

Lesion	Diagnosis to Be Considered
Comedo	Acne
Burrow	Scabies
Central depression in vesicle or papule	Viral disease
Black dots in callus	Verruca
Yellow crust	Pyoderma
Green nail	Pseudomonas infection
Pinch purpura: Compression or frictional force elicits purpura	Amyloidosis
Lichenification	Neurodermatitis
Papulopustules: nose, patient over 35	Rosacea
Koebner's phenomenon: Trauma to skin elicits new lesion after 10 days	Psoriasis, lichen planus
Bullae (widespread in older patient)	Bullous pemphigoid
Nikolsky's sign: Frictional force separates epidermis	Pemphigus
Christmas tree patterning of oval lesions on back	Pityriasis rosea
Solitary macule: Cycling red to brown	Fixed drug eruption
Darier's sign: Frictional force on lesion elicits local urticaria	Urticaria pigmentosa
Auspitz's sign: Pinpoint bleeding when scale is pulled off	Psoriasis
Follows nerve distribution	Herpes zoster

The atlases will teach you to recognize many diseases by their configuration (Table 6–3). The rings of tinea corporis, the plaques of mycosis fungoides, the bands of scleroderma, and the grouped vesicles of herpes zoster will all become as familiar and as recognizable as acne. And the atlases will teach you to think of specific diseases when you see lesions in

Table 6–3. Diagnostic clues obtained from configuration of lesions.

Annular lesions	Impetigo	Lichen planus
	Tinea corporis	Granuloma annulare
	Pityriasis rosea	Sarcoidosis
	Seborrheic dermatitis	Psoriasis
	Syphilis	Nummular eczema
	Urticaria	Erythema annulare centrifugum
Patches and plaques	Vitiligo	Elastosis perforans serpiginosa
	Albright's disease	Porokeratosis of Mibelli
	Mycosis fungoides	Leprosy
	Nevi	Erythema perstans
Linear patterning	Herpes zoster	Sebaceous nevi
	Verruca	Incontinentia pigmenti
	Linear scleroderma	Nevus unius lateris
	Lichen striatum	Lichen planus
	Contact dermatitis	Trichotillomania
	Dermographism	
Grouped vesicles	Herpes simplex	Dermatitis herpetiformis
	Herpes zoster	Lymphangioma circumscriptum

Table 6–4. Favored locations for skin diseases.

Scalp	Alopecia areata	Ectodermal defect
	Seborrheic dermatitis	Pediculosis
	Verrucae	Inclusion cyst (wen)
	Trichotillomania	Lichen simplex chronicus
	Epitheliomas	Nevi
	Folliculitis	Tinea capitis
	Psoriasis	
Face	Hemangioma	Sarcoidosis
	Herpes simplex	Rosacea
	Eczema herpeticum	Molluscum contagiosum
	Xanthelasma	Melasma
	Photosensitivity	Epitheliomas
	Scleroderma	Herpes zoster
	Vitiligo	Seborrheic keratosis
	Perioral dermatitis	Lentigines
	Verrucae	Lupus erythematosus
	Acne	Verrucae
	Furuncles	Dermatosis papulosa
	Impetigo	nigra
	Contact dermatitis	Actinic keratoses
Eyelids	Hordeolum	Amyloidosis
	Blepharitis	Dermatomyositis
	Verrucae	Syringoma
	Alopecia areata	Xanthelasma
	Basal cell epithelioma	Pediculosis
	Purpura	Acrochordon
	Edema	Vitiligo
	Contact dermatitis	Seborrheic keratoses
	Meibomian cyst	Behçet's syndrome
	Seborrheic dermatitis	
Trunk	Acne	Seborrheic dermatitis
	Keloid	Seborrheic keratoses
	Psoriasis	Pityriasis rosea
	Contact dermatitis	Tinea versicolor
	Darier's disease	Psoriasis
	Dermatitis herpetiformis	Urticaria
	Secondary syphilis	Varicella
	Paget's disease of	Kaposi's sarcoma
	breast	Actinic keratoses
	Miliaria rubra	
	Morphea	

Table 6–5. The history as a diagnostic aid.

Symptoms as a diagnostic aid

Itch	Contact dermatitis
	Scabies
	Dermatitis herpetiformis
	Lichen planus
Pain	
Unilateral	Herpes zoster
Muscle	Dermatomyositis
Focal	Infection
	Leiomyoma
	Glomus tumor

Associated diseases as diagnostic aid

Asthma or hay fever	Atopic dermatitis
Internal cancer	Erythema multiforme
Diabetes mellitus	Necrobiosis lipoidica
Focal infection	Psoriasis
	Erythema multiforme
	Erythema nodosum
	Urticaria

Miscellaneous factors as diagnostic aids

Environmental exposures	Actinic keratoses
	Contact dermatitis
	Photosensitivity
Tick bite	Erythema chronicum migrans
Occupational exposures	Contact dermatitis
Radiation therapy	Epitheliomas
Precise drug history	Drug eruption, urticaria
Detailed diet diary	Urticaria
Sexual contacts	Syphilis, scabies, herpes simplex
Homosexual contacts	Kaposi's sarcoma, scabies, herpes simplex

Association aids

Asian patient	Neurodermatitis
	Leprosy
Black patient	Keloid
	Sarcoidosis
Immunodeficiency or suppression	Severe herpes simplex
	Multiple viral infections of skin
Psychiatric illness	Factitial eruption
Travel	
Israel	Leishmaniasis
Caribbean beaches	Creeping eruption
Africa	Mycobacterial ulcer

Enrichment of diagnostic process by asking

Other physicians' views of the nature of this problem (eg, consultation with specialist).

Do previous diagnostic studies seem consistent with your diagnosis (eg, review diagnostic tests done by others)?

Do course, duration, and response to therapy favor your diagnosis?

specific areas (Table 6–4; Figs 6–1 and 6–2). Thus, seborrheic dermatitis and psoriasis favor the scalp. Rosacea and actinic keratoses are diseases of the face. Contact dermatitis commonly affects the eyelids, and seborrheic keratoses are an affliction of the older person's back. Atopic dermatitis uniquely involves the antecubital fossae.

Contact dermatitis is the most common hand problem. Fungal infection and warts can almost be predicted as the patient takes off his shoes and stockings. Thus, configurations and topographic findings prepare your mind to think of specific diagnoses.

Another way the mind is conditioned diagnostically is by the history (Table 6–5). If the cardinal symptom is localized itch, think of contact dermatitis. If it is generalized itch, think of scabies. Unilateral pain in a dermatome directs us to zoster and focal pain in a nodule to a glomus tumor. A history of asthma or hay fever suggests atopic dermatitis. Streptococcal pharyngitis suggests erythema

nodosum, even as a tick bite history points to erythema chronicum migrans associated with Lyme disease.

The experienced diagnostician, in searching for that diagnosis that eluded him in the first fraction of a second, takes a careful history; and this history centers on drugs—whether they be prescriptive, over-the-counter, or home remedies. It is hard to think of a

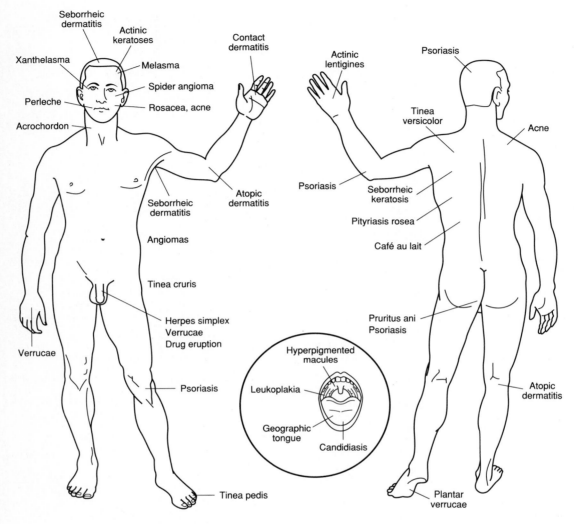

Figure 6–1. Diagnostic suggestions from the localization of lesions.

skin lesion that could not be drug-induced, as is so exquisitely demonstrated in Bork's text (1988).

Nothing can be ignored. That patient back from Israel could have leishmaniasis. The patient seeing a psychiatrist may have lithium-induced psoriasis or acne. And the black patient may have sarcoidosis. Get the history. Your diagnostic mind can but be refreshed by a good history. And the history can be amplified to your benefit on each visit.

But you've looked at the patient and you've looked in the atlases, you've considered the configuration and location, and you've taken a long history to no avail. What should you do next?

Take a biopsy, and let the dermatopathologist do the looking (Table 6–6). He or she can make diagnoses on histologic patterns as fast as you can on gross patterns. But give the dermatopathologist a

good specimen. It must be distinctive, representative—ideally a lesion you feel you should be able to recognize but cannot. If the patient has an extensive eruption, spend more time choosing the site than in taking the specimen. Be sure to send a brief history or differential diagnosis to the dermatopathologist along with the specimen.

And what to do when neither you nor the pathologist can make a diagnosis? It is time to turn to the clinical laboratory (Table 6–6). A lot of the laboratory findings are simply reassuring, but at times a clear diagnosis can be achieved in this way. Think of the positive serologic test for syphilis in that patient with ringed lesions on the face—the elevated blood urea nitrogen in that patient with pruritus—and the hematologic diagnosis of leukemia in the patient with previously unrecognized leukemids.

Table 6–6. Laboratory studies as diagnostic aids.

Test	Example	Test	Example
Microscopic		**Clinical laboratory**	
Scale (KOH)	Fungal infection	(*Continued*)	
Burrow	Scabies	ANA-ANTI-DNA-ENA	Lupus erythematosus
Sebum	Demodex infestation	Pemphigus antibodies	Pemphigus vulgaris
Smear (Gram stain)	Bacterial infection	Streptococcal antibodies	Erythema nodosum
Darkfield	Syphilis	Scleroderma antibody	Scleroderma
Perianal (cellophane tape	Pruritus ani (due to pinworm	Scl-70	
applied to skin)	infestation)	Deep fungal antibodies	Histoplasmosis
Histologic		Weil-Felix antibodies	Rickettsialpox
Tissue biopsy		T_3-T_4-TSH	Myxedema
H&E	Nevi	Long-acting thyroid stimula-	Pretibial myxedema
	Tumors	tor (LATS)	
	Lesions that appear clin-	RAST tests, IgE level	Atopic dermatitis
	ically distinctive but are	Complement profile	Vasculitis
	not clinically diagnostic	Immune complex profile	Vasculitis
		(C1q, Raji cell)	
Special stains		Lipid profile	Xanthoma
Brown-Hopp	Bacterial infections	Aldolase	Dermatomyositis
Hotchkiss-McManus	Deep fungal infection	Human chorionic gonado-	Papular dermatitis of preg-
Silver for spirochetes	Erythema chronicum mi-	tropin	nancy
	grans	Prolactin	Hirsutism
Acid-fast	Leprosy	Androgens	Hirsutism
Elastic tissue	Elastosis perforans ser-	Serotonin	Flushing carcinoid
	piginosa	Histamine	Mastocytosis
Immunofluorescence	Pemphigus vulgaris	Carcinoembryonic antigen	Erythema multiforme
	bullous pemphigoid	Chromosome analysis	Ataxia-telangiectasia
	Dermatitis herpetiformis	HLA-B27	Reiter's syndrome
	Lupus erythematosus	Serum vitamin A	Phrynoderma
	Vasculitis	Serum carotene	Carotenemia
Electron microscopy	Histiocytosis X	Serum vitamin B complex	Nutritional dermatitis
Clinical laboratory		Serum vitamin C	Scurvy
Complete blood count	Leukemia	Serum zinc	Acrodermatitis enteropathica
Sedimentation rate	Lupus erythematosus		Diabetic dermopathy
Automated channel chem-	Pruritus	Urinalysis	Porphyria cutanea tarda
istry		Urinary porphyrins	Melanoma
Platelet and coagulation	Purpura	Urinary melanin	Flushing of carcinoid
studies		Urinary 5-HIAA	
Serum proteins and electro-	Urticaria	**Microbiologic laboratory**	
phoresis		Culture and sensitivity stud-	Bacterial infections
Cryoglobulin, cryofibrinogen	Urticaria	ies (aerobic, anaerobic,	Viral infections
Cryoagglutinins	Urticaria	special media, long-term)	Fungal infections
C1 esterase inhibitor	Hereditary angioneurotic	Stool for ova and parasites	Urticaria
	edema	**Imaging**	
Hepatitis antigen	Urticaria	X-ray, CT scan, MRI	Tumors responsible for para-
Serologic test for syphilis	Syphilis		neoplastic lesions

And if the diagnosis still eludes you, it is time to check back on the "big five" causes of diagnostic confusion (Table 6–7). Recheck, reexamine, requestion for possible drugs, vitamins, or laxatives that could be the cause. Consider vasculitis again. Look for internal cancer. Ask yourself if these puzzling, bizarre lesions might be self-inflicted. And finally, remember that AIDS patients can have lesions that range from a telangiectatic macule to a large, deep

herpetic ulcer. The iatrogenically immunocompromised patient can display similar and at times unrecognizable infections in their extreme uncontrolled form.

But making the diagnosis is not enough. You must document it in your records, in reports, in correspondence, and even in conversation. Unfortunately, it is still not practical to do this photographically. One is reduced to using words to capture the visual image of what you have seen objectively. You must become dermatologically literate. You must acquire a vocabulary that allows you to describe the essential features of even the most complex skin changes. Even if you made the diagnosis in an instant, you must look at the patient again to label and record specifically the primary or significant lesions you saw.

Dermatologic literacy requires that you be able to

Table 6–7. Check list for puzzling skin problems.

Drug eruption
Vasculitis
Sign of internal cancer
Factitial eruption
AIDS

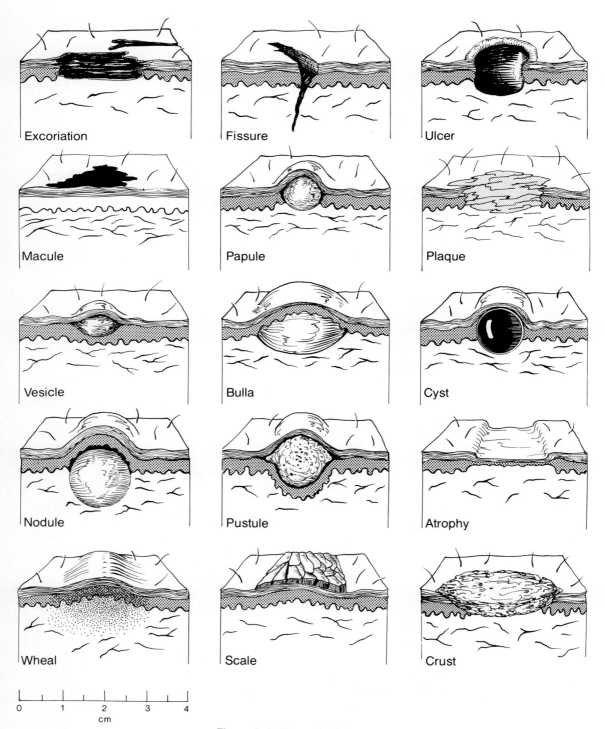

Figure 6–2. Types of skin lesions.

Excoriation

Fissure

Ulcer

Macule

Papule

Plaque

Vesicle

Bulla

Cyst

Nodule

Pustule

Atrophy

Wheal

Scale

Crust

0 1 2 3 4
cm

Table 6–8. Descriptive terms.

Impalpable Change	Palpable Mass	Free Fluid	Loss of Skin	Healing Stage	End Stage
Macule	Papule	Vesicle	Erosion	Scale	Atrophy
Patch	Nodule	Bulla	Ulcer	Crust	Scar
	Plaque	Pustule			
	Wheal	Abscess			

describe 16 essential changes in the skin (Table 6–8). These are not diagnoses but simply descriptive terms for objective findings. They describe, as it were, the features of the bird without naming the bird. You must familiarize yourself with these 16 terms. Knowing them allows you to look at the patient in a more discerning fashion. You begin to see what the skin disease is made of. These 16 terms will serve you well, not only in documenting the patient's problem but in seeing the parts of the puzzle that must be explained.

Knowing what one can see enables one to see it. As you progress, your vocabulary will expand, and with it an awareness of the in-depth nature of skin lesions (Figs 6–1 and 6–2). Acquiring this descriptive skill will enhance your diagnostic skill. Even description of an ulcer (Table 6–9) reveals diagnostic possibilities hidden to those who see only an ulcer.

Not only the ulcer but all of the other 15 basic skin lesions deserve to be fleshed out descriptively. You need to record the location, the patterning, the color, and the palpable features (Table 6–10). Fortunately, the terms used here are not foreign to you, but it takes effort to draw upon them. The written record is there to summon an accurate picture of the problem into the mind of the reader. How much better to describe pityriasis rosea as "widespread ovoid scaling erythematous lesions following the lines of change over the back" than to read simply, "a rash on the chest."

Finally, write it down. Table 6–11 gives an example of an orderly outline to follow in recording data,

no matter how haphazardly it has been acquired. Write it down legibly. You are creating an official record with legal significance, and what can't be read can be held against you. Writing down your findings as you sit with the patient establishes rapport and shows the patient you respect what you are being told. Leave space as you go for additions and emendations.

We leave you with 5 thoughts:

- Diagnosis is the art of recognition, not the science of cognition.
- The best diagnosticians are the ones with the best visual memories.
- The best history is taken by one who already knows the diagnosis.
- If puzzled, limit yourself to 3 working diagnoses.
- A good color atlas and a good dermatopathologist are your best friends. Take advantage of them.

Table 6–9. Appearance of ulcer as diagnositic aid.

Within white atrophic area	Infarct, atrophie blanche
Green pus	*Pseudomonas* infection Ecthyma gangrenosum
Raised edge	Cancer Granuloma
Undermined irregular edge	Meleney's ulcer
Arciform	Syphilis
In clusters	Vasculitis
Surrounded by pustules	Pyoderma gangrenosum

Table 6–10. Descriptive terms for skin lesions.

Distribution
Generalized	Multiple
Localized	Bilaterally symmetric
Scattered	Asymmetric
Patchy	Along cleavage lines
Single	

Arrangement
Discrete	Grouped
Confluent	Randomized

Configuration
Linear	Targetlike
Serpiginous	Polycyclic
Arciform	Reticulate
Annular	

Quality
Color: erythematous, blanched
Size
Border (distinct, indistinct margination)
Surface characteristics:
Dry	Purulent
Greasy	Bleeding
Moist	Verrucous
Oozing	

Assessment by palpation
Tenderness
Adherence of scale or crust
Consistency: soft, fluctuant, infiltrated, indurated
Fixation to underlying tissue

Table 6–11. General outline for dermatologic record (problem-oriented).

Chief complaint Nature, site, duration	**Menstrual history**

Present problem
  Details of onset
  Signs, symptoms, distribution
  Course
  Previous laboratory studies and diagnosis
  Treatments and their effects
  Factors: seasonal, occupational, menstrual, diet, diurnal, stress
  What patient thinks is cause or nature of problem
	Habits
	  Sleep
	  Diet
	  Alcohol
	  Smoking
	  Recreational drugs
	  Health aids: vitamins, minerals, laxatives, tranquilizers
	  Stress level

Past health
  Illnesses—include skin disease
  Medications
  Operations
  Allergies and idiosyncrasies:
    Atrophy?
    Drug intolerance?
    Keloids?
	Physical examination
	  Detailed description: (Tables 6–8 to 6–10); (Figs 6–1 and 6–2)
	
	Assessment of patient
	  Note if patient appears to be unreliable, confused, hypochondriacal, overreacting, withholding data, noncompliant, reluctant to accept therapeutic advice

Family history
  Parents, siblings, spouse, children
  Skin disease, asthma, hay fever, diabetes, melanoma, psoriasis
	Diagnosis or differential
	
	Laboratory studies to be done, including biopsy
	  Table 6–6

Occupation and hobbies Chemical compounds such as epoxy resins, chromium	**Prescriptions** **Interval until next visit**

REFERENCES

Beaven DW, Brooks SE: *Color Atlas of the Nail in Clinical Diagnosis.* Year Book, 1985.

Bhutani LK: *Color Atlas of Dermatology.* Mehta Offset Works, New Delhi, 1986.

Bhutani LK: *Colour Atlas of Sexually Transmitted Diseases.* Interprint New Delhi, 1986.

Bork K, Brauninger W: *Diagnosis and Treatment of Common Skin Diseases.* Saunders, 1988.

Bork K: *Cutaneous Side Effects of Drugs.* Saunders, 1988.

Buxton PK: *The ABC of Dermatology.* Taylor and Frameis, 1988.

Chessell GSJ et al: *Photo DX: An Aid for the Study of Physical Diagnosis.* Year Book, 1984.

duVivier A: *Atlas of Clinical Dermatology.* Saunders, 1986.

Fitzpatrick TB, Polano MK, Suurmond D: *Color Atlas and Synopsis of Clinical Dermatology.* McGraw-Hill, 1983.

Friedman-Kien AE: *Color Atlas of AIDS.* Saunders, 1989.

Habif TP: *Clinical Dermatology: A color Guide to Diagnosis and Therapy.* Mosby, 1985.

Jackson R: *Morphological Dermatology: A Study of the Living Gross Pathology of the Skin.* Thomas, 1979.

Jillson OF: Wood's light: An incredibly important diagnostic tool. Cutis 1981;28:620.

Lazarus GS, Goldsmith LA: *Diagnosis of Skin Disease.* Davis, 1980.

Lebwohl M (editor): *Difficult Diagnoses in Dermatology.* Churchill Livingstone, 1988.

Leider M, Rosenblum M: *A Dictionary of Dermatologic Words, Terms, and Phrases.* McGraw-Hill, 1968.

Levene GM, Galnan CD: *Color Atlas of Dermatology.* Year Book, 1974.

Levene GM, Goolamali SK: *Diagnostic Picture Tests in Dermatology.* Wolfe, 1986.

Lynch PJ: *Dermatology for the House Officer,* 3rd ed. Williams & Wilkins, 1987.

Marks R: *Skin Disease in Old Age.* Lippincott, 1987.

McLaren DS: *Nutritional Disorders.* Wolfe, 1981.

Pariser DM, Caserio RJ, Eaglestein WH: *Techniques for Diagnosing Skin and Hair Disease,* 2nd ed. Thieme-Stratton, 1986.

Pindborg JJ: *Atlas of Diseases of the Oral Mucosa,* 4th ed. Saunders, 1985.

Rassner G, Kahn G: *Atlas of Dermatology,* 2nd ed. Urban & Schwarzenberg, 1983.

Reeves JRT, Maibach HI: *Clinical Dermatology, Illustrated. A Regional Approach.* ADIS Health Science Press, 1984.

Rosen T, Martin S: *Atlas of Black Dermatology.* Little, Brown, 1981.

Soothill PW: Prenatal diagnosis of skin diseases. Arch Dis Child 1988;63:1175.

Weinberg S, Leider M: *Color Atlas of Pediatric Dermatology.* McGraw-Hill, 1975.

Winkelmann RK: Glossary of basic dermatologic lesions. Acta Dermatol Venereol 1987; Suppl 130:1.

Dermatopathology 7

Martin M. Black, MD, FRCP, Turner M. Caldwell III, MD,
& Mark V. Dahl, MD

HISTOLOGY OF THE SKIN

Martin M. Black, MD

SKIN BIOPSY

A skin biopsy is an important step in establishing a correct diagnosis of dermatologic disease. Until recently, there was a mistaken tendency among dermatologists to consider a skin biopsy as a last resort in diagnosis. It is now recognized that skin biopsy is an important extension of the clinical examination that provides specific and reliable information about diagnostic problems raised—for example—by "difficult" rashes. The dermatologist should therefore be prepared to biopsy more rather than less often than necessary.

Careful attention should be given to the selection of lesions for biopsy, as follows:

(1) The lesion should be representative of the eruption, unaltered by secondary changes due to topical applications, infection, trauma, etc.

(2) The stage of the lesion must be considered. Some lesions may require early biopsy (eg, vesicles), whereas in other instances it may be necessary to delay or repeat the biopsy (until evolutionary changes are characteristic, eg, cutaneous T cell lymphomas).

(3) Biopsy of lesions in areas of impaired circulation should be avoided when possible.

(4) Consideration should be given to cosmetic and functional aspects of the resulting wound scar. Lesions in noncosmetic and nonfunctional areas should be used for biopsy when possible.

Technique

Good biopsy technique is an essential prerequisite to the practice of dermatopathology. The biopsy must include all of the skin and some subcutaneous tissue and be large enough to contain skin structures such as hair complexes and sweat glands. In all but the simplest diagnoses the specimen should be sectioned serially to ascertain the consistency of any of the features present. The commonly employed 2–4 mm punch biopsy is usually not as satisfactory as an elliptical skin biopsy. In smaller lesions (1 cm or less) it is wise to resort to excisional biopsy so that the entire lesion is available for sectioning. Biopsies are often best taken from the active edge of a lesion. In lesions of variable or changing morphology multiple biopsies may be necessary. The area to be biopsied is anesthetized with 1% lidocaine, and a small cylinder of 2–4 mm diameter is removed with a cylindrical punch and forceps. Care must be taken not to crush the tissue. Immediately after biopsy the specimen is placed dermis down on a piece of paper to prevent curling in the formalin fixative. In his text, Mehregan details the pitfalls induced by artifactual changes to the biopsy which may lead to misinterpretation. The most widely used stain is hematoxylin and eosin (H&E) and enables many conditions to be diagnosed. However, H&E is not a complete stain since it does not elucidate important tissue components such as elastic fibers or mast cells, nor does it differentiate certain pigments or allow the demonstration of fungal mycelia. In dermatopathology the most commonly employed special stains are the periodic acid-Schiff (PAS) for demonstrating fungal mycelia and certain microorganisms, the orcein-Giemsa (O&G) for demonstrating the elastic tissue, and the alcian blue for demonstrating the presence of mucin. Immunoperoxidase stains can be used to identify specific structural components or specific infectious agents. For further details on special stains the reader is referred to the text of Luna.

Terminology

Just as one learns new terminology to describe a skin rash clinically, one has to learn a new terminology to describe the histologic changes encountered in dermatopathology. This subsection will define the more commonly encountered terms in dermatopathology. We have arbitrarily chosen to separate phenomena occurring in the epidermis from those occurring in the dermis.

A. Epidermal Changes:

1. Hyperkeratosis is an increase in thickness of the horny (cornified) layer. Hyperkeratosis may be "absolute"—ie, an actual increase in thickness of the horny layer—or "relative," in which it appears thicker in contrast to a thinner spinous layer.

2. Orthokeratosis is hyperkeratosis composed of cells that have cornified completely and have no retained nuclei.

3. Parakeratosis is hyperkeratosis in which pyknotic nuclei are retained in the squamous cells of the horny layer. Parakeratosis is usually seen in diseases where there is an accelerated rate of epidermal cell turnover (eg, psoriasis). A diminished or absent granular layer is usually found beneath areas of parakeratosis. In conditions such as chronic eczema, there may be areas of parakeratosis coexisting with serous exudates, causing a scale-crust over the surface of the epidermis.

4. Hypergranulosis is an increase in the number of keratinocytes in the granular layer, often associated with orthokeratosis.

5. Hypogranulosis is a decrease in the number of keratinocytes in the granular layer.

6. Hyperplasia is an increase in the number of keratinocytes that results in thickened epidermis. Characteristically, there are 4 patterns of epidermal hyperplasia: psoriasiform (evenly elongated rete ridges), irregular (unevenly elongated rete ridges), papillated (digitate upward epidermal projections), and pseudocarcinomatous (extreme hyperplasia that may resemble a well-differentiated squamous cell carcinoma). The term **acanthosis** denotes thickening of the spinous or prickle cell layer.

7. Hypoplasia is a decrease in the number of keratinocytes that results in a thinned epidermis.

8. Hypertrophy is an increase in size of keratinocytes that leads to a thickening of the epidermis.

9. Atrophy is a decrease in size of keratinocytes, resulting in a thinned epidermis.

10. Spongiosis is intercellular edema between the keratinocytes, resulting in widening of the intercellular spaces and later leading to a spongy appearance or an intraepidermal vesicle. Spongiosis is an important histopathologic sign of eczema.

11. Ballooning is intracellular edema of keratinocytes leading to loss of stain affinity (pallor) and later cellular rupture with formation of multiloculated intraepidermal vesicles. This is an important finding in herpes virus skin infections.

12. Acantholysis is a loss of cohesion between individual keratinocytes that may lead to cleft, vesicle, or bulla formation. Acantholysis is an important sign in the pemphigus group of disorders.

13. Spongiform pustule is an accumulation of neutrophils between epidermal cells that may lead to a spongelike appearance and even vesicle formation.

Spongiform pustulation is a characteristic accompaniment of certain forms of psoriasis (eg, pustular psoriasis).

14. Dyskeratotic cells are prematurely cornified keratinocytes that have eosinophilic cytoplasm and small dark-staining nuclei.

15. Necrosis is local death of cells. Necrosis can usually be identified because of the presence of nuclear fragmentation (karyorrhexis), nuclear ghosts (karyolysis), and nuclear shrinkage (pyknosis). In coagulative necrosis, all cellular detail may be lost apart from cellular outlines, but in caseation necrosis all cellular details are destroyed.

16. Vacuolar (liquefaction) degeneration of the basal cell layer is development of slitlike spaces above and below the basement membrane at the dermal-epidermal junction, which later leads to clefts and sometimes vesiculation.

B. Dermal Changes: Histologic changes in the dermis may be seen as alterations to the connective tissue or cellular infiltration (Table 7–1).

Histologic Reaction Patterns

Recognition of basic dermatopathologic patterns involves principles similar to those learned in recognizing the basic diagnostic pattern in clinical dermatology. For example, in clinical dermatology, viewing the patient from a moderate distance provides a diagnostically valuable perspective of the distribution of lesions (eg, flexural in atopy, extensor in psoriasis). The same advantage is gained in dermatopathology by viewing tissues from a distance (ie, low-power magnification). Ackerman (1978) had done much to popularize the method of facilitating diagnosis by using preliminary scanning power objectives (2.5–4×). The first step in evaluation is to note the location of the pathologic changes (ie, whether in the epidermis, dermis, subcutaneous fat, or a com-

Table 7–1. Types of histologic changes in the dermis.

Cellular infiltrates
Monomorphous: Cells of 1 type only.
Mixed: Cells of more than 2 types.
Lymphohistiocytic: Cells comprised of lymphocytes and histiocytes.
Lichenoid: A bandlike infiltrate of cells that extends across the upper dermis parallel to the epidermis, and tending to obscure the dermoepidermal interface.
Nodular: Well-circumscribed aggregates of cellular infiltrate.
Leukocytoclastic: Fragmentation (nuclear dust) of neutrophils, characteristically seen in allergic vasculitis.

Collagen hyalinization[1]
Fibrosis: Increased formation of collagen (often threadlike) with an increase in numbers of fibroblasts.
Sclerosis: Increased collagen, having a homogeneous and hyalinized appearance with a decreased number of fibroblasts.
Papillomatosis: Projections of the dermal papillae above the skin surface.

[1] Usually seen in degenerative states and characterized by a confluence and increased eosinophilic appearance of the collagen.

bination of sites). This greatly simplifies the more detailed study and interpretation of the various diagnostic histopathologic patterns.

Nine major histopathologic patterns have been identified by Ackerman (Table 7–2).

A. Superficial Perivascular Dermatitis: Nearly all the common inflammatory diseases of the skin (eg, eczema, psoriasis, lichen planus) affect the vessels of the superficial vascular plexus, which is situated in the upper reticular dermis. Superficial perivascular dermatitis can then be subdivided on the basis of accompanying epidermal changes as (1) perivascular without epidermal changes, (2) perivascular with obscuration of the dermal-epidermal interface (interface dermatitis), (3) perivascular with epidermal spongiosis (spongiotic dermatitis or eczematous tissue reaction), or (4) perivascular with epidermal hyperplasia (psoriasiform tissue reaction).

1. Eczematous tissue reaction (spongiotic dermatitis)– The prototype of this reaction pattern is the sequence of events that follow applications of irritants or contact allergens to the skin surface. The changes are characteristically epidermal and include intercellular edema, acanthosis, spongiosis, and parakeratosis, all in focal distribution. In subacute or acute eczema, these changes extend and lead to intraepidermal vesicles (Fig 7–1), which sometimes contain degenerating epidermal cells or other inflammatory cells (ie, in a process of exocytosis). The dermal changes are entirely secondary to the epidermal changes and consist of edema of the papillary dermis and a lymphohistiocytic infiltrate around the venules of the superficial papillary plexus. In less acute eczematous reactions, vesiculation is often absent and foci of spongiosis may be infrequent. The principal change in such cases is acanthosis, which may be irregular, psoriasiform, or even pseudocarcinomatous. Excoriations lead to serous exudates adjacent to parakeratotic foci or even full-thickness damage to the epidermis itself.

2. Psoriasiform tissue reactions– The principal features of psoriasiform reactions are suprapapillary exudate and focal parakeratosis. The exudate may contain edema fluid, leukocytes, or a mixture of both. The suprapapillary exudate stimulates epidermal mitosis. In chronic psoriasis, this leads to prominent

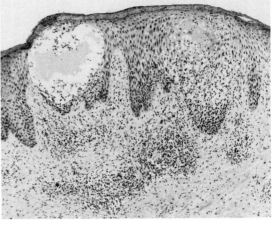

Figure 7–1. Eczematous tissue reaction. There is marked spongiosis within the epidermis, leading to microvesiculation. An accompanying superficial perivascular infiltrate is also present.

psoriasiform hyperplasia (Fig 7–2). Psoriasiform tissue reactions occur in psoriasis, seborrheic dermatitis, perioral dermatitis, nummular eczema, and Reiter's disease. In psoriasis, there is early acanthosis which later becomes psoriasiform. The suprapapillary areas become thinned, and the surface is covered by a lamellated scale with alternating layers of orthokeratotic and parakeratotic stratum corneum. Accumulations of pyknotic polymorphonuclear leukocytes are typically also found in the horny layer (Munro microabscesses). The papillary capillaries become congested and tortuous. In the more acute or pustular types of psoriasis, intact polymorphonuclear leukocytes may migrate through the epidermis to the horny layer (spongiform pustulation of Kogo). In pustular psoriasis, this process may lead to a massive collection of leukocytes just below the horny layer.

3. Interface dermatitis– Interface dermatitis can be subdivided according to whether vacuolar alteration (**vacuolar type**) or a cellular infiltrate (**lichenoid type**) is responsible for blurring of the dermal-epidermal interface.

a. Vacuolar type– In the vacuolar type, there is relatively little inflammatory infiltrate present. The major entity of this type is **erythema multiforme,** in which there is vacuolar alteration of the basal layer of the epidermis (Fig 7–3) associated with formation of necrotic keratinocytes and, later, confluent epidermal necrosis. There is edema of the papillary dermis and a sparse lymphohistiocytic infiltrate around the superficial papillary plexus.

b. Lichenoid type– In the lichenoid type, there is a dense bandlike infiltrate in the papillary dermis that tends to "hug" the rete ridges (Fig 7–4). The major entity of this type is **lichen planus,** in which the

Table 7–2. Major histopathologic patterns.[1]

1. Superficial perivascular dermatitis
2. Superficial and deep perivascular dermatitis
3. Vasculitis
4. Nodular and diffuse dermatitis
5. Intraepidermal vesicular and pustular dermatitis
6. Subepidermal vesicular dermatitis
7. Folliculitis and perifolliculitis
8. Fibrosing dermatitis
9. Panniculitis

[1]From Ackerman AB: *Histologic Diagnosis of Inflammatory Skin Disease: A Method by Pattern Analysis.* Lea & Febiger, 1978.

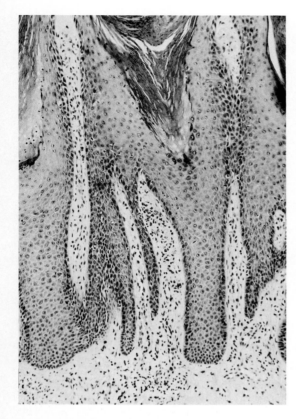

Figure 7–2. Psoriasis vulgaris. There is marked psoriasiform hyperplasia of the epidermis with absence of the granular layer and parakeratosis. Note the thinning of the suprapapillary areas and elongation of the capillaries in the papillary dermis.

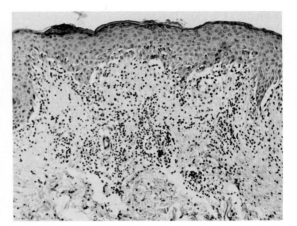

Figure 7–3. Erythema multiforme (early stage). Vacuolar liquefaction of the basal layer forms necrotic keratinocytes. The superficial perivascular infiltrate is only sparse.

changes of liquefactive degeneration of the basal epidermal layer excite a vigorous lymphohistiocytic inflammatory response that blurs the dermal-epidermal interface and in the fully developed stage becomes "bandlike" in the papillary dermis. Pink-staining homogeneous globs called **colloid bodies** occur focally or in clumps. These are degenerating dead keratinocytes. The granular layer becomes irregularly thickened, and there is uniform hyperkeratosis. The midepidermal cells appear larger, flatter, and paler than uninvolved keratinocytes, ie, they are pseudoacanthotic.

Lichenoid drug eruptions (eg, due to gold, anti-materials, and beta-blockers) are characterized by spongiosis and diffuse epidermal damage with colloid bodies "dotted" throughout the epidermis. The inflammatory infiltrate tends to be less dense, being mainly perivascular and sometimes containing several eosinophils.

B. Superficial and Deep Perivascular Dermatitis: In this pattern, the cellular inflammatory infiltrate surrounds the blood vessels of both the superficial and deep plexuses. Superficial and deep perivascular dermatitis may be subdivided into (1) primarily perivascular dermatitis, (2) interface dermatitis, (3) spongiotic dermatitis, and (4) psoriasiform dermatitis.

1. Perivascular dermatitis– In the perivascular subtype, the infiltrate may be lymphohistiocytic or mixed. A predominantly lymphohistiocytic infiltrate

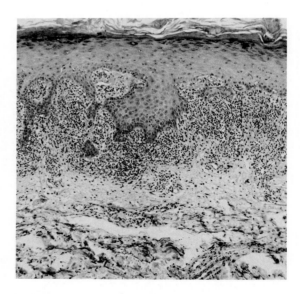

Figure 7–4. Lichen planus. There is a dense bandlike infiltrate obscuring the dermal-epidermal interface. Note the irregular acanthosis, relative hyperkeratosis, and hypergranulosis.

is classically seen in the erythemas such as those associated with lymphocytic infiltration (Jessner). There are no coexisting epidermal changes, and the infiltrate closely "cuffs" the blood vessels with a mixed inflammatory infiltrate. If eosinophils are prominent, various types of insect bite reactions should be strongly considered.

2. Interface dermatitis– The prototype of interface dermatitis of superficial and deep perivascular distribution is **discoid lupus erythematosus.** In this disorder, there is usually atrophy of the epidermis with relative hyperkeratosis and hypergranulosis and focal liquefaction degeneration of the basal layer. In some cases, the basement membrane region may become thickened and even "serpentine" in appearance on PAS staining. The follicular changes are usually conspicuous and consist of deep keratotic follicular plugs with atrophy of the pilar and sebaceous apparatus (Fig 7–5). There is usually marked edema, ectasia, and hyalinization of the papillary dermal region. The lymphocytic infiltrate characteristically involves the superficial and deep plexuses.

C. Vasculitis: All inflammatory processes involve blood vessels to some extent, but in vasculitis one sees organic damage to the vessel wall, such as necrosis, hyalinization, fibrinoid change (Fig 7–6), or

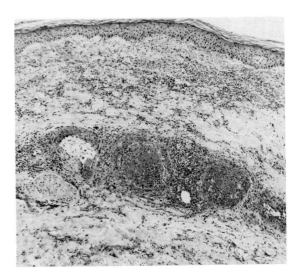

Figure 7–6. Leukocytoclastic vasculitis involving both smaller and larger vessels. There is extensive purpura with fibrinoid occlusion and thrombosis of larger vessels. The damaged vessels are surrounded by nuclear dust of degenerating neutrophils.

even granulomatous involvement. Vasculitis is conveniently divided histologically into small vessel and large vessel types. Large vessel vasculitis is less common and involves large muscular arteries and veins in the deeper dermis or subcutis (eg, **polyarteritis nodosa**). Small vessel vasculitis involves small blood vessels. Characteristically, neutrophils migrate through the damaged walls and degenerate. Fragmented leukocytic nuclei (nuclear dust) accumulate in and around the blood vessels—a process called leukocytoclasis. Edema and purpura develop in the upper dermis.

D. Nodular and Diffuse Dermatitis: Nodular dermatitis denotes discrete perivascular infiltrates within the dermis that are so large that they form histologic nodules. Diffuse dermatitis refers to a cellular infiltrate so dense that the dermal collagen may be obscured by it. Both nodular and diffuse dermatitis can be subdivided according to the predominantly inflammatory cell composition, eg, neutrophils, lymphocytes, plasma cells, histiocytes, mast cells, or mixed cells. The disorders encountered histologically by a nodular and diffuse dermatitis are too numerous to mention individually but include all the granulomatous reactions and the xanthomatoses.

E. Intraepidermal Vesicular and Pustular Dermatitis: There are 3 main ways in which intraepidermal vesicles may be formed: **intracellular edema (spongiosis), intracellular edema (ballooning),** and **acantholysis.** In some diseases, more than one of these features may coexist at the same time. Intracellular edema has already been discussed. Spongio-

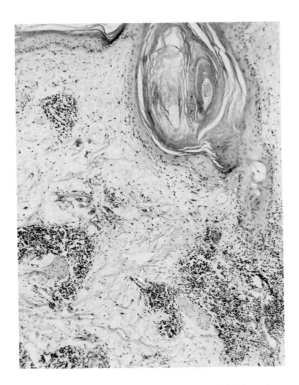

Figure 7–5. Lupus erythematosus (discoid). There is superficial and deep lymphohistiocytic infiltration and keratotic follicular plugging.

sis with neutrophils frequently progresses to formation of vesicopustules. This pattern overlaps with
psoriasiform tissue reactions but may also occur in
certain types of eczema.

1. Intracellular edema (ballooning)– Ballooning
vesicular changes are characteristically seen in certain viral infections (eg, with coxsackieviruses,
herpes simplex virus, and herpes zoster). Virus-
infected epidermal cells show such severe intraepidermal edema that they enlarge and round off (ie,
balloon). Multinucleated giant cells and acantholysis
are also commonly seen. Ballooned epidermal cells
soon die, so that the affected epidermis fills with
fluid, producing an intraepidermal vesicle, often with
a netlike appearance (reticular degeneration) (Fig 7–
7). In severe infections, this process can lead to complete epidermal necrosis.

2. Acantholysis– Acantholysis is the hallmark of
the pemphigus group of disorders, though the process
can occur in other vesicular disorders also (eg,
Hailey-Hailey disease, Darier's disease). It is convenient to subdivide acantholysis into the level of the
epidermis at which the split is occurring: suprabasal,
intraspinous, and subcorneal. The prototype of suprabasal acantholysis is **pemphigus vulgaris** (Fig 7–
8). Intraspinous acantholysis occurs in herpes virus
infections (see above). Subcorneal acantholysis occurs in the superficial forms of pemphigus (eg,
pemphigus foliaceus or pemphigus erythematosus).
The numbers of acantholytic cells are usually far
fewer in the subcorneal zone, but acantholytic cells
often coexist with neutrophils, so that the vesicles
later tend to become pustular.

F. Subepidermal Vesicular Dermatitis: In all of
these disorders there is a clean split between epidermis and dermis, so that the entire epidermis forms the

roof of the vesicle or bulla. The differential diagnosis
includes the subepidermal bullous diseases such as
bullous pemphigoid, cicatricial pemphigoid, linear
IgA bullous disease, herpes gestationis, dermatitis
herpetiformis, and others. Electronmicroscopy has
become an integral component of evaluating patients
with epidermolysis bullosa because it helps define the
ultramicroscopic site of bulla formation. In bullous
pemphigoid, subepidermal bulla formation is often
accompanied by an inflammatory infiltrate rich in
eosinophils (Fig 7–9).

G. Folliculitis and Perifolliculitis: Inflammation
involving the pilosebaceous complex can occur
around (perifollicular) or within the follicular complex. Both types can lead to destruction of hair follicles and permanent alopecia. Special stains can be
used to exclude fungal or bacterial infections. In
perifolliculitis, the inflammatory cells are situated
around the blood vessels of the perifollicular connective tissue. Lymphocytes predominate in keratosis
pilaris, lichen planopilaris, and discoid lupus erythematous. Histiocytes predominate in rosacea or
perioral dermatitis.

In contrast, the inflammatory cell infiltrate in folliculitis usually consists of neutrophils (Fig 7–10).
Folliculitis may be superficial or deep. Superficial
folliculitis presents as pustules, in which the neutrophils fill the entire infundibulum. Deep folliculitis
presents as papules or nodules that later may become
nodulocystic. If the follicle ruptures, the pattern of
inflammation may become granulomatous. Superficial folliculitis may occur in impetigo, tinea, or acne
vulgaris. Deep folliculitis occurs in furuncles, carbuncles, tinea, hidradenitis suppurativa, and the
deeper lesions of acne vulgaris.

H. Fibrosing Dermatitis: Fibrosis follows injury

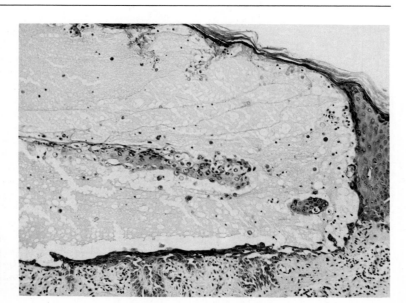

Figure 7–7. Herpes simplex vesicle. The large intraepidermal vesicle
has a netlike appearance and is
filled with clumps of acantholytic
ballooned epidermal cells.

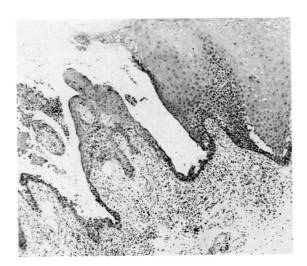

Figure 7–8. Pemphigus vulgaris. Suprabasal clefting and separation with clumps of acantholytic cells is well seen in this biopsy from the edge of an oral erosion.

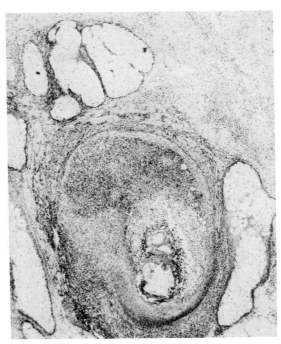

Figure 7–10. Folliculitis. A follicle is virtually completely destroyed and replaced by a neutrophilic abscess.

to the dermal collagen as a result of an inflammatory process. Destruction of collagen invariably involves a loss of elasticity. Fibrosing dermatitis may be hypertrophic (eg, hypertrophic scar, keloid, dermatofibroma), atrophic (eg, striae), or sclerotic (eg, lichen sclerosus et atrophicus). Important antecedents to fibrosis include ulceration, particularly if it involves the reticular dermis. Sclerosis of the papillary dermis produces white lesions (eg, lichen sclerosus et atrophicus) (Fig 7–11). Deeper sclerosing diseases may invoke either hyper- or hypopigmentation. In early scars, there is an increase in the number of fibroblasts, which may have a stellate appearance. Scarring, if severe enough, will eventually replace all adnexal structures such as follicles or sweat glands.

I. Panniculitis: The 3 major components of the subcutis—lipocytes, blood vessels, and fibrous trabeculae (septa)—are all continuous with the dermis, so that inflammatory processes in the deeper dermis are likely to involve the subcutis also. It is essential to take an adequate scalped incisional biopsy specimen, which obviously should extend deeply through the subcutis.

Unlike many dermatoses, most panniculitides are remarkably persistent, lasting for weeks or months. In general, for diagnostic purposes, the biopsy should be taken from an active lesion, ie, erythematous, indurated, and usually tender. The sequence of cellular events following injury to the subcutis is usually as follows: neutrophils → lymphocytes → histiocytes or macrophages (granulomatous) → fibroblasts (fibrosis).

The histologic findings will obviously differ depending on the age of the lesion biopsied. There are 4 main patterns of panniculitis: septal, lobular, and mixed panniculitis, and panniculitis with vasculitis.

Erythema nodosum is the prototype of septal panniculitis. The inflammatory process always involves

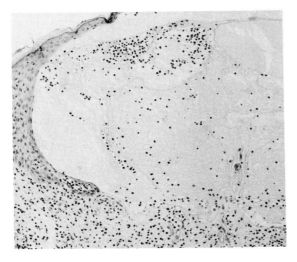

Figure 7–9. Bullous pemphigoid. A subepidermal bulla filled with fibrin is entrapping a few eosinophils.

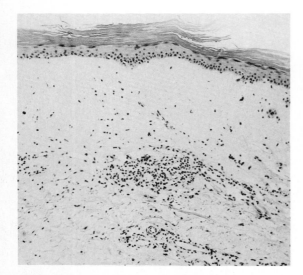

Figure 7–11. Lichen sclerosus et atrophicus. Although there is thinning of the epidermis, there is relative hyperkeratosis. Note the hyalinization of the collagen in the papillary dermis. A sparse perivascular round cell infiltrate is situated just below the sclerotic area.

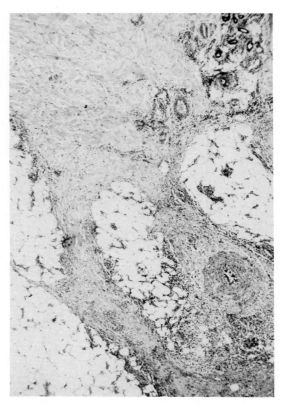

Figure 7–12. Erythema nodosum. The connective tissue septa are edematous and thickened, with a perivascular lymphohistiocytic infiltrate.

the overlying dermis. The septa become edematous and eventually widened, with transudation of neutrophils and later lymphocytes and histiocytes (Fig 7–12). Later, the inflammatory process in the septa becomes granulomatous, and eventually fibrosis supervenes.

The prototype of lobular panniculitis is **nodular panniculitis** (Weber-Christian). In this disorder, the fat lobules are infiltrated with inflammatory cells, mostly neutrophils. It is the later macrophage stage that is characteristic of nodular panniculitis. Macrophages ingest fat released from damaged lipocytes, and their cytoplasm appears foamy. Healing is by fibrosis. In pancreatic panniculitis, there is coagulative necrosis of the lipocytes, leading to "ghosts" of lipocytes and varying degrees of calcification. In infective panniculitis, focal areas of suppuration are found in the fat lobules. Special stains may identify the infective agent or its spores among the abscesses. In physical and factitial panniculitis, there is a focal necrosis of lipocytes with a mixed cellular infiltrate. The affected areas later tend to become "walled off" by fibrous tissue, and there may be calcification.

The prototype of mixed panniculitis is **lupus erythematous profundus.** In this disorder, there are dense "lymphoid" aggregates in the septa and characteristic hyalinization in the fat lobules.

Since the vasculature of the subcutis is housed in the fibrous septa, most vasculitis syndromes (particularly large vessel vasculitis) begin as a septal panniculitis with vasculitis and involve the fat lobules later.

HISTOCHEMISTRY

Turner M. Caldwell III, MD

STRUCTURAL HISTOCHEMISTRY

Histochemical techniques provide optical visualization of the morphologic features of a given tissue and its structural components—eg, proteins, carbohydrates, nucleic acids, lipids, pigments, and inorganic substances—on the basis of their staining properties. Hematoxylin and eosin (H&E), though relatively nonspecific in staining characteristics, are invaluable for routine histologic and histopathologic studies. Many other special histochemical stains may be utilized to reveal abnormal components of the skin not readily appreciated in routinely stained specimens.

Most of the commonly used histochemical procedures can be performed on routinely fixed and processed specimens, though there are important exceptions to that statement—an example being lipids, which require formalin-fixed *frozen* sections. Mucopolysaccharides and amyloid are best demonstrated in unfixed frozen sections. The clinician who is in doubt about the correct fixation or preservation of a tissue specimen should contact the pathologist or technician beforehand to determine how to handle the specimen.

The histochemical staining methods outlined in Table 7–3 are those most commonly used for studying skin. Except as noted, they can be performed on routinely fixed and processed specimens. Several processes stain more than one component, so that care in interpretation is necessary. For example, PAS stain colors glycogen, neutral mucopolysaccharides, and the walls of fungal organisms. The alcian blue reaction stains sulfated as well as nonsulfated acid mucopolysaccharides at pH 4.5 but only sulfated acid mucopolysaccharides at pH 0.5.

Table 7–3. Common used histochemical stains for the skin.

Stain	Component	Result
Hematoxylin and eosin	Routine	Blue: nuclei Red: collagen, muscle, nerves.
van Gieson	Collagen	Red: collagen Yellow: muscle, nerves
Masson's trichrome	Collagen	Blue: collagen Red: muscle
Verhoeff	Elastic fibers	Black
Acid orcein	Elastic fibers	Dark brown
Aldehyde fuchsin	Elastic fibers, mast cell granules, certain epithelial mucins	Deep purple
Silver nitrate impregnation	Reticulum fibers, nerves, melanin	Black
PAS and diastase	Glycogen, neutral mucopolysaccharides, fungi walls	Red (glycogen: diastase-labile)
Alcian blue (pH 4.5, 0.5)[1]	Acid mucopolysaccharides	Blue
Toluidine blue	Acid mucopolysaccharides	Purple (metachromatic)
Colloidal iron	Acid mucopolysaccharides	Blue
Von Kossa	Calcium	Black
Alizarin red	Calcium	Red-orange
Potassium ferrocyanide (Perls' stain)	Iron (hemosiderin)	Blue
Oil red O[2]	Lipids	Red
Sudan black[2]	Lipids	Greenish black
Ammoniated silver nitrate (Fontana-Masson stain)	Melanin	Black
Congo red (alkaline)	Amyloid	Red (green birefringence in polarized light)
Crystal violet	Amyloid	Red (metachromatic)
Gram	Bacteria	Blue: gram-positive Red: gram-negative
Fite	Acid-fast bacilli	Red
Methenamine silver (Grocott stain)	Fungi walls, Donovan bodies, Frisch bacilli	Black
Giemsa	(a) Mast cell granules (b) Leishmania	(a) Purple (metachromatic) (b) Red

[1] See text.
[2] Requires formalin-fixed, frozen sections.

ENZYME HISTOCHEMISTRY

The techniques of enzyme histochemistry provide methods of biochemical investigation of tissue structures that can be widely applied at both the light and electron microscopic levels. When these studies are done on cells, the term **enzyme cytochemistry** is sometimes used.

Routine handling may fail to preserve certain enzymes for study. Multiple fixatives are available, with aldehyde (formaldehyde or glutaraldehyde) fixation generally preferred, but the choice may vary with the enzyme being studied. Many enzyme stains require unfixed, fresh-frozen tissue sectioned on a cryostat.

Enzyme histochemical staining allows in situ identification and localization of enzymes by providing a substrate that becomes an insoluble "colored" compound. The various cellular organelles—eg, endoplasmic reticulum, lysosomes, mitochondria, Golgi apparatus, and plasma membrane—have relatively unique enzyme activities, but the level of activity can vary markedly. Different physiologic and pathologic conditions can change the usual "enzyme markers" of skin components, signifying the need for cautious interpretation of results in attempting to define the functional aspects of these components.

IMMUNOCYTOCHEMISTRY

Mark V. Dahl, MD

By the techniques of immunocytochemistry, antibodies are used to stain structures or antigens. A stain—either a fluorochrome, such as fluorescein, or a marker material, such as peroxidase—is attached to an antibody and allowed to react with the tissue. Antibodies have exquisite specificity and bind only to specific antigens in tissue. Therefore, these special stains can help identify specific cells or microorganisms when the usual methods based on inspection of morphologic features fails to do so or when the amount of antigenic material is small.

Many of the immunocytochemical reagents can be used to stain tissues that have been fixed in formaldehyde and processed through paraffin. Sometimes this fixing and processing destroys antigen. In some cases, therefore, a second biopsy must be done and fresh-frozen sections prepared to help the pathologist when it is critical to define the pathologic process more fully.

S100 protein is present in melanocytes, Langerhans cells, Schwann cells, and sweat glands. It can be used to differentiate a desmoplastic melanoma that contains the protein from a benign fibroblastic proliferation which does not. It can also help delineate the depth of cells at the lower border of a melanoma—cells that might otherwise be obscured by the inflammatory reaction.

The epithelial membrane antigen reacts with most epithelial neoplasms but not with lymphomas, melanomas, or most sarcomas. It therefore helps to identify a very pleomorphic squamous cell carcinoma.

Carcinoembryonic antigen (CEA) is present in eccrine and apocrine glands and in tumors arising from these sites. Leukocyte common antigen is found on B cells, T cells, thymocytes, macrophages, and granulocytes. Unique surface (CD) antigens are found on subsets of lymphocytes, such as CD4 on helper cells. Keratin is present in keratinocytes and therefore also in squamous cell carcinomas. Vimentin is found in melanomas and desmin in muscle cells such as leiomyomas. Lysozyme is present in cells of monocytic and histiocytic origin as well as in neutrophils and some epithelial cells. Staining for lysozyme helps to confirm a diagnosis of cutaneous malignant histiocytosis.

Specific monoclonal and polyclonal antibody stains have been used to identify various infectious agents in tissues. Antibody to human papillomavirus (wart virus) helps to distinguish warts from other verrucous keratoses. Other monoclonal and other immunocytochemical stains have been developed against herpesvirus, cytomegalovirus, and hepatitis virus.

Immunocytochemical stains are usually utilized when a specific diagnosis cannot be made from observation of strictly morphologic criteria. For example, anaplastic carcinomas cannot be distinguished morphologically from anaplastic melanomas or from anaplastic appendageal tumors. Melanomas stain with S100 protein and vimentin. Squamous cell carcinomas stain with keratin and epithelial membrane antigen. Appendageal tumors may contain epithelial markers such as carcinoembryonic antigen but may also express S100 protein.

REFERENCES

Ackerman AB: *Histologic Diagnosis of Inflammatory Skin Disease: A Method by Pattern Analysis.* Lea & Febiger,1978.

DeLellis RA (editor): *Advances in Immunohistochemistry.* Masson, 1984.

Hood AS et al: *Primer of Dermatology.* Little, Brown, 1984.

Junqueira LC, Carniero J, Kelley RO: *Basic Histology,* 6th ed. Appleton & Lange, 1989.

Lever WF, Schaumberg-Lever G: *Histopathology of the Skin,* 6th ed. Lippincott, 1983.

Luna LG (editor): *Manual of Histologic Staining Methods of the AFIP,* 3rd ed. McGraw-Hill, 1968.

Luna LG: *Manual of Histologic Staining Methods of the Armed Forces Institute of Pathology,* 3rd ed. McGraw-Hill, 1968.

Mehregan AH: *Pinkus' Guide to Dermatohistopathology,* 4th ed. Appleton-Century Crofts, 1986.

Kaye VN: Antigen-specific strains in dermatopathology. Curr Concepts Skin Dis 1987;**2**:5.

Miettinen M, Lehto VP, Virtanen I: Presence of fibroblastic type intermediate filaments (vimentin) and absence of neurofilaments in pigmented nevi and malignant melanomas. J Cutan Pathol 1983;**10**:188.

Montagna W, Parakkal PF: *The Structure and Function of Skin,* 3rd ed. Academic Press,1974.

Pearse AGE: *Histochemistry. Theoretical and Applied,* 4th ed. Churchill Livingstone, 1980.

Penny NS: Immunochemistry of adnexal neoplasms. J Cutan Pathol 1984;**11**:357.

8

Immunofluorescence

Beno Michel, MD & Mark V. Dahl, MD

Immunofluorescence is a technique that can detect antibodies in tissue sections or serum. Direct immunofluorescence is a histologic staining technique. Indirect immunofluorescence is a serologic technique and can be used to quantitate the amounts of antibody in serum or other body fluids.

Immunochemistry is a technique that uses monoclonal or polyclonal antibodies to stain specific chemicals in tissue sections.

THE IMMUNOFLUORESCENCE MICROSCOPE

To utilize immunofluorescence, a special microscope equipped with an ultraviolet light source is necessary. The light passes through appropriate filters and strikes the tissue section. Fluorescein or other fluorescent dyes are conjugated to antibodies that are used as stains. These dyes are excited by the ultraviolet radiation striking them, causing them to fluoresce. Light is emitted and passes through other filters so that extraneous ultraviolet radiation is filtered out.

In practice, a scope with a vertical illuminator is used. The ultraviolet radiation actually passes down onto the tissue section from above. Essentially, only the light emitted by the fluorescent dye is then detected, since other ultraviolet radiation passes through the microscope slide and is lost. When fluorescein is the fluorescent dye, antibodies in tissue sections are marked by an apple green color against a black background.

DIRECT IMMUNOFLUORESCENCE

Direct immunofluorescence is a histologic stain for antibody in tissue (Fig 8–1). A frozen section of skin is overlaid with a solution of fluorescein-labeled antihuman antibodies. If human antibodies are present in the tissue section, the fluorescein-labeled antihuman antibodies will bind to them and not wash off. When the biopsy specimen is observed under the fluores-

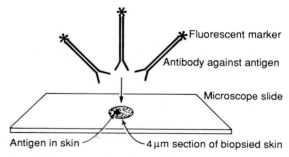

Figure 8–1. Direct immunofluorescence. Fluorescing antibodies are used to stain substances in skin biopsies. For example, fluorescein-labeled antihuman IgG will bind to IgG deposits along the basement membrane zone in skin from patients with bullous pemphigoid.

cence microscope, the site of antibody deposition is marked by green fluorescence.

Direct immunofluorescence can also be used to identify the type of the antibody in tissue by utilizing specific antihuman antibodies to IgG, IgM, IgA, or IgE. Fluorescein-labeled antibodies to complement, fibrinogen, albumin, and other reagents are also available for use in special circumstances. Since the technique is only qualitative, the exact amount of antibody cannot be determined. However, the relative brightness of the fluorescent areas gives some indication of the amount of antibody present.

INDIRECT IMMUNOFLUORESCENCE

In contrast, indirect immunofluorescence is a serologic technique used to detect and quantitate the amount of antibody in serum or other body fluids (Fig 8–2). Tissue sections of *normal* substrate are overlaid with serum from the patient for detection of antibodies against skin. The usual substrate is monkey esophagus, but normal human skin, guinea pig lip, esophagus, or other epithelial substrates may be used instead. If the serum contains antibody to a skin com-

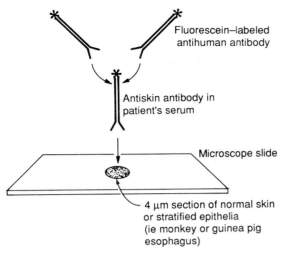

Figure 8–2. Indirect immunofluorescence: Fluorescing antibodies are used to mark where antibodies (if any) in patient serum are bound to normal skin in vitro.

ponent, the antibody will bind to the tissue section and will not wash off. Subsequently, fluorescein-labeled antihuman immunoglobulin is incubated with the section. If antibodies are present that bind to the substrate in the first step, the fluorescein-labeled antihuman antibodies will bind to these serum antibodies in the second step and be detected as green fluorescence under the fluorescence microscope.

Not only can indirect immunofluorescence be used to screen for the presence of antibodies, but the actual amounts can be quantitated by using serial dilutions of serum. Thus, for example, if antibodies may be detected at a 1:10 dilution but not at a 1:20 dilution, the antibody titer is 10.

THE BIOPSY

Because formalin alters protein, formalin-fixed tissue usually cannot be used for direct immunofluorescence. Instead, a biopsy is quick-frozen in liquid nitrogen or other cryogenic agent and kept frozen until it is processed by the laboratory. If the immunofluorescence laboratory is far away, the specimen can be placed in a special transport solution that preserves the antibodies. The specimen can then be sent unrefrigerated by regular mail to the immunofluorescence laboratory.

As with ordinary histology, detailed clinical information should be provided to aid the immunofluorescence microscopist in coming to a useful conclusion.

SERUM SPECIMENS

Serum specimens can be sent unrefrigerated by regular mail. Ordinarily, the blood is drawn, allowed to clot, and the serum is separated from the red blood cells by centrifugation. Serum is then removed from the clotted specimen and placed in a separate tube for mailing.

SITE OF BIOPSY

The exact site of biopsy depends upon the disease being studied. Only some general rules can be provided here; specific details are given in other chapters.

(1) For bullous diseases, never biopsy a blister. Biopsies of intact skin near to a blister are preferred.

(2) For help in diagnosis of lupus erythematosus, both involved and uninvolved skin are often sampled. Characteristically, immunoglobulins are found at the dermal-epidermal junction in lesions of patients with systemic or discoid lupus erythematosus. In contrast, only patients with *systemic* lupus erythematosus have deposits in *normal* skin. Therefore, biopsy of *lesional* skin can help establish the diagnosis of either form of lupus erythematosus and biopsy of *normal* skin can help differentiate discoid lupus erythematosus from systemic lupus erythematosus.

(3) For the diagnosis of *systemic* lupus erythematosus in normal skin, biopsies from sun-exposed areas are usually preferred, since the incidence of immunoglobulins in skin from these sites is higher.

(4) For biopsies of *involved* skin of patients with lupus erythematosus, biopsies should be from untreated lesions—preferably lesions more than 2 or 3 months old. Treated lesions and new lesions often fail to show immunoglobulin deposits.

(5) Although immunoglobulins are associated with immune complex vasculitis, the specificity and sensitivity of using immunofluorescence to diagnose this disease is very low. To make a diagnosis of vasculitis, ordinary histologic techniques are much preferred. However, if it is necessary to determine the **class** of immunoglobulin causing the immune complex vasculitis, biopsy of an early lesion of vasculitis is preferred. Immune complexes are typically destroyed within 18–24 hours by the necrotizing vasculitis itself.

OVERVIEW OF FINDINGS IN SPECIFIC DISEASES

The results of immunofluorescence studies for various diseases are discussed in appropriate chapters. A brief overview will be presented here.

Pemphigus

Antibodies bind to the intercellular area of stratified squamous epithelium (Fig 8–3). These antibodies are present both in skin and in serum of patients with pemphigus. The titer of antibodies in serum correlates with clinical disease activity, and serial titers may be useful in following the response to treatment in patients with this disease.

Bullous Pemphigoid

IgG or C3 (or both) is present along the basement membrane zone in essentially all patients with bullous pemphigoid provided the biopsy is from nonblistered skin (Fig 8–4). Serum from patients with bullous pemphigoid contains these antibodies approximately 70% of the time. Patients with bullous pemphigoid who do not have circulating antibody are somewhat more likely to have coexisting cancer.

Epidermolysis Bullosa Acquisita

The findings on direct and indirect immunofluorescence of patients with epidermolysis bullosa acquisita are identical to those of bullous pemphigoid. However, the antibody binds to a different level of the

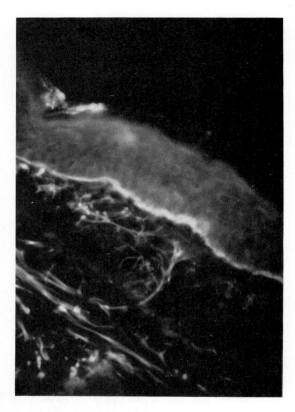

Figure 8–4. Bullous pemphigoid. Note the fluorescing deposits of IgG in linear array at the basement membrane zone.

basement membrane zone. Immunoelectronmicroscopy can provide an accurate diagnosis.

Herpes Gestationis

C3 is present in linear distribution along the basement membrane zone, as in bullous pemphigoid. Although circulating IgG antibodies may be present in low titer, ordinary indirect immunofluorescence is usually negative. Using a special technique called complement indirect immunofluorescence, C3 can be induced to bind at the basement membrane zone of normal skin substrates if serum from patients with herpes gestationis is applied to the substrate first.

Lupus Erythematosus

Thick linear and shaggy bands of immunoglobins occur at the epidermal-dermal junction in patients with hyperkeratotic and chronic atrophic lesions of both discoid and systemic lupus erythematosus. Thin or moderately thick linear bands are found in many inflammatory skin diseases besides lupus erythematosus, but bright fibrillar bands are more specific (Fig 8–5). Thin linear bands are seen in bullous

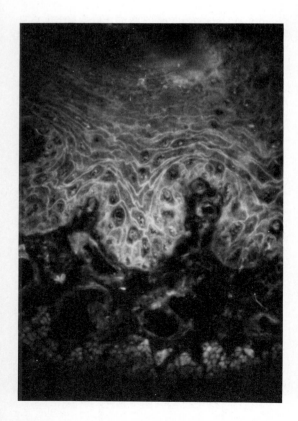

Figure 8–3. Pemphigus. Note the fluorescing deposits of IgG in the intercellular spaces of the epidermis.

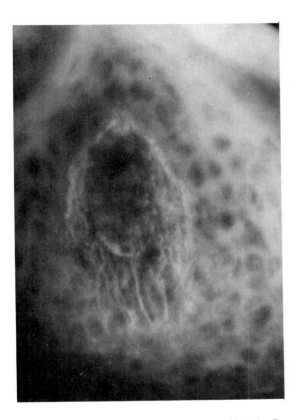

Figure 8–5. Systemic lupus erythematosus. Note the fluorescing fibrillar and granular deposits of IgG at and below the basement membrane zone.

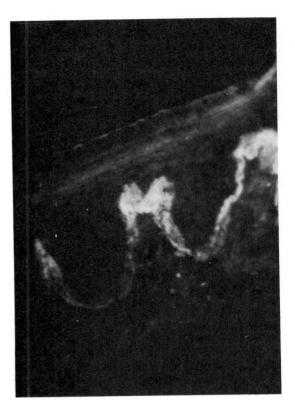

Figure 8–6. Dermatitis herpetiformis. Note the granular deposits of IgA at the dermal-epidermal junction and in the superficial parts of the dermal papillae.

pemphigoid and other bullous diseases. Granular bands are seen in both normal and abnormal skin of patients with systemic lupus erythematosus. Stippled deposits are sometimes superimposed upon bands of other configuration. Granular or stippled deposits of C3 at the dermal-epidermal junction are found in many disorders, and their presence is therefore nonspecific.

Dermatitis Herpetiformis

Normal skin from patients with dermatitis herpetiformis characteristically contains large granular deposits of IgA along the dermal epidermal junction and in the superficial papillary dermis (Fig 8–6). These deposits are particularly likely in dermal papillae and may be accompanied by deposits of C3.

REFERENCES

Beutner EH, Chorzelski TP, Bean AF: *Immunopathology of the Skin,* 3rd ed. Wiley, 1987.

Beutner EH, Chorzelski TP, Jablonska S: Immunofluorescence tests: Clinical significance of sera and skin: Bullous diseases. Int J Dermatol 1985;24:205.

Dahl MV: *Clinical Immunodermatology,* 2nd ed. Year Book, 1988.

Dahl MV: Immunoglobulin deposition in skin of patients with lupus erythematosus: Clinical correlates and indications for direct immunofluorescence. Adv Dermatol 1986;1:247.

Valenzuela R, Bergfield WF, Deodar SD: *Interpretation of Immunofluorescent Patterns in Skin Diseases.* ASCP Press, 1985.

Korman N: Bullous pemphigoid. J Am Acad Dermatol 1987;16:907.

Hall RP: The pathogenesis of dermatitis herpetiformis: Recent advances. J Am Acad Dermatol 1987;16:1129.

Shornick JK: Herpes gestationis. J Am Acad Dermatol 1987;17:539.

9

Electron Microscopy & Ultrastructure of the Skin

Alvin S. Zelickson, MD & Jess Mottaz, BS

THE ULTRASTRUCTURE OF THE SKIN

The electron microscope is used not only for basic research on the structure and function of the skin but also as an aid to diagnosis (see p 62).

Tissue for electron microscopic examination is usually obtained by punch biopsy. Great care must be taken not to crush the specimen. The cylinder of incised skin can be pulled out with a needle rather than a forceps so that crushing does not occur. The specimen is placed on a tongue depressor, cut into small (1 × 1 mm) rectilinear blocks with a new razor blade, and placed in 2% aqueous glutaraldehyde solution. The microscopist must know the purpose of the biopsy and the diagnosis or differential diagnosis in order to provide the needed information.

The ultrastructure of skin is complex and discussed in detail in Chapter 1 along with the functions of various organelles.

Basal Lamina

The epidermis is separated from the dermis by an electron-dense basal lamina consisting of a layer of connective tissue fibrils that run parallel to and follow the contour of the underside of the epidermis. In most cases this "membrane" is approximately 30 nm thick and is separated from the epidermis by a transparent structure called the lamina lucida (Fig 9–1). Beneath the basal lamina is a fairly broad, less dense zone containing many fine fibrils without apparent organization. These anchoring fibrils hold the epidermis on the dermis. Fibroblasts and bundles of collagen fibers are seen in this area and throughout the dermis.

Stratum Germinativum

The basal keratinocyte contains numerous and regularly oriented tonofilaments that stream into the cytoplasm from their location near the cytoplasmic surface of the desmosomes at the junctions of ker-atinocytes in the epidermis and hemidesmosomes at the dermal-epidermal junction. The cytoplasm of the basal keratinocyte also contains mitochondria, melanosome complexes, and a Golgi complex.

The basal keratinocytes have relatively straight lateral borders and are attached to one another by intercellular bridges (desmosomes) consisting of dense thickenings of adjacent epidermal cell membranes that appose one another. The tonofilaments originate near the internal or cytoplasmic surface of these attachment plaques and do not cross from cell to cell.

Stratum Spinosum

The keratinocytes in the stratum spinosum differ from those in the basal layer. The tonofilaments, loosely arranged in the stratum germinativum, are densely aggregated in the stratum spinosum. As the cell nears the stratum granulosum, it flattens, with its longest diameter becoming oriented parallel to the surface. Desmosomes are still visible and retain their characteristic internal structure. The tonofibrils appear less distinct at this level, lying parallel rather than perpendicular to the surface. The plasma membrane of the spinous keratinocyte is villous and attached to its neighbor by the desmosomes. Mitochondria and ribosomes are numerous throughout the cytoplasm and retain their normal structure. Melanosomes are present in smaller numbers and in complexes.

Numerous round, smooth-surface, thick-walled granules are present in the upper stratum spinosum and the stratum granulosum, but rarely in the stratum corneum. The granules appear relatively uniform in shape and diameter (100–200 nm). Termed membrane-coating granules (keratinosomes, Odland bodies), they have been found both extracellularly and intracellularly. They are increased in number in certain diseases and occur in keratinizing epithelium as well as in nonkeratinizing oral mucosa. After fusion with the plasma membrane, they empty their contents into the intercellular spaces. The contents of the granules

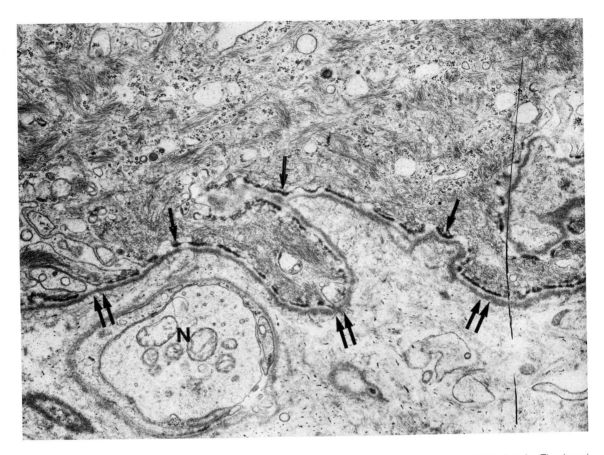

Figure 9–1. The basement membrane zone, including the lower epidermis and upper papillary dermis. The basal lamina is the dark continuous band indicated by the double arrows, and the lamina lucida is the light area above it. Above this are keratinocytes, which are attached to the basal lamina by the hemidesmosomes indicated by the single arrows. Below the basal lamina is the dermis. The main structure evident in the dermis is nerve tissue (N), located in the lower left of the micrograph.

spread over the surface of the cell membrane and form a thick cell envelope.

Stratum Granulosum

Electron-dense keratohyaline material is present in significant amounts in stratum granulosum. Keratohyaline granules are located throughout the cytoplasm; they increase in size and number as the cells approach the stratum corneum. Usually, keratohyalin is closely associated with the tonofilaments.

In the stratum granulosum, there is a continuation of differentiation. Present in smaller numbers are mitochondria, vesicles of the endoplasmic reticulum, melanosome complexes, and membrane-coating granules. Nuclei may still be present. The cell membrane has definite infoldings, and the desmosomes appear to be closer and more numerous than in the deeper layers.

Stratum Corneum

The stratum corneum is usually 10–15 cells thick.

The cells are flat and undulating, with a long axis parallel to the surface. A nucleus is no longer seen, nor are cytoplasmic structures, including melanin, mitochondria, endoplasmic reticulum, Golgi complexes, and the membrane-coating granules. Numerous round, unstained filaments, 10 nm in diameter, are seen embedded in an electron-dense cement substance (keratohyaline material). In some cells, the structural development of the stratum corneum is irregular, with individual cells at lower levels sometimes more "keratinized" than some nearer the surface. To prepare for desquamation, desmosomes change in a characteristic manner. An osmiophilic body forms in the intercellular space between the apposed cell membranes that make up the desmosome. When the cell is shed, the break in the desmosome occurs on either side of the intercellular body.

Melanocyte

Melanocytes arise from the neural crest and are

primarily located in the basal layer of the human epidermis between the epidermal keratinocytes. Melanin is attached to the protein matrix of the melanosome. These dendritic cells do not form a syncytium; their clear appearance is due to their relative lack of cytoplasmic filaments.

The melanocyte is distinguished from its neighbors by its dendritic appearance, lack of desmosomes, and relative lack of filaments (Fig 9–2). Mitochondria are abundant and dispersed throughout the cytoplasm. A well-developed endoplasmic reticulum is present. The Golgi apparatus is well developed and easily recognized; often it is located near the nucleus. Unlike the keratinocytes, the melanocyte has a plasma membrane that lacks desmosomes or other structural attachments to its neighbors or to the basement membrane, though periodic thickenings of the plasma membrane along the basement membrane may be seen.

The melanocyte produces pigment matrices known as melanosomes. The early melanosome has an organized protein matrix upon which melanin may be deposited. The earliest melanosome (stage I) is smaller than the mature form (stage IV). During development, spiral fibers join at the poles of the melanosome to form an oval structure (stage II). A unit membrane surrounds the melanosome. With further development, melanin synthesis starts (stage III). An osmiophilic material is deposited on the protein matrix of the stage II melanosome. As this process continues, each fiber becomes a thickened dark band. The spaces between the fibers become filled or partially filled, depending upon the color, and the melanosome becomes a fully developed stage IV melanosome. There is an inverse relationship between the amount of melanin formed and the tyrosinase activity present, ie, when the melanosome is fully developed there is no longer measurable tyrosinase activity.

As they mature, melanosomes migrate to the dendrites of the melanocytes. Portions of dendritic processes are phagocytosed by the adjacent keratinocytes, with the keratinocyte playing an active role in the process. After the portion of the dendrite is brought into the keratinocyte, the melanosomes are surrounded by the membrane of the melanocyte. The

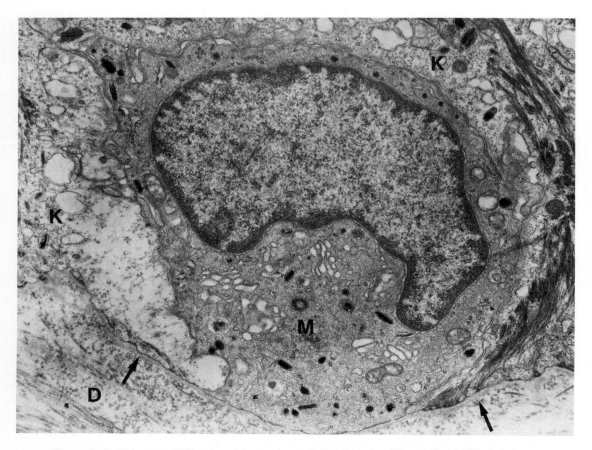

Figure 9–2. Melanocyte (M) on basal lamina (arrows). Keratinocytes (K) and dermis (D) also shown.

membrane eventually breaks down, and the melanosome contents are dispersed throughout the cell. In blacks, the melanosomes are usually dispersed singularly. In whites, they usually exist in groups of melanosome complexes.

The Langerhans Cells

These cells morphologically resemble melanocytes. The cell is dendritic and lacks desmosomes. The Golgi apparatus and the endoplasmic reticulum are well developed; mitochondria are numerous, but filaments are few. Langerhans cells also contain lysosomes, melanosomes, and lipid droplets. The Langerhans cell is distinguished from the melanocyte by its characteristic cytoplasmic granule (Langerhans granule) and by the convoluted appearance of its nucleus. Langerhans cells are found in the superficial, mid, and lower epidermis and in the dermis.

The Dermis

The papillary and the reticular layers of the dermis are distinct (Fig 9–3). The papillary layer lies just below the basal lamina and follows the contours of the rete ridge of the epidermis. The papillary layer contains fewer collagen fibers than the reticular layer, which is made up mostly of coarse collagenous fiber bundles, arranged generally parallel to the skin surface.

The dermis is approximately 25 times thicker than the epidermis and is composed primarily of cells, fibrous proteins, collagen, elastic and reticular fibers, and an amorphous ground substance. Except for the use of special stains, the amorphous ground substance is invisible to the electron microscope. Collagen fibers vary in diameter from 20 to 150 nm. Individual collagen fibers possess a characteristic and repeatable pattern. A longitudinal section of a collagen fiber presents a striated appearance that has an exact period of 64 nm. These striations or bands are separated by several interbands. The width of the fiber varies between the band and the interbands.

Elastic fibers are scattered throughout the dermis. Their appearance is slightly mottled and of varying electron density. The fibers are round or flat, branched, and vary greatly in size. Staining with phosphotungstic acid enhances their electron density. Electron micrographs of elastic tissue show amorphous elastin covering the elastic fibers. Reticular fibrils resemble collagen to some degree but lack its uniformity. In the dermis, reticular fibrils can most readily be identified in the area of the basal lamina. Ground substance is generally invisible to the electron microscope. It contains no fibrils but is an amor-

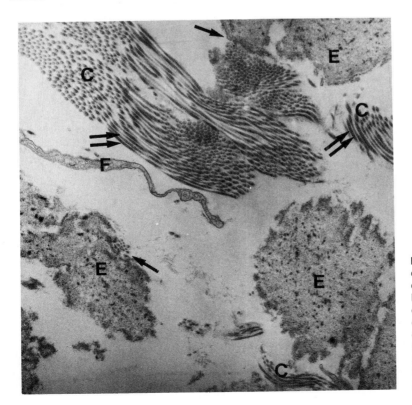

Figure 9–3. The reticular layer of the dermis. Present are 3 major dermal components: elastic tissue (E), collagen (C), and a portion of the cytoplasm of a fibroblast (F). Note the close intermixture of collagen and elastic tissue at the single arrows. Collagen can be seen in both cross and longitudinal section. The characteristic striations of collagen appear at the double arrows.

phous fluid that bathes the fibers and cells of the dermis.

The most prominent dermal cell is the fibroblast, which is responsible for production and maintenance of the connective tissue. This cell assumes a shape to fit its environment—ie, in the more densely packed reticular layer the cytoplasm becomes long and thin, whereas in the papillary layer the cytoplasm becomes confined and rounded. The nucleus of the fibroblast is round, with chromatin particles congregating mainly adjacent to the nuclear membrane. It contains one or more nucleoli. The endoplasmic reticulum is well developed, as is the Golgi complex, and a moderate number of mitochondria are found.

The next most prominent dermal cell is the mast cell, easily identified in an electron micrograph because it contains many highly specific granules with characteristic structures. The plasma membrane of the mast cell is characterized by a complex villiform surface. Other cells encountered in the dermis include Langerhans cells, plasma cells, histiocytes, macrophages, melanocytes, nerve cells, blood vessel cells, and cells composing hair bulbs, sweat glands, and sebaceous glands.

The electron microscope is a useful research tool. It demonstrates the ultrastructure of individual cells, and the workings of organelles can be observed.

CLINICAL USE OF THE ELECTRON MICROSCOPE AS AN AID IN THE DIAGNOSIS OF SKIN DISEASE

In the dermatopathology laboratory, the electron microscope is sometimes used to help diagnose tumors, abnormal pigment, defects of keratinization, blistering diseases, storage diseases, and certain viral infections. Characteristic ultrastructural changes often help confirm a clinical diagnosis. Listed below are a few areas where the electron microscope can aid in the diagnosis of skin disorders.

Disorders of Pigmentation

Vitiligo has no melanin or melanocytes. There is an increase in the number of Langerhans cells, especially along the basal cell layer.

Albinism will show numerous melanocytes that are structurally active but enzymatically inactive. Only stage I and stage II melanosomes are seen, and no complete melanosomes are formed.

Postinflammatory hypopigmentation—in contrast to albinism—shows decreased numbers of melanocytes, but some are still present. Melanin may be present in dermal macrophages.

Tuberous sclerosis (ash leaf macules) presents decreased melanogenesis, resulting in melanosomes that are fewer and smaller than normal.

Chédiak-Higashi syndrome is characterized by large abnormal melanosomes and large melanosome complexes in keratinocytes.

Neurofibromatosis will show giant melanosomes in café-au-lait patches. These are also found in multiple lentigines syndrome, nevus spilus, and Albright's syndrome. The clinical identification of a full-blown case of neurofibromatosis is easily made, but at times when only a few café-au-lait macules are present ultrastructural evaluation of the tissue for giant melanosomes is invaluable.

Drug deposits may impart a brown or gray color to skin that can be clinically confused with normal pigmentation. Chlorpromazine forms lysosome-like packages associated with melanosomes, and minocycline produces pigmented particles in the cytoplasm of dermal cells.

Papulosquamous Plaques

Discoid lupus erythematosus is usually diagnosed clinically and histologically. It can be clinically confused with polymorphous light eruption, seborrheic dermatitis, lymphocytic lymphoma, lymphocytoma cutis, and even psoriasis. The light microscopic picture may be helpful but not diagnostic. The ultrastructural finding of paromyxovirus-like inclusions in the endothelial cells of such patients can be diagnostic of lupus erythematosus (discoid or systemic).

Mycosis fungoides shows numerous mycosis fungoides cells in the epidermis as well as in the dermis. These are large lymphocytes with indented cerebriform nuclei. Probably the earliest way to diagnose mycosis fungoides is with the electron microscope. It is especially valuable in separating parapsoriasis en plaque from early mycosis fungoides.

Blistering Disorders

Epidermolysis bullosa consists of about 20 different hereditary disorders with varying hereditary patterns, clinical presentations, and prognosis. Electron microscopic changes in epidermolysis bullosa are not always characteristic of specific forms. However, the exact microscopic location of the bulla may aid in both the classification of the disease and in genetic counseling of the patient. Briefly, epidermolysis bullosa can be subdivided by the location of blister formation. Some develop within basal cells, others at the level of the lamina lucida, and still others below the lamina densa. Anchoring fibers may be absent (see Chapter 42). Biopsy is best done of normal unblistered skin. The trauma of the punch biopsy itself is usually sufficient to elicit a bulla.

Tumors

A neoplasm may be so anaplastic that the cell of origin cannot be identified by ordinary histologic examination. In these cases, identification of specific organelles may aid in the identification of tumors, ie, melanomas contain melanosomes and squamous cell carcinomas contain desmosomes.

REFERENCE

Zelickson AS: *The Clinical Use of Electron Microscopy in Dermatology,* 4th ed. Bolger, 1985.

10

Laboratory Evaluation of Immunity

Mark V. Dahl, MD

The immune system defends the body against infections, including infections of the skin. It also mediates inflammation. When it functions abnormally, disease may result. For these reasons, the immune system is often evaluated by laboratory tests. Some laboratory tests are easily performed and readily available at most hospitals and clinical laboratories. Others are more sophisticated and available only at specialized medical centers.

The most common indication for immunologic testing in dermatology is evaluation of patients with infections, dermatitis, and lupuslike syndromes for immunodeficiency. This chapter is mostly oriented to that end. Specific tests are often ordered when evaluating patients with specific skin diseases. This chapter serves as a guide to understanding these tests and interpreting their results.

EVALUATION OF HUMORAL IMMUNITY

Humoral immunity is mediated by antibodies. Widely available tests for evaluation of humoral immunity include quantitative determinations of immunoglobulin levels, isohemagglutinin titers, protein electrophoresis, measurement of levels of IgG antibodies to rubella and other infectious diseases, and quantifying the number of circulating B cells in peripheral blood.

QUANTITATIVE IMMUNOGLOBULIN LEVELS

The quantity of each class of immunoglobulins can be determined in serum and body fluids. Levels of IgG, IgM, and IgA are determined by radioim-

munodiffusion assays. The quantity of IgE is determined by radioimmunoassay. These tests measure the total amount of each class of antibody but do not show antibody specificity. Patients can be deficient in antibodies to specific agents yet have normal total immunoglobulin levels.

Tests for levels of antibodies to specific antigens are not widely available except for certain infectious organisms and various self-antigens. Easily obtained tests are for antibodies to antistreptolysin O (ASO), streptococcal DNase, herpesvirus hominis, varicella-zoster virus, and rubella virus.

The levels of immunoglobulins are age-dependent, tending to rise during childhood. The level of IgM tends to rise continuously from birth until late adolescence; that of IgG tends to drop soon after birth as maternally transferred antibody is consumed. After 3–12 months, levels begin to rise until adult levels are reached. Levels of IgA and IgE also rise during childhood. Levels that indicate an immunodeficiency among adults may be normal for a small child or neonate.

About 80% of patients with atopic dermatitis have high IgE levels. Determination of IgG levels may aid diagnosis of atopic dermatitis, but—since IgE may be elevated in patients with other diseases such as allergic rhinitis, asthma, and even other eczematous diseases—the results of these tests must be interpreted in the light of other clinical and laboratory findings as well.

ISOHEMAGGLUTININ TITERS

Isohemagglutinins are naturally occurring IgM antibodies against red blood cell antigens A and B. Levels are often low or absent during the first year or 2 and then rise during early childhood. Patients with IgM deficiency have only small amounts of isohemagglutinins. Because normal children under age 2 years often have low titers and patients with type AB blood have none, both the age and blood type of the patient must be considered in evaluating results of isohemagglutinin testing.

PROTEIN ELECTROPHORESIS

Protein electrophoresis can define classes of proteins in sera or other body fluids. Its use in evaluation of immune function lies in its ability to uncover a deficiency of all gamma globulins or an excess of one, such as a monoclonal paraprotein in a patient with myeloma or scleromyxedema. Patients with hypogammaglobulinemia have low total gamma globulin levels, but isolated deficiency of one or more immunoglobulin classes may not be detected by protein electrophoresis testing. Patients with multiple myeloma may have a functional immunodeficiency of humoral immunity despite high levels of gamma globulins from the paraprotein.

Immunoelectrophoresis depends on the precipitation of classes of immunoglobulins after they have migrated through agar under the influence of electrical charge. This test should not be used as a substitute for quantitative immunoglobulin levels.

Determination of Circulating B Cells

The number of circulating B cells can aid in evaluation of humoral immunity. These are the cells that secrete antibody and differentiate into plasma cells that secrete antibody. Normally, 10–25% of circulating lymphocytes are B cells. Because they have immunoglobulins on their surfaces, the number of B cells can be quantitated by direct immunofluorescence. A suspension of lymphocytes is incubated with a solution containing fluorescein-labeled antihuman IgG, IgM, IgA, and IgE. The percentage of fluorescing cells reflects the percentage of total B cells. The number of lymphocytes programmed to secrete specific immunoglobulin classes can also be quantitated by modifying this assay to incubate lymphocytes with fluorescein-labeled antibody against only that single specific class of immunoglobulin.

The presence of antibodies in serum is a marker of previous contact with antigen and some degree of immunocompetence. Many of the tests described above are static; they measure past immunologic capability. Measurement of a specific primary or secondary antibody response can assess current functional status. For example, a patient can be vaccinated with a neoantigen such as bacteriophage OX174. In practice, it is easiest to reimmunize with diphtheria, pertussis, and tetanus antigens (DPT booster). Blood is drawn before immunization and then weekly for 3–4 weeks. All specimens are submitted to the laboratory at the same time to minimize individual laboratory variation. Testing for antibodies following vaccination with live viruses or bacteria is not recommended because immunodeficient patients may develop clinical infection.

EVALUATION OF CELL-MEDIATED IMMUNITY

Cell-mediated immunity is mediated by T lymphocytes. In dermatologic practice, this limb of the immune system handles infections by viruses, fungi, and other pathogens that cause intercellular infections and directs the inflammatory response of allergic contact dermatitis.

TOTAL LYMPHOCYTE COUNTING

Because most circulating lymphocytes are T cells, the number of small lymphocytes reflects the total number of T cells. The normal lymphocyte count is more than 1500 cells per microliter. In practice, a simple white blood count and differential are usually sufficient. The peripheral blood smear may be examined in order to assess the morphology and number of small lymphocytes. The absolute numbers of T and B cells and the ratio of T helper cells to T suppressor cells in peripheral blood can be quantitated by immunofluorescence. Patients with AIDS have very low counts of T helper cells, and quantitation of T helper cells aids in the decision to institute prophylactic antimicrobial therapy.

INTRADERMAL SKIN TESTING

Intradermal skin testing is another convenient test for evaluation of cell-mediated immunity. Delayed hypersensitivity skin tests read 48 hours after injection evaluate recognition of antigen by the immune system, the ability of the cell-mediated immune system to mediate inflammation, and the ability of mediators and phagocytes to produce inflammation. Among recall skin test antigens in current use are antigens to *Candida,* tetanus toxoid, trichophytin, and tubercular purified protein derivative (PPD).

Small amounts of each antigen are injected intradermally, usually into the skin of the ventral forearm. Test sites are marked and evaluated at 30 minutes for an immediate wheal response and at 48 hours for a delayed hypersensitivity response. For evaluation of cell-mediated immunity, only the 48-hour reading is important. In general, if the area of induration is less than 5 mm in diameter (10 mm for PPD), the test can be considered negative. The criteria for positive and negative tests depend upon the quantity of antigen in the initial testing material as well as other factors. In the immunodeficient patient, any reaction might be significant.

Skin test antigens may cause titers of corresponding antibodies to rise following testing. Skin testing is of limited value in infants, because they have not encountered most antigens and therefore have no recall. Furthermore, immunizations and viral infections often depress reactivity.

TESTING FOR INFLAMMATORY RESPONSE

The susceptibility of skin to inflammation can be measured by applying a 24-hour closed patch test saturated with 10% aqueous solution of sodium lauryl sulfate to forearm skin. Be sure the patch is still wet when it is applied. This solution irritates the skin nonspecifically. The test site should be examined for erythema at least 1 hour after removal of the closed patch. If no erythema is present, the test should be repeated at another body site before concluding that the inflammatory response is blocked.

DINITROCHLOROBENZENE (DNCB) RESPONSE

Induction of allergic contact dermatitis to a previously unencountered chemical like dinitrochlorobenzene (DNCB) indicates a functioning cell-mediated immune system. Dinitrochlorobenzene can induce and elicit contact dermatitis in most persons. To induce allergy, 0.1 mL of 2% DNCB in acetone is applied to the skin of the upper arm, allowed to dry, and covered for 2 hours with nonocclusive paper tape. If a spontaneous flare does not occur by the 21st day, 0.1 mL of a 0.1% solution of DNCB in acetone is applied to a second site on the arm and evaluated 48 hours later. A positive test is marked by erythema and induration at the site of application.

Patients with severe combined immunodeficiency disease may lack adenosine deaminase or nucleoside phosphorylase. Levels in blood can be assayed.

TESTING FOR LYMPHOCYTE FUNCTION

Lymphocyte transformation evaluates the ability of lymphocytes to incorporate bases into new DNA, which they must be able to do in order to induce a cell-mediated immune response. In general, lymphocytes are incubated in suspension cultures with mitogens such as phytohemagglutinin (PHA), pokeweed mitogen (PWM), or concanavalin A (ConA). After 5 days, a radioactive nucleotide such as thy-

midine is added to the suspension. The amount of radioactivity emitted by these lymphocytes is a measure of blastogenic response. PHA and ConA are T cell mitogens. PWM stimulates both T and B cells. Lipopolysaccharide endotoxin (LPS), Epstein-Barr virus (EBV), and protein A of *Staphylococcus aureus* are B cell mitogens. For detecting immune deficiency, suboptimal concentrations of these mitogens should be used. This is best done by comparing dose-response curves of patients and controls.

Lymphokine production can be measured. There are about 100 functionally defined lymphokines. Assays can be functional or quantitative. Assays for quantitating the lymphokines interleukin-2 and gamma interferon are available commercially.

A variation of the lymphoblast transformation assay can also be used to determine the response of cells to individual specific antigens. In this situation, the suspension of lymphocytes is incubated with antigen instead of mitogen. Here only lymphocytes programmed to respond to the specific antigen will undergo blast transformation. A prolonged incubation with interleukin-2 and antigen is usually required.

TESTING FOR MIXED LYMPHOCYTE REACTION

In the mixed lymphocyte reaction (MLR), the stimulating antigens are cell-surface antigens on lymphocytes from a second individual. Responder lymphocytes undergo blast transformation if histocompatibility differences exist between them and the stimulator population.

QUANTITATION OF T CELLS

The number of T cells can be quantitated by immunocytochemical techniques. These monoclonal antibodies against determinants on T cells or their subsets can be labeled with peroxidase or immunofluorescent compounds like fluorescein or rhodamine. Markers on T cells are denoted by clusters of differentiation antigens (CD).

EVALUATION OF PHAGOCYTE FUNCTION

Phagocytes consist of neutrophils, eosinophils, basophils, and macrophages. Of these, the neutrophil and macrophage are the primary phagocytes involved in host defense. Evaluation of phagocyte function often requires the use of sophisticated laboratory techniques. In dermatologic practice, tests are indicated for patients with recurrent pyogenic infections, pyogenic infections that fail to respond to appropriate antibiotics, and infections caused by bacterial pathogens of low virulence.

TOTAL NEUTROPHIL COUNT

Simply measuring the number of neutrophils in the peripheral blood is a good screening test, because deficient numbers are the most common problem. Normally, more than 1000 polymorphonuclear leukocytes per microliter are present, and persistent counts between 200 and 300 cells/μL may be significant clues to a neutrophil deficiency state. In patients with active infection, counts are often higher. Neutropenia is an indication of phagocyte failure.

CHEMILUMINESCENCE TEST

When a cell phagocytoses a particle, it undergoes a "respiratory burst." The process generates a minute amount of light that can be detected by a liquid scintillation counter. Results are compared with normal values and simultaneous controls. Both the peak value and the duration of respiratory burst should be considered when interpreting the results.

A normal chemiluminescence response requires that (1) the particle must be opsonized properly, (2) the cell must phagocytose properly, (3) the cell must undergo a typical respiratory burst, and (4) the cell must generate superoxide. A normal chemiluminescence response ensures that all these steps have proceeded normally.

MEASUREMENT OF INTRACELLULAR ENZYMES

The levels of intracellular enzymes generating oxygen metabolites can be measured directly only in certain special laboratories. On the other hand, neutrophils can be stained for the presence of peroxidase and leukocyte alkaline phosphatase by rather simple techniques that are more widely available.

CHEMOTAXIS RESPONSE

Chemotaxis is the directed migration of phagocytic cells. When exposed to a gradient of chemotactic factor, a neutrophil or monocyte migrates preferentially toward increasing concentrations of that factor.

In the Rebuck skin window technique, normal skin is gently abraded and occluded with a glass coverslip. At various times, the coverslip is removed, stained, and examined for the presence of phagocytes. Normally, polymorphonuclear leukocytes appear early and mononuclear cells later. In the laboratory, chemotaxis can be evaluated by measuring the migration of phagocytic cells through filter paper or under agarose gel. Random migration can also be assayed by omitting chemotactic factors. Random migration refers to the nondirected migration of cells.

PHAGOCYTIC ADHERENCE TESTS

Cell adherence tests the stickiness of phagocytic cells to plastic or glass surfaces. Adherence is necessary for proper phagocytosis and chemotaxis. A suspension of cells is placed in a Petri dish or passed through glass wool. The percentage of cells that adhere to the solid phase is determined by cell counts.

EVALUATION OF COMPLEMENT FUNCTION

Complement consists of a series of plasma components that must be activated sequentially. The total hemolytic complement assay measures the functional integrity of the classic complement pathway. Antibody-coated red blood cells are added to patient sera. If all complement components are present, the red blood cells lyse. If a patient has a normal CH_{50} level, all components of the classic complement pathway are present in sufficient quantities.

Elevated levels of CH_{50} or individual components are nonspecific, because complement is an acute phase reactant. Low levels reflect decreased synthesis, increased consumption, dysfunctional protein, or utilization after venipuncture from improper handling, cryoglobulins, immune complexes, or coagulation.

The more common reason for checking complement levels is to determine if they are low because they are being consumed by an antibody reaction such as occurs in systemic lupus erythematosus and vasculitis. Low levels of CH_{50} are present in patients with an immunodeficiency of a specific complement component. In order to determine if a low CH_{50} reflects consumption or immunodeficiency, individual complement components can be quantitatively measured.

The functional activity of the alternative complement pathway is assessed by activating it with cobra venom in calcium-free, magnesium-enriched buffer. Generation of C5a is assessed by direct measurement or by measuring C5a-induced clumping of platelets in an aggregometer.

The ability of complement components to opsonize can be tested by a modification of the chemiluminescence assay. Here, patient sera is incubated with zymosan and phagocytes. If normal opsonization has not occurred, then the chemiluminescence response will be abnormal. The ability to opsonize can also be determined by measuring the number of opsonized latex particles that are phagocytosed by normal cells after incubation.

C1 esterase inhibitor is a protein that inhibits the action of C1 esterase (C1qrs). Patients with hereditary angioedema lack C1 esterase inhibitor, so serum levels are low. Some patients with normal levels of C1 esterase inhibitor still have hereditary angioedema. In these patients, the inhibitor is dysfunctional, ie, it is present in normal concentration levels but does not inactivate C1qrs properly. Patients with both deficiency and dysfunction of C1 esterase inhibitor have depressed levels of C4, because complement is consumed continuously.

IMMUNE COMPLEXES

Aggregates of antigens and antibodies comprise immune complexes. Circulating immune complexes can be detected by a number of assays. Some assays detect only specific types of complexes. For this reason, several different assays are often used simultaneously to screen for increased levels.

The C1q binding assay detects large complexes composed of IgM or IgG1. The monoclonal rheumatoid factor inhibition test utilizes radiolabeled rheumatoid factor (IgM against IgG) attached to latex beads. This assay detects IgG but not IgM complexes and is preferred to the C1q assay for detecting small complexes. The Raji cell test utilizes lymphoblastoid cells that have receptors to C3d, C3b, and Fc but not antibody. Levels are falsely elevated when anti-lymphocyte antibodies are present in serum.

CRYOGLOBULINS

Cryoglobulins are globulins that precipitate when cooled. Because of this, blood samples for cryoglobulin determinations must be kept warm from the time of venipuncture until they have clotted and serum has been separated from coagulated red blood cells. The specimen is then cooled to 4 °C for 72 hours and the amount of precipitate quantitated.

Cryoglobulins can be classified by rewarming separated cryoglobulins so that they dissolve. Type I cryoglobulins are composed of monoclonal IgG, IgM, IgA, or light chains. Type II cryoglobulins are composed of one monoclonal immunoglobulin and one or more polyclonal immunoglobulins of the same or different class. Type III cryoglobulins are made up solely of polyclonal immunoglobulins.

HLA ANTIGENS

HLA antigens may serve as genetic markers for inherited differences in immune response. As the influence of these genes and their function becomes clearer, the value of laboratory assessment may be enhanced.

Serologic cytotoxicity tests can determine the HLA antigen phenotype for class I and class II histocompatibility antigens. For HLA-A, HLA-B, and HLA-C, peripheral blood lymphocytes are incubated with various antisera to each specific HLA antigen type in separate test wells. Complement is added. Cells that react with antisera are lysed.

Serologic tests can also identify HLA-DR, HLA-DQ, and HLA-DP antigens. Before peripheral blood lymphocytes (which are mostly T cells) can be typed, the B cell population must be enriched by the removal of T cells.

Clinical uses of HLA typing are limited except to match donor and recipient for organ transplantation. HLA typing is helpful to adjudicate questions of paternity. As genetic markers, HLA antigens may aid genetic counseling through prenatal typing. In certain instances, HLA typing may increase or decrease the statistical probability that a given patient has a certain disease and thus aid diagnosis.

OTHER IMMUNOLOGIC TESTS

A wide range of other immunologically based tests are available for diagnosis. Many tests for antibodies to infectious agents or body tissues are discussed elsewhere. A few tests warrant special attention.

TESTS FOR ANTIBODIES TO SPECIFIC VIRUSES

Antibodies to specific viruses can be quantitated. People acquire viral infections usually because they do not have antibodies against the infecting virus. During the course of the disease, levels of virus-specific antibodies rise. Consequently, the appearance of antibody to a virus during the course of an illness or a sudden rise in the titer of such antibodies usually implicates that virus as the cause of illness.

TESTS FOR ANTIBODIES TO SPECIFIC BACTERIA

Antibody titers to specific bacteria also rise following bacterial infection. In contrast to viral infection, however, bacterial infection often occurs despite the presence of antibody. A 4-fold rise in antibody titer is often taken as presumptive evidence that specific bacteria are associated with the disease.

AUTOANTIBODY TESTING

A series of tests to detect autoantibodies in serum is also available. Most of these tests are performed by the indirect immunofluorescence technique. Serum from the patient is incubated with normal tissue sections. Following washing, the sections are incubated with fluorescein-labeled antihuman antibody, eg, antihuman IgG. Fluorescence occurs at the site of antibody binding when the tissue is examined under the immunofluorescence microscope. Using indirect immunofluorescence, autoantibodies can be detected against nuclei, nuclear constituents, mitochondria, smooth muscles, striated muscles, parietal cells, pancreatic islet cells, adrenal and parathyroid cortex cells, thyroglobulin, thyroid surface antigen, thyroid-stimulating hormone receptors, glomerular basement membrane, acetylcholine receptors, and other normal body constituents.

FLUORESCENT ANTINUCLEAR ANTIBODY TEST

The fluorescent antinuclear antibody test (FANA) detects autoantibodies to various nuclear constituents.

As performed today on human cell substrates, the FANA test is very sensitive and sometimes detects antibodies in normal young persons (2%) as well as elderly individuals and those with rheumatologic or nonrheumatologic disease.

If the FANA is positive, the specificity of the antibody should be determined if possible. Morphology of the ANA pattern is sometimes helpful, but one pattern may mask another, and there are many variations of speckled patterns.

Crithidia lucilliae are flagellates with a giant mitochondrion containing DNA with no histone. Only serum from patients with antibodies to native deoxyribonucleic acid (DNA) will cause the flagellate to fluoresce after processing by indirect immunofluorescence.

THE RAST TEST

The RAST (radioallergosorbent) test can measure the quantities of IgE antibodies against specific antigen. In this test, antigen is attached to a filter paper disk. Patient serum is incubated with the disk. Next, ^{125}I-labeled antihuman IgE is added to the suspension. The amount of radioactivity on the disk is proportionate to the number of IgE molecules present in the patient's sera. The ELISA assay is a modification of the RAST test that can be used to detect antibodies to specific antigens without radioimmunoassay.

DIRECT IMMUNOFLUORESCENCE

Direct immunofluorescence is a pathologic stain for antibody in tissue (see Chapter 9). Using this technique, tissue is incubated with fluorescein-labeled antihuman immunoglobulin, eg, IgG, IgM, IgA, or other immunoreactants such as C3, C4, C1q, or properdin. The presence of fluorescence marks the site of deposition of immunoglobulin or immunoreactant when frozen tissue sections are examined under the fluorescence microscope.

REFERENCES

Ahmed AR, Blose DA: Delayed-type hypersensitivity skin testing: A review. Arch Dermatol 1983;119:934.

Brody N: Laboratory tests to evaluate the immune system. Int J Dermatol 1981;20:301.

Dahl MV: Clinical Immunodermatology, 2nd ed. Year Book, 1988.

Roitt IM, Brostroff J, Male D: *Immunology.* Mosby, 1985.

Rose NR et al: *Manual of Clinical Laboratory Immunology,* 3rd ed. American Society for Microbiology, 1986.

Stites DP, Stobo JD, Wells JV (editors): *Basic & Clinical Immunology,* 6th ed. Appleton & Lange, 1987.

Stone J: *Dermatologic Immunology and Allergy.* Mosby, 1985.

Vyas GN, Stites DP, Brecher G: *Laboratory Diagnosis of Immunologic Disorders.* Grune & Stratton, 1975.

11 Psychogenic & Neurogenic Skin Disorders

Alan Lyell, MD

Although various internal changes (eg, increased peristalsis, vasodilatation) reflect the body's response to physical and mental forces, it is the skin that *visibly* responds to psychic influences, whether it takes the form of a blush or lichenified patches.

Skin diseases cannot be considered in isolation apart from psychologic factors: the mere existence of a skin lesion is an affront to the ego. The desire to look "normal" preoccupies not only those with diseased skin but also people with healthy skin who, for whatever reason, believe their skin to be abnormal. Almost all skin diseases are multifactorial in origin and cannot be ascribed to either purely physical or purely psychogenic causes. The psychogenic element varies in importance with the disease, the patient, and the situation; it is paramount in lichen simplex chronicus, neurotic excoriations, delusions of parasitosis, and dermatitis artefacta (factitial dermatitis). It may be slight and undetectable one time and may play a major role another time in diseases such as psoriasis, atopic dermatitis, urticaria, alopecia areata, lichen planus, rosacea, and acne vulgaris. Severe psoriasis may erupt during emotional stress or may develop regardless of any psychogenic influence.

Approach to the Patient

The physician's approach to the patient with skin disease is crucial in determining what sort of information will be obtained about the roots of the disorder. The notion that the physician has only to look at the skin to "know what is wrong" and therefore "what to do" is inaccurate. Assessment of the psychogenic element in skin disease must include conversing with the patient about work and other aspects of life in general. Such conversation is in itself a form of treatment. Although a disease may manifest itself in particular ways that serve to readily identify it, the factors causing the disease may not be so typical; eg, an inexperienced physician may recognize that the patient has psoriasis, but the experienced clinician discovers that one attack was precipitated by a urinary tract infection, the second by fear of losing a job, and the third by the death of a loved one.

What is appropriate for one patient may not be

suitable for another; cajoling may work with one person and explanation and reassurance with another. Some patients respond to neither, in which case psychiatric assessment may be indicated. Medication to allay anxiety or counteract depression may be useful but in general is prescribed too readily, so that the patient's problems may actually be compounded by drug-related factors.

Many of the diseases discussed in this chapter are not *caused* by psychiatric disease. Like many of the disorders discussed in other chapters, they may have a psychologic overlay that complicates or worsens the disease and interferes with successful treatment.

PRURITUS
(Itching)

Pruritus stems from a mixture of both physical and psychologic factors. It is a feature of many skin diseases and can be localized or generalized. Generalized pruritus without an obvious cause demands a searching physical examination, with special reference to sideropenia, polycythemia, liver or kidney disease, and lymphoma or occult neoplasm. Depression or psychologic factors such as repressed anger, hatred, disgust, sorrow, and frustrated ambition should not be accepted as a cause unless internal disease has been excluded.

A phlegmatic person, vaguely aware of an itch, scratches it and forgets; a more compulsive person, acutely aware of the discomfort, may pursue the itch by vigorous scratching and thus open the door to lichen simplex chronicus. The itch threshold varies in response to emotional and physical influences, being lowered by anxiety, frustration, lack of sleep, change of ambient temperature, and low humidity. Scratching, the natural response to itching, gives relief; but the itch returns, and there is further scratching. Scratching gives pleasure and is habit-forming, but engenders guilt. A scratch-itch cycle develops, and the guilt is reinforced by admonitions not to scratch.

Management is difficult unless a treatable cause can be identified. Antipruritic medicaments give limited relief but can cause diagnostic confusion. Soothing local applications are helpful (1% phenol in calamine lotion), but some are sensitizers (eg, the -caine group of local anesthetics) and should be avoided. The environment should be kept at a constant moderate temperature and the air kept humid. If the skin is dehydrated, especially in the elderly, aqueous cream should be applied routinely. Starch baths are useful.

LICHEN SIMPLEX CHRONICUS (Localized Neurodermatitis)

Essentials of Diagnosis

- Lichenified, poorly marginated, scaling, often slightly purple pruritic plaques.
- Site always reachable by the patient's fingers.
- Intense chronic rubbing or scratching of patches.
- Obsessive personality.

General Considerations

Lichen simplex chronicus is a common disorder that usually occurs in patients with obsessive personalities who focus most of their attention on the pruritic patches. Many are atopic and prone to spontaneous itching; in other patients, the disorder starts with some trivial event—eg, a cut, scratch, burn, pimple, or contact dermatitis—that fails to heal normally because it itches and is therefore rubbed repeatedly. Nervous tension increases the itching, as do heat and cold. Rubbing, which becomes automatic, relieves the itch temporarily but perpetuates the skin changes. Patients often deny rubbing the lesions, and an admission is best elicited by asking, "How do you rub your skin?" This usually prompts a demonstration. Fingernails used for rubbing will be polished, beveled, or worn down, or else they may be kept short deliberately to minimize skin trauma. Sticks or brushes may be used, and some patients seem to take a masochistic delight in hurting themselves.

Clinical Findings

A localized patch or patches of thickened and often pink or purple, hyperpigmented, scaling skin merge with surrounding normal skin. Lichenification (exaggeration of normal skin markings enclosing shiny, smooth facets of skin) is seen best in early lesions or in the margins of older, established lesions. Scratch marks are usually minimal, because the patient learns to avoid them by rubbing rather than scratching the skin. Lesions may be single or multiple and scattered, but they are always within reach of the fingers: no area of skin that the patient can reach is immune. Common sites are the nape of the neck, extensor surfaces of the elbows, flexor surfaces of the wrists, the ankles, the anogenital region, the external auditory meatus, and the palms and soles (where the correct diagnosis is often overlooked).

Differential Diagnosis

Lichen simplex chronicus must be distinguished from lichenified patches of psoriasis or dermatitis (particularly atopic dermatitis), lichen planus, or lichenoid drug eruption. Lichen simplex of the anogenital region and of the palms and soles must be distinguished from psoriasis and fungal infections; skin scrapings should be taken for microscopic examination and culture. Contact dermatitis may aggravate or initiate patches of lichen simplex, so that patch testing is sometimes indicated. Generalized lichenification occurs in severe atopic dermatitis and mycosis fungoides.

Treatment

A. General Measures: Antihistamines and tranquilizers are of questionable value. Vigorous exercise helps by using up excess physical energy that might otherwise be directed toward rubbing. Eliminating a cause of nervous stress may produce dramatic results.

Infection may be caused by autoinoculation of pyogenic organisms through rubbing and lead to cellulitis or abscesses; recurrent boils in the same area are likely to have such an origin and should be treated with systemic antibiotics.

B. Local Measures: Tar preparations such as 3% crude coal tar in petrolatum are messy but helpful; corticosteroid preparations are more acceptable cosmetically. They are helpful in proportion to their strength and, by extension, in proportion to their potential to cause skin atrophy. A reasonably potent one can be used to interrupt the itch-scratch-itch cycle and then a less potent one to sustain a remission. Topical antihistamines and -caine type (PABA-derived) local anesthetic preparations are contraindicated because of the risk of allergic reactions. Creams containing the topical anesthetic pramoxine are fairly free of this risk. Zinc oxide and castor oil creams and similar bland preparations may be useful. Occlusion of the itchy area so that the patient cannot reach it is often successful, but new areas of lichen simplex may appear, and panic may occur if the patient finds that proper scratching is no longer possible.

Prognosis

Lichen simplex tends to persist indefinitely, since if one area heals, new lesions tend to develop elsewhere. Areas that do heal regain normal appearance.

PRURITUS ANI, PRURITUS VULVAE, & OTITIS EXTERNA

Itching of the anus, vulva, and external ear canal includes an element of lichen simplex chronicus that may predominate, but other factors—eg, psoriasis, dermatitis, lichen sclerosus et atrophicus, leukoplakia, infections (due to dermatophytes, yeasts, bacteria, protozoa, or threadworms), infestations, diabetes mellitus, and allergy to medications or contraceptives—must always be considered.

The initial trigger in pruritus ani is often irritation of the skin by fecal contamination. The psychologic overtones of anogenital pruritus are significant, including the peculiar self-gratification resembling masturbation that may be derived from scratching this area and the protection from unwelcome sexual attention that pruritus vulvae affords. Psychosexual problems are common in patients suffering from anogenital pruritus, whereas patients with otitis externa are more likely to be experiencing mental stress at work. Treatment should address any component of lichen simplex, as well as any physical factors disclosed by investigation (diabetes mellitus, infections, etc). Pinworms should be ruled out. The skin of the anogenital area is particularly vulnerable to atrophy following the use of corticosteroid medications.

ACNE VARIOLIFORMIS

Acne varioliformis occurs in patients who have an itchy scalp with or without seborrheic dermatitis and who also carry a pathogenic strain of *Staphylococcus aureus*. Patients develop papulopustular lesions, especially along the hairline. The itching usually has a strong psychogenic element, and patients often demonstrate intense ambition. Treatment should include scalp care similar to that designed to prevent seborrheic dermatitis. Medications that eliminate staphylococci (eg, dicloxacillin, 250 mg 4 times daily for 10 days) may help. Application of bacitracin, neomycin, or mupirocin ointment to the nares after such treatment may prevent nasal carriage and lessen the chance of folliculitis. An antibiotic shampoo (eg, chloroxin [Capitrol]) and topical antibiotics (eg, clindamycin) to the scalp may also help.

NEUROTIC EXCORIATIONS

Essentials of Diagnosis
- Repeated picking at the skin.
- Distribution of lesions limited to accessible areas.
- Angular configurations to ulcers.
- Chronic course, with lesions present in all stages of development.
- Ulcers often arranged in lines or parallel lines.
- No primary lesions.

General Considerations
The skin does not necessarily itch in patients with neurotic excoriations. The patient picks at the skin in response to a feeling of restlessness that parallels the urge felt by chain smokers to light cigarettes one after another. The cause of tension is sometimes related to a specific situation, eg, a fear of cancer or family

problems. Picking at the skin enables such anxious patients to maintain their emotional balance.

Clinical Findings
Patients pick and gouge ulcers in the skin; when these heal, they leave whitish, round, papery scars that are clearly visible against a background of hyperpigmentation (Fig 11–1). Active, healing, and healed lesions can be seen simultaneously. Ulcers vary from 0.3 to 3 cm in size but are usually angular and small. Lesions may be found wherever the patient's fingers can reach but are usually maximal on the extensor aspects of the forearms and over the shoulders, where the ulcers are often rather linear and parallel. Although the lesions appear to be symmetrically distributed, close observation, especially in the shoulder blade region, discloses slight asymmetry because of the greater effectiveness of the dominant hand in scratching. With the patient standing with arms at the sides, palms directed dorsally, it can usually be demonstrated that there are more lesions on the front of the body than on the back. Such a pattern of distribution does not occur in most spontaneous eruptions. The affected areas along the upper shoulder region may have a distinct edge that is due to the limited reach of the contralateral hand over that shoulder, but this clear demarcation may be missing in supple individuals who can reach up from below.

Differential Diagnosis
Patients with delusions of parasitosis may have identical lesions; their rationale for picking at their skin is that they are trying to extract parasites. Neurotic patients seldom admit spontaneously to picking the skin but will agree reluctantly that they do so, though they believe they are treating some skin dis-

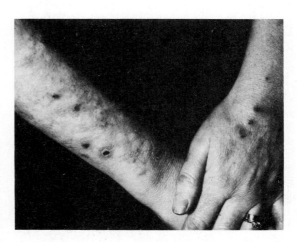

Figure 11–1. Neurotic excoriations. Scabbed active lesions, pale scars. (Reproduced, with permission, from Lyell A: Cutaneous artifactual disease. J Am Acad Dermatol 1979;1:391.)

ease by their actions. Patients with dermatitis artefacta deny interfering with the skin.

All other causes of pruritus must also be considered, including dermatitis herpetiformis, scabies, primary biliary cirrhosis, occult carcinoma, and lymphomas (Fig 11–2). Necrotic ulcers occur in pityriasis lichenoides et varioliformis acuta as part of a polymorphous eruption, but in this disorder primary lesions (papules, vesicles, or pustules) are present. Porphyria cutanea tarda and epidermolysis bullosa acquisita might rarely cause diagnostic confusion also.

Treatment

As a rule, patients with neurotic excoriations cannot stop picking. Attempts to occlude skin to prevent picking are not welcomed and, if the physician persists, may lead to panic reactions or depression. Efforts should be made to identify and eliminate specific causes of stress, but psychiatric consultation is usually nonproductive. Patients should be seen regularly by the physician and should be encouraged to minimize skin damage by paying attention to hygiene and by keeping the fingernails well trimmed.

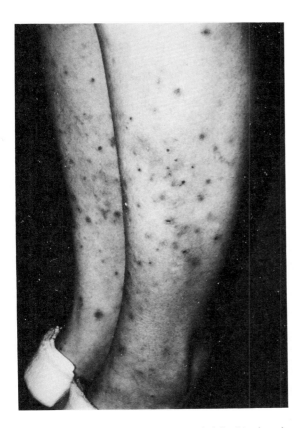

Figure 11–2. Neurotic excoriations mimicked by lymphadenoma.

ACNE EXCORIÉE & CUTANEOUS HYPOCHONDRIA

Some patients—most often women—constantly squeeze or pick at facial lesions, creating a rash that comes to resemble acne vulgaris. These patients are convinced that their activities will "cure" the lesions and do not realize the lesions are a direct result of their manipulations. The initial spot that attracts attention may be an acne lesion, a trivial pimple, or other slight blemish. Patients may not believe that they are responsible for making the initial lesion worse. If possible, the physician should attempt to have them discard their magnifying mirrors and divert their energies to applying harmless lotions rather than squeezing the pimples and overwashing the skin.

Acne excoriée is one of a group of disorders in which the patient has an exaggerated or perverted sense of what is abnormal. People vary in their ability to accept facial blemishes, but most accept a few pimples from time to time as normal. Adolescents are naturally sensitive about their appearance and tend to magnify their blemishes, whether perceived or real, but maturity usually brings a more relaxed attitude. Patients with cutaneous hypochondria complain inappropriately and importunately about their pimples, the greasiness of their skin, the distribution and quantity of their hair, the shape of their noses, and so forth. Commercial advertising aggravates or compounds the problem by focusing people's attention on the skin and by encouraging excessive washing and other forms of interference. Patients often seek plastic surgery but are almost always dissatisfied with the results. They may even commit suicide.

PRURIGO NODULARIS

Prurigo nodularis shares many characteristics with lichen simplex, but the lesions are bigger, the disorder is much rarer, and the itching is intense and distressing rather than pleasurable. The relationship of prurigo nodularis to emotional stress is much less clear-cut than that in lichen simplex, and the disease may represent some abnormality of cutaneous sensory innervation. The lesions are sparse, discrete nodules found mostly on the extensor surfaces of the limbs. They are usually flesh-colored, have a blunt, warty surface, and are surrounded by hyperpigmented skin. Sometimes the top of each nodule is surmounted by a small hemorrhagic crust. The disorder most commonly affects middle-aged women.

Hypertrophic lichen planus should be considered in the differential diagnosis. Prurigo nodularis resembles delusions of parasitosis in that "worms" may be extracted from the nodules; the worms are actually bits of dermal tissue or keratinous debris.

There is no uniformly successful method of treatment. Potent topical or intralesional steroids are commonly given. Some patients respond (albeit usually poorly and slowly) to a modified Goeckerman regimen consisting of tar ointments and daily exposure to ultraviolet radiation in the B spectrum (UVB). Cryotherapy may be successful.

DERMATITIS ARTEFACTA
(Factitial Dermatitis)

Essentials of Diagnosis

- Bizarre lesions.
- "Hollow" history.
- Emotional immaturity (hysterical personality).
- Patients frequently have paramedical background or employment.
- Stressful life situation.

General Considerations

Dermatitis artefacta, which occurs more commonly in women than in men, is the cutaneous manifestation of a general syndrome in which patients (who are often intelligent) are unable to deal maturely with emotional stress and react by engaging in self-mutilating activities. These patients act under an inner compulsion and may or may not be conscious of what they are doing.

The normal doctor-patient relationship is in abeyance, since the physician is regarded as an adversary. These patients "need" their illness and do not want to get better. They are often difficult, manipulative, evasive, untruthful, ungrateful, and, if cornered, vindictive.

The history lacks sincerity (so-called "hollow" history) because patients conceal or are unaware of the true nature of the lesions. They maintain that the lesions were fully developed when they first appeared. In the natural course of events, lesions start to heal, so that if illness is to continue, successive crops of new lesions must appear. The means for creating new lesions and the opportunity to do so must therefore remain available. Various methods are used, including applications of caustics such as phenol and silver nitrate, injection of foreign materials such as milk, burns from cigarettes and matches, application of ligatures, beating and hammering of the skin until it bruises, etc. The opportunity to produce lesions requires privacy, and if this is denied, other psychologic manifestations, eg, petit mal-like attacks, may replace the skin lesions.

The so-called hysterical personality that underlies this syndrome may have manifested itself in other ways, eg, transient paralyses, sensory loss of non-anatomic type (eg, glove-stocking distribution), deafness, aphonia, blindness, and unexplained abdominal pain. Fruitless investigation of hematuria, hemoptysis, hematemesis, or unexplained pyrexia may have been performed. Such studies tend to give negative or equivocal results, and the differential diagnosis may include rare and obscure diseases.

Clinical Findings

Signs may include erythema, blisters, ulcers, sinus tracts, abscesses, edema (from application of ligatures), superficial gangrene, and purpura. Lesions heal normally unless subjected to further manipulation by the patient. They are usually well-demarcated and occur in areas that can be reached by the patient's hands. The lesions look artifactual to the trained eye, because they are unlike those of recognized skin diseases and are scattered arbitrarily. They may assume bizarre rectilinear configurations. The patient may traumatize surgical scars and delay their healing. Effective occlusion of active lesions permits healing, but new lesions may appear on unoccluded skin.

Patients with Munchausen's syndrome (multiple hospitalizations, multiple surgical scars, dramatic illness) display the scars of previous operations or invent dramatic histories to explain scars that in reality have a commonplace origin. Some patients display an indifference to pain or a masochistic delight in suffering.

Differential Diagnosis

Patients who are malingering have a conscious motive for maintaining their illness and seek secondary gains such as narcotics, money, or avoidance of duty. Malingering occurs especially among members of the armed forces, prisoners, and those seeking monetary compensation for injuries. In neurotic excoriations, patients admit to traumatizing the skin. In acne excoriée, the patient seeks to "cure" the lesions by squeezing them. Patients with delusions of parasitosis dig openly in the skin for "parasites." Institutionalized patients develop behavioral disorders that may involve injury to the skin. Some psychotic patients find release for their nervous tension by cutting, scraping, burning, or otherwise damaging the skin.

In Munchausen's syndrome, which is commoner in men than in women, the artifactual element is the history; ie, the patient gives a usually dramatic history consistent with a known diagnosis. The unsuspecting physician may prescribe narcotics or conduct extensive investigations or surgery. Previous hospital admissions are likely to be concealed.

Treatment

Treatment must be individualized. The physician should refrain from directly confronting the patient with the artifactual nature of the lesions, because it is too difficult to do so without seeming accusatory. A discreet examiner should be able to convey indirectly without saying so outright that it is obvious the lesions are artifactual. Regularly scheduled appointments with an understanding physician may be of some help; medication, such as with tranquilizers, has little effect. A sympathetic psychiatrist is no better than a sympathetic dermatologist in caring for these patients.

Prognosis

The outlook varies with the patient's capacity to deal with emotion and the degree of stress to which he or she has been subjected. The prognosis is favorable in mature patients who have suffered a brief but traumatic experience; it is bad in immature individuals, who may adopt the production of artifactual lesions as a way of life.

DELUSIONS OF PARASITOSIS

Essentials of Diagnosis

- Crawling sensations in the skin.
- Conviction that cutaneous sensation is caused by parasites.
- Failure to find parasites on physical examination.

General Considerations

Any of the following may play a part in delusions of parasitosis: psychoses (schizophrenia, bipolar disorder), psychoneuroses, aging, arteriosclerosis, drug addiction (including alcoholism), certain toxic states (including some acute infections), anemia, vitamin B_{12} deficiency, pellagra and other nutritional deficiency states, diabetes mellitus, and diseases of the nervous system (eg, cerebrovascular disease and peripheral neuritis). Causative factors are usually more obvious in patients under age 50, in whom the sex incidence is equal, but two-thirds of patients are over age 50 and an overwhelming majority of these (3:1) are women. Some patients demonstrate monosymptomatic hypochondriac psychosis; ie, their mental abnormality is limited to their supposed infestation, which occurs against the background of a "normal" personality. The delusions are contagious in that other people who are close to the patient may come to believe in the existence of the "parasites" and may believe that they themselves are infested, a phenomenon known as "shared delusions." Patients are often intelligent, and medical personnel are often afflicted.

Patients may go to great lengths to purify themselves by washing frequently and applying antiseptics or parasiticides. They avoid contact with other people in order to prevent spreading the "contagion." They paint or renovate their houses to rid them of the "parasites"; or they change houses frequently to escape them. They destroy "infested" bedclothing and furniture, and they call on public health authorities and pest control firms for help.

Clinical Findings

Many patients have no visible skin abnormality, though they may insist that they do. Some penetrate the skin with their fingernails or needles to dig out "parasites." Lesions vary from insignificant scratch marks to severe excoriations (Fig 11–3). Specimens of the "parasites" are produced; these usually consist of bits of skin, hair, crusts, keratinous fragments, and assorted debris, but any available substance, including insects, may be used. Specimens should always be carefully examined with the naked eye and with the microscope. Patients reject any suggestion that there are no real parasites with disbelief, scorn, and bitterness, and advice that the patient should consult a psychiatrist is met with amazed refusal.

Differential Diagnosis

Genuine infestations must be excluded. Patients with neurotic excoriations do not believe they are infested with "parasites." Prurigo nodularis is similar to delusions of parasitosis in that patients pull "worms" of fibrillar tissue from the lesions. All other causes of pruritus must be considered in the differential diagnosis.

Complications

Complications are social rather than physical, since patients cut themselves off from other human contact because of their "infestation"; they also show paranoid traits that are often directed at members of the medical profession. Incessant attempts to cleanse the skin may cause irritant contact dermatitis. Suicide is possible.

Treatment

Opinions vary about whether the patient should be confronted with the delusion, with those in favor citing dramatic successes with this approach. Confrontation can be disastrous, however, since the patient is absolutely sure he or she is infested. Regardless of the approach used, the physician must never concur— though it is helpful to express concern and sympathy.

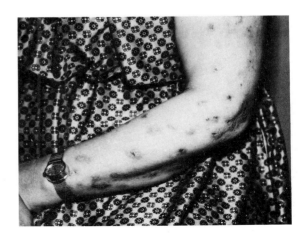

Figure 11–3. Delusion of parasitosis. The patient digs in the skin searching for imaginary parasites.

Antiparasitic lotions should not be prescribed. Depression should be treated.

Pimozide, 2–10 mg daily has helped many patients. Side effects include irreversible tardive dyskinesia, neuroleptic malignant syndrome, EKG abnormalities, drowsiness, and even death. Consultation with physicians familiar with the use of this drug is recommended.

Psychiatric consultation is required when paranoid or other psychotic traits become severe. Patients resist referral to psychiatrists.

Prognosis

The prognosis for patients with delusions of parasitosis was once thought to be universally hopeless, but a few have recovered. Chronic maintenance therapy with pimozide lets many patients live more normal lives.

NERVOUS HABITS & BEHAVIORAL DISORDERS

Children and anxious or tense adults may have certain nervous habits, including biting the nails, making hangnails or pulling at existing ones, picking at cuticles, picking the nose, pulling or biting the lips, and breaking off and rubbing the hair. Maturity may cure some habits, but others may start at this time, eg, abuse of tobacco, alcohol, or narcotics.

Confinement in an institution creates psychologic stresses stemming from loss of liberty. Pent-up nervous energy finds an outlet in repetitive movements or actions or in self-mutilating activities, eg, chewing, beating, or rubbing the skin.

TRICHOTILLOMANIA, ONYCHOTILLOMANIA, & TRAUMATIC NAIL DYSTROPHY

Manipulation of the hair or nails may be part of a behavioral disorder or nervous habit, may be due to habitual scratching, or may be a manifestation of delusions of parasitosis. In patients with trichotillomania, the bald patches are covered with healthy stubble (Fig 11–4), in contrast to the diseased, broken hairs seen in ringworm or the "exclamation point" hairs in alopecia areata. Some children eat their hair and are in danger of developing a hair ball in the stomach. Regrowth of hair is excellent once the patient stops twisting the hair.

Onychotillomania is usually a manifestation of delusions of parasitosis, in which the patient pares down the nails in a search for "parasites." Traumatic nail dystrophy (Chapter 29) is manifested as a column of short, transverse nail ridges running the length of the nail and is a nervous habit involving constant picking at a localized patch of cuticle.

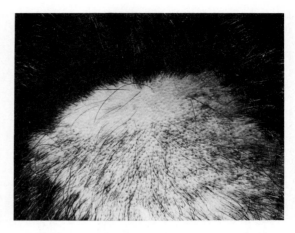

Figure 11–4. Trichotillomania. Stubble of broken but healthy hairs, best appreciated by running the finger against the grain of the hair.

NEUROGENIC SKIN DISEASE

TROPHIC LESIONS

The blue, cold, edematous, and often ulcerated flail leg of the patient who has recovered from poliomyelitis is now rarely seen. Perforating ulcers of the soles are now more often due to the peripheral neuropathy of diabetes mellitus than to syphilis. Indolent ulcers can develop in any area of anesthetic skin owing to nerve injury or diseases such as arteriosclerosis, diabetes, syringomyelia, leprosy, or syphilis. Diabetic patients should pay careful attention to their feet in order to prevent trophic ulcers. Anesthetic skin is more likely to be burned or otherwise traumatized in everyday activity, since the patient cannot feel that injury is occurring. Anesthetic skin is also subject to the risk of pressure sores, which are especially troublesome in spinal cord injuries. Sometimes strange sensations are felt in the skin, and patients may further damage the skin through self-mutilating acts performed in response to these sensations, as may occur on the face following trigeminal nerve damage. Denervated skin is dry (anhidrosis), and wound healing is poor.

Trophic ulceration occurs in patients with leprosy or congenital indifference to pain. The ulcers of radiodermatitis may mimic trophic ulceration.

Treatment consists of protecting the skin, especially from undue prolonged pressure, but healing is slow. All possible causes of delayed healing should be considered, including anemia, sideropenia, dietary and vitamin deficiencies, syphilis, tuberculosis, collagen disease, foreign body, or disease of underlying bone. Oral zinc sulfate has helped.

DISEASES SHARED BY THE SKIN & NERVOUS SYSTEM

Most neurocutaneous diseases are rare. Of practical importance are neurofibromatosis, tuberous sclerosis (epiloia), and hemangioma. All are discussed elsewhere.

CENTRAL NERVOUS SYSTEM DISEASE REFLECTED IN THE SKIN

Itching or paresthesias occasionally occur in multiple sclerosis. Blisters may appear in response to any type of intracerebral lesion, especially cerebrovascular accident, when pressure on the skin probably plays a large part, as it does in the blisters accompanying coma due to drug overdose, carbon monoxide poisoning, etc. "Seborrhea" of the cheeks occurs in postencephalitic parkinsonism. Acneiform lesions may be precipitated by trauma to the base of the skull, tumors in that region, or multiple sclerosis. Alopecia may be produced by brain stem lesions, and itching of the nostrils may be a symptom of cerebral tumor.

1. HORNER'S SYNDROME

Interruption of the sympathetic nerve supply to the face results in ipsilateral lack of sweating and vasodilatation, ptosis, a small pupil, and narrowed palpebral fissure on the affected side (Horner's syndrome).

2. CAUSALGIA

Causalgia is characterized by a severe burning pain in an area of skin supplied by a peripheral nerve that has been damaged by direct trauma or involvement in scar tissue. The pain tends to worsen during emotional stress and may become an all-consuming problem as the patient attempts to avoid the slightest stimulus that would elicit pain. Associated decalcification of underlying bone (Sudeck's atrophy) occurs occasionally. Causalgia may be due to interruption of sympathetic nerve fibers in the peripheral nerve. Other features include trophic ulcers, hyperhidrosis, edema, and atrophy of the skin. The eventual outcome is likely to be good, but full recovery may take many months. A 1-month trial of capsaicin cream 0.025%, applied 3 times daily, may be worthwhile, since capsaicin depletes substance P from nerves and alleviates the similar pain of postherpetic neuralgia.

3. SACRAL HAIR PATCH

A patch of long hair in the sacral region (fawn tail) often but not always overlies a bifid spinal cord. Since growth changes in the spinal column, especially at puberty, may result in traction damage to nerve tissue, children with a sacral hair patch should be thoroughly examined at an early age.

REFERENCES

Ayres S Jr: The fine art of scratching. JAMA 1964; 189:1003.

Butterworth T, Strean LP: Behavior disorders of interest to dermatologists. Arch Dermatol 1963;88:859.

Cotterill JA: Dermatological nondisease: A common and potentially fatal disturbance of cutaneous body image. Br J Dermatol 1981;104:611.

Crisp AH: Dysmorphophobia and the search for cosmetic surgery. Br Med J 1981;282:1099.

Fabisch W: Psychiatric aspects of dermatitis artifacta. Br J Dermatol 1980;102:29.

Gould WM, Gragg TM: Delusions of parasitosis: An approach to the problem. Arch Dermatol 1976;112:1745.

Koblenzer CS: Psychosomatic concepts in dermatology: A dermatologist-psychoanalyst viewpoint. Arch Dermatol 1983;119:501.

Lyell A: Cutaneous artifactual disease: A review, amplified by personal experience. J Am Acad Dermatol 1979; 1:391.

Lyell A: Delusions of parasitosis. Br J Dermatol 1983; 108:485.

Lyell A: The itching patient: A review of the causes of pruritus. Scott Med J 1972;17:334.

Pallis CA, Bamji AN: McIlroy was here: Or was he? Br Med J 1979;1:973.

Savin JA: Do systemic antipruritic agents work? Br J Dermatol 1980;103:113.

Sneddon I, Sneddon J: Self-inflicted injury: A follow-up study of 43 patients. Br Med J 1975;3:527.

Waisman M: Pickers, pluckers and impostors: A panorama of cutaneous self-mutilation. Postgrad Med (Dec) 1965; 38:620.

Section III:
Infections & Infestations

Bacterial Infections

12

Raza Aly, PhD, Howard I. Maibach, MD, Alan Lyell, MD, & Yehudi M. Felman, MD*

Skin infections due to bacteria may be conveniently divided for clinical purposes into primary and secondary types. **Primary infections** have characteristic morphologic features and courses of disease, start with infection by a single type of organism, and usually arise in normal skin. They are most frequently associated with coagulase-positive staphylococci or β-hemolytic streptococci. **Secondary infections** originate in areas of already damaged skin, and the bacteria present multiply and invade surrounding areas to aggravate and prolong the underlying skin disorder. Such secondary infections may occur when skin has been traumatized, infected with fungi, or altered by a noninfectious skin disease (eg, eczema). In such cases, infections tend to recur until the underlying disorders can be corrected.

PRIMARY BACTERIAL INFECTIONS

IMPETIGO

Impetigo is a contagious superficial infection of the skin initiated by *Staphylococcus aureus* or group A β-hemolytic streptococci. Two diverse forms are recognized on the basis of bacteriologic, clinical, and histologic findings: (1) In **superficial or common impetigo,** the lesions are characterized by a thick, adherent, and recurrent dirty yellow crusts with an erythematous margin (Fig 12–1). Superficial impe-

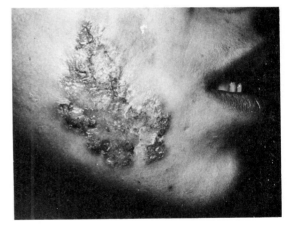

Figure 12–1. Impetigo. Note the superficial erosion of the skin and the crusts that are typically honey-yellow.

tigo is the most common skin infection of children. (2) **Bullous impetigo** is characterized by a superficial thin-walled bullous lesion that ruptures and develops a thin, transparent, varnishlike crust (Fig 12–2).

1. SUPERFICIAL OR COMMON ("STREPTOCOCCAL") IMPETIGO

Essentials of Diagnosis
- Itching of the face or other exposed areas.
- Thick honey-colored crusts covering superficial erosions surrounded by papular satellite lesions.

General Considerations
Common impetigo is more prevalent during hot, humid weather, which promotes the infection by pro-

*The sections on staphylococcal scalded skin syndrome and nonvenereal treponematoses were written by Dr Lyell and Dr Felman, respectively.

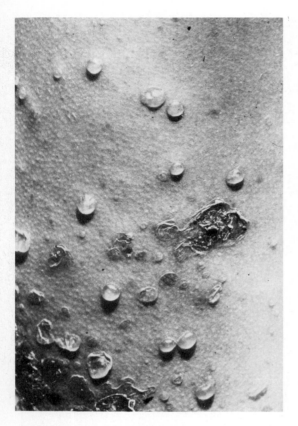

Figure 12–2. Bullous impetigo: Note the flaccid, fragile bullae on a noninflamed base.

viding greater opportunities for insect bites and other skin trauma on exposed extremities and by favoring bacterial growth on moist skin. Lack of personal hygiene and crowding are also predisposing factors.

Group A β-hemolytic streptococci and *S aureus* are found together or alone in common impetigo. Which organism is the primary pathogen remains controversial. One view is that common impetigo is streptococcal in origin with staphylococci as secondary invaders.

Early lesions are more likely to yield pure cultures of streptococci; later lesions are apt to yield mixed cultures. As the lesion ages, more staphylococci are present. The other view is that common impetigo is initiated by either *S aureus* or streptococci and that the *Staphylococcus,* being a more hardy organism, is encountered most frequently.

Clinical Findings

A. Symptoms and Signs: Most lesions are found on exposed areas, particularly the face, scalp, and extremities. The typical lesion begins as an erythematous papule in a traumatized area, such as an abrasion

or insect bite. Small transient vesicles may develop, but the lesion rapidly evolves to its crusted form. The crust is adherent; upon removal, a cloudy amber serous fluid exudes from the moist erythematous base. Punctate crusted satellite lesions may surround the central lesion. Lesions may be discrete and limited initially, but with time they become multifocal and coalescent. Scalp impetigo may become more extensive by the time the patient seeks medical help.

B. Laboratory Findings: The typical appearance of the thick, dirty-looking, honey-colored crust is almost pathognomonic of impetigo such that cultures generally are not needed before treatment is started. When the pus is aspirated from an intact pustule or vesicle, demonstration of organisms by Gram stain suggests a pathogenic relationship. Cultures and antibiotic sensitivity testing may be useful in evaluating patients who respond poorly to therapy.

Differential Diagnosis

Many skin diseases that weep may suggest impetigo. These include insect bites, eczematous dermatitis, and bullous diseases. *S aureus* is frequently isolated as a secondary invader. The history, distribution, and morphologic features of primary lesions provide the best help for diagnosis of these other conditions. Lesions of herpes simplex are localized to one anatomic site. Varicella has widely distributed lesions with uniform 2- to 3-mm vesicles.

Prevention

Cleanliness and prompt attention to skin trauma can help prevent impetigo. Patients with impetigo and their families should be taught to bathe regularly with soaps containing antibacterial agents and to apply topical antibiotics to insect bites, cuts, abrasions, and infected lesions as soon as they are noted. Impetigo in infants is highly contagious and serious and requires prompt treatment.

Treatment

Treatment for impetigo should be carried out with antistaphylococcal drugs because of co-existing *S aureus* infections in many circumstances. Oral dicloxacillin, cephalosporin, or erythromycin for 10 days have been demonstrated to be superior to local therapy. Dicloxacillin 500 mg orally every 6 hours for 10 days in adults is recommended. In children, 50 mg/kg/d, not to exceed 2 g per day, should be given in divided dosages every 6 hours. When the patient cannot tolerate dicloxacillin because of penicillin allergy, erythromycin 250 mg orally every 6 hours, can be substituted. Mupirocin (Bactroban) ointment, a new antibiotic, is recommended for the topical treatment of impetigo and pyodermas.

Prognosis

Superficial impetigo generally has a good prognosis. Poststreptococcal glomerulonephritis may occasionally follow impetigo. Certain nephritogenic streptococci (types 49, 2, 55, 56, and 31) have been prevalent in impetigo resulting in nephritis. The anti-DNase B level is significantly elevated in patients with streptococcal impetigo, especially those with nephritis, but the ASO titer is usually normal.

2. BULLOUS IMPETIGO (Staphylococcal Impetigo)

Essentials of Diagnosis
- Thin-walled, generally flaccid bullae ranging from 0.5 to 3 cm in diameter.
- Thin, varnishlike crust develops over ruptured bullae.

General Considerations
The etiologic agent is *Staphylococcus aureus*. The bullae are the result of the local action of epidermolytic toxin (exfoliatin) elaborated by *S aureus*, which causes dyshesion of keratinocytes.

Clinical Findings
The frequency of this disease has been increasing since 1970. The lesions are clinically characteristic. The bullae are thin-walled, usually flaccid, but occasionally tense. They are easily ruptured and contain fluid ranging from a thin, cloudy amber liquid to an opaque white or yellow pus. After rupture of the bullae, the moist erythematous base quickly dries to form a thin, shiny varnishlike veneer, which differs from the "stuck-on" thicker crust of common impetigo. Lesions are most often found in groups in a single region.

Differential Diagnosis
Bullous impetigo should be distinguished from other vesicular and pustular lesions.

Treatment
As in the case of impetigo, bullous impetigo should be treated with oral antistaphylococcal drugs (dicloxacillin, a cephalosporin, or erythromycin) because these are more effective than topical antibiotic therapy. See the section on treatment of impetigo, above. Local therapy is not necessary and may cause skin maceration or sensitization.

Prognosis
Impetigo typically resolves even without treatment. The prognosis is good with immediate therapy. Septic complications are rare.

ECTHYMA

Ecthyma is a deeper form of impetigo. The lesions occur commonly on the legs and other covered areas, often as a consequence of debility and infestation. Group A streptococci initiate the disease or complicate preexisting superficial ulcers.

The initial lesion is a vesicle or vesiculopustule with an erythematous base and surrounding halo, which enlarges and in a few days becomes thickly crusted. The ulcer has a "punched-out" appearance when crusts and purulent materials are removed. The lesions are slow to heal, leaving scars.

Erythromycin or dicloxacillin given orally is effective. (See above for dosage schedule.) Local treatment should consist of soaks and removal of crusts.

STAPHYLOCOCCAL SCALDED SKIN SYNDROME

Alan Lyell, MD

Essentials of Diagnosis
- Tender skin.
- Red, scalded appearance of skin.
- Skin may slough off with light lateral pressure (Nikolsky's sign).
- Intraepidermal separation of skin.
- Source of dermatopathic staphylococci (eg, impetigo, tonsillitis, ocular infection).

General Considerations
Staphylococcal scalded skin syndrome (Fig 12–3) occurs mainly in infants and children and only rarely in adults. In newborns, staphylococcal scalded skin syndrome has also been called Ritter's disease or the malignant form of pemphigus neonatorum; in children, it was formerly termed staphylococcal toxic epidermal necrolysis. Staphylococcal scalded skin syndrome is caused by dermatopathic strains of *Staphylococcus aureus* that elaborate an epidermolytic toxin which cleaves the epidermis longitudinally at the level of the stratum granulosum. These bacterial strains normally cause staphylococcal impetigo and its misnamed neonatal variant pemphigus neonatorum but not "characteristic" staphylococcal diseases, eg, boils, carbuncles, abscesses, osteomyelitis, and septicemia. Such strains often—not always—are members of phage group II (types 3A, 3B, 3C, 55, and 71); they can be identified with certainty by their ability to produce epidermolytic toxin. Experiments show that inoculation with living organisms results in impetigo, whereas injections of the isolated toxin cause localized "scalding." The cause of the red skin is not clear; the redness does not appear to be due to epidermolytic toxin.

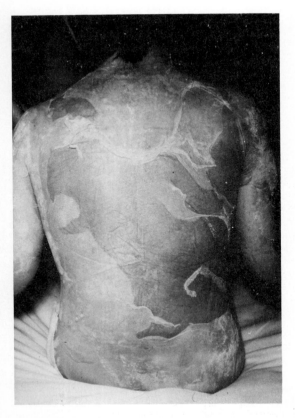

Figure 12–3. Staphylococcal scalded skin syndrome (formerly known as staphylococcal toxic epidermal necrolysis) in a child. (Reproduced, with permission, from Lyell A: Toxic epidermal necrolysis [the scalded skin syndrome]: A reappraisal. Br J Dermatol 1979;100:69.)

Clinical Findings

A. Symptoms and Signs: The skin suddenly becomes red and tender, often exquisitely so. The child usually cries and is apprehensive about being touched (Fig 12–4), so that an unwarranted impression of abuse is sometimes created. The skin begins to loosen, usually within hours, so that the outer layer can be easily pushed about by the finger (positive Nikolsky sign) and separated from the basal layer at the level of the stratum granulosum. The skin lies in wrinkles and resembles the skin on the surface of boiled milk. In places the skin peels away to expose a raw, red, tender, velvety surface. The skin around the mouth and genitalia and on the trunk is most commonly affected, but the process may occur anywhere, including the hands, where the skin may peel off like a glove. Exudation is minimal, and blisters seldom develop.

The source of the epidermolytic toxin is often obvious—eg, impetigo (especially around the nose or mouth), purulent conjunctivitis, or acute tonsillitis—

but occasionally no source is discernible. Other family members may have had impetigo or may be carriers of a dermatopathic strain of *S aureus.*

The child's general health is usually good, and experienced clinicians unfamiliar with staphylococcal scalded skin syndrome may have difficulty believing that staphylococcal toxemia is present.

Resolution is surprisingly rapid (within a week), probably because epidermal loss is only superficial. The skin heals completely, without scarring, pigmentary disturbance, or loss of hair.

In some patients, the initial redness does not lead to peeling in large sheets but is succeeded by a scaly desquamation.

B. Laboratory Findings: The skin splits intraepidermally, as shown by microscopic examination of frozen sections of recently peeled skin. Cytologic smears of cells on the surface of denuded areas show cells of the stratum granulosum (Tzanck smear). Cultures of the red skin may not be positive for dermatopathic strains of *S aureus,* because the causative infection is usually elsewhere; swabs of material should be taken from the nose, throat, conjunctiva, and any areas affected by impetigo. Isolates that are shown to be members of phage group II are more likely to elaborate epidermolytic toxin than those be-

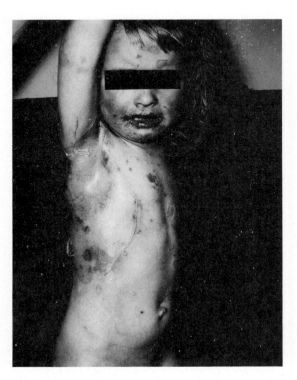

Figure 12–4. Staphylococcal scalded skin syndrome. Because the lesions so closely resemble scalds, mistaken allegations of child abuse have occasionally been made.

longing to another group or those that cannot be typed.

There may be a leukocytosis with neutrophilia on the peripheral blood smear.

Differential Diagnosis

Drug-induced scalded skin syndrome (drug-induced toxic epidermal necrolysis) occurs in children and adults and is a severe variant of "erythema multiforme" (Stevens-Johnson syndrome); it is characterized by stomatitis, conjunctivitis, and balanitis or vaginitis and by a blotchy red eruption. Areas of skin look scalded, are tender, and become denuded, so that the important differentiation from staphylococcal scalded skin syndrome by clinical criteria can be difficult. In staphylococcal scalded skin syndrome, the skin separates in the granular cell layer, but the separation occurs within the lower epidermis in the drug eruption. Inquiries should be made about a recent history of drug ingestion, but the crucial distinction is the level at which the skin splits.

Child abuse by thermal scalding is usually accompanied by other injuries such as bruises and fractures.

Rare causes of "scalding" include boric acid poisoning and skin contact with gasoline or kerosene. Kawasaki disease, toxic shock syndrome, and scarlet fever all have red exanthems, but the skin does not peel—at least not immediately—and then not in moist sheets.

Treatment

Treatment consists of administration of an oral penicillinase-resistant penicillin such as dicloxacillin, 50 mg/kg/d in 4 divided dosages to a maximum of 2 g per day, or parenteral oxacillin or nafcillin at a dose of 75–100 mg/kg/d in divided doses intravenously every 6 hours, not to exceed 8 g per day. Corticosteroids should be avoided since they can delay resolution of the process.

Prognosis

Death due to staphylococcal scalded skin syndrome is rare and usually results from some complicating illness such as streptococcal septicemia. Recovery is complete, and second attacks are rare.

FOLLICULITIS

Essentials of Diagnosis

- Itching and burning.
- Pustules in hair follicles.
- In sycosis barbae, inflammation of surrounding skin area.

General Considerations

Folliculitis is manifested by small erythematous follicular pustules without involvement of the surrounding skin. The scalp and extremities are favorite sites. Chronic recurrent folliculitis of the bearded area is termed sycosis barbae (barber's itch). Sycosis is usually propagated by the trauma of shaving and autoinoculation by fingers.

Clinical Findings

The symptoms are slight burning, itching, and pain on manipulation of hair. The lesions are pustules centered on hair follicles. Consequently, each pustule may be pierced by a centrally located hair. In sycosis, the surrounding skin becomes involved, resembling eczema with redness and crusting.

Differential Diagnosis

Folliculitis must be differentiated from tinea barbae by potassium hydroxide examination of hair or by culture. Acne vulgaris and bullous impetigo may occasionally cause confusion. The patient's age and absence of comedones suggest a diagnosis of folliculitis instead of acne. The lesions of impetigo are usually larger.

Treatment

The infected area should first be cleansed with a weak soap solution. This is followed by soaking or compressing affected skin with saline or aluminum subacetate twice daily. When skin is softened, one can gently open the larger pustules and trim away necrotic tissue. Extracting hairs from infected follicles is useful. Mixed ointment preparations containing polymyxin B, bacitracin, and neomycin can be effective when applied 2–4 times daily. Systemic antistaphylococcal antibiotics may be utilized if the skin infection is resistant to local treatment or if the scalp is involved.

Prognosis

The disease can become stubborn, lasting for months or even years.

FURUNCULOSIS & CARBUNCULOSIS

Essentials of Diagnosis

- Tender, round subcutaneous nodules.
- Usually fluctuant or capped with a small pustule.
- Typical spontaneous rupture, with discharge of pus.
- Carbuncles are deep, extremely painful infections of a group of contiguous follicles. *Staphylococcus aureus* is the causative agent.

General Considerations

A furuncle (boil) is an infection of the follicle with involvement of subcutaneous tissue (Fig 12–5). Most are infected with *S aureus*. The preferred sites of the furuncle are the hairy parts of areas exposed to friction and maceration. On the neck and upper back, multiple hair follicles may be involved, producing a carbuncle, which is a large, indurated, painful nodule

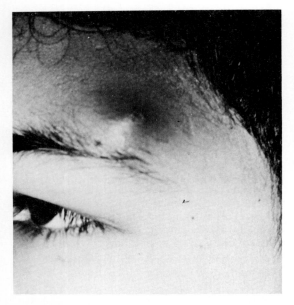

Figure 12–5. A furuncle is an abscess of a hair follicle.

with multiple draining sites. When infection occurs in the nasolabial area, extension via the vein draining into the cavernous sinus may lead to cavernous sinus thrombosis. Perinephric abscess, osteomyelitis, and similar hematogenous staphylococcal infection are other complications.

Clinical Findings

Tenderness and pain are due to pressure on nerve endings, particularly in areas where there is little room for swelling of underlying tissues. The pain, fever, and malaise are more severe with carbuncle than with a furuncle. The follicular abscess enlarges, becomes fluctuant, and then softens and opens spontaneously to discharge a core of necrotic tissue and pus.

Differential Diagnosis

Differentiate from vesiculopustules of virus infections, such as herpes simplex and vaccinia, and from other bacterial infections, such as anthrax and tularemia. Conglobate acne and hidradenitis suppurativa are infections of follicles, but the anatomic sites, multiplicity of lesions, and coexisting factors usually differentiate.

Treatment

A. Local Therapy: Local care and sometimes surgical drainage of pus are sufficient to cure a majority of furuncles. The application of moist heat to developing abscesses or pustules hastens localization and aids in early and spontaneous drainage. A daily bath with antimicrobial soap is advisable. Clothing, in-

cluding underwear, should be changed daily and laundered thoroughly.

B. Systemic Therapy: Knowledge of antibiotic sensitivity of the organism is desirable for the selection of treatment. About 80% of hospital strains of *S aureus* in the USA are resistant to penicillin. Oxacillin, dicloxacillin, nafcillin, and some cephalosporins are used in the treatment of these staphylococcal infections. Dicloxacillin, 500 mg orally every 6 hours for 10 days, is generally effective.

Prevention

Control of recurrent furunculosis can often be obtained by improving hygiene and by elimination of carriage with systemic antibiotics. Some advocate treatment by bacterial interference. After effective antibiotic therapy, a relatively avirulent strain of *S aureus* (502A) is deposited locally, preventing subsequent recolonization with a virulent strain. The procedure has been effective in controlling staphylococcal epidemics in newborn nurseries and in the management of patients with recurrent boils. The practice of painting the nares of carriers with antibacterials such as mupirocin (Bactroban) is occasionally a helpful strategy to prevent recurrences.

Prognosis

In some patients, prognosis cannot be reliably determined during the first attack. Recurrent boils may harass the patient for months or years.

ERYSIPELAS & CELLULITIS DUE TO STREPTOCOCCI

1. ERYSIPELAS

Essentials of Diagnosis

- The skin at the affected site is red, tender, and edematous.
- Erythema is sharply defined with or without vesicles.
- Fever, chills, malaise, and pain are common.

General Considerations

Erysipelas is an acute infection of the skin and subcutaneous tissues. It occurs on the face, scalp, hands, legs, and genitals. This disease is contagious but does not produce explosive epidemics like those of scarlet fever. Group A β-hemolytic streptococci are found in the edema fluid of the advancing margin and characteristically spread in subepidermal tissue.

Clinical Findings

Following an incubation period of 5–7 days, the abrupt onset of high fever is accompanied by headache, malaise, and vomiting. The skin at the affected site feels tense and uncomfortable, and this is followed by erythema and edema. The erythema is sharply marginated and may have vesicles or bullae near the advancing margin. Without effective treatment, bacteremia may develop.

Differential Diagnosis

Erysipelas should be distinguished from cellulitis, which has a less definite margin and involves deeper tissues. Erysipelas should also be differentiated from erysipeloid, an infection commonly seen in fishery workers and meat handlers (see below).

Treatment

Bed rest, application of hot packs, and aspirin for pain and fever are helpful. Penicillin is the drug of choice and should be given for 5–7 days (see cellulitis, below). Erythromycin is recommended when allergy to penicillin exists or is suspected.

Prognosis

Before the advent of antibiotics, the disease was life-threatening, particularly for infants and the elderly. With prompt treatment, it is now more readily controlled.

2. CELLULITIS

Cellulitis is diffuse inflammation of loose connective tissue, particularly subcutaneous tissue. Infection occurs generally through a breach in the skin surface, especially if tissue edema is present. Cellulitis, however, may arise in normal skin. Cellulitis presents as erythema and brawny edema that is tender with poorly defined borders. β-Hemolytic streptococci are most commonly responsible.

Treatment

Treatment is usually with penicillin. Penicillin V potassium, 250–500 mg orally every 6 hours for 10 days, should be given for adults and for children weighing over 40 kg; for children weighing less than 40 kg, give pencillin V potassium, 25–50 mg/kg/d in divided doses. Erythromycin and clindamycin are alternatives in the penicillin-allergic individual.

SCARLET FEVER

Essentials of Diagnosis

- Bright red exanthem of tiny red dots.
- Severe pharyngitis.
- Fever, malaise.
- Petechiae in body folds.

General Considerations

Scarlet fever is initiated by strains of group A streptococci that produce erythrogenic toxin in patients who lack antitoxin immunity. The disease follows streptococcal pharyngitis or tonsillitis. The ex-

anthem typically starts as an erythematous blush on the neck beneath the ear, on the chest, and in the axillas, quickly spreading to the abdomen, extremities, and face. Petechiae are present in creases of elbows, groin, and axillary folds (Pastia's lines). The pharyngeal area, including the tonsils, is edematous, red, and beefy in appearance. The tongue is usually coated white, with prominent bright red papillae, particularly on the lateral margin (strawberry tongue). Acute hemorrhagic glomerulonephritis and acute rheumatic fever are the most serious complications. A reliable diagnosis can be made on the basis of clinical findings. Positive streptococcal cultures along with antibody tests are confirmatory.

Treatment

Benzathine penicillin G and oral penicillin are preferred; erythromycin is the second choice. With benzathine penicillin G, adults are injected intramuscularly with 1.2 million units in a single dose; for older children, a single injection of 900,000 units; for infants and children weighing less than 27.3 kg, a single dose of 50,000 units/kg.

The use of penicillin V and erythromycin is discussed under bullous impetigo, above.

ERYSIPELOID

Infection due to *Erysipelothrix rhusiopathiae* (a gram-positive bacillus) must be differentiated from erysipelas and cellulitis. It is a usually benign infection commonly seen in fishery workers and meat handlers. The disease occurs in both humans and in swine. Two types of skin erysipeloid are recognized. In the localized form, a purple area of nonsuppurative cellulitis develops, usually on the back of the hand. In generalized erysipeloid, fever, arthralgia, and widespread cutaneous lesions are seen.

Treatment

Penicillin, 250–500 mg given orally every 6 hours for 5–7 days, is usually effective. Tetracyclines may also be useful. The dosage schedule of tetracycline hydrochloride in adults is 250 mg orally every 6 hours. Therapy should be continued for at least 1–2 days after signs and symptoms have subsided.

ERYTHRASMA

Erythrasma is a chronic superficial infection of the pubis, toe web, groin, axilla, and inframammary fold. Most lesions are asymptomatic but may cause mild burning and itching. The infected areas are irregularly shaped, circinate, dry, and scaly—initially pink but later brown. The widespread generalized form is more common in warmer climates. *Corynebacterium minutissimum* is the etiologic agent. The organism produces porphyrins and fluorescence in certain media and is responsible for the coral-red fluorescence in clinical lesions when examined under Wood's light.

Treatment

C minutissimum is extremely sensitive to many antimicrobials. Topical antimicrobials or keratolytic preparations are useful. Oral erythromycin, 250 mg every 6 hours for 7–10 days, is the treatment of choice in extensive erythrasma. Tolnaftate and Whitfield's ointment are also effective. Recurrences are common.

PITTED KERATOLYSIS

Pitted keratolysis is a noninflammatory infection of the plantar and occasionally palmar surfaces, producing punched-out pits or sulci in the stratum corneum. The pits may coalesce into irregularly shaped areas of erosion. The pits are produced by a "lytic" process that spreads peripherally. The areas most often affected are the heel, the ball of the foot, the volar pads, and the toes. Humidity and high temperature are frequent aggravating factors. Gram-positive coryneforms have been isolated from the lesions.

Treatment

The lesions may disappear spontaneously after the patient is removed from the moist environment or when drying agents such as antiperspirants are used. Whitfield's ointment applied twice daily or immersion of the foot in a solution of 4% formalin is usually effective. Topical application of 2% erythromycin solutions may stop the process and prevent recurrence if applied once or twice daily.

GRAM-NEGATIVE BACTERIAL INFECTIONS

In management of the 4 diseases described in this section, the affected areas must be kept dry. Depriving etiologic organisms of the moisture they require to flourish is probably critical. Systemic antibiotics should be chosen on the basis of culture and sensitivity tests.

1. ECTHYMA GANGRENOSUM

Ecthyma gangrenosum is characterized by necrotic ulcers generally located on the buttocks and ex-

tremities. This skin infection is a manifestation of underlying systemic *Peudomonas aeruginosa* bacteremia. Treatment should include intravenous therapy with piperacillin or another antipseudomonal penicillin in this group, combined with one of the aminoglycosides such as tobramycin.

2. FOLLICULITIS

Pseudomonas infections may also be acquired from contaminated swimming pools and hot tubs. These infections have been associated with a specific type of *P aeruginosa*. Whirlpool baths have been implicated in itchy folliculitis. The lesions are red with white centers and are mostly confined to the trunk and axillas.

Systemic antibodies are frequently not required, since some infections respond to simple topical treatments such as tretinoin, benzoyl peroxide, gentamicin cream, or 0.25% acetic acid compresses.

Patients receiving long-term antibiotic therapy for acne may develop "gram-negative folliculitis." Two types have been reported. One consists of superficial pustules, usually grouped around the nose, whose etiologic agent is either *Escherichia coli* or *Enterobacter aerogenes*. The other type consists of deep nodular and cystic lesions initiated by *Proteus* species. The organisms can usually be cultured from the nostrils and the lesions.

If feasible, the long-term antibiotic treatment should be stopped. Topical or systemic antibiotics can be used. Isotretinoin therapy may also be successful, but its use is generally limited to male patients because the drug is a teratogen.

3. TOE WEB INFECTION

Typically, toe web infections are characterized by hyperkeratotic white intertriginous toe lesions, which may show greenish discoloration from pigments elaborated by *P aeruginosa*. Wood's light examination reveals aqua-green fluorescence. Pseudomonal infection of toe webs is alleged to be more common in blacks. Secondary infections of toe webs are discussed below.

Topical therapy with gentamicin lotion or ointment should be initiated. Cotton can be inserted between the toes, and soaking the feet in Burow's solution may hasten healing. In refractory cases, ciprofloxacin, 750 mg orally twice daily can be considered. In the case of *Acinetobacter* infections, topical treatment with gentamicin lotion or ointment can be used.

SECONDARY INFECTIONS

Unlike the primary infections, secondary infections often show a mixture of organisms in culture, and it is often difficult to decide which of them plays the major etiologic role. The appearance of secondary lesions is not characteristic (in contrast to the primary infections initiated by these organisms); it is largely dependent on the nature of the underlying skin disease.

TOE WEB INFECTIONS

The diseases of the interdigital toe web space are commonly referred to as "athlete's foot." Most are infections by dermatophytic fungi. However, dermatophytes often cannot be cultured from or demonstrated microscopically in severe toe web lesions, because they are so heavily colonized with bacteria.

Although the dermatophytic fungi are the primary invaders that produce cutaneous damage, subsequent bacterial overgrowth contributes to the maceration and hyperkeratosis and resistance to treatment. The fungi, through the production of antibiotics, favor the growth of nonlipophilic coryneforms. Some of these bacteria produce various proteolytic enzymes, which then foster additional skin injury (Fig 12–6). If the feet remain damp for prolonged periods, gram-negative bacilli, always present, become the predominant flora, resulting in further damage to the toe webs. (See toe web infections, below.)

Treatment

Special strategies are required to combat toe web infection, because so many different types of organisms are involved. For simple dry, scaly lesions, topical antifungal agents are effective such as miconazole, clotrimazole, or ciclopirox olamine 1–2% cream applied twice daily. For wet macerated lesions, a systematic approach is required:

(1) Removal of excessive moisture (eg, not wearing closed shoes and separation of interspaces with cotton pads) is helpful. Compresses or daily treatment with 1% gentian violet, 20% alcoholic solution of aluminum chloride, or Castellani's paint helps to desiccate the involved skin.

(2) Use of broad-spectrum topical antimicrobial agents is adjunctive.

(3) Long-term use of a topical antifungal agent is required to avoid reinfection.

(4) Oral griseofulvin (adults: 250 mg ultramicrosize twice daily) or ketoconazole (adults: 200 mg/d) may be used in the treatment of resistant infections.

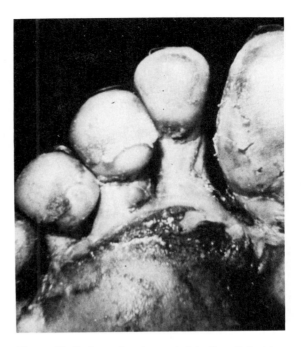

Figure 12–6. Spreading toe web infection. Note intensive maceration and hyperkeratosis due to secondary bacterial infections.

INTERTRIGO

This disorder is most common in chubby infants or obese adults. In the skin folds, heat, moisture, and friction produce erythema, maceration, or even erosions. Overgrowth of resident or transient flora is associated with this problem.

Treatment

The skin area should be kept clean and dry, guarding against overbathing. Powders or broad-spectrum antimicrobial creams (eg, 2% miconazole) applied twice daily usually help.

ACUTE INFECTIOUS ECZEMATOID DERMATITIS

This disorder arises from a primary exudative lesion, such as a boil or a draining ear or nose. A hallmark of this disease is a streak of dermatitis along the path of flow of the discharge material. Coagulase-positive streptococci are most frequently isolated.

Treatment

Compressing the involved areas may have a beneficial effect. Polymyxin B in combination with bacitracin is then applied to the infected skin. Also recommended is oral erythromycin, 0.25–0.5 g every

6 hours, or dicloxacillin, 0.25–0.5 g every 6 hours (adult doses).

PSEUDOFOLLICULITIS OF THE BEARD

This common disorder occurs most often in the beard area of black men who shave. See Chapter 52.

PYODERMA SECONDARY TO ECZEMA

The skin of atopic individuals is often colonized by *Staphylococcus aureus*. Over 90% of patients with chronic lichenified plaques carry this pathogen. The colonization of *S aureus* is even more pronounced in the acute exudative form of the disease, where the recovery rate of the organism is 100% with a mean density of 107 colony-forming units per square centimeter. This overgrowth of *S aureus* presents a threat not only to patients but also to those who come in contact with them.

Treatment

Because eczema is a multifactorial disease, several regimens are required to manage the infected lesions (see Chapter 40). Improvements in the underlying eczema are usually associated with decreasing bacterial colonization. Systemic antibiotics such as erythromycin or dicloxacillin, 250 mg 4 times daily (adults), is often indicated.

SYSTEMIC INFECTIONS INVOLVING THE SKIN

ACTINOMYCOSIS

Although human actinomycosis is usually associated with *Actinomyces israelii,* another agent, *Arachnia propionica,* is frequently isolated. Despite their filamentous appearance, these organisms are bacteria, not fungi. *Actinomyces* and *Arachnia* are members of the normal flora of the mouth and tonsillar crypts. These gram-positive, non-acid-fast organisms grow as filaments that fragment into bacillary and coccoid forms. In lesions, these filaments may be seen as a compact mass called a "sulfur granule." Actinomycosis is an infection of endogenous origin

that occurs when organisms normally found in the mouth are introduced into traumatized tissue.

Clinical Findings

Actinomycosis is divided into 3 clinical types: cervicofacial, thoracic, and abdominal. Cervicofacial infection is the most common; the infection usually follows injury to the mouth or jaw, such as a tooth extraction. Pulmonary infection may follow aspiration of infected materials from the mouth. Abdominal actinomycosis has been associated with abdominal surgery and accidental trauma. The organisms involved are probably residents of the oral cavity that have been swallowed. Actinomycosis from oral *A israelii* and *A propionica* has also been demonstrated following a human bite.

Cervicofacial actinomycosis develops slowly. Swelling of soft tissues of the face is not characteristic at first; the overlying skin, however, soon darkens to a deep red or purplish color. The swelling continues to a "wooden" type of hardness, and the surface appears uneven or lumpy. Abscesses develop, and multiple draining sinuses appear. Pain is minimal unless there is secondary infection. X-ray shows no involvement of bone initially but may reveal bony involvement in later stages of the disease.

Thoracic actinomycosis starts with a mild, irregular fever, cough, and sputum production. Involvement of the pleura may cause pleural pain. As the disease progresses, loss of weight and strength, anemia, spiking fever, and dyspnea occur. Multiple sinuses may bore through the chest wall. X-ray shows a smooth, massive area of consolidation typically in the lower half of the lung.

Abdominal actinomycosis is found usually in the ileocecal region, presenting a picture of acute or subacute appendicitis. As the disease advances, the patient loses weight, develops spiking fever, and may have night sweats and episodes of vomiting. X-ray may show enlargement of liver, spleen, or involvement of the vertebral bodies.

Diagnosis

Pus and other exudates are examined microscopically for the presence of granules, which appear as lobulate bodies composed of delicate branching gram-positive filaments with eosinophilic club-shaped ends. Anaerobic culture is necessary to distinguish *Actinomyces* species from the aerobic *Nocardia* species.

Treatment

Adequate surgical drainage is important. The general resistance of the patient should be supported by bed rest and a good diet. Lobectomy or pneumonectomy should be considered only in those cases that fail to respond to other therapy.

Penicillin is the drug of choice. The organism is highly susceptible to this antibiotic, but the disease resolves slowly. High doses of penicillin G are given parenterally for 4–6 weeks. A second antibiotic may be added to the regimen for secondarily infected lesions. To ensure cure, treatment should continue even after the clinical symptoms have subsided.

Prognosis

The prognosis of actinomycosis without treatment is generally grave, but the cervicofacial variety may remain localized for long periods. With penicillin and surgery, the prognosis is good.

NOCARDIOSIS

The microbial agent of nocardiosis is *Nocardia asteroides,* and the disease may simulate bacterial pneumonia, pulmonary abscesses, mycotic infection of the lungs, or tuberculosis. It may metastasize to the subcutaneous tissue or other organs of the body, especially the brain and meninges.

Nocardiosis has become increasingly prevalent in immunocompromised patients receiving antineoplastic or immunosuppressive therapy. Severe infection has occurred in renal and cardiac transplant patients.

Clinical Findings

Pulmonary nocardiosis presents as a pneumonia with cough and production of purulent sputum as the chief complaints. Consolidation of one or more lobes and involvement of the pleura are common. Sinus tracts may penetrate the chest wall. There is subsequent hematogenous spread. When fistulas open to the skin surface, they can be differentiated from those of actinomycosis by the lack of granules characteristic of actinomycosis and by the presence of partially acid-fast branching rods. Dissemination may involve any organ. Lesions in the brain and meninges are most frequent, and such spread may occur following any minor pulmonary lesion. Dissemination is frequent in debilitated patients.

Diagnosis

N asteroides grows in tissues as a widely spreading mycelium or as branching rods. The organism is aerobic, gram-positive, and partially acid-fast. *N asteroides* elicits an intense pyogenic tissue reaction characterized by small to massive, usually suppurative, abscesses within which the delicate branched filamentous rods are seen by Gram stain. Identification is confirmed by culture.

Treatment

Sulfadiazine has been recommended as the treatment of choice. Trimethoprim-sulfamethoxazole (TMP-SMX) has replaced this sulfonamide as the drug of choice in the minds of many investigators. In patients who are allergic to sulfonamides, sensitivity tests should be used to determine the appropriate anti-

biotic. Drainage or resection of abscesses may be required.

Prognosis

The prognosis is good with early diagnosis of the pulmonary disease before metastasis to the brain has occurred.

MYCOBACTERIAL SKIN INFECTIONS

1. SKIN TUBERCULOSIS

Skin tuberculosis is produced by the direct inoculation of *Mycobacterium tuberculosis* into the skin of persons not previously exposed to the agent or by the lymphatic or hematogenous dissemination with focal survival of the bacterium in individuals with tuberculosis. Skin tuberculosis in industrialized or developed countries is rare.

Clinical Findings

A. Localized Form: This follows after the introduction of tubercle bacilli into a wound in individuals with no previous immunologic experience with this agent. The course begins as an inflammatory nodule (the **tuberculous chancre,** containing bacilli) and is accompanied by regional lymphangitis and lymphadenitis. The course of the disease depends on the patient's resistance and the effectiveness of treatment.

In immune or partially immune hosts, 2 major groups of skin lesions are distinguished: tuberculosis verrucosa and lupus vulgaris. In **tuberculosis verrucosa,** inoculation of bacilli incites localized granulomatous papules or verrucose nodules containing few bacilli. **Lupus vulgaris** commences in early life. Patchy lesions studded with soft confluent tubercles appear as small, yellowish-brown "apple-jelly" nodules if the lesions are compressed by a glass microscopic slide (diascopy). New nodules develop at the periphery while the center undergoes atrophic scarring. Ulceration, edema, and hypertrophy due to lymphatic obstruction ensue. Tubercle bacilli are scarce. In temperate climates, the majority of lupus lesions are on the face, while those of tuberculosis verrucosa are on the hands. In tropical areas, the distribution of lesions may be different.

In **scrofuloderma,** tuberculosis of lymph nodes or bone is extended into the skin, resulting in the development of ulcers. Numerous fistulas may communicate beneath ridges of bluish skin. Tubercle bacilli can usually be isolated from the pus.

B. Disseminated Form: Bacteria, spread by the hematogenous route in patients with fulminating tuberculosis, initiate **miliary tuberculosis** in the skin. These lesions teem with tubercle bacilli. When hypersensitivity to tubercle bacilli is present, antigen spread via the blood produces tuberculids such as lichen scrofulosus. The strong immunologic reaction of tuberculids destroys mycobacteria, evoking a strongly positive tuberculin reaction. Papulonecrotic tuberculids occur in erratic crops on the face and extremities as symmetric eruptions of firm, acneiform papules, which undergo central necrosis that ends in small varicelliform scars.

Treatment

Although it is advisable to test the sensitivity of *M tuberculosis,* it is not usually necessary to wait for the results to initiate therapy. Isoniazid combined with rifampin is the initial treatment of choice.

2. INFECTIONS BY ATYPICAL MYCOBACTERIA

The atypical mycobacteria are acid-fast, like *M tuberculosis,* but their pathogenesis and cultural characteristics are distinctive. The following Runyon classification is based on cultural features:

Group I, the **photochromogens,** develop pigment only when growing cultures are exposed to light. *Mycobacterium marinum, M ulcerans,* and *M kansasii* are examples.

Group II, the **scotochromogens,** develop pigment in absence of light. They are infrequent pathogens in human disease.

Group III, the **nonchromogens,** include *M avium* and *M intracellulare.*

Group IV, the rapid growers, thrive at 37 °C and at lower temperatures still grow rapidly; there is no pigment production. Examples are *M fortuitum* and *M smegmatis.*

Infection Due to *M marinum*

Many cases occur in children and adolescents who have a history of swimming or cleaning fish tanks. Trauma often precedes the infection, but even in its absence, lesions are frequently on the sites most exposed to injury: the fingers, knees, elbows, and the bridge of the nose. The usually solitary lesion is a tuberculoid granuloma that rarely shows acid-fast organisms, though the skin tuberculin test is positive. Most cases can be left to resolve spontaneously. Hot compresses may be curative. Rifampin or sulfone drugs or minocycline may prove effective.

Infection Due to *M ulcerans*

In some tropical areas, chronic ulcers induced by this organism are common. Lesions are usually on the arms or legs but may occur elsewhere, except on the palms and soles. Most patients have a single painless cutaneous ulcer with characteristic undermined edges. Geographic association of the disease with swamps and water courses has been reported. On primary isolation, *M ulcerans* may not grow at 37 °C. This preference for a lower temperature may explain the restriction of lesions to the subcutaneous tissues. The organism is sensitive to a number of drugs in vitro, but the clinical results of chemotherapy have been disappointing. Excision and grafting are often necessary. Tetracyclines such as minocycline are often helpful.

LEPROSY

Like other members of genus *Mycobacterium, M leprae* is an acid-fast organism. It cannot be cultivated on artificial media nor in cell culture. The organism has been grown in the footpads of mice and armadillos. Humans are the only natural host.

Clinical Findings & Classification

The disease affects chiefly the skin, mucous membranes, peripheral nerves, and eyes. Skin lesions may occur as pale, anesthetic macular lesions, discrete erythematous nodules, or a diffuse skin infiltration. Neurologic disturbances are noted. In untreated patients, disfigurement due to infiltration and nerve involvement may be extreme.

Leprosy occurs in 3 forms plus a "borderline form," probably depending on the immunologic status of the patient:

A. Lepromatous Leprosy: The lepromatous form is characterized by nodular lesions with many bacilli. Nodules of the earlobes, extremities, and trunk may ulcerate and develop secondary infection. The lesions contain vast numbers of bacilli, and the patient is anergic.

B. Tuberculoid Leprosy: In tuberculoid leprosy, sparse macular lesions appear that are insensitive to pain, heat, and touch. Few or no bacilli are seen in the lesions, but the patient is lepromin-positive.

C. Intermediate Form: The intermediate (indeterminate) form is characterized by macular lesions with demonstrable bacilli.

D. Borderline Leprosy: In this variation, the clinical and histologic features of both tuberculoid and lepromatous leprosy are represented. Either of these forms can predominate in a patient.

Diagnosis

Diagnosis depends on demonstrating the bacilli in smears or tissue sections in lepromatous cases and on evaluation of the dermatologic, neurologic, and histologic features in the tuberculoid.

Treatment

Treatment is individualized depending on the form of the disease and the propensity of the infected individual to develop hypersensitive reactions to *M leprae* as treatment proceeds. In lepromatous leprosy, chemotherapy is continued as long as the patient lives, whereas indeterminate leprosy is commonly treated until 2 years after the disease becomes inactive. Borderline leprosy is treated for at least 10 years.

Patients with paucibacillary disease (intermediate and tuberculoid) are treated for 6 months with daily unsupervised dapsone, 100 mg, and monthly with supervised rifampin, 600 mg. The treatment is stopped and the patient remains under supervision for 2 years. Multibacillary patients (lepromatous and borderline cases) are treated for a minimum of 2 years or until skin smears are negative. This group is treated with daily dapsone, 100 mg, together with clofazimine, 50 mg, both unsupervised; and monthly with rifampin, 600 mg, together with clofazimine, 300 mg, both supervised. Multibacillary patients should remain under observation for 5 years after completion of the treatment.

Corticosteroids and thalidomide control the lepra reaction (one form of hypersensitivity to *M leprae*), during which the administration of sulfone is temporarily discontinued.

Appropriate surgical and other rehabilitative measures may be required.

Prognosis

Tuberculoid leprosy with localized skin lesions has an excellent prognosis. Many patients return to health spontaneously. Severe neuritis, even if treated, may result in varying degrees of numbness and paralysis. Prognosis is better for borderline leprosy near the tuberculoid end of the spectrum than for that toward the lepromatous end. The prognosis is usually good if lepromatous leprosy is treated in its early stages. With wide dissemination and damage to nerves, mucous membranes, and eyes, treatment may require 10 years or longer. Intermediate leprosy has a good prognosis. This disease is often seen in children who have been in contact with leprosy patients.

CUTANEOUS DIPHTHERIA

Essentials of Diagnosis

- Demarcated shallow ulcer with firm border.
- Gray-yellow or brown-gray membrane in early stages.
- The membrane may be peeled off intact, leaving a clean surface.
- Later, a black or brownish-black eschar appears.

General Considerations

Cutaneous diphtheria, common in tropical regions, also occurs in Canada and the southern USA. The infection is caused by *Corynebacterium diphtheriae*. The organism is an inhabitant of the mucous membranes of the nose and throat and probably occurs as transient flora on human skin. *C diphtheriae* strains differ in their toxin-producing ability. All strains are lysogenic for temperate phages; with loss of phage, the ability to produce toxin is also lost.

Clinical Findings

The early lesions are superficial ulcers with well-defined overhanging edges. Exudate from the ulcer floor forms a grayish membrane. Later, the diagnostic hallmark of the disease appears—a black or brownish-black adherent eschar. The eschar is removed with difficulty and is surrounded by a tender inflammatory zone. Regional lymph nodes may be affected. Faucial diphtheria is associated with adherent hemorrhagic crusts around the mouth and nose. Systemic involvement when present is mild, but in some cases it can be severe, especially in infants.

Differential Diagnosis

Cutaneous diphtheria must be differentiated from impetigo and eczema. The diagnosis may be suspected in patients with persistent ulcers with adherent membrane but must be confirmed bacteriologically.

Treatment

Combined therapy with a suitable antibiotic and specific antitoxin is effective. Penicillin V potassium orally may be used in mild cases without systemic involvement. Intravenous therapy with penicillin should be used in more severe cases and when there is any evidence of systemic involvement. Erythromycin for 2 weeks is an alternative. The agents will inhibit the bacteria but will not inactivate the toxin. Intramuscular injections of diphtheria antitoxin (20,000–50,000 units) will inactivate the toxin.

TULAREMIA

Essentials of Diagnosis

- History of contact with wild rodents, particularly with rabbits and muskrats, and bites of arthropods.
- Chills, fever, headache, and nausea.
- Ulcer at the site of inoculation.
- Enlargement of regional lymph nodes.
- Confirmation by culture of primary lesion, lymph node, or blood.

General Considerations

Tularemia is widespread in a number of natural hosts from which, by direct or indirect means, humans may contact the disease. The etiologic agent is *Francisella (Pasteurella) tularensis*. Tularemia is transmitted from animals to humans by contact with animal tissues, by the bite of deerflies or ticks, by eating infected uncooked food, or by drinking contaminated water. The disease is endemic to the USA and many parts of Europe.

Clinical Findings

The clinically observed manifestations depend on

the portal of entry in the skin, gastrointestinal tract, eye, or respiratory tract. In ulceroglandular or oculoglandular types, a papule at the site of inoculation develops and soon becomes ulcerated. Regional lymph nodes become enlarged and tender and may ulcerate. Pneumonia may develop. The typhoidal (an enteric form) and pulmonary forms are more fulminating. During toxemic stages of infections, skin lesions may develop; there may be a generalized eruption or maculopapular or profuse crops of nodules, usually on the limbs.

The organism may be cultured from ulcerated lesions, lymph nodes, or gastric or pharyngeal washings. The skin test is specific and remains positive after infection. An agglutination test is available.

Differential Diagnosis

In differential diagnosis, cat-scratch disease, rickettsial and meningococcal infections, infectious mononucleosis, and sporotrichosis must be excluded.

Treatment

Strepomycin is usually effective. Gentamicin intravenously may be an acceptable alternative. The tetracyclines are effective, but relapses may occur if treatment is stopped prematurely. Maintenance of fluid balance is essential, and oxygen may be required.

Prognosis

The mortality rate of untreated typhoidal and pulmonary forms is about 20%, and that of the oculoglandular form is 5%. Early treatment prevents fatality.

ANTHRAX

Anthrax is a zoonotic disease caused by *Bacillus anthracis*. The disease is transmitted to humans by entry through broken skin or mucous membranes or by inhalation or ingestion of spores.

Clinical Findings

Cutaneous anthrax ("malignant pustule") is characterized by development of a small erythematous papule that becomes vesicular. The vesicle ruptures, leaving a round sharp-edged ulcer crater containing a necrotic "black eschar." The area around the lesion is swollen or edematous. In severe untreated cases, high fever, malaise, and prostration terminating in death may occur. Hemorrhagic meningitis may also develop.

Differential Diagnosis

Anthrax should be distinguished from staphylococcal infections, cowpox, accidental vaccinia, cat-

scratch disease, North American blastomycosis, and sporotrichosis.

Treatment

Pencillin is the treatment of choice. The patient should be treated with high doses intravenously for 3–4 days until edema subsides. Oral therapy with penicillin V potassium 500 mg orally every 6 hours, can be substituted after the edema has subsided.

Prognosis

The prognosis is good in the cutaneous form of infection if promptly treated. Severe edema or toxemia has a poor prognosis.

GAS GANGRENE

Essentials of Diagnosis

- Pain and edema in the affected area.
- Brownish watery exudate with discolored skin surrounding the area.
- Crepitation from gas in the tissues.
- Fever, toxemia, shock, and death.
- Demonstration of organisms in culture and in smear of exudate.

General Considerations

Gas gangrene is caused by the infection of wounds with various species of *Clostridium*, alone or in combination with other bacteria. *Clostridium perfringens (C welchii), C novyi,* and *C septicum* are the important species, but many others may play a minor role. The clostridia are found in the soil and in the gastrointestinal tract of humans and other mammals. They grow and produce toxins in wounds under anaerobic conditions; alpha toxin (lecithinase) is the most potent.

Clinical Findings

The infection spreads in 1–3 days in deep dirty wounds in the muscular regions of the body. The affected areas become painful and swollen; this is accompanied by a fall in blood pressure and tachycardia. Body temperature may rise but not in proportion to disease severity. Wound swelling continues, and the surrounding skin becomes pale because of fluid accumulation beneath it. There is a development of crepitation in the subcutaneous tissue and muscle, with foul-smelling discharge, rapidly progressing necrosis, fever, toxemia, shock, and death.

In gas gangrene, mixed infection is common. In addition to toxin-producing clostridia, proteolytic clostridia and various gram-positive cocci and gram-negative bacteria are also present. The presence of large gram-positive spore-forming rods suggests gas gangrene clostridia. Spores may not be observed in the smear.

Differential Diagnosis

Peptostreptococci, *Bacteroides, Enterobacter,* and *Escherichia* may produce infection that can cause gas formation in the tissue.

Treatment

Prompt and extensive surgical debridement of all devitalized tissue is essential. High doses of penicillin are given parenterally. Polyvalent antitoxins are available, but their efficacy is uncertain.

Prognosis

In untreated cases, the mortality rate is high.

MENINGOCOCCAL INFECTIONS

Essentials of Diagnosis

- Fever, headache, vomiting, delirium, and convulsions (in meningitis).
- Stiffness of neck and back (in meningitis).
- Petechial or purpuric skin rash.

General Considerations

Meningococcal infections are caused by *Neisseria meningitidis,* an endotoxin-producing gram-negative diplococcus. The disease is transmitted by droplets from patients or healthy nasopharyngeal carriers. The disease tends to appear in winter and spring in enclosed populations and occurs in one of 3 forms: meningitis, acute meningococcemia, and chronic meningococcemia. The incubation period is 2–10 days.

Clinical Findings

In the fulminating stage, the fever is brief; in the chronic case, it may be predominant, and meningitic symptoms may not develop. If meningitis is present, fever, headache, vomiting, and delirium may be followed by convulsions. Stiffness of the neck and back is common.

Petechiae may vary from pinhead-sized rashes to large ecchymoses or extensive skin gangrene. Purpura is characteristic in the septicemic phase, occurring on the trunk, limbs, and mucous membranes but not in the nail beds. Extensive plaques of hemorrhagic gangrene are seen in some cases. Shock and disseminated intravascular clotting may be noted. Culture of blood, cerebrospinal fluid, or petechial aspiration is diagnostic.

Differential Diagnosis

Petechial rash should be distinguished from other bacterial infections (staphylococcal, *Haemophilus*) or rickettsial or echovirus infection.

Meningococcal meningitis should be differentiated from other meningitis.

Treatment

Treatment is with aqueous penicillin G, 24 million units every 24 hours for adults. Treatment should be continued for 7–10 days by the intravenous route or until the patient becomes afebrile for 5 days.

A vaccine for group A and group C meningococci is available. It has been found effective among military recruits and in civilian populations.

Supportive measures are essential, such as controlling temperature, maintaining fluid and electrolyte balance, and monitoring the clotting system (heparin therapy instituted when indicated).

LISTERIOSIS

Listeria monocytogenes is a short gram-positive rod that is aerobic to microaerophilic. Infected animals are common and are found worldwide. Listeriosis has a wide host range that includes mammals, birds, ticks, fish, and crustaceans.

Human infection occurs by handling animals and ingesting animal products. In the USA, most cases occur among urban residents.

Clinical Findings

The clinical picture is extremely variable in humans, the most common being meningoencephalitis or meningitis. The mortality rate among untreated patients is about 60–70%.

A less common but serious manifestation is perinatal septicemia (granulomatous infantiseptica), resulting from low-grade uterine infection in the mother. The disease in the newborn has a high mortality rate. The infant may be stillborn or premature and may develop a combination of respiratory and gastrointestinal symptoms, generalized erythema, and dark red or bluish papules, especially on the trunk and legs.

The diagnosis is established by blood culture, animal inoculation, and a rising serum agglutinin titer.

Treatment

Penicillin or ampicillin given intravenously in large doses is effective; erythromycin given intravenously is an effective alternative.

Prognosis

The prognosis without treatment is poor and fatality rates are high, but those forms resembling infectious mononucleosis are relatively benign.

RHINOSCLEROMA

Rhinoscleroma is caused by *Klebsiella rhinoscleromatis,* a gram-negative bacillus. The disease is chronic, infective, and somewhat contagious, occurring more commonly in rural areas when hygienic conditions are low. The disease occurs sporadically throughout the world. Rhinoscleroma has not been produced experimentally in laboratory animals or in volunteers.

Clinical Findings

The disease begins insidiously; the first manifestation is nasopharyngeal, with nasal catarrh and increased nasal secretion and encrustation. Gradually there is a nodular or diffuse sclerotic enlargement of the nose, upper lip, palate, or neighboring areas, giving rise to the so-called "Hebra nose."

Backward extension of the infection may produce obstruction of the respiratory tract, so that breathing becomes difficult and painful and tracheotomy may be required. The patient may die as a result of respiratory obstruction or intercurrent infections.

Differential Diagnosis

Rhinoscleroma is a distinct clinical entity and can be distinguished from other diseases involving nasal fossae and the upper respiratory tract. Its diagnosis depends on the basis of bacteriologic and serologic tests. Clinically, it can be confused with leishmaniasis, syphilitic gumma, sarcoid, nasal tuberculosis, leprosy, paracoccidioidomycosis, rhinosporidiosis, and nasal polyps.

Treatment

Rhinoscleroma is progressive and resistant to therapy. The sensitivity of the organism to various antibiotics should be determined. Gentamicin and tobramycin are drugs that have been found to be effective systemically. Ciprofloxacin, which is active against the organisms causing rhinoscleroma, may be an effective oral alternative, but this drug has not been extensively evaluated.

GLANDERS

Glanders is a disease of horses and cattle, rarely occurring in humans. The causative agent is *Pseudomonas (Malleomyces) mallei.* Humans are infected by direct contact with horses. The disease in humans is acquired by inoculation of bacteria through abraded skin or through the conjunctiva or nasal mucous membrane.

Clinical Findings

There is an inflammatory papule or vesicle at the site of inoculation, rapidly becoming nodular, pustular, and ulcerative. The regional lymphatics become swollen and tender, and the nodules along their course break down to form abscesses and sinuses. If there is an involvement of nasal or oral mucous membranes, extensive necrosis and destruction of the septum and palate are noted. Glanders may occur in an acute form—a rapidly fatal disease—or in a chronic

form that may linger for months or even years. Death probably results from nephritis, intercurrent infection, or exhaustion.

Diagnosis

Diagnosis is established by finding the gram-negative bacillus in a direct smear from the lesion or by serologic testing. Diagnosis is further aided by guinea pig inoculation and the demonstration of hypersensitivity of the animal to mallein (antigen prepared from a culture of the organism).

Treatment

There is no satisfactory treatment. Immediate surgical excision of the lesions and sulfonamide treatment are recommended. Tetracyclines, streptomycin, and chloramphenicol have been reported to be effective.

MELIOIDOSIS
(Whitmore's Disease)

Melioidosis is a specific infection of rodents caused by *Pseudomonas pseudomallei,* endemic in southeast Asia and Australia. The disease also occurs in sheep, cattle, swine, and horses. It is acquired by inhalation or by inoculation of abraded skin. The reservoir is soil or water, particularly rice paddies, where organisms can survive and grow.

Clinical Findings

In humans the disease may occur in 3 general forms: (1) an acute septicemic condition with diarrhea, (2) a subacute typhoidal form with pulmonary symptoms and local abscess formation, and (3) a chronic form. Its clinical characteristics are similar to those of disseminated fungal infections and tuberculosis. Severe urticaria has been noted with pulmonary melioidosis; it disappeared after treatment with tetracycline. More recent serologic tests indicate that the infection may be more common and milder than has been previously indicated.

The diagnosis is established by isolating the gram-negative organism or by the rise of antibody titer.

Treatment

The abscesses must be drained surgically. Effective therapy is determined by antibiotic sensitivity of the specific strain. Two to 3 g of tetracycline daily for at least 30 days is usually effective. Tetracycline in combination with chloramphenicol has been used with some success in prolonged treatment—1–5 months—to circumvent relapse. Piperacillin, gentamicin, and doxycycline have also been used.

RAT-BITE FEVER

There are 2 distinct kinds of rat-bite fever: (1) **sodoku,** caused by *Spirillum minus;* and (2) **septicemia,** produced by *Streptobacillus moniliformis* (erythema arthriticum epidemicum). Clinically, the 2 forms are very similar.

Clinical Findings

Following a bite by an infected rat, the original wound heals, but after an incubation period of 1–3 weeks it becomes swollen and painful. Fever, enlargement of lymph nodes, and skin eruptions occur, along with general malaise, anorexia, and pain in the joints.

Diagnosis

The diagnosis is confirmed by culturing the causative organism from the blood or joint aspirate. *S minus* is demonstrated by guinea pig or mouse inoculation. Large numbers of organisms are demonstrated in Wright-stained smears of the infected animals. *S moniliformis* is part of the resident flora in the rat's upper respiratory tract. The organism is gram-negative and pleomorphic and requires blood serum for growth in artificial media.

Rat bite fever should be differentiated from erysipelas, giant chancre, and leprosy.

Treatment

Penicillin G intravenously is effective for adults.

LEPTOSPIROSIS

Leptospirosis in humans is also known as Weil's disease, pretibial fever, and Fort Bragg fever.

Leptospirosis is an infection caused by the immunologically heterogeneous spirochetes of the genus *Leptospira*. Leptospires are parasites in lower mammals, including wild rodents and a variety of domestic animals. Human infection is acquired by direct contact with infectious urine or contaminated water containing infected urine or by direct contact with infected tissues.

Clinical Findings

After an incubation period of 1–2 weeks, Weil's disease starts with high fever followed by nausea, vomiting, headache, jaundice, petechiae and purpura on the skin and mucous membranes, and renal involvement, manifested by pyuria, hematuria, and azotemia. Severe conjunctivitis is a common diagnostic feature. *Leptospira icterohaemorrhagiae* is the etiologic agent.

Pretibial fever (Fort Bragg fever) is caused by *Leptospira autumnalis*. The disease is characterized by an acute exanthematous infectious erythema that appears on the fourth day of illness, generally on the skin. The erythema may exist over various parts of the body and may also become generalized. There is a polymorphonuclear leukocytosis of the peripheral blood.

Diagnosis

The diagnosis is established by a specific agglutination antibody titer, by demonstrating causative organisms in the blood, by dark-field microscopy, or by guinea pig inoculation.

Treatment

Treatment is mostly symptomatic. Penicillin in large intravenous dosages or tetracycline have been employed.

PLAGUE

Plague is primarily a disease of rodents caused by *Yersinia (Pasteurella) pestis,* a small gram-negative rod. The disease is transmitted from rodents to humans by flea bites. If a patient develops pneumonia, the infection can be transmitted by aerosols.

Clinical Findings

Following the flea bite, the bacteria spread through the lymphatics to the lymph nodes, which become painful and enlarged (bubo). The bacilli may then reach the bloodstream, involving most of the organs; with pneumonia or meningitis, the outcome is often fatal.

Cutaneous lesions occur in about 10% of cases in plague epidemics, but purpuric spots (black plague) have occurred in a high proportion of cases in some epidemics.

Primary cutaneous inoculation with plague bacilli occurs in sporadic cases but is not common.

Diagnosis

The organism may be found on smears of aspirates from buboes examined with Gram's or immunofluorescent stain. Cultures from blood, buboes, and sputum should be made.

Treatment

Streptomycin is the treatment of choice.

GRANULOMA INGUINALE

Granuloma inguinale (granuloma venereum, donovanosis) is a chronic granulomatous disease caused by *Calymmatobacterium (Donovania) granulomatis,* a gram-negative rod related to *Klebsiella* and other coliform bacilli. In Wright-stained smears from the lesions, the bacilli appear as oval bodies (Donovan bodies) in a large polymorphonuclear cell.

The exact mode of transmission of infection is not understood, but the role of sexual contact is not ruled out. The incubation period is 1–12 weeks.

Clinical Findings

Lesions occur on the skin or mucous membranes of the genitalia or perineal area. Extragenital lesions may also occur. The infection starts as a firm papule or nodule, breaking down into an ulcer with a sharply defined, overhanging edge. The lesions are relatively painless, and there is no adenitis. The lesions enlarge by autoinoculation and peripheral extension with satellite lesions. Scar formation and healing may occur along one border while the opposing side advances.

Secondary infection with spirochete-fusiform bacteria is common, thus complicating the clinical picture and treatment.

Differential Diagnosis

Granuloma inguinale must be distinguished from ulcers of the groin caused by syphilis and carcinoma and from lymphogranuloma of chlamydial origin.

Diagnosis

Smears from the lesions are obtained and examined for diagnostic Donovan bodies. The microorganism may be cultivated in the yolk sac of a chick embryo or on other specially enriched media.

Treatment

Treatment is with tetracycline, 500 mg 4 times daily, or ampicillin, 500 mg 4 times daily, until healing is complete. Gentamicin and chloramphenicol are effective drugs and cure most lesions within 3 weeks. Surgical correction may be required.

NONVENEREAL TREPONEMATOSES

Yehudi M. Felman, MD

Spirochetes of the genus *Treponema* are also responsible for certain diseases that resemble syphilis but do not carry the stigma of a venereal infection. These diseases include (1) nonvenereal syphilis (bejel), (2) yaws, and (3) pinta. All show a similar immune response and cannot be distinguished from one another by serologic reaction. All produce initial lesions followed by extensive secondary manifestations, and all exhibit the phenomenon of latency.

The major difference between these diseases and syphilis is the organs involved in the latter stages of infection. The worldwide distribution of venereal syphilis is in marked contrast to the endemic localization of the other treponematoses; the latter are found most frequently in children up to 15 years of age, and their transmission is strictly nonvenereal. These differences seem to be at least partially determined by the social and physical environment of the host.

Specific antitreponemal humoral antibodies are produced in individuals with bejel, yaws, and pinta, but the time of appearance of antibodies after onset of infection is variable, and seroactivity with nontreponemal antibody tests may take 4 times longer to develop in pinta than in syphilis. The fluorescent treponemal antibody absorption (FTA-ABS) test is a sensitive and specific diagnostic measure during all stages of the nonvenereal treponematoses but cannot differentiate the specific clinical disease. Cross-immunity between the various treponematoses exists, and individuals who have had yaws or pinta are relatively immune to syphilis.

Endemic Nonvenereal Syphilis (Bejel)

The causative organism of bejel is indistinguishable from *Treponema pallidum*.

Endemic syphilis is found today in the Middle East, in African countries bordering on the Sahara Desert, and in the northwestern Cape areas. Foci of endemic syphilis were present in Europe (Yugoslavia) even after World War II but have since been eradicated. Between the wars, the disease extended over wide areas of the southern USSR, Turkey, and Israel. There are also many historical examples, including "sibbens" of Scotland, "button scurvy" of Ireland, and the "radesyge" of Norway. Bejel has not been found in the Western Hemisphere.

Clinical Findings

The primary lesion usually is not observed but probably occurs in the mouth. The principal manifestations are mucous patches or a mucocutaneous lesion resembling the split papules or condylomas of secondary syphilis. Regional lymphadenopathy occurs, but generalized lymphadenopathy is unusual. The skin lesions usually disappear spontaneously within 1 year. Treponemes are abundant in the moist early lesions and in aspirates from regional lymph nodes. After a variable latent period, late lesions may develop. They consist of gummatous ulcerations of the mucous membranes, periostitis of the long bones, and hyperkeratosis of the plantar surfaces of the feet. Gummatous involvement of the mucous membranes of the nasopharynx is also seen.

Other complications of late venereal syphilis such as those of the cardiovascular or central nervous system occur rarely, if at all, in bejel. Individuals suffering from bejel always give positive serologic tests for syphilis.

Treatment

Treatment is similar for all treponematoses: benzathine penicillin G, 2.4 million units intramuscularly in adults, and half this dose (1.2 million units) in children. The result is rapid resolution of lesions.

Procaine penicillin in oil and 2% aluminum mono-stearate (PAM) has also been used. In persons allergic to penicillin, tetracycline hydrochloride, 500 mg 4 times daily for 21 days, is effective. In areas where less than 5% of the population has active disease, cases are managed on an individual basis. All contacts of infected persons are treated epidemiologically with full doses as the recommended treatment.

PINTA
(Mal del Pinto, Carate, Azul, Purpura)

Essentials of Diagnosis

- Enlarging papule at inoculation site.
- Regional lymphadenopathy.
- Later, pintids (papulosquamous).
- Resolve with depigmentation.
- Positive reaginic and antitreponemal antibody tests.

General Considerations

The etiologic agent, *Treponema carateum*, was demonstrated in 1938. Morphologically it resembles *T pallidum* but can be differentiated by specific serologic tests.

Pinta was the first treponematosis to evolve within the Afro-Asian land mass, from which it gained worldwide distribution, finally persisting among underprivileged peoples in more remote areas of Central America and the northern part of the South American continent, being most prevalent today in Mexico, Colombia, Peru, Ecuador, and Venezuela. About three-quarters of a million cases of pinta were believed to exist 29 years ago.

Pinta is almost exclusively limited to the pigmented races and is equally distributed between males and females. It usually affects persons between 10 and 25 years of age.

Clinical Findings

After an incubation period of 7–30 days, the primary lesion develops at the site of inoculation, more often on the extremities, face, neck, or buttocks. A papule increases slowly in size by peripheral extension and by coalescing with smaller satellite papules. Regional lymphadenopathy occurs. The secondary manifestation appears 1 month to 1 year after appearance of the primary lesion, consisting of macules and papules (called "pintids") that rapidly become confluent erythematosquamous plaques. The pintids are initially red but become deeply pigmented, reaching a slate-blue color after a variable period that is related to sun exposure. These pigmented lesions, known as "dyschromic macules," contain treponemes located principally in the epidermis in older lesions. Microscopic examination of these lesions shows increased pigment in the basal cells, with edema and mild inflammation composed of plasma cells and lymphocytes.

Numerous melanophores in the papillary dermis slowly disappear during the healing stage. Within 3 months to 1 year, most pintids show varying degrees of depigmentation, becoming brown and finally white, giving the skin a mottled appearance. The porcelain white achromic lesion represents the "late or tertiary" stage, in which the epidermis is atrophic and melanocytes and melanin are absent. With silver impregnation, spirochetes can readily be demonstrated in skin appendages and epidermis. Serologic reaginic and antitreponemal antibody tests are positive.

Treatment

Treatment is as for bejel (see above).

YAWS
(Frambesia, Pian, Bouba)

Essentials of Diagnosis

- Primary: rapidly enlarging raspberry-like plaque (mother yaw).
- Secondary: generalized scaling macules, papules, or nodules.
- Tertiary: destructive large ulcers.
- Positive reaginic and antitreponemal antibody tests.

General Considerations

The causative organism of yaws is *Treponema pertenue*, which is morphologically indistinguishable from *T pallidum*, though the experimental lesions in rabbits and monkeys are different.

Yaws may have evolved from pinta as a humid, warm environment developed in Afro-Asia. The new climate, resulting in much local moisture from sweating, favored production of exuberant skin lesions containing vast numbers of treponemes such as the papillomas and other infective manifestations characteristic of yaws. The surface lesions of yaws, like those of pinta, may remain infected for long periods. The absence of clothes with resultant exposure to minor trauma facilitates entry of the organism. Person-to-person contact of sweaty skins in a tropical environment facilitates spread among primitive communities and especially among children.

Yaws has been one of the world's most prevalent infections. It occurs mainly between the Tropics of Cancer and Capricorn, though with modern travel, an occasional case is encountered in temperate zones.

In the campaigns against the endemic treponematoses organized by WHO in 46 countries, a total of 160 million people have been examined and 50 million treated with penicillin as clinical cases of yaws or endemic syphilis, or as latent cases or contacts. The incidences of the diseases have been reduced to low levels in many areas, though continued seroactivity suggests that the disease continues in the community, probably subclinically.

Clinical Findings

The incubation period is 10–20 days. The primary lesion (the mother yaw) usually appears on an exposed portion of the body, most commonly the lower extremities, as a small papule that rapidly enlarges, reaching a diameter of several centimeters. It is encrusted, and beneath the crust is a dusky red, elevated, cauliflower-like lesion resembling a raspberry (frambesia). Microscopically, the lesion shows marked hypertrophy of the squamous cell epithelium, with hyperkeratinization and an intense inflammatory process containing polymorphonuclear leukocytes, lymphocytes, and plasma cells. Spirochetes are found in abundance in the lesion and in the regional lymph nodes, which may be enlarged. This lesion may heal spontaneously or persist and ulcerate. Two weeks to several months after the primary lesion appears, the secondary skin eruption occurs, consisting of scaly macules followed by follicular papules or typical frambesia-like nodules that measure 1–2 cm in diameter. The eruption is usually limited to the skin, especially the anogenital and circumoral regions, rarely involving mucous membranes. Occasionally, the lesions will ulcerate and be more destructive. Painful papules sometimes appear on the soles or elsewhere on the feet (crab yaws). This results in a peculiar crablike gait that may persist for life.

The histopathologic features of secondary stage lesions do not differ from those of the primary lesion. Other manifestations of early yaws include lymphadenopathy and nocturnal bone pain due to periostitis. Fever and other constitutional symptoms may occur. Infectious cutaneous relapses can occur at any time during the first 5 years.

Tertiary or late lesions of yaws may develop soon after or during the secondary stage and are responsible for severe disfigurement of some afflicted persons. Lesions consist of chronic ulcers on the face or extremities that heal with deforming scars and contractures. The histology shows endarteritis.

A destructive lesion involving the soft palate, nose, and pharynx is known as "gangosa" or rhinopharyngeal mutilans. Localized gummas on the tibia and radius accompanied by periostitis will produce saber shins and other bone deformities. "Gondou" is a peculiar exostosis of the maxillary bone that may interfere with vision. Hard periarticular nodes, composed of dense connective tissue and central necrosis, may occur near large joints.

Although not thought to have cardiovascular or neurologic complications or to be transmitted to the fetus, ocular abnormalities, raised immunoglobulin levels in the cerebrospinal fluid, and treponemes in the aqueous humor occur in some patients with late yaws.

T pertenue can be demonstrated by darkfield examination in early cutaneous lesions but should not be confused with other spirochetes found in tropical areas. The serum reagin antibody test becomes positive after 1 month, and the FTA-ABS test is also positive.

Treatment

Treatment is as for bejel (see above).

REFERENCES

Aly R, Maibach HI: *Clinical Skin Microbiology: Pathogenic Bacteria and Pathogenic Viruses.* Thomas, 1978.

Aly R, Maibach HI: Skin infections: Fungal and bacterial. In: *Hoechst Medication Update.* Institut Mensch und Arbeit, 1987.

Aly R, Shinefield HR (editors): *Bacterial Interference.* CRC Press, 1982.

Andersen KE: Painful, nonindurated chancre. Acta Derm Venereol (Stockh) 1978;58:554.

Anderson RH, Becker AE: *Cardiac Pathology.* Raven Press, 1983.

Antal GM, Causse G: The control of endemic treponematoses. Rev Infect Dis 1985;7(Suppl. 2):220.

Barksdale L: Leprosy vaccines. (Letter.) Int J Lepr 1983;51:107.

Brachman PS: Anthrax. In: *Clinical Medicine,* vol 11. Spitell JA Jr (editor). Harper & Row, 1980.

Brown JR: Human actinomycosis: A study of 181 subjects. Hum Pathol 1973;4:319.

Browne SF: Yaws. Int J Dermatol 1982;21:220.

Chapel TA: The variability of syphilitic chancres. Sex Transm Dis 1978;5:68.

Chemotherapy of leprosy. (Editorial.) Lancet 1988;2:487.

Clark EG, Danbold N: The Oslo study of the national course of untreated syphilis. Med Clin North Am 1964;48:613.

Collins FM: Mycobacterial disease immunosuppression and an acquired immunodeficiency syndrome. Clin Microbiol Rev 1989;2:360.

Dillon HC Jr: Topical and systemic therapy for pyodermas. Int J Dermatol 1980;19:443.

Eickhoff TC et al: *Pseudomonas pseudomallei:* Susceptibility to chemotherapeutic agents. J Infect Dis 1970;121:95.

Felman YM, Nikitas JA: Neurosyphilis. Sex Transm Dis 1976;3:12.

Felman YM, Nikitas JA: Syphilis serology today. Arch Dermatol 1980;116:84.

Fieldsteel AH, Cox DL, Moeckli RA: Cultivation of virulent *Treponema pallidum* in tissue culture. Infect Immun 1981;32:908.

Fitzgerald F: The great imitator, syphilis. West J Med 1981;134:424.

Fiumara NJ: Reinfection primary and secondary syphilis: The posttreatment serologic response. Sex Transm Dis 1977;4:132.

Fiumara NJ: Treatment of secondary syphilis: An evaluation of 204 patients. Sex Transm Dis 1977;4:96.

Fiumara NJ: Treatment of seropositive primary syphilis: An evaluation of 196 patients. Sex Transm Dis 1977;4:92.

Glassroth J, Robins AG, Snider DE Jr: Tuberculosis in the 1980s. N Engl J Med 1980;302:1441.

Guerrant RL et al: Tickborne oculoglandular tularemia: Case report and review of seasonal and vectoral associations in 106 cases. Arch Intern Med 1976;136:811.

Guthe T et al: Methods for the surveillance of endemic treponematoses and seroimmunological investigations of "disappearing" disease. Bull WHO 1972;46:1.

International symposium on yaws and other endemic treponematoses. Rev Infect Dis 1985;7(Suppl. 2):[Entire Issue].

Jaffe HW et al: Tests for treponemal antibody in CSF. Ann Intern Med 1978;138:252.

Jellard CH: Diphtheria infection in northwest Canada, 1969, 1970 and 1971. J Hyg 1972;70:503.

Kolar OJ, Burkhart JE: Neurosyphilis. Br J Vener Dis 1977;53:221.

Lal S, Nicholas C: Epidemiological and clinical features in 165 cases of granuloma inguinale. Br J Vener Dis 1970;46:461.

Leyden JJ, Kligman AM: Rationale for topical antibiotics. Cutis 1978;22:515.

Luxon LM: Neurosyphilis. Int J Dermatol 1980;19:310.

Maibach HI, Aly R (editors): *Skin Microbiology: Relevance to Clinical Infection.* Springer-Verlag, 1981.

Maibach HI, Aly R, Noble W: Bacterial infections of the skin. Pages 599–642 in: *Dermatology,* 2nd ed. Moschella SL, Hurley HJ (editors). Saunders, 1985.

Noble WC (guest editor): Cutaneous microbiology. Semin Dermatol 1982;1:91. [Entire issue.] a

Perine PL, Hopkins DR et al: *Handbook of Endemic Treponematoses.* World Health Organization, 1984.

Sparling PF: Diagnosis and treatment of syphilis. N Engl J Med 1971;284:642.

Young LS et al: Tularemia epidemic: Vermont, linked to contact with muskrats. N Engl J Med 1969;280:1253.

13

Sexually Transmitted Diseases

Stephen B. Webster, MD & Yehudi M. Felman, MD*

INTRODUCTION

The general term *sexually transmitted diseases (STD)* encompasses the broad or heterogeneous group of infectious diseases known to be associated with sexual activities. It is preferable to the older term *venereal diseases* that was largely limited to the traditional 5 sexually transmitted diseases: syphilis, gonorrhea, chancroid, lymphogranuloma venereum, and granuloma inguinale. The expanding spectrum of sexually transmitted diseases now includes at least 15 established clinical disorders, most of which involve the skin (see Table 13-1). While obviously not all of these conditions are spread exclusively through sexual contact, they frequently may be. The first 14 of these sexually transmitted diseases will be covered in this chapter; AIDS is covered in Chapter 15. Readers should consult the most current STD treatment guidelines (eg, Centers for Disease Control, 1989 Sexually Transmitted Diseases Treatment Guidelines, MMWR;38 [No. S-8]).

A significant increase in the number of patients with sexually transmitted diseases during the past 2 decades has been recognized almost universally. While exact numbers are impossible to determine, the sexually transmitted diseases are probably among the most common infectious diseases in the USA. The reasons for this increase are complex and may include changing attitudes and patterns of sexual behavior (the "sexual revolution"), increased emphasis on sex by the mass media and the motion picture industry, increased population mobility, complacent public belief in "quick cures," increased use of nonbarrier contraceptive measures, and the emergence of drug-resistant organisms.

There are important reasons why the clinician must be aware that a given patient's problems may be the result of sexual activity:

(1) Many of the sexually transmitted diseases can produce serious complications, and they must be diagnosed and treated as soon as possible. Prompt treatment will also prevent spread of the disease.

Table 13–1. Sexually transmitted diseases.

Gonorrhea	Herpes progenitalis
Nongonococcal urethritis	Molluscum contagiosum
Trichomoniasis	Condyloma acuminata
Candidal vaginitis and balanitis	Scabies
Sexual trauma	Pediculosis pubis
Chancroid	AIDS and Kaposi's sarcoma
Lymphogranuloma venereum	coma
Granuloma inguinale	Syphilis

(2) Sexual partners must be identified and promptly evaluated to make sure they receive the benefit of treatment, to prevent reinfection, and to prevent further spread through the community.

(3) A patient with one sexually transmitted disease is often at high risk for others. The patient with "crabs" (pediculosis pubis) or condylomata acuminata, for example, should be evaluated for the possibility of coexistent asymptomatic gonorrhea or syphilis.

(4) Pregnant women with sexually transmitted diseases can infect the fetus in utero or during parturition, often with serious or even fatal consequences.

(5) Safe sexual practices should be discussed with all patients with sexually transmitted diseases—both to prevent reinfection and to prevent the spread of AIDS.

A carefully elicited history of sexual contacts should be taken from all patients with suspected sexually transmitted disease in order to evaluate the total problem; it also provides essential information for public health purposes. The history should include the date of onset of symptoms, the date and nature of sexual exposure, and discussion of sexual partners. Much of this information is regarded as being of a highly personal nature and often is provided either reluctantly or not at all. To extract the most information, a physician should be both sensitive and professional.

No matter how lackadaisical or relaxed a patient may seem when discussing a sexually transmitted disease, this subject is generally associated with considerable anxiety and concern. Feelings of guilt and shame are not uncommon. The social stigma associ-

---

*Dr Felman wrote the section on syphilis for this chapter.

ated with "illicit," "promiscuous," or "unnatural" sexual activities (hence the old term "social disease") and name-case legal reporting requirements may add to the difficulty of obtaining necessary information.

Questioning must be carried out in privacy and in a considerate, objective, nonjudgmental, and non-threatening manner. The patient must be made aware of the necessity of providing such information. Naming contacts and bringing them in for treatment is thus a responsibility that must be shared by both patient and physician.

Although education associated with the AIDS epidemic has markedly changed the sexual practices of many homosexual men, others continue to be sexually active with many different and anonymous partners. Spread of sexually transmitted diseases in this group can be extensive.

An extensive discussion of homosexuality will not be attempted here, but several points are worthy of emphasis:

(1) There is no stereotypical homosexual individual.

(2) Although the homosexual subculture is becoming less hidden, more open, there are still barriers to effective physician-patient communication.

(3) Determining the patient's sexual orientation is an essential first step. Direct, relevant questioning is usually necessary and should convey empathy and understanding rather than homophobia.

(4) Objective, nonjudgmental elicitation of details about the type of homosexual activity engaged in (oral-genital, anal-genital, oral-anal), frequency of contact, number of partners, and dates of occurrence is required.

(5) Large numbers of homosexual patients are at particularly high risk for sexually transmitted infections. This is due to the prevalence of multiple anonymous contacts, difficulty in tracing contacts, and the high incidence of asymptomatic and multiple-site infections.

(6) If one infection is found in a homosexual patient, associated sexually transmitted diseases must be looked for.

The Physician's Role in Prevention of STDs

Considering the serious nature of the sexually transmitted diseases and the fact that some are difficult or impossible to cure, prevention becomes of the utmost importance. The physician should make every effort to discuss the basic principles of prevention of these infections with all patients at risk.

The most important feature of prevention that should be emphasized in discussions with patients is discriminating and fastidious selectivity of sexual partners. Besides limiting the number of sexual partners, it is important to know enough about every sexual partner to be able to evaluate whether he or she might be at risk for having contracted one or more

more STDs in the past. A suspect partner is one with a history of multiple indiscriminate liaisons, contact with bisexual or homosexual persons, or a history of use of intravenous drugs. While it may be difficult to know all the pertinent facts about a potential partner, it is foolhardy to enter into a sexual partnership if pertinent information of this sort is not available.

After emphasizing the importance of selection of sexual partners, the use of condoms as barriers should be discussed with the patient. Condoms are not absolutely protective but do offer some protection.

The CDC in 1988 listed recommendations for the proper use of condoms as follows:

(1) Latex condoms should be used because they offer greater protection against viral STD than natural membrane condoms.

(2) Condoms in damaged packages or those that show obvious signs of age (eg, those that are brittle, sticky, or discolored) should not be used.

(3) Condoms should be handled with care to prevent puncture.

(4) The condom should be put on before any genital contact to prevent exposure to fluids that may contain infectious agents. Hold the tip of the condom and unroll it onto the erect penis, leaving space at the tip to collect seminal fluid.

(5) Adequate lubrication is necessary. If exogenous lubrication is needed, only water-based lubricants should be applied to the condom. Petroleum- or oil-based lubricants (such as petroleum jelly, cooking oils, shortening, and lotions) should not be used because they weaken the latex.

(6) Use of condoms along with spermicidal jellies may provide some additional protection against STD.

(7) If a condom breaks, it should be replaced immediately. If ejaculation occurs after condom breakage, the immediate use of spermicide has been suggested. However, the protective value of postejaculation application of spermicide in reducing the risk of STD transmission is unknown.

(8) After ejaculation, care should be taken so that the condom does not slip off the penis before withdrawal; the base of the condom should be held while withdrawing. The penis should be withdrawn while still erect.

(9) Condoms should never be reused.

SYPHILIS

The treponemal diseases (treponematoses) are a group of diseases caused by spirochetal organisms of the genus *Treponema*. The 3 treponemes pathogenic to man are *Treponema pallidum,* the cause of venereal and nonvenereal syphilis; *Treponema pertenue,* the cause of yaws; and *Treponema carateum,* the cause of pinta.

The only known natural hosts for pathogenic treponemes are humans, higher apes, and rabbits, but all warm-blooded animals so far tested can be successfully infected with *T pallidum*. Lesions can be regularly produced in rabbits; avirulent strains of *T pallidum* are usually maintained in that species.

The treponematoses have been distributed during mass migrations, including religious pilgrimages and the African slave trade. The role of the seaman and soldier in the spread of syphilis and other sexually transmitted diseases is well known. Of no less importance in modern times are migrations of the unemployed in search of work and refugees fleeing from oppression; and the "travel explosion" of tourists who can spread these diseases anywhere in the world. All treponematoses are disabling diseases and should be eradicated by treatment. More than 100 million people still live in endemic areas where 30–40% of the population have treponemal infections.

General Considerations

Syphilis is a chronic systemic infection caused by *T pallidum* and characterized by the appearance, after an incubation period of 10–90 days (averaging 3 weeks), of a primary lesion (chancre) associated with regional lymphadenopathy; a secondary bacteremic stage associated with generalized mucocutaneous lesions and sometimes with lymphadenopathy; a latent period of variable duration—often many years—without clinical findings; and, in 30–40% of untreated cases, a tertiary stage characterized by progressive destructive mucocutaneous or parenchymal lesions, aortitis, or central nervous system diseases.

History

Although venereal disease has existed since recorded history, the first written reference to what has been diagnosed as syphilis dates from 1495, when French soldiers in Naples reported the existence of genital tumors. It is believed that the disease, endemic in the Americas, had been introduced to southern Spain by Columbus's returning sailors. The military upheavals in Europe helped spread syphilis with the virulence of a new plague. The history of syphilis since that time is of great interest, not only because of its clinical and social implications, but because of the succession of important discoveries having an impact on other aspects of medicine: demonstration of a causative spirochete (Schaudinn and Hoffmann, 1905); development of a diagnostic complement fixation blood test (Wassermann, 1906); and the first synthesis of a "specific" chemotherapeutic agent (Ehrlich, 1910).

Etiology

T pallidum is a thin, delicate, spiral organism with 6–14 spirals and tapered ends, measuring 6–15 μm in total length and 0.2 μin width. The cytoplasm is surrounded by a delicate inner mucopeptide layer (the periplast) that provides some structural rigidity, while the outer lipoprotein membrane is selectively perme-

able and osmotically sensitive. Under darkfield examination, it appears as a slowly moving spirochete that flexes and extends itself (whiplash motion) without undulating motion, rotating on its longitudinal axis. *T pallidum* stains with great difficulty, but when impregnated with silver it can be demonstrated in tissue and smears. It induces the production of 2 types of antibodies: reagin and antibodies directly related to the organism.

Outside the host, *T pallidum* is extremely susceptible to physical and chemical agents, which rapidly destroy it. Heat, drying, soap and water, and storage at refrigerator temperatures destroy the organism, though *T pallidum* has been preserved for years by freezing and storing at −78 °C.

Histopathology

Syphilitic infection occurs by penetration of the spirochetes through a microscopic break in the epithelial lining of the mucosa or the skin into the connective tissue. There they multiply and penetrate the lymphatics in the macular lesions.

Histopathologic examination of lesions in the tertiary stage of syphilis shows tissue destruction followed by a reparative inflammation. The tissue destruction may be diffused and not very evident, as seen in chronic degenerative and sclerosing lesions, or it may be massive, as seen in the gumma. The inflammatory response consists of endarteritis with vascular proliferation, perivenular infiltration of plasma cells, macrophages, and fibrosis.

Immunology

Despite centuries of interest in the clinical manifestations of syphilis, the nature of the immune response of the human host to infection with *T pallidum* remains poorly understood. Humans have no natural resistance to infection by pathogenic treponemes, but only about 50% of the named contacts of primary and secondary syphilis become infected. The rate of development of acquired resistance to *T pallidum* following natural or experimental infection is quantitatively related to the amount of antigenic stimulus, which depends upon both the size of the infecting inoculum and the duration of infection prior to treatment. Once the patient is treated, immunity to reinfection is relative and depends on the degree of immunity achieved before treatment and on the interval between treatment and reexposure. With time, there is a slow decline in the level of immunity in any treated patient. The cure of early infectious syphilis with penicillin is so rapid that in 24 hours one cannot detect *T pallidum* in surface lesions. As a consequence, the patient has little time to develop appreciable immunity, and reinfection with primary and secondary syphilis in patients treated with adequate doses of penicillin has been observed regularly. Even a patient previously treated for congenital syphilis, when reinfected years later, may develop darkfield-positive lesions of primary and secondary syphilis.

Both humoral and cellular immunity are involved in the response of the host to infection with *T pallidum*. Specific antibodies that attach to or immobilize *T pallidum* have been identified. Transfer of immune serum from animals or human subjects who have spontaneously recovered from syphilis confers partial protection on rabbits. These data suggest a protective role for antibodies in controlling or preventing infection. However, arguing against this concept are 2 major factors: (1) Syphilis progresses through primary and secondary stages despite the early development and persistence of these antibodies; and (2) very large amounts of serum have been required to protect rabbits against challenge with *T pallidum*, and the immunity conferred is only partial. The onset of this infection is delayed but not eliminated.

Cell-mediated immunity may be important. Delayed hypersensitivity—a reliable index of activation of cellular immunity—appears to treponemal antigen late in secondary syphilis, just prior to onset of latency. Tertiary lesions have a granulomatous appearance, similar to the reaction to organisms that promote a cellular immune response such as the tubercle bacillus or certain fungi. Immunization against challenge with *T pallidum* has required repeated injections of huge doses of killed organisms or inoculation with an attenuated treponeme (analogous to infections known to be mediated by cellular immunity such as brucellosis or tuberculosis).

Epidemiology & Mode of Spread

Since its first appearance in Europe, syphilis has always been largely an urban disease, the majority of cases occurring in cities with a population over 200,000. It is more frequent in young adults 20–24 years of age, followed in descending frequency by adults 25–29 years of age and then by adolescents 15–19 years of age.

The incidence of infectious syphilis is much higher in males than in females, particularly in the primary stage, when lesions may be hidden in the female. Sociologic factors may also be responsible, since the disorder can be spread by homosexual contact, and male homosexuals are more likely to have multiple sexual partners.

Infection is usually spread by sexual exposure, usually sexual intercourse, cunnilingus, or fellatio. Moist kissing can spread syphilis from the mouth. Prenatal transmission is responsible for congenital syphilis. Transfusions and accidental direct inoculations of organisms have also induced disease.

Laboratory Diagnosis

Diagnostic tests for syphilis include serologic tests, methods for demonstrating *T pallidum* in lesions by darkfield (phase contrast microscopy), or staining the treponemes with silver impregnation techniques (Levaditi's stain or Warthin-Starry stain). In the latter, spirochetes can be found in the dermis around capillary walls; these methods also stain reticulum fibers, which can be confused with spirochetes. Histologic examination of tissue using immunofluorescence for detecting treponemes may be fruitful in confirming the diagnosis if the darkfield examination is negative.

Serologic tests for syphilis are based on detection of several different antibodies and are classified by the type of antigen used, ie, nontreponemal (reagin) or treponemal. Nontreponemal tests use purified cardiolipin combined with lecithin to detect reagin in the sera of syphilitic patients and occasionally in individuals with other acute and chronic conditions. Treponemal tests use living or dead *T pallidum*, or fractions of these treponemes, as antigen sources to detect treponemal antibodies.

Quantitative nontreponemal tests are of value because they establish a baseline of reactivity against which future specimens may be compared. They serve as a guide to distinguish early latent from late latent syphilis and help in differentiating between congenital syphilis and passive reaginemia.

There are 2 types of nontreponemal tests for syphilis: flocculation and complement fixation. Although not absolutely specific for syphilis, they screen large populations and identify asymptomatic patients. The most widely used flocculation tests are the Venereal Disease Research Laboratory (VDRL) test, the rapid plasma reagin circle card test (RPR-CT), and the automated reagin test (ART). Complement fixation tests (eg, Wassermann, Kolmer) are no longer used in the USA. Nontreponemal tests are almost invariably reactive in untreated patients by the end of 4 weeks after appearance of the chancre. Approximately 25% of infected patients will be seroreactive 7 days after the appearance of the chancre.

Quantitative results may be obtained by diluting the serum in geometric progression to an end point. The titer is expressed in the highest dilution in which the test is fully reactive. The excessive production of antibody—particularly in the secondary stage of syphilis—occasionally results in the "prozone phenomena": undiluted specimens rarely will give a nonreactive or weakly reactive test result. Testing at higher dilutions, however, gives reactive test results.

A. False-Positive Reactions: Nontreponemal tests may sometimes be reactive in the absence of syphilis, the so-called biologic false-positive reaction. There are 2 types of biologic false-positive reactions: acute and chronic.

The acute reaction occurs in patients whose reagin blood test is reactive for less than 3–6 months. In general, any infectious disease and certain vaccinations and immunizations may be the cause of this reaction. Titers are generally positive at a level of less than 8 dilutions.

Chronic false-positive reactions occur in patients whose reagin blood test remains reactive for more than 6 months. Autoimmune (collagen) diseases commonly cause chronic false-positive reactions as well as viral hepatitis, lepromatous leprosy, metastatic liver disease, malaria, heroin addiction, etc.

Treponemal tests are used to confirm a diagnosis of syphilis. The treponemal antigen tests are more specific than the nontreponemal tests. The use of treponemal tests is clearly indicated for the following: (1) to distinguish reactions due to syphilis from false-positive reactions in nontreponemal tests; (2) to confirm a clinical impression of late syphilis in cases in which the nontreponemal antigen is nonreactive; (3) to resolve cases where there is epidemiologic evidence of syphilis in a marital partner and where repeated nontreponemal antigen tests are nonreactive; and (4) to assist in diagnosing syphilis in a mother who is nonreactive to the nontreponemal antigen test, who shows no clinical evidence of syphilis, and who has a congenitally syphilitic child. The most widely used treponemal test is the fluorescent treponemal antibody-absorption test (FTA-ABS). At present, the FTA-ABS test is the standard of sensitivity for the serodiagnosis of syphilis and is clearly more specific than the VDRL. Unlike the VDRL test, the FTA-ABS test often remains reactive despite adequate antibiotic therapy and therefore is not useful in following the serologic response to therapy. Although the FTA-ABS test is more sensitive than the VDRL in primary disease, this difference is not so great that the FTA-ABS should be ordered when primary syphilitic lesions are manifested. The finding of a clinically suspicious primary lesion and a reactive nontreponemal test are sufficiently specific for the diagnosis of primary syphilis.

An alternative method for detecting treponemal antibodies in serum is based on the ability of the serum to agglutinate tanned erythrocytes previously coated with antigen from *T pallidum*; this is the microhemagglutination test for *T pallidum* (MHA-TP). Like the FTA test, the hemagglutination test was modified to increase specificity by absorption of the serum with Reiter treponeme protein. This test is less sensitive than the FTA-ABS test in primary syphilis, but since treponemal tests are needed less often in primary disease than in other stages, this problem may be minor. Like the FTA-ABS test, the MHA-TP test tends to remain reactive despite antisyphilitic therapy.

B. Darkfield Fluorescent Antibody Test: An alternative to darkfield microscopy is the direct fluorescent antibody test for the identification of *T pallidum* (DFA-TP) in lesions. The few available studies suggest that the sensitivity of the DFA-TP relative to darkfield microscopy ranges from 80–100%.

C. FTA-ABS (IgM) Test: In response to various infections, including congenital syphilis, newborns and young infants have elevated serum levels of immunoglobulin M (IgM). IgM does not normally pass the placenta. The indirect fluorescent IgM test (IgM-FTA-ABS) is specific for congenital syphilis. However, it is not possible to detect IgM initially in the fetus when syphilis occurs late in pregnancy. Death may occur in infected neonates who do not demonstrate IgM levels, and high titers of IgM may develop in infants who do not have congenital syphilis.

D. Interpretation of the Low-Titer Reactive Serologic Test for Syphilis: In cases where the physical examination and history are negative, a low-titer reactive nontreponemal antigen test may be the only indication that a syphilitic infection exists. In evaluating a reactive serologic test with no corroborative evidence, 4 probabilities should be considered: (1) the reaction is due to syphilis and the patient was never treated or was inadequately treated; (2) the patient has had syphilis and was adequately treated in the past and has remained serofast; (3) the reaction is due to some condition or disease other than syphilis (benign false-positive); or (4) the laboratory is in error.

To evaluate a low-titer reactive serologic test, a suggested plan is as follows:

1. Repeat the nontreponemal test at weekly intervals to establish the presence of a static or rising titer.

a. If the second test is nonreactive and a history and repeated physical examination are negative, syphilis is not a likely diagnosis.

b. If the repeated tests show a rising titer of 2 or more dilutions, a diagnosis of syphilis is justified.

c. If the repeated tests show a static titer, the diagnosis is still questionable.

2. If, after repeated nontreponemal tests, the diagnosis is still questionable (the titer remains static or shows a one-dilution greater or lesser change), an FTA-ABS or MHA-TP test should be requested. If the result of the treponemal test is reactive, a diagnosis of syphilis is justified. However, this does not necessarily mean that the patient is infectious or needs treatment.

3. If early syphilis has been excluded, a reactive treponemal test indicates either untreated, inadequately treated, or adequately treated late syphilis. A properly performed nonreactive treponemal test indicates a false-positive treponemal test result. Keep in mind that no serologic test for syphilis is diagnostic by itself or can distinguish between active (never treated or inadequately treated) syphilis and inactive (adequately treated) syphilis. The diagnosis can be made only by considering serologic test results with a careful history and thorough physical examination.

1. PRIMARY SYPHILIS

Essentials of Diagnosis

- Chancre, usually single, painless, and indurated.

- Location usually on external genitalia but may occur elsewhere, including mouth, anus, cervix, or finger.
- *T pallidum* observed by darkfield examination of smears from chancre.
- Serologic test for syphilis usually becomes positive within 4 weeks.

Clinical Findings

A. Symptoms and Signs: Following an incubation period of 10–90 days (average 3 weeks), the primary lesion or chancre develops at the point of inoculation. Variability of the incubation period is related to the number of spirochetes in the inoculum; ie, the incubation period is inversely proportionate to the number of infecting organisms. Subcurative therapy during the incubation period may delay the onset of the primary lesions but does not prevent development of symptomatic disease.

The chancre is classically single and painless, with a smooth, clean base, raised indurated borders, and scanty yellow serous discharge. However, some patients have more than one chancre or indurated or painful chancres. The chancre is initially a papule (0.3–3.0 cm in diameter) that erodes, and the central portion often ulcerates. A grayish, slightly hemorrhagic crust may form. In most cases, the border is regular in outline, but occasionally there is an irregular lesion with indeterminate edges. Circling the margin of the ulcer may be a continuous or stippled line of hemorrhage.

Most chancres in heterosexual males occur on the penis. An intraurethral chancre may present as nongonococcal urethritis. Chancres may also appear on the base of the penis or on the scrotum. In homosexual males, the chancre is often found in the anal canal, within the mouth, on the lips, or on the external genitalia. In women, the most common sites are the labia, the fourchette, the urethra, and the posterior labial commissure. The cervix is probably more frequently involved than statistics indicate. Although most chancres appear on the genitalia, other sites of the body may be involved as a result of preliminary sex play (face, eyelids, breasts, fingers, etc).

Regional lymphadenopathy accompanies the primary lesion. This occurs within 7–10 days of the onset of the lesion in 60–80% of patients. The presence of unilateral or bilateral inguinal lymphadenopathy in primary syphilis is related to the duration of the chancre. Unilateral inguinal nodes accompany penile lesions of short duration, while bilateral adenopathy is associated with lesions of longer duration. Intraoral lesions are accompanied by unilateral lymphadenopathy of the submental and anterior cervical nodes, while chancres of the finger are associated with unilateral axillary nodes. The affected lymph nodes are enlarged, hard, and nonsuppurating.

The chancre heals spontaneously in untreated patients in 3–6 weeks, leaving a thin, atrophic scar, but lymphadenopathy may persist for months. The chancre will heal in patients who have received adequate treatment, usually within 2 weeks. Patients who have been inadequately treated develop a chancre redux (recurrence). Chancres will not develop if the mode of transmission is congenital or via transfusion or inoculation with a hypodermic needle.

B. Laboratory Findings: The diagnosis of primary syphilis can be made by darkfield examination of the early lesion, detecting *T pallidum* before the appearance of antibodies in the blood. Specimens may be taken from moist lesions, abraded dry lesions, and aspirates of regional lymph nodes. *T pallidum* may not be demonstrable in persons who have used topical medication or medicated themselves with antitreponemal drugs. A highly suspicious lesion may require darkfield examination on 2–3 successive days if the initial examination is negative. Concomitant chancroidal lesions or secondarily infected lesions may be treated with sulfonamides (other antibiotics should be avoided) without interfering with follow-up testing procedures for syphilis.

The syphilitic lesions of the primary stage of acquired syphilis are the chancre and regional lymphadenitis. The histopathology of the chancre consists of marked capillary proliferation and an inflammatory exudate composed of lymphocytes, plasma cells, and macrophages. Leukocytes are found mostly in the superficial areas. Spirochetes usually can be found in the dermis around the walls of capillaries with the use of silver staining. The number of spirochetes in the epidermis is small, in contrast to that seen with yaws and pinta. Histologic examination of swollen regional lymph nodes in primary syphilis is usually not done but can reveal a chronic inflammatory infiltrate containing many plasma cells, endothelial proliferation, and follicular hyperplasia. Spirochetes can be found in lymph node aspirates at times when they may not be found in the chancre.

Reagin serologic tests should become reactive in all untreated patients by 4 weeks after appearance of the chancre. Since it takes about 90 days for some chancres to manifest, serologic testing should be extended monthly for 4 months to reliably diagnose syphilis serologically.

The FTA-ABS test is sometimes positive in primary syphilis and can be useful for resolving false-positive reactions, but it is not recommended as a routine screening test for lesion syphilis (see serologic test for syphilis, above).

Differential Diagnosis

Primary syphilis must be differentiated from herpes simplex, chancroid, superinfected lesions (eg, secondarily infected scabies), fixed drug eruption, Behçet's syndrome, psoriasis, erosive balanitis or vulvitis, mycotic infections, squamous cell carcinoma, and other diseases characterized by marginated erythema or ulcers of the genitalia. Painful

Table 13–2. Treatment of Syphilis.

Early Syphilis (Primary, Secondary, and Early Latent)
  Best Choice:
    Benzathine penicillin G, 2.4 million units, 1 dose by IM injection.
  Alternatives for penicillin-allergic, nonpregnant patients:
    Doxycycline, 100 mg orally 2 times daily for 2 weeks, or tetracycline, 500 mg orally 4 times daily for 2 weeks.
  If compliance and follow-up are ensured:
    Erythromycin 500 mg orally 4 times daily for 2 weeks.
Late Latent Syphilis (More Than 1 Year Duration), Gummas and Cardiovascular Syphilis
  Best Choice:
    Benzathine penicillin G, 7.2 million units total, administered as 3 doses of 2.4 million units IM given once weekly for 3 consecutive weeks.
  Alternatives for penicillin-allergic nonpregnant patients (Use alternatives only after CSF examination has excluded neurosyphilis):
    Doxycycline, 100 mg orally 2 times daily for 4 weeks, or tetracycline, 500 mg orally 4 times daily for 4 weeks.
Neurosyphilis
  Best Choice:
    Aqueous crystalline penicillin G, 12–24 million units administered as 2–4 million units every 4 hours IV for 10–14 days.
  Alternatives (if compliance and follow-up are ensured)
    Procaine penicillin, 2–4 million units IM daily, plus probenecid, 500 mg orally 4 times daily, both for 10–14 days
  In addition, after treatment consider giving:
    Benzathine penicillin G, 2.4 million units IM weekly for 3 consecutive doses.
    Re-treat if pleocytosis in CSF has not decreased by 6 months or returned to normal by 2 years.
Follow-up
  Reexamine clinically and serologically at 3 and 6 months. If RPR has not declined by fourfold by 3 months with primary or secondary syphilis, or 6 months in early latent syphilis, or if signs or symptoms persist and reinfection is ruled out, consider CSF exam and re-treat appropriately. For late syphilis, if titers increase fourfold or a high titer fails to decrease, evaluate for neurosyphilis and treat appropriately.
  Testing for HIV infection and counseling are appropriate.

Adapted from 1989 STD Treatment Guidelines. MMWR Sept. 1, 1989;38:1.

anorectal lesions must be differentiated from nonspecific ulcers and fissures, carcinoma, and Crohn's disease.

Treatment (Table 13–2)

Currently penicillin G is the drug of choice for all stages of syphilis. Its antibacterial action affects actively multiplying treponemes. The antibiotic irreversibly binds to the treponeme and interferes with the synthesis of the glycopeptides that are essential constituents of the organism's wall, leading to death of the organism. The efficacy of penicillin treatment has not diminished over 35 years.

Treatment may alter the serologic picture of the patient in some stages or produce no change in other stages. Adequate treatment in the incubation stage of syphilis prevents seroconversion, and the nontreponemal test remains nonreactive. A small number of serologically nonreactive patients may develop tran-

sient reaginemia following penicillin treatment, reverting to seronegativity shortly after therapy. If treatment is given when patients are in the seroreactive-primary stage, seroreversal should be achieved within 1 year. The speed with which this seroconversion occurs depends on the duration of the primary lesions prior to treatment and on the height of the pretreatment titer. Patients with low titer before treatment become seronegative more rapidly than patients with high titers.

All patients who have been exposed to infectious syphilis within the preceding 3 months should be treated empirically, even if they show no evidence of being infected. Treatment is the same as for incubating syphilis.

Patients with syphilis should be re-treated (1) if treatment was suboptimal, (2) if it is not known what treatment has been given, (3) if treatment was with drugs other than those recommended, (4) if clinical signs or symptoms of syphilis persist or recur, (5) if there is a sustained 4-fold increase in the titer of a reagin test or (6) if an initially high-titer reagin test fails to decrease 4-fold within a year.

Prognosis

Cure occurs within a week if penicillin is given; without treatment, the disease usually goes on to clinical secondary syphilis.

2. SECONDARY SYPHILIS

Essentials of Diagnosis

- Often a history of chancre, or the lesion may still be present.
- Generalized lymphadenopathy.
- Typical discrete, sharply demarcated symmetric plaques (papulosquamous).
- Eruption involves trunk and extremities, including palms and soles.
- Low-grade fever, sore throat, headache, arthralgias.
- "Moth-eaten," nonscarring patchy alopecia, condylomata lata, mucous membrane plaques.
- Reactive serologic test for syphilis and FTA-ABS.

Clinical Findings

A. Symptoms and Signs: The secondary stage develops 6–8 weeks after the chancre and usually 6 weeks to 6 months following the original infection. The primary lesions will still be present in over one-third of patients with secondary syphilis, but a latency period often occurs following resolution of the chancres before the appearance of secondary syphilis. Any organ system of the body may be affected during the secondary stage.

Constitutional symptoms may precede or accompany skin and mucous membrane lesions. The patient may complain initially of an influenzalike syndrome with low-grade fever, headache, malaise, sore throat, arthralgias, or myalgias. Generalized lymphadenopathy is characteristic and often precedes the cutaneous manifestations. The lymph nodes may be enlarged, nontender, hard, rubbery, and nonsuppurative. The inguinal, epitrochlear, axillary, cervical (anterior and posterior), suboccipital, submental, and posterior auricular nodes may be enlarged.

Skin lesions of secondary syphilis may mimic any skin disorder, but certain characteristics should suggest syphilitic origin. The eruption is usually generalized, painless, nonpruritic (with the exception of the follicular type), bilateral, and symmetrically distributed in early secondary syphilis. In later stages, the palms and soles are often involved. The lesions are discrete, sharply demarcated, and reddish-brown in color, with intensification of color in the center of the lesion. Four main groups of lesions may be seen in secondary syphilis: macular, papular, papulosquamous, and pustular. Vesicular or bullous lesions are rare in acquired syphilis but occur in congenital syphilis.

Macules are the first type of secondary lesions to appear. Individual lesions are nonpruritic, noninfiltrated, or scaling. On black skin, macular lesions appear darker than the surrounding skin. Macular syphilids may resolve in a few days, progress and disseminate and last for several months, or develop into papular syphilids.

Papules often develop before the macules disappear (maculopapular eruption). They may appear all over the body, be confined to the palms and soles, or localize at other sites. In moist areas of the body with opposing skin surfaces, papular syphilids become rounded, flat-topped, macerated masses (condylomata lata). These lesions are teeming with spirochetes and are highly infectious. They are pink or red except when covered with a mucoid exudate (due to necrosis, in which case they are grayish white). Condylomata lata should be differentiated from venereal warts.

Papular lesions may be follicular. On the scalp, these cause moth-eaten, nonscarring alopecia beginning in the occipital area. Hair loss is not permanent; hair will regrow whether or not the patient is treated. The eyebrows may also lose hair.

Papulosquamous lesions evolve from papules when they begin to scale. Usually the scales are fine and pityriasiform, but they may be so marked as to suggest psoriasis.

Pustules are rare and are usually seen only in patients with a debilitating disease. Deep central necrosis of the papule causes it to be covered by discolored crusts of tissue (rupia). These along with other pustules may suggest chickenpox or generalized impetigo, but drainage of the central lesion elicits very little or no pus.

Mucous membrane lesions (mucous patches) are round, flat, focal white patches surrounded by a red areola. The lesion becomes fissured when located at the angle of the mouth. On the surface of the tongue, the mucous patch appears as an oval or round plaque where the papillae have been flattened. Mucous membrane lesions and condylomata lata are the most infectious lesions of syphilis because of the large number of treponemes in each lesion.

Annular syphilis may be macular, maculopapular, or papular and appears most frequently in black patients at the angles of the mouth, in the nasolabial area, on the chin, and on the mid face. In these locations, the plaques look like rings.

Hyperpigmentation may occur in early secondary syphilis on the skin of the neck and is known as the "collar of Venus." Hyperpigmentation, fading gradually, may also occur as the papules resolve.

Other organs may also be involved in secondary syphilis. Hepatitis may be manifested as an enlarged liver or abnormalities of liver function tests, especially elevation of alkaline phosphatase, without symptoms. Membranous glomerulonephritis is manifested as the nephrotic syndrome. Involvement of the vocal cords may cause hoarseness. Periostitis is uncommon, affecting the anterior tibia, and is characterized by bone pain, particularly at night, and exacerbated by immobilization. Iritis is rare.

B. Laboratory Findings: Darkfield examination of secondary lesions usually demonstrates *T pallidum*. The reagin test should be reactive at a titer usually greater than 1:16, except for the "prozone phenomenon" (see serologic test for syphilis, above) that occurs in less than 1% of patients with secondary syphilis. Occasionally, histologic examination of tissue using immunofluorescence for detecting treponemes may be fruitful in confirming the diagnosis if darkfield examination is negative. The FTA-ABS test is always positive at this stage.

The histopathology of the secondary lesions is similar to that of the primary chancre but with more pronounced capillary damage followed by capillary proliferation. Large macrophages appear, occasionally forming giant cells resembling the Langerhans type of giant cells found in tuberculosis. Spirochetes are demonstrable in papular lesions—especially condylomata lata—but not in the macular lesions.

Differential Diagnosis

Syphilis has been called "the great imitator," and with good reason. Syphilis can mimic most other dermatologic diseases, especially in its secondary stage, depending upon morphology. Among these diseases are pityriasis rosea, tinea versicolor, tinea corporis, psoriasis, parapsoriasis, lichen planus, drug reactions, and scabies. Pustular forms suggest varicella, acne, impetigo, iododerma, and pyoderma. Annular forms suggest sarcoidosis, granuloma annulare, and erythema multiforme. The alopecia, mucous patches, and condylomata lata also have differential diagnoses, but usually the combination of skin lesions with these conditions helps establish a diagnosis of syphilis.

Treatment

If treatment is given during the secondary stage, seronegativity should be achieved within 2 years. The results of treatment in the latent or late stages of syphilis vary, but as a rule the response is better if treatment is instituted earlier in the course of the disease.

Some other general comments on treatment and follow-up are given later in this chapter.

3. LATENT SYPHILIS

Latent syphilis is that stage of untreated disease in which there are no clinical signs or symptoms, the spinal fluid is negative, and serologic tests for syphilis are reactive. All syphilis is latent at some time during its course; some cases may be latent for the duration of the disease or the life of the patient. The diagnosis of latent syphilis is made on the basis of repeated reactive serologic tests in the absence of concurrent disease that may produce a false-negative reaction. A treponemal test (FTA-ABS) is indicated to establish the syphilitic nature of the serologic test reactivity.

4. LATE SYPHILIS

Latent syphilis is classified in early and late stages. It is early latent syphilis when the patient has a history of—or lesions consistent with—primary or secondary syphilis within the preceding year or a nonreactive serologic test for syphilis within the preceding 4 years. In 1972, early latent syphilis was subclassified by the World Health Organization as "early latent syphilis under 1 year" and "early latent syphilis of 1–4 years." Early latent syphilis is potentially infectious sexually because of the frequency of relapsing secondary syphilis during this period. Approximately 25% of untreated patients will experience one or more subsequent generalized or localized mucocutaneous relapses at some time during the first 2–4 years after infection.

Late latent syphilis begins 4 years after infection in the untreated patient; it is associated with immunity to infectious relapse and with resistance to reinfection. *T pallidum* may still intermittently seed the bloodstream during this stage, and pregnant women with latent syphilis may infect the fetus in utero. Untreated late latent syphilis may have 3 possible outcomes: (1) it could persist throughout the life of the individual; (2) it could develop into late syphilis; or (3) it could end with spontaneous cure of infection with reversion of

the serologic test to negative. However, although 50–70% of untreated patients with late latent syphilis never develop clinically evident late syphilis, most experts doubt the possibility of spontaneous cure.

5. TERTIARY SYPHILIS

Essentials of Diagnosis

- Neurosyphilis: convulsions, diplopia, deafness, hemiplegia or coma, general paresis, tabes dorsalis, Argyll-Robertson pupil, Charcot joints.
- Cardiovascular: coronary artery disease, aortic valvular insufficiency, aortic aneurysm, cardiac failure.
- Skin: Solitary, indurated, chronic, destructive annular nodules or deep-seated plaque (gumma).

General Considerations

Untreated late syphilis may present a tremendous range of signs and symptoms, varying from none to those indicating severe damage to one or more body systems. One-third of patients with untreated latent syphilis develop clinically apparent tertiary disease.

Clinical Findings & Diagnosis

A. Neurosyphilis: One of the most severe forms of tertiary syphilis is neurosyphilis. The classic course of untreated syphilis is documented by the Oslo study (1891–1951). Neurosyphilis is more frequent in males than in females.

1. Symptoms and signs– Early in syphilis, even before the primary lesion appears, treponemes disseminate through blood and lymphatics to all tissues, including the brain. In spite of the presence of slight change in the cerebrospinal fluid, there are usually no symptoms until the tertiary stage. In a small number of cases (about 10%), meningitis occurs with neck stiffness, headache, and marked cerebrospinal pleocytosis. Cerebrospinal fluid findings invariably return to normal when the patient is treated with standard penicillin regimens. Cerebrospinal fluid examination is not recommended for cases of syphilis that are known to be under 1 year's duration.

Neurosyphilis may be classified into 3 groups: (1) asymptomatic, (2) meningeal and vascular or cerebrospinal, and (3) parenchymatous.

In symptomatic neurosyphilis, patients with latent syphilis show no neurologic abnormalities but the cerebrospinal fluid shows pleocytosis, elevated protein levels, or a positive cerebrospinal fluid serologic test for syphilis (STS). Untreated asymptomatic neurosyphilis may spontaneously remit, persist in latent form, or progress to symptomatic neurosyphilis. The probability of progression to clinical neurosyphilis in patients with untreated asymptomatic neurosyphilis is about 20% in the first 10 years of infection and increases with the passage of time. If treatment is instituted in the asymptomatic stage, progression to symptomatic involvement is usually prevented.

Although symptomatic neurosyphilis is described as having distinct clinical entities, it is likely that they are all part of continuing destructive luetic syphilitic meningovascular disease. In meningovascular neurosyphilis, there are definite signs and symptoms of central nervous system damage resulting from cerebrovascular occlusion, infarction, and encephalomalacia. Focal neurologic signs vary with the size and location of the lesion. In some cases, arachnoiditis and inflammation of leptomeninges can obstruct the foramen of Luschka and Magendie with resultant hydrocephalus and Argyll-Robertson pupils. Convulsions, focal seizures, strokes, hemianopia, diplopia, deafness, hemiplegia, and coma are common.

Parenchymatous neurosyphilis represents a mixture of an inflammatory and degenerative process due to destruction of nerve cells, principally in the cerebral cortex. Its manifestations are as follows: (1) Paresis, whose manifestations include psychiatric changes, dementia, memory loss, affect disturbances, speech disorders, tremors, convulsions, or paralysis. Without treatment, this form of neurosyphilis leads to death. Unlike other forms of neurosyphilis, 60–70% of patients with paresis may continue to progress despite adequate therapy. (2) Tabes dorsalis (progressive locomotor ataxia) with ataxia (Romberg's sign is classically present), visceral crisis, loss of reflexes, and impaired sensation (vibratory, temperature, position, deep pain). The loss of pain sensation may result in trophic degenerative joint disease (Charcot's joints). Perforating ulcers (mal perforans) on the soles and toes may be associated with loss of deep pain. Pupillary abnormalities include the Argyll-Robertson pupil (normal reaction to accommodation, complete absence of response to light). Optic atrophy and sensory neural deafness may also occur. Tabetic crises are lightning pains of the legs and trunk lasting 1 or 2 seconds and following the path of the dorsal nerve roots.

2. Diagnosis– The diagnosis of neurosyphilis is based on clinical evidence (neurologic or psychiatric abnormalities), serologic tests, and examination of the cerebrospinal fluid. The classic symptoms and signs described above currently are seen less frequently due to increased use of antibiotics for unrelated illness. Reagin (VDRL) testing of the cerebrospinal fluid establishes the diagnosis of asymptomatic neurosyphilis and differentiates symptomatic neurosyphilis from other diseases with similar clinical findings. A reactive cerebrospinal fluid reagin (VDRL) test is usually an indication of neurosyphilis. However, false-positive reactions may occur, though much less often than serologic biologic false-positives. Meningococcal, benign lymphocytic, and tuberculous meningitis, subarachnoid hemorrhage, cerebral malaria, and neoplasms may cause false-positive cerebrospinal fluid serologic tests. Ad-

ditionally, cerebrospinal fluid (with reactive blood serum) contaminated by a bloody lumbar puncture containing sufficient blood to be microscopically visible can produce a false-positive cerebrospinal fluid serologic reaction.

Since cerebrospinal fluid reagin tests do not distinguish between past untreated or inadequately treated infection and present infection, they cannot be used to reflect activity of neurosyphilis. Activity of neurosyphilis is usually determined by other criteria, usually the pleocytosis (> 5 lymphocytes/μL) and elevated protein (> 40 mg/dL). Following effective treatment of active neurosyphilis, the cell count is the first test to become normal (within 6 months); then the increased protein values (2 years) and the VDRL (many years) become negative, though the usefulness of the cerebrospinal fluid reagin test following response to therapy is diminished. Patients with active progressive neurologic disease and reactive serologic tests of cerebrospinal fluid or serum may have normal cerebrospinal fluid cell counts and normal total protein values. In such cases, activity of neurosyphilis may be determined by the presence of plasma cells in the cerebrospinal fluid, increased concentration of cerebrospinal fluid IgG, immunoelectrophoretic abnormalities of cerebrospinal fluid IgG, and an increased serum level of IgM. Conversely, nonreactive results may be found in patients with late neurosyphilis of the tabetic type.

Cerebrospinal fluid reagin tests are rather insensitive and may be falsely nonreactive in many cases of neurosyphilis. The diagnostic value of the cerebrospinal fluid FTA tests in patients with neurosyphilis is unclear. These tests may be reactive in patients with symptomatic neurosyphilis as well as syphilitic patients with no evidence of neurosyphilis. Conversely, nonreactive results may be found in patients with late neurosyphilis. The diagnosis of neurosyphilis thus should not be made on the basis of a single laboratory test but should be based on a critical evaluation of all clinical and laboratory investigations.

B. Cardiovascular Syphilis:

1. Symptoms and signs– The onset of cardiovascular symptoms occurs 10–40 years after infection with *T pallidum*. The cardiovascular manifestations are caused by damage to the vessels that provide the blood supply to the heart. Involvement usually begins as an arteritis in the supracardiac portion of the aorta (ascending and transverse segment of the arch) and progresses to cause the following: (1) narrowing of the coronary ostia, with resulting decreased coronary circulation, angina, cardiac insufficiency, and acute myocardial infarction; (2) scarring of the aortic valves, producing aortic insufficiency, with an aortic diastolic murmur, frequently an aortic systolic murmur, cardiac hypertrophy, and eventually cardiac insufficiency; and (3) weakness of the aortic wall, with saccular aneurysm formation and pressure symptoms (dysphagia, hoarseness, back pain).

Syphilitic aneurysms are usually saccular, occasionally fusiform, and do not lead to dissection. Asymptomatic syphilitic aortitis may be suspected if linear calcification of the ascending aorta is demonstrated on chest x-ray, since arteriosclerotic disease seldom produces the sign. About one in 10 aortic aneurysms of syphilitic origin involves the abdominal aorta, usually above the renal artery, whereas arteriosclerotic abdominal aneurysms usually are found below the renal artery. The nervous system is also affected in 40% of patients with cardiovascular syphilis. Cardiovascular complications are common and occur at an earlier age in men than in women, and more often in blacks than in whites.

2. Diagnosis– Serologic tests for syphilis are usually reactive in cardiovascular syphilis. Since the treponemal tests are more sensitive than the reaginic tests in late syphilis, the FTA-ABS or MHA-TP tests in serum should be part of the diagnostic workup.

C. Late Lesions of the Eyes: Iritis associated with pain, photophobia, and dimness of vision or chorioretinitis can occur during secondary syphilis and also as a relatively common manifestation of late and tertiary syphilis. Adhesions of the iris to the anterior lens (synechiae) may produce a fixed pupil—not to be confused with Argyll-Robertson pupil. Optic atrophy may cause blindness.

D. Late Benign Syphilis: The essential lesion of late benign syphilis is a granuloma, the gumma. The term "benign" is used because these lesions seldom result in total physical incapacity or death, though when gummas occur in the brain or other vital organs, the word benign is misleading. Gummas may be multiple or diffuse but are usually solitary lesions varying from microscopic in size to several centimeters in diameter and are probably the result of cellular hypersensitivity to relatively few treponemes. In areas where syphilis is endemic in childhood, when one member of a household acquires a fresh infection, other members who become reinfected develop gummas. Experimental inoculation of *T pallidum* into individuals with latent or late syphilis also sometimes results in gumma formation at the inoculation site. The most commonly involved sites are the skin, skeletal system, mouth and upper respiratory tract, larynx, liver, and stomach, but any organ may be involved.

Skin lesions tend to form violaceous indurated circles or segments of circles, are destructive and chronic, and tend to heal centrally and extend peripherally. They respond rapidly to a therapeutic trial of penicillin. Bone lesions are usually marked by periostitis with associated new bone formation or by gummatous osteitis with bone destruction. Gummas of the upper respiratory tract can lead to perforation of the nasal septum or hard palate. In late benign syphilis serologic tests are almost always reactive and usually of high titer.

Treatment

If treatment is given in late latency, 20–30% of the patients are nonreactive within 5 years. Treatment of late syphilis may also be followed by a serologic decline in titer over a period of time. As in late latent syphilis, not more than 20–30% of the patients become nonreactive within 5 years after penicillin treatment. In the majority of cases of latent and late syphilis, the posttreatment titer changes little or not at all; it should not be used to gauge adequacy of treatment. However, if there is a sustained 4-fold increase in the titer of a nontreponemal test, the disease is active and treatment should be reinstituted.

Careful posttreatment follow-up of patients with neurosyphilis is important. Clinical evaluation and cerebrospinal fluid examinations should be done at 6 weeks, 3 months, and 6 months following completion of therapy. Additionally, annual cerebrospinal fluid examinations should be performed for several years after treatment to determine inactivity of the disease.

Patients with advanced neurosyphilis may present special problems in management. Optic atrophy and eighth nerve deafness require both penicillin and corticosteroid therapy. If there is a progression of the disorder, higher doses of corticosteroids (30–60 mg daily) may be beneficial. Cases of tabes dorsalis with atonic bladder may require catheterization or the teaching of bladder drill. Lightning pains are often controlled with codeine, but for intractable pain, corticosteroids, phenytoin, or carbamazepine may be indicated if necessary. In severe cases, cordotomy should be considered. Charcot's arthropathy may cause severe joint destruction, necessitating orthopedic supports. Cases of general paralysis may require long-term institutional care if clinical progression continues (in spite of repeated penicillin therapy) and severe mental derangement occurs.

6. CONGENITAL SYPHILIS

Essentials of Diagnosis

- Vesicles or bullae.
- Snuffles (rhinitis), with white or blood-tinged discharge.
- Lymphadenopathy or hepatomegaly.
- Osteochondritis or periostosis, seen by x-ray examination.
- Later, nerve deafness, interstitial keratitis, notched incisor teeth and maldeveloped molar teeth, and Clutton's joint.

General Considerations

The chances of a fetus becoming infected with congenital syphilis depend on the stage of maternal infection, the duration of the disease in the mother, and when treatment is started. The mother with untreated primary or secondary syphilis represents a greater hazard to her fetus than one with latent syphilis, but an infected and untreated mother can infect her fetus long after she is no longer infectious to a sex partner. The longer the mother has had the disease, the less chance of fetal infection, but the possibility of fetal infection is never entirely eliminated.

Treponemes cross the placenta as early as 8–9 weeks' gestation. The earliest syphilitic lesions become apparent after the fetus becomes immunocompetent (18–24 weeks' gestation).

Clinical Findings & Diagnosis

The clinical manifestations of congenital syphilis have been divided into early manifestations (appearing in the first 2 years of life) and late manifestations (any time thereafter). Late congenital syphilis is not infectious.

There are no lesions in congenital syphilis corresponding to the primary stage in acquired syphilis. When a chancre is present, it is acquired when passing through the birth canal.

A. Early Congenital Syphilis: Skin manifestations are similar to those seen in acquired secondary syphilis. The eruption usually appears 2 or more weeks after birth. Vesicles and bullae are associated with a poor prognosis when they appear on the palms and soles. Snuffles (rhinitis) produces a whitish and sometimes blood-tinged nasal discharge. Lymphadenopathy is common. Hepatosplenomegaly can be present; jaundice may be severe. Before osseous involvement is shown radiologically, movement of an infant's extremity causes pain so severe that the child will not move it (Parrot's syphilitic pseudoparalysis). Roentgenographic changes in the bone (osteochondritis and periostitis) are of great diagnostic value, especially when serologic and clinical findings are ambiguous. The changes are usually present at birth but may appear in the first few weeks of life.

Two clinical forms of renal involvement have been described: the nephrotic syndrome and acute glomerulonephritis. Abnormalities in the cerebrospinal fluid include mononuclear pleocytosis, increased protein, and a positive VDRL test.

B. Late Congenital Syphilis: The classic Hutchinson's triad consists of eighth nerve deafness, interstitial keratitis, and hutchinsonian incisors (notched barrel-shaped central incisors). Mulberry molars or Moon's teeth (maldevelopment of the cusps of the first molars) are also characteristic of congenital syphilis. Deciduous teeth are not deformed. Involvement of the eighth cranial nerve may occur without other detectable central nervous system changes and can lead to deafness. Any part of the skeletal system may be involved. Bones may be sclerotic (tibial osteitis), producing the characteristic anterior-curving saber shin, or be lytic due to gummas. Clutton's joint is syphilitic symmetric synovitis

of the knees without bone or cartilage involvement. Perioral dermatitis leads to atrophic fissures and the characteristic "rhagades."

If the many signs and symptoms pointing to early congenital syphilis are considered, there is little or no difficulty in diagnosing the disease. The asymptomatic mother and infant with reactive blood tests, however, may pose diagnostic problems. All pregnant women should have a VDRL test performed during the first and third trimesters. If the VDRL test is reactive, an FTA-ABS test should be done to confirm the diagnosis. If syphilis is suspected on the basis of the history and physical signs, the prospective mother should have VDRL and FTA-ABS tests done simultaneously.

If the FTA-ABS test has been positive in the past, a repeat test will not help because it remains positive for life, even with adequate treatment. For the woman with a history of syphilis or of positive serologic tests for syphilis, the clinician must ascertain the nature of previous treatment and the clinical and serologic responses to it. If the mother has been adequately treated before this pregnancy and is still VDRL-positive, passive transfer of reagin (IgG) to the infant commonly occurs. When investigating possible infection in the infant, perform an initial quantitative reagin test in both the baby and mother. Weekly quantitative tests are done on the infant for the first month. If there is passive reagin transfer with no infection, there will be a drop in the quantitative blood test titer, in which case the infant's blood should be tested every 2 weeks during the second month. The blood test usually becomes negative by the end of the third month. The passive transferred reagin (VDRL) antibody usually declines in titer before the passively acquired FTA antibody disappears. Since the IgM-FTA-ABS test findings may be false-positive or false-negative, they should not be used as a screening tool.

Treatment

Treatment of the pregnant woman with syphilis before the eighth to 18th weeks of gestation will prevent the stigmas of congenital syphilis. Treatment is not necessary if there is documented evidence of adequate prior treatment for syphilitic infection and clinical laboratory evidence to rule out a relapsing state. If there is any doubt as to adequacy of prior treatment or evidence of a clinical or serologic relapse, re-treatment should be administered.

Although erythromycin is the drug of choice in the treatment of pregnant women who are allergic to penicillin, this drug has poor placental transfer and erratic absorption. Plasma levels of erythromycin in the fetus are about 6–20% of the maternal plasma levels; close follow-up of clinical manifestations and serologic tests are important in both the mother and neonate.

In congenital syphilis, the recommended follow-up should begin with repeated clinical examinations to document resolution of active lesions. A pretreatment quantitative VDRL test establishes a baseline titer. For children under age 2 years, a quantitative VDRL test on serum is recommended at monthly intervals for 6 months, then at 3-month intervals for 1 year. Generally, in children under age 2 years, lesions heal rapidly with treatment, and the VDRL reverts to non-reactive. However, loss of reactivity in the spinal fluid takes many months to occur. Skeletal changes may not disappear radiographically for a long time, even when the mother received an adequate course of therapy during pregnancy. Untreated early congenital syphilis frequently subsides, but *T pallidum* can persist in the tissues. The infant soon becomes noncontagious. However, a congenital syphilitic female can transmit syphilis to her offspring. In late congenital syphilis, antibiotic therapy is generally similar to that for early congenital syphilis, but interstitial keratitis will require additional treatment with topical corticosteroids and cycloplegics. In cases presenting with interstitial keratitis, optic atrophy, chorioretinitis, and iritis, ophthalmologic consultation is mandatory.

Jarisch-Herxheimer Reaction (Therapeutic Shock)

This is a dramatic reaction occurring within the first 12 hours of treatment with any antitreponemal agent. There is a rise in temperature (38.3–38.9 °C [101–102 °F]) with chills, malaise, and arthralgia, accompanied by exacerbation of symptoms. Symptoms usually subside within 24 hours. Herxheimer reactions are most marked in stages in which treponemes are abundant (secondary stage and general paresis). Although the reaction is benign in secondary syphilis and indicates a favorable response to treatment, in neurosyphilis—particularly in paresis—the Herxheimer reaction may in rare cases be severe. Convulsions, rapid deterioration of paresis, progression of optic atrophy, exacerbation of lightning pain, or hemiplegia may occur. In such cases, it is customary to administer corticosteroids by mouth to alleviate or minimize the reaction (5 mg of prednisone every 6 hours).

The pathogenesis of the Herxheimer reaction may involve release of endotoxin in tissue. Patients should be warned to expect such symptoms, which usually can be managed with bed rest and aspirin.

GONORRHEA

Essentials of Diagnosis
- Dysuria and yellowish, thick urethral discharge in the male.

- Female patients are often asymptomatic but may present with symptoms of pelvic inflammatory disease.
- The possibility of asymptomatic urethral infection in the male should be considered.

General Considerations

Gonorrhea is an infection produced by the gram-negative diplococcus *Neisseria gonorrhoeae* (gonococcus). About 3 million persons are infected with this disease organism each year in the USA. The incidence is highest in the age group from 20 to 24, but gonorrhea is increasing most rapidly in the 15- to 19-year-old age group. Gonorrhea is more common in males than in females.

The bacterium lives in the genital tract, anal canal, and oropharynx and is thus primarily spread sexually from these sites. The most common spread is by genital-to-genital contact. However, anal-genital contact can produce gonococcal proctitis, and oral-genital contact can produce gonococcal pharyngitis. The organism can survive in moist, warm areas away from the body for a short period, but transmission from these areas is extremely infrequent.

The gonococcus is a gram-negative diplococcus that can tolerate oxygen but requires 2–10% CO_2. It is a glucose fermenter, is oxidase-positive, and lives intracellularly. Pathogenic gonococci possess pili, tiny filamentous surface structures that allow them to adhere to the mucosal cells of the host. As the bacteria die, they release an endotoxin that elicits the purulent discharge.

Clinical Findings
A. Symptoms and Signs:
1. Symptomatic infection in the male– The average incubation period is 3–5 days, with a range of 1 day to 2 weeks. The first symptom is moderately severe burning with urination. A thick yellowish-brown urethral discharge is usually present and tends to be most abundant in the morning. Inguinal adenopathy occurs, especially in very active persons. Epididymitis, seminal vesiculitis, and prostatitis may occur but usually develop much later.

2. Asymptomatic infection in the male– Some men have infections without discharge or other symptoms. The diagnosis depends on isolating the organism by culturing material taken from the urethral meatus. A sexually active male with asymptomatic infection can nevertheless transmit the disease to unsuspecting females who in turn may remain asymptomatic for long periods. Certain strains of the gonococcus are more likely to cause asymptomatic infection. Ten percent—perhaps as many as 15% of infected males are asymptomatic and thus represent a significant reservoir for the spread of the disease.

3. Uncomplicated infection in the female– Fifty to 60 percent of females with endocervical gonorrhea are asymptomatic. Uterine tube infection can produce pelvic inflammatory disease. Nonspecific symptoms such as vaginal discharge, dysuria, and abnormal uterine bleeding may occur. Urethral infection in the female is unusual.

4. Pelvic inflammatory disease– Pelvic inflammatory disease (PID), primarily salpingitis or endometritis, occurs in at least 20% of females with gonorrhea. The infection results from ascending infection from the endocervical area and usually develops 1–2 months after the initial infection. The risk is greater in patients with an intrauterine contraceptive device. Only about half of all cases of pelvic inflammatory disease are due to *N gonorrhoeae*.

The symptoms of pelvic inflammatory disease are fever, lower abdominal pain, and pain during intercourse or gynecologic examination when the cervix is moved. There is usually adnexal tenderness and sometimes an adnexal mass.

5. Disseminated gonococcal infection– Disseminated gonococcal infection frequently has its onset during menstruation. Commonly presenting as the dermatitis-arthritis syndrome, patients suddenly develop chills, fever, and joint pains, especially in the joints of the hands and feet. This early joint involvement is basically a tenosynovitis.

The skin eruption starts as an inflammatory macule that becomes purpuric, pustular, and eventually necrotic (Fig 13–1). The skin lesions are usually acral in location and often occur on the lateral aspects of the fingers and toes. The classic pustulonecrotic skin lesions, fever, and tenosynovitis are seen early in the bacteremic stage of disseminated gonococcemia,

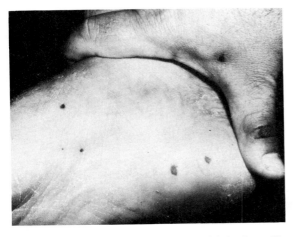

Figure 13–1. Disseminated gonococcal infection with the typical necrotic hemorrhagic lesions on the hands and feet.

which may last 3–5 days. Culture of blood may isolate gonorrhea at this time.

As the infection progresses, the skin lesions resolve, but the patient may develop monarticular septic arthritis. This usually involves the large weight-bearing joints, which can become exquisitely tender, red, and swollen. Gonococcal arthritis is the most common cause of acute arthritis in young adults.

6. Anorectal gonorrhea– Infection of the anal area is usually the result of anal-genital sexual activity. On occasion, a woman with endocervical gonorrhea may infect the rectum directly without anal sexual contact. Anal gonorrhea is usually asymptomatic, but approximately 10% of patients have symptomatic proctitis with rectal bleeding, discharge, and tenesmus.

7. Oropharyngeal gonococcal infection– Among patients with gonorrhea, pharyngeal infection is seen in approximately 20% of homosexual men, 10% of women, and 3% of heterosexual men. Most such cases are asymptomatic, but a small percentage may be associated with sore throat with erythema of the pharynx and occasionally a purulent exudate on the tonsils.

B. Laboratory Findings: The diagnosis of gonorrhea is made by direct smear and by culture. In the symptomatic male with a purulent urethral discharge or gonococcal proctitis, material may be collected from the urethra or anal canal and spread on a glass slide, heat-fixed, and stained with Gram's stain. The gram-negative intracellular diplococcus can be easily identified in the polymorphonuclear leukocyte (Fig 13–2). In gonorrhea involving virtually all other areas, culture of the exudate is necessary because the smear is insensitive and of limited value.

Thayer-Martin medium is used for culture. This is an enriched "chocolate" agar containing antimicrobial agents to prevent bacterial contamination and overgrowth. It is available commercially in plates and in packages that contain a source of CO_2, so the culture plate can be readily sent through the mail. It is often advantageous to culture several anatomic sites of infection regardless of presenting symptoms. The culture is taken from the endocervix (not the vagina), pharynx, or rectum with a cotton-tipped applicator and inoculated on the plate. Menstruation is not a contraindication to the examination; actually, cultures are more apt to be positive during the first 5 days of the cycle. For the male urethra, the small calcium alginate-tipped swab should be inserted 2–4 cm into the urethra to obtain the specimen. The plate is then inoculated with either the calcium alginate swab or the ordinary cotton swab and is then placed in a CO_2 atmosphere and incubated at 35–37 °C. Commercial culture systems with self-contained CO_2 atmosphere are incubated in a similar manner and can be sent through the mail to the laboratory. Properly done, the culture is a sensitive test, but the gonococcus is a delicate, fastidious bacterium, so care must be taken

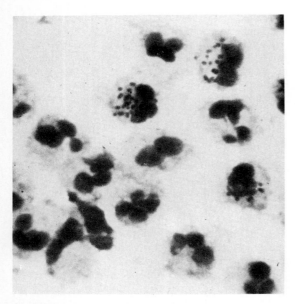

Figure 13–2. The gram-negative intracellular diplococcus, *Neisseria gonorrhoeae,* in the exudate of a male patient with urethral gonorrhea.

to warm the plate to room temperature, obtain the specimen correctly, and place the inoculated plate in a CO_2 atmosphere as quickly as possible.

Blood cultures may be positive in the early bacteremic stage of the dermatitis-arthritis syndrome, but this is not common. A specific fluorescent antibody test can be utilized to detect *N gonorrhoeae* in blood and skin lesions, and a solid phase enzyme immunoassay test is now available (Gonozyme) that may offer help in some clinical situations.

Differential Diagnosis

In the symptomatic male, gonorrhea must be differentiated from nongonococcal urethritis. A smear reveals the gram-negative intracellular diplococcus in gonorrhea. Other microbial agents cause pelvic inflammatory disease in about 50% of cases (eg, chlamydia, anaerobes, and virtually any organism indigenous to or normally a member of the lower vaginal or intestinal flora).

Complications

The male with untreated gonococcal urethritis may develop prostatitis, seminal vesiculitis, epididymitis, urethral stricture, and sterility. In the female, the most serious complication is sterility due to tubal scarring associated with salpingitis. Spread into the bloodstream may cause fever, septic arthritis of one or more joint, and infective pustules, often on the fingers.

Prevention

Sexual contact with an infected individual should be avoided. The condom offers some—but not complete—mechanical protection if used properly. Intravaginal spermicidal creams may reduce the risk of infection.

Treatment

The current guidelines for treatment of sexually transmitted diseases as published by the Centers for Disease Control should be followed. Ceftriaxone, 250 mg intramuscularly once, plus doxycycline, 100 mg orally 2 times a day for 7 days, is currently recommended for uncomplicated gonorrhea in adults. Long-acting penicillin is not used, because it does not produce adequate blood levels. Amoxicillin, 3 g, or ampicillin, 3.5 g, with 1 g of probenecid orally can be given as a single oral dose.

Sexual partners of patients with gonorrhea should be examined, cultured, and treated with one of the therapeutic regimens outlined above. The most current recommendations for the therapy of gonorrhea as published by the CDC should be consulted for specific situations.

Follow-Up, Course, & Prognosis

An initial serologic test for syphilis should be obtained at the time of diagnosis, because the patient with one sexually transmitted disease is at risk for having other sexually transmitted diseases. If the initial serologic test is negative, it does not have to be repeated in patients treated with penicillin, because penicillin will also cure incubating syphilis. In patients treated with other antibiotics, the serologic test should be repeated in 3 months.

Follow-up cultures should be done in 4–8 days to test for cure. The patient should abstain from sexual activity until the culture has been shown to be negative.

The patient with gonorrhea must be reported to the local public health department. The sexual partners must be identified and treated. This is the responsibility of the physician who treated the initial patient.

CHLAMYDIAL INFECTIONS (Nongonococcal Urethritis)

Essentials of Diagnosis

- Dysuria and a whitish, mucoid discharge from the urethra.
- Microscopic examination of the discharge shows many polymorphonuclear leukocytes but no bacteria.
- Culture on Thayer-Martin medium of the exudate is negative.
- No skin lesions unless another sexually transmit-

ted disease is present with cutaneous manifestations.

General Considerations

Nongonococcal urethritis is a sexually transmitted disease that mimics the symptoms of gonorrhea, but the gonococcus is not present. It is a common condition and may be the most common sexually transmitted disease.

Several different organisms have been associated with nongonococcal urethritis. *Chlamydia trachomatis* is the agent responsible in 40–50% of cases. Other organisms that may rarely be factors include *Ureaplasma urealyticum* (T-strain mycoplasmas), *Corynebacterium genitalium, Trichomonas vaginalis, Candida* sp, herpes simplex virus, and cytomegaloviruses.

Clinical Findings

A. Symptoms and Signs: The incubation period is usually 1–3 weeks. The discharge is clear or white and tends to be mucoid but may be quite thin. It is most noticeable in the morning. Burning with urination is usually mild, though on occasion it may be severe. Most cases in females are asymptomatic.

B. Laboratory Findings: Smear of urethral discharge is important in the diagnosis and will show few inflammatory cells and no organisms on a gram-stained smear. Culture of the urethra should be performed on Thayer-Martin medium to rule out gonorrhea. Culture for *Chlamydia* is a cell culture technique and is expensive. Many laboratories can supply a fluorescent antibody test that utilizes fluorescent-conjugated monoclonal antibodies and has high sensitivity.

Differential Diagnosis

A negative culture for gonorrhea and a negative Gram stain in a patient with urethral inflammation establishes the diagnosis. In unusual cases, *Candida, Trichomonas,* or herpes simplex virus need to be considered.

Complications

C trachomatis may cause acute epididymitis, nongonococcal pelvic inflammatory disease, nongonococcal ophthalmia neonatorum, and neonatal pneumonia.

Prevention

Use of a condom and scrupulous washing will aid in prevention. It appears that 70% of female contacts of men with the disease are asymptomatically infected.

Treatment

Tetracycline is the drug of choice. The usual course of therapy is 500 mg of tetracycline 4 times daily for 7–14 days. Longer courses of therapy have been recommended, but additional benefit is not proved. Doxycycline, 100 mg twice daily for a similar duration, has the benefit of requiring only twice-daily administration. Penicillin is ineffective, but erythromycin base or stearate, 500 mg orally 4 times daily for 7 days, is an alternative treatment.

Mixed infections with *C trachomatis* and *N gonorrhoeae* occur fairly commonly, and if penicillin is used for the gonorrhea infection, the nongonococcal infection will present as a postgonococcal urethritis and require tetracycline as described. The use of tetracycline as the primary therapy for gonorrhea will treat nongonococcal infection satisfactorily. The sexual partner should be treated with tetracycline outlined for the primary patient, both to cure the partner and to prevent recurrence in the patient.

VAGINAL INFECTIONS

1. TRICHOMONIASIS

Essentials of Diagnosis

- Symptoms are seen chiefly in women, with vaginal burning, pruritus, and a greenish-yellow, foamy vaginal discharge.
- In men, the organism is found in the urogenital tract, primarily the prostate.
- Symptoms of mild urethritis are seen in only about 20% of infected male patients.
- The skin is not affected.

General Considerations

Trichomoniasis occurs chiefly in women. About 25% of US women harbor the protozoon *Trichomonas vaginalis* in their vaginas. Transmission is primarily via sexual intercourse, though remote infections can be acquired by contact with inanimate objects such as douche nozzles, bath towels, and moist bathing suits.

T vaginalis is a unicellular protozoan flagellate up to 15 μm in length. It grows optimally at 35–37 °C in a moist environment with a slightly acid pH. The vagina and prostate are perfect environments for growth.

Clinical Findings

A. Symptoms and Signs: The primary finding in *T vaginalis* vaginitis is yellow leukorrhea with a gray to greenish-yellow discharge that may be profuse. The discharge tends to be foamy. The odor is offensive, and the discharge is usually associated with vaginal discomfort, pruritus, and burning. Dyspareunia is not uncommon.

The vaginal mucosa is diffusely red, with scattered petechiae. The posterior fornix may have a red granular appearance referred to as "strawberry vagina." The labia may be erythematous and edematous.

The organism in the male may rarely cause symptoms of urethritis with a mucoid discharge and dysuria.

B. Special Examination: A drop of the discharge is placed on a warm slide, diluted with normal saline, and covered with a coverslip. Examination under the moderately high-power microscope with a low light source reveals undulating protozoan organisms propelled by 4 flagella. In 20% of men harboring the organism, it can be found in prostatic secretions.

Differential Diagnosis

Other causes of vaginitis include candidiasis, herpes simplex infection, and infections with *Haemophilus vaginalis* and other bacteria. In men, rare cases of *Trichomonas* urethritis must be differentiated from gonorrhea gonococcal and nongonococcal urethritis.

Complications

Epididymitis and prostatitis may rarely occur.

Prevention

Good personal hygiene is important, but avoidance of contact with an infected person is of primary importance. Condoms offer protection. Sexual partners of infected women must be treated.

Treatment

A single dose of metronidazole 2 g orally is effective, but it may be associated with gastrointestinal upset. An alternative regimen is metronidazole 500 mg twice daily for 7 days. The drug should not be used in the first trimester of pregnancy, because it may be mutagenic and carcinogenic. Alcohol should not be taken during the treatment period because of the disulfiram effect of metronidazole. Sexual partners should be treated. Warm sitz baths offer symptomatic relief.

Course & Prognosis

Metronidazole is highly effective. The possibility of reinfection should always be considered.

BALANITIS & CANDIDAL VAGINITIS

The yeast organism *Candida albicans* can cause vaginitis in the female and balanitis in the male. Certain conditions predispose to the infection, including diabetes, pregnancy, antibiotic therapy, oral contraceptive agents, and obesity. It can be transmitted by the hands, towels, clothing, and inanimate objects. It can also be spread by sexual contact, and it is imperative that both sexual partners be treated at the same time.

Candidiasis is covered in detail in Chapter 16.

NONSPECIFIC VAGINITIS

Nonspecific vaginitis is a poor name for bacterial vaginitis usually caused by *Gardnerella (Haemophilus) vaginalis,* an organism that is recovered from 95% of women with nonspecific vaginitis but can also be found in asymptomatic women—so that its etiologic role is still in question. Women with nonspecific vaginitis appear to have a complex alteration in their vaginal microbial flora so that other organisms, especially anaerobic bacteria, may proliferate and combine with *G vaginalis* to produce the symptoms.

Symptoms include a gray to white discharge associated with a fishy amine odor that is often the most troublesome complaint. A vaginal smear will usually show **clue cells,**—vaginal epithelial cells with indistinct borders owing to the large number of organisms attached to them. Clue cells are virtually pathognomonic for *Gardnerella*-associated vaginitis.

The most effective therapy is metronidazole, 500 mg twice daily for 7 days. An alternative treatment regimen is clindamycin, 300 mg orally twice daily for 7 days. Sulfonamide-containing vaginal creams are not effective.

SEXUAL TRAUMA

Physical trauma causes abrasions and tears involving the penis and vagina or the anal verge in both sexes may result from sexual trauma. The young, sexually inexperienced female may have vaginal tears, especially if lubrication is not adequate. Anal intercourse, because of the anatomy and limited extensibility of the anal verge, can result in tears in the homosexual patient or in the female practicing anal sex. Sexual paraphernalia or other foreign bodies can also cause trauma in the vaginal or anal areas.

In the male, trauma to the penis may be associated with lack of adequate lubrication. The pubic hair or vaginal orifice can abrade the penis during intercourse (slang term: "haircut"). During oral sex, teeth can cause abrasions or lacerations to the penis (Fig 13–3). These lesions are usually linear and do not resemble infectious disease. Genital restraints and apparatus can also cause injury. The geometric appearance of these lesions is often the hint that they are traumatically induced. There may be edema or allergic or contact dermatitis. Lesions can become sec-

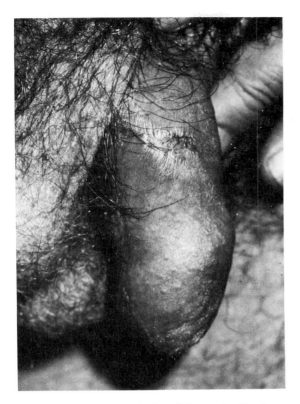

Figure 13–3. Traumatic lesion of the penis. The linear, crusted lesion on the shaft of the penis was the result of a human bite.

ondarily infected, which may make their identification more difficult.

Victims of sexual assault, both men and women, must be cared for in a professional yet compassionate manner. The appropriate authorities should be consulted. Suspicion of sexual abuse in children usually requires reporting and consultation with social workers specially trained in dealing with abused children and their families.

Differential Diagnosis

Abrasions and lacerations of the genitals must be differentiated from primary syphilis, herpes progenitalis, chancroid, granuloma inguinale, and pyodermas.

Treatment

Treatment of psychologic trauma requires insight and understanding of the patient's fears and anxieties. Help the patient talk about it. It is not the physician's place to judge the patient. Medical evaluation and therapy must in no way be compromised when dealing with these patients. Social services should be contacted in cases of sexual assault or abuse.

Physical trauma requires recognition of the cause and discussion with the patient of the ways in which trauma can be avoided or minimized. Often adequate lubrication with an appropriate jelly is the only addition necessary. Other sexually transmitted diseases must be looked for and appropriate cultures and blood tests performed. The areas must be kept clean; if secondarily infected, antimicrobial therapy should be administered. In this regard, it is best not to use erythromycin or other broad-spectrum antibiotics that alter tests for syphilis. Sulfisoxazole is a reasonable choice, as this will not kill the treponemal organism.

CHANCROID

Essentials of Diagnosis

- Isolated or multiple genital ulcers.
- Ulcers tend to be ragged, necrotic, deep, and painful to touch.
- Painful, suppurative adenopathy.

General Considerations

Chancroid is an ulcerating condition caused by the gram-negative bacillus *Haemophilus ducreyi*. It is spread almost solely by sexual contact, and extragenital lesions are rare. The disease is 20 times more common in men, and it has been suggested that women may act as asymptomatic carriers. It is seen primarily in poorer, underdeveloped urban areas, especially in Africa, Asia, and South and Central America, but it has been reported worldwide. It is relatively uncommon in the USA.

H ducreyi is a short gram-negative bacillus with rounded ends. It has been classified as a streptobacillus. In culture it forms chains, but in tissue the organisms are usually in clusters resembling a "school of fish."

Clinical Findings

A. Symptoms and Signs: The incubation period is usually 3–5 days. The initial lesion is a pustule that appears most commonly on the shaft of the penis. This rapidly breaks down to form a ragged undermined ulcer with a grayish exudate (Fig 13–4). It is exquisitely tender and painful. Autoinoculation causes new ulcers in skin surfaces opposite the primary ulcer. These lesions are referred to as "kissing ulcers."

Regional inguinal adenopathy develops within a week in about 50% of cases, especially in individuals who are physically active. The adenopathy is usually unilateral and tends to form tender, matted nodes that may suppurate to form draining sinuses.

Systemic symptoms are usually absent except for occasional low-grade fever and malaise.

B. Laboratory Findings: Smears are best taken from the undermined edge of the ulcer. Pinch a small

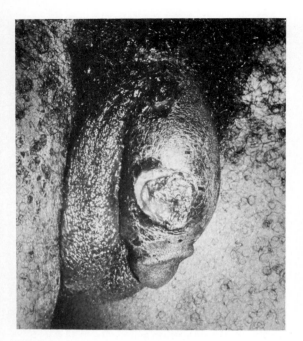

Figure 13–4. Chancroid in a black male. The lesion presents as a dirty, crusted, ragged, painful ulcer.

bit of the ulcer base between 2 glass slides, spread it on the slide, heat-fix it, and stain it with Gram's, Giemsa's, Wright's, or Unna-Pappenheim stain. Gram-negative short bacilli can be seen in up to 88% of properly done smears. A fluorescent stain is available in some medical centers to aid in identification. Material aspirated from a bubo can be similarly examined.

Histopathologic examination shows 3 different layers in the ulcer base—distinctive enough to establish the diagnosis in some difficult cases.

This rather fastidious organism can be isolated on rabbit blood agar or fetal bovine serum agar supplemented with vancomycin. This "ECA-V" enriched chocolate agar containing vancomycin is available in most laboratories or can be relatively easily prepared. The organism can also be cultured in fresh defibrinated and clotted rabbit blood and in autologous human blood and requires a heat-stable factor from erythrocytes for growth.

Differential Diagnosis

The differential diagnosis includes primary syphilis, granuloma inguinale, herpes progenitalis, trauma, and other bacterial infections. Chancroid forms a ragged, often large, painful ulcer with satellite lesions. The primary chancre of syphilis tends to be nonpurulent and nonpainful, and the genital ulcer of granuloma inguinale does not have an undermining edge. Herpes progenitalis usually shows a few vesicles, and traumatic lesions are usually angular.

Complications

Balanitis, phimosis, and swelling can develop. The suppurating lymph nodes can cause persistent draining sinuses. The initial ulcer may become infected with fusospirochetal organisms and produce an extensive phagedenic ulcer.

Prevention

Abstinence from sexual contact with an infected individual is obviously recommended. A condom offers some protection if properly used, as will thorough washing after intercourse, though this protection is not absolute.

Treatment

Ceftriaxone, 250 mg intramuscularly as a single injection, is recommended by the CDC, but extensive experience with ceftriaxone is lacking in this country. Either trimethoprim-sulfamethoxazole, 1 double-strength tablet (160 mg TMP, 800 mg SMZ) orally twice daily, or erythromycin, 500 mg by mouth 4 times daily, can be used. Erythromycin-resistant cases have been reported in China. Therapy should be continued for at least 10 days and until ulcers and lymph nodes have healed. Appropriate serologic studies for syphilis should be performed initially and in 2 months.

Penicillin has no effect on chancroid and should not be used.

Course & Prognosis

The disease usually responds well to therapy, which should be continued until the lesion clears totally. Early diagnosis and therapy are important to shorten the course. The patient should be observed for the development of other sexually transmitted diseases.

LYMPHOGRANULOMA VENEREUM

Essentials of Diagnosis

- Initial lesion is a transient, painless, nonindurated, superficial ulcer on the genitals, often unnoticed.
- Painful inguinal adenopathy is the usual presenting complaint.

General Considerations

Lymphogranuloma venereum is spread primarily through sexual contact, though there are reports of accidental inoculation on extragenital locations. It is more commonly found in the tropics than in the USA and is more common in men than in women. The disease is caused by *Chlamydia trachomatis* serovars L1, L2, and L3. A complement fixation test is available that depends on a lipoprotein carbohydrate antigen common to all *Chlamydia* species and is therefore only group-specific. The specific serovars of *C trachomatis* can be differentiated in the laboratory.

Clinical Findings

A. Symptoms and Signs: Lymphogranuloma venereum is considered a disease of the lymphatic system. The initial lesion occurs on the genitals 3–6 weeks after infection; it is a small, nonindurated papule or vesicle that ulcerates. It is painless and usually heals within 2–3 days. It is not often seen by the physician, as it is usually not sufficiently alarming to bring the patient to a medical facility.

Inguinal adenopathy develops usually 2–3 weeks after the primary lesion. It is generally unilateral, but one-third of cases are bilateral. Men are more commonly affected. The nodes initially are firm and tender and fixed to the overlying skin. The skin over the lymph nodes has an edematous, dusky red appearance. The nodes become fluctuant and break down to form multiple ragged and draining sinuses. The nodes above and below Poupart's ligaments are frequently involved, and the ligament may produce a cleft between the involved nodes called the "sign of the groove" (Fig 13–5). The patient may have some constitutional symptoms of fever, chills, malaise, and headache. The duration of the disease is usually 8–12 weeks.

Women develop a more indolent, shallow ulcer that lasts longer than the transient lesion seen in the male. Anorectal involvement may be due to infection by anal intercourse, by extension from the vagina, or by lymphatic anastomosis between the inguinal nodes and the perianal nodes. Inguinal adenopathy is rare in women because the lymphatic drainage pattern is different from that in men. Anorectal involvement may be seen in male homosexuals. The patient will experience a bloody mucopurulent discharge but generally has little discomfort. The rectal mucosa is red and edematous, with superficial ulcerations. The ragged

mucosal pattern in some cases is pseudopolypoid. Extensive granulation tissue may develop later, leading eventually to fibrosis with scarring and rectal strictures associated with considerable pain along with constipation.

B. Laboratory Findings: The lymphogranuloma venereum complement fixation test becomes positive 1 week after infection. A titer of 1:16 is significant but is not correlated with disease activity. As noted previously, this test depends on a lipoprotein carbohydrate antigen that is common to all *Chlamydia* species; therefore, the test is only group-specific, not type-specific. A microimmunofluorescence test is available but only at a few medical centers. A fluorescent-conjugated monoclonal antibody has been used to identify the organism in smears taken directly from pus. The chlamydial organism can be grown in cell culture. Chick embryo yolk sac is commonly used, though the culture is difficult and not generally done clinically.

C. Special Examinations: The Frei skin test uses an antigen prepared from the yolk sac culture of the chlamydia organisms. It is an intradermal test and is read at 48 hours with an inflammatory indurated reaction of at least 5 mm considered positive. It is generally positive 2 weeks after infection. A control site using only material from the chick embryo should be applied.

Differential Diagnosis

The early inguinal lymphadenopathy is to be differentiated from the lymphadenopathy caused by chancroid, severe herpes progenitalis, and syphilis. The skin lesions will usually differentiate these diseases. Multiple draining sinuses can be distinctive for lymphogranuloma venereum. A malignant lymphoma also needs to be considered.

The anorectal syndrome can resemble rectal polyposis, condylomata acuminata, gonococcal proctitis, ulcerative colitis, Crohn's disease, hidradenitis suppurativa, and carcinoma.

Complications & Sequelae

The scarring and disruption of the lymphatic drainage may lead to elephantiasis of the genitalia in both male and female patients. Chronic ulcers of the swollen, edematous genitals can develop. Rectal strictures can cause severe pain, tenesmus, and rectovaginal fistulas. The chronic inflammatory changes may be associated with malignancy in the bowels. Erythema multiforme and erythema nodosum may develop in response to this infection. Meningoencephalitis has also been reported.

Treatment

The drug of choice for lymphogranuloma venereum is doxycycline, 100 mg orally twice daily for 21 days. Alternative regimens include tetracycline, 500 mg orally 4 times a day for at least 21 days;

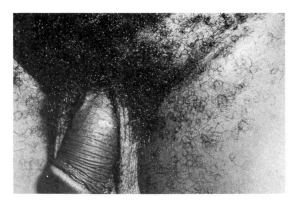

Figure 13–5. Lymphogranuloma venereum with enlarged lymph nodes above and below Poupart's ligament, representative of the "sign of the groove."

erythromycin, 500 mg orally 4 times a day for 21 days; or sulfisoxazole, 500 mg orally 4 times a day for 21 days. The antimicrobial therapy will prevent late sequelae and halt progression of the disease, but the enlarged lymph nodes require 4–6 weeks to resolve. Fluctuant lymph nodes should not be incised and drained but should be aspirated with a large-bore needle as often as necessary to avoid spontaneous drainage and the development of sinus tracts.

Course & Prognosis

The duration of the adenopathy may be quite prolonged, lasting as long as 8–12 weeks. Early therapy is important to prevent late scarring.

GRANULOMA INGUINALE

Essentials of Diagnosis

- An irregular ulcer of the genitals with an exuberant granulating base.
- Secondary lesions in the warm, moist folds of the perineum.

General Considerations

Granuloma inguinale is a chronic inflammatory disease caused by *Calymmatobacterium (Donovania) granulomatis.* It involves chiefly the genital organs. Sexual contact appears to be the major means of transmission, but the disease is not very contagious. *C granulomatis* is primarily an enteric inhabitant and produces disease by autoinoculation, sexually through a vagina contaminated by enteric bacteria, or possibly by anal intercourse.

The disease is most common in the sexually active age groups, more common in men than in women, much more common in blacks, and much more frequent in tropical and subtropical regions. It is relatively infrequent in the USA, occurring most commonly in the southern states.

C granulomatis is a plump gram-negative enteric bacillus showing bipolar staining. Organisms exist both intra- and extracellularly, most commonly in mononuclear cells, and have been grown in chick embryo yolk sacs.

Clinical Findings

A. Symptoms and Signs: The incubation period ranges from 1 to 12 weeks. The initial lesion is a soft, elevated painless nodule with a bright-red granulomatous surface. The nodule is commonly found on the genitals—on the shaft of the penis or on the labia majora. Satellite lesions develop in areas of skin opposition, and the plaques tend to show polycyclic borders with extensions down the folds and creases of the perineum. Extensive areas may be involved, but the lymph nodes are not. Subcutaneous granulomas in

the inguinal area may present as pseudobuboes. Plaques tend to be chronic, and older lesions show areas of scarring, hypopigmentation, and erosion with new active areas of granulation tissue. The process is relatively painless. Systemic symptoms are rare. Variants of granuloma inguinale can be classified in the following groups:

1. Ulcerovegetating– The nodular granulomatous lesions break down into ulcers, often with a rolled border and a foul sanguineous discharge. This is a common variant.

2. Cicatricial– The cicatricial form shows areas of hypertrophic scarring.

3. Hypertrophic– The hypertrophic form shows massive edema and elephantiasis due to impairment of the lymphatic channels by pressure.

B. Laboratory Findings and Special Examinations: The diagnosis is established by histopathologic demonstration of the organism. A small amount of tissue from the active border or the granulomatous lesion can be obtained with a sharp curette. In some cases, a punch biopsy can be used to obtain tissue, which is crushed between 2 glass slides, alcohol-fixed, and stained with Wright's or Giemsa's stain. Donovan bodies show up as plump bacilli with bipolar staining in mononuclear cells. They stain bright red with Giemsa's stain but are not well demonstrated with routine hematoxylin-eosin stains.

Differential Diagnosis

The early bright-red granulomatous lesion is distinctive and not usually confused with other conditions. Very early lesions could resemble condylomata acuminata, and on the glans the lesions could resemble erythroplasia of Queyrat (carcinoma in situ). Later lesions should be differentiated from deep mycosis, cutaneous tuberculosis, hidradenitis suppurativa, pyoderma gangrenosum, and carcinoma.

Complications

Elephantiasis of the genitalia has been mentioned. Urinary tract infection may develop in chronic cases, and phimosis may occur. Lesions in bones, joints, and viscera have been reported. Hemorrhage may develop if a large vessel is eroded by the primary lesion. The possibility of development of carcinoma should always be considered in chronic cases.

Prevention

The organism has a low rate of infectivity. Careful personal hygiene is of primary importance in prevention.

Treatment

Tetracycline hydrochloride, 500 mg orally 4 times a day, is the most commonly used drug therapy. This treatment needs to be continued until the lesion is completely healed, which often requires 3 weeks or longer. Resistance to tetracycline has been noted in the USA and elsewhere, and trimethoprim-sulfamethoxazole (TMP 160 mg, SMZ 800 mg), 1 tablet twice daily orally for 2–4 weeks, is an effective alternative. Chloramphenicol, 500 mg orally 3 times a day, or gentamicin, 1 mg/kg intramuscularly 2 times a day for 2–4 weeks, has also been used.

Course & Prognosis

Untreated granuloma inguinale progresses for at least 10–20 years and ultimately can cause extensive destruction of the genitalia. Response to therapy is adequate, but recurrences are common.

HERPES PROGENITALIS: GENITAL INFECTION WITH HERPES SIMPLEX VIRUS (Herpes Genitalis) (See also Chapter 14.)

Essentials of Diagnosis

- Early lesions show grouped vesicles on an erythematous base in the genital area.
- The vesicles rapidly rupture to form superficial shallow ulcerations.
- Primary infection tends to be associated with more pain, inflammation, and regional adenopathy.
- Recurrent lesions tend to be associated with fewer symptoms.

General Considerations

Herpes progenitalis is an infection of the genitals with herpes simplex virus (HSV). The antigenic type 2 strain of the herpesvirus (HSV-2) is more common in genital infections than the type 1 strain. Herpes progenitalis is spread primarily through intimate personal contact, most commonly sexual intercourse. The incubation period is 3–7 days. The primary infection is often associated with a severe inflammatory disease. The recurrent lesions generally show fewer symptoms and less alarming signs. Herpes simplex infections are also discussed in detail in Chapter 14, so the discussion here will be brief.

Clinical Findings

A. Symptoms and Signs:

1. Primary infection– Some initial infections may be virtually asymptomatic, while others are quite severe. The infection tends generally to be less severe in men than in women. Localized burning and paresthesias may develop before the lesions actually develop. The lesions are initially vesicles on an erythematous base. These vesicles rapidly rupture to form superficial ulcers that are often painful. Smaller scattered ulcers may coalesce to form large, extensive ones. Swelling of the labia and ulcerations

about the urethra can cause severe dysuria, even to the extent of producing urinary retention. Urethritis may develop, associated with a purulent watery discharge. Constitutional symptoms include fever, chills, malaise, headache, and regional and generalized adenopathy. These symptoms last up to 1 week, but the entire course of the primary complex may last 4–6 weeks.

2. Recurrent infections– Probably less than 10% of patients are plagued with recurrent lesions occurring more than 4 times a year for over 2 years; however, with the large number of herpesvirus infections, this represents a sizable population. The virus persists in the body in latent form, and activity can be triggered by a number of stimuli such as trauma of sexual intercourse, other infectious diseases, fever, menstruation, emotional stress, and apparently many other factors. The recurrent lesions tend to be less severe than the primary infections. Grouped vesicles rupture to form superficial erosions on the genitals (Fig 13–6). There is only minimal discomfort and usually no adenopathy. The eruption generally lasts 7–10 days and heals completely.

3. Asymptomatic infection– The main reservoir is the female cervix. Viral shedding in asymptomatic women has been reported in 4% of individuals, and the percentage may be higher. Thus, the possibility of passing the virus on to sexual partners is a serious problem. In the male, the rate of asymptomatic HSV infection, primarily urethral, is about 1%.

4. Herpes simplex infection and the neonate– Perhaps the most serious consequences of HSV-2 infection occur in the fetus and neonate. Infection of the neonate can result in disseminated disease with a

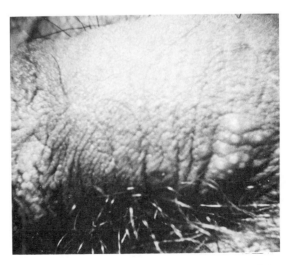

Figure 13–6. Genital herpes. Note the grouped vesicles on an erythematous base in the midportion of the shaft of the penis.

mortality rate as high as 60%. Significant neurologic or ocular sequelae occur in at least 50% of survivors. The infection occurs in neonates exposed to genital infection of the mother during parturition. Neonatal infection will usually develop in the first 2 weeks of life and is 4–5 times more common in premature infants and in infants born to mothers with a primary infection at or near delivery. (Strategies for managing pregnant patients and their offspring are given in Chapter 14.)

B. Laboratory Findings: An easily and rapidly performed diagnostic test is the Tzanck smear—cytologic examination of material taken from a fresh lesion. An early intact vesicle is opened with a No. 15 scalpel. The base of the vesicle is scraped with the blade, and the cells are spread on a glass slide. The slide is dried in air or with heat and then stained with Wright's or Giemsa's stain (Fig 13–7). With this technique, multinucleated giant cells from infected epidermal cells can be seen in viral disease, but this result is not specific for herpes simplex infection since the cells are also seen in infection with varicella-zoster virus. The test thus lacks specificity, and other tests are necessary for positive diagnosis.

Immunofluorescent studies utilize direct smears taken from vesicles. Viral culture of intact vesicles is relatively easy and shows characteristic cytopathic changes in 12 hours to 4 days.

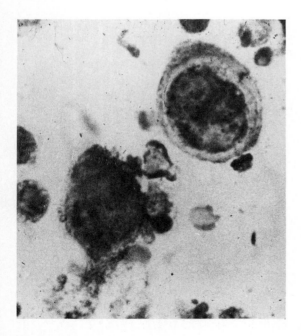

Figure 13–7. Multinucleated giant cells in a smear from the base of a vesicle of herpes simplex stained with Wright's stain. Note the marginal chromatin pattern in the nuclei.

Differential Diagnosis

The differential diagnosis can be varied, depending on the stage on the lesion. Considerations should include syphilis, trauma, bacterial infection, contact dermatitis, and other viral infections.

Complications

Two significant complications include secondary bacterial infection and urinary retention. The possibility of infection of the neonate can also be viewed as a complication. Other complications include genital neuralgia, urethral stricture, labial fusion, and lymphatic suppuration. Anorectal HSV infection can produce extensive perianal ulceration with severe pain and lumbosacral radiculomyelopathy. This may be manifested by neurologic symptoms such as paresthesias and neuralgia in the buttocks and by urinary dysfunction.

Prevention

Recurrent lesions of herpes progenitalis are contagious for at least 5–7 days, and sexual contact should be avoided until the lesions are healed. Primary lesions can be contagious for up to 3 weeks. Precautions are usually unnecessary in the absence of active lesions, but if a partner has a past history of genital herpes, condom prophylaxis may be recommended because virus can be shed without signs or symptoms.

Recurrences may be prevented with acyclovir, 200 mg orally 3 or 4 times a day, as discussed in Chapter 14.

Treatment

For the primary infection, symptomatic care is indicated. Therapy depends on the severity of the inflammatory reaction. Patients with severe infection are usually women; bed rest should be recommended and topical anesthetic agents utilized to relieve discomfort. A female patient with periurethral ulceration may have extreme dysuria and difficulty with urination that can be made easier by voiding in a warm sitz bath. A Foley catheter may be required.

Acyclovir inhibits viral DNA replication. It is indicated in the management of primary herpes simplex infection and in recurrent herpes simplex infections in immunosuppressed patients. Both oral and intravenous administration of acyclovir are effective in initial and recurrent herpes simplex infections in the immunocompromised host and in the severe initial episode of herpes progenitalis in the nonimmunocompromised patient. Details of treatment are discussed in Chapter 14.

For primary (first episode) genital herpes, acyclovir, 200 mg, can be given orally 5 times a day for 7–10 days or until clinical resolution occurs. For the first clinical episode of herpes proctitis, the dose of acyclovir is 400 mg orally 5 times a day for 10 days or until clinical resolution occurs. Most recurrent episodes do not benefit from therapy with acyclovir unless it is started during the prodrome or within 2 days after onset.

MOLLUSCUM CONTAGIOSUM

Essentials of Diagnosis

- Pinkish-white, dome-shaped, smooth, umbilicated papules.
- Most commonly seen in children with nonsexual spread; spread by sexual activity in adults is common.

General Considerations

Molluscum contagiosum is a mildly contagious but relatively common skin disorder caused by a poxvirus. It is worldwide in distribution and occurs most frequently as a non-sexually transmitted disease in children; spread is apparently by close contact among schoolchildren. The disease is less common in adults, and transmission is usually through intimate sexual contact with lesions in the genital area.

Molluscum contagiosum virus is a member of the poxvirus group, a DNA virus that is large, measuring 200×300 nm. In the human host cell, it forms large, typical intracytoplasmic inclusion bodies.

Clinical Findings

A. Symptoms and Signs: The asymptomatic lesions are usually 2–6 mm, pinkish-white, smooth, and dome-shaped, usually with central umbilication. Giant lesions measuring 1.5–2 cm have been reported. The extremities are more commonly involved in children, while in adults the pubic and genital areas are chiefly affected. Multiple lesions are usually present. The incubation period, based on experimental transmission in humans, is 2–7 weeks.

B. Laboratory Findings and Special Examinations: The clinical picture is usually diagnostic. The central core of the lesion can be expressed and smeared and crushed between 2 glass slides. Wright's or Giemsa's stain can be used to demonstrate the large cytoplasmic inclusion bodies.

Biopsy of the lesion reveals epidermal cells containing Feulgen-positive intracytoplasmic inclusion bodies pushing the nucleus to one side. There is downgrowth of the infected cells to form a pouch (the central umbilication seen clinically), and the cells are sloughed off into the central pouch to form the soft, mushy material that can be expressed from the core.

Differential Diagnosis

The differential diagnosis included warts, lichen planus, papillomas, varicella, basal cell carcinoma, and even pyoderma manifesting as small pustules. Extensive infections are often seen in patients with AIDS.

Complications

Complications include pruritus, secondary bacterial infection, and secondary eczematous changes. These are relatively rare. The association with other sexually transmitted diseases must be kept in mind and investigated by appropriate means.

Prevention

Prevention consists of avoidance of contact with infected individuals.

Treatment

The simplest and probably most effective therapy is to remove the lesion with a sharp curette. The lesions are soft and easily removed. Simple pressure on the base will control the minimal bleeding that occurs after expression. Expression of the central plug with a small needle and a comedo extractor may remove the lesion. Freezing with liquid nitrogen or light electrocautery is also effective, and topical tretinoin has reportedly been useful, especially in younger patients. It is often necessary to have the patient return for re-treatment as new lesions develop.

The patient's sexual partner should be examined and treated appropriately.

Course & Prognosis

Most cases resolve spontaneously in 6–9 months, though some cases persist much longer.

CONDYLOMATA ACUMINATA

Essentials of Diagnosis

- Warty, heaped-up lesions in the moist anogenital area.
- Lesions are frequently pedunculated.
- Lesions are seen on both skin and mucous membrane.

General Considerations

Condylomata acuminata are a variety of wart or verruca. The verrucae are papillomas that occur on the skin and mucous membranes. They are due to infection with the human papillomavirus (HPV), an epidermotropic DNA virus. HPV serotypes 6 and 11 are most commonly associated with genital condylomas. The incidence of condylomata acuminata is not known, but the diagnosis is common in sexually transmitted disease clinics. It is worldwide in occurrence and is readily spread by sexual contact. The condylomas are seen primarily in moist genital folds and creases, moisture probably making them more susceptible to spread.

Clinical Findings

A. Symptoms and Signs: Condylomata acuminata form verrucoid papillomatous growths, reddish or dirty gray in color (Fig 13–8). In men, they can occur anywhere in the anogenital area, including the prepuce, the glans penis, the shaft of the penis, the urethral meatus, and the anus. In women, they may be seen on the labia, vagina, urethral orifice, and anal area. Involvement of the external labia and perianal areas should alert the physician to the possibility that lesions are present on the internal mucous membrane surfaces.

The lesions may be discrete and single, but more commonly they cluster to form large cauliflowerlike masses. They grow much more luxuriantly in moist areas. They may be traumatized and bleed, but in general they are painless. Women who are pregnant or taking oral contraceptives tend to have a more exuberant growth of these warts.

Venereal warts can sometimes be flat and nearly invisible. Flat warts (verrucae planae) are more easily visualized by compressing the skin for 15 minutes with 5% acetic acid. The warts appear white after such treatment.

Differential Diagnosis

The verrucoid lesions of condyomata acuminata are quite distinctive, but condyloma latum of secondary syphilis needs to be differentiated. Condylomata lata are generally flat-topped papules with a smooth surface, as opposed to the roughened, heaped-up lesions of condylomata acuminata. On occasion, molluscum contagiosum, pyoderma, lichen planus, and squamous cell carcinoma need to be considered. Flat

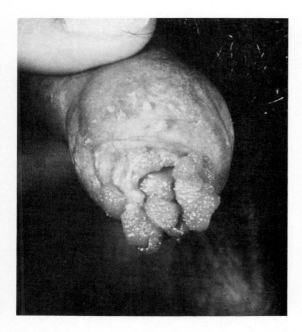

Figure 13–8. Vegetating, heaped-up condylomata acuminata in an uncircumcised male.

warts on the penis may resemble seborrheic keratoses.

Complications & Sequelae

Giant condylomata acuminata can become locally invasive (Buschke-Löwenstein tumor). Histopathologic examination shows a relatively benign-appearing tumor with hypertrophic epithelial changes. Rarely, these lesions may develop into squamous cell carcinoma. Irritation and secondary infection may occur in ordinary condylomata acuminata. Bleeding may occur in larger, heaped-up lesions in women, especially during pregnancy. Other sexually transmitted diseases may be present.

Bowenoid papulosis presents as brownish-red, elevated, verrucoid papules and plaques that on histologic examination show atypical cells resembling squamous cell carcinoma in situ. Bowenoid papulosis is associated with HPV types other than the types 6 and 11 mentioned above. HPV types 16 and 18 are often involved with these lesions. Early biopsy of any such lesion on the genitalia is advisable.

There is strong epidemiologic and immunologic evidence supporting a relationship between genital warts and genital cancer, especially cervical cancer. Human papillomavirus DNA has been found in 90% of cervical cancer biopsies. HPV types 16, 18, and 31 are the types most commonly associated with cancer, with types 35 and 39 mentioned in some cases.

Prevention

These moist warts are easily spread, and patients should abstain from sexual contact.

Treatment

No known treatments eradicate human papillomavirus from skin. The viral genome has been demonstrated in adjacent tissue even after laser treatment. Recurrence is common. The effect of genital wart treatment on human papillomavirus transmission and the natural history of infection is largely unknown. The goal of treatment is therefore to simply remove exophytic warts and ameliorate the signs and symptoms of the disease. Expensive toxic or severe treatments should be avoided, especially those that might result in permanent scarring. Sexual partners should be examined for warts. Patients with anogenital warts should use condoms to help reduce transmission.

Most lesions in moist areas can be treated with application of 25% podophyllum resin (podophyllin) in tincture of benzoin. This is carefully painted on the lesion, sparing the surrounding skin, and then allowed to dry. The patient is instructed to wash the material off in 2–8 hours, or sooner if burning develops. Extensive areas, especially on mucous membranes, should not be treated at one time as toxic absorption can occur. For the same reason, pregnant women should not be treated. Dry lesions respond less well to podophyllum resin. Treatment with 25% podophyllum may be repeated up to 5 times.

Cryotherapy using liquid nitrogen is often effective. Cryotherapy is nontoxic, does not require anesthesia, and—if used properly—usually does not scar. Similarly, under local anesthetic, electrodesiccation and curettage can be successfully used.

Human leukocyte interferon (alpha interferon) is available for treatment of resistant condylomas but is not generally recommended because of its relatively low efficacy, high incidence of toxicity, and high cost. The carbon dioxide laser and conventional surgery are useful in the management of extensive warts, particularly for patients who have not responded to other treatments.

The pregnant woman is difficult to treat successfully; cryotherapy is most effective. Women taking oral contraceptives often must stop taking them before the condyloma can be successfully treated. Persistent lesions after repeated courses of therapy should be biopsied to rule out malignant transformation.

SCABIES
(See also Chapter 18.)

Scabies is transmitted sexually. Although it is a generalized eruption, one should keep in mind its rather typical appearance in the genital areas. Especially on the penis, the appearance is one of inflammatory, often excoriated papules. Secondary bacterial infection is common. The possible association with other sexually transmitted diseases must be kept in mind. These patients may need a serologic test for syphilis and a culture for *N gonorrhoeae*.

PEDICULOSIS PUBIS
(See also Chapter 18.)

Pediculosis pubis is a common sexually transmitted disease. The severe pruritus often brings the patient in to see the physician. The finding of pediculosis pubis usually indicates a sexually active individual, and so a search should be instituted for other sexually transmitted diseases.

REFERENCES

Antal GM, Causse G: The control of endemic treponematoses. Rev Infect Dis 1985;7(Suppl 2):220.

Baker DA: Herpesvirus. Clin Obstet Gynecol 1983;26:165.

Blom I et al: Long-term oral acyclovir treatment prevents recurrent genital herpes. Dermatologica 1986;173:220.

Browne SF: Yaws. Int J Dermatol 1982;21:220

Burns M et al: Preliminary evaluation of the Gonozyme test. Sex Trans Dis 1983;10:180.

Centers for Disease Control: Condoms for prevention of sexually transmitted disease. MMWR 1988;37:133.

Chuang TY: Condyloma acuminatum. J Am Acad Dermatol 1987;16:376.

Ellis RE: Chlamydial genital infections: Manifestations and management. South Med J 1981;74:809.

Eron LJ et al: Interferon therapy for condyloma acuminatum. N Engl J Med 1986;315:1059.

Felman, YM, Nikitas JA: Sexually transmitted molluscum contagiosum. Dermatol Clin 1983;1:103.

Fiumara NJ, Rothman K, Tang S: Diagnosis and treatment of chancroid. J Am Acad Dermatol 1986;15:939.

Fraiz J, Jones RB: Chlamydial infections. Ann Rev Med 1988;39:357.

Guthe T et al: Methods for the surveillance of endemic treponematoses and seroimmunological investigations of "disappearing" disease. Bull WHO 1972;46:1.

Handsfield MM: Gonorrhea and non-gonococcal urethritis. Med Clin North Am 1978;62:925.

Hart G: Chancroid, donovanosis, and lymphogranuloma venereum. Dermatol Clin 1983;1:75.

Hume JC: Trichomoniasis, candidiasis, and *Gardnerella vaginalis* as sexually transmitted diseases. Dermatol Clin 1983;1:137.

International Symposium on Yaws and Other Endemic Treponematoses. Rev Infect Dis 1985;7(Suppl 2): [Entire issue.]

Jarratt M: Genital herpes simplex infection. Dermatol Clin 1983;1:85.

Kampmeier RH: Granuloma inguinale. Sex Trans Dis 1984;11:318.

Kraus SJ, Reynolds GH, Rolfs RT: Therapy of uncomplicated gonorrhea due to antibiotic-resistant *Neisseria gonorrhoeae*. Sex Trans Dis 1988;15:234.

Krieger JN et al: Diagnosis of trichomoniasis. JAMA 1988;259:1223.

1989 STD Treatment Guidelines. MMWR September 1, 1989;38:1.

Ostrow DG: Homosexuality and sexually transmitted disease. In: Holmes KK et al (editors): *Sexually Transmitted Diseases*. McGraw-Hill, 1984.

Owen WF Jr: Sexually transmitted diseases in the homosexual community. Dermatol Clin North Amer 1983;1(1):123.

Owen WF Jr: The clinical approach to the male homosexual patient. Med Clin North Am 1986;70(3):499.

Rosen T et al: Granuloma inguinale. J Am Acad Dermatol 1984;11:435.

Shah KV, Busclema J: Genital warts, papillomavirus, and genital malignancies. Ann Rev Med 1988;39:371.

Silva PD, Micha JP, Silva DG: Management of condyloma acuminatum. J Am Acad Dermatol 1985;13:457.

Stone KM, Grimes DA, Magder LS: Personal protection against sexually transmitted diseases. Am J Obstet Gynecol 1986;155:180.

Tam MR et al: Culture-independent diagnosis of *Chlamydia trachomatis* using monoclonal antibodies. N Engl J Med 1984;310:1146.

Treatment of Sexually Transmitted Diseases. Med Lett Drugs Ther 1988;30(757):5.

Wolner-Hanssen P et al: Clinical manifestations of vaginal trichomoniasis. JAMA 1989;261:571.

Zur Hausen H: Genital papillomavirus infection. Proc Med Virol 1985;32:15.

Viral Infections*

14

Michael T. Jarratt, MD & Mark V. Dahl, MD

Viral infections are a common cause of skin disease. Some skin eruptions, such as warts, are infections of the skin alone, while others, such as the exanthem of measles, are manifestations of systemic viremias.

HERPES SIMPLEX

Michael T. Jarratt, MD

Essentials of Diagnosis

- Painful grouped vesicles.
- Rapid evolution into erosions with crusts.
- Localized to one anatomic site.
- Lesions recur periodically in the same area of skin or mucous membrane.

General Considerations

Herpes simplex virus is a member of the herpesvirus family that includes varicella virus (herpes zoster virus), cytomegalovirus, and Epstein-Barr virus (infectious mononucleosis virus). Herpes simplex viruses are divided into 2 groups, type 1 (HSV-1) and type 2 (HSV-2), distinguished in the laboratory by several techniques. HSV-1 virus tends to cause disease above the waist, whereas (HSV-2) virus occurs most frequently below the waist. Either type, however, can infect any site on the skin or mucous membranes.

Herpes simplex virus infection is acquired through close personal contact. Infectious viral particles gain access to new hosts via mucous membranes and traumatized epithelia. Primary infection occurs most commonly in childhood between ages 1 and 5 years, when children are exposed through close personal contact with infected adults or other children. Primary infection in adulthood is usually acquired from sexual contact by kissing or intercourse.

Primary herpes simplex infection occurs in persons with no previous exposure to the virus and, consequently, no immunologic protection. The primary infection is severe and prolonged, sometimes requiring 2–6 weeks for complete healing. During primary infection, herpes simplex virus establishes latent infection in cranial nerve ganglia or spinal dorsal root ganglia from which it periodically reactivates, traverses peripheral nerves back to the skin or mucous membrane, and induces the characteristic focal recurrent herpetic lesion.

Clinical Findings

A. Symptoms and Signs:

1. Primary herpetic gingivostomatitis– The severity of primary herpetic gingivostomatitis ranges from mild and inapparent to severe and painful. The incubation time from exposure to clinical disease is 3–10 days. The onset of severe primary gingivostomatitis is characterized by sore throat and fever followed by extremely painful vesicles and erosions on the tongue, palate, pharynx, gingivae, buccal mucosa, and lips. Vesicles on the mucous membranes evolve within hours to coalescing erosions covered with a yellowish membrane (Fig 14–1). In children with severe gingivostomatitis, painful oral

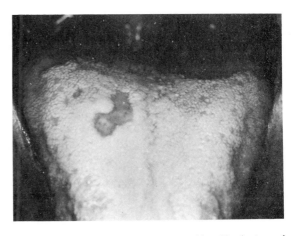

Figure 14–1. Primary herpetic stomatitis with clusters of punched-out geometric erosions on the tongue and pharynx.

erosions are associated with drooling, fetid breath, fever, malaise, and striking regional lymphadenopathy. Extreme sensitivity of the eroded oral mucous membranes may interfere with feeding and fluid intake, so that hospitalization with intravenous fluid support may be required. Severe primary gingivostomatitis persists for 2–6 weeks before resolving spontaneously.

The key to early clinical diagnosis is recognizing early vesicles and discrete erosions in characteristic clustered or grouped configuration before they coalesce into ulcers.

Primary herpetic gingivostomatitis must be distinguished from Stevens-Johnson syndrome, streptococcal pharyngitis, diphtheria, Vincent's infection, coxsackievirus infection, extensive candidiasis, pemphigus vulgaris, severe aphthous stomatitis, and Behçet's syndrome.

2. Recurrent herpes labialis– After primary gingivostomatitis, the patient is subject to periodic localized recurrences on the vermilion border of the lip. Recurrent herpes labialis is characterized by the familiar 1- to 2-cm vesicular and crusted lesion known commonly as a "fever blister" or "cold sore," which may in fact be composed of confluent vesicles or ulcers. Recurrent lesions usually heal in 5–7 days and normally are not associated with systemic toxicity. Recurrences may be frequent after primary infection but usually become less frequent 1–5 years later. Recurrences, though unpredictable in frequency, may be precipitated by trauma to the lips or by sunburn, emotional stress, fatigue, menstruation, or upper respiratory tract infections.

Herpes labialis must be distinguished from aphthous ulcers, erythema multiforme, and impetigo.

3. Herpetic whitlow– Herpetic whitlow is a recurrent herpes simplex infection of the fingers and hands. Two to 5 percent of the normal adult population periodically shed infectious herpes simplex virus in the saliva. Consequently, doctors, nurses, dentists, and dental technicians who work in and around the mouths of patients may inoculate the virus into the skin of their fingers and hands. The incubation time from inoculation to onset of primary infection is approximately 5–7 days. Painful, deep, clustered vesicles give a honeycombed appearance and sometimes coalesce to form a large bulla (Fig 14–2). During the 2- to 6-week primary infection, regional nodes are enlarged and tender. Fever and toxicity may occur.

After resolution of the primary infection, fingers and hands are subject to periodic, recurrent focal lesions identical to herpes labialis or herpes genitalis. Recurrent lesions are characteristically painful and associated with regional lymphadenopathy. Fever and toxicity are usually absent with recurrent disease.

Recurrent herpetic whitlow must be distinguished from bacterial cellulitis, acute paronychial abscesses, sporotrichosis, atypical acid fast bacterial infection, and erysipeloid.

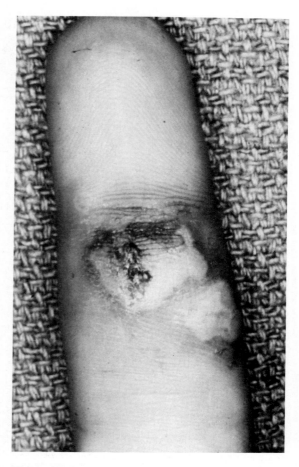

Figure 14–2. Herpetic whitlow with large pustules superimposed on erythema and edema of the finger.

4. Eczema herpeticum– Kaposi's varicelliform eruption is the general term used to denote widespread cutaneous infection with herpes simplex virus or vaccinia virus. Eczema herpeticum is the specific term for Kaposi's varicelliform eruption caused by herpes simplex virus.

Most cases of eczema herpeticum occur in patients with atopic dermatitis. Atopic patients, even without active skin disease, are susceptible to disseminated cutaneous herpetic infection. Other cutaneous diseases subject to development of eczema herpeticum are Darier's disease, pemphigus, and epidermolytic hyperkeratosis. Approximately 10 days after primary inoculation of herpes simplex virus into the skin of a patient with underlying cutaneous disease, vesicles erupt rapidly and coalesce into large erosions (Fig 14–3). Lesions may be confined to previously abnormal skin or may disseminate widely. Pustulation and intravesicular hemorrhage occur frequently. The face in particular may become grossly edematous. Gener-

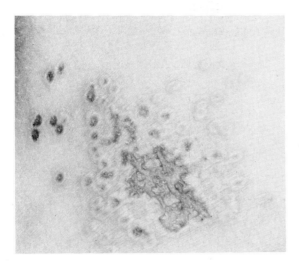

Figure 14–3. A patch of eczema herpeticum composed of umbilicated vesicles with central large erosion.

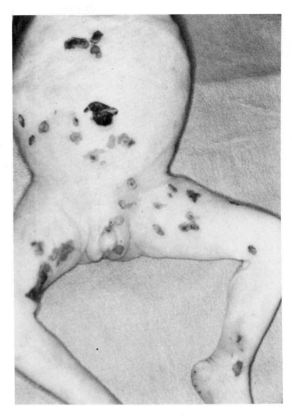

Figure 14–4. Disseminated neonatal herpes simplex manifested as generalized cutaneous erosions and crusts (Courtesy of L Golitz, MD.)

alized tender lymphadenopathy is present. High fever and severe toxicity are common. Large eroded areas frequently become secondarily infected by bacteria. After the primary infection, patients with chronic skin diseases may have milder recurrent attacks, usually unassociated with systemic symptoms.

Eczema herpeticum caused by herpes simplex virus is to be distinguished from widespread impetigo and from Kaposi's varicelliform eruption caused by vaccinia virus. Sometimes the ulcerated vesicles mimic excoriations of atopic dermatitis, but the patient will usually complain of pain.

5. Herpetic keratoconjunctivitis– Herpes simplex virus infection of the eye causes recurrent, painful erosions of the conjunctiva and cornea. The earliest and least severe form is superficial dendritic keratitis. With multiple recurrences, however, deeper ameboid ulcers develop, sometimes resulting in deep stromal keratitis and blindness.

Herpetic keratoconjunctivitis is to be distinguished from herpes zoster, adenovirus infection, vaccinia, and chlamydial conjunctivitis.

6. Genital herpes– The primary eruption usually occurs 5–10 days after sexual exposure. Painful small vesicles occur on the penis, vulva, or anus. After 2–4 days, vesicles rupture and burst, and healing is usually complete in 2 weeks. Some infections are asymptomatic, and others are associated with fever, headache, fatigue, and lymphadenopathy. Recurrences are common but of shorter duration. Asymptomatic shedding of virus carries a risk for transmission of infection. Genital herpes is discussed in detail in Chapter 13.

7. Neonatal herpes simplex– Clusters of vesicles and bullae erode rapidly and become crusts (Fig

14–4). The presenting fetal part—ie, the scalp in a normal cephalic delivery or the buttocks in a breech delivery—may be the first site for herpetic vesicles to appear. An infant that survives the disseminated infection may experience widely scattered focal recurrent lesions for several years.

Asymptomatic genital shedding of herpes simplex virus at parturition may cause neonatal infection of the infant. In a recent study of women who delivered herpes simplex virus-infected newborns, 70% (39 of 56) were without signs or symptoms of genital herpes simplex virus infection. One-third of these women were considered high-risk mothers because of a past history compatible with herpes genitalis or a sexual partner with herpes genitalis.

Neonatal herpes simplex may be fatal. At least half of the survivors have significant neurologic or ocular sequelae. About 75% of isolates from affected neonates are HSV-2; 25% are HSV-1. The incubation period for neonatal infection is usually less than 2 weeks but may be as long as 4 weeks. Skin vesicles alone are the presenting sign of infection in approximately 70%. Progression to systemic infection from isolated skin vesicles occurs in 70%; thus, the recovery of herpes simplex virus from the skin of a newborn is an indication for therapy with intravenous acyclovir.

8. Recurrent herpes simplex and erythema multiforme– In a small percentage of patients with recurrent herpetic infections, erythema multiforme follows the onset of the herpetic lesion by 7–10 days. Herpes labialis is the most common recurrent herpetic syndrome to precipitate erythema multiforme. In patients susceptible to erythema multiforme, the hypersensitivity reaction occurs regularly for months or years after each episode of herpes labialis.

Erythema multiforme following herpes labialis is usually limited to the palms, wrists, forearms, feet, elbows, knees, and the dorsal surfaces of the hands. Occasionally, painful erosions appear on the buccal mucous membranes. The earliest lesions are pruritic, dusky-red macules or papules that increase in size centripetally to reach a diameter of 1–2 cm in 48 hours. The periphery remains red, and the center becomes violaceous or purpuric to form the characteristic iris or target lesion (see Chapter 35). New lesions appear in successive crops for a few days and fade away in 1–2 weeks, leaving postinflammatory hyperpigmentation. Occasionally, recurrent bullous erythema multiforme with painful erosions in the mouth is a debilitating disease.

9. Herpes simplex in the immunologically suppressed– In patients immunosuppressed by chronic disease or chemotherapy, herpes simplex virus induces chronic progressive cutaneous ulcers and occasionally disseminates to internal organs. Dissemination has occurred with pemphigus, ataxia telangiectasia, mycosis fungoides, multiple myeloma, leukemia, and organ transplantation. The poorly understood immunosuppressed state of pregnancy also predisposes to severe disseminated herpes simplex infection.

Disseminated herpes simplex may present clinically as pharyngotonsillitis, esophagitis, gastritis, fulminant hepatitis, or a generalized varicelliform eruption.

B. Laboratory Findings: The quickest and least expensive laboratory test for diagnosis of cutaneous herpes simplex is the Tzanck smear. An intact vesicle or fresh erosion is gently scraped with a No. 15 surgical blade. Epithelial debris from the base of the lesion is smeared thinly onto a glass slide and allowed to dry in air before staining. The hematoxylin and eosin (H&E) stain is easiest to read, because the cytoplasm of the multinucleated giant cells stains pink around the large blue-staining nuclei.

A quick, single-step office stain is the toluidine blue-basic fuchsin stain. Wright's and Giemsa's stains are also useful.

The cytopathogenic effect of herpes simplex virus is manifested as giant, multinucleated epithelial cells

2–5 times the diameter of normal epithelial cells.

A positive Tzanck smear from a focally recurrent, erosive lesion is diagnostic of herpes simplex. The Tzanck smear is not positive after the third or fourth day of a recurrent lesion. Herpes zoster and varicella also produce a positive Tzanck smear, but they are usually distinguishable from herpes simplex on clinical grounds.

Herpes simplex virus can be cultured on live tissue culture, but the process is expensive and unavailable in many areas. Typing is generally done by neutralization procedures, adding considerably to laboratory expense.

Serum antibodies to herpes simplex virus are of little diagnostic value because their presence indicates previous exposure to the virus; ie, a positive antibody test does not prove that a current or recent clinical lesion is due to herpes simplex virus. Furthermore, the titer of serum antibodies to herpes simplex virus does not vary with the activity of recurrent disease. Therefore, acute and convalescent sera are not helpful diagnostically.

Treatment

Herpes simplex infection is treated with acyclovir, 15 mg/kg/d intravenously, or with 200 mg orally 5 times a day. Recurrences can be prevented by prophylactic administration of three or four 200-mg tablets daily. The drug has an excellent therapeutic ratio, and side effects are rare in patients who have good renal function and who are not dehydrated. The primary side effect is nephrotoxicity.

A. Primary Gingivostomatitis: Acyclovir, 200 mg orally 5 times a day, decreases the severity and shortens the duration of primary gingivostomatitis. Pain is ameliorated with frequent mouth washes of sodium bicarbonate in warm tap water. Further relief is achieved with topical anesthetic agents such as viscous lidocaine held in the mouth. Systemic analgesics may be used if the infection is severe and protracted. Hospitalization for intravenous fluid and electrolyte maintenance and for treatment with acyclovir, 5 mg/kg intravenously over 1 hour every 8 hours, may be required.

B. Recurrent Herpes Labialis: Topical acyclovir ointment, idoxuridine ointment, and vidarabine ointment do not shorten the duration of recurrent herpes labialis. Nonspecific remedies encourage drying and crusting and prevent secondary bacterial infection. Burow's solution applied with a cotton ball, chlorhexidine tincture, erythromycin solution, and clindamycin solution applied 3 times daily may prevent secondary bacterial infection.

Immunization with smallpox, influenza, or poliovaccine for the treatment of recurrent herpes simplex is ineffective and risky.

Some patients claim that prolonged application of

an ice cube to a fresh lesion relieves pain and aborts development of the lesion.

Patients with frequent recurrent herpes labialis or frequently recurring herpes simplex infections elsewhere are candidates for treatment with oral acyclovir.

C. Herpetic Whitlow: Herpetic whitlow is sometimes mistaken for bacterial cellulitis and treated inappropriately by incision and drainage and by systemic antibiotics. Oral acyclovir, 200 mg 5 times daily, can be given, until resolution is complete. Systematically administered analgesics should be given as needed.

D. Eczema Herpeticum: For severe life-threatening infection, intravenously administered acyclovir (5 mg/kg infused over 1 hour every 8 hours) may be indicated. Less serious infections may be managed with oral acyclovir or topically with Burow's compresses followed by application of acyclovir ointment (Zovirax) to decrease viral shedding and minimize autoinoculation. If secondary bacterial infection ensues, appropriate oral or intravenous antibiotics are indicated.

E. Herpetic Keratoconjunctivitis: An ophthalmologist should see and follow the patient. Superficial dendritic ulcers may be topically anesthetized and mechanically debrided. Frequent instillation of ophthalmic antiherpetic agents are helpful. Topical corticosteroids are contraindicated in the treatment of dendritic and ameboid herpetic corneal ulcers. For more details, see Chapter 49.

F. Genital Herpes: See Chapter 13.

G. Neonatal Herpes Simplex: Because neonatal herpes simplex infection is associated with high morbidity and mortality rates, immediate treatment with intravenous vidarabine or acyclovir is indicated at the earliest sign of cutaneous or internal infection. The dose of acyclovir is 250 mg/m² body area infused over a 1-hour period every 8 hours.

H. Recurrent Herpes Simplex and Erythema Multiforme: In mild cases, symptomatic relief may be achieved with oral antihistamines and topical corticosteroids. Although systemically administered corticosteroids abort the development of erythema multiforme, their routine use is not recommended. Prophylactic treatment with oral acyclovir, 200 mg 3 times a day, usually prevents both the recurrent herpes infection and the erythema multiforme.

I. Herpes Simplex in the Immunologically Suppressed: Systemically administered oral or intravenous acyclovir or vidarabine may be required for destructive progressive lesions. Acyclovir is preferred. Burow's compresses and antibiotic creams decrease secondary bacterial complications but have no effect on the progressive viral infection. Acyclovir ointment (Zovirax) decreases viral shedding and pain but has little effect on duration of lesions.

VARICELLA & HERPES ZOSTER

Michael T. Jarratt, MD

Varicella and herpes zoster are caused by the same DNA herpesvirus: varicella-zoster virus (VZV). The dual role of VZV was confirmed in clinical studies when fluid from herpes zoster vesicles was inoculated into children who subsequently developed varicella. Strains of VZV isolated from varicella and from herpes zoster are serologically identical. Isolates of VZV from patients with varicella and zoster form identical DNA bands when subjected to restrictive enzyme cleavage.

1. VARICELLA

Essentials of Diagnosis

- Usually occurs in childhood but may be delayed until adulthood.
- Generalized eruption of 4- to 6-mm vesicles with red bases involving the skin and mucous membranes.
- Vesicles become pustules, umbilicate, rupture, and crust.
- New crops of lesions occur over 3–5 days, so that lesions in all stages of development and resolution are present simultaneously.

General Considerations

During the viremic phase of varicella, varicella-zoster virus hematogenously seeds the skin, subsequently spreading centripetally along peripheral nerves to dorsal root ganglia, where it establishes latent infection. Trauma, immunosuppression, and unknown factors cause reactivation of latent ganglionic varicella-zoster virus, subsequently returning to the skin via peripheral nerves to induce the characteristic bandlike herpes zoster, usually limited to one or 2 dermatomes.

Clinical Findings

Following an incubation period of 14–21 days, varicella often begins with low-grade fever and malaise followed promptly by a generalized vesicular eruption, though many children seem well. Vesicles are concentrated on the trunk and distributed more sparsely on the extremities. Mucous membranes are involved. Individual lesions evolve rapidly from erythematous macule to papule to umbilicated vesicle to umbilicated pustule to crusted ulcer. Recurrent crops of new lesions appear during the first 3–5 days. Lesions in all stages of evolution are present simultaneously (Fig 14–5). In 6–8 days, fever declines, new lesion formation ceases, and old lesions crust.

Differential Diagnosis

Varicella may be confused with impetigo, scabies,

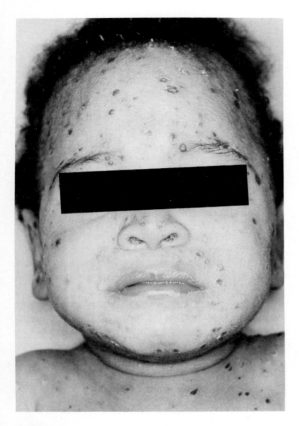

Figure 14–5. Chickenpox lesions of all ages (vesicle to crust) are present simultaneously.

eczema herpeticum, dermatitis herpetiformis, insect bites, and papular urticaria.

Complications & Sequelae

Varicella in childhood is usually benign and well tolerated. Occasionally, temperatures may reach 40.6 °C (105 °F), and severe involvement of oral and genital mucous membranes may be painful. Varicella in adults is usually accompanied by more systemic toxicity with high fever, headache, malaise and anorexia.

In immunocompromised patients, varicella may progress to disseminated infection with potentially fatal pneumonitis or encephalitis. The skin lesions may become hemorrhagic and deeply necrotic.

Neonatal varicella may occur when mothers have varicella 4 days or less before delivery. Neonatal infection may result in severe or fatal disseminated disease.

Maternal infection during the first trimester may result in the **congenital varicella syndrome**, characterized by low birth weight, one hypotrophic limb bearing a zosteriform scar, eye abnormalities (microphthalmia, cataracts, optic atrophy, chorioretini-

tis), and central nervous system damage with mental retardation.

Prevention

Zoster immune globulin (ZIG) administered intramuscularly within 3 days after exposure ameliorates subsequent clinical disease. Immunized persons will experience either subclinical exposure manifest only by seroconversion or mild clinical infection. Zoster immune globulin has no effect when administered after clinical signs of varicella have appeared. It has no effect on disseminated infection in immunocompromised patients.

Treatment

The pruritus of varicella may be controlled with oral antihistamines such as diphenhydramine or hydroxyzine. Skin and mucous membrane vesicles and erosions may be soothed by tap water baths or by compresses of Burow's solution 1:20 followed by application of zinc oxide shake lotion. Acetaminophen may control fever. Aspirin is contraindicated because of its potential for induction of Reye's syndrome.

Neonates or immunocompromised children with disseminated varicella may be treated with intravenously administered vidarabine or acyclovir. Higher doses of acyclovir are needed than with herpes simplex (eg, 10 mg/kg infused over 1 hour every 8 hours).

Severe varicella in an adult with high fever (> 102 °F) and malaise may be treated with oral or intravenous acyclovir.

2. HERPES ZOSTER

Essentials of Diagnosis

- Usually occurs in later adulthood but may occur in childhood.
- Eruption of painful clusters of 4- to 6-mm umbilicated vesicles limited to a bandlike dermatomal distribution.
- Deep aching pain may precede the eruption by 1–3 days.
- Residual pain (postherpetic neuralgia) may persist for weeks, months, or years.

General Considerations

Herpes zoster occurs most frequently in elderly persons or in patients of any age immunocompromised by illness or chemotherapy, but it may occur in otherwise healthy adults and children as well. In children, it runs a benign course, with minimal pain and no postherpetic neuralgia.

Clinical Findings

The first manifestation of herpes zoster is usually deep aching pain with associated tenderness and hyperesthesia of the involved dermatome. Pain may precede the eruption by 3 or 4 days. The eruption begins as clusters of red papules, rapidly evolving into vesicles and pustules forming in a continuous or interrupted dermatomal distribution (Fig 14–6). Mucous membranes in the infected dermatome may be involved. New clusters of lesions continue to erupt within the involved dermatome for 2–4 days. Low-grade fever, headache, and malaise may accompany the cutaneous eruption. Pain and cutaneous hyperesthesia may be severe. Lesions resolve in 2–4 weeks.

In approximately 5% of patients, lesions similar to those of varicilliform lesions may occur on the body outside the involved dermatome. The appearance of a dozen or so such lesions is not unusual and does not imply disseminated zoster or a poor prognosis.

Differential Diagnosis

Herpes simplex occasionally takes a zosteriform distribution. Since herpes zoster and herpes simplex cause a positive Tzanck smear, the 2 can be distinguished sometimes only by viral culture.

Complications & Sequelae

Postherpetic neuralgia, the most common sequela, increases in incidence and severity with age, occurring most commonly in patients over 40 years of age. It is unusual in childhood. The neuralgia is most frequent and severe in trigeminal nerve distribution. Protracted, constant, or intermittent pain may be disabling.

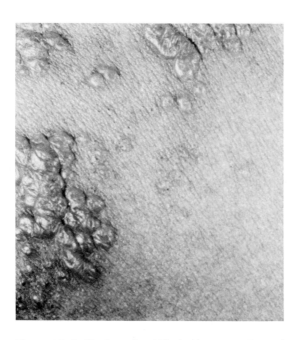

Figure 14–6. Clusters of umbilicated herpes zoster vesicles erupt in linear, dermatomal patterns.

Trigeminal zoster may cause shedding of teeth and may be accompanied by VZV meningitis. Lactation may accompany herpes zoster pectoralis. Some cases of Bell's palsy may be due to VZV. Herpes zoster may cause paralytic ileus, dysfunction of urinary bladder detrusor muscles or perianal sphincters, and paralysis of limbs.

Prevention

Recurrent episodes of herpes zoster are precipitated by spinal injury, by anesthetic manipulation of spinal ganglia, and by immunosuppression.

Treatment

The acute pain may be managed with simple analgesics or with narcotics as indicated. Burow's compresses 1:20 followed by application of zinc oxide shake lotion soothes and dries lesions.

Acyclovir, 800 mg orally 5 times daily for 5–10 days, accelerates healing and may decrease the severity of postherpetic neuralgia.

Systemic corticosteroids during the acute infection have been claimed to prevent postherpetic neuralgia in patients over 40, though a recent well-controlled study (Huff, 1988) suggests that this may not be true. Two recommended treatment schedules are as follows: (1) prednisone, 60 mg/d orally for 7 days, 30 mg/d for 7 days, and then 15 mg/d for 7 days; or (2) triamcinolone, 16 mg orally 3 times daily for 7 days, then 8 mg 3 times daily for 7 days, and then 8 mg twice daily for 7 days.

In order to prevent postherpetic neuralgia, corticosteroid must be administered early during the acute attack. Because of the risks of corticosteroids and the controversy regarding their effectiveness, chronically ill or immunocompromised patients should *not* be treated with corticosteroids.

Zoster immune globulin is not useful in the treatment of herpes zoster.

Disseminated herpes zoster may be treated with intravenous acyclovir, 10 mg/kg infused over 1 hour every 8 hours.

Painful trigger zones of postherpetic neuralgia may be relieved by local intracutaneous injections of triamcinolone, 2 mg/mL in lidocaine, or by topical application of capsaicin 0.025% cream 3 times a day for 4–6 weeks or more.

Excision of neuralgic scarred skin may provide pain relief.

WARTS

Michael T. Jarratt, MD

Essentials of Diagnosis

- Hyperkeratotic, steep-shouldered, skin-colored papules with velvety verrucous surfaces.

- Asymmetric; may occur anywhere on skin or mucous membranes.
- Lesions assume varied shapes depending on location and viral type.

General Considerations

Warts are caused by human papillomavirus, a member of the papovavirus family. Warts assume many clinical forms, including common warts, plantar warts, flat warts, filiform warts, paronychial warts, genital warts (condylomata acuminata), and oral and laryngeal papillomas. Different clinical lesions are caused by different human papillomaviruses.

Human papillomavirus infection is spread directly by person-to-person contact or indirectly by contact with public shower floors, swimming pools, etc. The virus may be autoinoculated from one area of the body to another. Incubation from inoculation of virus to appearance of clinical lesions is approximately 3 months.

Between ages 6 and 12 years, children commonly go through a period lasting several months during which multiple warts develop. All or most of the warts then resolve spontaneously. About 65% of warts in children disappear spontaneously within 2 years.

Human papillomavirus has worldwide prevalence. The peak incidence of warts is between 12 and 16 years of age. Ten percent of school children under age 16 have one or more warts.

Clinical Findings

A. Common Warts: Ordinary warts are most common on the hands and distal forearms. They begin as deep-seated, translucent, shiny papules developing over weeks into steep-shouldered, skin-colored, verrucous, hyperkeratotic papules 0.25–1 cm in diameter. Within the verrucous papules are multiple small black dots representing thrombosed capillary loops.

B. Periungual Warts: Especially in nail-biters and cuticle-pickers, the wart virus is autoinoculated into periungual areas, causing persistent and troublesome verrucous lesions under and around the fingernails (Fig 14–7).

C. Flat Warts: Multiple flat warts are common on the face (Fig 14–8), neck, forearms, knees, and the backs of the hands. They are flat, flesh-colored, 2- to 4-mm papules that may number in the hundreds.

D. Filiform Warts: Slender, fingerlike warts are common on the face, particularly around the eyes and on the eyelids; they measure 1 or 2 mm in width but may reach 0.5 cm in length.

E. Condylomata Acuminata (Venereal Warts): Anogenital warts occur on the penis and around the anus (Fig 14–9) and vagina, where they may cluster densely and become white and macerated from moisture and occlusion. Condymomata acuminata are usually sexually acquired in adults. Perianal or vaginal warts in children should raise a suspicion of sexual abuse.

F. Plantar Warts: Warts on the plantar surface begin as deep-seated, translucent papules. Because of weight-bearing pressure, the raised, verrucous hyperkeratotic lesions common on the hands do not develop on the plantar surface. They are flush with—but extend deeply into—the plantar surface. Isolated solitary lesions (Fig 14–10) may have smooth keratotic surfaces, making them difficult to distinguish from corns or calluses. Surgical paring of a wart reveals multiple capillary bleeding points from the base of the lesion, whereas a corn has a white friable center and a callus consists of solid, translucent keratin to the base of the lesion. Plantar warts may seed to adjacent skin, giving rise to small satellite lesions. In some cases, centrifugal spread results in confluent, large hyper-

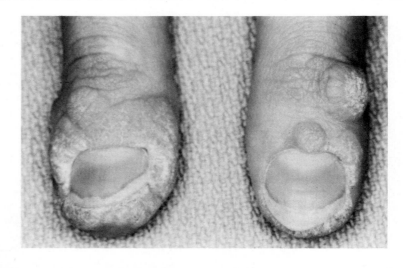

Figure 14–7. Periungual warts.

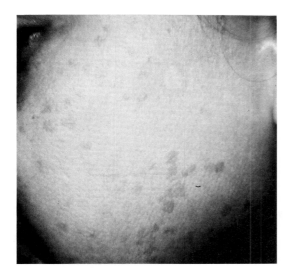

Figure 14–8. Flat warts on the face.

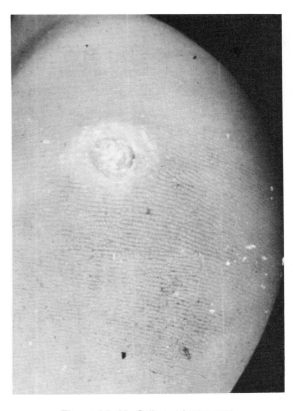

Figure 14–10. Solitary plantar wart.

keratotic plaques called **mosaic warts,** which generally are not as deep and painful as isolated, solitary plantar warts.

Differential Diagnosis

Common warts may be mistaken for actinic keratoses, seborrheic keratoses, squamous cell carcinoma, and keratoacanthoma. Flat warts on the face may resemble actinic or seborrheic keratoses, syringoma, adenoma sebaceum, basal cell carcinoma, and trichoepithelioma. Plantar calluses overlying the metatarsal heads may be mistaken for plantar warts. Large plantar warts and plantar verrucous carcinomas can be distinguished only by biopsy.

Complications & Sequelae

Immunocompromised patients with lymphoma, cancer, sarcoid, AIDS, or severe atopic eczema may develop generalized infection with thousands of cutaneous and mucosal warts. Infants born to mothers with vaginal condylomata acuminata may acquire human papillomavirus infection of the larynx, developing large, rapidly growing laryngeal papillomas with airway obstruction. Large genital and anal condylomata acuminata occasionally undergo malignant change to squamous cell carcinoma. Small, flat genital warts may have an atypical histologic appearance suggestive of squamous cell carcinoma in situ (bowenoid papulosis). Human papillomavirus has been implicated as a cause of cervical cancer.

Treatment

A. Surgical Procedures: Simple excision and

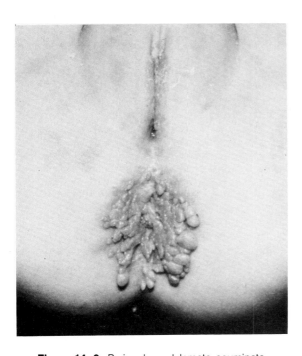

Figure 14–9. Perianal condylomata acuminata.

electrodesiccation with curettage are standard and effective means of treating common warts and condylomata acuminata but may leave a scar. Caution should be used with surgical treatment of plantar warts, since the resulting scar may be as painful as the wart and lasts longer.

B. Liquid Nitrogen: Freezing with liquid nitrogen on a cotton-tipped applicator with or without prior local anesthesia is quick and efficient treatment for most warts. Liquid nitrogen freezing of plantar or palmar warts may cause painful hemorrhagic blisters.

C. Salicylic Acid: Salicylic acid 40% plasters are produced commercially in 4×2 pads from which a patch the size of the plantar wart may be cut and applied nightly under occlusive tape. A combination of salicylic acid and lactic acid in flexible collodion (Duofilm) or salicylic acid in quick-drying base (Occlusal) may be applied daily to common warts, periungual warts, and flat warts without occlusion and to plantar warts with occlusion. Condylomata acuminata should not be treated with salicylic acid preparations.

D. Cantharidin: Cantharidin 0.7% in acetone and flexible collodion (Verr-Canth) may be applied daily with good results on periungual and common warts but may spread warts centrifugally, causing larger annular warts.

E. Podophyllum Resin: Moist and macerated perianal and vaginal warts may resolve after topical application of 25% podophyllum resin in tincture of benzoin. The drug is applied sparingly to lesions and the area is powdered with talc to decrease spread to adjacent normal skin. It should be washed away thoroughly with soap and water after 2–6 hours. Application may be repeated every 4–7 days depending on the amount of residual chemical irritation. Repeated applications are usually required for 6–8 weeks. Podophyllum resin is contraindicated in pregnancy, and systemic toxic reactions have been reported after application of large amounts to vaginal warts.

F. Fluorouracil: Topically applied fluorouracil 5% cream may induce the resolution of facial flat warts after 6–8 weeks of treatment. Fluorouracil cream is less useful for common warts, periungual warts, and plantar warts.

G. Dinitrochlorobenzene (DNCB) Sensitization: Patients with multiple or resistant warts may be sensitized with DNCB 2% in acetone applied under a perforated bandage strip for 24 hours. After sensitization, warts are carefully painted with DNCB 0.1% cream or solution. With daily treatments, warts have been seen to resolve within 7 days to 4 months. Generalized autosensitization reactions have been seen in 5–10% of treated patients, and the treatment is still considered experimental.

H. Laser: Photocoagulation of condylomata acuminata with the CO_2 laser is often successful.

I. Miscellaneous Therapies: Salicylic acid 6% in propylene glycol gel (Keralyt) applied daily for 2–3 months has induced resolution of facial flat warts.

Formalin 40% in Aquaphor applied daily to common warts and periungual warts, may induce resolution after several weeks of therapy. Allergic contact sensitization to formalin is a therapeutic risk. Condylomata acuminata may be injected repeatedly with interferon alfa-2b (Intron A).

ORF

Michael T. Jarratt, MD

Essentials of Diagnosis

- Large umbilicated pustules with central crusting, usually on the hands.
- Center white, edge red, with purple hue in between.
- Acquired by contact with sheep or goats.
- Spontaneous healing in 3–6 weeks.

General Considerations

Orf is caused by a virus belonging to the paravaccinia subgroup of poxviruses. The disease is distributed worldwide in sheep and goats. Young lambs are at high risk for infection and are a common vector for infection of humans. Human lesions usually result from direct inoculation of infected material from animals or animal products. Veterinarians, farmers, shepherds, and butchers are at particular risk. The primary infection conveys lasting immunity.

Clinical Findings

After an incubation period of 5–7 days, a firm erythematous papule appears and enlarges over 2–4 days into a large umbilicated, hemorrhagic pustule with central crusting. Fully developed lesions measure 2–5 cm in diameter. Lesions are usually solitary or few, localizing on the fingers, hands, forearms, and occasionally on the face. Lymphangitic streaking and regional lymphadenopathy may be associated with low-grade fever. The lesions heal spontaneously in 3–6 weeks.

Diagnosis is made by inspection. Electron microscopic examination of a biopsy specimen of the lesion demonstrates the characteristic cylindric poxvirus with its distinctive woven pattern.

Differential Diagnosis

Orf must be distinguished from milker's nodule, anthrax, sporotrichosis, and staphylococcal furunculosis.

Complications & Sequelae

Erythema multiforme occasionally occurs during the second or third week of infection.

Prevention

Animal handlers should be alert to orf lesions

around the mouths of sheep and goats. Human-to-human infection has not been reported.

Treatment & Prognosis

No treatment is required other than antiseptic procedures to prevent secondary infection. The disease heals spontaneously in 3–6 weeks and confers lasting immunity.

MILKER'S NODULE

Mark V. Dahl, MD

Essentials of Diagnosis

- Tricolored, occasionally painful nodule (black, white, and red).
- Usually occurs on fingers of people who milk cows.

General Considerations

Milker's nodule is caused by a poxvirus called paravaccinia virus, endemic to cattle. Lesions often occur on cows, where they are called pseudocowpox. Infection occurs from contact of human skin with these lesions.

Clinical Findings

A. Symptoms and Signs: A single asymptomatic or slightly painful nodule often develops on the finger. Multiple lesions may occur.

Initially, the lesion is an erythematous macule appearing 4–7 days after infection. It becomes papular and then papulovesicular. At this stage, it characteristically has 3 colors. The center is often a crust and is surrounded by a somewhat white-appearing vesiculopustule, which in turn is surrounded by an erythematous base. If the crust is not present, the center is often yellow or black, so the lesion looks like a target.

B. Laboratory Findings: The brick-shaped poxvirus may be seen by electron microscopy.

Differential Diagnosis

The disorder closely resembles orf, but the contact with cows instead of sheep usually makes the distinction. Cowpox, herpetic whitlow, furuncle, pyodermas, anthrax, tularemia, tuberculosis verrucosa cutis, atypical mycobacterial infections, sporotrichosis, chancre of syphilis, pyogenic granulomas, and vaccinia are all in the differential diagnosis. Many of these can be ruled out by other tests. (See clinical and laboratory findings in appropriate chapters.)

Prevention

Infected animals should be isolated. Protective gloves may confer some degree of protection as well.

Treatment & Prognosis

There is no specific therapy. The typical lesion heals spontaneously without sequelae but may leave a scar. Topical antibiotics such as bacitracin may be applied in hope of minimizing the chance of secondary infections.

RUBEOLA
(Measles)

Mark V. Dahl, MD

Essentials of Diagnosis

- Generalized morbilliform (netlike) exanthem.
- High fever.
- Cough, coryza, and conjunctivitis.
- Koplik's spots precede rash.
- Photophobia.

General Considerations

Measles is a highly contagious infectious disease caused by a paramyxovirus. It usually affects infants and children and spreads rapidly in populations without antibodies. It is more likely to occur in the winter or spring. Infection is spread by contact or inhalation of infectious droplets. Patients are contagious from 2 days prior to symptoms until 4 days after the exanthem appears.

A live attenuated measles virus vaccine has been available in the USA since 1963. Because widespread immunization programs have dramatically reduced the incidence of measles, many physicians have never seen a classic case.

Clinical Findings

A. Symptoms and Signs: Measles is usually preceded by a prodrome of coryza, conjunctivitis, and cough. The coryza suggests a severe common cold. The conjunctivitis is associated with photophobia and affects especially the lid margins. The cough is dry and may be quite severe. Fever often reaches 40 °C (104 °F). Generalized lymphadenopathy is common.

Approximately 1–7 days after the onset of prodromal symptoms, the rash occurs. It begins over the forehead and face and spreads down over the neck and trunk. This progression is rather slow. It usually takes at least 3 days for the eruption to reach the hands and feet.

The morphologic appearance is of a reticulated erythema, especially over the upper body (morbilliform rash), that blanches easily on pressure. Lesions on the leg are more likely to remain as localized macules. As the disease continues, pigment cells are stimulated so that the skin has a slightly yellow hue when blanched with a diascope. The skin begins to desquamate with very fine dustlike scales.

Koplik's spots are irregular, blue-white pinpoint elevations of the mucosa. They usually look like grains of sand on a red base. They often disappear at about the time the rash develops. Lesions are typically clustered on the buccal mucosa near the second molars. Occasionally, Koplik's spots are seen on the inner canthus or palate.

B. Laboratory Findings: The diagnosis is usually made on clinical grounds. Virus isolation is technically difficult. A rise in antibody titer between acute and convalescent serum specimens confirms the diagnosis, albeit usually after the disease has resolved.

Biopsy of skin occasionally shows necrotic epidermal cells with multinucleated giant cells.

Differential Diagnosis

The differential includes rubella (German measles), atypical measles, scarlet fever, toxic shock syndrome, Rocky Mountain spotted fever, enteroviral infections, and drug-related eruptions. Kawasaki syndrome may also be confused with measles. The combination of characteristic rash and prodromal signs and symptoms usually is sufficient to make a clinical diagnosis. The presence of Koplik's spots confirms the diagnosis. Cultures and antibody tests will confirm the diagnosis in the laboratory but are not usually done. Other disorders can often be ruled out by clinical findings, appropriate laboratory tests, or the history.

Complications & Sequelae

Encephalitis occurs in about one out of every 1000 cases and may cause death. Most patients recover completely, but some have permanent brain damage. Purpura is often associated with thrombocytopenia and may be severe and cause "black measles" associated with extreme toxicity, gastrointestinal bleeding, respiratory tract bleeding, high fevers, and death. Occasionally, a few red blood cells will leak through dilated blood vessels and be visible in fair-skinned children, but this does not warrant great concern since it is usually benign. Bacterial superinfection can occur and lead to sepsis.

Measles depresses the cell-mediated immune system and may aggravate or exacerbate tuberculosis. Skin tests are characteristically negative within 2 weeks after infection.

Subacute sclerosing encephalitis is a rare degenerative complication with seizures and intellectual impairment.

Prevention

Measles is preventable by immunization with live attenuated measles virus vaccines. Immunization is usually delayed until around the age of 15–18 months, because maternal antibodies passively transferred into the infant can interfere with appropriate immune responses if the vaccine is given earlier. Immune globulin (0.25–0.5 mL/kg, up to a total of not more than 15 mL) may prevent measles in a suscepti-

ble person if given within 6 days after exposure. This means of prevention is reserved especially for infants and immunosuppressed individuals who cannot be vaccinated with live virus vaccines.

Treatment & Prognosis

There is no specific antiviral therapy for measles. Fever can be suppressed with antipyretic agents. Aspirin is not recommended for children. Antitussive medications may suppress cough. The skin eruption requires no treatment. The appearance of desquamation can be masked with emollients if desired. The disease usually resolves within 10 days without problems. Poor nutrition and immunosuppression predispose to complications.

RUBELLA
(German Measles)

Mark V. Dahl, MD

Essentials of Diagnosis

- Morbilliform eruption initially involves the face, then spreads to the neck, arms, and trunk and fades on the face and upper body by the time the eruption appears on the feet.
- Rash lasts only a day or 2 in any anatomic area.
- Generalized lymphadenopathy.
- Mild systemic symptoms of low-grade fever, headache, conjunctivitis, sore throat, rhinitis, and cough.

General Considerations

Rubella is a common infectious viral disease of children caused by a rubivirus of the togavirus family. It is acquired through direct or droplet contact and usually resolves spontaneously. However, if contracted by a woman during pregnancy, it can cause significant congenital malformations of the fetus.

Clinical Findings

A. Symptoms and Signs: The incubation period is 2–3 weeks. The rash usually appears without any prodromal symptoms. Characteristically, it occurs first on the face and rapidly spreads to the neck, arms, trunk, and legs. It looks like measles but spreads rapidly over the body and is usually clearing on the face by the time it reaches the feet. Red, pinhead-sized, punctate macules may be present over the soft palate.

The lymphadenopathy is generalized. Suboccipital adenopathy is characteristic. The suboccipital, post-auricular, and anterior and posterior cervical nodes are usually markedly enlarged and tender. The adenopathy may persist after the rash has cleared.

Fevers, arthritis, and arthralgias are usually mild and are more common in adults than children.

B. Laboratory Findings: Culture of swabs taken from the throat or rectum isolates the virus, and serologic tests showing rises in antibody titer confirm the diagnosis. The diagnosis is usually made clinically, but a laboratory diagnosis should be made in pregnant women and newborn infants.

Differential Diagnosis

Rubella must be differentiated from rubeola, scarlet fever, infectious mononucleosis, toxoplasmosis, roseola, erythema infectiosum, enteroviral infections, and drug-related eruptions.

Complications & Sequelae

Most patients recover uneventfully. Large and small joints may occasionally become swollen, and joint effusions may rarely occur. Thrombocytopenic purpura may cause bleeding.

Approximately 50% of mothers who develop rubella during the first trimester of pregnancy deliver infants with signs of congenital rubella. These signs include low birth weight, microcephaly, mental retardation, cataracts, nerve deafness, patent ductus arteriosis, ventricular septal defect, bony abnormalities, and other abnormalities of the heart, eye, and central nervous system.

Prevention

A live attenuated rubella vaccine is available and is usually administered as a single injection after the age of 15 months. All women should be immunized prior to pregnancy. Congenital rubella syndrome has not been observed after vaccination during pregnancy, but pregnant women should not be given rubella vaccine. Pregnant mothers who develop rubella during the first trimester should consider abortion, because 50% of offspring will be afflicted.

Treatment & Prognosis

There is no specific antiviral treatment for rubella. Patients usually do well and require no treatment. The disease usually lasts about a week, and the prognosis is generally excellent.

ATYPICAL MEASLES

Mark V. Dahl, MD

People who have been immunized with the heat-killed rubeola vaccine may have only partial immunity. In these patients, active infection produces an atypical clinical presentation. The lesions are often purpuric and located primarily on the arms and legs.

Atypical measles is frequently accompanied by fever, malaise, myalgias, nausea, vomiting, coryza, conjunctivitis, dry cough, photophobia, and pleuritic pain. Chest x-ray films show abnormalities in more than 75% of patients and include interstitial infiltrates.

The measles virus usually cannot be isolated by cultures, but serologic tests often demonstrate extremely high titers of antibodies to measles and a 4-fold rise in antibody titer between acute and convalescent specimens.

Because purpura is common, the differential diagnosis includes Rocky Mountain spotted fever, varicella, scarlet fever, meningococcemia, infectious endocarditis, secondary syphilis, typhoid fever, typhus, coccidioidomycosis, disseminated intervascular coagulopathy, drug-related eruption, erythema multiforme, and dengue.

There is no specific therapy. Treatment is supportive and symptomatic. The condition usually resolves spontaneously in 7–10 days.

EXANTHEM SUBITUM
(Roseola Infantum)

Mark V. Dahl, MD

Essentials of Diagnosis

- High fever lasting 3–5 days with rapid defervescence.
- Onset of rash occurs at the time the fever lessens.
- Morbilliform eruption of discrete and confluent small pink macules.

General Considerations

Exanthem subitum is an infectious disease of young children between the ages of 6 months and 6 years. It is rare in other age groups. A member of the herpesvirus group called HSV-6 is the likely cause.

Clinical Findings

A. Symptoms and Signs: The fever is high and constant and usually lasts 3–5 days. Children usually appear well otherwise. Occasionally, the fever can be high enough to cause convulsions. Onset of skin rash coincides with disappearance of fever. The rash is morbilliform and consists of small, 3- to 5-mm, pink, discrete and confluent macules. It does not desquamate or become pigmented and lasts only a few hours in most cases.

B. Laboratory Findings: There may be mild leukopenia. No serologic or culture tests are indicated.

Differential Diagnosis

The differential diagnosis includes German measles, nonspecific viral exanthems, and drug-related eruptions. The course is usually suggestive enough so that the diagnosis can be made clinically.

Complications & Sequelae

Neurologic complications have been reported.

Treatment & Prognosis

There is no specific therapy. Antipyretic agents can be used to reduce fever. The prognosis is generally excellent.

ERYTHEMA INFECTIOSUM
(Fifth Disease)

Mark V. Dahl, MD

Essentials of Diagnosis

- Red patch on face ("slapped cheek").
- Circumoral pallor.
- Reticulated eruption of the arms and upper trunk after 1–4 days.
- Mild or no prodromal symptoms.

General Considerations

Erythema infectiosum is caused by a parvovirus and affects primarily children. It tends to occur in epidemics, especially in winter or spring.

Clinical Findings

A. Symptoms and Signs: The prodrome is usually absent or mild. Headache, malaise, nausea, and muscular aches are most common. The eruption occurs as pink macules or papules on the cheeks, which coalesce to form a confluent erythematous patch resembling a slapped cheek, hot to the touch but not tender. The area around the mouth is not involved (circumoral pallor). After a day or 2, this rash clears and the characteristic reticulated exanthem occurs on the arms and upper trunk. These lesions are evanescent and recurrent but fade after 6–10 days.

B. Laboratory Findings: A mild leukocytosis may occur. Eosinophilia and lymphocytosis may develop later. Specific laboratory diagnosis is difficult. Demonstration of the virus by DNA hybridization or electron microscopy is possible, and a rise in antibody titers to parvovirus also establishes the diagnosis.

Differential Diagnosis

Flushing, chapping, irritant dermatitis, cellulitis, erysipelas, scarlet fever, rubeola, rubella, sunburn, lupus erythematosus, and drug-related eruptions are all in the differential diagnosis. The physician can usually eliminate these entities on the basis of the history and the course of the disease and make a relatively certain diagnosis from the clinical features alone.

Treatment & Prognosis

Only symptomatic treatment is available. The prognosis is excellent.

PAPULAR ACRODERMATITIS
(Gianotti-Crosti Syndrome)

Mark V. Dahl, MD

Essentials of Diagnosis

- Affects children.
- Skin-colored or slightly pink papules.
- Lesions symmetric on face, extremities, and buttocks.
- The patient is usually otherwise well but may have fever and malaise.
- Frequent association with hepatitis B virus infection.

General Considerations

Papular acrodermatitis can result from several viruses, especially hepatitis B. Other viruses that have caused the eruption include hepatitis A virus, Epstein-Barr virus, coxsackievirus A16, parainfluenza virus, respiratory syncytial virus, and even poliovaccine enterovirus.

Clinical Findings

A. Symptoms and Signs: The child is usually well but may have diarrhea or an upper respiratory infection. Jaundice is rare. The skin suddenly erupts with skin-colored to slightly pink monomorphic papules, and additional papules may appear in crops. Symmetry is common, and most lesions occur on the face, extremities, and buttocks. Individual lesions last 3–8 weeks and resolve spontaneously.

B. Laboratory Findings: Skin biopsy shows nonspecific heavy infiltration of the dermis with lymphocytes and histiocytes, with mild epidermal spongiosis, acanthosis, and occasionally parakeratosis. Cultures or serologic tests can identify the viral cause. A test for hepatitis B surface antigen should always be done. Liver function tests are usually only slightly elevated.

Differential Diagnosis

Papules of lichen planus, lichen nitidus, and lichenoid drug reactions are the hardest to differentiate clinically, but biopsy distinguishes these disorders from papular acrodermatitis. Papular generalized granuloma annulare or sarcoid may occasionally also cause confusion clinically.

Treatment

No specific treatments are available. If pruritus is present, antipruritic lotion (eg, menthol 0.124% in 10% urea lotion), weak topical corticosteroid lotions (eg, 1% hydrocortisone), or systemic sedating antihistamines (eg, hydroxyzine) may be helpful.

Course & Prognosis

Individual lesions last 3–8 weeks and resolve spontaneously. New crops of papules can occur. The disorder clears spontaneously. Although liver function tests may be abnormal, most patients do not develop jaundice. Occasionally, children become chronic carriers of hepatitis B virus.

DENGUE

Mark V. Dahl, MD

Dengue presents as classic dengue or hemorrhagic dengue. It is caused by group B togavirus, transmitted to humans by the *Aedes* mosquito.

In classic dengue, the rash appears on the elbows and knees. Two to 5 days later, a morbilliform or scarlatiniform rash appears on the chest and spreads distally. Most patients have fever, headache, eye pain, conjunctivitis, backache, muscle and joint pain, adenopathy, and fatigue. During the last days of fever, petechiae may occur on the skin or mucous membranes in about half of cases. In hemorrhagic dengue, the hemorrhagic manifestations are more marked and include petechiae, purpura, and ecchymosis. Diffuse hemorrhage into serous cavities and disseminated intravascular coagulation may occur.

The virus can be isolated by culture and acute and convalescent serum for antibodies to dengue virus are available.

Treatment is supportive. The possible role of systemic steroids in the treatment of dengue hemorrhagic fever is controversial.

The prognosis for classic dengue is good. Symptoms usually resolve in 5–7 days. In hemorrhagic dengue, the prognosis is more guarded. Hemorrhagic shock may cause death.

REFERENCES

Boxer RJ, Skinner DG: Condylomata acuminata and squamous cell carcinoma. Urology 1977;9:72.

Brunell PA, Gerson AA: Passive immunization against varicella-zoster infections and other modes of therapy. J Infect Dis 1973;127:415.

Carey L, Spear PG: Infections with herpes simplex viruses. N Engl J Med 1986;314:686.

Centers for Disease Control: Rubella and congenital rubella: United States 1983. MMWR 1984;33.

Cherry JD: Viral exanthems. Curr Probl Pediatr 1983;13:1.

Crum CP et al: Human papillomavirus type 16 and early cervical neoplasia. N Engl J Med 1984;310:880.

Draelos ZK, Hansen RC, James WD: Gianotti-Crosti syndrome associated with infections other than hepatitis B. JAMA 1986;256:2386.

Eaglstein WH, Katz R, Brown JA: The effects of early corticosteroid therapy on the skin eruption and pain of herpes zoster. JAMA 1970;211:1681.

Epstein E: Treatment of zoster and post-zoster neuralgia by the intralesional injection of triamcinolone. Int J Dermatol 1976;15:762.

Esterly NB: Viral exanthems: Diagnosis and management. Semin Dermatol 1984;3:140.

Guinan ME et al: The course of untreated recurrent genital herpes simplex infection in 27 women. N Engl J Med 1981;304:759.

Huff JC et al: Therapy of herpes zoster with oral acyclovir. Am J Med 1988;85(Suppl 2A):84.

Massing AM, Epstein WL: Natural history of warts. Arch Dermatol 1963;87:306.

Moore RM Jr.: Human orf in the United States, 1972. J Infect Dis 1973;73:731.

Pierard-Franchiment C, Legrain A, Pierard GE: Growth and regression of molluscum contagiosum. J Am Acad Dermatol 1983;9:669.

Plummer FA et al: An erythema infectiosum-like illness caused by human parvovirus infection. N Engl J Med 1985;313:74.

Robinson AJ, Peterson GU: Orf virus infection of workers in the meat industry. N Engl J Med 1983;96:81.

Smith EB, Raimer SS: Common viral infections of the skin and their treatment. Med Clin North Am 1982; 66:807.

Spector SA et al: Treatment of herpes virus infections in immunocompromised patients with acyclovir by continuous intravenous infusion. Am J Med 1982; 73(1A):275.

Thin RN et al: Value of Papanicolaou-stained smears in the diagnosis of trichomoniasis, candidiasis, and cervical herpes simplex virus infection in women. Brit J Vener Dis 1975;51:116.

Weller TH: Varicella and herpes zoster: Changing concepts of the natural history, control, and importance of a not-so-benign virus. N Engl J Med 1983;309:1362.

Whitley RJ et al: The natural history of herpes simplex virus infection of mother and newborn. Pediatrics 1980;66:489.

Williamson AP: The varicella-zoster virus in the etiology of severe congenital defects. A survey of eleven reported instances. Clin Pediatr 1975;14:553.

Young EJ, Killam AP, Greene JR Jr.: Disseminated herpesvirus infection: association with primary genital herpes in pregnancy. JAMA 1976;253:2731.

15

Acquired Immune Deficiency Syndrome

Bijan Safai, MD, DSc, David J. Gross, MD, & Mark V. Dahl, MD

I. THE BIOLOGY & EPIDEMIOLOGY OF AIDS

The human immune deficiency virus (HIV), one of the more recently discovered human retroviruses, is the causative agent of the acquired immune deficiency syndrome (AIDS). The virus has spread rapidly among various high-risk populations and has achieved pandemic status. Infection occurs from sexual contact with an infected person, from transfusion or heavy contact with contaminated blood or blood products, or transplacentally in infants born to infected mothers.

The virus kills helper T lymphocytes, rendering the patient immunodeficient. As a consequence, the patient may develop opportunistic infections and various types of cancer.

Epidemiology

Most patients with AIDS are homosexual or bisexual men who have had multiple sexual liaisons in which they have been the anal receptive partner. Genital ulcerative diseases have been found to increase the risk for infection in all sexually active groups.

Drug abusers comprise the second largest group of individuals who develop AIDS. Drug abusers are more likely to be black or Hispanic, whereas homosexuals in the USA are mostly white. Other groups reported more likely to develop AIDS include Haitians, hemophiliacs, transfusion recipients, infants whose mothers were prostitutes or drug abusers, female sexual partners of men with AIDS or at high risk for AIDS, and black Africans.

Most women with AIDS are intravenous drug users, but a significant number contract AIDS by intimate heterosexual contact with infected partners. Infected women are not necessarily symptomatic at the time of delivery and can give birth to infected infants who may then become symptomatic before they themselves do. The efficiency of viral transmission in utero has been estimated to range from 35% to 65%, and the number of children with AIDS will rise in tandem with the growing number of infected women.

By the end of 1988, the cumulative number of AIDS cases in the USA as reported by the CDC was almost 81,500 for adults and adolescents and 1346 for children. Of the adult and adolescent cases, 50,325 involved homosexual or bisexual men; 16,151 cases occurred among intravenous drug users; and 5874 cases involved homosexual men who were also intravenous drug users. Among affected children, 83 had hemophilia or other coagulation disorders, and 1044 were born of parents with AIDS or at risk for AIDS.

The present trend is for increasing numbers of intravenous drug users to develop AIDS, while homosexual and bisexual men are being diagnosed as having AIDS less frequently.

Etiology

The human immunodeficiency virus (HIV), a member of the retrovirus family, is the cause of AIDS. (The counterpart in sheep in lentivirus.) It is an RNA virus requiring a special enzyme—reverse transcriptase (RT)—for replication. Reverse transcriptase is responsible for the transcription of viral RNA into proviral DNA, and it is this double-stranded DNA that can become integrated into the host cell DNA. As the host cell DNA replicates, so does the integrated DNA copy of viral RNA. The proviral DNA can either replicate along with host cell DNA and remain silent, or it can be transformed into active virus depending on as yet undetermined signals. It may be that secondary infections such as those with cytomegalovirus, Epstein-Barr virus, etc, might activate viral replication and cause more rapid progression of HIV infection toward clinical manifestations of AIDS.

The virus contains at least 8 genes, including *pol*

(polymerases), *env* (envelope), *gag* (core), various positive and negative regulatory products, and other products of undetermined significance.

The infected individual forms antibodies to viral antigens, including envelope gene products (gp160, gp120, and gp41), core gene products (p55, p24, and p17), and polymerase gene products (p66, p51, and p3) (Table 15–1). Antibodies to envelope gene products are the most frequent ones detected, followed next by polymerase antibodies and lastly by antibodies to the core gene products. Diminishing antibody titers to core gene products occur as the disease progresses.

The most frequently employed methods for serologic antibody testing to HIV include the enzyme immunoassay (EIA), indirect immunofluorescence (IF), and Western blot (WB) techniques. WB or IF methods are used to verify results on specimens that have been found to be reactive using the EIA technique. In high-risk groups, IF and WB yield comparable results, but in unselected low-risk groups it is best to validate EIA results using WB rather than IF. New "second-generation" EIAs may be as sensitive as WB, so HIV antigen will rarely be found in the absence of antibody using this revised technique. The polymerase chain reaction (PCR) technique is perhaps the most sensitive method for detecting the virus.

The envelope precursor glycoprotein gp160 appears as gp41 (transmembrane envelope protein) and gp120 (outer membrane envelope protein) in finished form. HIV is able to infect helper T cells because of the specific interaction between the viral envelope (gp120) and the CD4 antigen present on the surface of T4 cells.

For most other viral diseases, antibodies directed against viral envelope antigen are completely protec-tive, but this is not true in the case of HIV. It remains unclear, however, if the presence of neutralizing antibodies provides some partial protection against the virus or influences the course of the infection.

II. THE CLINICAL SYNDROMES OF AIDS

Essentials of Diagnosis

- Opportunistic infections.
- Kaposi's sarcoma or extranodal lymphoma.
- Weight loss, often with diarrhea.
- No other cause of immunodeficiency.
- Antibodies to HIV in serum.

CLASSIFICATION OF HIV-RELATED DISORDERS

Infection with HIV has varied consequences ranging from asymptomatic infection to life-threatening opportunistic infections or cancers that appear after immunosuppression has become sufficiently severe (Table 15–2). A classification system for diseases associated with HIV is presented in Table 15–3.

The acute infection (group I) often presents as a mononucleosis-like illness that occurs at the time of seroconversion. Prior to seroconversion, the infected individual is asymptomatic.

Table 15–1. Description of major gene products of human immunodeficiency virus (HIV).[1]

Gene Product[2]	Description
p17	Gag protein
p24	Gag protein
p31	Endonuclease component of pol translate
gp41	Transmembrane env glycoprotein
p51	Reverse transcriptase component of pol translate
p55	Precursor of gag proteins
p66	Reverse transcriptase component of pol translate
gp120	Outer env glycoprotein
gp160	Precursor of env glycoprotein

gag = core, pol = polymerase, env = envelope
[1]Reproduced, with permission, from CDC.
[2]Number refers to molecular weight of the protein in kilodaltons; measurements of molecular weight may vary slightly in different laboratories

Table 15–2. Opportunistic infections encountered in patients with AIDS.

Fungi	*Candida* sp *Cryptococcus neoformans* *Histoplasma capsulatum* *Aspergillus* sp *Sporothrix schenckii*
Parasites	*Pneumocystis carinii* *Toxoplasma gondii* *Cryptosporidium* sp
Viruses	Cytomegalovirus Herpes simplex Varicella-zoster Epstein-Barr virus Papovavirus-JC Adenovirus
Bacteria	*Mycobacterium* sp *Nocardia asteroids* *Salmonella* sp *Listeria monocytogenes* *Streptococcus pneumonia* *Haemophilus influenza* *Staphylococcus aureus* *Clostridium perfringens* *Shigella* sp

Table 15–3. Summary of classification system for human immunodeficiency virus

Group I	Acute infection
Group II	Asymptomatic infection[1]
Group III	Persistent generalized lymphadenopathy[1]
Group IV	Other disease
Subgroup A	Constitutional disease
Subgroup B	Neurologic disease
Subgroup C	Secondary infectious diseases
Category C-1	Specified secondary infectious diseases listed in the CDC surveillance definition for AIDS[2]
Category C-2	Other specified secondary infectious diseases
Subgroup D	Secondary cancers[2]
Subgroup E	Other conditions

[1]Patients in Groups II and III may be subclassified on the basis of a laboratory evaluation.
[2]Includes those patients whose clinical presentation fulfills the definition of AIDS used by CDC for national reporting.

The incubation period for the development of perinatally acquired AIDS averages 6–8 months, while the mean incubation period is 28 months for adolescents and adults.

Asymptomatic patients (group II) may already have had a mononucleosis-like illness and become seropositive, or the patients may never have been ill and yet show evidence of HIV infection upon serologic testing.

Patients with persistent generalized lymphadenopathy fall into group III in this classification. These individuals have had enlarged lymph nodes in 2 or more extrainguinal sites for more than 3 months without explanation. In the homosexual and bisexual populations, persistent generalized lymphadenopathy occurs about 9 times more frequently among seropositive individuals as compared to seronegative ones. Persistent generalized lymphadenopathy in the absence of symptoms does not indicate the severity of immune compromise; however, there are estimates that at least 50% of seropositive persistent generalized lymphadenopathy patients will develop AIDS within 5 years.

Group IV (other disease) consists of several subgroupings that are self-explanatory (see Table 15–2).

The current CDC surveillance case definition for AIDS includes AIDS-indicative diseases such as the HIV wasting syndrome or HIV encephalopathy and allows the presumptive diagnosis of AIDS-indicative diseases without confirmatory evidence from the laboratory.

AIDS in children presents in slightly different ways. Common findings in children with AIDS include failure to thrive, hepatosplenomegaly, chronic interstitial pneumonitis, and progressive neurologic disease that can manifest itself, for example, as loss of developmental milestones. When one is dealing with pediatric AIDS cases, the possibility of a primary immunodeficiency disease must be ruled out.

DERMATOLOGIC MANIFESTATIONS OF AIDS

For many AIDS patients, entry into the health care system occurs in the office of a dermatologist. The dermatologic manifestations of AIDS can range from a severe form of a normally self-limited eruption to unusual lesions such as Kaposi's sarcoma and oral hairy leukoplakia. Cosmetically disturbing skin conditions can be the first signal of systemic immunosuppression, indicating perhaps that the patient is infected with HIV.

Skin Infections & Infestations (Table 15–4)

A. Viral Infections:

1. Herpes simplex– The frequency of attacks of herpes simplex is greater in AIDS patients than in the general population. Furthermore, the lesions are more likely to be deep, painful, and nonhealing, especially around the perianal area. Acyclovir resistance has been detected in HSV-2 isolates from several AIDS patients, and foscarnet or vidarabine are therapeutic options in such situations.

2. Herpes zoster– The occurrence of herpes zoster in a member of a high-risk group indicates that the probability of being infected with HIV is quite high and the development of AIDS likely. Chronic varicella-zoster infection can also occur in AIDS patients.

3. Molluscum contagiosum– Papules of molluscum contagiosum are common in patients with AIDS and often appear on the face, are numerous, and are refractory to treatment.

4. Warts– Both common warts and condylomata acuminata are common among patients with AIDS. Warts in the anal area can become huge and require surgical excision or laser destruction. Warts can also become widely disseminated.

5. Oral hairy leukoplakia– This skin lesion is rather specific for AIDS and is presumed to be due to a combined infection by human papillomavirus and Epstein-Barr virus. Candidal infection is often present. The lesions appear as white, fine, vertical linear areas on the sides of the tongue, though they may also be found elsewhere. Histologically, they show acanthosis, parakeratosis, and hyperkeratosis. Balloon cells may appear in the stratum corneum.

B. Bacterial Infections:

1. Syphilis– Because AIDS is sexually transmitted, many patients with AIDS have also had syphilis. The clinical presentation of secondary syphilis may

Table 15-4. Mucocutaneous findings with AIDS.

Hair	Alopecia areata AIDS trichopathy (hair becomes smoother, lighter, softer, and silkier)
Nails	Yellow nail syndrome Purple nail bands secondary to AZT
Mouth	Thrush Kaposi's sarcoma Hairy leukoplakia

Skin	Generalized granuloma annulare
	Eosinophilic pustular folliculitis
	Kaposi's sarcoma
	Psoriatic exacerbation
	Severe and inflammatory seborrheic dermatitis
	Ichthyosis
	Xerosis
	Flesh-colored papular eruption
	Infections including:
	    Exaggerated scabies
	    Herpes zoster: dermatomal, disseminated, chronic varicella zoster
	    Molluscum contagiosum: large, numerous
	    Herpes simplex: recurrent, disseminated, deep ulcerations
	    Dermatophytosis
	Papulonodular demodicidosis
	Cat-scratch disease
	Cutaneous cryptococcosis
	Disseminated warts
	Bacillary epithelial angiomatosis

be atypical. The eruption may be extensive, and serologic tests have occasionally been nonreactive in the early secondary stage, making diagnosis much more difficult. Furthermore, one dose of benzathine penicillin may not cure early syphilis in AIDS patients.

2. Cat-scratch disease– Disseminated cat-scratch disease with angiomatous nodules closely resembling epidemic Kaposi's sarcoma has been observed in AIDS patients.

3. Mycobacterial infections– Disseminated tuberculosis has occurred in AIDS patients. Atypical mycobacterial infections can occur, particularly with *Mycobacterium avium-intracellulare*. These may present as ecthymatous ulcers or as nodules.

4. Other bacterial infections– In addition to opportunistic bacterial infections, both staphylococcal and streptococcal infections are common. These include ecthyma, cellulitis, abscesses, impetigo, folliculitis, staphylococcal scalded skin syndrome, and bacillary epithelioid angiomatosis..

C. Fungal Infections:

1. Candidiasis– Oral candidiasis is very common in patients with AIDS. White patches occur on the tongue or other areas of the mouth. If the esophagus becomes involved, it may be painful. *Candida* can disseminate widely. Candidal infections of the nails are common also.

2. Superficial fungal infections– Dermatophyte fungal infections are common, including tinea cruris

and tinea pedis. Odd forms and locations have been reported, including tinea faciale and hyperkeratotic tinea pedis of the soles.

3. Cryptococcosis– Systemically disseminated cryptococcal infection may present as a single skin ulcer or as herpetiform ulcers and even as multiple skin papules and nodules. It can also resemble papules of molluscum.

4. Histoplasmosis– Disseminated histoplasmosis may present as papules with a central keratotic plug. Clinically, the papules may resemble molluscum contagiosum, but they can be distinguished histologically.

D. Amebiasis: A nonspecific amebic papule or ulcer may occur in the perirectal area.

E. Scabies: Scabies in AIDS patients may be severe and atypical. Crusted (Norwegian) scabies has occurred, as might be expected in patients with profound immunosuppression.

Skin Neoplasms

A. Kaposi's Sarcoma: This disorder is discussed in greater detail at the conclusion of this section on the dermatologic manifestations of AIDS. Lesions often begin as purple or brown macules that enlarge slowly to become purple nodules, plaques, and tumors. The plaques tend to be oval and often elongate along skin lines in a configuration resembling pityriasis rosea. Involvement of the upper trunk, head, neck, and upper extremity is usual. Visceral involvement is common.

B. Lymphomas: Both Hodgkin's disease and non-Hodgkin's B cell lymphoma may involve the skin with nodules and papules.

C. Squamous Cell Carcinomas: Both oral and anal squamous cell carcinomas have occurred in patients with AIDS.

Miscellaneous Skin Manifestations

A. Drug Eruptions: For some reason, patients with AIDS receiving trimethoprim-sulfamethoxazole are more prone than others to development of drug reactions. Of course, other drugs can cause exanthems in patients with AIDS.

B. Psoriasis: Explosive psoriasis or sudden flare of preexisting psoriasis can occur in AIDS. The use of methotrexate to treat psoriasis in patients with AIDS has been associated with a poor prognosis, because methotrexate further depresses the immune and inflammatory systems. Zidovudine (AZT) has been used with some success.

C. Seborrheic Dermatitis: Patients with AIDS often develop severe seborrheic dermatitis not only of the scalp but also of the face, axillas, chest, groin, and genitals. The center of the face is commonly affected.

D. Dry Skin: Acquired ichthyosis and xerosis have been found in AIDS patients.

E. Nutritional Deficiencies: Patients with AIDS may develop pellagra or zinc deficiency dermatitis.

F. Papular Eruption of AIDS: Several hundred 2- to 5-mm skin-colored or slightly red papules may develop over the head and neck, upper trunk, and extremities. These lesions may be single or coalesce and are often pruritic.

G. Angular Cheilitis: Fissuring at the corners of the mouth is often associated with oral candidiasis.

H. Eczematous Dermatitis: An atopic-like dermatitis has occurred in up to 50% of children with AIDS.

I. Granuloma Annulare: Disseminated papules showing necrobiotic granuloma on histologic examination have been described.

J. Pruritus: Some patients develop intractable pruritus without evidence of other skin disease.

K. Eosinophilic Pustular Folliculitis: This is a very pruritic eruption often helped by UVB phototherapy.

Hair Abnormalities

A relationship between alopecia areata and AIDS has been proposed. Hair changes, such as smoother, lighter, softer, and silkier hair, have been reported with disease progression.

Nail Changes

A yellow nail syndrome has been reported in AIDS patients. The nails display yellow discoloration distally. Nails with the appearance of transverse bluish bands coinciding with time of zidovudine administration have been described.

LABORATORY FINDINGS IN AIDS

Laboratory tests indicative of immune deficiency in AIDS patients include diminished reactivity to skin tests or delayed hypersensitivity to common antigens and an inability to be sensitized by topical application of solutions of dinitrochlorobenzene (DNCB). Severe lymphopenia and helper T cell subset depletion have become hallmarks of the disease, resulting in reversal of the normal T4/T8 ratio of 2. Not only is there a quantitative defect in the T4 subset, but qualitative defects exist as well.

A comparison of well seropositive homosexuals with well seronegative homosexuals revealed lower T4 cell levels in the former group. Among the seropositive subjects, 2 patterns of serial T4 cell counts emerged. One pattern showed a low normal but stable pattern of T4 cells with minimal clinical disease; the other showed a progressive fall of T4 cell count along with clinical deterioration. Frequently, the number of T helper cells is higher and the degree of immunologic derangement is less in patients whose initial manifestation of AIDS is Kaposi's sarcoma rather than an opportunistic infection.

Natural killer cell activity is depressed, and B cell function is altered. The hypergammaglobulinemia that is frequently present is perhaps secondary to spontaneous polyclonal activation of B cells, and the B cells have been rendered refractory to various T cell-independent B cell mitogens.

DIAGNOSTIC STANDARDS FOR AIDS

For purposes of national reporting, AIDS is defined as an illness characterized by one or more of the following "indicator" diseases, depending on the status of laboratory evidence of HIV infection.

I. Without Laboratory Evidence Pertaining to HIV Infection

If laboratory tests for HIV were not performed or gave inconclusive results and the patient had no other cause of immunodeficiency (listed in I.A, below), then any disease listed in I.B indicates AIDS if it is diagnosed by a definitive method.

A. Causes of Immunodeficiency That Disqualify Diseases as Indicators of Aids in the Absence of Laboratory Evidence for HIV Infection:

1. High-dose or long-term systemic corticosteroid therapy or other immunosuppressive cytotoxic therapy less than 3 months before the onset of the indicator disease.

2. Any of the following diseases diagnosed less than 3 months after diagnosis of the indicator disease: Hodgkin's disease, non-Hodgkin's lymphoma (other than primary brain lymphoma), lymphocytic leukemia, multiple myeloma, any other cancer of lymphoreticular or histiocytic tissue or angioimmunoblastic lymphadenopathy.

3. A genetic (congenital) immunodeficiency syndrome or an acquired immunodeficiency syndrome atypical of HIV infection, such as one involving hypogammaglobulinemia.

B. Indicator Diseases Diagnosed Definitively:

1. Candidiasis of the esophagus, trachea, bronchi, or lungs.

2. Cryptococcosis, extrapulmonary.

3. Cryptosporidiosis with diarrhea persisting more than 1 month.

4. Cytomegalovirus disease of an organ other than liver, spleen, or lymph nodes in a patient more than 1 month of age.

5. Herpes simplex virus infection causing a mucocutaneous ulcer that persists longer than 1 month; or bronchitis, pneumonitis, or esophagitis of any duration in a patient more than 1 month of age.

6. Kaposi's sarcoma in a patient under 60 years of age.

7. Lymphoma of the brain (primary) in a patient under 60 years of age.

8. Lymphoid interstitial pneumonia or pulmonary lymphoid hyperplasia ("LIP-PHL complex") in a child under 13 years of age.

9. Disseminated *Mycobacterium avium* complex or *Mycobacterium kansasii* infection (ie, at a site other than or in addition to lungs, skin, or cervical or hilar lymph nodes).

10. *Pneumocystis carinii* pneumonia.

11. Progressive multifocal leukoencephalopathy.

12. Toxoplasmosis of the brain in a patient over 1 month of age.

II. With Laboratory Evidence of HIV Infection

Regardless of the presence of other causes of immunodeficiency, any disease listed above (I.B) or below (II.A) justifies a diagnosis of AIDS if there is laboratory evidence for HIV infection.

A. Indicator Diseases Diagnosed Definitively:

1. Bacterial infections, multiple or recurrent (any combination of at least 2 within a 2-year period) of the following types affecting a child under 13 years of age: septicemia, pneumonia, meningitis, bone or joint infection, or abscess of an internal organ or body cavity (excluding otitis media or superficial skin or mucosal abscesses) caused by *Haemophilus, Streptococcus* (including pneumococcus), or other pyogenic bacteria.

2. Coccidioidomycosis, disseminated (at a site other than or in addition to lungs or cervical or hilar lymph nodes).

3. HIV encephalopathy (also called "HIV dementia," "AIDS dementia," or "subacute encephalitis due to HIV").

4. Histoplasmosis, disseminated (at a site other than or in addition to lungs or cervical or hilar lymph nodes).

5. Isosporiasis with diarrhea persisting more than 1 month.

6. Kaposi's sarcoma in a patient of any age.

7. Lymphoma of the brain (primary) in a patient of any age.

8. Other non-Hodgkin's lymphoma of B cell or unknown immunologic phenotype and the following histologic types:

a. Small noncleaved lymphoma (Burkitt's or non-Burkitt's).

b. Immunoblastic sarcoma (equivalent to any of the following, though not necessarily all in combination: immunoblastic lymphoma, large-cell lymphoma, diffuse histiocytic lymphoma, diffuse undifferentiated lymphoma, high-grade lymphoma).

Note: Lymphomas are not included here if they are of T cell immunologic phenotype or their histologic type is not described or is described as "lymphocytic," "lymphoblastic," "small cleaved," or "plasmacytoid lymphocytic."

9. Any disseminated mycobacterial disease caused by mycobacteria other than *Mycobacterium tuberculosis,* (ie, at a site other than or in addition to lungs, skin, or cervical or hilar lymph nodes).

10. Extrapulmonary *M tuberculosis* infection (ie, involving at least one site outside the lungs, regardless of whether there is concurrent pulmonary involvement).

11. Recurrent *Salmonella* septicemia other than typhoid fever.

12. HIV wasting syndrome (emaciation, "slim disease").

B. Indicator Diseases Diagnosed Presumptively:

Note: Given the seriousness of diseases indicative of AIDS, it is generally important to diagnose them definitively—especially when therapy may have serious side effects or when definitive diagnosis is needed for eligibility for antiretroviral therapy. Even so, there are times when a patient may not permit the performance of definitive tests or when accepted clinical practice is to diagnose presumptively based on the presence of characteristic clinical and laboratory abnormalities.

1. Candidiasis of the esophagus.

2. Cytomegalovirus retinitis with loss of vision.

3. Kaposi's sarcoma.

4. Lymphoid interstitial pneumonia or pulmonary lymphoid hyperplasia ("LIP-PLH complex") in a child under 13 years of age.

5. Disseminated mycobacterial infection (acid-fast bacilli with species not identified by culture) (ie, involving at least one site other than or in addition to lungs, skin, or cervical or hilar lymph nodes).

6. *Pneumocystis carinii* pneumonia.

7. Toxoplasmosis of the brain in a patient over 1 month of age.

III. With Laboratory Evidence Against HIV Infection

With laboratory test results negative for HIV infection, the diagnosis of AIDS for surveillance purposes is ruled out unless *both* III.A and III.B apply:

A. All other causes of immunodeficiency listed above (I.A) have been excluded.

B. The patient has had *either* of the following:

1. *Pneumocystis carinii* pneumonia diagnosed by a definitive method.

2. Any of the other diseases indicative of AIDS listed above in I.B diagnosed by a definitive method *and* a T helper/inducer (CD4) lymphocyte count less than 400/μL.

PREVENTION OF AIDS

Both homosexuals and heterosexuals should limit the risk of contracting AIDS. Physicians can help by counseling.

The number of sexual partners should be limited.

Knowing a partner well may decrease the risk of AIDS by avoiding intercourse with men known to be bisexual and with male or female prostitutes or intravenous drug abusers. Noninsertive sex is safe; mutual masturbation, touching, and massaging are less risky than oral sex or intercourse. Condom use decreases the risk but is not completely safe. Use of a spermicide with a condom may provide protection greater than use of a condom alone. Guidelines for condom use are presented in Chapter 13. The presence of sores on the genitals increases the risk of infection through intercourse.

Antibody testing, donor self-deferral, and heat-treatment of factor concentrates have done much to limit the spread of AIDS from transfusions of blood components.

Women at high risk should be tested for HIV antibodies prior to becoming pregnant.

No one should use illicit intravenous drugs. Drug abusers should always use clean syringes and needles. Sharing needles can transmit HIV infection.

TREATMENT OF AIDS

Agents have been developed that can interrupt the viral replicative process at any number of steps. The most successful drug therapy to date affects the integrity of the viral reverse transcriptase enzyme. Zidovudine (AZT), a derivative of thymidine, is the most common agent used in HIV infection. Following triphosphorylation, AZT is polymerized into DNA by HIV reverse transcriptase and causes the premature termination of DNA synthesis.

The present recommended dose for initiation of AZT therapy is 200 mg every 4 hours (in a 70-kg man, 2.9 mg/kg). In addition to its use for patients with AIDS, it is being administered to HIV-infected persons with T helper cell counts below $200/\mu L$, and some advocate administering the drug to other infected asymptomatic patients as well. Some institutions have even developed protocols for house staff and ancillary personnel who have been stuck with needles from patients infected with HIV.

Hematologic abnormalities attributable to AZT have been substantial, though toxicity is less severe in patients with early disease. Caution is advised when prescribing this drug for patients with evidence of bone marrow compromise as demonstrated by granulocyte counts less than $1000/\mu L$ or hemoglobin concentrations less than 9.5 g/dL. Once AZT treatment is begun, however, therapy should proceed uninterrupted, since cessation of therapy has been associated with enhanced viral replication.

AZT has been used successfully in combination with acyclovir to treat a small group of patients with AIDS or ARC. The dose of AZT used in this combination is half the usual dose, since acyclovir poten-

tiates the anti-HIV activity of AZT in vitro without adding to its hematologic toxicity.

KAPOSI'S SARCOMA

Essentials of Diagnosis

- Early: red, blue, purple, or red-brown macules occurring anywhere on the skin surface or mucous membranes.
- Later: burgundy-purple plaques, nodules, and tumors.
- Usually otherwise asymptomatic.
- Mucous membranes may be involved.
- Usually more than one lesion.
- Diagnostic histologic findings.
- Usually positive HIV test.

General Considerations

Prior to the AIDS epidemic, physicians in the USA were familiar with Kaposi's sarcoma in its classic form as an indolent disease of older people, usually of European ancestry, characterized by the appearance of reddish-purple to dark-blue maculopapular or nodular lesions, most commonly on the lower extremities. Patients with classic Kaposi's sarcoma can live for years with their disease.

Kaposi's sarcoma is endemic in certain parts of Africa, where its behavior varies greatly depending on morphology, presenting in nodular, florid, infiltrative, or lymphadenopathic forms. The disease has occurred also among renal transplant recipients and patients with autoimmune disorders following the initiation of immunosuppressive therapy, with reported regression of Kaposi's sarcoma in some cases after discontinuing the immunosuppressive drugs.

Kaposi's sarcoma has appeared frequently among AIDS patients, especially white homosexual men. In fact, the AIDS epidemic was initially recognized by the increased frequency of this cancer among the homosexual and bisexual population. It has been reported in all high-risk groups but with lower frequencies than among homosexuals. Cofactors along with HIV infection that may account for this phenomenon are under investigation.

It is of interest that there has been a decline in the incidence of Kaposi's sarcoma among patients being diagnosed with AIDS in the USA.

Clinical Findings

A. Symptoms and Signs: Although relative immunodeficiency is usually present when Kaposi's sarcoma develops, many patients are otherwise subjectively well. The initial lesions are rather banal-appearing pink to brown-red macules occurring anywhere on the skin or mucous membranes. The lesions enlarge and elongate, with the long axis often following the skin lines. As they enlarge, the macules usually thicken and turn more purple. In advanced cases, many burgundy-colored, irregular nodules, plaques, and tumors are present.

B. Laboratory Findings: Skin biopsy is the diagnostic procedure of choice. In the dermis, vascular channels are filled with erythrocytes. The channels are lined by spindle-shaped to plump endothelial cells, and surrounding macrophages are usually laden with hemosiderin. The strands of endothelial cells form fascicles that intertwine among the red blood cells. Early lesions are less diagnostic, and the histologic appearance may suggest granulation tissue.

Differential Diagnosis

The clinical differential diagnosis of early macular lesions is vast but includes dermatofibromas and macules of subtle inflammatory diseases. In its plaque and nodular forms, the diagnosis is usually obvious, but biopsy to confirm the diagnosis is recommended in all cases. Disseminated cat-scratch disease needs to be excluded.

Treatment

Radiation or laser therapy (photodynamic therapy) can be used if lesions are few or if lesions affect the face or cause obstruction.

Recombinant interferon alfa-2b (Intron A) can be administered subcutaneously or intravenously at high dosages, ie, $20-30$ million IU/m^2 daily or 3 times a week. The average time for response is about 2 months. Patients with more intact immune system (ie, with relatively high numbers of CD4 cells) seem to do better. Almost all patients develop adverse side effects, especially flulike symptoms. There may be synergistic adverse effects when interferon is given with AZT—especially proneness for neutropenia. White blood cell counts should be monitored (see prescribing information).

REFERENCES

Armstrong D et al: Treatment of infection in patients with acquired immunodeficiency syndrome. Ann Intern Med 1985;103:738.

Bowen DL, Lane HC, Fauci AS: Immunopathogenesis of the acquired immunodeficiency syndrome. Ann Intern Med 1985;103:704.

CDC: Classification system for human immunodeficiency virus (HIV) infection in children under 13 years of age. MMWR 1987;36:225.

CDC: Classification system for human T-lymphotropic virus type III/lymphadenopathy-associated virus infections. MMWR 1986;35:334.

CDC: Revision of the CDC surveillance case definition for acquired immunodeficiency syndrome. MMWR 1987; 36(Suppl 1S):3S.

Cooper DA et al: Acute AIDS retrovirus infection. Lancet 1985;1:537.

Goodman DS et al: Prevalence of cutaneous disease in patients with acquired immunodeficiency syndrome (AIDS) or AIDS-related complex. J Am Acad Dermatol 1987;17:210.

Guinan ME, Hardy A: Epidemiology of AIDS in women in the United States 1981–1986. JAMA 1987;257:321.

Hoxie JA: Current concepts in the virology of infection with human immunodeficiency virus (HIV): A view from the III International Conference on AIDS. Ann Intern Med 1987;107:406.

Kaslow RA et al: Infection with the human immunodeficiency virus: Clinical manifestations and their relationship to immune deficiency. Ann Intern Med 1987; 107:474.

Koop CE: *Surgeon General's Report on Acquired Immune Deficiency Syndrome.* US Government Printing Office, 1986.

Lange W et al: Clinical, immunologic and serologic findings in men at risk for acquired immunodeficiency syndrome: The San Francisco Men's Health Study. JAMA 1987;257:326.

Matis WL et al: Dermatologic findings associated with human immunodeficiency virus infection. J Am Acad Dermatol 1987;17:746.

Pahwa S et al: Spectrum of human T-cell lymphotropic virus type III infection in children: Recognition of symptomatic, asymptomatic, and seronegative patients. JAMA 1986;255:2299.

Ranki A et al: Neutralizing antibodies in HIV (HTLV-III) infection: Correlation with clinical outcome and antibody response against different viral proteins. Clin Exp Immunol 1987;69:231.

Richman DD et al: The toxicity of azidothymidine (AZT) in the treatment of patients with AIDS and AIDS-related complex: A double-blind, placebo-controlled trial. N Engl J Med 1987;317:192.

Safai B: Kaposi's sarcoma: A review of the classical and epidemic forms. Proc NY Acad Sci 1984;437:373.

Safai B et al: The natural history of Kaposi's sarcoma in the acquired immunodeficiency syndrome. Ann Intern Med 1985;103:744.

Warner LC, Fisher BK: Cutaneous manifestations of the acquired immunodeficiency syndrome. Int J Dermatol 1986;25:337.

Winkelstein W et al: Sexual practices and risk of infection by the human immunodeficiency virus. The San Francisco Men's Health Study. JAMA 1987;257:321.

16

Fungal Infections

Henry Earl Jones, MD

The noninvasive cutaneous mycoses—tinea versicolor, dermatophytosis, etc—parasitize only the cornified components of the skin, hair, and nails. It is rare when one of these fungi invades vascularized living skin, subcutaneous tissue, or other organs. These infections have been referred to as the dermatomycoses, or superficial infections, but the term **noninvasive** more precisely distinguishes them from more pathogenic fungi.

The invasive cutaneous mycoses—chromomycosis, maduromycosis, etc—result from direct penetration of viable epidermis, dermis, subcutaneous, and deeper tissues. Spread within the skin and deeper tissues is by contiguous extension. *Sporothrix schenckii,* a pathogen of this group, may occasionally disseminate from the original cutaneous focus and, albeit uncommonly, may even produce primary pulmonary infection.

The systemic mycoses (eg, coccidioidomycosis and blastomycosis), almost always begin as invasive pulmonary infections that may spread by contiguity within the lung and adjacent tissues but more typically disseminate through the bloodstream. Apparently the etiologic agents are transported as intracellular pathogens within blood-borne phagocytic cells. Thus, the systemic mycoses disseminate discontiguously to other tissue, including, frequently, the skin and mucous membranes. Some fungi, particularly the dermatophytes, *Coccidioides immitis,* and *Histoplasma capsulatum,* may also produce sterile allergic signs in the skin—eg, dermatophytids, erythema multiforme, and erythema nodosum.

The United States National Health Survey of 1971–1974 estimated the prevalence of all cutaneous mycoses at 88 per 1000 persons. These mycoses were the second most prevalent skin condition in the US population. Although the available data do not reveal the prevalence of each cutaneous fungal infection, more than 90% were noninvasive cutaneous mycoses.

Worldwide, the cutaneous mycoses are common causes for seeking medical care. An average of 7% of all outpatient visits in 9 large dermatology clinics on 5 continents were for cutaneous fungal infection.

These data provide an incomplete but reasonable

picture of the relative frequency of cutaneous fungal infection. The noninvasive cutaneous mycoses are extremely common, accounting for more than 90% of all fungus-related doctor-patient encounters. These pesky problems plague both the patient and the physician and result in major expenditures of time and money and much morbidity but few or no deaths.

The deep mycoses, on the other hand, have a great medical, economic, and social impact. Some of them—eg, histoplasmosis in the midwestern USA and coccidioidomycosis in the southwestern USA—are common serious medical problems in their endemic areas. In industrialized western countries, the invasive cutaneous and systemic mycoses are increasingly important causes of disease because they (1) have occult clinical presentations that make diagnosis difficult; (2) produce considerable morbidity and mortality; (3) are increasing in frequency in hospitalized, immunosuppressed, and medicated patients; and (4) affect persons from endemic areas who are increasingly traveling to Western countries.

Host Resistance Factors

The host-parasite struggle is influenced by factors peculiar to both participating parties. Little is known regarding fungal virulence factors and potential differences in the pathogenic potential of different fungal species, subspecies, and variants. More is known about the host's role in this struggle. Competent T cell immunity, phagocytosis, and complement function are important host defense mechanisms against pathogenic fungi. Transferrin and lactoferrin may play roles, but antibody appears to be of little importance. A vigorous inflammatory response is in general a reliable sign that the host defenses are good.

Defective host defense is often reflected by an inability to mount or sustain an inflammatory response to fungal invasion. Most host-parasite interactions produce polar degrees of inflammation, ie, highly inflamed or minimally inflamed infections. Since the level of inflammation produced is so readily visible in the skin, one may, by noting its intensity, predict (within limits) the clinical manifestations and outcome of many cutaneous fungal infections (Table 16–1).

Table 16–1. The degree of inflammation within involved skin determines the character of cutaneous fungal infection.

Inflammation	Pathology	Microbiology	Signs and Symptoms	Extent (Surface Area)	Response to Therapy
Present and intense	Acute dermatitis	Generally few fungi	Tenderness, pain, intensely inflamed vesicles, oozing, weeping, crusting, indurated nodules	Focal, limited	Good
Minimal or indolent	Chronic dermatitis, with or without granuloma formation, pseudoepithelomatous hyperplasia, fibrosis and scarring	Organism plentiful	Dryness, pruritus, pain, mild erythema, scaling, hyperkeratosis, verrucous keratosis, fissures, with or without pustules, erosions, ulcerations, abscesses, sinus formation.	Widespread	Poor

Irrespective of whether the infection is classified as noninvasive, invasive, or systemic, most cutaneous infections follow one of the 2 courses. Infections confronted by intact host defenses follow a self-limited course. Acute ringworm, lymphangitic sporotrichosis, and primary inoculation cutaneous blastomycosis are good examples of these infections that are each briskly inflamed, focal, and characterized by an acute self-limited course. Infections met with inadequate host resistance produce less inflammatory lesions that usually spread locally or disseminate and typically have a chronic or progressive course. Chronic mucocutaneous candidiasis, mycetoma, and disseminated cutaneous coccidioidomycosis are good examples. Both the pathogen's virulence and the host's defenses determine the outcome.

DIAGNOSTIC TECHNIQUES FOR THE CUTANEOUS MYCOSES

Direct Microscopic Examination

In addition to the clinical history and physical signs, the physician will find direct microscopic examination for fungi the most useful laboratory test. Samples of involved skin, hair, nails, pus, grains, tissue fluids, etc, are placed on a glass slide and treated with 10–20% potassium hydroxide (KOH) to optically clarify the specimen ('KOH test'). Examination with reduced substage lighting will reveal fungal elements that may be accentuated by selective staining or counterstaining. KOH tests readily demonstrate fungi causing dermatophytosis, candidiasis, and tinea versicolor (Table 16–2). The less common pathogens causing tinea nigra, chromomycosis, eumycotic mycetoma, blastomycosis, paracoccidioidomycosis, cryptococcosis, and occasionally coccidioidomycosis can also be identified by KOH examination. The noninvasive infections can usually be distinguished on a KOH slide except when the hyphae of *Candida* are not accompanied by budding spores or typical chlamydospores. In such instances, the hyphae of *Candida* and dermatophytes cannot be distinguished. In fact, all *Candida* species plus the numerous species of the 3 dermatophyte genera may have an identical appearance on KOH examination.

Clarification of thick specimens—eg, blister tops, nail, and hair—in KOH solution may take 30 minutes or more, but gentle heating or inclusion of dimethyl

Table 16–2. Identification of the common noninvasive cutaneous mycoses.

Type of Infection	Synonyms	Causative Organism	Microscopic Appearance in Smears From Lesions	Growth on Sabouraud's Dextrose Agar
Dermatophytosis	Tinea, ringworm	*Trichophyton, Epidermophyton, Microsporum* spp	Branched, septate hyphae	2–3 weeks as filamentous molds[1]
Candidiasis	Candidosis, moniliasis	*Candida* spp	Branched, septate hyphae with or without budding yeast forms	1–3 days as moist yeasts[2]
Tinea versicolor	Pityriasis versicolor	*Pityrosporum orbiculare*	Short, curved hyphae plus clumps of spores	No growth[3]

[1]Slow growth producing white to tan thallus, often with colored obverse side
[2]Differentiation of *Candida albicans* from other species requires further tests.
[3]Growth occurs when lipid (eg, olive oil) is added to agar.

sulfoxide (DMSO) in the solution will accelerate the process.

Mycologic Culture

With a few exceptions, only culture permits definite identification of the genus and species of the pathogen. This is absolutely true of *Candida* and the dermatophytes. A positive direct KOH smear or demonstration of fungal elements in histopathologic specimens should be confirmed and the organism identified by culture. For sporotrichosis and histoplasmosis, mycologic culture may be the only way to establish the diagnosis. Specimens should be inoculated onto both simple nutritive agar (eg, Sabouraud's dextrose) and selective agar (eg, Mycosel) for primary isolation. Selective media alone are inadequate because the cycloheximide or other additives inhibit growth of some pathogenic and many opportunistic species such as *Cryptococcus neoformans, Blastomyces dermatitidis,* and *Histoplasma capsulatum.* Addition of chloramphenicol to selective media inhibit growth of *Actinomyces* and *Nocardia.*

Histopathology

Fungi may be detected in biopsy tissue by routine hematoxylin and eosin staining, but a greatly increased yield is obtained with special stains such as periodic acid-Schiff (PAS) and Gomori-methenamine silver (GMS). Direct immunofluorescence histopathology may be helpful in identifying fungal elements in tissue. Tissue biopsy is usually indicated only for certain invasive cutaneous and systemic mycoses, but occasionally a noninvasive infection not suspected on clinical grounds is diagnosed histopathologically. The form of the fungal elements in tissue may strongly suggest a specific pathogen, but a definitive etiologic diagnosis cannot usually be made on this basis.

Wood's Light

Examination of affected skin and hair in a darkened room by 360-nm ultraviolet light (Wood's light) may be helpful in detecting or delineating tinea capitis and tinea versicolor infection. Formerly, the Wood's light was the main tool for screening patients and groups of school children for epidemic tinea capitis caused by *Microsporum audouini.* Wood's light is of little value in screening for tinea capitis today in the USA, because this organism has been supplanted as the principal pathogen by nonfluorescent *Trichophyton tonsurans.*

Skin Testing

Skin testing with fungal antigen is infrequently indicated. The principal use for skin testing in the mycoses today is in epidemiologic and clinical investigations. For the systemic mycoses, a skin test may have a "booster effect" and produce a nonspecific rise in complement-fixing antibody that cross-reacts with serologic tests for all the systemic mycoses. Delayed-type hypersensitivity (DTH) is the typical skin test reaction exhibited by most humans infected with non-invasive, invasive, and systemic fungal pathogens. IgE-mediated, immediate "urticarial" reactions are obtained especially in individuals with chronic, widespread dermatophytosis.

Serologic Tests

Serologic testing is of diagnostic and prognostic value in the systemic mycoses and perhaps in certain invasive cutaneous mycoses. Serology has no clinical value in any type of noninvasive infections.

GENERAL PRINCIPLES OF THERAPY

Symptomatic treatment is important in therapy of fungal infection of the skin. The clinical findings dictate what is to be done. Acute, severely inflamed infections should be treated like any acute dermatitis. Soothing compresses (eg, Burow's solution 1:40 for 10 minutes every 1–2 hours) sometimes produce more symptomatic relief (and resolution of the infection) than a specific antifungal agent. Chronic hyperkeratotic, indolent lesions may respond to keratolytic agents such as Whitfield's ointment and aggressive debridement more rapidly than to specific antifungal treatment.

The anatomic location of the infected part must be considered. Involvement of the skin of the lower leg may require elevation or bed rest. Strong and irritating topical medications cannot be applied to eroded or ulcerated skin nor to the thin, delicate skin of the genitalia and eyelids. The presence of superinfection with pyococci necessitates local or systemic antibiotic therapy. Allergic manifestations such as erythema multiforme and erythema nodosum may require ancillary anti-inflammatory therapy for best results.

The mainstay for treatment of all forms of cutaneous fungal infections are the topical, oral, and parenteral antifungal medications (Table 16–3). The primary indications for each medication are shown. Many of the factors clinicians consider in selection of an antifungal agent for a particular clinical situation are listed in Table 16–4.

Topical Agents

A. Cyclopiroxolamine (Loprox): This substituted pyridine is available as a 1% cream that inhibits the growth of dermatophytes, *Candida albicans,* and the agent causing tinea versicolor. It is generally applied twice daily.

B. Haloprogin (Halotex): Haloprogin is available as a 1% cream or solution with antifungal activity against dermatophytes and to a lesser extent *Candida* species and *Malassezia furfur.* It is generally applied 2 or 3 times daily.

Table 16–3. Some antifungal drug formulations and infections for which they are primarily indicated.

| Medication | The Common Noninvasive Cutaneous Mycoses | | | Invasive | |
	Tinea Versicolor	Dermatophytosis	Candidiasis	Cutaneous Mycoses	Systemic Mycoses
Topical agents					
Moderate potency					
Castellani's paint	...	+	+	...	...
Gentian violet	...	+	+	...	...
β-Hydroxyquinoline	...	+	+	...	...
Selenium sulfide	+	...	...	...	...
Sodium thiosulfate	+	...	...	...	...
Whitfield's ointment	...	+	...	...	...
Zinc pyrithione	+	...	...	...	...
Higher potency					
Cyclopiroxolamine	+	+	+	...	...
Amphotericin B	...	...	+	...	...
Haloprogen	...	+	...	...	...
Nystatin	...	...	+	...	...
Tolnaftate	...	+	...	...	...
Pimaricin	...	...	...	+ (keratitis)	...
Clotrimazole	+	+	+	...	...
Miconazole	+	+	+	...	...
Ketoconazole	+	+	+	...	...
Oxiconazole	+	+	+	...	...
Spectinazole	+	+	+	...	...
Sulconazole	+	+	+	...	...
Butaconazole	+	+	+	...	...
Naftifine	+	+	+	...	...
Systemic agents					
Orally administered					
Flucytosine	...	...	+	+ (chromo)	+
Griseofulvin	...	+	...	...	...
Ketoconazole	+	+	+	+	+
Fluconazole	...	+	+	+	+
SSKI	...	...	...	+ (sporo)	...
Intravenous					
Amphotericin B	...	...	+	+	+
Miconazole	...	+	+	+	+
Hydroxystilbamidine	...	...	...	...	+ (blasto)

C. Imidazoles: This enlarging family of drugs now includes the following FDA-approved compounds: butaconazole, clotrimazole, ketoconazole, miconazole, oxiconazole, spectinazole, and sulconazole. They have fungistatic activity against dermatophytes, *Candida albicans,* and tinea versicolor. Most are available in cream or solution formulations at 1% or 2% concentrations. These topical agents are generally very effective, but no studies have shown any one of them to be superior to the rest. They are usually applied twice daily, but certain compounds are approved for usage in a single daily application. Ketoconazole and fluconazole—approved for oral usage—will be discussed separately.

An imidazole-steroid combination has been introduced, ie, clotrimazole and betamethasone valerate (Lotrisone). Unfortunately, it has been overused and abused. The steroid is a potent one, and this has produced cutaneous atrophy, striae, secondary infections, and other side effects.

D. Naftifine (Naftin): This new allylamine antifungal agent shows activity against the dermatophytes and *Candida* species when applied topically. An oral dose form is being studied but is not available at this time.

E. Nystatin (Mycostatin, Nilstat): Nystatin is available in creams, ointments, powders, and suspensions and in combination with topical steroids. The concentration is usually 100,000 U/g. It has both fungistatic and fungicidal activity and is indicated for the treatment of cutaneous or mucocutaneous infections caused only by *Candida albicans* and other *Candida* species. For this reason, this medication should not be used to treat dermatophytosis or tinea versicolor.

F. Tolnaftate (Tinactin): This medication, which is active only against dermatophytes, is available as a cream, solution, and powder.

G. Undecylenic Acid: This agent has been used for decades but is marginally effective and more irritating than the imidazoles and hence is being prescribed less frequently.

Table 16–4. Some factors physicians consider in selecting antifungal agent for a cutaneous mycosis.

1. Category of the infecting organism; eg, dermatophyte versus *Candida* versus invasive or systemic pathogen.
2. Anatomic area(s) affected: foot, trunk, neck, etc.
3. Component of skin involved: nail, hair, stratum corneum, panniculus, mucosa, etc.
4. Intensity of inflammation and degree of skin damage.
5. Extent of the infection, ie, percentage of skin surface affected.
6. Duration of the infection, ie, weeks, months, years, and number of previous episodes.
7. Exact genus and species of the pathogen.
8. Antifungal sensitivities on the pathogen isolated.
9. Effectiveness of previous therapy.
10. Patient's age, sex, habitus, occupation, etc.
11. Health status and concurrent medications.
12. Adverse effects previously experienced from antifungal agents.
13. Anticipated acceptability and compliance for each possible therapeutic agent, formulation, and route of administration.
14. Cost of a full course of treatment.

H. Whitfield's Ointment: This age-old ointment contains benzoic and salicylic acid and can be applied twice daily and is useful for treating the hyperkeratotic, moccasin type of tinea pedis, since it has keratolytic activities as well. It may irritate sensitive skin and intertriginous areas.

Systemic Antifungal Agents

A. Potassium Iodide: This simple chemical has been used for almost 100 years to treat lymphatic sporotrichosis with good success. The saturated solution of potassium iodide (SSKI) is prescribed in a slowly increasing dose beginning with 3 drops 3 times daily until limited by adverse effects or until a clinical response is achieved—or until a maximum of roughly 90 drops per day is reached. It is interesting that SSKI shows no activity in vitro against sporotrichosis, and it is not effective in any other fungal infection. Side effects are common and include acneiform eruptions, nausea, vomiting, parotiditis, and even hypothyroidism.

B. Griseofulvin (Fulvicin, Griseofulvin, Grisactin): Griseofulvin is an antifungal antibiotic that inhibits mitosis by inhibiting microtubular function. The drug is effective orally against dermatophytes but is ineffective against bacteria, *Candida* species, and the agent that causes tinea versicolor. In general, it is the systemic treatment of choice for dermatophyte infection, including tinea capitis, tinea corporis, and tinea pedis. The drug is absorbed more quickly and completely with a fatty meal and is generally tolerated better by the patient when taken in this manner.

Griseofulvin is available in both a microcrystalline and separate ultramicrocrystalline form. The dosage is different depending on which formulation is used. Therefore, the form of medication must be specified by the prescribing physician or confusion and perhaps overdosing can result. The usual oral dose of microcrystalline griseofulvin for adults is 500 mg daily in a single or divided dose. One gram or more daily can be used in special situations. The dose for children is 10 mg/kg/d.

The normal adult dose of the ultramicrocrystalline form is 330 mg daily as a single dose or in divided doses. The dose can be doubled in special situations. The usual oral dose for children is approximately 7 mg/kg/d. The duration of treatment is variable depending upon which condition is being treated. Details of its use in various conditions is discussed later.

Headaches and gastrointestinal disturbances are the most common side effects, but leukopenia, granulocytopenia, and hepatitis, though less common, are nevertheless among the more serious adverse effects. Other side effects include dyschezia, dry mouth, arthralgia, peripheral neuritis, vertigo, fever, syncope, blurred vision, photosensitivity, insomnia, serum sickness, hepatitis, angioedema, confusion, lapses of memory, impaired judgment, and estrogen-like side effects. The drug is contraindicated in patients with acute intermittent porphyria because it may precipitate an acute abdominal attack. Because it induces microxidase enzymes involved in the metabolism of warfarin and barbiturates, the dosage may have to be increased when griseofulvin is given to patients receiving either of these drugs. Griseofulvin may interact with oral contraceptive pills, especially the triphasic type, and produce breakthrough bleeding or permit unwanted pregnancy.

C. Ketoconazole (Nizoral): Ketoconazole is an imidazole that interferes with the biosynthesis of ergosterol, which is part of the cell membrane of fungi. The drug is used to treat dermatophytosis, yeast infections, and tinea versicolor as well as several invasive and systemic mycoses (see below).

The usual adult dose is 200 mg or 400 mg once daily in the morning. The dose for children is 50 mg if the child weighs less than 20 kg, 100 mg if the child weighs 20–40 kg, and 200 mg for children over 40 kg.

Gastric acid is important for dissolution of the tablets and for absorption and bioavailability of the drug. For this reason, antacids and H_2 histamine blocking agents should not be given concomitantly. Drug interactions are important and must be considered: the combination of ketoconazole with rifampin, isoniazid, warfarin, cyclosporine, or phenytoin can have serious consequences.

The most common side effects are nausea and itching, but headache, dizziness, abdominal pain, constipation, diarrhea, somnolence, and nervousness have been reported. Urticaria and anaphylactoid reactions have been observed with the first dose of ketoconazole, but no fatal reactions have been reported. Less common but potentially more serious adverse effects include endocrine suppression and hepatotoxicity.

Gonadal sterol synthesis is transiently blocked with each dose of ketoconazole, and in the male patient reduced testosterone levels can produce gynecomastia and impotence. Transient adrenal suppression is also produced in a similar manner, but at ordinary dosage schedules the endocrine effects are not clinically significant. It is for this reason that ketoconazole should always be prescribed as a single daily dose to be taken in the morning.

Ketoconazole can cause a chemical hepatitis in roughly one in 10,000 patients adequately exposed to the drug. The hepatitis is usually reversible, but if developing hepatitis is not detected and the drug is not discontinued, a potentially fatal massive hepatic necrosis may occur. For that reason appropriate monitoring of liver function tests is indicated during therapy, and the drug should be stopped immediately if jaundice develops.

D. Amphotericin B (Fungizone): This antifungal agent must be given intravenously to treat systemic mycoses such as blastomycosis. It is a polyene antibiotic that binds to fungal cell membranes, affecting their permeability. It is indicated in the treatment of almost all systemic fungal infections (see below). A topical cream formulation is also available, but given the availability of superior agents it is seldom used today.

The dosage of amphotericin B must be individualized by considering factors such as the disease being treated, the age and tolerance of the patient, and the availability of effective alternative medications. The usual dose is 0.25 mg/kg infused over 2–4 hours. The dose may be increased slowly over several days to a maintenance level of 0.4–0.6 mg/kg/d.

Amphotericin B has numerous side effects. Acute febrile reactions are common during infusions and may be relieved by the simultaneous intravenous infusion of hydrocortisone sodium succinate 25 mg. Wheezing and hypoxemia may develop, but true anaphylaxis is rare. Most patients develop a dose-dependent azotemia. Permanent renal damage may occur, especially when patients need large doses for long periods. Patients often develop mild anemia. Vomiting, anorexia, and weight loss are common. Sclerosis and phlebitis often affect the veins used for intravenous therapy.

E. Flucytosine (Ancobon): This synthetic fluorinated pyrimidine interfaces with fungal RNA synthesis and may block DNA synthesis, both of which produce fungistasis. These effects may be overcome rapidly, with resulting fungal resistance and relapse of infection. The drug is usually prescribed in combination with amphotericin B or ketoconazole when indicated for chromoblastomycosis, disseminated candidiasis, or cryptococcosis.

NONINVASIVE CUTANEOUS INFECTIONS (Tinea)

The term "tinea" refers to all noninvasive cutaneous mycoses except those caused by *Candida* species, which are termed candidiasis or moniliasis. In addition to tinea, the appropriate Latin term—eg, capitis, pedis, cruris, etc—is added to designate the anatomic location of the infection. Tinea versicolor is an exception to this rule.

The noninvasive cutaneous mycoses may be subdivided into 3 distinct subgroups based on the pathogenic potential of the fungi and the degree of host reaction provoked, namely, superficial infections, dermatophyte infections, and candidiasis.

SUPERFICIAL INFECTION

Tinea versicolor, tinea nigra palmaris, and piedra are conditions of the skin surface in which the causative organism proliferates only on the surface or infects only the soft keratin of the stratum corneum. These fungi are not capable of penetrating the hard keratin of hair and nails, and the infections will be characterized here as superficial. The signs and symptoms they produce are caused (1) by accumulation of bulk, eg, piedra; (2) by alteration in skin color, eg, tinea nigra and tinea versicolor; and, less commonly, (3) by eliciting an inflammatory reaction, eg, tinea versicolor.

1. TINEA VERSICOLOR

Essentials of Diagnosis

- Hypo- or hyperpigmented macules that fail to tan with sun exposure.
- Follicular papules, scaly patches, or plaques
- Involvement of trunk, neck, and shoulders.
- Mild pruritus, especially when perspiring or wet.
- Microscopic demonstration of spores and hyphae in skin scales.

General Considerations

Tinea versicolor (pityriasis versicolor) is one of the most superficial fungal infections. It is caused by the dimorphic lipophilic yeast *Pityrosporon orbiculare,* which grows in sebaceous gland-rich areas of human skin. In the follicular infundibulum, it grows predominantly in the yeast phase *(P orbiculare),* whereas on the skin surface, away from the follicle, it grows as short, thick hyphae. *Malassezia furfur* is an admixture of these 2 morphologic forms that is seen microscopically in KOH-treated skin scales which look like "spaghetti and meatballs." KOH is sufficient for diagnosis; mycologic culture is not usually obtained, because the diagnosis is usually evident clinically and by KOH and because culture requires special media.

The pathogenic organism can be isolated from the skin of 90% of the nonaffected normal population. No age is exempt from infection, though the very young and the very old present less frequently for medical care than individuals between the second and fourth decades. Men and women are equally susceptible, though women may—because of greater cosmetic concerns—present more frequently. Tinea versicolor is worldwide in distribution. In temperate climates, there are more symptomatic patients during the summer months, a result of increased environmental temperature and humidity. Similarly, tinea versicolor is more prevalent in semitropical or tropical regions of the world. In some groups—eg, South Sea Island people, where, in addition to climatic factors, it is the custom to apply coconut oil to the body—tinea versicolor is present in every man, woman, and child.

The associated hypopigmentation may be produced by the inhibition of tyrosinase or melanocyte cytotoxicity due to dicarboxylic acids (particularly azelaic acid) biosynthesized by the fungi from human lipids. As the name versicolor implies, hyperpigmentation is also seen, but the mechanism is unclear.

Microbiology & Immunology

Not enough is known of the immunology of tinea versicolor to determine if immunologic mechanisms are relevant to its clinical manifestation. Since the organism in yeast form is a normal skin inhabitant, a ridding immune reaction probably does not occur.

Clinical Findings

A. Symptoms and Signs: Complaints of changes in pigmentation dominate—especially hypopigmentation. Mild itching may be exacerbated by sweating or bathing.

Typically, chamois-colored, finely scaling macules or papules, varying from a few millimeters in diameter to large confluent areas, are present on the trunk and neck (Fig 16–1). Involvement may be reticulate or confluent. Light scraping with the fingernail generally produces a characteristic abundance of fine scale, helpful in differential diagnosis. Affected areas may be either hypo- or hyperpigmented. Some patients may have papular or inflammatory follicular infections.

Lesions of tinea versicolor may appear on the forearms, face, scalp, fingers, groin, and legs, but the upper torso, neck, and proximal upper extremities are more commonly affected. The palms, soles, and mucous membranes are never affected.

B. Laboratory Findings: Large, blunt, somewhat

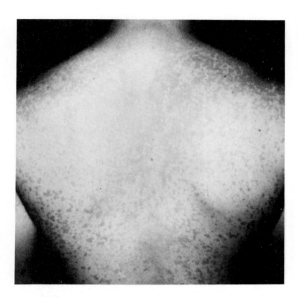

Figure 16–1. Tinea versicolor. Typical brownish, scaling macules in a reticulated pattern over back.

distorted hyphae admixed with clusters of thick-walled budding spores—the so-called spaghetti and meatballs pattern—in direct microscopic examination is virtually diagnostic.

Differential Diagnosis

The presence of scaling in hypo- or hyperpigmented areas should distinguish tinea versicolor from disorders of pigmentation, eg, vitiligo, café-au-lait spots, etc. It is sometimes more difficult to differentiate tinea versicolor from some papulosquamous diseases, especially seborrheic dermatitis, pityriasis rosea, and the chronic dermatitides such as allergic contact dermatitis, but KOH examination of scales helps. The follicular form may mimic acne.

Complications & Sequelae

Typically there are no complications, though persistent hypopigmentation in a darkly pigmented individual, especially in certain countries or ethnic groups, may take on medical, social, and economic importance. In this sense, it should be mentioned that *M furfur* and certain related species, eg, *Malassezia pachydermatis,* may serve as opportunist pathogens in humans, especially premature infants (see Cutaneous Signs in Fungal Septicemia at the end of this chapter).

Prevention

Since *P orbiculare* is common on normal skin of healthy individuals, the disease is not considered contagious. If the cutaneous microenvironment is suitable, the organism proliferates over the skin surface from the follicles to produce clinical signs and symptoms. It is not possible nor practical to prevent the spread of the organisms from person to person.

Treatment

A. Specific Measures: Several antifungal shampoos can be used: selenium disulfide, zinc pyrithione, etc (see Table 16–3). One should consider the region of the body involved, the extent of the infection, etc, in selection of therapy. Shampoos should be used for 2 weeks: left on the skin for 5–10 minutes daily and then removed by shower or bath. Alternatively, they may be left on overnight for several nights, but irritation may occur.

The topical imidazole creams applied twice daily may be helpful but are much more expensive.

Tinea versicolor does not respond to oral griseofulvin.

Most patients respond to topical treatment and do not require systemic therapy. Ketoconazole, 400 mg as a single dose for just 1 or 2 days, can be used to treat widespread infections recalcitrant to topical agents.

B. General Measures: Encourage good skin hygiene, and prepare the patient to expect the hypo- or hyperpigmentation to lag behind therapy by weeks or months, depending on suntanning exposure, skin color, and other factors.

Course & Prognosis

The natural course for the majority of patients with tinea versicolor, especially in temperate zones, is good and follows Course A (Fig 16–2). There are a few patients, however, whose course, even with aggressive topical therapy, is to retain widespread recalcitrant or relapsing infection for years.

2. TINEA NIGRA PALMARIS

Essentials of Diagnosis

- Single brown to black macule on palm or sole.
- Centrifugal enlargement of the pigmented area.
- Brownish-green hyphae in skin scales.
- Mycologic culture of *Cladosporium (Exophiala) werneckii*.

General Considerations

Tinea nigra is a superficial fungal infection of the stratum corneum, usually of the palms, though plantar skin may be affected also. The brownish to black nonscaling macules tend to spread centrifugally.

The condition occurs worldwide but is uncommon in North America. Both sexes and all age groups may be affected. Compared to the other noninvasive cutaneous mycoses, the prevalence and incidence are low, even in South America.

The thick keratinized and cornified stratum corneum of the palm or sole is penetrated by the thick, short hyphae of *C werneckii*. Penetration into the viable epidermis does not occur, but there is slow lateral spread within the stratum corneum. There is little or no inflammatory reaction to the organism, but there may be slight acanthosis and hyperkeratosis.

Microbiology & Immunology

Almost nothing is known regarding host predisposition, microbiology, and immunology of tinea nigra.

Clinical Findings

A. Symptoms and Signs: These brownish to black macules are asymptomatic. Typically, there is a single brownish to black macule with irregular mottling of the dark hues. The infected area is usually sharply marginated, macular, and nonscaly. The palmar aspect of the fingers or the palm is typically affected. There may be more than one focus or several large, irregularly shaped macules.

B. Laboratory Findings: Direct microscopic examination of epidermal scrapings digested with 10–20% KOH reveals the brownish to green, thick-walled, septate hyphae and budding yeast-like elements. KOH examination is usually sufficient for diagnosis. Direct smear could perhaps be confused morphologically with that seen with tinea versicolor or candidiasis. The fungal elements of *P orbiculare* are colorless, as are those of *Candida albicans*. Hence, the pigmented elements of *C werneckii* are usually diagnostic.

Mycologic culture produces a slow-growing, adherent yeast-like colony, initially light in color,

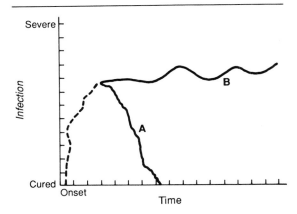

Figure 16–2. Schematic diagram of the divalent, polar courses most cutaneous fungal infections follow. Dotted line represents the developing infection. **Course A** is characteristic of highly inflammatory infections that generally heal spontaneously. **Course B** is characteristic of the minimally inflamed infections that remain stabilized for years or progressively become more severe and extensive.

rapidly becoming green to brown to black, identifying *C werneckii*.

Differential Diagnosis

Junctional nevi and melanoma, especially the acral lentiginous form, may mimic tinea nigra. Incipient trauma and hemorrhage into the palm or sole may produce similar dark pigmentation called "black heel." Silver nitrate, ammoniated mercury, paraphenylenediamine, and certain organic or chemical dyes may produce similar brown to black stains. Systemic aberrations in the pigment system such as Addison's disease may also mimic tinea nigra, but the pigmentation is more generalized over the entire palm or sole.

Complications & Sequelae

Although not associated with significant morbidity or mortality per se, tinea nigra may mimic malignant melanoma and, through misdiagnosis, result in amputation or surgical mutilation and debilitation.

Treatment

The brownish to black macules can be removed with keratolytic agents such as Whitfield's ointment, Keralyt gel (salicylic acid 6%), or 40% urea. Removal of fungus by physical scraping with the edge of a glass slide or an emery pad is an effective adjunct. Topical application of imidazole creams (eg, Lotrimin, Monostat-Derm) may help also. There is no established oral antimycotic therapy; surgical measures are contraindicated.

Course & Prognosis

Most infections respond to treatment. Recurrence is rare.

3. PIEDRA (Trichosporosis)

Piedra is a distinctive condition of the hair shaft characterized by firm, irregular nodules composed of the elements of the causative fungus. These surface hair concretions may be black, caused by *Piedraia hortai*, or white, caused by *Trichosporon cutaneum*.

The best treatment is to remove the affected hairs by clipping or shaving them off.

DERMATOPHYTE INFECTION

In contrast to fungi that produce the superficial infections, the various species of the *Trichophyton*, *Epidermophyton*, and *Microsporum* genera have the capability to infect all cornified components of the skin, including the hair and nails. Actual invasion of the viable epidermis and vascularized dermis is unusual.

The important clinical aspects of dermatophytosis will be discussed for each of the common clinical and anatomic infection syndromes. The relative frequency of these syndromes is shown in Table 16–5, prepared from the proportionate rates observed in 200,000 US Army dermatology clinic visits.

Although there are numerous dermatophytes, 7 species cause more than 90% of all infections. Their relative frequency, microbial characteristics, and clinical-anatomic syndromes produced are set forth in Table 16–6.

1. TINEA PEDIS

Essentials of Diagnosis

- Hyperkeratosis and scaling of the entire plantar surface.
- Scaling, maceration, or blistering in the toe web spaces.
- Blisters on the sole or instep area.
- Pruritus, intense at times.
- Pain associated with blisters, cracks, or fissures.
- Demonstration of septate branching hyphae in skin scales.
- Recovery of a dermatophyte on culture.

General Considerations

Tinea pedis is by far the most prevalent fungal infection (Table 16–5). Although the term tinea pedis is used for any dermatophyte infection of the foot, clarity of diagnosis is enhanced by an addendum specifying (1) interdigital, (2) vesicular, or (3) hyperkeratotic erythrodermic moccasin. Interdigital involvement typically does not spread beyond the intertriginous confines and is distinct in its presentation and natural course from the other 2 forms of tinea pedis (Fig 16–3A). The intensely inflammatory vesicular infections occur anywhere on the foot, typically with vesicles and bullae in foci or clusters (Fig 16–3B). The third distinct type is the minimally inflammatory infection, characterized by a dull erythema, dryness, scaling, and hyperkeratosis (Fig 16–3C), usually not focal nor limited to the interdigi-

Table 16–5. Dermatophytoses: The proportional rates for the common clinical-anatomic infection syndromes.

Clinical-Anatomic Infection Syndrome	Percentage Each Syndrome Contributes to the Total for All Forms of Dermatophytosis
Tinea pedis	44
Tinea unguium	16
Tinea cruris	15
Tinea corporis	13
Tinea manuum	5
Tinea barbae, faciae, majocchis, etc.	4
Tinea capitis	3

Table 16–6. The frequency, microbial characteristics, and clinical-anatomic syndromes produced by the 7 common dermatoses.

Genus and Species	Frequency of Isolation	Identifying Characteristics on Sabouraud's Dextrose Agar		Common Clinical-Anatomic Syndromes				
		Colony	Microscopic	Capitis	Corporis	Cruris	Pedis	Unguium
Trichophyton rubrum	Very common	White cotton; red reverse	Sparse	—	+	+	+	+
Trichophyton mentagrophytes	Common	White cotton, or cream to tan powder	Abundant microaleuriospores	Ectothrix	+	+	+	+
Epidermophyton floccosum	Moderate	Fuzzy; tan, yellow, green	Fanlike micro-aleurisospores	—	+	+	+	+
Trichophyton tonsurans	Moderate	Flat, powdery, or suedelike; yellow	Sparse	Endothrix	+	—	—	—
Microsporum canis	Moderate	Woolly, yellow-white	Typical micro-aleuriospores	Ectothrix*	+	—	—	—
Microsporum audouinii	Low	White, tan, silky to furry	Sparse	Ectothrix*	+	—	—	—
Trichophyton verrucosum	Low	Folded, heaped; gray-white	Branched coarse hyphae	Ectothrix	+	—	—	—

*Involved hair fluoresces a brilliant green.

tal area but affecting the entire plantar skin of both feet in sandal or moccasin distribution.

Any subtype of tinea pedis may be produced by several of the dermatophytes. The *Trichophyton* species, ie, *Trichophyton rubrum* or *Trichophyton mentagrophytes,* are common; *Epidermophyton floccosum* is less common, and the *Microsporum* species are rarely involved. The natural source of the pathogen and the reasons for their epidemiologic features are not clear. Some organisms may be anthropophilic, passed from human to human by fomites or perhaps, more commonly, on floors in public facilities. Others—eg, *T mentagrophytes* var *granulare,* which has been chiefly associated with inflammatory infection—frequently have a zoophilic origin.

No form of tinea pedis is common before the pubertal years at which time boys—but not girls—begin to experience dermatophyte infections of the feet.

Tinea pedis knows no geographic restriction; it is less common in areas where footwear is not used. The hyperkeratotic erythrodermic moccasin type of tinea pedis has a stabilized, type B natural course (Fig 16–2); this distinctive form of tinea pedis contributes largely to the high prevalence of tinea pedis in the USA. *T rubrum* is frequently isolated from moccasin tinea pedis. The inflammatory vesicular form of tinea pedis, likely to have a type A natural course, may have a high annual incidence but a lower prevalence. The interdigital type of tinea pedis may have either a type A or type B natural course. The latter is more frequent.

Pathogenesis

After the skin is colonized, the dermatophyte hyphae penetrate into the stratum corneum until approximately the granular layer of the epidermis is reached. There, vertical penetration halts. There is continuing spread laterally through the cornified stratum corneum.

One of the chief determinants of the clinical manifestations and course of the infection is the host's immune response to the infecting organism and its exocellular antigens.

During a primary infection, specifically sensitized T cells appear in the living layers of the skin immediately below fungus-infected stratum corneum. In instances where the T-effector cell response to fungal antigen is vigorous, an inflammatory reaction ensues, and the skin becomes intensely inflamed. Histopathologic examination shows a spongiotic dermatitis; frank intraepidermal vesiculation may be present on clinical examination.

When the T cells do not respond to the dermatophyte antigen (there are many explanations for lack of response), little cutaneous inflammation results, and the epidermis is not sufficiently damaged to disrupt the anatomic integrity of the stratum corneum. Centrifugal spread of the fungus within the stratum corneum continues until limited by other factors. For example, noninflammatory interdigital infection is for unclear reasons delineated by the boundary of the intertriginous skin. In the erythrodermic moccasin type of tinea pedis, the entire sole becomes infected. Yet the glabrous skin of the dorsum of the foot does not become involved. The general principles of the host-parasite struggle (Table 16–1 and Fig 16–2) apply to tinea pedis.

The most important dermatophyte antigen appears to be cell wall glycopeptides, which are chemically complex. The immune response to the polysaccharides and peptides are distinct. The dominant host immune response to the polysaccharides is humoral. Production of specific IgA, IgG, and IgM antibodies is poor. Antibodies of the IgE class are produced in

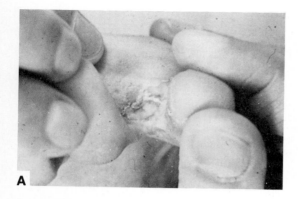

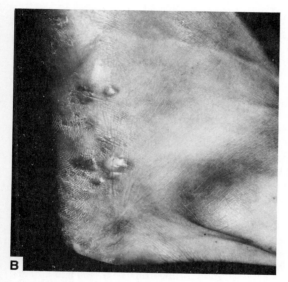

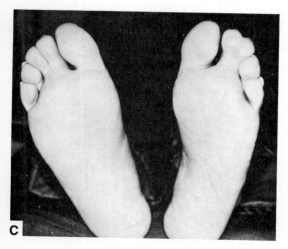

Figure 16–3. A: Interdigital tinea pedis: Maceration is prominent. **B:** Vesicular tinea pedis: Grouped vesicles on the lateral aspect of the foot at the plantar-glabrous skin junction. **C:** Erythrodermic hyperkeratotic moccasin tinea pedis: Typical confluent involvement of the entire plantar surfaces.

relatively greater quantity, and this tendency explains the frequency of the immediate, anaphylactic type of skin test reaction observed in humans tested with *Trichophyton*. The occurrence of the immediate IgE-type anaphylactic type of skin test reaction to *Trichophyton* antigens is associated with chronicity of infection and, in general, heralds a poor prognosis.

The fungal peptides appear to be the target of the human T cell response. Experimental digestion of the protein component of the crude glycopeptide antigen significantly reduces the delayed hypersensitivity response. The presence of vigorous T cell-mediated immune responsiveness to the fungal antigen is documented by a marked reaction 48 hours after intradermal injection of *Trichophyton* antigens.

In addition to immune-produced inflammation, the skin can be damaged by other mechanisms, including, for example, complement activation by fungal polysaccharides with PMN attraction and production of pustules.

Clinical Findings

A. Symptoms and Signs: The symptomatology varies from patient to patient, depending chiefly on which clinical-anatomic infection syndrome is present and the host immune response. Itching, burning, and stinging of the third and fourth web spaces are usually present in the interdigital type of infection. Itching and pain from the vesicles and bullae of the intensely inflammatory type of tinea pedis is the rule. The erythrodermic moccasin tinea pedis may produce complaints of pruritus and dryness as well as tenderness, pain, and bleeding from fissures and cracks. Symptoms may also result from superinfection or lymphangitis.

The physical findings depend on the particular clinical-anatomic syndrome and immune response. Scaling and hyperkeratosis in the web spaces may produce macerated white folds of skin that fissure, become denuded, and hurt. Inflammatory vesicular infection typically produces grouped vesicles, often in the instep area or anywhere on the plantar skin. The moccasin type of tinea pedis gives the plantar stratum corneum a powdery white to pinkish-red hue, but scaling and hyperkeratosis are marked.

B. Laboratory Findings: Skin scrapings from the interdigital area or any portion of the plantar stratum corneum in the moccasin type of tinea pedis or the blister roof of vesicular tinea pedis will reveal fungal hyphae on direct microscopic examination. One or a few typical hyphae may be seen, or an arborized mycelium may be found. Mycologic culture on Sabouraud's dextrose agar and Mycosel (or other reliable media) is necessary for confirmation that a dermatophyte is present. Culture and perhaps subculture on special media are necessary for speciation (Table 16–6). Remember that *Candida* species may have an identical appearance on KOH examination, and only culture will definitively identify the pathogen.

Differential Diagnosis

The web space form of tinea pedis must be distinguished from nonspecific dermatitis or bacterial intertrigo, which is extremely common. Intertrigo and not dermatophytes causes most interdigital "athlete's foot." The vesicular form of tinea pedis may be confused with cellulitis, pyococcal infection, eczema, and contact dermatitis, to mention only a few. The erythrodermic hyperkeratotic moccasin form of tinea pedis is characteristic but may be confused with "dry feet," psoriasis, lichen planus, some forms of ichthyosis, and numerous other conditions including manifestations of the graft-versus-host reaction.

Complications & Sequelae

Secondary bacterial infection with ascending lymphangitis and lymphadenitis is not uncommon.

Prevention

Little is known about effective preventive measures aside from good hygiene and minimizing footwear friction, wetness, and maceration.

Treatment

Cellulitis, lymphangitis, and lymphadenitis require emergency measures including systemic antibiotics, bed rest, and elevation of the affected foot.

For interdigital infections, a topical agent and formulation should be chosen that is compatible with the nature of infection being treated and which will provide the most acceptable answer to the considerations in Table 16–4. After the prescribed course of therapy, a maintenance antifungal or absorbent powder is recommended. Remember that bacterial intertrigo may not respond to specific antifungal therapy. Topical application weekly of aluminum chloride 20% in alcohol may be helpful by decreasing sweating in interdigital areas in intertrigo but may sting if fissures are present and may irritate the skin if used daily.

The inflammatory, vesicular form of tinea pedis will generally require oral antifungal therapy. Griseofulvin equivalent to 500 mg of the microsized preparation administered twice daily is recommended. Topical antifungal applications may be helpful if compatible with the state of the skin (ie, not fissured). Oral ketoconazole is an alternative to griseofulvin.

The erythrodermic moccasin tinea pedis is the most difficult therapeutic opponent. The time-honored topical antifungal preparations such as Whitfield's ointment may be of benefit, but the newer topical imidazole antifungals are superior. Topical agents alone rarely cure this form of tinea pedis, however; an oral antifungal is usually needed.

Before embarking on oral therapy, obtain a mycologic culture for confirmation of the exact dermatophyte responsible for the infection.

Irrespective of whether griseofulvin or ketoconazole is chosen as oral therapy, the drug should be given daily for 2–3 months. When ketoconazole is used, it is important to obtain pretreatment liver function tests and repeat them at monthly intervals for the first 6 months of therapy in order to detect idiosyncratic ketoconazole hepatitis. If ketoconazole hepatitis occurs, the drug should be immediately discontinued.

Course & Prognosis

The natural course and prognosis of each of the 3 types of tinea pedis can be predicted from Table 16–1 and Fig 16–2. The most stubborn, chronic form of infection is erythrodermic moccasin tinea pedis. Some patients remain in a stabilized relationship with their fungus for so long that they begin to accept the symptoms and signs as normal.

The inflammatory vesicular form of tinea pedis has the best prognosis, especially if there is a solitary group of vesicles on the sole. For reasons that are not clear, some individuals who have grouped vesicles in the instep area may have recurrent or relapsing infection over months or years. Table 16–1 and Fig 16–2 would not, given the degree of inflammation observed, enable one to predict the recurrence and recalcitrance of the instep vesicular tinea pedis.

Interdigital tinea pedis may, depending on the intensity of the host's immune-mediated inflammation, have a short course or tend to recur. Hygienic measures, especially use of an absorbent powder, appear to alter the natural course and ultimate prognosis of the interdigital type of infection.

2. TINEA UNGUIUM

Essentials of Diagnosis

- Dry, brittle, friable nails.
- Thickened, hypertrophic, dystrophic toenails.
- Discolored, opaque, white to yellow, lusterless nails.
- Both demonstration of dermatophyte hyphae in nails and recovery of dermatophyte on culture are necessary for definitive diagnosis.

General Considerations

Definitive diagnosis of tinea unguium is more difficult than with most other tineas. Fingernail infection presents less of a diagnostic problem than infection of the toenails. Among shoe-wearing populations, there is, with advancing age, an increased frequency of dystrophic toenails, especially nail of the great toe. Many dystrophic nails are not due to fungal infections, however, and the term tinea unguium refers only to dermatophyte infection of the nails. Since fungi other than dermatophytes may be primary nail pathogens or secondary invaders, tinea unguium is a diagnosis that requires microbiologic proof. Tinea unguium is common (Table 16–5). It affects both sexes with increasing frequency after age 35.

The pathogenesis of nail infection is not clear. *Trichophyton rubrum*, *Trichophyton mentagrophytes*, and *Epidermophyton floccosum* are the most common microbial agents. The organism usually invades under the free margin of the nail. Invasion sets up a reaction pattern that produces increasing hyperkeratosis of the nail plate and progressive dystrophy of the nail. When invasion occurs through the nail per se, there are often white, cloudlike discolorations of the nail surface. Opaque, whitish-yellow discoloration of the affected portion of the nail is common, as is the brittle, dystrophic state of the nail. Nail infections are almost always noninflammatory. Nail destruction is probably due to mechanical or enzymatic action of the fungus. The hyperkeratosis is a host reaction, but the stimulus and response are poorly understood.

Clinical Findings

A. Symptoms and Signs: Unsightly disfigurement is the most common complaint, especially in fingernail infection. Involvement of the fingernails cosmetically disables a physician, dentist, waiter, or other person whose hands are viewed by the public. There are usually few other symptoms. Pain or discomfort may occasionally be present. The nails may catch on fabrics, and handling of papers may be more difficult.

The patient's nails may be thick, hypertrophic, dystrophic, brittle, white-yellow, opaque, and lusterless. One or several nails may be involved, and sometimes all 20 fingernails and toenails will be affected.

B. Laboratory Findings: Dermatophyte infection must be definitively established to protect the patient from being mistakenly given oral antifungal therapy for months or years. Scrapings of the affected hyperkeratotic nail material should be soaked in hot 20% potassium hydroxide for 1–2 hours or longer if necessary to achieve adequate clarification for examination. The mere demonstration of fungal hyphae does not prove the presence of a dermatophyte, as there are several nondermatophyte species, eg, *Scopulariopsis brevicaulis*, *Hendersonella tortuloidea*, *Aspergillus* spp, *Cephalosporium* spp, and *Candida* spp, which can grow in dystrophic nails. Although these may serve as primary pathogens, only the isolation of a dermatophyte on mycologic culture serves to substantiate the diagnosis of tinea unguium.

Differential Diagnosis

The other fungal infections and colonizations mentioned above—plus psoriasis, lichen planus, trauma, and onychogryposis—may mimic tinea unguium. Dystrophy may also result from trauma.

Complications & Sequelae

Thick hyperkeratotic nails may interfere with wearing of shoes and may lead to secondary infection or lymphangitis.

Prevention

Treatment of tinea pedis and tinea manuum—especially the erythrodermic, hyperkeratotic moccasin form, which frequently precedes the development of nail infection—would be important measures in the prevention of tinea unguium.

Treatment

Treatment of dermatophyte nail infections is difficult. There are no topical antifungal agents of proved efficacy. Local measures have included physical paring down of thickened hypertrophic nail, chemical debridement or removal using 40% urea plasters, and surgical debridement. Oral antifungal therapy with griseofulvin has been the treatment of choice. Griseofulvin in full doses—500 mg of microsized, twice daily or more often, for 6–12 months—produces a favorable response in 30–50% of patients with fingernail infections. The response is lower in toenail infections—17% or less—even when griseofulvin is given for 1–2 years.

The efficacy of ketoconazole in nail infections is equivalent but not superior to that of griseofulvin, and ketoconazole thus remains a secondary drug for nail infection. It could not be recommended for tinea unguium at this time unless the patient required treatment and was known to be infected with a griseofulvin-resistant, ketoconazole-sensitive strain.

Course & Prognosis

Tinea unguium of the toenail is chronic. Many patients apparently maintain their infection for life.

3. TINEA CRURIS

Essentials of Diagnosis

- Pruritic dermatitis characterized by minimal to severe inflammation limited to the inguinal, crural area.
- Central clearing, marked activity at the peripheral margin.
- Thigh involved, but adjacent scrotal skin spared.
- Branching septate hyphae in direct smear.
- Dermatophyte isolated on culture.

General Considerations

Dermatophytosis of the intertriginous skin of the inguinal and crural area is often imprecisely referred to as jock itch. Other skin problems mimic tinea cruris.

Tinea cruris occurs worldwide. Moisture, maceration, CO_2 tension, and perhaps friction contribute to the localization of dermatophyte infection to the groin. Tinea cruris may be caused by any of the dermatophytes, with *Trichophyton rubrum*, *T mentagrophytes*, and *Epidermophyton floccosum* predominating. The condition may be more common in the obese or those who, for reasons of occupation, avocation, or work environment, perspire heavily. Tinea cruris usually afflicts adult men. At all ages, women have much less tinea cruris.

The pathogenesis and pathology of tinea cruris do not differ significantly from what has been described above for dermatophyte infection of the feet.

Microbiology & Immunology

See discussion in the section on tinea pedis.

Clinical Findings

A. Symptoms and Signs: Markedly pruritic dermatitis is limited to the intertriginous crural skin. The erythematous to eczematous skin lesion shows central clearing and a well-demarcated active border. The intensity of inflammation produces a spectrum of changes ranging from a light pink erythema through brisk, violaceous erythema. Mild scaling may dominate, or, with intense dermatitis, vesicles and pustules may be present.

B. Laboratory Findings: Skin scales obtained from the border and examined with a microscope after preparation with 10–20% potassium hydroxide reveal typical dermatophyte hyphae. Culture will identify the dermatophyte (Table 16–6). Since the hyphae of *Candida albicans* may appear identical, one must resort to mycologic culture to definitively distinguish between *Candida* and the dermatophytes in crural infection not clinically characteristic and in which *Candida* chlamydospores are not demonstrated in direct smears.

Differential Diagnosis

Inverse psoriasis and seborrheic dermatitis mimic tinea cruris, including central clearing and activity at the peripheral margin. Nonspecific intertrigo and candidiasis as well as irritant and allergic contact dermatitis can mimic tinea cruris but usually involve the scrotum. Contact dermatitis to topical medicaments used to treat a primary tinea cruris can lead to diagnostic error. Erythrasma is less inflamed and fluoresces red with Wood's light. Neurodermatitis is distinguished on the basis of its indistinct borders and lichenification. Rarely, Bowen's disease or extramammary Paget's disease can occur asymmetrically in the groin and require biopsy to confirm. These diseases should be suspected when the plaque is asymmetric or when it has undulating borders.

Complications & Sequelae

Secondary infection and lymphangitis occasionally develop.

Prevention

Proved methods of prevention are not available; however, most physicians believe that the use of absorbent powders or prophylactic topical antimycotic agents reduces the incidence of infection.

Treatment

A topical antifungal in a lotion or cream base is generally satisfactory therapy. In recalcitrant or recurrent infections, oral antifungal therapy with griseofulvin or ketoconazole is occasionally necessary. Measures to remove excess moisture and dry the affected skin are helpful.

Course & Prognosis

Most patients respond to therapy, though some will have a tendency for relapses or recurrences.

4. TINEA CORPORIS

Essentials of Diagnosis

- Erythematous, scaling eczematous dermatitis with central clearing or large, geographic papulosquamous plaques.
- Sometimes concentric red, scaly rings.
- Sometimes vesicles and pustules, especially at follicular orifices.
- Branching septate hyphae on microscopic examination.
- Dermatophyte recovered on culture.

General Considerations

Children may present with tinea corporis, but the prevalence in American children is low. Tinea corporis is more common in adults of both sexes. In humid, tropical areas of the world, extensive tinea corporis is common. The zenith is reached in tinea imbricata, which in certain foci in Central American, South American, and the South Pacific Islands affects virtually 100% of the skin surface of 100% of the population.

Trichophyton rubrum is the most common cause of tinea corporis today. *T mentagrophytes, Epidermophyton floccosum, Trichophyton tonsurans, Trichophyton verrucosum,* and other dermatophytes are occasional etiologic agents of tinea corporis. The pathogenesis and resulting pathology are similar to that described for tinea pedis.

Microbiology & Immunology

See discussion in the section on tinea pedis.

Clinical Findings

A. Symptoms and Signs: For the acute, highly inflammatory infection, pruritus is the dominant symptom, but there may be pain and tenderness. The chronic widespread form of tinea corporis produces much itching and scaling.

Depending on the nature of the host-parasite relationship, focal inflammatory infection or widespread, noninflammatory infection will be found (Table 16–1). Focal infection may produce vesicular, pustular, tender boggy areas that represent glabrous skin kerions. Tinea barbae is not uncommonly of the inflammatory type, and other acute ringworm on the legs and trunk may produce the same picture.

Widespread, minimally inflamed but scaling plaques on the torso, thighs, legs, and arms are typical in the noninflammatory type of infection (Fig 16–4). Follicular involvement may produce isolated inflammatory papules and pustules even in the noninflammatory type. Fungal activation of complement and PMN chemotaxis is a plausible explanation of how such pustules are formed.

B. Laboratory Findings: The demonstration of fungal hyphae and the recovery of a dermatophyte on mycologic culture are necessary for diagnosis (Tables 16–2 and 16–6).

Differential Diagnosis

The acute, highly inflammatory focal form of dermatophyte infection may mimic pyoderma or even furunculosis. The chronic, widespread scaly form of tinea corporis may mimic psoriasis, parapsoriasis, seborrheic dermatitis, allergic contact dermatitis, and other chronic pruritic, scaling eczematous conditions.

Complications & Sequelae

Chronic, scaly ringworm may be associated with severe or potentially severe underlying medical problems such as thymoma, lymphoma, and immunologic deficiencies.

Prevention

No effective preventive measures are known.

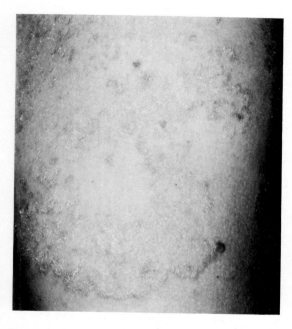

Figure 16–4. Tinea corporis. Typical papulosquamous plaque on the arm in chronic, widespread dermatophytosis.

Treatment

Topical application of an antifungal cream twice daily is usually satisfactory, especially for the acute inflammatory ringworm infection. If inflammation is sufficient to have denuded the skin or to have produced kerions or pustules, an oral antifungal would be appropriate. For the chronic, widespread noninflammatory form of tinea corporis, therapy is more difficult. One should isolate the infecting organism and use griseofulvin or ketoconazole for a minimum of 60–90 days or 1 month past the disappearance of clinical signs and symptoms.

Course & Prognosis

The acute, inflammatory form of ringworm is generally self-limited. The chronic, widespread form is problematic, and recurrence or relapse is the rule. In some patients, maintenance antifungal therapy may be necessary.

5. TINEA MANUUM

Essentials of Diagnosis

- Powder-like dryness of a palmar surface.
- Only a single palm involved.
- Branching, septate hyphae in direct smears.
- Recovery of a dermatophyte on culture.

General Considerations

In some ways, tinea manuum is analogous to the erythrodermic hyperkeratotic moccasin type of tinea pedis. It is not clear why the erythrodermic hyperkeratotic hand is essentially the only variant of dermatophyte infection that occurs on the palm. Plantar skin, which is otherwise similar, exhibits a variety of clinical manifestations, eg, vesicles and bullae. Furthermore, it is not clear why only one hand is frequently infected. The patient with unilateral hand infection will often have coexistent moccasin form tinea on both feet. Such patients often maintain an enigmatic infection of two feet and one hand for decades.

Like all glabrous skin infections, infections of the dorsum of the hand are considered analogous to tinea corporis.

Microbiology & Immunology

See discussion under tinea pedis.

Clinical Findings

A. Symptoms and Signs: Patients usually complain of dryness of the involved hand and, occasionally, symptoms attributable to the hyperkeratosis, ie, insensitivity in handling paper, pins, and other small objects.

The entire palmar surface of the affected hand is usually dry, scaly, and dull red. The infectious process rarely spreads to the dorsal surfaces.

B. Laboratory Findings: See discussion under tinea pedis.

Differential Diagnosis

Psoriasis, allergic contact dermatitis, pityriasis rubra pilaris, and plane xanthoma may rarely mimic tinea manuum, but the diagnosis of tinea manuum is usually strongly suspected from clinical appearance.

Treatment & Prognosis

Treatment is as for the erythrodermic hyperkeratotic moccasin form of tinea pedis. Response to therapy is somewhat better.

6. TINEA CAPITIS

Essentials of Diagnosis

- Bald patches, scaling scalp.
- Tender, oozing, weeping, pustular eruptions in scalp.
- Similar problems in playmates or siblings.
- Branching, septate hyphae in hair.
- Recovery of dermatophyte on culture.

General Considerations

Tinea capitis or ringworm of the scalp was formally a major public health problem. With the advent of improved personal hygiene, public health control measures, and griseofulvin, tinea capitis has become less common. Today, most tinea capitis is caused by *Trichophyton tonsurans*. Tinea capitis has always been much more common in prepubertal children than any other age group and is the most common fungal infection in children. *T tonsurans* is more common in black children and lower socioeconomic groups. *Microsporum canis* is the second most frequent cause of tinea capitis, whereas *Microsporum audouini* is rare today. The proportional rate of tinea capitis in outpatient clinics (Table 16–5) is low.

Two forms of tinea capitis due to *T tonsurans* are seen today. One, the so-called dry, scaly type, mimics dandruff, seborrheic dermatitis, and psoriasis. In contrast, the more inflammatory form of tinea capitis is characterized by an acute inflammatory exudative called a kerion. Both are caused by *T tonsurans;* the nature of the host response determines the clinical presentation.

There are 2 forms of hair invasion. *M canis, M audouinii, T verrucosum, T mentagrophytes,* and occasionally other species penetrate only the surface and subsurface of the hair—ectothrix hair invasion. Invasion all the way into the medulla of the central hair shaft is characteristic of *T tonsurans, T violaceum, T schoenleinii,* and occasionally *T rubrum* as well as the African dermatophytes *T yaoundei, T gourvillii,* and *T soudanense*—endothrix hair invasion.

Microbiology & Immunology

Much of what is known about the invasion and pathogenesis of dermatophytosis in the stratum corneum applies to tinea capitis. The dry, lusterless state of invaded hair must be an effect of fungal enzymes, etc. The host response produces the cutaneous inflammation. It is not known why certain forms of tinea capitis resolve spontaneously at puberty.

Clinical Findings

A. Symptoms and Signs: Persistent "dandruff" unrelieved by dandruff shampoos, itching of the scalp, patchy complete or partial hair loss, and tender, boggy infected areas are all symptoms that may cause patients to seek medical attention.

The physician should look for evidence that hairs are broken off at or just above the scalp. Alopecia, papulosquamous plaques, and tender, boggy kerions may each be present, but rarely or never would all be present simultaneously in the same patient.

B. Laboratory Findings: Several involved hairs should be plucked out of the follicles for microscopic examination after treatment with 10–20% KOH. Mycologic culture of fluorescent hairs or those otherwise demonstrated to be infected is the definitive laboratory test (Table 16–6). Cultures do not always isolate fungi from kerion infections because the infectious agents are sparse and the inflammation is overwhelming.

C. Special Examinations: Examination with Wood's light may be useful. This procedure was formerly of great value because most infections were caused by *M audouinii* and *M canis,* which, along with *M ferrugineum,* fluoresce bright green. In addition, *T verrucosum, T schoenleinii,* and *T simii*—as well as *M distortum* and several other species—may fluoresce. The emergence of *T tonsurans* as the principal cause of tinea capitis has reduced the importance of Wood's light, which thus has no value today in screening schoolchildren for tinea capitis caused by *T tonsurans.*

Differential Diagnosis

Dandruff, seborrheic dermatitis, the alopecias (especially alopecia areata), psoriasis, and pyoderma must be considered in the differential diagnosis.

Complications & Sequelae

The development of a kerion can through scarring lead to permanent alopecia. Allergic id reactions may be associated with kerions, but ids do not produce permanent sequelae.

Prevention

Sharing hats, combs, or brushes of an infected individual is to be avoided.

Treatment

There are no effective topical measures. Oral

griseofulvin is the time-honored treatment, and its efficacy is well established in *M audouinii* infections. For children, the dose is 10 mg/kg/d (microsize) up to 250 mg twice daily. If tinea capitis due to *T tonsurans* does not respond to griseofulvin, ketoconazole appears effective at a dose of 5 mg/kg/d up to 200–400 mg/d. Treatment should be continued until no fungi can be isolated by culture. Daily shampoo with selenium sulfide 2.5% (Exsel, Selsun) seems to help. If kerions are present, systemic steroids such as prednisone, 1 mg/kg/d orally, may be used for several weeks to suppress the scarring inflammation while the fungal elements are being eliminated.

Course & Prognosis

Tinea capitis due to *T tonsurans,* especially the dry, scaly type, may have a protracted course. The prevalence and ultimate impact of the *T tonsurans* carrier state is unknown.

7. ALLERGIC DERMATOPHYTIDS

Essentials of Diagnosis

- Erythematous, papular, eczematous, and, on the palm, vesicular eruptions.
- Urticaria or erythema annulare centrifugum (EAC)
- No fungi within the erythema annular centrifugum, eczematous, or urticarial eruptions.
- Demonstration of dermatophyte infection elsewhere on the body.

General Considerations

Dermatophytids are mycologically sterile skin eruptions caused by dermatophyte infection of another anatomic site that are mediated through immune mechanisms.

The prevalence and incidence of allergic dermatophytids are unknown. The lesions are allergic manifestations that can usually be correlated with the type of immune response the host exhibits to fungal antigen (trichophytin), ie, urticarial dermatophytids occur only in individuals with IgE-mediated type 1 hypersensitivity reactions to trichophytin. Erythema annulare centrifugum-type ids can only be reproduced experimentally around a positive trichophytin delayed-type hypersensitivity skin test reaction. The erythematous papular eczematous ids may be associated with delayed-type hypersensitivity reactions to trichophytin, but it is not clear if this immune mechanism produces the eruption. Especially on the palms, the eczematous dermatophytid will often produce vesicles reminiscent of those produced on the foot at the site of the primary infection (Fig 16–5).

Clinical Findings

A. Symptoms and Signs: The signs and symptoms are those to be expected from eczema, urticaria, and erythema annulare centrifugum.

The focus of dermatophyte infection should be similar in intensity of inflammation to that exhibited by the eruption thought to represent an id, eg, a patient with an erythematous papular eczematous eruption on the hands could not be correctly diagnosed as having an allergic id eruption if the only evidence of dermatophyte infection were a banal, minimal interdigital tinea pedis. The presence of a highly inflammatory vesicular tinea pedis would, on the other hand, make the finding of the erythematous papular eczematous or vesicular eruption on the hands consistent with an id reaction. Similarly, urticaria could not be considered a dermatophytid if the patient did not have an immediate IgE-mediated urticarial reaction to trichophytin. Patients having urticarial ids will probably have a minimally inflammatory chronic infection of the feet or the torso.

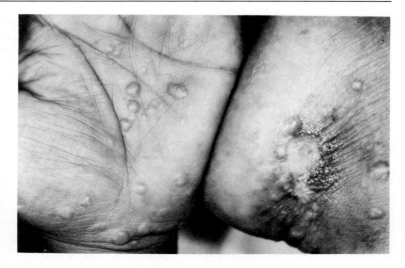

Figure 16–5. Allergic dermatophytid. Vesicular-bullous id eruption (KOH-negative) on palm with the responsible and, for comparison, the similar-appearing focus of vesicular-bullous infection (KOH-positive) on the foot.

B. Laboratory Findings: The allergic id eruption is by definition always negative on smear and culture for dermatophytic fungi. An active dermatophyte infection must be present elsewhere, typically in a site anatomically remote from the site of allergic id eruption.

C. Skin Testing: One of the few uses for the trichophytin skin test is in evaluation of the allergic dermatophytids. A positive immediate or delayed-type hypersensitivity (DTH) skin test does not establish the diagnosis. The test results must be interpreted in light of the clinical situation. In certain situations, a positive test may be consistent with a clinical diagnosis, or a negative test may negate the diagnosis.

Differential Diagnosis

Dermatophytids must be distinguished from dermatophyte infection per se and from numerous other causes of eczema, urticaria, and erythema annulare centrifugum. One of the most difficult differential diagnostic exclusions is that of conditioned hyperirritability (autoeczematization or absorption reaction). Inflammatory tinea pedis or tinea capitis may produce both. Distinguishing between them is of more academic than clinical value. The trichophytin skin test response should correlate with the type of allergic id reaction. Since more than half of adult males develop reactions to trichophytin 48 hours after injection, the clinical value of the skin test is greatest when a negative delayed hypersensitivity reaction excludes the possibility of an id reaction.

Treatment

Specific therapeutic measures should be directed against the primary focus of dermatophyte infection. Topical or oral therapy should be used. Symptomatic therapy with topical corticosteroids may be helpful in erythema annulare centrifugum and erythematous, papular, eczematous eruptions. Antihistamines may help in urticarial ids.

Course & Prognosis

Id reactions are typically episodic, and recurrences are relatively common.

CANDIDA INFECTION*

Candida has the greatest pathogenic potential of the "noninvasive" cutaneous pathogens. Although less adept than the dermatophytes at attacking hair and nails, *Candida* thrives in moisture and frequently exists as a commensal or transient inhabitant in the human gastrointestinal tract. *Candida* produces skin disease by invasion through the keratinized epidermis. Invasion of the viable epidermis and dermis—

particularly the mucous membranes—has been infrequently documented. In some forms of chronic mucocutaneous candidiasis, especially candidal granuloma formation, invasion of the dermis and subcutaneous tissue occurs. *Candida albicans* and certain other species may affect diseased heart valves, produce organ parenchymal infections, and cause septicemia. However, the vast majority of *Candida* infections are of the noninvasive cutaneous type discussed herein.

1. CUTANEOUS CANDIDIASIS

Essentials of Diagnosis
- Beefy red, weeping areas with satellite pustules.
- Involvement often limited to intertriginous skin.
- Rarely, dry, scaly, ringworm-like infections.
- Demonstration of hyphae in pustule top or skin scale.
- Recovery of *Candida* species on culture.

General Considerations

Candidiasis of the glabrous skin has a strong predilection for the intertriginous areas of the inguinal folds, intergluteal cleft, axillae, inframammary folds, and umbilicus. The intradigital space of the hand, particularly the third such space, seems predisposed. In uncircumcised males, balanitis from *C albicans* is not uncommon.

Cutaneous candidiasis occurs when there are precipitating factors, such as moisture from any source that, because of anatomic factors, cannot evaporate. Factors such as obesity, pendulous breasts, or an abdominal apron increase the natural occlusion and contribute to infection.

Diabetes is a frequent clinical association, as is the use of antibiotics, corticosteroids, and immunosuppressive medications. Factors that affect occlusion and moisture in the intertriginous areas and not one's sex or age determine when one contracts candidiasis. The moist intertriginous skin is colonized from the host's own gastrointestinal or mucosal sources, which normally harbor the organism. An increase in body weight and relaxation of tissues make the elderly prone to cutaneous candidiasis. Bedfastness and immobility, especially when associated with fevers, perspiration, and incontinence, may be triggering factors. In such patients, the areas involved will often be the occluded skin.

Microbiology & Immunology

C albicans invades the stratum corneum in the hyphal form, penetrating into or just below the granular layer. Activation of complement is critical to the formation of vesicles and pustules in cutaneous candidiasis. The alternative complement pathway is activated by the fungal elements that penetrate below the stratum granulosum or by soluble *Candida* mannans.

*Oral (mucosal) candidiasis is discussed in Chapter 48.

Complement component attracts polymorphonuclear leukocytes to the site of invasion, which results in pustule formation. Experimental infection of complement-depleted animals is followed by invasion at the same or deeper levels of the skin, but pustule formation is absent.

The role of antibody and T-effector cells in production of clinical lesions and host defenses is less clear.

Delayed-type hypersensitivity to *Candida* skin test antigen is present in most healthy adults; lack of sensitivity is characteristic of deficient cellular immunity and chronic recalcitrant mucocutaneous *Candida* infections.

Clinical Findings

A. Symptoms and Signs: Burning, stinging, and itching occur on the intertriginous skin of the groin, axilla, or other affected sites.

Typical acute changes are a beefy red, scalded skin with an irregular margin and satellite pustules (Fig 16–6). A chronic, scaling form of candidiasis may be occasionally seen. Any skin surface may be involved, and the infection appears much like dermatophytosis.

B. Laboratory Findings: Removal of the roof of a vesicle or pustule for direct microscopic examination will reveal mycelial elements within the stratum corneum. It is useless to examine scrapings from the beefy red scalded area or base of the pustule, as the organisms never invade to that depth. Mycologic culture of a satellite pustule should yield a creamy mucoid colony within 48–72 hours. Definitive speciation requires demonstration of typical chlamydospores or carbohydrate fermentation testing. There are several *Candida* species that may produce cutaneous infections, and they must be distinguished from *C albicans*.

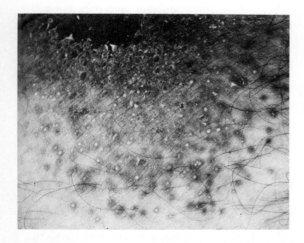

Figure 16–6. Cutaneous candidiasis. Intertriginous candidiasis in a female, showing denuded center and discrete satellite pustules in the periphery.

Differential Diagnosis

Nonspecific intertrigo, allergic contact dermatitis, primary irritant dermatitis, and psoriatic intertrigo are the most common conditions misdiagnosed as cutaneous candidiasis. A variety of other problems may be considered in the differential diagnosis, including dermatophytosis. In the inguinal-crural area, tinea cruris almost never involves the scrotum, which is commonly involved in candidiasis. In addition, candidiasis is usually much redder. Pityriasis rosea and Hailey-Hailey disease may also mimic candidiasis.

Prevention

Patients who are bedfast, febrile, and perspiring heavily should minimize moisture, occlusion, maceration, and irritations from soaps used for bed baths.

Treatment

Treatment should include nonspecific measures, especially removal of moisture, maceration, and occlusion factors that precipitate the infection. Diabetes should be controlled and corticosteroids and antibiotics discontinued, if possible.

Topical nystatin in a cream vehicle applied 3 times a day is excellent therapy in most instances. Addition of 1% hydrocortisone provides more rapid relief. Alternatively, one may use one of the topical imidazole antifungal agents. Primary irritation or allergy to the topical medication may occur in occluded body surfaces and thus worsen the clinical problem. Compresses with Burow's solution, aeration, or infrared heat lamp drying of affected parts may be helpful. If topical preparations cannot be applied because of sensitivity of the denuded skin—or if there is widespread infection—ketoconazole, 200 or 400 mg/d orally as a single dose, is effective for adults.

Course & Prognosis

Most cutaneous candidiasis is acute or subacute. Chronic cutaneous infection is rare, usually occurring in patients who have chronic mucocutaneous candidiasis.

2. *CANDIDA* PARONYCHIA

Essentials of Diagnosis

- Red, swollen, tender paronychia and fingertip.
- Acute, subacute, or chronic involvement of one or a few nails.
- History of repeated wetting of hands.
- Demonstration of *Candida* species on direct smear and recovery on mycologic culture.

General Considerations

Candida paronychia is a common form of candidiasis that, because of the anatomy of the fingernail and paronychial skin, presents a distinct clinical-anatomic infection syndrome. These infections are common in people who frequently immerse their hands in water, eg, dishwashers, housewives, mothers of diaper-age children, and people whose hobbies involve wetting of their hands. The acute lesion is a reddened, bulbous swelling of the nail folds and distal phalanx of the finger. The acute process often looks like an early abscess.

It is presumed that this is an autoinfection contracted from commensal *Candida* in the intestinal tract or moist mucosal surfaces. The nail fold becomes colonized, and *Candida* proliferates in the hyphal form and invades the lateral and proximal nailfold. The anatomy of the nail fold provides a cleft for moisture to accumulate and the organism to thrive. In subacute and chronic infections, the paronychial tissue and the nail progressively become hard, thick, yellowish brown, discolored, and chronically inflamed. The nail is not directly destroyed, as in tinea unguium. Rather, the nail matrix and supporting tissues are destroyed, leaving a dystrophic nail.

Microbiology & Immunology

See section above under cutaneous candidiasis.

Clinical Findings

A. Symptoms and Signs: The patient usually complains of a red, swollen, tender finger and fingernail area. Tenderness may interfere with employment and other activities.

The distal phalanx for as much as 2 cm from the affected nail is swollen, erythematous, and tender to palpation. There may be a serous or purulent discharge from the nail fold, though discharge is more common in bacterial paronychia. Usually only one or a few nails are affected. Toenail involvement is less common unless the paronychiae are part of chronic, mucocutaneous candidiasis.

B. Laboratory Findings: Direct smear and culture of material from the lateral nail groove should demonstrate *C albicans*.

Differential Diagnosis

Nail infection by dermatophytes usually involves the distal free margin of the nail plate, with proximal progression, and the nail folds are not so markedly inflamed. Onychomycosis due to infection with non-dermatophytic fungi directly affects the nail, producing roughness and thickening. These changes are late signs in *Candida* paronychia if they occur at all. There are few entities that closely mimic chronic *Candida* paronychia, bacterial paronychia being most common. Psoriatic nail dystrophy or pachyonychia congenita should be considered.

Onycholysis may be caused by *C albicans*. The clinical picture is virtually indistinguishable from onycholysis due to psoriasis, but culture establishes the diagnosis.

Complications & Sequelae

Chronic *Candida* paronychia can result in scarring of the nail matrix with resulting lifelong nail dystrophy.

Prevention

Persons with a predisposition for *Candida* paronychia should avoid immersing the fingertips and, if they become wet meticulously dry them.

Treatment

Soaking the finger or nail or compressing with Burow's solution 1:40 for 10 minutes 4 times a day are helpful in treatment of acute paronychia. Topical imidazole antifungals in a solution or cream vehicle can be used with some success, especially if the affected part can be kept dry. Combination preparations such as Lotrisone—ie, an imidazole antifungal (clotrimazole) plus a corticosteroid (betamethasone)—are useful. A drop of 4% thymol in chloroform or absolute alcohol applied to the nail fold twice daily is a time-honored method of treatment.

Oral ketoconazole, 200–400 mg/d for 3–4 weeks, has helped. Ketoconazole is less effective in chronic paronychia, and the best results are obtained by combined oral and topical treatment.

Course & Prognosis

If the affected parts cannot be kept dry, development of subacute or chronic paronychia may be expected.

3. CHRONIC MUCOCUTANEOUS CANDIDIASIS

Essentials of Diagnosis

- Oral candidiasis of greater than 3 months duration.
- Multiple chronic *Candida* paronychiae.
- Foci of chronic cutaneous candidiasis—groin, scalp, face, or elsewhere.
- Demonstration of *Candida* on direct smear.
- Recovery of *Candida albicans* on culture.

General Considerations

Chronic mucocutaneous candidiasis is a group of infection syndromes characterized by chronic and persistent *Candida* infection of the mucous membranes, skin, and nails. Males and females appear equally affected. Although most become infected during the first years of life, the syndrome may begin at any age. Chronic mucocutaneous candidiasis is divided into 5 distinct groups. In group 1, the clinical manifestations are limited to chronic oral candidiasis, though some patients develop chronic esophageal involvement with esophageal stricture. Group 2 includes patients with the candidiasis endocrinopathy syndrome. These infections usually begin in childhood, and the most frequently observed endocrinopathies include hypoadrenalism, hypoparathyroidism, and hypothyroidism, although many patients have polyendocrinopathies.

The third group includes patients with chronic, localized (exophytic) candidiasis and has been termed the *Candida* granuloma group. Infections in these patients involve the mucous membranes, skin, and nails and frequently cause marked hyperkeratosis and disfigurement.

The fourth group, chronic diffuse mucocutaneous candidiasis, typically has widespread, mucosal, skin, and nail infection. Infection typically begins in childhood. Although there are no related endocrine disorders, the tendency to develop this problem may be inherited. It is important in these patients to distinguish candidiasis of glabrous skin from chronic tinea corporis, which may accompany chronic mucocutaneous candidiasis and may present an almost identical picture.

The fifth group is comprised of patients with adult-onset candidiasis affecting the mucous membranes, skin, and nails. Most patients are men and have associated thymomas, myasthenia gravis, aplastic anemia, neutropenia, hypogammaglobulinemia, AIDS, or lupus-like syndromes.

Thus, chronic mucocutaneous candidiasis is a disorder of many causes. The predisposition for 2 chronic mucocutaneous candidiasis syndromes is inherited as autosomal recessive, but in other families there is evidence of other modes of transmission, perhaps autosomal dominant.

The infection begins as mucosal candidiasis, paronychia, or cutaneous candidiasis and progresses from the acute to the subacute to the chronic phase, where its treatment-resistant nature validates the term chronic mucocutaneous candidiasis. In spite of the extensive involvement of the skin and mucous membranes, there is virtually no predisposition of patients with chronic mucocutaneous candidiasis to develop *Candida* sepsis or infection of visceral organs.

Microbiology & Immunology

One-half or more of chronic mucocutaneous candidiasis patients have other chronic or recurrent significant infections, suggesting unusual susceptibility. Chronic mucocutaneous candidiasis has been described in patients with a variety of immunologic deficiency syndromes, with immunologic defects limited to the T cell system or involving both the T cell and the B cell systems. In contrast, chronic mucocutaneous candidiasis is not found in patients with immunologic defects limited to the immunoglobulin producing system. Thus, it appears that T cell-mediated immunity is critical for host defenses against *Candida* and, when appropriately compromised, may lead to chronic mucocutaneous candidiasis. A variety of clinical and laboratory abnormalities of cell-mediated immunity have been demonstrated in these patients.

Clinical Findings

A. Symptoms and Signs: Patients complain of itching, stinging, and burning of the affected mucosal surfaces and other areas.

All mucosal surfaces may be affected or only one, eg, chronic oral candidiasis. A chronic *Candida* paronychia is commonly present on one to several digits. Perlèche (infection at the ends of the lips) is common, and infection may extend onto the nasolabial folds, face, cheek, and scalp. Infected areas may be continuous or discontinuous. Involvement of the groin or glabrous skin elsewhere may occur. Many of these patients also develop widespread tinea corporis due to *Trichophyton rubrum* or *Epidermophyton floccosum* and cutaneous bacterial infections.

B. Laboratory Findings: Diagnosis can be firmly established only by demonstration of the fungal elements of *C albicans* or other *Candida* species in direct smears from affected sites and by recovery of the organism on mycologic culture. For involvement of the nails, scalp, and glabrous skin, direct smears and cultures should be done to rule out possible concomitant dermatophyte infection. Mycologic culture identifies the etiologic agent.

Differential Diagnosis

Chronic mucocutaneous candidiasis is usually not difficult to diagnose, though it may be mimicked by pachyonychia congenita, acrodermatitis enteropathica, glucagonoma syndrome, essential fatty acid deficiency, and iatrogenic zinc deficiency from hyperalimentation.

Complications & Sequelae

Perhaps the most common complication is involvement of the esophagus, which leads to strictures, stenosis, and perhaps perforation, mediastinitis, and death. Elective surgical juxtaposition of an intestinal segment in place of the diseased esophagus has been successful in some patients. Failure to identify the associated endocrinopathies—eg, thymoma, myasthenia gravis—could lead to serious complications.

Prevention

No prevention is known. There is an early indication from several centers that early treatment with an effective systemic antifungal like ketoconazole may spare development of the full-blown syndrome.

Treatment

Treatment of esophageal, mucosal, cutaneous, or nail candidiasis in these patients has been notoriously difficult. Effective systemic therapy with amphotericin B has usually been associated with an excellent short-term remission rate, but there is usually rapid relapse of the chronic mucocutaneous infection. Adjunctive immunotherapy with transfer factor combined with antifungal antibiotics has proved helpful in selected patients.

The introduction of ketoconazole has made it possible to manage most chronic mucocutaneous candidiasis patients in the outpatient setting. The administration of 200–400 mg/d orally—or, in selected cases, slightly higher doses—has made it possible to control the esophageal, mucosal, cutaneous, and nail infections. The initial response is within days to weeks, and most patients clear completely or improve more than 75% in the first 6 months of therapy. When the drug is discontinued, relapse is likely. Maintenance therapy schedules may involve taking as little as 100 mg of ketoconazole every other day, but the maintenance schedule for each patient should be individualized.

Course & Prognosis

This is a stubbornly chronic disorder. The patient's condition is generally fairly stable. Progressive worsening may occur. Esophageal involvement is serious and may lead to difficulties in swallowing, weight loss, cachexia, and death.

THE INVASIVE CUTANEOUS MYCOSES

In contrast to the infections discussed thus far, the invasive cutaneous mycoses almost always begin at a point focus within the skin. Frequently this is a site of trauma, and a foreign object may have penetrated the skin.

Chromomycosis, mycetoma, mucormycosis, and sporotrichosis all share the trait of spreading from the primary focus by direct extension through skin, lymphatics, and other contiguous tissues. Sporotrichosis is the only member of this disease group caused by a single organism, *Sporothrix schenckii*. This pathogen is also the only member of the group that can disseminate to visceral organs and produce primary pulmonary infection.

CHROMOMYCOSIS (Chromoblastomycosis)

Essentials of Diagnosis

- Warty sores that develop following trauma.
- Verrucous, foul-smelling plaque on the lower extremity.
- Involvement of a single extremity without sinus tract formation or dissemination.
- Demonstration of brown fungal elements in smears or tissue.

General Considerations

Chromomycosis involves the viable layers of the epidermis and dermis. Numerous species of the *Fonsecaea*, *Phialophora*, and *Cladosporium* genera are the obligatory etiologic agents. There may be contiguous local spread within the skin, and involvement of an entire extremity or even more generalized infection is occasionally encountered. There is little tendency for invasion of the musculoskeletal system lying directly beneath the focus of infection. Dissemination to visceral organs is rare.

Chromomycosis is principally a tropical infection by a group of closely related molds that have in common a dark mycelium. These fungi grow as filamentous, saprophytic organisms in the soil, where they extract nutrients from decaying vegetation. Individuals involved in manual labor with soil or its products contract chromomycosis. A history of trauma is usually elicited. Though typically on lower extremities, the trauma may be on the upper extremities or elsewhere.

It is not clear why chromomycosis is a disease of tropical or semitropical areas of the world. It is speculated that in northern climates, individuals must wear shoes, and that perhaps it is the shoeless state of the poor, rural, tropical laborers that leads to the high frequency of infection. Even in the tropics, however, chromomycosis is uncommon.

The taxonomy of the obligatory pathogens of chromomycosis can best be characterized as confusing and unsettled. The steps by which these fungi produce clinical disease is unknown. It is not clear which host defense mechanisms check the invasion of these organisms. The complex host-parasite interaction that follows inoculation of the fungus is characterized by pseudoepitheliomatous hyperplasia, scarring, etc. Histopathologically, the tissue reaction ranges from acute to subacute to chronic and includes both polymorphonuclear leukocytes and granulomatous reactions with foreign body giant cells. The fungus is visible in unstained or stained tissue sections as brown fungal bodies sometimes called sclerotic cells. Hyphal elements may also be seen. These dematiaceous fungi take special stains such as Gomori-methenamine silver and appear black, as do other fungi.

Microbiology & Immunology

The microbiology of the *Fonsecaea*, *Phialophora*, and *Cladosporium* organisms is not well characterized. The immunologic response of various hosts to these organisms has been studied; no diagnostic serologic tests are available.

Clinical Findings

A. Symptoms and Signs: The earliest changes are an itching, warty papule or perhaps an ulcer on the lower extremity. Patients often present much later in the evolution of the infection with foul-smelling, putrid, verrucous plaques covering a palm-sized area of the foot, ankle, knee, elbow, or hand.

The infection causes a papule, or sometimes an ulcer, that slowly enlarges over months or years. A rough exophytic, papillomatous and verrucous surface develops. As the process slowly spreads within the skin, the central area of infection becomes noticeably scarred. There may be admixed hypertrophic scars or even keloids. An infected papule or plaque may have black dots within its verrucous surface. Minute abscesses may be present. Spread may occur along the lymphatics.

Many patients develop secondary bacterial infection, with a resulting foul odor. Symptoms are remarkably few, and many patients delay for years seeking medical attention. Elephantiasis of the lower extremity may result if fibrosis and obstruction of the lymph channels occur.

The presence of verrucous papules, nodules, or plaques (Fig 16–7) on an extremity should alert the physician to chromomycosis as a possible diagnosis. The presence of black dots or microabscesses within the verrucous surface is a helpful diagnostic sign, but this sign also occurs in other fungal infections and conditions characterized by pseudoepitheliomatous hyperplasia. Centrifugal spread, atrophy, and scarring in the central area is suggestive of chromomycosis. Infection in more than one anatomic site can occur, especially in long-standing infection. Direct extension along the lymphatic channels—but within the skin—is common.

B. Laboratory Findings: Specimens should be collected from a black dot or microabscess within a verrucous nodule and smeared for KOH examination. Brown branching hyphae are presumptive evidence of chromomycosis. The organisms may also be seen in biopsy specimens. Mycologic culture is confirmatory; speciation should be done.

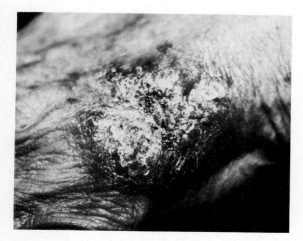

Figure 16–7. Chromomycosis. Typical crusted, hyperkeratotic, indurated plaque on dorsum of hand.

Differential Diagnosis

Chromomycosis must be distinguished from other conditions characterized by pseudoepitheliomatous hyperplasia, including other fungal infections, and squamous cell carcinoma. The overall picture is usually distinct from verruca vulgaris, lupus erythematosus, lichen planus, and tuberculosis verrucosa cutis. In endemic areas, cutaneous leishmaniasis, mycetoma, elephantiasis, and yaws may be in the differential. Histoplasmosis, blastomycosis, coccidioidomycosis, sporotrichosis, and some forms of chronic mucocutaneous candidiasis may produce a similar picture. The diagnosis will ultimately be established by direct examination of scrapings, tissue biopsy, and mycologic culture.

Complications & Sequelae

Considerable morbidity may be produced by the disease process. Involvement of a foot may limit ambulation. If the hand is affected, the manual dexterity of a person whose livelihood is probably earned by manual labor is compromised. The development of elephantiasis further complicates matters. The most serious complication is the development of squamous cell carcinoma in an area of chronic chromomycosis. Since the infection itself looks like carcinoma, diagnosis of this complication is often delayed.

Prevention

Wearing of shoes or other protective footwear is an excellent preventive measure.

Treatment

Nonspecific measures include bed rest, elevation of the affected part, and antibiotic therapy for control of secondary infection. Specific therapeutic measures may include surgical excision or destruction of the affected tissue or medical therapy with potassium iodide, flucytosine, thiabendazole, ketoconazole, and topical heat, each of which has been used with some success. It would appear that topical flucytosine 10%, oral ketoconazole, and focal hyperthermia are the 3 most efficacious treatments. Management of each patient should be individualized.

Course & Prognosis

The course is invariably chronic, often lasting years; many cases go on for decades. The prognosis is good unless there is maiming or dissemination.

MADUROMYCOSIS
(Mycetoma)

Essentials of Diagnosis
- Nodular, tumorous, fibrotic deformity of the foot or hand.
- Sinus tracts.
- White, tan, or brightly colored grains in draining fluid.

- Demonstration of true fungal elements in the grains.
- Consistent recovery of the pathogen in mycologic culture.

General Considerations

Mycetoma is the general name of a clinical syndrome caused by either bacteria or fungi. Mycetomas caused by true fungi have traditionally been referred to as maduromycosis, or eumycotic mycetoma. Eumycotic mycetoma accounts for approximately half of all mycetomas.

Most cases occur in the tropical or subtropical areas of the world that share a similar climate with the Sudan, Mexico, South India, certain areas in South America, the Mediterranean basin, and Oceania.

The etiologic agents of both the bacterial mycetomas and the eumycotic mycetomas are associated with nature, chiefly the soil, debris, and vegetation. Individuals working in rural areas, therefore, are at greatest risk; manual laborers, farmers, and others who are male and in mid-life have the larger share of these infections. Typically, there is a history of trauma from a thorn, stone, or other sharp object followed by a quiescent period (months to years) before the active disease process begins. There is insidious swelling that becomes focal, producing a nodule or a painless tumorous process that eventually breaks down and begins to drain to the surface. The organism spreads through similar invasive sinus tracts in the fascial planes into the subcutaneous tissue and within the ligaments, bones, nerves, and muscles. The nerves are usually spared; however, the muscle is often directly invaded.

The fungi that cause eumycotic mycetoma are numerous: *Allescheria boydii* is the most common cause, especially in certain geographic areas, but *Madurella* species, *Phialophora,* and others are also isolated. It is not clear why the disease develops so slowly during the period following inoculation or what, if anything, is wrong with relevant host defense mechanisms. The actinomycotic mycetomas are of bacterial origin and tend to produce a more pyococcal reaction and purulent, grain-laden discharge from sinus tracts. *Nocardia, Actinomyces,* and *Streptomyces* species tend to be destructive, with muscle invasion and sometimes marked destruction of bone. In eumycotic mycetoma, the pathologic process quickly becomes subacute and chronic, with granuloma formation, a foreign body giant cell reaction, and fibrosis dominating.

Microbiology & Immunology

Knowledge of the microbiology of these organisms and the immunology of the host response is limited.

Clinical Findings

A. Symptoms and Signs: The patient usually complains of a painless, rather indolent process slowly destroying the affected part. Since this is typically the foot or the hand, the patient usually becomes concerned when the mycetoma interferes with manual labor, walking, etc. The discharge is bothersome; there may be associated pain.

The physician must look for the triad of (1) sinus tracts draining to the skin surface; (2) discharge fluid-containing grains that range from white to red to black; and (3) a nodular, tumorous, fibrotic swelling. The foot or hand may be grotesquely distorted, and ambulation may be impossible. Occasionally—especially in actinomycotic mycetoma—there will be numerous miniature volcano-like papules, each containing in its center the opening of a sinus tract. This finding suggests that an actinomycete is present. Any site on the body into which the organism is traumatically implanted may become involved—commonly the neck, chest, and buttocks.

B. Laboratory Findings: Laboratory diagnosis depends upon clinical and laboratory examination of the grains, tissue biopsy, and culture. Excessive emphasis has been placed on the importance of grain color in determining which organism is involved. The nature of the grain, including its texture, color, and size, is helpful. In addition to examination of grains, culture for fungi on a simple, nonselective medium free of cycloheximide (which may inhibit the eumycotic agents) is critical to diagnosis. Sabouraud's agar is satisfactory. Grains should be crushed and inoculated onto nutritive bacterial agar such as blood agar and incubated both anaerobically and aerobically, or the anaerobic actinomycetes such as *A israelii* may be missed.

A deep tissue biopsy may help in that histopathologic examination may show sinus tracts containing typical grains, perhaps in instances where surface fungal or bacterial contamination may cloud the clinical picture.

C. Imaging Studies: An experienced radiologist may, upon finding typical roentgenographic changes, suggest the clinical diagnosis of mycetoma. The x-ray pattern, however, is not specific and will not decrease the need for determining the microbiologic etiology.

Differential Diagnosis

In the early phase, the pathologic findings are indeterminate and can mimic many conditions from trauma to tumors. Later, the disease becomes more characteristic. Pyococcal infection with staphylococci (in a distinctive syndrome called botryomycosis) may closely mimic mycetoma. Chromomycosis, some forms of sporotrichosis, and even blastomycosis and coccidioidomycosis may have similar clinical presentations. Other infections such as yaws, syphilis, and tuberculosis verrucosa cutis may be in the differential diagnosis. Noninfectious conditions such as hidradenitis suppurativa, dermatofibrosarcoma protuberans, and gross chronic edema may mimic mycetoma.

Complications & Sequelae

Destructive fibrosis, tumefaction, and swelling to the point of elephantiasis may render the foot, hand, or other body part useless and necessitate amputation. Hematogenous spread is rare. Actinomycotic mycetomas disseminate more frequently, particularly if the primary focus is on the torso.

Treatment

Nonspecific measures are often helpful, especially if there is superinfection of the surface with other bacteria or fungi that produce purulence. These would include soaking the infected part in tap water and administration of antibiotics based on culture of surface organisms.

Specific therapeutic measures largely depend upon whether the mycetoma is actinomycotic or eumycotic. Actinomycotic infections can for the most part be successfully managed using trimethoprim-sulfamethoxazole or dapsone. Medications are given for at least several months after a clinical cure is obtained to prevent relapses.

Specific therapy for the maduromycoses is inadequate. Antifungals have been used from the iodides through amphotericin B. There is little promising information on the role of ketoconazole therapy, and itraconazole or another of the newer oral azole will perhaps have greater efficacy. Sulfones may be occasionally effective.

Surgical drainage of abscesses and debridement by an orthopedist may help, but amputation is often necessary, especially in advanced cases.

MUCORMYCOSIS

Mucormycosis, zygomycosis, and phycomycosis are the clinical terms applied to invasive infections caused by fungi belonging to the genera *Rhizopus, Mucor, Absidia,* and *Cunninghamella.* These infections are uncommon. Mucormycosis is usually opportunistic, with most patients having serious medical problems ranging from metabolic acidosis, usually diabetic in origin, to leukemia and lymphoma, often complicated by iatrogenic immunosuppression.

The rhinocerebral form of mucormycosis may rapidly invade major arteries and the brain and be fatal within hours to days. Other forms include the pulmonary-thoracic form, the gastrointestinal form, and the abdominal-pelvic form. Skin involvement in mucormycosis is even less common.

Primary invasion of the skin and subcutaneous tissues may occur. There are no consistent physical findings that suggest the diagnosis. Infection often occurs in injured and necrotic tissue such as that associated with vascular infarcts and burns. Nosocomial cutaneous infections have been transmitted by contaminated dressings for superficial wounds.

SPOROTRICHOSIS

Essentials of Diagnosis

- Chancriform complex on an upper extremity.
- A fixed plaque of verrucous papules, erosion, and ulceration.
- May have musculoskeletal or chronic pulmonary involvement.
- Paucity of organisms in smears and tissue.
- Recovery of *Sporothrix schenckii* on mycologic culture.

General Considerations

Sporothrix schenckii infection typically follows trauma and usually causes a painful ulcerated nodule. Fixed cutaneous sporotrichosis may present as scaly papules that make up an indurated plaque. The papules may become hyperkeratotic and verrucous, erode, and form indolent, chronic ulcers.

Sporotrichosis disseminated through hematogenous entry via the skin may produce several clinical manifestations. In addition to primary pulmonary infection, the organism may affect the eye, nervous system, or other organs as a true systemic mycosis. The skeletal system may also be affected, leading to destructive arthritis, tenosynovitis, and lesions in the major bones of the extremities as well as the ribs, phalanges, carpals, and tarsals. In this way the infection, though classified as an invasive cutaneous infection, can, albeit rarely, produce systemic mycotic infection.

Both sexes and all age groups are affected, and the disease is worldwide. Individuals who through vocation or avocation contact soil, vegetation, untreated plant products, or decaying vegetable matter are at greatest risk. Trauma to the fingers, hand, or arm, as from a rose thorn or other puncture wound, is a typical inciting event. In children, inoculation and infection are usually on the face. The incidence, prevalence, and proportional rates are low.

The vast majority of patients develop the acute chancriform or lymphangitic type of infection, and dissemination and systemic involvement is rare. It is puzzling why so few organisms are present in smears and biopsy material, even from acute primary lesions. Culture of tissue, however, usually is positive. The histologic picture of the clinical lesion is dependent upon the stage—acute, subacute, or chronic—and the clinical form—chancriform, fixed, disseminated, etc. Reactions may be pyogenic, granulomatous, verrucous, or fibrotic.

Microbiology & Immunology

Considerable work has been done on the immunology of sporotrichosis. A skin test antigen is chiefly useful in epidemiologic surveys, and delayed-type hypersensitivity develops in endemic areas. Individuals with no clinical symptoms, signs, or history suggestive of infection may exhibit a positive skin test. A variety of serologic procedures have been used in the clinical diagnosis and management of patients with sporotrichosis. There is considerable controversy about which technique is best and especially as to clinical interpretation.

Strongly reacting antisera have been developed that can be used in a direct immunofluorescence diagnostic procedure utilizing biopsy material. The fluorescent technique can even be applied to hematoxylin and eosin-stained histopathologic material (but not to PAS- or methenamine silver-treated specimens) by removing the stain first.

Clinical Findings

A. Symptoms and Signs: The symptoms are directly attributable to the form of the clinical disease. In the chancriform infection, the patient will complain of a tender, sometimes painful nodule on the finger or hand, accompanied by tender epitrochlear and axillary lymphadenopathy. The fixed cutaneous plaques and ulcers may be tender and painful, and occasionally in verrucous lesions pruritus may be present. Cutaneous symptomatology in pulmonary, musculoskeletal, and disseminated sporotrichosis is not present unless the skin is affected. Painful hard subcutaneous nodules or tender areas overlying involved bones and joints may be present.

Chancriform sporotrichosis presents the highly suggestive findings of an acral ulcer with an ascending lymphangitic chain of nodules or ulcers leading to enlarged, tender lymph nodes. The typical clinical picture, accompanied by supporting historical information, is extremely suggestive of the diagnosis. The lesions in fixed cutaneous sporotrichosis are more polymorphic and less diagnostic; this type may be unsuspected clinically and histopathologically only to be identified when the organism is recovered on microbiologic culture. Skin lesions in disseminated sporotrichosis may suggest a systemic fungal infection but are not specific for sporotrichosis. Patients with musculoskeletal lesions typically have cutaneous or subcutaneous lesions, but those with pulmonary sporotrichosis usually do not have cutaneous involvement.

B. Laboratory Findings: The salient laboratory findings are the paucity of organisms in histologic material and the importance of mycologic culture. Smears from suspected lesions are almost always negative and play little role in the diagnosis of this particular mycosis. An organism in the histopathologic material may be identified by fluorescent antibody staining techniques.

The organism may be cultured on any mycologic medium with Sabouraud's dextrose agar or on more selective media being used for primary isolation of the organism. The colonial morphology and microscopic appearance of the organism are characteristic.

Differential Diagnosis

For chancriform sporotrichosis, other primary inoculation mycoses and certain bacterial infections such as nocardiosis may present a similar picture. Primary inoculation blastomycosis and coccidioidomycosis, the latter usually occurring in laboratory investigators, may resemble chancriform sporotrichosis. Mycobacterial infection, particularly with atypical mycobacteria (eg, *Mycobacterium marinum*), may present a similar picture.

Fixed cutaneous sporotrichosis is mimicked by many more conditions. Chromomycosis, tuberculosis verrucosus cutis, cutaneous leishmaniasis, syphilis, halogenoderma, and the ulcerative form of lupus erythematosus or lichen planus may have a similar appearance. Depending on the morphologic features and the anatomic location of the fixed cutaneous lesions—as well as the clinical setting—numerous other infections and conditions including dermatitis factitia must be considered in the differential diagnosis. Similar comments apply to the cutaneous lesions associated with musculoskeletal sporotrichosis.

Complications & Sequelae

Dissemination, albeit rare, is a serious complication and may lead to death.

Treatment

Specific measures differ depending on the form of sporotrichosis. Lesions of chancriform sporotrichosis appear to heal spontaneously, but this has not been established in controlled studies. It is therefore advisable to treat patients with chancriform sporotrichosis. Iodides—particularly saturated solution of potassium iodide (SSKI)—have been the preferred therapy. The mechanism of action of SSKI is poorly understood, but the absence of any in vitro effect on *S schenckii* suggests that the drug augments host defenses. SSKI contains approximately 1 g of potassium iodide per milliliter. The initial dose is 3 drops 3 times daily diluted in a flavorful liquid such as orange juice. The daily dose should be increased slowly every second to third day until 10–15 drops—or, in resistant cases, up to 20 drops—are being given 3 times daily. Administration in this manner minimizes side effects such as parotitis and acneiform eruptions and iododermas. Therapy should be continued 4–6 weeks past clinical cure.

Amphotericin B, flucytosine, and ketoconazole have also been used in the treatment of chancriform sporotrichosis. More recently, clinical trials of itraconazole have led to excellent clinical results. If itraconazole's apparent safety is confirmed, it will likely become the treatment of choice for sporotrichosis.

The fixed cutaneous form of sporotrichosis is less responsive to SSKI treatment, and this appears true also for the rare lesion that affects the mucocutaneous surfaces. SSKI is not effective in musculoskeletal sporotrichosis and pulmonary sporotrichosis.

The standard therapy for musculoskeletal, pulmonary, and systemic infection is amphotericin B. Ketoconazole does not appear particularly effective in sporotrichosis. Itraconazole may become the treatment of choice.

Course & Prognosis

The prognosis for chancriform sporotrichosis is usually excellent. The fixed forms of sporotrichosis and the cutaneous lesions that may accompany musculoskeletal sporotrichosis have a more chronic course and a guarded prognosis. Pulmonary and systemic sporotrichosis, especially the latter, have a more guarded prognosis and may lead to death.

PROTOTHECOSIS

Protothecosis is actually not a fungal disease but an infection of the skin caused by saprophytic achloric algae. This uncommon infection is mentioned here only for completeness, as these verrucous, nodular, ulcerative to granulomatous lesions may mimic invasive cutaneous fungal infection.

ACTINOMYCOSIS
(See Chapter 12.)

Actinomycosis is actually a bacterial infection caused by *Actinomyces israelii* and *Actinomyces bovis*. It is included here because it must be differentiated from many of the fungal infections mentioned above, particularly those associated with draining sinuses, fibrosis, and scarring.

NOCARDIOSIS

Nocardia asteroides and *Nocardia brasiliensis* are infections with bacteria similar to the actinomycetes and produce a similar disease process. Nocardiosis is mentioned here because it may mimic not only invasive cutaneous mycoses but also skin lesions produced by the systemic mycoses.

RHINOSPORIDIOSIS

Rhinosporidium seeberi is the etiologic agent of this distinctive but uncommon mycosis. The skin lesions per se are minimal. Lesions of the nose, eyes, and mouth clinically resemble nasal polyps or other polypoid tumors, including condylomata acuminata and hemangiomas. The disease has been seen in many countries throughout the world but chiefly in India and Ceylon.

CUTANEOUS INVOLVEMENT IN THE SYSTEMIC MYCOSES

Cutaneous involvement in the systemic mycoses differs fundamentally from the noninvasive and invasive cutaneous mycoses. The systemic mycoses essentially all begin in the lung, and the course from that point on varies tremendously from organism to organism and from patient to patient. The clinical manifestations may be limited to the lung or may reflect dissemination to other viscera, the brain, the musculoskeletal system, or the skin. Cutaneous manifestations are a result of allergic manifestations or hematogenous dissemination into the skin. The reader is referred to other sources for comprehensive information on noncutaneous manifestations of these infections.

Four of the systemic mycoses—blastomycosis, coccidioidomycosis, histoplasmosis, and paracoccidioidomycosis—have many clinical and pathologic similarities and produce similar cutaneous or mucocutaneous lesions. Cryptococcosis and the opportunistic fungi that produce fungal septicemia will be discussed separately.

CUTANEOUS MANIFESTATIONS OF COCCIDIOIDOMYCOSIS

Essentials of Diagnosis
- Flu-like syndrome ("valley fever").
- Erythema multiforme or erythema nodosum.
- Verrucous, granulomatous nodules.
- Subcutaneous abscesses, sinus tracts, and cutaneous ulcers.
- Suggestive x-ray and serologic tests.
- Demonstration of the organism in histopathologic sections.
- Isolation of *Coccidioides immitis* on mycologic culture.

General Considerations
Coccidioides immitis is a mold that grows only in dry areas of the world—ie, where there are 10 inches or less per year of rainfall, most of which falls in one season, and in which there is a hot summer and a mild winter. When wind and weather conditions are optimal, the organism becomes airborne along with dust particles; a high percentage of persons who inhale the fungus develop primary pulmonary infection.

About 60% of primary infections are subclinical and are appreciated only in retrospect when the patient is found to have a positive coccidioidin skin test. The remaining patients have varying symptomatology during the acute primary infection. Fewer than 1% probably disseminate, and—for reasons that are not clear—dark-skinned people are at a greater risk. American Blacks, Filipinos, and dark-skinned Mexicans appear to develop dissemination 10 times more frequently than northern European Caucasians.

Microbiology & Immunology

C immitis is a dimorphic organism that grows in nature as a mold and in the human principally as spherules and endospores, though mycelium may be seen.

All coccidioidomycosis is caused by a single species, *C immitis*.

Serology is useful in diagnosis and prognosis. Precipitin test is usually positive early. Complement-fixing antibodies appear later but persist longer. A rising complement fixation titer is a bad prognostic sign, especially if accompanied in the early phase by an eosinophilia.

Clinical Findings

A. Symptoms and Signs: Symptoms are attributable to the clinical manifestations in the patient. Itching may accompany erythema multiforme; pain and tenderness may accompany erythema nodosum. The verrucous, granulomatous nodules may be asymptomatic or somewhat pruritic. Abscesses, ulcers, and sinuses may be tender or painful.

Erythema multiforme appears during the acute primary pulmonary infection. The erythema multiforme associated with coccidioidomycosis distinctively involves the upper half of the body, with the neck, face, upper back, and chest principally affected. It may subside and recrudesce in a second wave.

Erythema nodosum appears early during the primary pulmonary infection and may accompany erythema multiforme. The eruption is not distinctive and affects the anterior surface of the lower extremities in the usual manner.

Secondary cutaneous involvement through hematogenous dissemination from a primary pulmonary focus may assume any of several forms. In an endemic area, the dermatologist must stay alert for the diagnosis because there is no specific morphology, configuration, or anatomic distribution that permits diagnosis of all forms of cutaneous infection. Perhaps the most characteristic lesion is a verrucous papule or nodule about the central face, scalp, or neck (Fig 16–8). Histopathologically, these nodules are granulomatous, and the overlying epidermis is involved in a marked pseudoepitheliomatous hyperplasia that produces the characteristic verrucous surface. These papules or nodules may expand or multiply rapidly, and the patient may or may not be systemically ill. Resolving lesions may produce significant scarring. The nonwarty cutaneous lesions are often associated with dissemination and deteriorating general health. There may be erythematous areas, acne-like lesions,

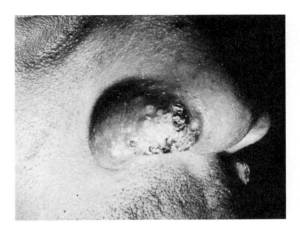

Figure 16–8. Coccidioidomycosis. Typical verrucous nodule on nose in disseminated infection.

ulceration, abscess formation, and drainage from sinus tracts.

B. Imaging Studies: X-ray of the chest and bones and CT scans are helpful in delineating cavities and cysts.

C. Special Examinations: Coccidioidin skin testing is a useful epidemiologic tool and may be helpful in the clinical evaluation of patients outside endemic zones. Diagnostic serologic testing should precede the antigenic stimulation of a skin test.

Differential Diagnosis

A variety of clinical conditions may mimic the cutaneous manifestations of coccidioidomycosis. The skin lesions of all the invasive cutaneous mycoses and systemic mycoses may be similar, since they all develop pseudoepitheliomatous hyperplasia. This process may represent an attempt on the part of the skin to transepidermally eliminate foreign elements that host defense mechanisms cannot destroy. Nonfungal infections such as keratoacanthoma, squamous cell carcinoma, elastosis perforans serpiginosa, and tuberculosis cutis may produce a similar picture.

Complications & Sequelae

Skin lesions have no particular sequelae except scarring. The systemic disease, when disseminated, is a serious medical problem.

Prevention

Avoid breathing dust-laden air in endemic zones. Limited clinical trials suggest that vaccination against coccidioidomycosis may be possible.

Treatment

Specific and nonspecific measures should be used as indicated. Of the specific measures, amphotericin B is the standard of therapy, and it is reasonably effective in all forms of the disease except the severe, disseminated form. Ketoconazole appears effective in many patients.

Course & Prognosis

Coccidioidomycosis is generally a benign condition. Dissemination is common in dark-skinned individuals, and the prognosis is grave if any patient is unresponsive to amphotericin B therapy and the complement fixation titer is rising.

CUTANEOUS INVOLVEMENT IN NORTH AMERICAN BLASTOMYCOSIS

Essentials of Diagnosis

- Hyperkeratotic warty papules, nodules, and plaques on the face, torso, and extremities.
- Cough and weight loss.
- Demonstration of broad-based budding yeasts in smears or tissue sections.
- Isolation of *Blastomyces dermatitidis* by culture.

General Considerations

This uncommon disease is most frequent in the Ohio and Mississippi River Valley area of the United States. Men between the ages of 30 and 50 are most often affected. Subclinical cases are uncommon. Blastomycosis occurs in mini-epidemics in relation to certain occupations or sites. The reservoir for the organism may be the soil. Pigeon droppings have been incriminated in the spread of the organism; there is evidence that canine blastomycosis may share a similar geographic distribution with human blastomycosis.

A large percentage of such infected patients have a benign course. Some may recover from predominantly cutaneous blastomycosis without specific antifungal therapy.

Skin lesions almost always result from dissemination of a primary pulmonary focus. The changes in the skin—like those in coccidioidomycosis and other invasive cutaneous and systemic fungal infections—often have pseudoepitheliomatous hyperplasia as their dominant feature.

Microbiology & Immunology

North American blastomycosis is caused by a single species, *Blastomyces dermatitidis*. The immunology, virulence factors of the organism, and relevant host defense mechanisms are poorly understood. There is a serologic complement fixation test that is useful clinically, but its value may be negated by prior skin testing with blastomycin antigen. For that reason—and because skin tests are frequently negative in early infection—skin testing is generally not recommended except in epidemiologic studies.

Clinical Findings

A. Symptoms and Signs: The presenting complaint of most patients with blastomycosis is either skin involvement or cough. Skin lesions are apparently present in 60–90% of patients. In an endemic area, a suggestive skin lesion plus cough, hemoptysis, and chest pain are highly suggestive of North American blastomycosis. Genital and urinary system complaints, hoarseness, night sweats, and painful joints may also be reported.

Typical verrucous papules, nodules, and plaques develop on the face, neck, or upper torso. Lesions on the torso are often elliptic (Fig 16–9). One or a few lesions may be present, or, in more severe, chronic cases, numerous lesions may be present (Fig 16–10). Lesions on the extremities and on the buttocks and thigh area are less common. Ulcers on the mucous membranes, draining sinuses, and nonspecific skin changes may be present.

B. Laboratory Findings: The demonstration of broad-based, budding yeast forms on direct microscopic examination of material from skin lesions establishes a presumptive diagnosis. Demonstration of broad-based budding spores on histopathologic examination of tissue is even more highly suggestive. Definitive diagnosis of blastomycosis must be made by isolation of the organism. Sabouraud's unmodified medium should be used, since the organism will not grow if the medium contains cycloheximide. Growth

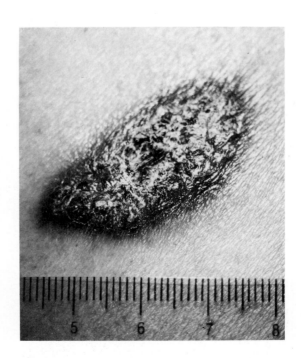

Figure 16–9. Blastomycosis. Typical solitary plaque on back with hyperkeratotic, crusted surface. Note elliptic shape.

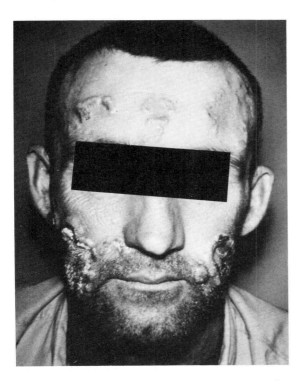

Figure 16–10. Blastomycosis. Multiple chronic scarring plaques.

is slow and may take at least 3–5 weeks. If cultures are negative but the organism can be demonstrated in tissue sections, direct immunofluorescence using antisera prepared in rabbits may be helpful in establishing an etiologic diagnosis.

C. Imaging Studies: Roentgenographic examination of the chest and bones may be helpful.

Differential Diagnosis

All of the deep mycoses may produce similar morphologic changes in the skin, and each must be considered in the differential diagnosis. A typical expanding verrucous plaque with ulceration and clearing in a scarred center is suggestive of the diagnosis, especially if black dots are found near the margin of the verrucous plaque. Cutaneous lesions may also suggest squamous cell carcinomas.

Treatment

Some investigators today believe that some patients with blastomycosis heal spontaneously without medical or surgical treatment. Until prospective studies delineate the natural course of infection, it would be prudent practice to treat all infected persons. Treatment for North American blastomycosis has traditionally included a variety of agents, but intra-venous amphotericin B has been the standard. Ketoconazole has worked well in many patients and may be the treatment of choice. Potassium iodide, hydroxystilbamidine, and intravenous miconazole have been used with variable results.

Course & Prognosis

The course of treated cutaneous blastomycosis is variable—subacute to chronic—but the disease resolves in most individuals.

CUTANEOUS MANIFESTATION OF PARACOCCIDIOIDOMYCOSIS

Essentials of Diagnosis

- Nonhealing, progressive ulceration of the oral pharynx.
- Massive cervical lymphadenopathy.
- Gastrointestinal and pulmonary symptoms.
- Weight loss, cachexia.
- Microscopic demonstration of the organism in secretions or tissue.
- Recovery of *Paracoccidioides brasiliensis* in culture.

General Considerations

Paracoccidioidomycosis, also known as South American blastomycosis, is not related to infection with *Blastomyces dermatitidis* or *Coccidioides immitis*. The organism is found in the soil, and the infection in the vast majority of patients is contracted by inhalation. The primary pulmonary infection is usually mild and subclinical. Like coccidioidomycosis and histoplasmosis, a large percentage of the population in endemic areas have positive skin tests. Ninety percent of all paracoccidioidomycosis patients are men, and most are in the productive mid-life years. All cases reported have been contracted in South America, usually in the warm, rainy, low mountain forests. Although several thousand cases have been described, epidemiologic studies have not defined the exact prevalence and incidence of subclinical or overt infection.

Primary infection in the lung is usually not locally progressive. Rather, the primary site subsides or stabilizes, and lesions then appear in the oropharyngeal area. Dissemination may be by respiratory secretion or hematogenous spread.

Clinical Findings

A. Symptoms and Signs: The most common presentation of paracoccidioidomycosis is oropharyngeal ulceration. Patients may present early in the disease but more often later, after significant pain, distress, and disfigurement are present. Patients may complain of papules, nodules, and verrucous plaques on the skin, principally on the face or neck. Massive cervical lymphadenopathy may lead to painful abscesses and draining sinuses.

A patient who has a nonhealing oral ulceration—particularly on the tongue, palate, uvula, or epiglottis—and who was born or has lived in rural South America where paracoccidioidomycosis is endemic—may have this disease. Massive lymphadenopathy with minimal or advanced oropharyngeal disease is highly suggestive.

Papules or vesicles form, and erosion occurs. The initial lesions are painless and may go unnoticed. Failure to heal and extension of the ulcerations cause distress and pain. Eating may become difficult. Extensive vegetations, ulceration, and fibrosis may destroy the tongue, soft palate, uvula, and epiglottis.

The disease may spread to the mucocutaneous surface, nose, or lips, causing extensive destruction and disfigurement. Eating becomes difficult, and the resulting cachexia is debilitating. Discrete lesions may appear on the skin; systemic involvement, especially in the gastrointestinal tract, is common. Widespread dissemination to other viscera, including the central nervous system and musculoskeletal system, is less common.

Primary pulmonary paracoccidioidomycosis is usually benign but may be progressive. Extensive scarring may compromise pulmonary function. After primary pulmonary paracoccidioidomycosis has resolved, the lungs may be reinfected in progressive systemic paracoccidioidomycosis.

B. Laboratory Findings: Direct examination of KOH-prepared sputum, scrapings from an ulcer or skin lesion, or discharge from a draining sinus may reveal typical yeast cells that possess multiple narrow connections to daughter buds. Mycologic culture should be obtained for confirmation. Histopathologic material will show a chronic granulomatous disease with remarkable involvement of lymphoid tissues. Special stains may be diagnostic if the pathognomonic "pilot wheel" budding yeast cell is seen in tissue sections. A paracoccidioidin skin test material is available. Clinical serologic tests are available and appear useful in diagnosis and prognosis.

C. Imaging Studies: Dramatic x-ray abnormalities of the lungs may be present, but minor changes analogous to those of histoplasmosis are more common in the subclinical infections.

Differential Diagnosis

Since the presentation of most patients with paracoccidioidomycosis is with the oropharyngeal ulceration, other causes of oropharyngeal ulceration such as lethal midline granuloma or Wegener's granulomatosis should be considered. Lesions on the skin or mucocutaneous junction will mimic chromomycosis, sporotrichosis, blastomycosis, histoplasmosis, tuberculosis, leishmaniasis, yaws, syphilis, etc. Squamous cell carcinoma may produce similar physical findings. The massive lymphadenopathy

of cervical nodes may simulate lymphoma, particularly Hodgkin's disease.

Complications & Sequelae

Progressive destruction of the structures of the mouth and oropharynx may result in inability to eat, weight loss, and cachexia. Dissemination, progressive systemic disease, and death may follow.

Treatment

Specific treatment has consisted of administration of sulfonamides and amphotericin B until recently, when ketoconazole was found to produce dramatic cures in more than 90% of patients. The dosage is 200 or 400 mg/d for approximately 6 months. Ketoconazole is especially valuable because it is an oral medication that can be used on an outpatient basis, allowing men to continue working.

Course & Prognosis

Most infections are subclinical. Until ketoconazole became available, the mucocutaneous form was chronic, progressive, and mutilating. Disseminated systemic paracoccidioidomycosis follows a progressive course.

CUTANEOUS MANIFESTATIONS OF HISTOPLASMOSIS

Essentials of Diagnosis

- Ulcer on the mucosal surface.
- Appropriate clinical setting.
- Suggestive histopathologic features.
- Demonstration of *Histoplasma capsulatum* on culture.

General Considerations

Histoplasmosis is caused by the dimorphic fungus, *Histoplasma capsulatum,* which is present worldwide. Ecologic factors and, apparently, the density of birds—especially starlings—affect the prevalence of human infection. The organism is especially prevalent in the Ohio and Mississippi River Valleys, where human infection is frequently associated with exposure to bird droppings. The disease—especially the chronic pulmonary form—is more frequent in men. Fulminant histoplasmosis occurs mainly in children of either sex.

Histoplasmosis is acquired through inhalation of the organism, and the resulting primary pulmonary infection is usually subclinical. More than 90% of the population at risk may be skin test positive.

H capsulatum is an intracellular pathogen in monocytic phagocytes. The organism disseminates hematogenously from the primary pulmonary focus of infection. Histoplasmosis has 3 clinical forms: (1) acute, (2) acute progressive, and (3) chronic progressive. Skin lesions other than ulcers of the mucous membranes of the body, particularly the tongue and oropharynx, are uncommon.

Microbiology & Immunology

The histoplasmin skin test is a useful epidemiologic tool, but in endemic areas it has no diagnostic value. Serologic tests may be of diagnostic and prognostic value, especially if serial determinations can be obtained.

Clinical Findings

A. Symptoms and Signs: Skin lesions are uncommon, with chronic ulcerative lesions of a mucosal surface being by far the most typical and frequent mucocutaneous manifestation. Although the rectal and genital mucosa may be affected, it is more typically the oropharynx or tongue that suffers.

A nonhealing ulcer of the tongue, oropharynx, or other mucocutaneous surface is the most suggestive physical finding. Verrucous or granulomatous lesions, pustules, abscesses, and draining sinuses have been described on the skin, but all are rare.

B. Laboratory Findings: The histopathologic features may be suggestive of histoplasmosis. The granulomatous findings in histoplasmosis are reminiscent of tuberculosis. Mycologic culture is necessary for definitive diagnosis.

C. Imaging Studies: The pulmonary parenchyma often contains multiple typical calcific densities from which an experienced radiologist can, without additional information, predict that the patient has resided in an endemic area.

D. Special Examinations: Histoplasmin skin testing is a useful epidemiologic test but has little clinical value.

Differential Diagnosis

The differential diagnosis of mucocutaneous ulceration is broad and must include carcinoma, syphilis, and other infectious ulcerations—including other fungal infections and, especially in endemic areas, blastomycosis, *Candida (Torulopsis) glabrata* infection, and paracoccidioidomycosis.

Treatment

Treatment is not necessary in acute uncomplicated pulmonary histoplasmosis. Treatment is essential in progressive histoplasmosis. Amphotericin B has been the standard of therapy, but results with ketoconazole have been impressive in at least some forms of histoplasmosis. Ketoconazole is the treatment of choice for at least chronic pulmonary histoplasmosis.

Course & Prognosis

Primary histoplasmosis is usually subclinical but may follow an acute, progressive course that is especially rapid and relentless in children. Chronic progressive histoplasmosis follows a much more indolent course reminiscent of tuberculosis.

CUTANEOUS MANIFESTATIONS OF CRYPTOCOCCOSIS

Essentials of Diagnosis

- Panniculitis, ecchymoses, acneiform to ulcerative lesions.
- Appropriate clinical setting.
- Microscopic demonstration of the organism in smears or tissue sections.
- Isolation of *Cryptococcus neoformans* on mycologic culture.

General Considerations

Cryptococcosis is caused by *Cryptococcus neoformans,* an encapsulated budding yeast. The organism is found worldwide, closely associated with birds that harbor and spread the organism through their droppings. Infection may occur at any age, though most patients are adults—especially those who are already ill from lupus erythematosus or lymphoma or compromised through iatrogenic immunosuppression. Clinically significant primary cryptococcosis in an otherwise healthy individual is an unusual clinical presentation. The incidence and prevalence, though unknown, must be low. Skin infections are usually secondary and not particularly common nor distinctive.

Cryptococcus neoformans is a yeast with a thick polysaccharide capsule, making it a distinctly different pathogen in comparison with other systemic mycotic agents. The pathogenesis and clinical pathologic features are different in many ways from those of other fungal infections. It is thought that the thick capsular polysaccharide, which is not highly antigenic, reduces the host response compared to that seen in other fungal diseases. In many cryptococcal infections, there is a paucity of host response, and in some only gelatinous abscesses form. Some manifest a more granulomatous process characteristic of the mycoses.

For reasons that are not clear, this organism has a strong predilection for the central nervous system, and the presence of meningitis in a debilitated, immunosuppressed patient should suggest cryptococcosis. This is especially true in patients with lupus erythematosus, malignant lymphomas, and AIDS.

Microbiology & Immunology

C neoformans is the only species involved in cryptococcosis. The capsular polysaccharide antigen is soluble in host tissue fluids. The presence of capsular antigen has led to the development of diagnostic tests that measure antigenemia in tissue fluids such as the blood and spinal fluid.

Clinical Findings

A. Symptoms and Signs: There are no characteristic symptoms of cutaneous cryptococcosis. Primary cutaneous ulcers have been alleged to occur, and ac-

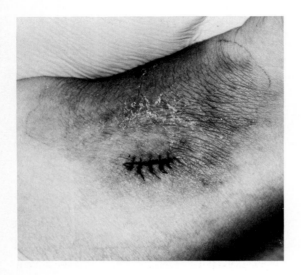

Figure 16–11. Cryptococcosis. Indolent panniculitis on thigh.

neiform lesions are still mistakenly thought by some to be characteristic. In fact, a variety of morphologic lesions have been reported, including abscesses, tumor-like masses, draining sinuses, panniculitis (Fig 16–11), papules, nodules, and ulcerations. Cryptococcosis may mimic a bacterial cellulitis or molluscum contagiosum in immunosuppressed patients and patients with AIDS.

B. Laboratory Findings: Demonstration of a remarkably thick-walled budding yeast in smears from lesions or in histopathologic sections is virtually diagnostic. Recovery of *C neoformans* on culture is the definitive laboratory test.

Complications & Sequelae

The development of meningitis is a grave sign.

Treatment

Specific therapeutic measures include intravenous amphotericin B and oral flucytosine. Ketoconazole has limited efficacy because it fails to penetrate the blood-brain barrier. Fluconazole, which freely penetrates into the central nervous system tissues, is more effective, and if further studies confirm its efficacy and safety, this now experimental azole will probably become the treatment of choice.

Course & Prognosis

In a debilitated patient, especially one with lupus erythematosus, lymphoma, AIDS, or iatrogenic immunosuppression, cryptococcosis may be progressive and fatal.

CUTANEOUS SIGNS IN FUNGAL SEPTICEMIA (See Chapter 32.)

Fungal septicemia in hospitalized patients has become more common recently. These infections can, for the most part, be considered opportunistic infections that develop because of debilitation and iatrogenic or nosocomial factors. Organisms ordinarily not pathogenic may be involved, as may fungal pathogens discussed earlier.

REFERENCES

Andre J, Achten G: Onychomycosis. Int J Dermatol 1987;26(8):481.

Artis WM, Odle BM, Jones HE: Griseofulvin-resistant dermatophytosis correlates with in vitro resistance. Arch Dermatol 1981;117:16.

Barnetson RS, Milne LJ: Mycetoma. Br J Dermatol 1978;99:227.

Batres E et al: Transepithelial elimination of cutaneous chromomycosis. Arch Dermatol 1978;114:1231.

Campbell GD, Chapman SW: Blastomycosis. Semin Respir Med 1987;9(2):164.

Curry WA: Human nocardiosis: A clinical review with selected case reports. Arch Intern Med 1980;140:818.

Daniel CR III, Lawson LA: Tinea unguium. Cutis 1987; 40(4):326.

Dennis JE et al: Nosocomial *Rhizopus* infection (zygomycosis) in children. J Pediatr 1980;96:824.

Dismukes WE: Azole antifungal drugs: Old and new. Ann Intern Med 1988;109:177.

Faergemann J: A new model for growth and filament production of *Pityrosporum ovale (orbiculare)* on human stratum corneum in vitro. J Invest Dermatol 1989; 92(1):117.

Goodfield MJD, Saihan EM, Crowley J: Experimental folliculitis with *Pityrosporum orbiculare:* The influence of host response. Acta Derm Venereol (Stockh) 1987;16(3 part 1):554.

Greer DL: Topical treatment for moccasin-type tinea pedis. J Am Acad Dermatol 1987;16(3 part 1):554.

Grossman ME, Silvers DN, Walther RR: Cutaneous manifestations of disseminated candidiasis. J Am Acad Dermatol 1980;2:111.

Gueho E et al: Association of *Malassezia pachydermatis* with systemic infections of humans. J Clin Microbiol 1987;25(9):1789.

Hanifin JM, Tofte SJ: Itraconazole therapy for recalcitrant dermatophyte infections. J Am Acad Dermatol 1988; 18(5 part 1):1077.

Hay RJ, Clayton YM, Moore MK: A comparison of tioconazole 28% nail solution versus base as an adjunct to oral griseofulvin in patients with onychomycosis. Clin Exp Dermatol 1987;12(6):175.

Hay RJ: Recent advances in the management of fungal infections. Q J Med 1987;64(244):631.

Hoeprich PD, Jordan MC (editors): *Infectious Diseases: A Modern Treatise of Infectious Processes,* 4th ed. Lippincott, 1989.

Johnson ML: *Skin Conditions and Related Need for Medical Care Among Persons 1–74 Years: United States, 1971– 1974.* US Department of Health, Education, and Welfare, 1979.

Johnson PC, Sarosi GA: Histoplasmosis. Semin Respir Med 1987;9(2):145.

Jones HE, Simpson JG, Artis WM: Oral ketoconazole: An effective and safe treatment for dermatophytosis. Arch Dermatol 1981;117:129.

Jones HE: *Ketoconazole Today: A Review of Clinical Experience.* ADIS Press, 1987.

Kalter DC et al: Genital white piedra: Epidemiology, microbiology, and therapy. J Am Acad Dermatol 1987; 14(6):982.

Kaplan MH, Rosen PP, Armstrong D: Cryptococcosis in a cancer hospital: Clinical and pathological correlates in forty-six patients. Cancer 1977;39:2265.

Kariya H, Iwatsu T: Statistical survey of 100 cases of sporotrichosis. J Dermatol (Tokyo) 1979;6:211.

Lehrer RI et al: Mucormycosis. Ann Intern Med 1980; 93:93.

Lesher JL Jr, Smith JG Jr: Antifungal agents in dermatology. J Am Acad Dermatol 1987;17(3):383.

Levine BE: Coccidioidomycosis. Semin Respir Med 1987; 9(2):152.

Leyden JJ, Kligman AM: Interdigital athlete's foot: The interaction of dermatophytes and resident bacteria. Arch Dermatol 1978;114:1466.

MacCarthy KG, Dahl MV: Inhibition of growth of *Trichophyton rubrum* by the myeloperoxidase-hydrogen peroxide-chloride system. J Invest Dermatol 1989; 92(4):639.

Mahgoub ES: Medical management of mycetoma. Bull WHO 1976;54:303.

Martinez-Roig A, Torres-Rodriquez JM, Bartlett-Coma A: Double blind study of ketoconazole and griseofulvin in dermatophytoses. Pediatr Infect Dis J 1988;7(1):37.

Mayou SC et al: Deep (subcutaneous) dermatophyte infection presenting with unilateral lymphoedema. Clin Exp Dermatol 1987;12(5):385.

McDaniel PA, Caldroney RD: Oral contraceptive and griseofulvin interaction. (Correspondence.) Drug Intell Clin Pharm 1986;20(5):384.

McGinnis MR: Chromoblastomycosis and phaeohyphomycosis: New concepts, diagnosis, and mycology. J Am Acad Dermatol 1983;8:1.

Nazzaro-Porro M, Passi S: Identification of tyrosinase inhibitors in cultures of *Pityrosporum.* J Invest Dermatol 1978;71:205.

Prevost E: Nonfluorescent tinea capitis in Charleston, SC: A diagnostic problem. JAMA 1979;242:1765.

Radentz WH et al: Opportunistic fungal infections in immunocompromised hosts. J Am Acad Dermatol 1989; 20(6):989.

Rasmussen JE, Ahmed AR: *Trichophyton* reactions in children with tinea capitis. Arch Dermatol 1978;114:371.

Restrepo A et al: Estrogens inhibit mycelium-to-yeast transformation in the fungus *Paracoccidioides brasiliensis:* Implications for resistance of females to paracoccidioidomycosis. Infect Immun (Nov) 1984;46(2):346.

Restrepo A et al: Itraconazole therapy in lymphangitic and cutaneous sporotrichosis. Arch Dermatol 1986; 122(4):413.

Restrepo A et al: The gamut of paracoccidioidomycosis. Am J Med 1976;61:33.

Rippon JW: *Animal Models of Experimental Dermatophyte Infections.* Vol 3 of: *Experimental Models in Antimicrobial Chemotherapy.* Academic Press, 1986.

Rippon JW: *Medical Mycology: The Pathogenic Fungi and the Pathogenic Actinomycetes,* 2nd ed. Saunders, 1982.

Roberts DT et al: Comparison of ketoconazole and griseofulvin in the treatment of tinea pedis. J Med Vet Mycol 1987;25(5):347.

Robertson LI: Itraconazole in the treatment of widespread tinea versicolor. Clin Exp Dermatol 1987;12(3):178.

Ron E, Modan B, Boice JD: Mortality after radiotherapy for ringworm of the scalp. Am J Epidemiol 1988; 127(4):713.

Roth RR, James WD: Microbiology of the skin: Resident flora, ecology, infection. J Am Acad Dermatol 1989; 20(3):367.

Schupbach CW et al: Cutaneous manifestations of disseminated cryptococcosis. Arch Dermatol 1976;112:1734.

Shama SK, Kirkpatrick CH: Dermatophytosis in patients with chronic mucocutaneous candidiasis. J Am Acad Dermatol 1980;2:285.

Singer C, Kaplan MH, Armstrong D: Bacteremia and fungemia complicating neoplastic disease: A study of 364 cases. Am J Med 1977;62:731.

Sudman MS: Protothecosis: A critical review. Am J Clin Pathol 1974;61:10.

Svejgaard E, Christophersen J, Jelsdorf H: Tinea pedis and erythrasma in Danish recruits. J Am Acad Dermatol 1986;14(6):993.

Wallace RJ Jr, Musher DM: Actinomycosis: An update. Int J Dermatol 1977;16:185.

Walling DM et al: Disseminated infection with *Trichosporon beigelii.* Rev Infect Dis 1987;9(5):1013.

Weitzman I: Saprophytic molds as agents of cutaneous and subcutaneous infection in the immunocompromised host. Arch Dermatol 1986;122:1611.

Zaias N: *The Nail in Health and Disease.* Spectrum, 1980.

17   Rickettsial Infections

David S. Feingold, MD

The rickettsiae are obligate intracellular parasites that resemble gram-negative bacteria and, except for *Coxiella burnetii*, the agent of Q fever, are carried to humans by arthropod vectors from animal reservoirs. The rickettsial infections can be conveniently grouped as the spotted fevers (Rocky Mountain spotted fever, other tickborne fevers, rickettsialpox), the typhus group (epidemic or louseborne typhus, endemic or murine typhus, scrub typhus), Q fever, and trench fever.

Epidemiologic aspects of the various rickettsial diseases differ. The details are included with discussions of the specific diseases; however, certain generalizations can be made.

With the exception of Q fever, arthropods are involved at some stage of transmission of all rickettsial diseases in nature. The arthropods may be both reservoir and vector when the organisms are passed from one generation to the next transovarially or spread among the arthropods, as with ticks and *Rickettsia rickettsii*. Some arthropods harbor rickettsiae only temporarily and are purely vectors, spreading disease from animal to human (eg, fleas transmitting murine typhus) or from human to human (eg, lice transmitting epidemic typhus). In the rickettsial infections other than epidemic typhus and trench fever, humans only accidentally intrude into the natural cycle and are "dead-end" hosts.

Organisms are inoculated into humans at the time the arthropod vector penetrates the skin. Local proliferation and bacteremia follow. In rickettsialpox, scrub typhus, and some of the eastern hemisphere spotted fevers, a lesion—often an eschar—develops at the inoculation site. The rickettsiae then parasitize the endothelial cells of small blood vessels, with resultant endothelial proliferation and necrosis. The pathologic picture is that of necrotizing vasculitis. This is the hallmark of all rickettsial diseases: The vasculitis is responsible for most of the clinical signs and symptoms. The skin vessels are often most heavily infected, which accounts for the rash. Although the early phases of vasculitis result from rickettsial multiplication, a later second phase of vascular damage is caused by immunologic mechanisms.

Rickettsial toxins have been demonstrated in experimental animals; it is likely that toxins are responsible for some of the clinical features.

MICROBIOLOGY & IMMUNOLOGY

Organisms of the family Rickettsiaceae are small coccobacillary bacteria which, except for *Rochalimaea quintana,* share the requirement for an intracellular milieu for growth. Under the electron microscope, they resemble gram-negative bacteria. Three genera are pathogenic for humans: *Rickettsia, Coxiella,* and *Rochalimaea.* Organisms that cause the typhus group of diseases grow freely only in the cytoplasm of the cells. The spotted fever group of organisms grow in the nucleus and the cytoplasm. *C burnetii* also grows only in the cytoplasm, but each organism is enclosed in a host cell membrane vesicle. *R quintana* grows in cell-free systems. Demonstration of typical organisms in endothelial cells on biopsy of skin lesions is one basis for positive diagnosis in the acute phase of rickettsial infections.

Immunity to rickettsial infections is solid and long-lasting except in the case of epidemic typhus and scrub typhus. The mechanisms of immunity are unknown. Antibodies to rickettsiae can be detected 1 week after the onset of clinical disease. With severe rickettsial infection, treatment should be instituted before immunologic confirmation of the diagnosis is possible. Thus, the serologic diagnosis is for retrospective diagnosis and for epidemiologic surveys.

The Weil-Felix agglutination test is based on the sharing of polysaccharide antigens by many rickettsiae and the rough *Proteus* species OX19, OX2, and OXK. The test may help in the diagnosis of epidemic and endemic typhus (OX19), the spotted fever group (OK19 or OX2), and scrub typhus (OXK). The specific tests below are preferable when available.

A complement fixation test is available in the USA through most state health departments. The test has disadvantages: frequent anticomplementary activity of serum in spotted fever, resulting in false negatives; cross reaction among various rickettsial diseases; and relative insensitivity compared with some of the newer serologic tests.

The complement fixation test is being replaced by indirect immunofluorescence antibody and ELISA tests. The serodiagnosis of acute diseases is based on detection of antirickettsial IgM, and epidemiologic studies depend on detection of antirickettsial IgG.

CLINICAL & EPIDEMIOLOGIC FEATURES

The rickettsioses, except for Q fever, are characterized by fever, headache, and rash. The morphology, distribution, and evolution of the skin eruption differ among the various specific entities. The clinical manifestations of rickettsial infections are often not typical. Rash may be absent, and arthropod association may be obscure. In such case, differentiation from innumerable other febrile conditions cannot be made except retrospectively by serologic tests. Fortunately, when the disease is severe enough to be life-threatening, a rash is almost always present, and biopsy can yield definite diagnosis leading to treatment early in the course of the acute disease.

THE SPOTTED FEVER GROUP

1. ROCKY MOUNTAIN SPOTTED FEVER

A recent tick bite history is almost always present in Rocky Mountain spotted fever. The ixodid ticks are both major reservoir and vector for *R rickettsii*. The role of infected small mammals in this zoonosis is unclear. It is a disease of the temperate regions of North and South America. The highest incidence is in early summer, reflecting the height of tick activity and of human exposure to ticks. Human-to-human transmission does not occur. Over 70% of the cases in the USA occur near the East Coast, between Maryland and Georgia, where the dog tick *Dermacentor variabilis* is the important ixodid.

The typical clinical picture is distinctive. After an incubation averaging 7 days, there is an abrupt onset of fever, chills, malaise, headache, and myalgias. Shorter incubations are often associated with more severe disease.

Two to 4 days later, a pink, macular, blanchable eruption occurs near the wrists and ankles. In 1–3 days, the rash develops a papular component and spreads centrally, involving the trunk and face; the palms and soles are also involved. A petechial component soon develops, and the rash no longer blanches on pressure. In severe cases, small areas of gangrene occur in the periphery and on the genitalia, reflecting the vascular obstruction. When large ecchymoses are seen, one must be concerned that disseminated intravascular coagulation is taking place.

Central nervous system vasculitis presents as headache; however, in severe cases, delirium, coma, or convulsions can be seen. Other signs and symptoms may include edema, conjunctival infection, arthralgias, vomiting, or diarrhea.

Untreated, the fever persists 2–3 weeks and gradually subsides. The mortality rate in untreated cases has been estimated at 20%, with most deaths occurring in the elderly. Because patients with milder disease do not arrive at medical centers or elude diagnosis, the overall mortality rate is probably exaggerated.

Antibiotic treatment is effective; the estimated 5% mortality rate in treated cases may reflect late diagnosis or treatment.

2. OTHER TICKBORNE RICKETTSIOSES

In foci on every continent there are ixodid ticks infected with organisms that share a group antigen with *R rickettsii* and cause diseases similar to but usually milder than Rocky Mountain spotted fever. The best-defined of these are North Asian tick typhus (*Rickettsia sibirica*) and boutonneuse fever (*Rickettsia conorii*). However, there are probably several other rickettsial species capable of causing similar tickborne infections. As with Rocky Mountain spotted fever, wild rodents may be an important reservoir.

In Queensland tick typhus and boutonneuse fever, the first sign is usually a local lesion at the site of the tick bite. This is an indurated lesion that becomes a necrotic ulcer about 5 mm in diameter with a red areola; this eschar is also termed the *tache noire* ("black spot").

3. RICKETTSIALPOX

Rickettsialpox is an urban disease transmitted to humans by the mite of the common house mouse. Reported from several urban centers since its description in New York in 1946, the etiologic organism, *Rickettsia akari,* belongs to the spotted fever group based on shared antigens and growth in nucleus as well as cytoplasm of parasitized cells.

One to 3 weeks following the mite bite, a local lesion develops, first as an erythematous papule that becomes vesicular and breaks down into an eschar. The eschar may be up to 1.5 cm in diameter and associated with local lymphadenopathy. Within a week after onset of the local lesion, the patient has fever, chills, headache, and myalgias. This is followed in a few days by a generalized maculopapular rash that evolves into a vesicular eruption resembling chickenpox, unique for rickettsial disease. The eruption may be sparse, and the disease is generally mild and self-limited.

THE TYPHUS GROUP

1. EPIDEMIC (LOUSEBORNE) TYPHUS

The body louse becomes infected with *Rickettsia prowazekii* following a blood meal on a bacteremic person. The louse dies of the infection in 2–3 weeks but during this period is infectious for humans. This louse-human-louse cycle is the major route for the disease. The infection occurs in sharp epidemics, which distinguishes epidemic typhus from other rickettsial diseases. Major epidemics occur in association with war and other types of human misfortune that predispose to lousiness. Epidemic typhus has been a scourge of civilization and has decisively affected military campaigns, as dramatically described by Zinsser in his classic work, *Rats, Lice and History.*

Because the lice cannot fly or jump, crowded conditions are necessary for spread; colder climates in which people wear heavy clothes for prolonged periods are favored. The disease occurs endemically in Central and South America, especially in Andean villages, as well as in highland areas of Africa and central Asia. *R prowazekii* infects flying squirrels in the eastern USA. Transmission from this reservoir to humans may occur, but the importance of the zoonosis is unclear.

In general, the disease is less severe than Rocky Mountain spotted fever. The incubation period is 1–2 weeks. A mild prodrome is followed by the abrupt onset of fever to 41 °C (105.8 °F), chills, a severe and unremitting headache, and generalized myalgias. The rash develops less than 1 week after onset of fever. It may begin as cutaneous erythema. Pink-red macules in severe cases progress to a hemorrhagic eruption. Rarely does the rash have a papular component. It begins in the axillas and on the trunk, spreading within a few days to the extremities but sparing the face, palms, and soles. A variety of complications may be observed, including peripheral gangrene, con-

junctival suffusion and photophobia, cough, altered mental states, hypotension, and azotemia. Untreated sustained high fever lasts about 2 weeks. The mortality is 10–50%, highest in the elderly and frail.

Recrudescence of typhus (**Brill-Zinsser disease**) may occur months to years after the original infection. It is caused by persistence of virulent organisms in lymphoid tissue of the host. The disease is similar to but milder than epidemic typhus, with less fever and a sparse or absent rash. As with other rickettsial diseases, the diagnosis can be made by demonstrating the organisms in the vascular endothelial cells on skin biopsy. In Brill-Zinsser disease, the Weil-Felix test is negative, and the early antibody response is IgG rather than the IgM seen with primary infection.

2. ENDEMIC (MURINE) TYPHUS

Endemic typhus is worldwide in distribution, and its importance as a disease in humans is probably grossly underestimated. It is caused by *Rickettsia mooseri* and is a zoonosis primarily in rat populations and also some other small mammals, spread by the rat flea and occasionally transmitted to humans. It occurs around harbors, grain elevators, and places where rats and humans have contact. In the USA, most cases have been reported in the Southeast and Gulf Coast regions.

The disease is milder than epidemic typhus but can be debilitating. An incubation period of 1–2 weeks is followed by abrupt fever, severe headache, and myalgias. On day 3–5, a macular to maculopapular nonpruritic eruption develops first on the trunk and then on the extremities. The mortality rate is negligible, with deaths occurring mainly in debilitated patients. Confusion may at times exist between endemic typhus and Rocky Mountain spotted fever; agglutinins of Proteus OX19 may develop in both. However, the tick bite history is lacking, and the evolution of the rash differs.

3. SCRUB TYPHUS

Scrub typhus is an acute, febrile rickettsial infection whose importance probably has been underestimated. The main reservoir and vector are rodent mites. The chigger (larval mite), which has been infected transovarially, bites and infects humans and also spreads a zoonosis among rats and wild rodents. Scrub typhus was named in the belief that the disease is only acquired in terrain with secondary or scrub vegetation. The disease is also called **chiggerborne typhus,** and by local names such as tsutsugamushi disease or Japanese river fever. It is restricted to rural areas of Southeast Asia, the Indian subcontinent, Japan, eastern USSR, and the islands of the South and West Pacific.

The etiologic agent, *Rickettsia tsutsugamushi,* shares no antigens with other rickettsiae, though it may elicit antibodies that agglutinate Proteus OXK. *R tsutsugamushi* includes several different serotypes. Infection with one serotype generates only limited cross immunity to others. Thus, one can have multiple attacks of scrub typhus, and strains may differ in virulence. Recent studies in endogenous areas suggest that scrub typhus may account for a large proportion of "fevers of unknown origin" with absent rash, eschar, and Proteus OXK agglutinins. The diagnosis can be made only by complement fixation or indirect immunofluorescent antibody testing using several different serotype antigens of *R tsutsugamushi*.

One to 3 weeks following the chigger bite, the patient experiences the classic symptoms of rickettsial disease: fever, chills, and severe headache. At the site of the bite, an indurated and sometimes vesicular lesion develops late in the incubation period. This undergoes necrosis and becomes an ulcer with a black center. About 1 week after the onset of fever, a red macular or maculopapular rash develops on the trunk, spreads to the extremities, and fades within a few days. Also characteristic is the occurrence of generalized lymphadenopathy—not seen with other rickettsioses. Focal involvement results in meningoencephalitis, associated with various central nervous system signs and symptoms, myocarditis, and interstitial pneumonitis. Defervescence is seen after about 2 weeks. In infected American troops in Vietnam, only 46% developed an eschar and 34% had generalized rash.

Q FEVER

Q fever is a rickettsial disease of worldwide distribution caused by *Coxiella burnetii*. It differs from other rickettsial diseases in several important respects. It is transmitted to humans primarily by inhaled dust, causing pneumonitis in the majority of patients. Q fever must be considered in patients with pneumonitis, hepatitis, endocarditis, or "fever of unknown origin" if they have been in contact with sheep, cattle, goats, or their excreta. No characteristic rash has been reported. The organism is infrequently recovered from patients, but antibodies to *C burnetii* phase 2 develop regularly.

TRENCH FEVER
(Quintana Fever, Shin Bone Fever)

Like epidemic typhus, this self-limited rickettsial infection has a louse-human-louse cycle. Epidemics

have been reported in both world wars; recently, endemic foci have been reported from Mexico. The infecting organism, *Rochalimaea quintana,* is unique in that it can be grown on cell-free media, eg, blood agar containing 10% fresh blood. It has been isolated from previously infected patients years after the acute illness. The presenting symptoms and signs, occurring 1–4 weeks postexposure, are recurrent fevers, weakness, headache, back and leg pains, and photophobia. After the initial fever remits, several relapses may occur. The rash consists of erythematous macules or papules primarily on the trunk in 70% of infected patients. The rash occurs at the time of the fever and may wax and wane with the fever. The duration of disease may be prolonged, with up to 8 fever relapses.

DIAGNOSIS & DIFFERENTIAL DIAGNOSIS

The tickborne spotted fevers must be differentiated from meningococcemia. In the latter disorder, the rash appears earlier and does not show the characteristic progression seen in spotted fevers. However, the eruptions can be morphologically identical. Occasionally, the neisseriae can be seen on Gram's stain of an aspirate from a lesion.

The most helpful diagnostic test is examination of biopsies of skin lesions; both will show necrotizing vasculitis with neisseriae on Gram's stain in meningococcemia and rickettsia on Giemsa's stain in the spotted fevers. In practice, it is often wise to treat both infections until the correct diagnosis is confidently made. If an eschar is present, one of the eastern hemisphere tick typhuses is favored. Other conditions to be considered include measles, atypical measles (measles in a partially immune host), leptospirosis, enteroviral infections with exanthems, and necrotizing vasculitis of various etiologies.

Chickenpox may pose a differential diagnostic problem in rickettsialpox. In chickenpox, there is no initial lesion, the vesicles appear in crops, and the rash comes with the fever. The vesicle in rickettsialpox occupies only part of a papule; the vesicle is the total lesion as chickenpox evolves. Tzanck smears show multinucleated giant cells in chickenpox.

Because louseborne typhus occurs in sharp epidemics, the diagnosis is usually clear-cut. It is not possible to differentiate on clinical grounds among mild cases of louseborne typhus, recrudescent typhus, and murine typhus. Scrub typhus may be confused with the tick typhus infections associated with eschar that overlap in geographic distributions. In endemic areas, scrub typhus may present as "fever of unknown origin," with or without lymphadenopathy, and as such is one of a legion of diagnostic possibilities.

PREVENTION OF RICKETTSIAL INFECTIONS

Preventive measures are directed primarily against the arthropod vectors. With the tickborne rickettsioses, control of the tick vector in the wild is not feasible, though the ticks can perhaps be controlled in domestic dogs. Exposed individuals should carefully examine the whole body twice daily and remove ticks. It is likely that there is a grace period of several hours between arrival of the tick and transmission of rickettsiae.

Proper louse control will abort epidemics of typhus. Simple hygienic measures are helpful, as are insecticides. Rat and flea control for murine typhus and mite (chigger) control for scrub typhus are the only preventive measures available.

Vaccines have been developed for Rocky Mountain spotted fever and epidemic typhus. They are not currently available in North America. The killed vaccines tried for Rocky Mountain spotted fever are of dubious value. Use of killed vaccine for epidemic typhus lessens its severity. Live vaccines are being field-tested. The vaccines may be helpful in endemic foci of typhus.

TREATMENT

Therapy for rickettsial infections includes specific antibiotics, supportive measures such as fluid and electrolyte administration, nursing care to prevent complications, and prompt treatment of complications.

Tetracyclines (at least 25 mg/kg/d) and chloramphenicol (at least 50 mg/kg/d) are effective for most rickettsioses. One can expect a response within 24 hours and defervescence within 1–4 days. Therapy should be continued until 14 days after the onset of fever and for at least 2 days after defervescence. Development of the long-acting lipophilic tetracyclines has dramatically altered treatment for epidemic and scrub typhus. In these infections, one treatment with 200 mg of doxycycline may be curative. This is probably not the case with Rocky Mountain spotted fever. Tetracycline- and chloramphenicol-resistant *R prowazekii* have been reported from Africa.

Brief treatment with glucocorticoids has improved the outlook for neurologic complications of the rickettsial infections. When steroids are given along with appropriate antibiotics, they have not adversely affected the course of the disease. Heparin therapy may be lifesaving if disseminated intravascular coagulation has been triggered.

REFERENCES

Assaad F: Rickettsioses: A continuing disease problem. Bull WHO 1982;60:157.

Burgdorfer W, Anacker RL (editors): *Rickettsiae and Rickettsial Disease.* Academic Press, 1981.

Murray ES: Rickettsiae. In: *Microbiology,* 3rd ed. Davis BD (editor). Lippincott, 1980.

Wisseman CL Jr: Rickettsial disease. In: *Cecil Textbook of Medicine,* 17th ed. Wyngaarden JB, Smith LH Jr (editors). Saunders, 1985.

Parasitic Infections & Infestations

18

Karen C. McKoy, MD, Samuel L. Moschella, MD, Milton Orkin, MD, & Howard I. Maibach, MD*

Parasitic infections are endemic in many developing countries. In these reservoir areas, poverty, poor hygiene, and inadequate sanitary facilities create favorable conditions for infection. Rapid transportation permits movement of people from endemic regions, eliminating the natural quarantine of earlier long journeys. Immigrants, foreign students, and diplomats from such areas bring tropical medical problems into the USA. American diplomats, technical assistants, missionaries and their families, and religious and government-sponsored volunteers assigned to endemic areas may acquire parasitic infections. The crowding of immigrants in cities increases potential infectivity.

Control of parasitic diseases requires a multifaceted approach: (1) diagnosis and treatment when disease occurs, (2) education of patients and the community in preventive measures, (3) improvements in community sanitation, and (4) control of reservoir hosts and vectors.

Medical parasitology has 3 main divisions: (1) diseases due to protozoa (single-celled animals), (2) diseases due to helminths (worms), and (3) diseases due principally to arthropods.

I. PROTOZOAL INFECTIONS

Protozoal infections with dermatologic manifestations include leishmaniasis, African trypanosomiasis, South American trypanosomiasis, amebiasis, trichomoniasis, and toxoplasmosis.

LEISHMANIASIS

Essentials of Diagnosis

- Ulcers, nodules, or verrucous or vegetative plaques.
- Histopathologic demonstration of *Leishmania* in biopsy tissue.
- Culture on Nicolle-Novy-MacNeal (NNN) medium.
- Positive monoclonal antibody studies.

General Considerations

Leishmaniasis, a complex of infections, is found on all continents except Australia and Antarctica; it is absent in southeast Asia, the USA (except Texas), and large tracts of tropical Africa. The intracellular obligate parasite belongs to the genus *Leishmania* (subkingdom Protozoa, order Kinetoplastida, family Trypanosomatidae), whose life cycles are completed in 2 different hosts: a vertebrate and an insect. Vertebrate hosts are principally mammals, though some species are found in reptiles.

As a rule, there is a well-balanced host-parasite relationship in the natural vertebrate host, where the parasite is scattered in the macrophages of the skin, viscera, and blood; but in unusual hosts, such as humans, an inflammatory reaction results in skin, mucous membrane, or visceral lesions. In the macrophage, the organism is the amastigote (*Leishmania* stage) measuring $1.5-3 \times 3-6.5$ μm in diameter, depending on the species. The cytoplasm of the parasite stains pale blue with Giemsa, Wright, Feulgen, and Romanovsky stains, and the intracellular rod-shaped kinetoplast and single nucleus stain reddish purple. The amastigote multiplies by binary fission in the macrophage. The promastigote (*Leptomonas* stage) is in the insect vector and cultures and has a distinct flagellum.

The disease is transmitted by the bite of the sandfly, mainly of the genera *Phlebotomus*, *Lutzomyia*, and *Psychodopygus*, distributed in tropical and subtropical regions of the Eastern and Western Hemispheres.

In most geographic areas of infection, leishman-

---

*Section III, Ectoparasitic Diseases, is by Milton Orkin, MD, and Howard I. Maibach, MD.

iasis is a zoonosis. The reservoirs are sylvatic rodents, dogs, and other mammals. Humans are an occasional host in the cycle and in certain areas—India and Bangladesh, for example—the sole host.

The old classification of leishmaniasis—cutaneous, mucocutaneous, and visceral, due (respectively) to *L tropica, L brasiliensis,* and *L donovani*—is oversimplified. The great variety of clinical presentations and the complex pathologic picture require understanding of the significance and virulence of the responsible species and also the host immunologic response. Understanding the different geographic strains of the parasites is essential. For a current classification of leishmaniasis, considering the species of the organism, the geographic region, the nature of the area, the reservoir host, the principal vector, and the clinical characteristics, see Moschella and Hurley (1985).

Natural immunity due to subclinical infection exists in endemic areas in both the Old and New Worlds. There is lack of cross-immunity between various strains of parasites causing Old World and New World (South and Central America, Texas) leishmaniasis. During active infection, reinoculation by the same organism will reproduce a lesion resembling the clinical stage of the existing primary.

Clinical Findings

A. Symptoms and Signs: The clinical manifestations of Old World and New World cutaneous leishmaniasis may be classified as follows: (1) localized—acute, chronic, and recidivans; and (2) generalized—multiple lesions, anergic disseminated cutaneous leishmaniasis, and leishmanids.

On the exposed inoculation site, the localized acute lesion presents initially as a papule resembling an insect bite; it grows firmer and larger and may ulcerate. Satellite lesions may appear. Satellite lymphadenitis and lymphangitis (especially of the lower leg) with lymphedema rarely occur. The lesions may become vegetative, a result of secondary infection of skin and local lymphatics. Depending on the immunologic response of the infected patient, the lesion may become chronic and resemble cutaneous tuberculosis (lupus vulgaris-like) both clinically and histologically. These lesions can have a verrucous, keloidal, or psoriasiform component. In the Old World form, leishmaniasis recidivans is characterized by peripheral red-brown papules around existing scars, producing circinate plaques. The localized mucocutaneous lesion is unusual in Old World leishmaniasis but endemic (incidence of 15–80%) in the New World, especially in Venezuela, Brazil, and Peru; it is characterized by an infiltrative mutilatory process of nasopharyngeal and adjacent skin. This can be complicated by sepsis and by respiratory and swallowing problems.

Widespread lesions limited to exposed areas may result from multiple local inoculations by the vector.

Leishmanids are a manifestation of hypersensitivity. They are a rare cutaneous complication resulting from hematogenous dissemination of the parasite. A regional or generalized lichenoid eruption reveals tuberculoid granulomas with necrosis and absence of demonstrable organisms upon histopathologic examination.

Anergic disseminated cutaneous leishmaniasis (diffuse cutaneous leishmaniasis, disseminated cutaneous leishmaniasis, leishmaniasis cutanea pseudolepromatosa) is a rare disseminated form of cutaneous leishmaniasis that is chronic and progressive and resists treatment. Clinically, it resembles lepromatous leprosy.

Post-kala-azar (or postvisceral) dermal leishmaniasis is a late cutaneous complication that occurs in patients with kala-azar that has become chronic or has relapsed after incomplete treatment. The dermatologic manifestations of post-kala-azar dermal leishmaniasis are hypopigmented macules, an erythematous butterfly rash, and nodules (resembling those of lepromatous leprosy) that can be widespread or localized to the face.

Laboratory Findings: The leishmanin (Montenegro) skin test, consisting of an intradermal skin test of a phenolized suspension of promastigotes, has relatively high sensitivity and specificity and is a valuable tool for epidemiologic studies and for the diagnosis of lesions that are *Leishmania*-poor, such as leishmaniasis recidivans and the late mucocutaneous forms of American leishmaniasis. A positive test consists of a tuberculin type delayed hypersensitivity reaction interpreted in 24–72 hours. The leishmanin skin test becomes positive in nearly all cases of Old World and New World leishmaniasis; however, in the rare cases of disseminated anergic leishmaniasis, it remains negative; patients with kala-azar develop a positive skin test after cure has been effected. Parasites may be demonstrated by direct examination, culture, or inoculation into hamsters.

Material for culture is inoculated into NNN medium. Histopathologic sections are stained with hematoxylin and eosin and Giemsa stains. Hamsters inoculated with aspirates in the nose and feet reproduce lesions.

Differential Diagnosis

Leishmaniasis mimics many diseases. The acute localized ulcerative lesions on exposed areas must be differentiated from ulcerative ecthymatous or vegetative pyodermas, chancriform lesions (syphilis, tuberculosis, nocardiosis), yaws (initial lesion), insect bites, myiasis, tropical ulcer, Buruli ulcer (*Mycobacterium ulcerans* infection), sporotrichosis, and chromomycosis. Diseases that may resemble chronic lupoid leishmaniasis are lupus vulgaris, sarcoidosis, leprosy, lupus erythematosus, and tertiary syphilis. The disseminated nodular lesions of disseminated anergic leishmaniasis and postvisceral dermal leishmaniasis may be confused with those of lepromatous leprosy, xanthoma tuberosum, and a generalized nodular type of keloidal blastomycosis (Jorge Lobo disease). Mucocutaneous leishmaniasis, a potential mutilatory rhinopharyngopathy, must be differentiated from the late expression of the treponematoses (syphilis, yaws, bejel), lepromatous leprosy, South American blastomycosis, histoplasmosis, granuloma inguinale, cancrum oris, nasal myiasis, rhinophyma, basal or squamous cell carcinoma, pyoderma gangrenosum, midline lethal granulomas (lymphomatoid or granulomatous hypersensitivity angiitis), and lymphoma. The chiclero ulcer of leishmaniasis, a localized form seen especially in the Yucatan Peninsula and Guatemala, is confined to the ears and may resemble other destructive auricular diseases such as leprosy, Jorge Lobo disease, epitheliomas (basal and squamous cell carcinoma), melanoma, and lymphoma.

Treatment

Appreciation of the varied expressions of the different geographic strains of parasites is essential in the management of cutaneous leishmaniasis. Because we do not understand the pathogenesis of the chronic, recidivous, mucocutaneous, and disseminated anergic forms from a primary inoculation, all primary localized types of lesions should be treated unless the patient is from an endemic area where only the classic, self-healing primary localized type of cutaneous leishmaniasis exists. Even in the latter situation, however, treatment may be indicated—eg, for lesions on the face, to minimize unsightly scarring or drainage to eyelids and mucosal surfaces. Vaccination in the unexposed areas of the body (not covered by clothing) with live homologous strains of organisms (promastigotes) is practiced in endemic areas to prevent disfigurement. All types of cutaneous leishmaniasis with secondary bacterial infection should be treated with appropriate antibiotics.

Glucantime (meglumine antimonate) is the most widely used pentavalent antimonial. It is injected intramuscularly or intravenously daily until the lesion is gone. An alternative drug is sodium stibogluconate (Pentostam). The pentavalent antimonials tend to accumulate and are excreted slowly. Treated patients require close observation for cardiac, hepatic, renal, and cerebral drug toxicity as well as for anaphylactoid reaction. In the chronic lupoid form of leishmaniasis, brief courses of intralesional steroid or systemic corticosteroids may be helpful.

In antimony-resistant localized mucocutaneous and disseminated anergic leishmaniasis, amphotericin B is recommended. Among the side effects are nausea, vomiting, fever, nephrotoxicity (the main limiting factor), phlebitis, and cardiotoxicity.

Other drugs used with varying success include metronidazole, levamisole, dehydroemetine, and rifampin.

Prevention

For the control of leishmaniasis, measures to eliminate vectors and reservoirs could be helpful. Ideally, a simple effective polyvalent vaccine could be developed. No effective chemoprophylaxis has been developed.

TRYPANOSOMIASIS

Two distinct types of infection by protozoans of the genus *Trypanosoma* exist: the African and American forms.

1. AFRICAN TRYPANOSOMIASIS

Trypanosomal disease is endemic in a belt across central Africa in the region between 15 degrees N and 15 degrees S. Disease is transmitted by the bite of the tsetse fly.

Cutaneous lesions are usually limited to the site of the initial fly bite. In the first stage, the trypanosomal nodule or "chancre" develops at the entry site 4–10 days after the tsetse fly bite. The lesion is a painful red nodule measuring 7–10 cm in diameter; it is usually on the head or limbs and often accompanied by regional lymphadenopathy. Examination of fluid aspirated from this lesion or involved lymph nodes demonstrates trypanosomes. The nodule resolves spontaneously within 2 weeks, at which time the second stage of disease is usually evident. This stage correlates with bloodstream invasion of the protozoon and is characterized by irregular fever and symmetric adenopathy. **Winterbottom's sign** (posterior cervical adenopathy) is frequent in Gambian disease. Caucasians more frequently develop an eruption consisting of transient erythematous annular or serpiginous plaques that may be poorly marginated and extensive. Another common manifestation is transient painful edema of the hands, feet, and eyelids. Erythema nodosum may occur.

Suramin and pentamidine are effective but toxic agents for the treatment of African trypanosomiasis. Involvement of the central nervous system is best treated with the combination of melarsoprol (an arsenic compound) and suramin.

2. AMERICAN TRYPANOSOMIASIS

Essentials of Diagnosis

- Chagoma: boardlike induration, erythema, and tenderness at site of bite.
- Asthenia, fever, lymphadenopathy, cardiopathy.
- Demonstration of the parasite in blood smears or tissue or by culture techniques.

- Serologic tests for antibodies to *Trypanosoma*.
- Xenodiagnosis.

General Considerations

American trypanosomiasis (Chagas' disease) occurs only in the Western Hemisphere; it is caused by the protozoon *Trypanosoma cruzi*. The disease is a major health problem in rural South and Central America.

Many types of animals serve as natural reservoirs (dogs, cats, rodents, pigs, bats, and armadillos); raccoons and opossums are important wild reservoir hosts in the USA. The infection is transmitted from human to human and from animal to human by an intermediate host, the reduviid bug (genus *Triatoma*), known as the "kissing bug" because of its habit of biting the faces of sleeping victims. Trypanosomes multiply in the gut of the bug and are excreted in the feces. The bug's habit of defecating while feeding on the host is an important factor in disease transmission. Human infection occurs through the skin as a result of contamination of the bite wound or preexisting skin lesions with trypanosome-laden feces. Infection may also occur via the mucous membranes of the mouth or conjunctiva. Congenital infection due to transplacental transmission may occur; blood transfusions are another source. Poor socioeconomic conditions contribute to disease frequency, because the insect vectors thrive in primitive housing of adobe, mud, and thatch.

Two stages of disease are usually seen. The initial infection may be occult or acute, spontaneously subsiding in 1–4 months. The infection then enters a chronic stage with asymptomatic periods as long as 12 years before symptoms evolve from damage to the myocardium or intestinal walls. About 10% of serologically positive individuals develop overt chronic disease.

Clinical Findings

A. Symptoms and Signs: The primary stage of infection is characterized by the "chagoma of inoculation," fever, and lymphadenopathy, with hematogenous dispersion of the parasites. This chagoma, the most distinctive feature of this stage, is usually on the face or other exposed area. Variable edema, erythema, and tenderness are present at the site of inoculation. Boardlike induration is often present, associated with regional adenopathy. Romaña's sign (the oculoglandular syndrome) is frequent, with unilateral eyelid edema, conjunctivitis, and preauricular adenopathy. The chagoma of inoculation lasts 2–3 months, then gradually resolves, leaving hyperpigmentation and occasional depression. Ulceration and scarring may occur. Rarely, disease may begin without a primary chagoma. Hematogenous or secondary chagomas may be seen, especially in children under 3 years of age; these are slightly tender indurated areas, 1–3 cm in diameter, usually over the trunk and proximal extremities. Other less specific cutaneous changes may be seen in the acute stage, including erythema multiforme, urticaria, exanthems, and generalized edema.

Most patients survive the acute phase, but death may occur, especially in children, owing to myocarditis or severe central nervous system involvement. As acute symptoms resolve, organisms disappear from the blood and localize in the tissues, particularly the myocardium and intestines. Symptoms include asthenia, fever, and lymphadenopathy. The clinical picture is usually dominated by cardiac arrhythmias and cardiac failure; megacolon and megaesophagus may occur secondary to damage of the intestinal autonomic ganglia.

B. Laboratory Findings: Histologic examination of a specimen taken from the site of inoculation shows a severe inflammatory reaction characterized by neutrophils, lymphocytes, and edema. Intracellular leishmanial forms are seen within histiocytes; the fat cells are often invaded, leading to lipogranulomas. The hematogenous chagomas show a similar reaction in the subcutaneous tissue. After hematogenous dissemination, organisms may be found in any tissue, but they seem to prefer cardiac and skeletal muscle, the nervous system, and reticuloendothelial cells.

The diagnosis of Chagas' disease is based on demonstration of the parasite in blood smears or tissue or by culture techniques. In the acute stages, trypanosomes may be found in fresh blood smears or on Giemsa-stained thick smears. Culture of organisms and inoculation in laboratory animals are difficult. Xenodiagnosis (infection of laboratory-reared reduviid bugs by allowing feeding on the suspected patient) is the most sensitive method but not readily done in the USA. Indirect fluorescent antibody, hemagglutination, and complement fixation tests are useful serologic methods. Serologic positivity persists for life in untreated patients.

Treatment & Prevention

There is no effective specific therapy; treatment is symptomatic. The only effective drugs are nifurtimox and benznidazole, both of which may be toxic.

Prophylaxis consists chiefly of avoidance of the insect vector. Better housing and community public health measures are crucial to eliminate breeding places.

AMEBIASIS

Essentials of Diagnosis

- Painful ulcer with undermined edge.
- Demonstration of motile trophozoites.
- Demonstration of amebas in histopathologic sections of tissue.
- Serologic tests (indirect immunofluorescent, hemagglutination, and gel diffusion precipitin tests).

General Considerations

Infection with the protozoan parasite *Entamoeba histolytica* is worldwide; prevalence varies between 5% in temperate areas to 80% in some tropical countries. In the USA, prevalence has been estimated at 3–10%.

The life cycle of *E histolytica* involves 2 stages of the parasite. Trophozoite forms live and multiply in the human cecum and colon, evolving into cysts passed in the feces. Amebiasis is transmitted by food and drink contaminated with cysts.

Disease is often asymptomatic and usually confined to the gastrointestinal tract lumen. Factors predisposing to invasive disease of the bowel and extraintestinal sites are poorly understood; the strain of parasite, host nutritional status, and intestinal bacterial flora are believed to be related to invasiveness. Systemic corticosteroid use and AIDS have been linked with fulminant disease. Other genera of amebas may rarely become invasive; *Acanthamoeba* has been reported with ulcerating skin lesions and systemic invasion.

Infections with *E histolytica* in the USA are primarily in asymptomatic carriers. Amebic dysentery with mild to fulminant bloody diarrhea and hepatic abscess formation occur most commonly in homosexual men.

Cutaneous amebiasis is an uncommon complication, usually found in patients with active intestinal or hepatic disease. The skin may be invaded by several routes: (1) direct extension of amebic bowel disease to adjacent skin areas following surgical procedures; (2) direct extension of amebic hepatic abscess, either spontaneously or following surgical procedures; or (3) direct implantation of trophozoites on the skin, with or without preexisting skin lesions.

Direct extension to the perianal or genital region from colonic disease is the most frequent form. Ulcers may develop on the abdominal wall after surgical procedures to drain a hepatic amebic abscess or in incisions or colostomies of patients with unsuspected amebic intestinal disease. Direct inoculation seems responsible for some cases of penile amebiasis in men whose partners have rectal or vaginal amebic lesions. Cutaneous ulcers in sites remote from the gastrointestinal tract probably start after direct inoculation. A history of diarrhea is not essential in making the diagnosis of cutaneous amebiasis.

Clinical Findings

A. Symptoms and Signs: The usual cutaneous lesion is a painful ulcer with a necrotic purulent base, distinct undermined borders, and an erythematous rim. Considerable tissue destruction may expose muscle and sometimes bone. The duration of lesions varies from 10 days to 2 years; rapid severe destruction occurs more commonly in children.

B. Laboratory Findings: Diagnosis may be made by examination of fresh nonnecrotic material curetted from the edge of the ulcer. Tissue fragments are immediately suspended in saline and examined; motile trophozoites are diagnostic. A biopsy of the ulcer edge less reliably demonstrates amebas; a periodic acid-Schiff (PAS) stain may help localize trophozoites. Multiple fresh stools may need to be examined by an experienced laboratory to find organisms. Antibiotics, barium, and antidiarrheal preparations may interfere with stool examination. Serologic tests such as indirect hemagglutination and indirect immunofluorescence tests remain positive for several years; they are of value as screening tests in area of low endemicity. A gel diffusion precipitin test is highly specific for active clinical disease. All serologic tests are more sensitive for extraintestinal amebiasis (nearly 100%) than for intestinal disease (70% sensitivity).

Differential Diagnosis

The differential includes lymphogranuloma venereum, granuloma inguinale, cutaneous tuberculosis, carcinoma, and phagedenic ulceration. Urticaria may occur as a manifestation of intestinal amebiasis.

Treatment

Treatment varies with the site of infection. Combinations of drugs may be necessary, because some are more effective in the gut lumen (metronidazole, emetine, and dehydroemetine) and others are active systemically (diiodohydroxyquin, diloxanide, and tetracyclines). Chloroquine is often given as supportive treatment for liver abscesses. In patients with cutaneous disease (extraintestinal infection), metronidazole is probably the safest drug. In most cases, 750 mg is given 3 times daily for 10 days. Treatment failures have been reported. Metronidazole may be more effective when given as a single daily dose of 1.4 g/d for 3 days. Diiodohydroxyquin (650 mg 3 times daily for 20 days) or tetracycline (250 mg 4 times daily for 10 days) may also be given for concomitant intestinal disease. Emetine and dehydroemetine are effective but more toxic amebicides. Dehydroemetine is given intramuscularly in a dosage of 1.5 mg/kg to a maximum of 90 mg/d for 10 days. Cutaneous lesions usually respond rapidly, with improvement occurring in 4–5 days. Without treatment, the disease may be fatal, particularly in infants.

II. HELMINTHIC INFECTIONS

Parasitic worms infect humans worldwide. Helminthic infections are particularly common in tropical countries, where a warm, humid climate creates favorable conditions for worm survival and poor so-

Table 18–1. Helminths.

Organism	Disease
Nemathelminthes	
Nematoda	
Intestinal roundworms	
Enterobius (Oxyuris) vermicularis	Pinworms, oxyuriasis
Strongyloides stercoralis	Strongyloidiasis, larva currens
Necator americanus	Human hookworm disease, uncinarial dermatitis, ground itch
Ancylostoma duodenale	
Ancylostoma braziliense	Animal hookworm disease, cutaneous larva migrans, "creeping eruption"
Ancylostoma caninum	
Uncinaria stenocephala	
Bunostomum phlebotomum	
Toxocara canis	Toxocariasis, visceral larva migrans
Gnathostoma spinigerum	Gnathostomiasis
Tissue roundworms	
Wuchereria bancrofti	Filariasis
Brugia malavi	
Onchocerca volvulus	Onchocerciasis
Loa loa	Loiasis, Calabar swellings
Dipetalonema streptocerca	Streptocerciasis
Dipetalonema perstans	Acanthocheilonemiasis, dipetalonemiasis
Dirofilaria sp	Dirofilariasis
Dracunculus medinensis	Dracunculosis, guinea worm disease
Trichinella spiralis	Trichinosis
Platyhelminthes	
Trematoda	
Schistosoma japonicum	Visceral schistosmiasis
Schistosoma haematobium	
Schistosoma mansoni	
Schistosomes of the genera *Schistosoma, Trichobilharzia, Gigantobilharzia, Ornithobilharzia*	Cutaneous schistosomiasis, swimmer's itch
Cestoidea	
Taenia solium	Cysticercosis, pork tapeworm infection
Echinococcus granulosus	Hydatid disease, echinococcosis
Spirometra mansonoides	Sparganosis
Spirometra mansoni	
Multiceps sp	Coenurosis

cioeconomic circumstances and primitive hygiene foster disease transmission.

There are 2 main groups: roundworms (Nemathelminthes) and flatworms (Platyhelminthes). A single class of Nemathelminthes causes disease (Nematoda). There are 2 important classes of Platyhelminthes: Trematoda (flukes) and Cestoidea (tapeworms). An outline of helminths causing disease of importance to dermatologists is presented in Table 18–1.

NEMATODA

Nematodes that are parasitic in humans may be intestinal or tissue roundworms. The life cycles vary in complexity; transmission to a new host depends on ingestion of infectious eggs or larvae or penetration of the skin or mucous membranes by the larvae.

INTESTINAL ROUNDWORMS

1. ENTEROBIASIS
(Pinworms)

Essentials of Diagnosis

- Nocturnal, perianal, and perineal pruritus, especially in children.
- Demonstration of worm on preparations of cellophane tape.

General Considerations

Enterobius vermicularis occurs worldwide and is the most common helminth infecting humans. Estimates of prevalence are 30% in children and 16% in adults. Infection rates may approach 100% in institutions, where overcrowding facilitates transmission.

E vermicularis is a threadlike white worm 1 cm in length. After ingestion of embryonated eggs by the host, adult worms of both sexes develop and take up residence in the lumen of the cecum. At the end of the life cycle (2–8 weeks), the dying gravid female migrates from the anus, especially at night, and deposits numerous sticky eggs in the perianal area. An infective larval stage develops in hours.

Mature infective eggs may remain viable for up to 20 days under cool, moist conditions; they may be found in great numbers on bedclothes and in house dust. The most common means of infection occurs via the anus-hand-mouth route in children. Eggs may be ingested also with contaminated food. Retrograde infection may occur, with hatching of the larvae on the perianal skin and migration back up the anus into the cecum.

Clinical Findings

A. Symptoms and Signs: The primary symptom of pinworm infection is perianal and perineal pruritus, usually nocturnal and intense. It seems related to the passage of the gravid female worm or the sticky outer egg coat. Insomnia and irritability, perineal intertrigo, and superinfected excoriations may be prominent. *E vermicularis* does not normally invade tissue.

B. Laboratory Findings: Female worms may occasionally be observed at night by vigilant parents of an infected child and are rarely observed on toilet paper. Eggs are rarely demonstrated by stool examination. To best demonstrate the eggs, the sticky side of a 2-inch strip of cellophane tape is pressed against the perianal skin at night or on awakening. (This procedure is facilitated by placing the tape around a tongue depressor or test tube.) The sticky side of the tape is then placed over a drop of toluene on a microscopic slide and examined for the characteristic eggs—24 × 54 μm, oval in shape, flattened on one side. A single test detects 50% of infections and 5

tests will detect 99%. All family members should be examined.

Treatment

Mebendazole as a single oral dose of 100 mg (all ages) gives cure rates of 90–100%. There is minimal absorption of this drug, which seems to be relatively free of side effects. Pyrantel pamoate is a satisfactory alternative. Either drug should be given a second time after 2 weeks.

Reinfection is common from the contaminated environment or from asymptomatic household members.

2. HUMAN HOOKWORM DISEASE

Essentials of Diagnosis

- Most infections are asymptomatic.
- Dermatitis on soles or toes for 1–2 weeks after infection.
- Anemia and growth retardation.
- Eosinophilia.
- Demonstration of eggs in feces.

General Considerations

Hookworms infect approximately 25% of the world's population. Disease occurs in nearly all subtropical and tropical countries. *Necator americanus* is the principal cause in the Western Hemisphere; *Ancylostoma duodenale* is prevalent in southern Europe and northern Africa. There is considerable overlap of these organisms, particularly in Asia. Most hookworm infections in the USA are caused by *N americanus* and occur in the southeastern states. The disease caused by both is similar, except that dermatologic manifestations are less common with *Ancylostoma*.

Adult worms live attached to the small intestinal mucosa. Eggs passed in the feces reach the soil, where, under favorable conditions of moisture and warmth, they hatch into rhabditiform larvae (about 0.3 mm in length). These larvae migrate into the soil, undergo metamorphosis (double their size), and become infective or filariform larvae. Where sanitation is lacking—especially where people habitually use the same area for defecation—opportunities for exposure are great.

The parasites like warmth and for that reason readily penetrate the skin, where the temperature is greater than that of soil. The parasites reach the bloodstream, are carried to the alveoli of the lungs, and migrate up the trachea and down the esophagus to reach feeding and breeding grounds in the small intestine. Alternatively, the larvae may be ingested with food and drink. In the absence of reinfection, immunity develops, causing a gradual reduction in the intestinal worm load, with total elimination in 5–7 years.

Clinical Findings

A. Symptoms and Signs: Skin penetration by filariform larvae of *N americanus* often causes local dermatitis ("ground itch" or "dew itch"). Edema, erythema, and a papular, vesicular, or bullous eruption develops, usually on the toes and soles. An urticarial eruption and ankle edema may be present. The eruption, rare in *A duodenale* infections, is transient, subsiding spontaneously in 2 weeks unless complicated by secondary bacterial infection. Definitive diagnosis of the transient cutaneous eruption is all but impossible, resting entirely on circumstantial evidence. The inflammatory skin response is usually more marked in reinfections.

Larval migration to the lungs may be associated with cough, wheezing, and eosinophilia. After the larva reaches the intestine, most infections are asymptomatic. The severity of symptoms depends upon the duration and intensity of infection as well as the nutritional status of the host. Heavy infections may result in iron deficiency anemia, growth retardation in children, and gastrointestinal complaints. Severe anemia and hypoproteinemia may develop in the malnourished patient.

B. Pathologic and Laboratory Findings: Larvae cannot be demonstrated at the site of cutaneous invasion. Edema, hyperemia, and an infiltrate of neutrophils and eosinophils predominate. The diagnosis is made by demonstrating eggs in the stool. The eggs of the 2 organisms are indistinguishable.

Treatment & Prevention

The cutaneous lesions are treated symptomatically; bacterial superinfection may require antibiotics. Several drugs may be used for intestinal infection. Mebendazole, 100 mg twice daily for 3 days; or albendazole, 200 mg/d for 3 days, is highly effective against both *A duodenale* and *N americanus.* Pyrantel pamoate, bephenium hydroxynaphthoate, and tetrachlorethylene are alternative drugs but are now used less often than previously.

Prophylaxis of hookworm disease is based on sanitary disposal of human excreta and prevention of soil contamination.

3. STRONGYLOIDIASIS

Strongyloides stercoralis is a roundworm with worldwide distribution, most commonly in warm, wet climates. The life cycle is similar to that of hookworm.

Entry of the larvae through the skin may cause a mild itch similar to but rarely as marked as that of the human hookworm. Local erythema, edema, urticaria, or petechiae may develop with pruritus, usually subsiding within 2 days. When the infective larva penetrates the perianal skin of the host, skin lesions, typically within a 25-cm radius from the anus, extend down the thighs or across the buttocks or abdomen as pruritic urticarial bands. The genitalia are spared. These may extend as rapidly as 10 cm/h (in contrast to animal hookworm larvae, which migrate at the rate of 1–2 cm/d). These lesions may be recurrent for years; the individual lesions usually last 40 hours.

In immunosuppressed patients, hyperinfection with massive numbers of worms may occur, with diarrhea, malabsorption, pulmonary symptoms, encephalopathy, meningitis, and eosinophilia.

Treatment

Thiabendazole, 25 mg/kg orally twice daily for 2 days, is the drug of choice. Albendazole and mebendazole have also been used.

4. CUTANEOUS LARVA MIGRANS ("Creeping Eruption")

There is considerable confusion about the disorders included under this heading, because several different parasites produce similar clinical pictures. The distinctive feature of creeping eruption is the migratory urticarial bands corresponding to the parasite movements in the skin. "Stationary" lesions—abscesses, furuncles, nodules, etc—caused by infection with a variety of fly larvae or helminths are not larva migrans. The lesion (or the parasite) must creep or migrate. The "creeping" entities can usually, but not always, be separated on clinical grounds, for each parasite tends to produce its own peculiar lesions.

Creeping eruption may be divided into 2 etiologic groups: (1) migratory helminthiasis secondary to nematodes (Table 18–2) and (2) migratory myiasis caused by various fly species, which is discussed in Chapter 19.

The terms "creeping eruption" and "cutaneous larva migrans" usually denote the disorder caused by cat or dog hookworm larvae.

Ancylostoma braziliense is the most common cause in South America, the southeastern USA, and many tropical countries. *Ancylostoma caninum* is a less frequent cause. In Europe, the dog hookworm, *Uncinaria stenocephala,* produces a milder type of eruption. The cattle hookworm, *Bunostomum phlebotomum*, is an uncommon cause. *Capillaria* species and *Strongyloides* species of nutria and raccoon are rare reported causes. *Strongyloides stercoralis* infection results in a type of creeping eruption.

Creeping eruption occurs wherever human skin comes into contact with soil contaminated with cat or dog feces. Shaded, moist, sandy areas provide the best conditions for larval development; beaches, children's sandpiles, and areas underneath houses are favorable environments. Eggs passed in animal feces hatch into infective larvae that penetrate human skin (even through beach towels) and begin an aimless wandering in the lower epidermis. Unable to penetrate the human dermis, they cannot complete their

Table 18–2. Causes of cutaneous larva migrans secondary to helminths.

Species	Clinical Features
Ancylostoma braziliense (cat, dog hookworm)	Threadlike, pruritic migratory burrow; may persist for months; moves 1–2 cm/d.
Ancylostoma caninum (dog hookworm)	Papular, rarely linear lesions; disappear in 2 weeks.
Uncinaria stenocephala (European dog hookworm)	Similar to *Ancylostoma braziliense.*
Bunostomum phlebotomum (cattle hookworm)	Papules with few millimeters' migration; clear in 2 weeks.
Strongyloides stercoralis	Urticarial band in perianal or buttock area; rapid migration up to 10 cm/h; chronic and intermittent for years.
Strongyloides myopotami (Nutria parasite)	Maculopapular serpiginous lesions.
Capillaria sp	Linear tract; severe pruritus.
Gnathostoma sp (cat, dog, pig, and wild feline nematodes)	Intermittent episodes of red, edematous subcutaneous nodules; limited migration of individual lesions; may be recurrent for years.

usual life cycle. Humans are, therefore, a dead-end host. In the appropriate animal host, the life cycle is similar to that of human hookworm.

Clinical Findings

A. Symptoms and Signs: Cutaneous lesions typically occur in areas in frequent contact with the soil (buttocks, feet, hands). A transient reddish papule usually occurs within a few hours after larval penetration. After an incubation period of a few days to a few months, the larva begins to migrate. A 2- to 4-mm wide, red, slightly elevated, intensely pruritic threadlike line develops; vesicles may be superimposed. *A braziliense* usually forms a continuous line; *A caninum* may form an interrupted track with itching papules up to 1 cm apart. The 0.5-mm larva is situated ahead of the track in seemingly normal skin within a radius of 1–2 cm. As the larva proceeds through the skin at a rate of several millimeters or a few centimeters daily, the older portion of the tunnel becomes crusted. An amazing variety of tortuous loops, curves, and lines may be created, particularly when multiple larvae are tunneling in unison. Because of severe pruritus, the patient can rarely refrain from frenzied scratching; bacterial superinfection and excoriation may obscure the original tunnellike lesions. In severe infections, some larvae may succeed in leaving the skin and producing eosinophilia and transitory pulmonary symptoms (Löffler's syndrome).

B. Laboratory Findings: The diagnosis is made from the clinical appearance and history. Biopsies are impractical. Serum IgE levels are elevated.

Differential Diagnosis

Differential diagnosis includes larva currens, gnathostomiasis, and migratory myiasis.

Treatment & Prognosis

Thiabendazole is the drug of choice. Topical thiabendazole is best for mild infections; a 10% aqueous suspension (Mintezol) may be applied 4 times daily for 1 week (98% clearing of tracks). This should be applied to the tracks and to normal-appearing skin surrounding the lesions, because the larva is outside the area of the visible lesion. Systemic thiabendazole is also effective, though associated with a high incidence of side effects (dizziness, nausea and vomiting); 25 mg/kg twice daily for 2 days gives a 99% cure rate.

Older methods of treatment—freezing of the advancing track with ethyl chloride, carbon dioxide, and liquid nitrogen—are traumatic and unreliable.

The disease is self-limited. About 50% of larvae die within 12 weeks regardless of treatment.

5. GNATHOSTOMIASIS

Gnathostomiasis is a form of larva migrans caused by the nematode *Gnathostoma spinigerum*, an organism widely distributed in southeast Asia, particularly Thailand. Humans are a dead-end host; the parasite fails to mature and wanders through body tissues for as long as 10 years. Almost any tissue may be invaded; the usual route of migration leads from stomach to liver, skeletal muscles, and subcutaneous tissue.

The parasite usually chooses to wander in the subcutaneous tissue. Intermittent circumscribed palmsized swellings with mild erythema, pruritus, and tenderness appear anywhere on the body but are most frequent on the chest and abdomen. The edema usually lasts a few days and spontaneously disappears. There may be abscess formation or small hemorrhagic spots. Rarely, the worm may emerge spontaneously from the lesion. Systemic symptoms indicate migration through other organs.

Surgical removal, if possible, is the treatment of choice.

TISSUE ROUNDWORMS

Nematodes that parasitize the extraintestinal tissues of humans include the filarial worms, guinea worm (*Dracunculus medinensis*), and *Trichinella* (*Trichina*) species.

The filarial infections (filariasis, onchocerciasis, and loiasis) are major health problems in many parts of the world. Viviparous female worms of the superfamily Filarioidea give birth to prelarval microfilariae. After these microfilariae are ingested from blood or tissues by a bloodsucking insect, they develop into filariform larvae in the intermediate insect host. These infective larvae are transmitted to humans by the insect's bite, after which they migrate to a location specific for the given species (eg, lymphatics for *Brugia malayi*) and develop into the adult worm. The adult female, after mating, produces numerous microfilariae to complete the cycle.

1. FILARIASIS
(Elephantiasis)

Essentials of Diagnosis
- Lymphangitis, lymphatic obstruction, and lymphedema.
- Demonstration of microfilariae in blood or body fluids.
- Lymph node or blood vessel biopsy.
- Serologic tests.

General Considerations
Bancroftian and Malayan filariasis (known simply as filariasis) are similar diseases caused by the nematodes *Wuchereria bancrofti* and *Brugia malayi*. About 200 million people are affected. *W bancrofti* is widespread throughout tropic and subtropic areas of South America, Africa, Asia, and the Pacific. *B malayi* is more restricted, occurring primarily in southeast Asia. Humans are the only host for *W bancrofti*; *B malayi* has been found in primates and felines (features of clinical disease are nearly identical).

The bite of a mosquito injects larvae of the parasite, which migrate to the lymphatics and lymph nodes and develop within about 1 year into mature worms. The adult threadlike white worms measure $40–100 \times 0.1–0.25$ mm. The fertilized female discharges microfilariae that circulate in the blood, available for the mosquito's next blood meal to complete the cycle. In bancroftian filariasis particularly, the microfilariae are released in periodic nocturnal showers usually corresponding to the biting habit of the vector mosquito.

Damage to the host is due to the presence of adult worms in the lymphatics; microfilariae may be present in huge numbers in the blood without causing symptoms.

Elephantiasis usually develops only after prolonged residence in an endemic area; the diagnosis is unlikely if a patient has not visited such an area.

Clinical Findings
A. Symptoms and Signs: Many infections are asymptomatic. The clinical phases of filariasis may be divided into inflammatory and obstructive; symptoms of both may be concurrent.

The initial inflammatory symptoms occur after an incubation period of 3 months to 1 year and last only a few weeks at most. Local lymphangitis with swelling, redness, and pain occurs in an extremity or in the scrotum, usually with regional lymphadenopathy. The lymphadenitis may occur independently of lymphangitis. Other manifestations include orchitis, funiculitis (lymphangitis of the spermatic cord), epididymitis, and filarial fever. Abscesses may occur, caused by a combination of dying worms and secondary bacterial infection. These inflammatory episodes frequently are recurrent before gradual progression to the chronic obstructive phase. Other cutaneous findings include urticaria and erythema nodosum-like swellings.

Repeated inflammatory episodes and gradual fibrosis in the lymphatics lead to lymphatic obstruction with varices and lymphedema, particularly in the genital and leg areas. Less frequently, the arms and breasts may be affected. Chronic edema stimulates growth of dermal connective tissue, causing massive permanent enlargement and deformity ("elephantiasis"), particularly of the leg or scrotum. Other obstructive complications include hydrocele, chyluria (secondary to thoracic duct obstruction), and lymph scrotum. Fortunately, elephantiasis occurs in only a small proportion of patients after years of infection. Microfilariae are usually not demonstrable in the blood by the time elephantiasis develops.

B. Laboratory Findings: On histopathologic examination, adult worms are observed in dilated lymphatics or lymph node sinuses. A caseating granulomatous reaction develops around degenerating worms. Later biopsies show fibrous obliteration of lymphatics.

Microfilariae in blood or body fluids (urine or hydrocele) are diagnostic. Microfilariae may not be present in early stages of the disease. Blood should be drawn at midnight. A lymph node or vessel biopsy may demonstrate the adult worm in 25% of specimens. Biopsies may aggravate lymphatic obstruction. Serologic tests are not highly specific (not differentiating among many nematodes) but may be suggestive in patients from nonendemic areas.

Treatment
Diethylcarbamazine rapidly reduces the number of circulating microfilariae and may affect adult worms. Reactions to dying parasites are common, with fever, malaise, nausea, and vomiting. Because of this, lower initial doses are given. The drug is given for a 3-week course as follows: day 1, 50 mg; day 2, 50 mg 3 times; day 3, 100 mg 3 times; days 4–21, 2 mg/kg 3 times daily. Oral antihistamines may help control urticarial reactions, and elastic stockings may help control edema. Treatment will not reverse elephan-

tiasis. Surgery may be required for hydrocele or massive scrotal enlargement.

2. ONCHOCERCIASIS
(River Blindness)

Essentials of Diagnosis

- Onchocercoma: firm, nontender subcutaneous nodules.
- Blindness.
- Skin snips contain microfilariae.
- Positive skin test and complement fixation test.

General Considerations

Onchocerciasis is a chronic filarial worm infection affecting 40 million people in rural Africa and South America. The causal organism is *Onchocerca volvulus,* a nematode transmitted by blackflies of the family Simuliidae. These 1- to 5-mm day-biting insects—also known as "buffalo" or "turkey" gnats—breed on the banks of turbulent rivers and streams. Onchocerciasis is widespread in tropical Africa; endemic centers are in Central America, Guatemala, and Mexico, particularly on the western slopes of the Sierras. The disease is common in Venezuela, Colombia, and Yemen.

Infective larvae, inoculated into the skin by the female fly's irritating bite, grow into adult worms in the subcutaneous tissue. The males (20–40 cm long) and females (35–50 cm) are found coiled together in fibrous nodules where they may survive for up to 15 years. Each female produces enormous numbers of microfilariae (150–350 μm long) that migrate through the subcutaneous tissues and eyes for up to 2 years. These microfilariae are ingested by flies during a bite; infective larvae develop after 2 months in the thoracic muscles of the insect. Humans are the only definitive host. Infection may occur at any age; severe aspects of the disease correlate with more intense infections seen in long-term residents of endemic areas. Travel or short visits in endemic areas rarely results in infection that develops into severe disease.

Clinical Findings

A. Symptoms and Signs: There are 3 cardinal features: subcutaneous nodules, pruritic dermatitis, and ocular lesions that may produce blindness. The first sign of infection is usually the subcutaneous nodule, followed by the dermatitis. In some cases, dermatitis may be present in the absence of nodules.

Onchocercomas are firm, nontender subcutaneous nodules 0.5–10 cm in diameter. They may adhere to one another, forming lobulated masses, occasionally attaching to the periosteum. These nodules containing the adult worms typically form over bony prominences. In Africa, they are most common on the lower body over the rib cage, iliac crest, femoral trochanters, and sacrum. In Central and South America, nodules are more common on the head. Lesions are sometimes deep in muscle or fascia. The number of onchocercomas is variable, ranging from 10 to over 100. The nodules are usually asymptomatic except for discomfort due to pressure over bones.

Onchocercal dermatitis may present several clinical appearances depending on geographic location and chronicity. Symptoms and signs are related to the wanderings of the microfilariae in the dermis. Itching—not always present—is usually the earliest symptom and may be the only one in lightly infected patients. Scratching frequently leads to secondary infection. Subtle pigmentary changes may also be present in this early stage, with macular irregular areas of hyperpigmentation (rarely hypopigmentation). The dermatitis tends to be more common in areas adjacent to nodules. Pruritus, papular eruptions, edema, pigmentary changes, and late atrophy are the primary manifestations.

In the Central and South American form of onchocerciasis, cutaneous lesions are more likely on the upper body and head. The term "mal de morado" denotes localized purplish edematous lichen planus-like plaques. "Coastal erysipelas" is an acute facial erysipelas-like eruption associated with fever, headache, and photophobia. This syndrome is probably a secondary bacterial infection but may be allergic; it is reproduced by treatment with diethylcarbamazine.

Late cutaneous changes occur with long-standing onchocerciasis. Atrophy is common, with thin, wrinkled, dry, shiny skin hanging in redundant folds. There may be prominent localized spotty depigmentation, giving a "leopard skin" appearance, particularly on the shins and genitals.

Firm, nontender lymphadenopathy is common in onchocerciasis; the nodes involved usually drain areas of onchocercal dermatitis. "Hanging groin" may occur in African patients with loose atrophic pouches of skin containing large fibrotic nodes. Genital elephantiasis in Zaire and Chad has been attributed to onchocerciasis.

Decreased visual acuity and blindness remain the most feared results. The eye may be examined for microfilariae directly or with a slit lamp. Disabling eye involvement usually develops with chronic infection and heavy worm loads. In some areas, blindness secondary to *Onchocerca* affects 5–20% of the adult population. In general, ocular disease is more prominent in patients with nodules on the head (the adult worms serve as a source for a higher density of microfilariae); the changes are therefore particularly common in Central America. Onchocercal eye disease usually appears late, with advanced damage found in middle-aged or older patients. Eye damage results from tissue reaction to the death of microfilariae, which can migrate to any part of the eye. The cornea, iris, ciliary body, retina, choroid, and optic nerve may be invaded.

B. Pathologic and Laboratory Findings: On histopathologic examination, cutaneous nodules consist of living or dead adult worms encased in a fibrous capsule; fibrosis may permeate the nodule, or there may be a soft center with granulation tissue and a polymorphous infiltrate of neutrophils, eosinophils, plasma cells, lymphocytes, and giant cells. Microfilariae are seen within the nodules as well as in the adjacent skin in great numbers. The density of microfilariae falls as the distance from the nodule increases.

Microfilariae may be demonstrated in the skin by use of the "skin snip," usually done on the buttocks and legs in Africans and the shoulder and buttocks in Central America. Excision of nodules demonstrates the adult worms.

Urine and sputum may demonstrate microfilariae, particularly after diethylcarbamazine treatment. The Mazzotti test has been used as a diagnostic aid; a few hours after a small dose of diethylcarbamazine, patients with onchocerciasis develop itching and a papular eruption. Because of occasional severe reactions in heavily infected patients, this test should be used with caution.

Although immunologic tests for onchocerciasis are not always reliable for sensitivity or specificity, the filarial skin test and complement fixation test with antigens from adult *Onchocerca* may be useful. Eosinophilia is frequent.

Differential Diagnosis

Differential diagnosis of the dermatitis includes scabies, streptocerciasis (in Africa), and other causes of pruritus and lichenification. The nodules may be mistaken for sebaceous cysts, lipomas, ganglia, or enlarged lymph nodes.

Treatment

Treatment is aimed at eliminating microfilariae and adult worms. The lack of adequate vector control programs in many endemic areas virtually ensures reinfection. Many patients are asymptomatic and do not require therapy. Treatment is usually given to patients with acute pruritic skin lesions and those whose vision may become impaired.

Surgical removal of nodules is partially effective. Many nodules are deep and difficult to find. Head nodules should be removed because of the higher risk of eye involvement. Drugs in use for onchocerciasis are diethylcarbamazine, which kills only microfilariae; suramin, which is effective against adult worms and some microfilariae; and ivermectin, a new drug that kills microfilariae slowly and is the current drug of choice. Trichlorphon and the combination of mebendazole and levamisole are alternatives but are not usually recommended.

Diethylcarbamazine frequently causes severe ("Mazzotti") reactions in the skin and eyes due to the death of microfilariae; these include marked itching, a papular edematous dermatitis with desquamation, regional lymphadenitis, conjunctivitis, iritis, fever, arthralgias, malaise, and anorexia. Corticosteroids may help control these reactions. Diethylcarbamazine is used for mild symptomatic cases that do not warrant the risks of suramin and when ivermectin is unavailable.

Suramin will kill the adult worms and most microfilariae but must be given intravenously and may cause idiosyncratic reactions or severe kidney damage. Eye involvement is an indication for suramin treatment.

Ivermectin has a strong but slow microfilaricidal effect; yearly treatments keep microfilarial counts at a low level and prevent tissue damage.

3. LOIASIS

Essentials of Diagnosis
- Worm passage seen in the eye or skin.
- Calabar swellings (transient edema) of the extremities.
- Microfilariae in the blood.
- Serologic tests for filarial infections.

General Considerations

Loiasis is a chronic nematodal infection limited to the rain forests of central and west Africa. In some endemic areas, 90% of the population may be infected.

Loa loa is a restless roundworm migrating as an adult through the subcutaneous tissues, producing transient "calabar" or "fugitive" swellings. The adult—a white threadlike worm measuring 30–70 mm—usually migrates continuously through the subcutaneous tissues at a maximum rate of 1 cm/min. Adults may live for 4–17 years. The gravid female liberates microfilariae that appear in the bloodstream during the day and inhabit the capillaries of the lungs and other deep organs at night. The disease is transmitted from human to human by the bite of several species of tabanid or "deer" flies belonging to the genus *Chrysops*. Microfilariae, taken up with blood during the fly's bite, develop into infective larvae and are transmitted to humans with a subsequent bite. The larvae mature slowly into adult worms; symptoms do not usually appear until 1 year after infection, when the adult worm begins its nomadic migrations. Microfilariae may not be found in the blood until 18 months after inoculation.

Clinical Findings

A. Symptoms and Signs: Diagnostic findings include Calabar swellings, a worm seen crossing the eye, a subcutaneous outline of the worm, and microfilariae in the peripheral blood smear.

The most distinctive findings and complaints center

on the Calabar swellings—edematous worm "tumors" that may appear anywhere but have a predilection for the wrists and ankles. Lesions emerge suddenly, attain the size of a small hen's egg, and disappear in 2–3 days. Pain may precede the edema and hamper function of an extremity. Recurrence at the same site is common. The swellings are most likely an allergic response to the passage of the worm.

Adult worms may sometimes be found within Calabar swellings; they may be found in the skin or eye without an edematous reaction. Worms are most easily noticed in the eye when migration beneath the bulbar conjunctiva causes pain, itching, and edema. The parasite has been found beneath the skin of the finger, trunk, scalp, and penis. Wanderings of the worm may be associated with a sensation of prickling or creeping; many patients are asymptomatic until the worm is noticed crossing the eyeball. Urticaria, fever, and generalized pruritus may be present; less common complications include peripheral neuritis, meningoencephalitis, retinopathy, and glomerulopathy.

B. Pathologic and Laboratory Findings: On histopathologic examination, migrating worms usually are not associated with inflammatory changes; dying worms provoke intense inflammatory reactions in the deep dermis, with subsequent granulomatous changes and fibrosis. Microfilariae may sometimes be seen in skin biopsies in capillaries.

Because of the diurnal periodicity of microfilaremia, blood samples are best drawn at noon; hemoconcentration techniques may be helpful in demonstrating microfilariae. In light infections, microfilariae may not be found. Eosinophilia of up to 7000/μL is common. Skin tests and complement fixation tests with dirofilarial antigens are usually positive but cross-react with other filarial infections.

Treatment

Diethylcarbamazine provides effective treatment, killing the adults and microfilariae. The dosage is the same as for filariasis. Side effects are few, but there may be marked allergic reactions to the death of the parasite, including Calabar swellings, pruritus, diffuse papular eruptions, fever, arthralgias, and malaise. Prophylaxis with diethylcarbamazine (5 mg/kg/d orally for 3 days once a month) is effective for visitors or residents in endemic areas.

Low-dose mebendazole has also been used as treatment for loiasis in a dosage of 100 mg 3 times daily for 45 days.

4. STREPTOCERCIASIS

Dipetalonema streptocerca is restricted to the tropic rain forest areas of western and central Africa,

where it occasionally causes a chronic dermatitis similar to that of onchocerciasis.

5. DIROFILARIASIS

Several species of filarial nematodes of the genus *Dirofilaria* normally infect animals, but some species may cause pulmonary "coin lesions" in humans and, rarely, subcutaneous nodules. *Dirofilaria tenuis* is a natural subcutaneous parasite of the raccoon in the USA and is responsible for most human cases, which are reported primarily in the southeastern region. Subcutaneous nodules occur in many body areas. *D tenuis* has a predilection for the eyelid or periorbital region; rarely, the worm may be visible in the conjunctiva. Subcutaneous nodules are usually solitary, 1–2 cm in diameter, movable, and sometimes tender and red. The lesion develops slowly over a period of several weeks and may rarely migrate. Proptosis may be prominent in patients with orbital disease.

On histopathologic examination, nodules usually contain a single, coiled, dead or degenerating worm. In early lesions, the worm is located in an abscess with eosinophils and neutrophils; late lesions show a granulomatous reaction with eosinophils, epithelioid cells, and giant cells.

Excision of nodules is the only treatment.

6. DRACUNCULIASIS

The adult female dragon worm or guinea worm (*Dracunculus medinensis*) lives in human subcutaneous tissue and may reach the astonishing length of more than 120 cm. The worm's habit of extruding itself through the skin for the purpose of liberating its larvae produces the only significant manifestation of the disease: a localized skin lesion. The worm is encountered in western and eastern Africa, India, and parts of the Middle East.

There are no symptoms during the long incubation period. As the female worm's head nears the cutaneous surface, pronounced prodromal symptoms develop: local erythema, generalized urticaria, itching, dyspnea, gastrointestinal disturbances, and sometimes mild fever. Occasionally there are asthma-like symptoms, giddiness, and syncope. Several hours after the onset of these systemic prodromes, a papule appears that soon becomes surmounted by a vesicle. During the next day or 2, the vesicle enlarges to a firm bulla situated on an inflammatory indurated base 2–6 mm in diameter. The blister ruptures, leaving a small ulcer or erosion, in the center of which the head of the parasite may often be seen. Usually the worm becomes palpable in the tissue and may be seen by oblique illumination as a tortuous stringlike structure. All toxic symptoms subside when the blister ruptures, but owing to secondary bacterial infection, local lesions may become inflamed and painful. Multiple infections are not uncommon. Abscesses and chronic ulcerations may persist for months when many worms are present; sometimes this leads to permanent disability from ankylosis of joints or contracture of limbs.

Calcified dead worms may be demonstrated on roentgenologic examination.

The objective of treatment is to remove or destroy the worm. The worm may also be removed by surgical excision under local anesthesia. Surgery is particularly necessary when abscesses form near a joint or in the extradural space.

Chemotherapy reduces inflammation and allows easier removal of the worm. Equally effective drugs are metronidazole, 400 mg/d for 10–20 days or 30–40 mg/kg 3 times daily for 3 days; and thiabendazole, 50 mg/kg/d in 2 divided doses for 3 days.

New worms may emerge later because the drugs do not kill immature worms.

TRICHINOSIS

Trichinosis is a self-limited infection caused by the small roundworm *Trichinella spiralis*. It is widespread throughout temperate regions and is endemic in the USA, Central and South America, and Europe.

Cutaneous manifestations are often the initial physical signs of muscle invasion. Periorbital edema is the initial sign in more than 80% of cases; edema may involve the entire face. Subconjunctival and subungual splinter hemorrhages may be seen in severe cases. A maculopapular or petechial eruption is seen in 10% of patients. Other symptoms include fever, myalgias and muscle tenderness, headache, cough, dyspnea, and dysphagia. Cardiac, neurologic, and urologic symptoms are occasionally seen in severe infections. Fatalities occur in 2% of symptomatic patients owing to interstitial myocarditis, encephalitis, or pneumonia.

In many cases, the diagnosis is presumptive based on the clinical features and supporting serologic tests. Diagnosis is definitively made only by demonstrating larvae in striated muscle. Muscle biopsy (from the biceps or gastrocnemius muscle) may not show infection until 3–4 weeks after infection. Laboratory investigation shows peripheral blood eosinophilia and positive serologic tests (ELISA, bentonite flocculation).

Mebendazole has proved larvicidal (20 mg/kg divided into 4 daily doses for 2 weeks) and may need to be repeated in severe infections. Systemic corticosteroids may be necessary to attenuate the allergic reactions associated with muscle invasion.

Thiabendazole appears to be effective in the intestinal phase only. Albendazole may also be effective for the tissue phase.

TREMATODA

SCHISTOSOMIASIS

There are 2 types of human schistosomiasis: (1) cutaneous schistosomiasis (cercarial dermatitis, swimmer's itch), a purely cutaneous infection due to nonhuman schistosomes for which humans are an abnormal host; and (2) visceral schistosomiasis, a serious systemic disorder (with inconsequential occasional cutaneous manifestations) due to the human blood flukes *Schistosoma mansoni*, *S japonicum*, and *S haematobium*. When human blood flukes penetrate the skin during the invasive stage of visceral schistosomiasis, an eruption is occasionally provoked that may mimic swimmer's itch due to nonhuman schistosomes. This circumstance has occasioned some confusion with respect to the terminology used in distinguishing these 2 different diseases. The generic term "schistosomal dermatitis" includes both, unless qualifying phrases such as "schistosomal dermatitis due to human flukes" are used to define the cause. The terms "swimmer's itch" and "cutaneous schistosomiasis," however, refer exclusively to the eruption caused by nonhuman schistosomes.

1. CERCARIAL DERMATITIS (Cutaneous Schistosomiasis)

Essentials of Diagnosis
- Itching after swimming or contact with bodies of water harboring ducks and snails.
- Wheals, papules, occasionally vesicles.
- May spare areas covered by clothing.

General Considerations
Cutaneous schistosomiasis (cercarial dermatitis, "swimmer's itch") is a distinctive papular eruption produced by the cercariae of nonhuman schistosomes. In some areas of the world, it may affect large numbers of people and is known by a variety of colloquialisms: "Clamdigger's itch" is seen on the saltwater tributaries of Long Island Sound, while "sawah itch" or "duck-feces dermatitis" may plague the rice-paddy worker in Malaysia or China. Humans are an abnormal "dead-end" host for these flukes; while the cercariae can enter the skin, further development cannot occur and the parasite dies in the skin without gaining access to the circulation and deeper tissues. Sensitization rapidly develops and is the basis of the clinical inflammatory reaction.

Cercarial dermatitis is a potential hazard whenever humans share an aquatic area with animal and molluscan species capable of harboring schistosomes. The cercariae of approximately 20 species of schistosomes have been implicated; the usual animal hosts are either birds (waterfowl, especially ducks, and passerine birds) or small mammals (mice, moles, and muskrats). Many species of freshwater and marine mollusks serve as intermediate hosts.

Cercarial dermatitis occurs in the Great Lakes area of the USA and Canada and in several widely scattered parts of the world. Disease is usually reported in freshwater lake areas but may occur in saltwater coastal regions. In the USA, the worst outbreaks occur in the lake regions of Wisconsin, Michigan, and Minnesota, where numerous lakes attract crowds of bathers in the summer months.

The life cycle of nonhuman schistosomes is similar to that of human schistosomes. Being positively phototactic, the cercariae are attracted to the surface layer of water; thus, contact with swimmers is more likely. The cercariae penetrate the skin as the water evaporates, as if to escape the obvious threat of desiccation, but penetration can occur during immersion as well.

Clinical Findings

After exposure to water inhabited by cercaria, the patient experiences a prickling or itching sensation lasting for a few minutes to 1 hour while the cercariae are entering the skin. Small erythematous macules soon form at the sites of entrance, but occasionally there may be a diffuse erythema with some swelling or, in highly sensitized persons, wheals. These immediate lesions usually disappear within a short time, to be replaced after 10–15 hours by the signs that typify the disorder: discrete, highly pruritic papules surrounded by a zone of erythema. Vesicles that may become pustules frequently form 1–2 days later, surmounting each papule. The lesions gradually subside within 1 week, leaving small pigmented spots.

The different clinical responses are related to the degree of sensitization, and this in turn depends on the number of exposures or the magnitude of the exposure, as well as on the constitutional capacity to become sensitized. On first exposure, the delay of 1 week or so before inflammatory signs appear is the time required for sensitization to take place. Upon reexposure, the host reaction is accelerated and more intense, causing the disappearance of the cercariae in about 3 days and resulting within 12–16 hours in the formation of highly inflammatory, pruritic papules.

Prevention & Treatment

The best and most practical method of control is destruction of snails. Treatment of the water with a mixture of copper sulfate and carbonate—or with sodium pentachlorophenate—has proved successful in reducing or eradicating swimmer's itch in lakes large and small, where the application has been in expert hands. A thick coating of almost any grease or wearing tightly woven clothing offers protection, but such methods are obviously unsuitable for bathers. Some degree of protection may be given by bathing with a hexachlorophene soap before exposure. Five percent hexachlorophene in lanolin or petrolatum may also be effective in repelling cercariae. Vigorous rubbing with a towel after swimming may remove some organisms. Local and systemic antipruritic preparations such as calamine lotion and oral antihistamines are used to tide the patient over until the lesions spontaneously disappear in a few days.

2. VISCERAL SCHISTOSOMIASIS

Essentials of Diagnosis

- Transient dermatitis or urticarial reactions.
- Warty or ulcerating genital lesions or nodular trunk lesions.
- Eggs in urine, stool, or tissue biopsy.
- Serology.

General Considerations

Three species of the genus *Schistosoma* are responsible for disease in more than 200 million people in 71 countries. Infection is usually limited to the urinary and gastrointestinal tracts but may occasionally involve the skin.

The human host infected with *Schistosoma mansoni* and *Schistosoma japonicum* excretes eggs in the feces—and in the urine in the case of *Schistosoma haematobium*. Coming in contact with water, these eggs hatch into free-swimming miracidia. The miracidia invade certain species of snail and end in the liberation of fork-tailed cercariae, the free-swimming form infective for the human host. The cercariae penetrate the skin of persons bathing, washing, wading, or working in infected water, particularly as the water evaporates after immersion. Penetration occurs in less than 30 minutes, probably with the aid of lytic substances secreted by the cercariae. The parasite passes rapidly through the epidermis, gaining access to the venous circulation in less than 24 hours. Because the cercariae do not stay in the skin, cutaneous reactions in visceral schistosomiasis are minor or absent. The larvae pass through the heart and lungs, eventually localizing in the tributaries of the intrahepatic portion of the portal system, where the flukes mature. Finally, they pass out of the liver via the portal system, working their way down toward the finer portal radicles of the intestine or bladder, where the eggs are laid in the mucosa and submucosa. The egg escapes into the lumen of the gut or bladder; there it is excreted with the urine or feces, completing the life cycle.

Clinical Findings

Only the cutaneous aspects of disease will be considered. Cutaneous manifestations reflect different stages of the host-parasite relationship and include (1) schistosomal dermatitis due to skin penetration by cercariae, (2) urticarial reactions associated with acute infections, and (3) cutaneous lesions due to the deposition of ova in the skin.

A. Symptoms and Signs: The relatively minor

and inconstant reaction of the skin to penetration by cercariae—causing visceral schistosomiasis—stands in sharp contrast to the marked dermatitis of "swimmer's itch" provoked by nonhuman schistosomes. On the other hand, some individuals develop a dermatitis that closely mimics "swimmer's itch," especially if there has been prior exposure. Sensitivity is established that enables the skin to become more reactive with repeated exposures. Shortly after exposure, pruritic, hivelike swellings appear and become itchy papules in about 24 hours. The eruption subsides spontaneously in a few days unless there is secondary infection.

Another cutaneous manifestation occurs during the acute initial stages about 4–8 weeks after penetration of the skin by the cercariae. Characteristically, there are fever, malaise, chills, joint pains, abdominal cramps, diarrhea, and enlargement of the spleen and liver. During this period, which may be prolonged, an urticarial eruption commonly emerges, particularly characteristic and frequent in *S japonicum* and less so in the other 2 types. The reaction is believed to be due to circulating immune complexes that form after the release of large amounts of antigenic material in the form of eggs.

Cutaneous lesions due to the presence of eggs in the skin may occur in the genital and perineal areas or as papular ectopic lesions of the trunk. Asymptomatic deposition of eggs in the anogenital area may be a frequent occurrence.

In endemic areas, genital and perigenital lesions due to eggs of *S haematobium* and *S mansoni* are not uncommon. These are typically nontender, soft, warty, vegetating masses that vary from flesh color to dark brown or pink. These may be associated with honeycombing fistulous tracts of the perineum and buttocks. Ulceration, secondary infection, and malignant change to squamous cell carcinoma are common complications.

Extragenital (or ectopic) lesions are much less frequent and are usually on the trunk, occasionally in zosteriform distribution. Most cases are due to *S haematobium*. The primary lesion is an asymptomatic, firm, flesh-colored papule 2–3 mm in diameter. Papules coalesce slowly into irregular plaques that may darken, become scaly, and rarely ulcerate. Lesions usually evolve over 1–2 months and may take 5 months to resolve under treatment.

B. Pathologic and Laboratory Findings: The characteristic eggs may be found in urine, feces, or rectal biopsy. Their presence is also diagnostic when found in the skin, either in lesions or in clinically normal anogenital skin. A variety of immunodiagnostic tests are helpful but secondary to the demonstration of ova; the intradermal and complement-fixation tests are useful. Eosinophilia is common.

Treatment

There is no specific treatment for schistosomal dermatitis or acute urticarial reactions. Praziquantel is active against all species of schistosomes and is the drug of choice. Alternative drugs are oxamniquine for *S mansoni* and metriphonate for *S haemotobium*.

SEABATHER'S ERUPTION

Essentials of Diagnosis

- Bitelike papules with central crust.
- Localized to skin covered by bathing suit.
- History of contact with salt water (usually swimming).

General Considerations

The cause of this disorder has not been established. Similar lesions have been produced experimentally by marine cercariae. Many agents have been implicated in causing saltwater eruptions, including the nematocysts of jellyfish, pteropods, diroflagellates, and algae.

The disease has been encountered principally in persons bathing off the Atlantic or Gulf Coast areas of Florida. It has a strict seasonal incidence from March to September. Outbreaks are sporadic and unpredictable, occurring in large numbers on certain days and not at all at other times, sometimes not for years.

Clinical Findings

There are significant points of difference, which are sufficient to justify their separation as clinical entities, between seabather's eruption and swimmer's itch.

The eruption ensues within a few hours after bathing and consists of pruritic erythematous wheals or papules lasting a few days and involuting spontaneously. The lesions are often capped with a slight serous crust appearing as a central punctum; most have a follicular distribution. Individual lesions closely resemble insect bites. A characteristic feature is localization of the eruption to areas covered by the bathing suit. Usually no discomfort is noted until itching develops several hours after leaving the water. In children with extensive eruptions, fever of 38.3–38.8 °C may occur.

Two features of seabather's eruption distinguish it clinically from swimmer's itch: (1) it occurs predominantly in the bathing suit area, while the latter is on exposed portions; and (2) it is limited to salt water, whereas swimmer's itch is characteristically, but not invariably, a freshwater disease.

Treatment

A shower after seabathing may help prevent the eruption. Palliative treatment with antihistamines is usually sufficient, as the eruption resolves within 7–10 days.

CESTODIA

CYSTICERCOSIS

Taenia solium, the pork tapeworm, causes 2 distinct types of infection in humans: (1) taeniasis, in which adult tapeworms infect the intestinal tract; and (2) cysticercosis, in which larval forms of the parasite are present in the tissues. Disease is most common in regions of the world with low public health standards. Infection is rare in North America but common in eastern Europe, Central and South America, Africa, and Asia.

While adult worms in the intestine cause little or no reaction, cysticerci in tissues incite inflammatory reactions, followed by fibrotic encapsulation. They lodge most frequently in the skin and subcutaneous tissues, brain, eye, skeletal muscles, liver, lungs, and heart, producing tumorlike nodules that may seriously interfere with function in accordance with their position. The nodules may subsequently caseate and calcify, sometimes being detectable by x-ray examination of soft tissues.

Biopsy of involved tissue may reveal the parasite. Serologic tests for antibodies to cestodes are positive. Examination of feces may show eggs if taeniasis is present simultaneously.

In the skin, the disease is known as *Cysticercus cellulosae cutis.* The nodules are firm, elastic, rounded, painless tumors, ranging from the size of a pea to that of a walnut, sharply demarcated, and persisting unchanged for years. There may be one or many, usually on the trunk or extremities and sometimes associated with cysticerci elsewhere on the body, although these may be difficult to locate.

The most effective treatment for cysticercosis is surgical removal. Praziquantel is now used for cerebral cysticercosis but should be used only in hospital under expert neurologic supervision and corticosteroid coverage.

ECHINOCOCCOSIS
(Hydatid Disease)

Two species of the tapeworm *Echinococcus* may parasitize humans. *Echinococcus granulosus* may cause the more common unilocular hydatid cysts, while *Echinococcus multilocularis* causes the more destructive alveolar form of disease. Infection with *E granulosus* is prevalent in sheep-raising countries around the world.

Cutaneous involvement is rare. Hydatid cyst of the liver and lungs is the most common expression of the disease.

In the skin, the tumors are soft, fluctuant, rounded masses of inconstant size, causing no distress and not altering the overlying skin. After a variable period of years, the cysts may degenerate, become resorbed, or calcify.

Surgical excision is the best treatment.

SPARGANOSIS

Sparganosis is an infection caused by tapeworm larvae of the genus *Spirometra* invading human tissue. Disease in humans is usually benign, with encystment of the larva in the subcutaneous tissue.

Most cases are described in Asia; however, scattered instances are known throughout the world, and 65 cases have been reported in the USA, particularly in the southeastern states.

Diagnosis is usually made after excision of a subcutaneous mass or nodule. These are usually slowly growing, tender, and rarely migratory nodules about 2 cm in diameter. Cutaneous lesions may resemble acnelike nodular pustules. The nodules may lie more deeply in the musculature and have rarely been found in the eye, brain, lung, epididymis, urethra, and intestine.

Surgical removal of spargana is the treatment of choice.

III. ECTOPARASITIC DISEASES

Milton Orkin, MD & Howard I. Maibach, MD

SCABIES

Essentials of Diagnosis

- Severe itching, often worse at night.
- Several members of a family or group with itching rash (contact cases).
- Generalized eruption of excoriated papules.
- Short, wavy lines (burrows), especially on finger webs, wrists, elbows, and penis.
- Mites, ova, or fecal pellets demonstrable microscopically.

General Considerations

The itch mite, *Sarcoptes scabiei* var *humanus,* was described in 1687, making scabies one of the first diseases in humans with a known cause. Epidemics of scabies historically occurred in 30-year cycles, with a 15-year gap between the end of one epidemic and the beginning of the next. The current cycle began in the mid 1960s; however, it is continuing.

Scabies occurs worldwide, in both sexes, and in any age group. The disease accounts for 2–4% of all dermatologic visits in the USA.

Scabies is an itching dermatosis transmitted by skin-to-skin contact. Sexual transmission is common (scabies frequently coexists with other sexually transmitted diseases), but nonsexual spread occurs in family groups. The greater the number of parasites on an individual, the greater the likelihood of transmission. When several members of a family or group complain of a pruritic eruption, scabies is a likely diagnosis. Fomites are relatively unimportant in its transmission.

Clinical Findings
(Table 18–3)

A. Symptoms and Signs:

1. Classic scabies– Itching is characteristically nocturnal. Lesions are bilateral and often begin on the hands, particularly in the finger webs and on the sides of the digits. The flexor surfaces of the wrists, the elbows, and the anterior axillary folds are commonly involved.

At most sites, small, erythematous, often excoriated papules are present. The pathognomonic burrow is a short, wavy, dirty-appearing line (Fig 18–1). The areolar areas of the female breasts may have eczematous changes. Papular lesions are usually present around the umbilicus. Penile involvement is characteristic: nodules, chancriform ulcers, or pyoderma (Fig 18–2). The disease may affect the lower buttocks. Secondary eczematization and infection may overshadow other features.

2. Special forms of scabies– Scabies frequently occurs in special forms that may present diagnostic difficulties.

a. Scabies in clean persons– There is a definite increase in the incidence of scabies in clean individuals. The disease is easily misdiagnosed, because lesions are sparse and burrows more difficult to find.

b. Scabies incognito– Corticosteroid administra-

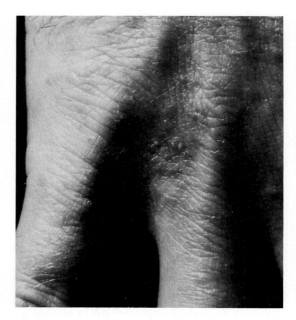

Figure 18–1. Multiple burrows and papules are present on the finger webs. (Courtesy of Axel Hoke, MD.)

tion (topical or systemic) may mask symptoms and signs of scabies, though the infestation remains freely transmissible. This often results in unusual clinical presentations such as atypical and wide distribution, in some instances closely imitating other conditions.

c. Nodular scabies– This is characterized by reddish-brown pruritic nodules (Fig 18–3) on covered parts (most frequently the male genitalia, groin, and axillary regions) and probably represents a hypersensitivity reaction to retained mite parts or antigens. Mites are seldom found, and the lesions are not contagious.

d. Scabies in infants and young children– Misdiagnosis is frequent because of low index of suspicion and secondary eczematous changes. In contrast to adults, lesions may occur on the head, neck, palms, and soles. Vesicles are common, as is secondary infection.

e. Animal-transmitted scabies– Puppies are the major source. Humans are infested by direct or indirect contact, and transmission occurs more readily than from humans. Scabies contracted from animals has a different distribution pattern (frequently the trunk, arms, and abdomen; rarely, the fingerwebs and genitalia) and a shorter incubation period. There are no burrows, because the animal mites do not complete their life cycle on humans.

f. Crusted (Norwegian) scabies– This rare condition is highly contagious because of the myriad of mites in the exfoliating scales. Local or regional epidemics of more typical forms of scabies may spread

Table 18–3. Diagnosis of scabies.

Suggestive

Distribution: Hands, wrists, elbows, anterior axillary folds, areolas of female breasts, abdomen, genitals, buttocks
Morphology: Small, excoriated papules are prominent. Burrows are pathognomonic.
Nocturnal pruritus.
Contact cases: This is highly suggestive.
Skin biopsy, compatible with bite reaction.

Diagnostic

Identification of the mite (success rate varies with experience and persistence).
Microscopic study: Skin scrapings or other technique.
Skin biopsy (performed in difficult cases): Sections may reveal mites or fecal pellets.

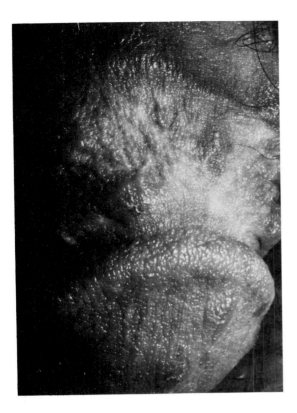

Figure 18–2. Pyoderma of the penis is highly suggestive of scabies. (Courtesy of Axel Hoke, MD.)

made by microscopic identification of the mites, eggs, or fecal pellets. One should try to verify the diagnosis, because this infestation may be underdiagnosed (scabies may mimic any pruritic dermatosis) or overdiagnosed (resulting in treatment of other conditions with scabicides). Techniques for diagnosis are as follows:

1. Skin scrapings– Burrows or unexcoriated papules are located with the help of a hand lens or loupe. Mineral oil is dropped onto a sterile scalpel blade and allowed to flow onto the lesions. Vigorous scraping with the blade about 6 or 7 times removes the tops of burrows or papules. The oil and scraped material are then transferred to a glass slide and covered with a coverslip and examined under low power. The diagnosis is confirmed by noting the presence of the mite (any stage), eggs, or the typical fecal pellets, which outnumber the living organisms (Fig 18–4).

2. Curettage (dermal curet)– Superficially curet the long axis of a burrow or across the summit of a papule, and deposit the material on a clean slide. Then place 1 or 2 drops of mineral oil on the material and cover with a coverslip and examine under low power. This technique is particularly valuable in infants, small children, or anxious or uncooperative patients of any age as well as patients suspected of having HIV/AIDS.

Differential Diagnosis

Scabies can be confused with almost any pruritic

from an individual case, usually in hospitals or other institutions. The condition is a psoriasiform dermatosis of the hands and feet, with dystrophy of the nails and a variable erythematous scaling eruption that may be generalized. Itching is minimal. It occurs in mentally retarded or physically debilitated persons or those who are immunologically deficient for any reason. Failure to scratch or failure to develop hypersensitivity allows the mites to proliferate profusely.

Atypical (crusted or "exaggerated") scabies may occur in patients with human immunodeficiency virus (HIV). This association will become much more common, ie, another opportunistic infection and cutaneous manifestation of HIV-AIDS disease.

g. Scabies in the elderly– In the elderly, the reaction to the mite is muted, but the patient itches severely. The vivid inflammatory reaction seen in young people is usually absent. Scabies is frequently not recognized, and instead the itching is attributed to "senile pruritus," dry skin, or anxiety. For elderly patients in nursing homes and other extended-care facilities—particularly those who are bedridden for long periods—there may be involvement of the back (unique for adults with scabies).

B. Laboratory Findings: Definitive diagnosis is

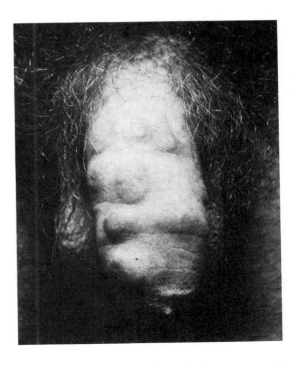

Figure 18–3. Nodular scabies. Multiple nodules are present on the penile shaft.

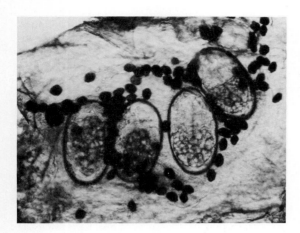

Figure 18–4. Skin scrapings of burrows disclose large eggs and numerous fecal pellets. (Courtesy of Axel Hoke, MD.)

dermatosis but most commonly with atopic dermatitis, papular urticaria, pyoderma, insect bites, and dermatitis herpetiformis.

Complications

Secondary bacterial infection may occur. Nephritogenic streptococcal strains colonizing scabietic lesions and leading to acute glomerulonephritis have been reported mainly in tropical areas, but the potential is universal.

Most patients with secondarily infected scabies do not require systemic antibacterial therapy; the pyoderma clears with scabicidal therapy. When bacterial infection is extensive, some physicians prefer to utilize oral antibacterial agents such as erythromycin. Systemic antimicrobials do not alter the likelihood of developing secondary renal disease.

Treatment

A. Principles of Therapy: There have been few controlled trials of scabicides. The choice of drug should be based on considerations of efficacy and potential toxicity. Treatment may be preceded by a tepid bath. Patients tend to apply the drugs more frequently and over longer periods than prescribed. Limiting the quantity prescribed prevents dermatitis caused by overtreatment, which the patient may mistake for persistence of scabies, and minimizes percutaneous penetration. Approximately 30 g (1 oz) of a topical preparation adequately covers the trunk and extremities of the average adult. Scabicides should be applied thinly but thoroughly from the neck downward to all areas, with special attention to the hands, feet, intertriginous areas, and under the fingernails.

Selective treatment of asymptomatic family members at high risk for acquiring the infestation from a confirmed case may be appropriate. The physician should exercise good judgment; for example, if the patient routinely shares a bed with another person, the probability is high that transmission to that person has already occurred, and therefore treatment of the asymptomatic bed partner is justified. Sexual contacts should also be treated simultaneously. It is less significant to treat those with minimal skin-to-skin contact with an afflicted family member.

At the conclusion of therapy, intimate articles of clothing, bed linen, and towels should be machine-washed and dried, using the hot cycle of each machine. It is not necessary to clean outerwear or furniture, because the mites survive only briefly away from the human host.

B. Specific Scabicides:

1. Lindane– Lindane is the most frequently used scabicide and the most thoroughly studied. Lindane lotion is easy to use and usually effective. Many physicians prefer to use lindane lotion in older children and nonpregnant adults. An application of the lotion is left on for 8 hours and washed off thoroughly. The lotion should be kept away from the eyes and mucous membranes. A second application is appropriate only when there is failure of compliance, reinfestation, or resistance.

Ten percent of lindane applied to the skin can be recovered in the urine. Clinical central nervous system toxicity has occurred only with misuse related to abuse, overuse, failure of the patient to comprehend warning instructions, and similar factors not under the control of the prescribing physician or pharmacist. Scabicides other than lindane are preferred for infants, young children, pregnant or nursing women, and patients with seizure disorders or other neurologic disease.

The mite of scabies appears to be developing some resistance to lindane.

2. Sulfur– Used for centuries, sulfur is generally prescribed as precipitated sulfur (6%) in petrolatum, applied nightly for 3 nights and washed off thoroughly 24 hours after the last application. Patients find it less acceptable than modern scabicides because of its odor, messiness, and staining. Precipitated sulfur is the preferred treatment for infants, small children, and pregnant or lactating women as well as for patients with seizure disorders or other neurologic diseases.

3. Permethrin– Permethrin 5% dermal cream, a synthetic pyrethroid, is a recently approved scabicide. Because of low mammalian toxicity, it is likely to enjoy wide usage. A single application is removed after 8–14 hours.

4. Crotamiton cream– Crotamiton is not a highly effective scabicide. Five daily applications may be better than the 2 currently recommended, but current data are inconclusive.

C. Treatment of Some Special Forms of Scabies:

1. Nodular scabies– These pruritic, hypersensitivity nodules do not respond to scabicides. They clear spontaneously but may persist for months to more than a year. They may improve or clear with topical applications of corticosteroid creams. The nodules frequently subside with nightly applications of 5% tar gel for 2–3 weeks.

2. Animal-transmitted scabies– This condition is self-limited (several weeks) if the animal is cured or separated from the human. The animals should be treated by a veterinarian skilled in veterinary dermatology. The condition is not contagious between humans.

3. Crusted scabies– Therapy for crusted scabies is similar to that for the more common types, though the former responds more slowly and may require sequential use of lindane, sulfur, and crotamiton. The organisms may find refuge and protection from treatment under the free edge of the nail plates. In addition to the usual regimen, it may help to keep the fingernails trimmed very short and brush the scabicide under the free edge of the nail for several consecutive days. (This may also help in the treatment of scabies in nursing home patients.)

D. Antipruritic Medications: An oral antipruritic medication such as an antihistamine may blunt the pruritus that characteristically lingers after adequate antiscabietic therapy. Topical 1% hydrocortisone cream may provide symptomatic relief in adults, and a lubricating agent or emollient may be helpful in infants and young children.

In the rare instance of incapacitating posttreatment itching in an adult, a short course of systemic corticosteroid therapy, such as a 7- to 10-day course of prednisone at an initial dosage of 40 mg/d, gives prompt, dramatic relief.

Prognosis

Treatment as described above is usually effective but may fail if the patient does not follow instructions. Reinfestation from an outside source does not occur commonly except in sexual transmission. Resistance can be proved only by demonstrating the mites again in patients in whom there is reasonable assurance that the medication has been properly applied.

PEDICULOSIS
(Louse Infestation)

Infestations of humans by lice have been documented for thousands of years. The insects themselves have been in existence for several million years. The head louse was present in the New World long before its discovery.

More deaths have occurred from diseases transmitted by lice than from any insect-borne disease other than the malaria mosquito. The major louse-borne diseases of the past (epidemic typhus, murine typhus,

and trench fever) have largely been brought under control through improved standards of hygiene (the most important being the ability to wash and change clothes), the development of more effective pediculocides, and the availability of antibiotics to treat the rickettsial diseases carried by the lice.

Lice are wingless, dorsoventrally flattened, blood-sucking insects of the order Anoplura. Three species of lice infest humans: *Pthirus pubis* (the crab louse), *Pediculus humanus capitis* (the head louse), and *Pediculus humanus humanus* (the body or, more accurately, the clothing louse).

Body lice and head lice are similar in appearance. The body of the crab louse is much shorter and is almost as wide as it is long.

Lice have 3 pairs of legs. In the crab louse, the first pair of legs terminate in a slender claw, while the second and third pairs have well-developed claws; this anatomy is perfectly adapted to grasping the coarse, widely spaced hairs of the pubis, axilla, beard, and occasionally the eyelashes. Unlike head lice and body lice, which are highly mobile (traveling up to 23 cm/min), pubic lice are sluggish and travel a maximum of 10 cm/d.

The egg incubation period is about 6–10 days; the time required for the development of the egg to the adult is 17–25 days in head and body lice and 22–27 days in crab lice. The organisms survive away from the human host 1–7 days for body lice, 6–20 hours for head lice, and 12–48 hours for pubic lice.

Microbiology & Immunology

The bites of lice are relatively painless and can only rarely be detected, even under close observation, as a slight tickling sensation. The host is often unaware that lice are feeding.

The clinical signs and symptoms arise from the reaction of the host to the saliva or anticoagulant injected by the louse, at the time of feeding, into the dermis. Depending on the degree of sensitivity and previous exposure, the sites of feeding may produce small 2- to 3-mm erythematous macules or papules, which erupt in hours to days after feeding, or an acute hivelike immediate reaction with typical flare-and-wheal formation. The hallmark of all types of pediculosis is intense pruritus, compelling the sufferer to scratch, particularly at night.

1. PEDICULOSIS CAPITIS

Essentials of Diagnosis

- Usually in children.
- Pruritus and crusted excoriations.
- Nits (eggs) on hairs of the posterior scalp.

General Considerations

Pediculosis capitis is a current and possibly growing problem in the USA and other advanced countries. Official reports underestimate the prevalence. In recent years, no area of the USA has been free of pediculosis capitis. Head lice can infest people in all levels of society and most ethnic groups, with the notable exception of the black population of North America (not true in Africa), in which the prevalence is very low.

Persons with head lice are seen more commonly by school nurses, public health personnel, and family physicians and less commonly by dermatologists.

Transmission of pediculosis capitis is most efficient by head-to-head contact. Particularly in the tropics and over most of the USA in the summer months, inanimate objects (shared towels, brushes, and combs) play a significant role. Head lice are more common in girls than in boys, though length of hair is not an important factor. The most common age group for pediculosis capitis is 3–10 years, probably reflecting the greater degree of personal contact and sharing of common items of headgear and grooming aids in these age groups.

Clinical Findings

A. Symptoms and Signs: Head louse infestation is more common in children but occurs also in adults (and sometimes in the elderly). Most cases in schools in the USA are detected by observation of head scratching by one or more children. Newly acquired infestation may produce no symptoms until several weeks have passed—the time required for sensitization.

Well-groomed children with head lice in more economically advanced societies usually have only a dozen or so eggs and rarely more than 20 lice. Brushing and combing of the hair and manual grooming seem to play a role in reducing the number of lice and eggs on such children.

Pediculosis capitis is typically confined to the scalp—particularly the occipital region (Fig 18–5)—and to a lesser extent the postauricular region; it rarely involves the beard or other hairy areas. Erythema and scaling may be present, and there may be linear excoriations at the periphery of the hairy areas. Occasionally, there is an urticarial eruption over the neck and shoulders and a variable maculopapular rash on the trunk resembling German measles. Pruritus of varying degree is a cardinal symptom but does not always occur. Excoriations frequently lead to pyoderma, with the hairs matted by the exudate. Cervical lymphadenopathy (especially posterior) and febrile episodes are not uncommon.

B. Laboratory Findings: As with pubic lice, there are few adult organisms, but there are myriad oval nits (eggs) cemented to the hairs. The diagnosis is confirmed by plucking a hair, placing it on a slide, and studying it under the microscope (Fig 18–6). This differentiates the nits from seborrheic scales, hair casts, and artifacts on the hair (eg, hair spray).

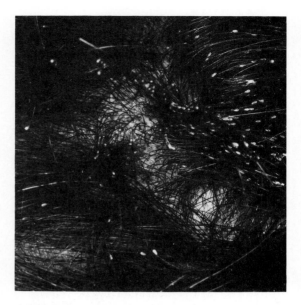

Figure 18–5. Pediculosis capitis. Myriads of nits are attached to hair on occipital scalp. Erythematous, excoriated patches are noted. (Courtesy of Axel Hoke, MD.)

Differential Diagnosis

Pyoderma at the back of the scalp or neck should not be diagnosed until pediculosis capitis has been excluded. Tinea capitis, seborrheic dermatitis, eczema, psoriasis, and contact dermatitis are also differential considerations.

The nits of head and crab lice are firmly cemented to the hair of the host. Unlike dandruff, the egg casings cannot be pulled from the hair by the fingers.

Treatment

A. Principles of Therapy: Other children and adults in the household should be examined, but only those infested need be treated; the exception might be another person who shares a bed with the infested individual. (Some authors suggest routinely treating the entire family simultaneously.)

With any of the specific products listed below, if there is a question about whether the infestation is persisting and the medication is not working or if there is a possibility of resistance, it is valuable to pluck some hairs again and examine them under the microscope to see if any persisting nits are viable. This gives objective evidence of the status of the infestation.

After treatment has been given, infested individuals should put on clean clothing and machine-wash and tumble-dry (hot cycle) all washable clothing, towels, bed linen, and headgear with which they have been in contact. Clothing that is not washable (coats, hats, scarves, sweaters) should be dry-cleaned. Items that can be taken out of use may be placed in plastic

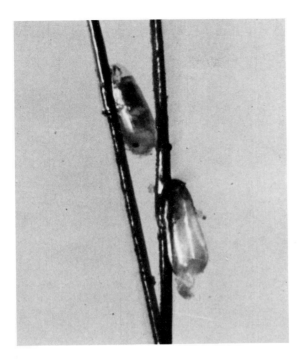

Figure 18–6. Pediculosis capitis. Upper hair shows non-viable nit (empty with operculum raised); lower hair shows intact, viable, unhatched nit (embryo with eye spot and claws). (Courtesy of Professor David Taplin and Terri Meinking. Reproduced, with permission, from Curr Concepts Skin Dis 1989;10:6.)

bags and left in a warm place (75–85 °F) for 2 weeks. Combs and brushes may be washed in hot water (130 °F) for 10–20 minutes. Some authors prefer to coat combs and brushes with the pediculicide for 15 minutes and then wash them in hot soapy water. Floors, play areas, and furniture should be thoroughly vacuumed to remove hairs that may have been shed with viable eggs attached.

B. Specific Pediculocides:

1. Lindane– Lindane shampoo is elegant and simple to use. Physicians should estimate and prescribe the specific amount, specifying "no refills," so that the patient does not utilize the material more frequently than desirable. The patient should shampoo the scalp thoroughly for 4 minutes with 30–40 mL (depending on the thickness of the hair). The hair is then rinsed thoroughly and dried. Remaining nits should be removed with a fine-tooth comb. The shampoo is repeated in 1 week only if viable eggs persist or if new eggs appear at the hair-skin junction. (Some authors routinely prescribe a second treatment in 1 week to kill any newly hatched nymphs.)

Concern has been expressed over the potential for topical lindane products to cause central nervous system toxicity. Most such reports have been related to overuse or accidental ingestion. If it is used as directed, the likelihood of convulsions or clinical signs of central nervous system toxicity following a single treatment with lindane shampoo is remote, but the potential for abuse and overuse exists. Blood levels of lindane increase with repeated use.

Reports of increased tolerance of head lice to lindane have been noted in the UK, Panama, the Netherlands, and Egypt.

Lindane shampoo offers no advantage in pediculocidal or ovicidal activity when compared with several over-the-counter synergized pyrethrin products.

2. Synthetic pyrethroid (1% permethrin cream rinse)– The hair is first shampooed and toweled dry. Sufficient permethrin cream rinse is added to coat the hair thoroughly and is left on for 10 minutes, followed by a clean water rinse. The hair is usually easier to comb after this treatment, and nit removal is facilitated. Combing of the nits is not required but may be done for cosmetic purposes. A single treatment is usually sufficient; residual amounts of medication are bound to the hair.

The product has low mammalian toxicity. It has ovicidal (incomplete) properties. The most frequent adverse reaction is pruritus.

Permethrin 1% cream rinse has been shown to be as effective as or more effective than lindane shampoo in controlled studies in 3 countries.

3. Synergized pyrethrins– Synergized pyrethrins (eg, Rid) are over-the-counter preparations. They should be applied undiluted until the scalp is entirely wet and allowed to remain on the area for 10 minutes. The scalp and head is then washed thoroughly with warm water and shampooed and dried. To remove nits completely, comb the hair with the fine-tooth comb that accompanies the package. A second application is used in 7–10 days to kill any newly hatched nymphs from eggs that may have survived the first treatment.

Note: Some pediculocides contain refined kerosene or distillates that may cause eye irritation. Care must be exercised in the use of these products to avoid contact with the eyes; quickly irrigate the eyes with tap water if accidental contact does occur.

2. PEDICULOSIS PUBIS

Essentials of Diagnosis

- Pruritic eruption of a hairy area, especially pubic hair.
- Nits can be seen clinging to hairs.

General Considerations

Pediculosis pubis has become epidemic in the USA and western Europe. The condition is typically transmitted sexually and frequently coexists with other sexually transmitted diseases, particularly gonorrhea and trichomoniasis and to a lesser extent scabies, nongonococcal urethritis, genital warts, candidiasis, and syphilis. As in gonorrhea, pediculosis pubis is more common in females than in males in persons aged 15–19 years; the sex distribution is reversed in persons over age 20. While pediculosis capitis is far more common in American white children than in black children, there is no racial difference in the distribution of pediculosis pubis in North American adults. Patients with pubic lice are encountered commonly at venereal disease clinics and student health services.

Clinical Findings

When pediculosis pubis involves portions of the body other than the pubic region, the diagnosis may be difficult. This infestation should be suspected in any pruritic eruption of the hairy area. Diagnosis at times may be established more easily by examination of the axillas and locations other than the pubic region, because the patient may already have eradicated the pruritic groin eruption with self-medication prior to consulting the physician but will be less likely to treat other sites.

A. Symptoms and Signs: As the name implies, the most common site affected is the pubic region (Fig 18–7). Although the organisms do not move much from the initial site of contact, involvement may occur, especially in hairy individuals, on the short hairs of the thighs and trunk and occasionally on the beard and moustache.

Involvement of the eyelashes and the periphery of the scalp occurs mainly in children, with transmission likely from close contact with an infested mother; however, this can occur rarely in adults of all ages. Eyelash infestation is particularly difficult to diagnose, because seborrheic or infectious eczematous blepharitis may be simulated; careful examination reveals that the "crust" consists of parasitic organisms. *Pthirus pubis* on the eyelashes or hair of children should alert the physician to the possibility of sexual abuse, but other modes of transmission occur.

Excoriations may lead to pyoderma (which may mask the parasites), with lymphadenitis and febrile episodes. Characteristic but not frequently present are the maculae ceruleae (sky-blue spots)—asymptomatic bluish or slate-colored macules located on the trunk and thighs, fading within short periods.

B. Laboratory Findings: Adult organisms are few. Although initially difficult to observe on the patient, the parasite becomes more discernible after a blood meal, when it becomes rust-colored. The diagnosis is more frequently made by identifying the more numerous nits attached by a cement substance to the pubic hair, initially at the junction with the skin. Because the ova grow out with the hair, the approximate duration of the infestation can be judged by the distance of the ova from the cutaneous surface (also true of pediculosis capitis). Although the nits can be seen with the naked eye, they can be confused with kinks and knots in the hair or flakes of seborrheic dermatitis (which can be brushed off); it is desirable to confirm the diagnosis by plucking the hair, placing it on a slide, and demonstrating the nit under the microscope.

Differential Diagnosis

Common misdiagnoses are pyodermas, impetigo, neurotic excoriations, pruritus vulvae, folliculitis, seborrheic dermatitis, psoriasis, contact dermatitis, seborrheic blepharitis, and atopic blepharitis.

Treatment

A. Principles of Therapy: Treatment preparations are applied to the infested and adjacent hairy areas, with particular attention to the pubic mons and perianal regions. In hairy individuals, applications include the thighs, trunk, and axillary regions because of frequent involvement at these sites. (A common cause of treatment failure is treating only the pubic area in hairy individuals.) Sexual contacts should be treated simultaneously. Other uninfested household members need not be treated. At the conclusion of therapy, infested individuals and sexual partners should use new underclothing, nightwear, sheets and pillowcases, and these articles should be machine-washed and tumble-dried or laundered by boiling and then ironed.

B. Specific Agents: Although extensive comparative studies of pediculicides have not been done, a recent study comparing lindane and synergized

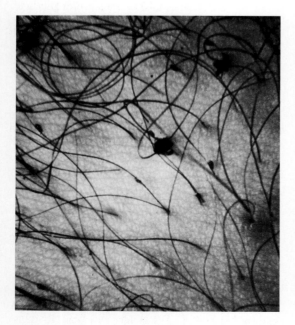

Figure 18–7. Pediculosis pubis. Adult lice are present, as well as numerous nits attached to pubic hair. (Courtesy of Axel Hoke, MD.)

pyrethrins produced similar results in patients with pubic lice.

No resistance of pubic lice to insecticides has been noted. Therapeutic inefficiency is usually due to failure to follow instructions, neglecting to treat sexual contacts, or reinfestation. Persistent itching may be caused by irritation of the pediculicide (usually too frequent use) or patient anxiety. Parasitophobia is fairly common and difficult to deal with.

1. Lindane– Lindane shampoo should be lathered into the affected sites for 5 minutes, then rinsed thoroughly and towel-dried. The remaining nits should be removed with a fine-tooth comb or forceps. One application is usually sufficient; the second application is repeated in 1 week if viable eggs persist or if new eggs appear at the hair-skin junction. (Some authors routinely prescribe a second treatment in 1 week to kill any newly hatched nymphs.)

2. Synergized pyrethrins– Synergized pyrethrins (eg, Rid) are over-the-counter products that appear to be safe and effective in the treatment of lice infestations. They are applied undiluted until the infested areas are entirely wet and allowed to remain in place for 10 minutes; then the area is washed thoroughly with warm water and shampooed and dried. A fine-tooth comb (provided in some trade packages) permits removal of dead lice and eggs. A second application is used in 7–10 days to kill any newly hatched nymphs from eggs that may have survived the first treatment.

C. Eyelash Involvement: Therapy for eyelash involvement consists of applying petrolatum thickly twice daily for 8 days, followed by manual removal of any remaining nits.

3. PEDICULOSIS CORPORIS

Essentials of Diagnosis

- Purpura at site of bites.
- Vertical excoriations, especially on trunk and neck.
- Crusted papules.
- Postinflammatory hyperpigmentation.
- Nits in seams of clothing.

General Considerations

The prevalence of pediculosis corporis does not seem to be changing. It is rare in the Western World except in indigent vagabonds and those with low intelligence and poor hygiene. The infestation is transmitted chiefly by contaminated clothing or bedding. It is treated mainly in public hospitals.

Clinical Findings

Early lesions consist of hemorrhagic macules or papules at the site where the louse punctures the skin to obtain blood. The characteristic eruption, however, consists of numerous vertical excoriations due to intense itching, especially on the trunk and neck. Crusts and, at times, pus or serum may stain the underclothing. Transitory wheals and bacterial infections may complicate the process. Postinflammatory pigmentation is common. The pigmentation of "vagabond's disease" may be due to heavy infestation with body lice but also to poor nutrition, poor hygiene, and scratching.

There are few or no adult organisms; numerous nits are found in seams of clothing (particularly around the armpits, the belt line, and collars), where they cling while feeding on the human host. Parasites may be absent from the body except in heavily infested persons.

Treatment

Therapy consists mainly of proper hygiene, bathing, use of clean underclothing and bedding, and proper nutrition. Previously used underclothing and bedding should be laundered with hot water or boiled. Dry cleaning destroys lice on wool garments. Pressing woolens at home is also satisfactory, but special attention should be paid to the seams.

Lindane lotion may be applied as a single treatment from head to toe and left on for 8 hours, then washed off thoroughly. All likely contacts (members of the household, close contacts in institutions) should be examined and treated if there is evidence of infestation.

The body louse has been shown to be resistant to lindane, DDT, and malathion in other countries but not as yet in the USA.

REFERENCES

Buck AA (editor): *Onchocerciasis: Symptomatology, Pathology, Diagnosis.* World Health Organization, 1974.

Ciba Foundation Symposium 20: *Trypanosomiasis and Leishmaniasis, With Special Reference to Chagas' Disease.* Excerpta Medica, 1974.

Drugs for parasitic infections. Med Lett Drugs Ther 1988;30:15.

Duke B: Treatment of onchocerciasis. Pages 46–52 in: *Research and Control of Onchocerciasis in the Western Hemisphere.* Pan American Health Organization, 1974.

Epstein E Sr, Orkin M: Scabies: Clinical aspects. In: *Cutaneous Infestations and Insect Bites.* Orkin M, Maibach HI (editors). Marcel Dekker, 1985.

Font RL, Neafie RC, Perry HD: Subcutaneous dirofilariasis of the eyelid and ocular adnexa: Report of six cases. Arch Ophthalmol 1980;98:1079.

Fujita WH, Barr RJ, Gottschalk HR: Cutaneous amebiasis. Arch Dermatol 1981;117:309.

Gratz NG: The current status of louse infestations throughout the world: The control of lice and louse-borne diseases. In: *Proceedings of the International Symposium on the Control of Lice and Louse-Borne Diseases.* Pan American Health Organization, 1973.

Grove DI, Warren KS, Mahmoud AA: Algorithms in the diagnosis and management of exotic diseases. 6. The filariases. J Infect Dis 1975;132:340.

Hawking F: Diethylcarbamazine and new compounds for the treatment of filariasis. Adv Pharmacol Chemother 1979;16:129.

Hubler WR Jr et al: Loaiasis: A case report and review of the literature. Arch Dermatol 1973;108:835.

Immunology of Chagas' disease. Bull WHO 1974;50:459.

Katz R, Ziegler J, Blank H: The natural course of creeping eruption and treatment with thiabendazole. Arch Dermatol 1965;91:420.

Kirschenbaum MB: Swimmer's itch: A review and case report. Cutis 1979;23:212.

Manson-Bahr PE, Bell DR (editors): *Manson's Tropical Diseases,* 19th ed. Bailliére Tindall, 1987.

Marsden PD: Current concepts in parasitology: Leishmaniasis. N Engl J Med 1979;300:350.

Moschella SL, Hurley HJ (editors): *Dermatology,* 2nd ed. Saunders, 1985.

Muller R: Guinea worm disease: Epidemiology, control, and treatment. Bull WHO 1979;57:683.

Orkin M: Special forms of scabies. In: *Cutaneous Infestations and Insect Bites.* Orkin M, Maibach HI (editors). Marcel Dekker, 1985.

Orkin M, Epstein E, Maibach HI: Treatment of today's scabies and pediculosis. JAMA 1976;236:1136.

Orkin M, Maibach HI: Scabies. In: *Sexually Transmitted Diseases,* 2nd ed. Holmes KK et al (editors). McGraw-Hill, 1990.

Orkin M, Maibach HI: Treatment of today's pediculosis. Pages 213–217 in: *Cutaneous Infestations and Insect Bites.* Marcel Dekker, 1985.

Osment LS: Update: Seabather's eruption and swimmer's itch. Cutis 1976;18:545.

Sacks HN, Williams DN, Eifrig DE: Loiasis: Report of a case and review of the literature. Arch Intern Med 1976;136:914.

Smith JD, Goette DK, Odom RB: Larva currens: Cutaneous strongyloidiasis. Arch Dermatol 1976;112:1161.

Stone OJ: Systemic and topical thiabendazole for creeping eruption. Tex Rep Biol Med 1969;27(Suppl 2):659.

Taplin D, Meinking T: Infestations. Pages 1465–1515 in: *Pediatric Dermatology.* Churchill Livingstone, 1988.

Taplan D, Meinking TL, Porcelain SL: Permethrin 5% dermal cream: A new treatment for scabies. J Am Acad Dermatol 1986;15:995.

Taylor HR, Greene BM, Langham ME: Controlled clinical trial of oral and topical diethylcarbamazine in treatment of onchocerciasis. Lancet 1980;1:943.

Torres VM: Dermatologic manifestations of *Schistosoma mansoni.* Arch Dermatol 1976;112:1539.

Warren KS, Mahmoud AA: Algorithms in the diagnosis and management of exotic diseases. 5. Enterobiasis. J Infect Dis 1975;132:229.

Woody NC, Woody HG: American trypanosomiasis. J Pediatr 1961;58:568.

Zinsser H: *Rats, Life, and History.* Little, Brown, 1935.

Dermatoses Caused by Animals & Arthropods

19

Karen C. McKoy, MD & Samuel L. Moschella, MD

Animals and bugs may injure the skin by biting, stinging, or in other ways. Injury results from trauma or from chemical reactions, including both toxic and immunologic forms of inflammation. In most cases the diagnosis is obvious and treatment not necessary. In others, the severity of the reaction, the possible transmission of infectious agents, or the possibility of parasitosis dictates specific therapeutic interventions. Since the skin is the site of attack, it is the organ most commonly affected. Dermatologists as well as other physicians may be consulted.

I. ARTHROPODS

No group of animals has been more successful in evolving vast numbers of species than the arthropods; their extraordinarily diverse members have tormented humankind for ages.

Arthropods are inimical to humans in the following ways.

1. They serve as vectors or intermediate hosts for viral, bacterial, rickettsial, and parasitic diseases.

2. They cause envenomation by injection of poisonous or allergenic substances.

3. They infect with larvae. For example, fly larvae may take up residence in human skin (myiasis).

4. They cause dermatoses by living parasitically in or on the skin (pediculosis, scabies) or through transient contacts in which the host is bitten, provoking reactions of irritation or hypersensitivity.

5. Secondary infection with bacteria is a frequent complication of insect bites.

The phylum Arthropoda includes numerous species; only those of significant dermatologic importance are considered here.

DISORDERS DUE TO ARACHNIDS

The 3 medically important orders of the class Arachnida include scorpions, spiders, ticks, and mites.

SCORPIONS

Essentials of Diagnosis
- History of scorpion bite.
- Local pain, edema, and erythema.
- Occasional systemic symptoms.

General Considerations
Scorpions are found in tropical and subtropical areas of the world; of the many species, only a few inject sufficient venom to cause concern. Venomous species are found in arid areas of the southwestern USA and Mexico (*Centruroides* spp). Death from a scorpion sting is rare in the USA but common in Mexico, usually in children. Scorpion venoms are complex mixtures of peptides producing neurotoxic, cardiotoxic, and hemolytic effects. Scorpions feed at night on insects and hide during the day in moist, cool, shady places beneath stones and logs or in crevices in the ground or walls; in houses, they may rest in shoes or clothing.

Clinical Findings
Manifestations vary according to the scorpion species. Most scorpions produce only local pain, edema, and erythema of variable degree. Local reactions are not prominent when the scorpion is of a neurotoxic species. Necrosis of skin may rarely occur. Systemic reactions may include signs of sympathetic nervous

system stimulation (restlessness, roving eye movements, hypertension, nausea, abdominal cramps, salivation, sweating, and convulsions), bradycardia, respiratory depression, electrocardiographic changes, pulmonary edema, disseminated intravascular coagulopathy, pancreatitis, and hemolysis.

Treatment

Local treatment is rarely necessary. Pain may be relieved with topical lidocaine ointment. Intermittent applications of ice packs may alleviate pain. Early administration of specific antivenom has been advocated. Morphine and opiates are contraindicated, as they may increase venom toxicity. Hypnotic doses of barbiturates can prevent death from convulsions but may intensify respiratory depression.

SPIDERS

Two species are responsible for most of the serious spider bites in the USA: widow spiders (*Latrodectus*) and the nocturnal band-spinning spiders (*Loxosceles*).

1. WIDOW SPIDERS

Essentials of Diagnosis
- Transient local pain.
- Rapid onset of systemic symptoms (muscle cramps, sweating, nausea).
- History of spider bite (may not be noticed).

General Considerations

Latrodectus envenomation of humans is a medical problem in many parts of the world. Widow spiders are recognized by the black, gray, or brown globose abdomen with a ventral red, orange, or yellow hourglass marking. Female bodies are about 12 mm long; the males are smaller. Of principal importance, the black widow spider, *Latrodectus mactans,* is found over most of the USA, frequenting stone walls, trash piles, barns, and outdoor toilets.

Clinical Findings

The bite may not be noticed; local moderate burning pain usually develops and disappears promptly. Symptoms of general toxemia appear after a short latent period (usually about 10 minutes). The most characteristic symptoms are muscle spasms and cramps, particularly of the abdomen, legs, chest, and back. The marked abdominal rigidity may simulate acute appendicitis, a perforated ulcer, or other abdominal emergency. Other symptoms and signs include cutaneous hyperactive tendon reflexes, headache, sweating, and nausea. Eyelid edema and a diffuse macular rash may be seen. Acute symptoms last 24–48 hours. The bite may be fatal in the very young or old or in those with hypertension.

Treatment

Intravenous calcium gluconate (10 mL of 10% solution) is usually effective in relieving muscle cramps, but its action is brief. Other muscle relaxants such as methocarbamol give longer relief. Specific antivenom, if given promptly, relieves symptoms and speeds recovery.

**2. *LOXOSCELES*
(Brown Recluse Spider Family)**

Essentials of Diagnosis
- Small papules to large necrotic ulcer.
- Systemic reactions may occur (hemolysis, nausea, fever).
- History of bite by brown spider with violin-shaped markings.

General Considerations

Two species of *Loxosceles*, one in South America (*Loxosceles laeta*) and the other in the USA (*Loxosceles reclusa*), cause necrotic arachnidism with extensive gangrenous sloughing at the bite site; this may be accompanied by systemic signs and symptoms.

L reclusa (the Missouri brown spider), reported from nearly half the United States, is most numerous in central and south central USA. These secretive spiders hide in storage spaces, under boxes, in closets, and behind clothing and pictures hanging against walls. The 10- to 15-mm long yellow-brown spider is identified by the dark brown violin-shaped marking extending from the eyes posteriorly on the cephalothorax. Venoms of the recluse spiders possess dermonecrotic and hemolytic activity.

Clinical Findings

A. Symptoms and Signs: Reactions to the brown spider bite are extremely variable, probably reflecting the amount of venom injected, the patient's age, and the immune and medical status of the patient. Two basic reactions occur: (1) cutaneous injury, from a small papule to a huge necrotic ulcer; and (2) a systemic reaction consisting of intravascular hemolysis, hemoglobinuria, renal failure, and anemia, which may develop within the first 48 hours after envenomation. Nausea, vomiting, fever, and severe malaise may be present. Severe systemic reactions with death are most frequent in children. Fortunately, severe envenomation is rare; nearly all brown recluse spider bites have a benign course.

The local cutaneous reaction may be minor, with mild pruritus and an urticarial plaque or with a small area of necrosis resolving spontaneously within 3–5 days. In patients who presumably have more venom injected, a more severe reaction occurs. A blue-gray halo of vasoconstriction is initially present at the puncture site; after 12–18 hours, a small blister develops, with a surrounding zone of erythema and edema. The blister ruptures, and the erythema becomes violaceous; after 5–7 days, the skin becomes necrotic and the base forms a thick black eschar that separates slowly over several weeks. A generalized transient, erythematous macular rash may develop with mild or severe bites.

B. Laboratory Findings: Specific diagnosis is made by identification of the spider. The lymphocyte blast transformation test using venom antigen offers confirmatory evidence 4–6 weeks after envenomation; a serodiagnostic test has been described for earlier diagnosis.

Treatment

Optimal therapy for necrotic arachnidism is not established. Small bites usually require no more than cold compresses, elevation, control of pain, tetanus prophylaxis, and reassurance. Dapsone, 100–200 mg/d, may help prevent necrosis. Although corticosteroids are often used for larger lesions, their efficacy is not proved. Antibiotics may prevent secondary infection. Heparin may benefit the rare patient with disseminated intravascular coagulation. Local excision of necrotic bite areas over 1 cm has been suggested, but wound healing is often impaired, and the overall clinical result may be worse.

TICKS

Essentials of Diagnosis

- Asymptomatic or mildly pruritic papules.
- Occasionally, persistent nodules.
- History of tick bite at site.

General Considerations

Ticks are more important as vectors than as primary causes of skin disease. They may transmit Rocky Mountain spotted fever and related rickettsioses, tick-borne relapsing fever, Lyme disease (see Chapter 35), Colorado tick fever, tularemia, and other diseases.

Clinical Findings

The tick feeds by embedding its head into the skin, an act that ordinarily goes unnoticed. The parasite becomes enormously engorged with blood, swells to many times its normal size, and remains in situ for days. Occasionally—most often in children and infants—the feeding tick releases a toxin that causes a progressive ascending lower motor neuron paralysis which resolves promptly when the parasite is removed. A generalized urticaria associated with toxic symptoms sometimes develops.

Ordinarily, no harm is done by the tick bite, but

persistent dermal nodules or papules (0.5–2.5 cm in diameter) occasionally develop. These reactions are more likely to follow attempts at forced removal, which detaches the head of the tick, leaving the mandibles as a foreign body in the skin. Other cutaneous reactions include papular urticaria-like lesions due to multiple bites, patchy scalp alopecia following a bite, painful local edema, ecchymosis and ulceration (with species of *Ornithodoros*), and erythema chronicum migrans (in Lyme disease).

Treatment

Excision of nodules is often necessary. Persistent bite reactions, however, have occurred despite excision.

Removal of ticks requires care. Time-honored methods include touching the tick with a lighted match or cigarette, or applying gasoline, kerosene, camphorated phenol, 0.6% pyrethrins in methyl benzoate, or soft paraffin, which irritate the tick so much that it withdraws its head. Gently pulling on the tick parallel to its long axis can often remove it intact.

Among the better tick repellents are diethyltoluamide, butopyronoxyl, and benzyl benzoate.

MITES

There are more than 30,000 species of mites; most are free-living, but many parasitize plants, animals, and occasionally humans. Mites have been associated with transmission of disease (scrub typhus, rickettsialpox, murine typhus, and, rarely, tularemia and plague), allergic rhinitis, asthma, and eczema (house dust mite), and dermatitis.

Mites of dermatologic importance include (1) the sarcoptic mites, including human and animal scabies (see Chapter 18); (2) the trombiculid (harvest) mites; and (3) a large group of "fortuitous" mites, normally present on animals or food products, which may take up temporary residence on human skin.

Human scabies is discussed in Chapter 18. Animal scabies and other mites are discussed below.

ANIMAL SCABIES

Essentials of Diagnosis

- Small crusted pruritic papules.
- No burrows.
- Lesions resolve when infested pets are removed or treated.

General Considerations

Parasites closely related to the human scabies mite cause scabies in a host of animals. Under conditions of intimate contact, humans may suffer a self-limited but uncomfortable eruption. Humans are not a suitable host, and parasites do not become firmly entrenched. Domestic animals that may become infested with *Sarcoptes scabiei* include swine, cattle, horses, mules, sheep, camels, goats, and dogs. *Cheyletiella* species (nonburrowing mites) infesting dogs, cats, and rabbits have been increasingly recognized as a source of human skin disease. The most commonly encountered problems are those with canine scabies and *Cheyletiella* species.

Clinical Findings

In canine scabies, lesions in the dog are variable and characterized by small reddish papules, scaling, crusting, and lichenification. There may be spotty areas of hair loss due to rubbing. The eruption is usually most severe on the ears, elbows, and axillary and inguinal areas. Humans in contact with the dog develop small crusted papules particularly on the forearms, abdomen, and lower legs; children may show facial lesions. Vesicular or urticarial lesions may occur.

The signs of *Cheyletiella* infestation in animals are often subtle, with only a tendency to dandruff and skin hyperesthesia and pruritus. Not all persons exposed develop cutaneous lesions. In about one-third of infected patients, a characteristic response pattern may be seen of crops of small red macules that develop into 2- to 4-mm papules that become vesicular and then crusted; old lesions may show a central area of necrosis. Lesions occur on the arms, neck, and trunk, discretely or in groups. Individual lesions resolve in about 3 weeks, but pigmentary changes may remain for 3–6 months. Other cutaneous reactions include papular urticaria, bullae, generalized pruritus, urticaria, and lesions simulating erythema multiforme and dermatitis herpetiformis. Mites are rarely demonstrable on patients.

Treatment

Human disease remits upon removal or treatment of the pet with various pesticides. A veterinarian should be consulted. Patients may be treated symptomatically with antihistamines. In *Cheyletiella* infestations, the animal's bedding must also be disinfested.

HARVEST MITE

Essentials of Diagnosis

- Itchy papules of legs, belt line, and pressure areas of clothing.
- Usually affect people who live in or visit rural areas.

General Considerations

The family Trombiculidae has many members with worldwide distribution, but in the USA only a few species are important. *Eutrombicula alfreddugési,* the common chigger (red bug, harvest mite), is particularly prevalent in the southern United States during summer and fall. The parasites live on grasses, shrubs, vines, and stems of grains; they infest farmers, hunters, berry pickers, harvesters, and others in rural enterprises. The larvae do not burrow into the skin but partake of a blood meal, falling off when engorged.

Clinical Findings

Lesions are most abundant on the legs above the shoes but also at the belt line and in other areas of pressure from clothing. Papules form in a few hours; they are notoriously itchy and often enlarge to form nodules. Sometimes the red mites can be seen in the center of the lesions, but usually they drop off after inflammation begins. In severe cases, an "id" reaction of eczematous lesions ensues, complicating the picture. The lesions regress slowly in a week or two.

Prevention

If exposure is anticipated, the skin should be covered with tightly woven clothing, snug at the wrists and ankles. Insect repellents may help to prevent bites. Protection from the chiggers may be obtained by treating the clothing with dimethyl phthalate, ethohexadiol, diethyltoluamide, or any agent used for protection against ticks.

Treatment

Treatment consists of local antipruritic agents and corticosteroids and occasionally systemic steroids.

FORTUITOUS MITES

Numerous species of animal, grain, and food mites may cause transient symptoms in humans. The most commonly encountered in the USA include the tropical rat mite *(Ornithonyssus bacoti),* avian mites *(Dermanyssus gallinae),* and the grain itch mite *(Pyemotes tritici).* Lesions are typically papules or wheals, often surmounted by vesicles or a slight crust, frequently grouped like other insect bites. Eruptions are self-limited. Palliation may be obtained with antipruritic medications. Insect repellents offer some protection when impregnated in clothing.

INSECTS

Of the many orders of insects, only a few have significance for dermatologists. These are (1) Diptera (flies), (2) Siphonaptera (fleas), (3) Hymenoptera (bees and wasps), (4) Anoplura (lice) (see Chapter 18), (5) Hemiptera (bugs), (6) Coleoptera (beetles), and (7) Lepidoptera (butterflies and moths).

Individuals vary widely in their responses to the bite of a particular insect, but for the most part the bites of different species have a high degree of similarity. It is difficult—often impossible—to determine the responsible species from the appearance of the lesion. There are, however, important clues that a particular eruption is probably the work of an insect.

In this section, biting insects are considered—those that produce reactions chiefly through substances contained in the saliva and those that elicit reactions in other ways, such as stinging (bees and wasps) or releasing irritant body fluids (blister beetles, moths, and caterpillars). Mites, ticks, and spiders are not insects and are considered elsewhere.

Generally speaking, chemicals contained in the salivary fluids of common pests (mosquitoes, fleas, bedbugs, lice, etc) are not very toxic; individuals bitten for the first time respond mildly or not at all. The increasingly severe and often highly troublesome reactions that emerge as individuals continue to be bitten are hypersensitivity reactions. Allergens in the saliva are responsible, and sensitization evolves in stages. The large amount of information on mosquito bite reactions is presented as an example.

Following the initial bite, there is an incubation period during which sensitization develops, ranging from 1 week to several weeks depending on the frequency of exposure. The delayed papular reaction (tuberculin type response) is the first expression of hypersensitivity. With continued biting, the pattern of reaction evolves. An immediate wheal appears within a few minutes after the bite, followed by the delayed papular reaction 24–72 hours later. As biting continues and sensitization deepens, this transitional stage combining the immediate and delayed reactions gives way to a stage in which the bite produces only an immediate wheal. Individuals arrested in the transitional stage of this progression are the ones in whom insect bites produce papular urticaria. Complete desensitization occurs occasionally in individuals who continue to be bitten massively over years by fleas, mosquitoes, biting flies, chiggers, etc. Such individuals do not react to insect bites. The tolerance is maintained only as long as the individual continues to be bitten; reactivity returns when exposure stops.

Although insect bite reactions are generally transient, papules and nodules occasionally persist for long periods, sometimes as a result of unrestrained scratching, being essentially a neurodermatitis initiated by the bite. Sometimes the protracted irritation is a foreign body reaction due to some portion of the biting apparatus left in the skin. The response to bites is somewhat dependent upon the body site—those on the lower legs tending to be worse and more persistent.

Even without the obscuring influences of scratching and eczematization, the diagnosis of insect bites is not always obvious. Not only do reactions to the same insect show great individual variation, but a legion of different insects may prey on the skin. Knowledge of local fauna, the recent work and play situations of the patient, the degree of domestic cleanliness, and the presence of similar eruptions among intimate contacts may provide clues. Flying insects (mosquitoes) attack exposed parts. Crawling ones (fleas, bedbugs) attack almost any area but frequently choose those where their movement is obstructed by clothing. The bites may be single, with no tendency toward grouping, as with mosquitoes that feed at one spot until satiated, or in clusters, as with fleas and bedbugs that prefer to sample different spots, taking a small meal at each. The most frequent lesions produced by insects are discrete papules and wheals, often having a central punctum; however, intensely inflammatory bullae occasionally develop, as well as hemorrhagic papules, nodules, and ulcers. The histologic variability of insect bite reactions matches the wide clinical spectrum. Sometimes insect bites even suggest lymphomas or granulomas.

General Principles of Treatment of Insect Bites

Therapy is directed at protection from bites, relief of pruritus, and control of secondary infection.

Itching is the primary complaint. Simple applications of topical preparations containing menthol, phenol, or camphor may give temporary relief, as may oral antihistamines. Topical steroids may help inhibit the hypersensitivity reaction to bites. Patients with multiple bites and a severe reaction may require bed rest and a short course of systemic steroids. Secondary infection may be controlled with topical or oral antibiotics.

Prevention of bites is the most effective therapy. If the patient is unable to identify the offending insect, its identity may be suspected from the location and grouping of bites, a knowledge of the patient's environment, and a familiarity with the local insect fauna. Examination of brushings from the patient's clothing, pets, and house may help. An empirical disinfestation routine with the help of local pest exterminators may produce dramatic results even if the source of infestation is not apparent. The habits and life cycles of suspected insects should be kept in mind when selecting insecticides and locations for their use.

Insect Repellents

In cases in which it is impossible to limit exposure to insects, application of insect repellents to the skin may offer temporary protection. Insect repellents differ from insecticides in that they do not kill insects but discourage them from biting or landing on protected areas. A good repellent should be nontoxic, nonirritant, nonallergenic, harmless to clothing, without an offensive odor, easily applied, inexpensive, and effective against multiple insects; it should also offer protection for several hours under variable weather conditions. The ideal repellent has not yet been developed, but research during World War II provided a number of effective agents.

The most effective insect repellent is diethyltoluamide. Others include dimethyl phthalate, ethohexadiol, butopyronoxyl, and benzyl benzoate (primarily for clothing). A combination of 2 or 3 repellents may be more effective than one. All repellents may damage paints, varnishes, and some plastics to varying degrees; some will damage synthetic cloth (rayon but not nylon), fingernail polish, or plastic watch crystals. Ethohexadiol is the least injurious in this respect. Most repellents are toxic if taken internally but safe if used as recommended. Some may cause contact dermatitis; most cause discomfort when applied to mucous membranes.

Repellents are effective only when present on the skin and clothing in relatively large quantities. It is critical that all exposed areas be coated with repellent; nontreated areas a few centimeters away may be bitten. The use of clothing repellents does not eliminate the need for skin application.

PAPULAR URTICARIA

Papular urticaria is a misnomer, since the primary lesion is a papule rather than a wheal. The disorder is caused by a hypersensitivity reaction to insect bites—especially to those of fleas of dogs, cats, humans, and birds and less commonly to those of bedbugs, mosquitoes, and dog lice.

Atopic children aged 2–7 years are chiefly affected; the disease is rare in the newborn and uncommon in adults. The lesions may appear anywhere but tend to be distributed on exposed areas, especially the face and extensor surfaces of the extremities. They may or may not be grouped.

The characteristic lesions are papules, but even more definitive transitional forms suggest a combination of a wheal and a papule. The lesions are usually not numerous but evolve into inflammatory, increasingly hard, red or brownish, persistent papules. As with other types of insect bites, highly sensitized persons may present, in addition, vesicles and bullae. Bacterial superinfection and excoriations often obscure the primary lesions.

Practitioners who live in flea-infested areas have no hesitation in making a diagnosis of flea bites when confronted with a case of papular urticaria. In the eastern USA, the disorder occurs almost exclusively in the summer, when insect life flourishes, but on the West Coast the disorder tends to occur throughout the year. When carefully questioned, many patients remember having been bitten. Persons in the lower eco-

nomic strata are the principal victims, owing to a higher exposure to fleas and bedbugs. Bites of chiggers, flies, and mosquitoes can also cause papular urticaria.

MOSQUITOES & FLIES (Order Diptera)

By sheer numbers of species and the extraordinary variety of means of contributing, directly or indirectly, to human disease or discomfort, this group dominates all others in medical importance. Flies attack skin in one of 2 ways: (1) The adults bite to obtain nourishment, releasing toxins and allergens that incite inflammatory lesions, and (2) the larvae or grubs establish themselves within the skin, producing the offensive maggot infestation myiasis.

1. THE BITING DIPTERA

Family Ceratopogonidae (Heleidae)

Known variously as "no-see-ums," midges, or punkies because of their extraordinarily small size (1–5 mm), species of the genus *Culicoides* are the most important pests of this family. In the southern United States bordering the Atlantic Ocean and the Gulf of Mexico, life may be made miserable on warm evenings because of the ability of these insects to slip through wire mesh. The bites cause intense itching and papular or vesicular reactions that may persist for days.

Family Simuliidae

These small (1- to 5-mm) humpbacked flies (black flies, buffalo gnats, turkey gnats) are distributed throughout the world. They are vicious biters, attacking all exposed areas;, some species are particularly dreaded because of a preference for the eyes, ears, and nostrils. The ensuing lesions are painful and often attended by considerable swelling, at times face-distorting. Fever and intestinal reactions may add to the victim's distress. Ulceration may be a complication. A swarm can kill domestic and game animals. Black flies may appear in enormous numbers in subarctic and north temperate climates. They are most numerous in areas of rapidly flowing streams, where breeding occurs. Some species serve as vectors for onchocerciasis.

Family Psychodidae (Sand Flies)

Species of the genus *Phlebotomus* are of great medical importance, serving as vectors of kala-azar, cutaneous leishmaniasis, and Carrión's disease. They confine their biting to the night. By preference, they attack the ankles, wrists, knees, and elbows. Numerous bites may cause constitutional reactions. A polymorphous eruption called harara or urticaria multiformis endemica is seen in infants and adults newly arrived in Israel or neighboring countries. The lesions, like most insect bites, represent hypersensitivity reactions; after patients are in the area for a while, spontaneous desensitization may take place, providing immunity. The lesions consist variously of firm red papules, vesicles, urticoid wheals, and papular wheals, mostly on the exposed parts, resembling papular urticaria. Impetiginization is common, as is hemorrhage into the blisters.

Family Culicidae
(Mosquitoes)

In any competition for honors conferred for causing human misery, mosquitoes must receive serious consideration. There are 2600 species with worldwide distribution. Their biting habits make them intolerable pests and transmitters of human diseases. Mosquitoes are able to bite through thin, loosely woven clothing; they are attracted by warmth, moisture, and dark clothing. Human sweat may release substances attractive to mosquitoes; anhidrotic patients are less attractive. Bites tend to be irregularly distributed over exposed areas; reactions vary in severity depending on the sensitivity of the patient.

2. CUTANEOUS MYIASIS
(Disorders Due to Infestation of
the Skin by Diptera Larvae)

Myiasis is uncommon in areas of high standards of personal hygiene. Fly larvae may infest not only the skin but also the gastrointestinal and genitourinary tracts, usually accidentally, as well as the eyes, nose, and ears. For certain species such as the human botfly to complete their life cycle, the larvae must spend a certain period in the tissues of an animal host, a condition of obligate parasitism known as **specific myiasis.** Others, such as flesh flies, can develop in living or in nonliving tissue, depending on opportunity **(semispecific myiasis).**

Cutaneous myiasis may be migratory or nonmigratory. In the former, the larvae wander in the tissues, exciting a mobile pattern of inflammation corresponding to the parasites' migrations. In nonmigratory myiasis, the larvae produce a fixed lesion. The larvae may either burrow into normal skin or infest an antecedent wound, ulcer, or draining lesion. The maggots do not necessarily do any harm but may "clean up" the wound. In preantibiotic days, maggots were deliberately introduced into necrotic foci, such as osteomyelitic lesions, for purposes of debridement.

Myiasis Due to Family
Gasterophilidae (Botflies)

The larvae of botflies of horses and asses normally live in the gastrointestinal tract. On occasion, especially in warmer climates, flies lay eggs on human skin; the emerging larvae burrow into the skin, wandering about producing a pattern simulating classic creeping eruption due to dog hookworm. Botfly larvae may survive for months in human skin, creating a tortuous, telltale inflammatory ridge or line marking their migrations. The important causative species belong to the genus *Gasterophilus*, especially *Gasterophilus intestinalis*. A drop of mineral oil just in advance of the visible line of inflammation generally reveals the parasite. Surgical extraction of botfly larvae with a sharp needle is then easily accomplished.

Myiasis Due to Family Oestridae
(Botflies)

The larval stages ordinarily attack animals—cattle most commonly, humans rarely. The human botfly, *Dermatobia hominis,* a native of Central and South America, causes a characteristic fixed form of myiasis. The eggs reach human skin indirectly, being deposited there by some carrier insect, mosquitoes or other flies, to whose abdomens the female *Dermatobia* has fastened her eggs. After hatching, the larvae descend into the skin. Entrance of the larvae into the skin is usually not perceived, but following a week of pruritus, a serous exudate appears and a furunclelike lesion gradually evolves, becoming painful by about the fourth week. The swelling is typically open at the top, from which a serous or suppurative exudate issues continuously. The lesion may continue to expand, attaining 2.5 cm or so in diameter. After 2–3 months of comfortable development within the skin, the larvae, considerably fatter and larger, forsake the lesion and drop to the ground to pupate. This painless process is followed by spontaneous involution of the lesion.

Muscle stiffness and soreness are a frequent complaint, sometimes associated with drowsiness. Movements of the larvae within the lesion may produce excruciating pain. Local tissue necrosis may be massive, with associated lymphangitis and regional adenitis.

Treatment consists of incising the lesion and removing the larvae with forceps.

Usually the maggots of the head botfly of sheep, *Oestrus ovis,* work their way into the nasal and frontal sinuses of sheep and goats, but on occasion the adult flies deposit larvae in the human eye, producing ophthalmomyiasis that may lead to loss of vision. This disorder is relatively common among shepherds of Middle Eastern countries. The head botfly of horses and asses in Europe, Africa, and Asia causes a similar condition.

Human infestation from cattle botflies or ox warbles is rare but distressing. The larvae are restless and nomadic, wandering deeply in the skin but generally upward. The chief signs of infestation are muscle soreness and swellings, sometimes hernialike, shifting from place to place in accordance with the capricious larval movements. Larvae inadvertently approaching the surface become sluggish. Perforation of the skin permits removal of the parasite. Surgical extirpation is the treatment of choice.

Family Calliphoridae (Blowflies)

Cordylobia anthropophaga (the tumbu fly), confined to Africa, produces furunclelike lesions similar to those caused by the human botfly. Children are more affected than adults. Tumbu fly myiasis can occur in any part of the body. Early removal of larvae is best done surgically and later by manual extraction after the application of mineral oil.

Species of *C* occur in the Western Hemisphere, where their larvae are known as screwworms. *Cochliomyia hominivorax*, the outstanding screwworm of animals and humans in the southern USA and South American tropics, is the most important though not the commonest species. Infestation may be serious, causing some deaths. The adult flies are attracted by an open wound or discharging orifice, particularly the nose. The larvae, unable to penetrate intact human skin, get their start in diseased tissue; however, they do not remain in such necrotic foci but burrow deeply into living tissue, even cartilage and bone. Infestations of the nose and ears are dangerous owing to the possibility of penetration of the brain. Deep suppurative lesions of an extremely malodorous nature are typical. Localization within the nose is most common, causing swelling and intense pain, together with a sensation of "crawling." Mature larvae are about 20 mm in length and may usually be seen if looked for carefully. The larvae may be removed by forceps under local anesthesia.

FLEAS (Order Siphonaptera)

The order Siphonaptera contains 2 families of dermatologic importance: (1) Members of Pulicidae are responsible for bothersome flea bites, a frequent cause of papular urticaria; and (2) The family Tungidae is represented by the chigoe flea, *Tunga penetrans.* Fleas of other families may serve as vectors for plague and murine typhus.

Members of the family Pulicidae include the ubiquitous human flea, *Pulex irritans;* the cat and dog fleas, *Ctenocephalides felis* and *Ctenocephalides*

canis; and a number of other species parasitizing other mammals and sometimes birds. All of these species are capable of feeding on humans. Adult fleas are amazingly hardy and can live for several months without taking a blood meal. Eggs are laid in cracks between floor boards or in dusty areas. Larval periods vary in duration, and pupae can remain viable for months. Eradication efforts must be directed against both larval and adult stages. *Pulex irritans* inhabits crevices in floors and walls, furniture, refuse heaps, sand, and earth.

The human flea is a wingless, reddish brown insect, 2–4 mm long. The flea likes to sample several adjacent spots while feeding, so that bites typically occur in clusters. The lesions are usually wheals and papules and various transitional forms combining the features of both, depending on the stage of sensitization of the host. The wheals may even evolve into bullae in highly susceptible persons, and in extreme sensitivity, ulceration may occur. Impetiginization from scratching and bacterial infection with lymphangitis are possible sequelae. In the center of the urticarial lesions, a tiny hemorrhagic punctum is often present. The repeatedly bitten host gradually becomes sensitized. Newborns do not react. Newcomers to a flea-infested area quickly become sensitized and are greatly bothered by bites for the first year or so. Continuous exposure has its compensations, however, especially in regions of mild temperatures where fleas breed all year, as in California. Most individuals become desensitized.

Elimination of fleas and larvae in the environment may be accomplished with thorough use of insecticides directed into crevices of furniture, beneath rugs, into beds, and in all other areas of possible concealment. Damp basements or subways are favorite haunts, especially in warm climates. Breeding places such as rubbish and sandpiles should be removed. Pets must be dusted with insecticide powders and re-treated every 2 weeks during the summer months. DDT in powder form is effective for home, clothing, and pets. Impregnation of clothing with diethyltoluamide or benzyl benzoate is most effective. Desensitization against fleabites with injections of commercially available flea antigens is probably not worthwhile, since spontaneous desensitization with continued exposure occurs anyway.

A member of the family Tungidae is responsible for tungiasis. *Tunga penetrans* (the burrowing flea, chigoe, sand flea, or jigger) is widely distributed in South America, the West Indies, and Africa. The lesion is produced by the female, which, as soon as she is impregnated, seeks any available mammal or bird, burrowing diagonally into the skin until only her posterior segment protrudes. Deeply ensconced, she sucks blood and gradually undergoes an enormous increase in size, reaching the dimensions of a small pea as a consequence of prodigious ovulation. The eggs are then ejected to the ground. The gestating female buried in the skin causes a hard, slightly raised, itchy, red nodule the center of which presents a dark plug, representing her posterior. Inevitably there is suppuration, resulting in a pustule formed about the distended body of the pest. One or many females may reside in the skin. If there are many, the pustules are numerous and, when close enough, become aggregated into solid plaques with a well-defined honeycomb appearance. The lesions are usually situated between the toes, on the soles, or even under the toenails. From sitting or lying on the ground, scantily clothed natives and others may be affected.

If the burrowing flea is not removed, the expanding suppuration eventually ruptures the pustule and expels the insect, leaving a pitlike ulcer. Neglect may lead to deep ulceration, gangrene, lymphangitis, and septicemia. Fatalities from these complications are not rare.

Adequate prophylaxis requires use of appropriate footwear (preferably high boots), meticulous daily foot inspection, and cleaning of infested areas by fire or with DDT, dimethyl phthalate, diethyltoluamide, or lindane. After the flea has burrowed into the skin, it must be extracted intact, preferably in the earliest stage. A chloroform or ether-soaked pledget will kill the pest when applied to the lesion. The pustule is incised and the flea shelled out with sterile instruments. Local or parenteral antibacterial therapy may be indicated.

BEES & WASPS
(Order Hymenoptera)

Essentials of Diagnosis
- Reactions vary in severity from anaphylaxis to local edema.
- Anaphylaxis may occur.
- Venom skin test most specific.

General Considerations
More than half of deaths due to venomous animals are a result of Hymenoptera stings. Three superfamilies of Hymenoptera are significant: (1) the Apoidea, including the honeybee and bumblebee; (2) the Vespidae, including wasps, hornets, and yellow jackets; and (3) the Formicoidea, including several species of ants (see next section). Hymenopterans are social insects; they live in large colonies and often attack in groups. Hornets, honeybees, and wasps usually live in trees or shrubs, while yellow jackets nest underground. The stinging apparatus is a modified ovipositor; only the honeybee leaves its barbed stinger with attached venom sacs in the wound.

Hymenoptera venoms are complex mixtures of allergenic proteins and pharmacologically active amines and peptides; complete characterization of all

components has not yet been achieved. An individual's reaction to a sting is a combination of the local and (rarely) systemic effects of the pharmacologically active peptides and amines and of the degree of the person's hypersensitivity to the allergenic proteins of the venom.

Clinical Findings
Reactions may be divided into immediate (within 2 hours) and delayed types (over 2 hours). Immediate reactions are the most common and may be characterized by local, extensive local, or systemic reactions. The majority of (nonallergic) responses to stings are cutaneous, with local edema, erythema, transient pain, and pruritus. This reaction usually subsides within a few hours. In some patients with hypersensitivity to venom, the local reaction is marked by more severe and prolonged edema and redness. Systemic reactions may be mild or severe enough to be fatal. Milder reactions are manifested by urticaria, pruritus, malaise, or angioedema. More severe reactions may be accompanied by nausea, vomiting, dizziness, and wheezing. The most severe (anaphylactic) reactions involve hypotension and respiratory difficulty due to laryngeal edema or bronchospasm. Anaphylactic reactions usually occur within the first 10–30 minutes after the sting; speed of onset correlates with severity of reaction. Death due to hypersensitivity reactions may be due to respiratory compromise (with massive edema and secretions) or vascular changes (with massive vascular engorgement, hemorrhage, hemolysis, or coronary occlusion). Delayed reactions are uncommon; they include local skin necrosis, serum sickness, thrombocytopenic purpura, nephrotic syndrome, necrotizing angiitis, neurologic changes, and hepatorenal syndrome.

The diagnosis of Hymenoptera allergy is presently imperfect. The only sure way is to assess the reaction after a sting; even this method is not foolproof, since a test sting may lead to increased sensitivity. The most sensitive and specific test is the venom skin test. The radioallergosorbent test (RAST) is useful in patients who cannot be skin-tested but not as specific for sensitivity as the skin test. Even with a clinical history of a systemic reaction and a positive venom skin test, only 60% of patients react to future stings.

Treatment
Treatment for insect sting consists of local care for mild reactions, emergency measures against anaphylaxis, and hyposensitization for patients with a history of severe systemic reactions. In honeybee stings, the stinger and attached venom sac should be scraped from the skin; forceps should not be used because pressure on the venom sac can inject more venom. Ice, elevation, and oral antihistamines minimize local pain and swelling. In delayed local reactions appearing after 24 hours, a 4- to 5-day course of systemic steroids may be effective.

Individuals known to be allergic should be given an emergency kit that must be readily available to them at all times. Commercial bee-sting kits include a tourniquet, syringe, ampule of epinephrine (1:1000), and antihistamine tablets. Epinephrine (0.1–0.5 mL of 1:1000) should be given subcutaneously and repeated every 5–15 minutes if necessary. Anaphylaxis is a medical emergency and requires prompt physician care; airway support, intravenous fluids, vasopressors, aminophylline, and oxygen all may be necessary.

Hyposensitization is recommended for patients with a history of a severe systemic reaction and a positive venom skin test. Immunotherapy with venom is 95% effective.

ANTS

True ants (superfamily Formicoidea) can sting severely; fire ants, harvester ants, and numerous tropical species are especially feared. The fire ant is most commonly encountered in the USA. Two South American species, *Solenopsis richteri* (black) and *Solenopsi invicta* (red), now occupy more than 150 million acres in the southern USA after importation into Alabama around 1930. The fire ant is important as an agricultural pest; it causes a characteristic local bite reaction and occasional systemic allergic reactions similar to those caused by other Hymenoptera species.

The method of stinging produces a typical cluster of cutaneous lesions. The fire ant grasps the skin with its mandibles and simultaneously inserts the abdominal stinger. It pivots about the head, stinging at multiple sites in a circular pattern. Two hemorrhagic puncta may be seen at the attachment of the mandibles, and a circular pattern of surrounding pustules can be seen at the sites of stinging.

In nonsensitive individuals, there is a predictable sequence of responses to a sting. Immediate pain quickly subsides, but a 2- to 10-mm wheal develops. Within 4 hours a vesicle forms that becomes cloudy and sometimes umbilicated; a typical lesion at 24 hours is an umbilicated sterile pustule on a red, edematous base. This usually takes several days to heal, sometimes with hyperpigmentation, a residual fibrotic nodule, scarring, and on occasion severe secondary infection. Occasionally, individuals may suffer multiple stings and present with thousands of pustules; this is particularly common in heavy drinkers who fall asleep on fire ant mounds. Systemic allergic reactions similar to bee stings may rarely be encountered.

There is no specific effective treatment for the local reaction. Treatments are based on symptoms. Hyposensitization appears worthwhile in patients with a history of severe systemic reactions.

TRUE BUGS
(Order Hemiptera)

1. BEDBUGS

The 2 common species of bedbugs are *Cimex lectularius* in temperate areas and *Cimex hemipterus* in the tropics, especially Asia.

The bedbug is a clandestine bloodsucker, foraging at night and hiding during the day in crevices of walls, bedding, floors, and furniture. It is reddish-brown and about 6–7 mm in length. Customarily, the bug sucks blood from several sites in close proximity, thereby creating groups of discrete lesions, a telltale sign. Usually, the host is not awakened from sleep and does not feel the bite. The bug lives about 6 months, during which time the female may lay 200–500 eggs. Bedbugs feed upon other animals when unable to reach humans.

Soon after the bite, the usual reaction is a pruritic, burning wheal with a central hemorrhagic punctum. The purpuric reaction helps differentiate the lesion from an ordinary wheal. The bedbug wheal may become variably erythematous and firm, or it may evolve into a bulla, particularly in children. The wheal ordinarily subsides within a short time, but it sometimes lasts for hours. The bites often appear 2–3 in a line. The favored sites are the back, neck, face, ankles, wrists, buttocks, or wherever the body touches the bed, enabling the bug, which is wingless, to crawl onto the skin. Scratching and secondary infection corrupt the initially discrete lesions, so that the final appearance may be decidedly different, presenting pustules, vesicles, eczematized plaques, purpuric blotches, and thickened patches.

Bedbugs are easily killed with malathion, lindane, pyrethrins, and DDT. Professional exterminators are best at making sure that all inaccessible crevices frequented by bedbugs are sprayed.

2. KISSING BUGS
(Assassin Bugs)

Members of the family Reduviidae are known chiefly because of their role in transmitting South American trypanosomiasis. However, about 15 species of kissing bugs of the genus *Triatoma* are found in the southwestern USA and are known by a variety of names (assassin bugs, kissing bugs, cone-nose bugs, Walapai tigers, and Mexican bedbugs). The bugs usually remain near their natural hosts (rodents, armadillos, and opossums) but can adapt to living in houses and feeding on humans.

The feeding bite is painless, occurring at night on uncovered body areas (face, neck, shoulders, and arms). There is usually a clustering of bites in a small area. Reactions depend upon the degree of host sensitization; the usual reaction is a 2- to 3-cm urticarial nodule or plaque with severe pruritus, lasting from 2 to 7 days. Vesicular, hemorrhagic, and giant urticarial reactions have been described; anaphylactic reactions may occur.

BEETLES
(Coleoptera)

1. VESICATING BEETLES
(Blister Beetles)

The best-known of the blister beetles are members of the family Meloidae. In Europe, the Spanish fly *(Cantharis vesicatoria)* is found in great numbers in France and Spain. Of more than 200 species of blister beetles, most occur in the southeastern and western USA, the commonest belonging to the genus *Epicauta*. Blister beetles are 10–15 mm in length, soft, long-legged, and very agile. In the USA, they mature in the summer and disappear in the winter, accounting for a strictly seasonal incidence. They contain the potent vesicant cantharidin throughout their bodies. Little or no cantharidin is excreted if the beetle walks undisturbed across the skin, but with the slightest pressure the beetle's body exudes a clear amber fluid from the knee joints, prothorax, and genitalia. A mild tingling may develop in 10 minutes, followed in 8–12 hours by a flaccid bulla without surrounding inflammation. A large bulla may develop if the insect is crushed on the skin. Often the victim "brushes off" an insect without knowing it, later showing surprise at the appearance of blisters that seem to have come from nowhere. Blister beetles contact the skin mostly at night, so that the patient discovers the blisters in the morning. The blisters occur on exposed parts, frequently in a line. Since the beetles feed on various flowering plants, potatoes, clover, and soybeans, agricultural workers are commonly affected.

Rove beetles of the family Staphylinidae (genus *Paederus*) occur in Asia, Africa, and South America. These produce a vesicating substance different from cantharidin.

There is no specific treatment for beetle vesication. Large blisters should be drained. Topical corticosteroids and oral antihistamines are of little value.

2. BUTTERFLIES & MOTHS
(Order Lepidoptera)

Several species of caterpillars (the larval form of moths and butterflies) may cause cutaneous lesions; less commonly, the adult or cocoon stage may be incriminated. Most of the trouble comes from the hairy caterpillars that may possess 2 types of hairs. Some merely cause mechanical irritation. The more damaging (or "urticating") hairs are hollow and associated with venom glands or cells. The bristly hairs easily penetrate skin. Some slender hairs may be readily detached and left where they fall or blown distances by wind. Not much is known about lepidopteran venoms, as they have been difficult to obtain in pure form.

The most notorious of caterpillars in the USA is the puss caterpillar *(Megalopyge opercularis)*, also known as the woolly slug, possum bug, Italian asp, and el perrito (Spanish for "little dog"). This caterpillar occurs in the southern USA and Mexico; it is particularly common in Texas, where thousands of cases of dermatitis have occurred in a season. The saddleback caterpillar *(Sibine stimulea)*, the tree asp *(Euclea delphinii)*, the large, showy caterpillar of the io moth *(Automeris io)*, and gypsy moth caterpillar *(Lymentria dispar)* are well-known species in the eastern USA. Pine caterpillars *(Thaumetopoea)* and processionary caterpillars *(Ctenocampa)* are important in Europe and the Mediterranean. The brown-tail moth caterpillar *(Nygmia phaeorrhea)* causes trouble in both Europe and the USA. Adult moths of the genus *Hylesia* are responsible for epidemics of dermatitis in South America.

Agricultural workers, entomologists, and children playing outdoors are most likely to suffer. Hairs can be transferred easily from the hands to the face or eyes. Hairs can be swept about in airborne clouds or rain down from trees on people below.

Clinical manifestations vary according to the species and the intensity of exposure. Contact with *Megalopyge* is characterized by severe immediate pain, followed by prolonged pruritus. Erythematous macules appear quickly and are succeeded by firm wheallike red papules, the color disappearing under diascopic pressure. Individual lesions last from a few hours to days. When few, the lesions are discrete, but confluence of many lesions creates patches that may be intensely pruritic but rarely become eczematous. The toxin of the puss caterpillar seems particularly potent, for when penetrated by many hairs, the patient may experience nausea and fever, with numbness and swelling of the affected part.

Detached spines landing in the eyes can cause painful ophthalmia. In a few cases, an intractable endophthalmitis may necessitate removal of the eye.

Local treatment has little effect on stings by caterpillars; prompt application of adhesive tape removes many spines. Intravenous calcium gluconate has been reported effective in severe *Megalopyge* envenomation. Narcotic analgesics help relieve acute pain.

CLASS CHILOPODA
(Centipedes)

Centipedes are wormlike arthropods with a pair of poisonous claws on the first segment used for defense and in killing prey. Bites are painful and frequently followed by lymphangitis and lymphadenitis. Swelling and tenderness may persist for up to 3 weeks; necrosis may occasionally occur. Pain may be relieved by injection of local anesthetics into the vicinity of the bite.

CLASS DIPLOPODA (Millipedes)

Millipedes do not bite, but many species may exude toxic or repugnant substances onto the body surface when disturbed. Human injury from millipedes is infrequent, but eye and skin lesions from contact with millipedes may occur. Cutaneous lesions resemble a chemical burn. There is an initial discoloration of yellow to purple-brown, subsequent blister formation, and exfoliation of the area of contact. When the eyes are exposed, there is intense lacrimation and burning, with subsequent chemosis and conjunctivitis. Treatment involves copious rinsing of the affected areas with water.

CRUSTACEA

Small marine crustaceans—cymothoids (sea lice)—live in shoal waters of temperate and tropic seas and feed upon higher marine animals but will attack humans. The underwater bites are rapid and sharp and cause punctate hemorrhages at the sites, which a few hours later become small ulcers with indurated, erythematous halos. The eruption—sea louse dermatitis (cymothoidism)—heals in 5–6 days without residua.

II. NOXIOUS OR VENOMOUS INVERTEBRATES

COELENTERATES (Coelenterata)

Essentials of Diagnosis
- Local stinging with subsequent edematous, papular lesions.
- Associated variable systemic reactions.

General Considerations
Approximately 100 species of the phylum Coelenterata are capable of inflicting injuries on humans.

Three major classes are responsible: (1) Hydrozoa, which includes the Portuguese man-of-war and hydroids; (2) Scyphozoa, which includes the true jellyfish; and (3) Anthozoa, which comprises the sea anemones and corals. Almost all coelenterates possess nematocysts or "sting capsules" containing venom largely concentrated on the tentacles of the organism. Each nematocyst contains a spirally coiled thread with a barbed end. On contact, this thread is uncoiled and ejected with the venom capsule into the skin. Both chemical and mechanical factors such as fresh water and friction trigger the discharge of nematocyst venom. The nature of most coelenterate venoms is poorly characterized; many inhibit nerve activity by altering ionic permeability.

Swimmers, fishermen, surfers, scuba divers, and shell collectors are exposed. The injurious effects depend on the species of the coelenterate, the type of nematocyst, the penetrating power of the nematocyst, the inoculated skin site of the victim, and the sensitivity of the individual to the venom. Almost all the coelenterates of medical importance occur in subtropical or tropical salt water.

Most coelenterate stings are characterized by a local reaction consisting of a stinging or burning sensation followed by a linear or papular eruption with erythema and edema. In most cases, this disappears within a few hours to days without sequelae. Systemic reactions may occur with some species, due to venom toxicity or to host hypersensitivity; these include urticaria, pruritus, edema, dyspnea, cramps, vomiting, paralysis, cardiac arrest, and death.

1. HYDROZOA

Physalia physalis (the Portuguese man-of-war) is the best-known hydrozoan; it inhabits temperate to tropic water zones from the Atlantic to the Mediterranean. Each man-of-war is actually a colony of hydroids consisting of a bladderlike sac from which are suspended numerous fishing tentacles containing beadlike batteries of nematocysts. Tentacles may reach lengths of 30 m and may remain venomous for weeks after the organism has died on shore.

A hapless swimmer, engaging a tentacle, receives numerous stings at once, which quickly show up as a row of erythematous lesions spaced a few millimeters apart. The affected area quickly swells, becoming red and painful. Severe systemic effects may result within 1 hour: anxiety, muscular pains and cramps, dyspnea, prostration, and occasionally death. Anaphylactoid reactions with cough, coryza, and urticaria may appear in highly sensitive persons.

Other hydrozoans that may cause problems include Calycophora (or "glassy nectophore" because of its transparency), which may cause a pruritic eruption, and species of the order Leptomedusae ("feather hydroids"), which may cause immediate urticarial lesions or delayed papular reactions in characteristic 20-cm "bands." Erythema multiforme or generalized morbilliform eruptions may be associated, as may systemic symptoms of anxiety, muscle spasms, diarrhea, and fever. *Millepora alcincornis* (stinging or fire coral) is not a true coral; it causes a tender, red, burning lesion on contact.

2. SCYPHOZOA

Certain species of true jellyfish may be deadly. Many deaths off northern Australia have been due to *Chironex fleckeri* (the sea wasp). Other species such as *Chrysaora, Cyanea* (sea nettles), and *Rhizostoma* cause painful skin lesions that may be accompanied by dyspnea, cough, cramps, and vomiting.

3. ANTHOZOA

Sea anemones are sessile coelenterates with a flowerlike appearance; several species may cause variable cutaneous reactions. The most common species is *Sagartia*, which causes "sponge diver's disease"; this small anemone (4 cm) attaches itself to the base of the sponges and, on contact with the diver's skin, causes a burning sensation followed by edema, erythema, and vesicles. Headache, nausea, vomiting, fever, and muscle spasms are frequently associated.

Coral cuts and ulcers are a constant threat to those in contact with living coral. The injuries are not especially painful, but they heal slowly and frequently suppurate. The pathogenesis is not well understood, but a foreign body reaction with secondary bacterial infection appears to be the primary process. Coral cuts should be vigorously scrubbed, cleansed with hydrogen peroxide and alcohol, and sprinkled with an antibiotic powder.

Treatment

Several general precautions should be observed in treating nematocyst dermatitis. Contact with fresh water and rubbing of the affected area should be avoided. Nematocysts may be inactivated by applying liquid of a high alcohol content (spirits, rubbing alcohol, or cologne). Acidic toxins may be neutralized by rinsing with mildly alkaline solutions of baking soda or ammonia. Rubbing papain (meat tenderizer) on the site may occasionally be helpful. Tentacles clinging to the skin should not be pulled off but instead scraped off with dry sand or a paste of seawater and baking soda or flour. Treatment of severe stings may be difficult because of the rapid progression of symptoms. One should be prepared to treat shock with the usual supportive measures. Parenteral antihistamines may be helpful, along with epinephrine, intravenous calcium gluconate, and systemic steroids. Narcotic analgesics may be necessary for pain. Stings from the deadly sea wasp may require the use of antivenin.

ECHINODERMATA

Essentials of Diagnosis

- History of contact with a sea urchin.
- Delayed reaction with nodules or induration.
- Lesions in areas of trauma from spines.

General Considerations

Sea urchins are spheric organisms with a calcareous skeleton enclosing a soft body; the shell is studded with movable brittle spines of calcium carbonate covered with pigmented epithelium. The spinal epithelium in some species may contain unidentified toxins. Venom glands may be associated with other appendages called pedicellariae, which have hooklike jaws able to inject venom; pedicellarial envenomation is infrequent and usually results from allowing the urchin to crawl on the skin.

Clinical Findings

Most sea urchin injuries are due to inadvertent contact, leading to puncture wounds from the brittle spines, which break off easily in the skin. Reactions may be immediate or delayed. Most punctures do not produce pain out of proportion to the mechanical injury. With some species, an immediate severe burning pain with or without edema may persist for several hours. Profuse bleeding may occur. With other species, pain may be minimal. The puncture wound is often dark and surrounded by a purplish ring due to dyes in some spines. This may sometimes give the impression that a spine is present; x-rays will detect the presence of spines.

Delayed reactions may occur 2–12 months after injury and may be one of 3 types: (1) epidermal inclusion cysts, which may form from fragments of epithelium implanted in the depth of the wound; (2) foreign body granulomas, which may form around fragments of spines, usually healing after extrusion of these fragments; and (3) sarcoidlike granulomatous lesions in which no foreign bodies can be demonstrated. These lesions are probably due to a hypersensitivity reaction, as they have been reproduced with intradermal tests to spine extracts. Two types of lesions may be seen. The nodular variant consists of firm nodules—flesh-colored, pink, or brown, 2–4 mm in diameter—that may be umbilicated. The diffuse variant occurs primarily on the fingers and toes, where a bluish-red fusiform induration deforms the digit; there may be focal bone or joint destruction. Both types may be stubbornly persistent, with rare spontaneous resolution.

Treatment

Treatment for immediate injuries consists of application of topical antibiotic creams and the removal of any easily seen spines (difficult to remove because of brittleness). Delayed sarcoidal reactions may improve after injections of intralesional corticosteroids. The diffuse fusiform digital lesions may require systemic steroids and antibiotics.

Surgery is indicated if x-rays reveal spines in delayed reactions. X-rays should document suspected spines before surgical exploration is attempted.

MOLLUSKS

Mollusks are soft-bodied, unsegmented invertebrates, and most of them secrete protective shells. The mollusks most dangerous to humans are the cone shells. Most stings have been reported off the coasts of Australia and New Guinea, but venomous species are also found off California and possibly Florida. Variable local pain or burning may occur with the sting; swelling or numbness may ensue. Systemic symptoms of serious poisoning include diplopia, slurred speech, numbness, muscular weakness and paralysis (respiratory paralysis), and terminal coma. Death may occur within 6 hours after the sting.

There is no specific treatment. Supportive measures with oxygen and a respirator may be lifesaving.

SPONGES

Sponges are stationary animals living attached to the sea bottom. Although sponges lack special structures for venom injection, the tissues of some species contain toxic substances; other species possess small spicules that may be irritating.

Tedania ignis (the fire sponge) is abundant in the Miami and Florida Keys coastal areas. If handled, the sponge causes an acute reaction with itching, followed within a few hours by swelling, stiffness, pain, and an acute eczematous dermatitis. Symptoms usually subside within 2 days. Erythema multiforme has resulted after fire sponge contact. *Fibula nolitangere* (the poison bun sponge) in the West Indies may cause an even more severe reaction than *Tedania*. The red sponge, *Microciona prolifera,* may cause a similar acute dermatitis in oyster fishermen of the northeastern USA; if not treated, the eruption may persist for several months.

Treatment of sponge reactions is nonspecific. Weak acid solutions such as vinegar are said to give some relief from immediate reactions. Corticosteroids (topical or systemic) and oral antihistamines are helpful in delayed reactions.

Some sponges produce traumatic injury with spicules made of silicon dioxide or calcium carbonate, which may break off in the skin. These are difficult to remove; the application of adhesive tape to the affected area may remove some spicules.

LEECHES & MARINE WORMS

Leeches are wormlike, bloodsucking animals of the phylum Annelida, class Hirudinea. Species may be marine, freshwater, or terrestrial.

In sucking blood, the leech secretes an anticoagulant, hirudin, which may cause prolonged bleeding and extensive blood loss even after the leech has dropped off. Secondary infection of bites is common. Sensitization to leeches is manifested by an urticarial or bullous bite reaction.

Protection against terrestrial leeches is best afforded by protective clothing (trousers tucked inside socks in properly laced boots) and insect repellents applied to skin and clothing.

Leeches may be detached from the skin by the application of alcohol, table salt, strong vinegar, or heat. If pulled off, the jaws may remain in the wound. Bleeding may be stanched with a styptic pencil.

Marine annelids may produce wounds from bites or an irritant dermatitis from bristles. The blood worm (*Glycera dibranchiata*) is taken as a bait worm along the Atlantic coast of the USA and Canada; its bite is followed by pain and swelling lasting up to 2 days. Several species of bristle worm (*Chloeia, Eurythoe,* and *Hermodice*) have chitinous spines filled with an uncharacterized venomous fluid. These worms are particularly common in Malaya, Australia, the West Indies, the Gulf of Mexico, and the Gulf of California. Contact with the spines produces burning pain, swelling, and an erythematous papular eruption followed by numbness and itching that may last several weeks. Necrotic lesions have occasionally occurred. The spines are easily detached and may need to be removed from the skin with forceps or adhesive tape. Cold compresses or alcohol may be soothing.

III. NOXIOUS OR VENOMOUS VERTEBRATES

FISH

Fish produce cutaneous injury primarily by lacerations with spines equipped with venom-producing glands. A few species of fish may produce irritant dermatitis by contact with noxious material on its skin.

1. INJURY DUE TO VENOMOUS FISH SPINES

Essentials of Diagnosis
- History of contact with fish.
- Intense pain, swelling, and redness.
- Slow-healing variable systemic symptoms.

General Considerations
The term **ichthyoacanthotoxism** denotes injury from venomous fish spines. The more commonly encountered types of venomous fish include stingrays, scorpion fish (lionfish, stonefish, bullrout, rock cod), weeverfish, catfish, toadfish, stargazer, rabbitfish, Norway haddo

Clinical Findings
Persons with fish spine wounds suffer intense pain lasting several hours. Swelling and redness around the puncture site may simulate bacterial cellulitis; blistering and necrosis may occur. The wounds are typically slow to heal and easily become secondarily infected. Systemic symptoms may occur (particularly with the stingray, scorpionfish, and weevers), with nausea, vomiting, salivation, headache, fever, chills, abdominal pain, sweating, dyspnea, cardiac arrhythmias, convulsions, muscular paralysis, and death.

Treatment
Treatment of wounds includes local debridement, attempts to minimize effects of the venom, and treatment of pain, systemic symptoms, and secondary infection. The wound should be promptly washed to remove any fragments of venom-containing tissue. Because fish spine venom is heat-labile, injured areas should be immersed in water as hot as can be tolerated for 30–90 minutes. Pain is often relieved by this maneuver. In severe envenomation, a loosely applied tourniquet may slow venous return; local suction as for snakebites has been suggested for scorpionfish stings. Narcotic analgesics or intralesional lidocaine should be used for severe pain. Treatment for shock with cardiac and respiratory support may rarely be necessary. Tetanus prophylaxis should be given; antibiotics are used for secondary infection. Antivenin for stonefish poisoning is available in Australia.

2. IRRITANT DERMATITIS FROM FISH

Contact with the soapfish, *Rypticus saponaceus,* in the Virgin Islands and Puerto Rico produces dermatitis; an irritant called grammistin is present in the soapy mucus secreted when the fish is disturbed. Several scombroid fish (tuna, skipjack, and bonito) may cause dermatitis in those handling them without gloves. Mackerel that have eaten "red feed" (a red crustacean of the *Calanus* species) may also cause dermatitis when handled.

HUMAN & ANIMAL BITES

Human bites, particularly to the hand, are a common injury. Soft tissue infection with oral flora may have disabling consequences; a high complication rate with tenosynovitis, septic arthritis, or osteomyelitis has been noted. Bacterial cultures usually reveal gram-positive cocci, principally *Staphylococcus aureus,* which is often penicillin-resistant. *Streptococcus* species and occasional associated gram-negative organisms may be isolated. Uninfected or superficially infected injuries should be thoroughly cleansed and then soaked and elevated frequently for 48 hours. Wounds should be left open; oral antibiotics are generally prescribed. Patients with moderately to severely infected injuries may require local debridement, hospitalization, and intravenous antibiotics. Wound drainage should be cultured and gram-stained. Cephalosporins are a rational initial antibiotic choice, since *S aureus* has been cultured from the majority of bite wounds and is strongly associated with most complications. Hepatitis B has been transmitted.

Cat and dog bites may transmit rabies as well as lead to secondary bacterial infection. Dog bites are a common problem in the USA, with at least 1 million people bitten each year. The average dog's mouth harbors more than 60 species of bacteria, including *S aureus* and *Pasteurella multocida.* Most bites sustain the same infection rate as that of simple lacerations (6%). Certain risk factors define a population more likely to become infected; these include age over 50 years, a delay of more than 24 hours in seeking treatment, puncture wounds, and hand wounds. Wounds should be thoroughly irrigated, debrided, and sutured (unless on the hand). Tetanus prophylaxis should be given. Hand lesions should be elevated, immobilized, and treated with prophylactic antibiotics. A penicillinase-resistant penicillin or cephalexin is probably the best choice; erythromycin or tetracycline is indicated for patients allergic to penicillin. Treatment of established infections should be guided by Gram stain and culture results.

Pasteurella infections after dog or cat bites typically present as an acute cellulitis at the bite site, with regional adenopathy, discharge, and low-grade fever. Tenosynovitis or septicemia may be a secondary complication. Penicillin, tetracycline, and cephalothin are effective treatment.

REFERENCES

Baden HP, Burnett JW: Injuries from sea urchins. South Med J 1977;70:459.

Best WC, Sablan RG: Cymothoidism (sea louse dermatitis). Arch Dermatol 1964;90:177.

Brothers WS, Heckmann RA: Tungiasis in North America. Cutis 1980;25:636.

Burgdorfer W, Keirans JE: Ticks and Lyme disease in the United States. Ann Intern Med 1983;99:121.

Callaham M: Dog bite wounds. JAMA 1980;244:2327.

Cohen SR: Cheyletiella dermatitis; A mite infestation of rabbit, cat, dog, and man. Arch Dermatol 1980;116:435.

Fisher AA: *Atlas of Aquatic Dermatology*. Grune & Stratton, 1978.

Fisher AA: Water-related dermatoses: 2. Nematocyst dermatitis. Cutis 1980;25:242.

Manowitz NR, Rosenthal RR: Cutaneous-systemic reactions to toxins and venoms of common marine organisms. Cutis 1979;23:450.

Hewitt M et al: Pet animal infestations and human skin lesions. Br J Dermatol 1971;85:215.

Hewitt M, Walton GS, Waterhouse M: Pet animal infestations and human skin lesions. Br J Dermatol 1971;85:215.

King LE Jr, Rees RS: Dapsone treatment of a brown recluse spider bite. JAMA 1983;250:648.

Lehman CF, Pipkin JL, Ressmann AC: Blister beetle dermatosis. Arch Dermatol 1955;71:36.

Maibach HI et al: Use of insect repellents for maximum efficacy. Arch Dermatol 1974;109:32.

Maibach HI, Khan AA, Akers W: Use of insect repellents for maximum efficacy. Arch Dermatol 1974;109:32.

Malinowski RW et al: The management of human bite injuries of the hand. J Trauma 1979;19:655.

Manowitz NR, Rosenthal RR: Cutaneous-systemic reactions to toxins and venoms of common marine organisms. Cutis 1979;23:450.

Manson-Bahr PEC, Bell DR (editors): *Manson's Tropical Diseases*. Bailliere Tindall (London), 1987.

Minton SA Jr: *Venom Diseases*. Thomas, 1974.

Morgan RJ et al: Myiasis. Arch Dermatol 1964;90:180.

Patterson JW et al: Localized tick bite reaction. Cutis 1979;24:168.

Rees RS et al: The management of the brown recluse spider bite. Plast Reconstr Surg 1981;68:768.

Patterson JW, Fitzwater JE, Connell J: Localized tick bite reaction. Cutis 1979;24:168.

Rook A: Papular urticaria. Pediatr Clin North Am 1961;8:817.

Strassburg MA et al: Animal bites: Patterns of treatment. Ann Emerg Med 1981;10:193.

Wasserman GS, Siegel C: Loxoscelism (brown recluse spider bites): A review of the literature. Clin Toxicol 1979;14:353.

Weber DJ et al: "Pasteurella multocida" infections: Report of 34 cases and review of the literature. Medicine 1984;63:133.

Yunginger JW: Advances in the diagnosis and treatment of stinging insect allergy. Pediatrics 1981;67:325.

Section IV:
Disorders of Structure & Function

Genodermatoses

20

Lowell A. Goldsmith, MD

PHENOTYPIC APPROACH TO THE DIAGNOSIS OF GENETIC SKIN DISEASE

To diagnose and eventually treat genetically caused skin disease, an operational scheme is useful. In Table 20–1, the major phenotypic categories of genetic skin diseases are listed, and the entities are discussed in this chapter, with cross-reference where appropriate to other parts of this text. The reader should note that many genetic diseases belong to more than one of these artificial categories and that in this text the individual entities will be discussed under its major phenotypic change.

The ichthyotic and hyperkeratotic disorders are discussed in Chapter 21; genetic pigmentary disorders of the skin in Chapter 22; and nail defects in Chapter 29.

Many of the diseases discussed in this chapter have important internal manifestations that must be considered in any patient evaluation.

PRENATAL DIAGNOSIS OF SKIN DISEASES

Prenatal diagnostic procedures have been used to diagnose some serious genetic disorders. For the diagnosis of these diseases, study of fetal biopsy by electronmicroscopic techniques has been frequently used as well as biochemical analysis. In Table 20–2, the diseases in which fetal skin biopsy has been successful are listed. False-negatives are a problem in skin biopsies.

Disorders of keratinization may be difficult to diagnosis since complete epidermal keratinization occurs at 18–20 weeks while fetal biopsy is often done early during pregnancy. Chorionic villus sampling and use

of genetic probes will allow earlier diagnosis. Abortion of an affected fetus would prevent disease.

HAIR DEFECTS

An approach to the classification and diagnosis of genetic hair defects is presented in Fig 20–1. Several of the diseases causing hair defects are discussed below.

DECREASED HAIR

1. HIDROTIC ECTODERMAL DYSPLASIA

Essentials of Diagnosis
- Sparse to absent hair on body and scalp.
- Autosomal dominant inheritance.
- Diffuse hyperkeratosis of palms and soles.
- Lifting of the nails off the nail beds (onycholysis).

General Considerations
Patients with this not uncommon genetic disease usually present because of sparse hair. Although most common in eastern Canada, New York, and New England, the disease is worldwide in distribution. Onset is in childhood, and both sexes are equally affected.

The molecular mechanism of the defect is un-

Table 20–1. Major phenotypic categories of genetic skin disease.

Hyperkeratosis
  Universal
  Palm/sole predominating

Nail defects
  Nail plate
  Nail bed

Pigmentary defects
  Hypopigmentation
  Hyperpigmentation

Hair defects
  Decreased
  Morphologically abnormal
  Increased

Blistering

Photosensitivity

Urticaria and edema

Connective tissue defects

Multiple new skin growths
  Vascular
  Benign neoplasms
  Malignant neoplasms
  Perforating transepidermal elimination diseases

Skin ulceration

Sweating defects
  Anhidrotic epidermal dysplasia
  Cystic fibrosis
  Dysautonomia

known, though a decrease in hair cysteine and alteration of hair peptides have been noted.

Clinical Findings

A. Symptoms and Signs: Diffuse to complete nonscarring hair loss often begins in childhood and is lifelong. The remaining hair is often lighter in color than that of other individuals of the same racial group. Loss of scalp hair is most obvious, and typically the outer two-thirds of the eyebrows are thinned. Axillary and pubic hairs are also involved. Palmar and plantar hyperkeratosis increases with age and is accentuated on weight-bearing surfaces or with occupationally related pressure (eg, pushing a broom or weight lifting leads to localized calluslike hyperkeratosis on top of diffuse, velvety hyperkeratosis). The nail plates have a yellow hue and are recessed far beyond the tip of the nail pulp, and prominent papules appear around sweat duct openings near the fingertip. These papules represent proliferation of the cells of the terminal part of the sweat gland. Diffuse hyperpigmentation occurs. Bilateral premature cataracts rarely occur.

Apparent wide variation of the skin manifestations within families is due to differences in expression. The trait is usually found to be fully penetrant when all members of a family are examined carefully.

B. Laboratory Findings: Biopsy of fingertips

shows increased terminal sweat glands, which suggests the diagnosis.

C. Imaging Studies: Tufting of the distal phalanges on x-ray confirms the diagnosis.

Differential Diagnosis

The various causes of nonscarring hair loss should be considered (Fig 20–1), as should the causes of diffuse hyperkeratosis. The nail findings may be minimal but are important in distinguishing this disorder from others such as pachyonychia congenita. Normal teeth and sweating distinguish this disorder from anhidrotic ectodermal dysplasia.

Complications & Sequelae

The major sequelae are psychologic. They are decreased or prevented by early diagnosis and use of a wig.

Prevention

Prenatal diagnosis has not been reported. Affected individuals would prevent the disease by not reproducing, but genetic counseling with that objective is not warranted considering the nature of the defects.

Treatment & Prognosis

Wigs and hairpieces are advised for cosmetic purposes. Palmar and solar hyperkeratosis responds to mild keratolytics with occlusion, eg, 6% salicylic acid (Hydrisalic, Keralyt). The course is lifelong, but no interference with normal life is implied by the diagnosis. Reassurance is both appropriate and important.

2. ANHIDROTIC ECTODERMAL DYSPLASIA

Essentials of Diagnosis

• Decrease in or absence of sweating.

Table 20–2. Skin disorders diagnosed prenatally.

By electron microscopic studies
  Harlequin fetus
  Epidermolytic hyperkeratosis
  Sjögren-Larsson syndrome
  Dystrophic recessive epidermolysis bullosa
  Junctional epidermolysis bullosa
  Oculocutaneous albinism

By biochemical studies of fetal or amniotic cells
  Epidermolytic hyperkeratosis
  Fabry's disease
  Mucopolysaccharides II (Hunter's syndrome)
  Lesch-Nyhan syndrome
  Menkes' disease
  X-linked ichthyosis with sterility

By DNA repair studies or special karyotypic studies
  Bloom's syndrome
  Xeroderma pigmentosum

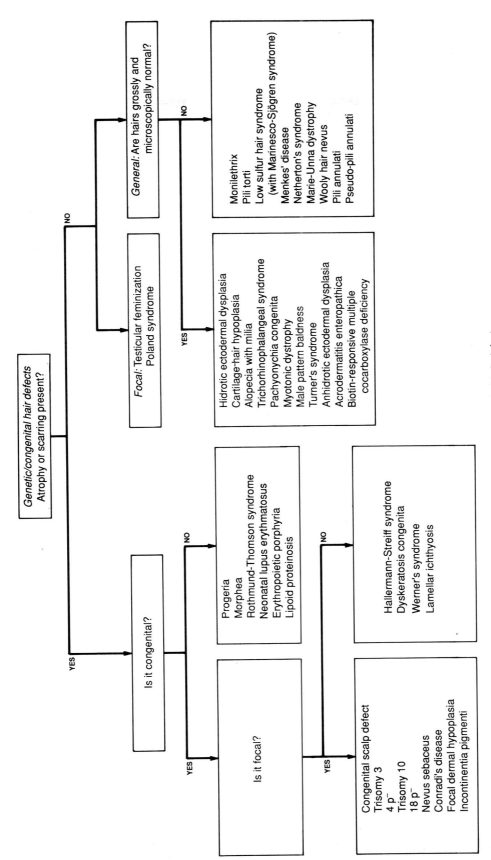

Figure 20–1. Genetic and congenital hair defects.

- Decrease in scalp hair and eyebrows.
- Abnormal or hypoplastic dentition.
- Midfacial (maxillary) hypoplasia.

General Considerations

This syndrome is characterized by decreased sweating and dental abnormalities as its most characteristic features. Both the basic defect and the true incidence are unknown. Because infants may have severe hyperthermia, fevers of unknown origin, and possible sudden death, recognizing the disease is important. The classic (and most common) form of the disease is transmitted by an X-linked inheritance pattern, with males predominantly affected. Individual diseases with autosomal recessive or dominant transmission are included in the syndrome.

Clinical Findings

A. Symptoms and Signs: Hair may be sparse, light in color, coarse, or strawlike at the time of birth or early in childhood. Abnormal hair patterning with a frontal upsweep suggests abnormal growth of the scalp during fetal development. Premature balding occurs. Eyelashes and eyebrows are often quite sparse.

Anhidrosis or hypohidrosis leads to pyrexia, especially in warm climates or in heavily clothed children. Absence of perspiration may be noted in infants, but it is not unusual for the sweating abnormality to go unrecognized for years. Exercise results in flushing or easy fatiguing. An atopiclike dermatitis frequently accompanies the syndrome, as do allergic rhinitis and asthma.

Midfacial hypoplasia leads to similar facial features—but variable in degree—among affected individuals. Frontal bossing, a depressed nasal bridge, pouting lips, and ears protruding from the head are characteristic. There is decreased size and activity of lacrimal, nasal, and salivary glands. In the mouth, there are decreased alveolar ridges, hypodontia, adontia, and conical incisors, canines, and bicuspids.

In women, the breasts may be hypoplastic or absent.

B. Laboratory Findings: Decreased sweat gland openings on the epidermal ridges can be seen with a magnifying glass; using a dissecting microscope, they can easily be photographed and quantified. Eccrine glands are absent to markedly decreased in affected males. In carrier females, glands are decreased but no mosaic distribution is present as might be expected from X-chromosome inactivation. Sweat tests with starch-iodide or reagents to detect amino acids (eg, ninhydrin) can be used to find areas of anhidrosis or hypohidrosis.

In patients with both atopic dermatitis and anhidrotic epidermal dysplasia, there are increased levels of serum IgE and altered responsiveness to tests for delayed hypersensitivity.

C. Imaging Studies: Dental x-rays are valuable for detecting minor tooth defects—including small or congenitally missing teeth—in affected individuals and carriers.

Differential Diagnosis

Hidrotic ectodermal dysplasia is often confused with anhidrotic ectodermal dysplasia; the differentiation is based on the presence in the former of involved nails and hyperkeratosis of palms and soles and in the latter by decreased sweating. The ectrodactyly-ectodermal dysplasia-clefting (EEC) syndrome is dominantly inherited and is marked by lobster-claw abnormalities of the hands or feet, cleft lip or palate, sparse and fine hair, and hypopigmentation. The skeletal abnormalities distinguish this disorder from anhidrotic ectodermal dysplasia.

Rarer syndromes often classified as ectodermal dysplasia have been exhaustively reviewed by Solomon (1980, 1987).

Prevention

Specific prenatal diagnosis has been possible by fetal skin biopsy, showing absent appendages.

Treatment

A. Emergency Treatment: Acute hyperthermia must be treated with environmental control and cool baths or sprays, which the body heat can then evaporate.

B. General Management: Education of the patient and family about the tendency to hyperthermia is necessary. Drugs such as chlorpromazine, anticholinergics, and diazepam, which can interfere with temperature control, should be avoided, especially during hot weather.

The accompanying atopic dermatitis can be treated with antihistamines such as hydroxyzine—which has weak anticholinergic effects—emollients, and topical corticosteroids.

Course & Prognosis

This is a lifelong condition to which people can adjust and still enjoy productive full-time schooling and employment.

3. CARTILAGE-HAIR HYPOPLASIA

Short-limb dwarfism is present at birth, and x-ray evidence of metaphyseal dysostosis establishes the diagnosis. The hairs are thinner than normal and hypopigmented. Defective T cell function is associated with recurrent respiratory infections and severe varicella; inheritance is autosomal recessive.

There is no treatment.

4. TRICHORHINOPHALANGEAL SYNDROME

This autosomal dominant syndrome (type I) is characterized by sparse scalp and lateral eyebrow hair, a prominent pear-shaped nose, and a long infranasal groove (philtrum). The phalanges have cone-shaped epiphyses. There may be associated lax skin. In type II of the syndrome, in addition to the above defects, there is bony exostosis, apparent by examination and confirmed by x-rays.

5. BIOTIN-RESPONSIVE CARBOXYLASE DEFICIENCY

Complete alopecia may start early in the second year of life and be accompanied by lethargy, spasticity, candidiasis of the nails, and keratoconjunctivitis. Severe acidosis is present, and urine chromatography reveals increased levels of the derivatives of branched-chain amino acids. Lifelong treatment with biotin, 10 mg/d, is curative in the forms of this disease due to a defective enzyme in branched-chain amino acid metabolism.

A similar disorder has occurred during parenteral hyperalimentation with solutions lacking biotin. In autosomal recessive vitamin D-resistant rickets due to a defective 1,25-dihydroxycholecalciferol (vitamin D_3) receptor, an alopecia totalis syndrome results.

6. MARIE-UNNA HAIR DYSTROPHY

This autosomal dominant disease is characterized at birth by absence of eyebrows, eyelashes, or body hair. During childhood, the hair is coarse and twisted. Hair loss begins again at puberty.

The hair is twisted and ribbonlike, with intracellular fractures and increased interfibrillary matrices. Milia (epidermal inclusion cysts) may be present. Milia are a feature of the hypotrichosis-milia syndrome, a disease in which the hair is sparse, hypopigmented, and not twisted.

7. CONGENITAL SKIN DEFECT (Bart Syndrome, Aplasia Cutis)

At birth, there is a single ulcer (rarely more than one) that may extend to the bone. The scalp is a common site. The ulcer heals to leave a scar without appendages. Autosomal dominant inheritance is often present and associated with chromosomal abnormalities and other somatic features.

8. CHONDRODYSPLASIA PUNCTATA (Conradi's Disease)

Chondrodysplasia punctata is associated with a peculiar facial appearance, congenital cataracts, and, in 30% of cases, skin abnormalities. Autosomal dominant and recessive forms exist. At birth, an ichthyosiform dermatitis is present that progresses to atrophic skin, especially around hair follicles. Cica-

tricial alopecia may occur. X-rays show punctate changes in the epiphyses.

9. INCONTINENTIA PIGMENTI

This is a rare X-linked hereditary disease of unknown biochemical cause seen chiefly in females because the trait is usually lethal in males. In the neonatal period, vesicles and bullae containing eosinophils are present for weeks to months. Later in the first few months of life, warty verrucous papules are present, and, in the third to twelfth months of life, artistic swirls of hyperpigmentation suggesting the chocolate swirls in marble cake develop while bullous and verrucous lesions disappear. Atrophy and scarring alopecia occur. Microcephaly, convulsions, mental retardation, and eye defects—including coloboma—and blindness occur. Peg-shaped incisors and other dental defects occur.

10. FOCAL DERMAL HYPOPLASIA

Females are predominantly affected in this disease; the mode of inheritance suggests an X-linked dominant trait, usually lethal in males. Papillomas develop near mucosal-cutaneous junctions. The hypoplastic dermis allows herniations through it of subcutaneous fat and causes soft outpouching of the skin. Scalp hair is focally absent, thin, or sparse and brittle. Skeletal defects include kyphoscoliosis, syndactyly, and claw hands. Hypoplastic dermal ridges occur. Eye defects range from strabismus to colobomas and even anophthalmia.

11. OCULOMANDIBULODYSCEPHALY WITH HYPOTRICHOSIS (Hallermann-Streiff Syndrome)

This congenital disease is usually not hereditary, and the children are considered bird-headed dwarfs because of the brachycephaly with frontal and parietal bossing. Manifestations are midfacial hypoplasia, dental hypoplasia, or aplasia; a small nose, microphthalmia, and often bilateral congenital cataracts.

Hypotrichosis affects especially the anterior scalp. The skin is atrophic—again, especially on the scalp —and scalp veins are prominent.

MORPHOLOGIC DEFECTS OF HAIR

1. LOW-SULFUR HAIR SYNDROMES

Essentials of Diagnosis
- Friable hair with a low sulfur and cysteine content.
- Alternating bands of birefringence and complete extinction seen on polarizing microscopy of hair.

General Considerations

Several clinical types of low-sulfur hair syndromes have been described. The basic biochemical defect is unknown; the inheritance pattern of all these diseases is autosomal recessive. Many structural proteins in hair are decreased.

Clinical Findings

A. Symptoms and Signs: The hair is friable and often short. Ichthyosis resembling lamellar ichthyosis is sometimes present, and nail plates may be thinned. Associated features in some families have included short stature, mental retardation, and decreased fertility. Some families have had only the hair defect. In one of the severe forms, Marinesco-Sjögren syndrome, there is short stature, congenital cataracts, cerebellar ataxia, and horizontal and vertical nystagmus.

B. Laboratory Findings: With light microscopy, sharply delineated breaks in the hair are present. With polarizing microscopy, one sees alternating bands of birefringence and complete extinction of light showing as dark bands.

The sulfur content of the hair is decreased by one-third to one-half; the cysteine content to about one-half of normal. Electrophoresis of affected hairs shows decreases in the high-sulfur proteins. On mechanical testing, the affected hairs break at lower stresses than normal.

Differential Diagnosis

In argininosuccinicaciduria, the hair is friable and has a distinctive nodular appearance (trichorrhexis nodosa). Hepatomegaly, increased blood ammonia, and signs of liver failure accompany this severe disease.

In Menkes' disease, an X-linked disorder, the hair is thin, highly twisted, and hypopigmented. Hypothermia, physical and mental retardation, and tortuous blood vessels are present. A defect of copper transport and metabolism causes low ceruloplasmin levels and increased copper storage in some tissues.

In hereditary pili torti, the twisted hairs may be accompanied by hearing or tooth defects. Acquired pili torti is a vexing but harmless disease that occurs during adolescence.

Monilethrix is characterized by irregularly beaded hairs that easily break and remain very short. Scalp and neck papules are frequently present. In Netherton's disease, there are bamboolike nodes on the hair, best seen with dissecting microscopy. Ichthyosis and atopy accompany this disease.

Ringed hair (pili annulati) is a harmless change in the hair. Prominent highlights caused by air-filled spaces in the hair cortex forming dark and light bands are reflected from the hair.

Localized areas of tightly curled hairs (woolly hair nevus) occur rarely.

Treatment

There is no treatment.

Prognosis

Prenatal diagnosis is not possible. In the low-sulfur hair syndrome with associated severe systemic defects, genetic counseling is appropriate, emphasizing that each prospective sibling has a 25% chance of being affected.

INCREASED HAIR

1. HYPERTRICHOSIS LANUGINOSA

Hypertrichosis lanuginosa is transmitted by an autosomal dominant inheritance pattern and usually is noticeable at birth. White, silky hair up to 10 cm long is present over large areas of the body, including the face. Rarely, some teeth are absent. The disease has cosmetic and psychologic implications that should be handled sympathetically.

Acquired forms of this disease are invariably associated with internal cancer of epithelial surfaces, including the lungs, lower gastrointestinal tract, and urinary bladder.

BLISTERING DISORDERS

Blistering is a unique reaction pattern of lesions limited to the skin and a few other epithelia. Blistering diseases are discussed in Chapter 42. The discussion in this section is limited to genetic blistering diseases. An approach to their diagnosis is presented in Fig 20–2.

The porphyrias, characterized by blistering and photosensitivity, are discussed in Chapter 38.

EPIDERMOLYSIS BULLOSA

This is a heterogeneous group of genetically determined disorders with several modes of inheritance and variations in the degree of clinical severity. In all forms, blisters are induced by trauma (see Chapter 51).

ACRODERMATITIS ENTEROPATHICA

Essentials of Diagnosis

- Periorificial and acral skin eruptions.

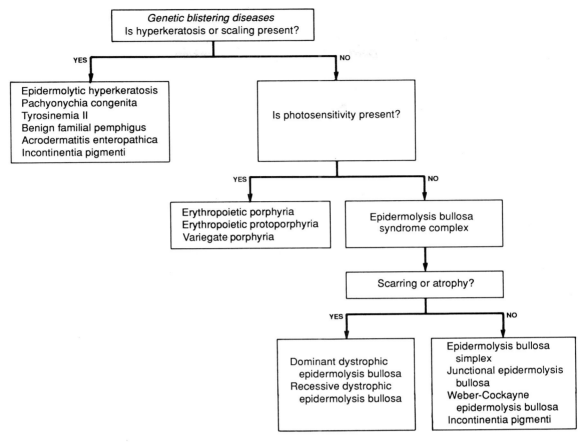

Figure 20–2. Genetic blistering diseases.

- Alopecia.
- Onset in infancy.
- Growth retardation.
- Diarrhea with intestinal candidiasis.
- Decreased serum zinc concentrations.
- Autosomal recessive inheritance.

General Considerations

This disorder is caused by low levels of zinc in the skin due to an abnormality of zinc metabolism.

After weaning from breast milk, symptoms occur in infants of both sexes. Human breast milk contains a ligand permitting zinc absorption even in the absence of the intestinal factor deficient in this rare genetic disease. Picolinic acid, a tryptophan derivative, has been implicated as the deficient ligand. Increased dietary zinc overcomes the genetic defect and restores normal health.

Clinical Findings

A. Symptoms and Signs: This disorder begins 4–10 weeks after birth in infants who are not breast-fed or after weaning in breast-fed infants. Failure to thrive and diarrhea with candidal infections may be observed. Vesicles, pustules, or erosions develop around the mouth, anus, elbows, knees, and fingers. Alopecia and nail dystrophies are common. Blepharitis, conjunctivitis, and photophobia occur. The child is emotionally unstable and has decreased appetite. Spontaneous improvement at puberty is usually seen. The disease may persist into adult life and resemble psoriasis.

B. Laboratory Findings: Serum zinc levels below 50 μg/dL are diagnostic. (**Note:** Rubber stoppers contain high zinc levels that may contaminate specimens. Use acid-washed tubes with special stoppers.)

Differential Diagnosis

Epidermolysis bullosa and combined immunodeficiency syndrome with candidiasis may have clinical presentations similar to that of acrodermatitis enteropathica. Similar lesions may occur in patients requiring parenteral hyperalimentation or receiving a diet deficient in essential fatty acids. Incomplete amino acid diets used for treating some metabolic defects may also induce similar lesions.

Complications & Sequelae

The disease may rarely lead to septicemia, inanition, and death if unrecognized and untreated.

Treatment

Zinc dietary supplements rapidly restore normal health and reverse all features of the disease. The usual dose of zinc gluconate or zinc sulfate is 5 mg/kg/d orally in divided doses. The drug is usually well tolerated but may cause nausea. Absorption is inhibited, however, by taking with food, especially bread.

In the past, breast milk and dihydroxyquinolone were reasonably effective therapies—the latter complicated rarely by optic neuritis.

Course & Prognosis

The disease is lifelong. Prenatal diagnosis is not yet possible. Proper treatment leads to complete remission and presumably a normal life span.

TYROSINEMIA TYPE II

Hepatic tyrosine aminotransferase deficiency is an autosomal recessive disease associated with tyrosinemia. In infancy, there is keratitis and then vesicular, erosive, and hyperkeratotic lesions on the palms and soles. Mild mental retardation may accompany the disease. Blood and urinary tyrosine levels are elevated; tyrosine and its metabolites in the urinary tract can be determined by the α-nitrosonaphthol test.

Lifelong treatment with a low-tyrosine, low-phenylalanine diet (Mead Johnson 3200 AB) is curative of the skin and eye lesions but will not reverse mental retardation.

PACHYONYCHIA CONGENITA

Essentials of Diagnosis

- Thickening of the nail plates due to massive subungual hyperkeratosis.
- Palmar and plantar hyperkeratoses, with hyperhidrosis and blistering.
- White plaques on mouth and tongue.
- Autosomal dominant inheritance.

General Considerations

This is a rare dominantly inherited disorder of keratinization characterized by thickening of the nail bed and irregular involvement of skin, hair, mouth, and eyes. The disease begins in childhood; early recognition helps focus on treatment, prognosis, and genetic counseling. Skin biopsy is not diagnostic. Morphologic evidence suggests an abnormality in keratinization, but the basic molecular defect is unknown. Families with pachyonychia congenita and eye involvement with steatocystoma multiplex have been reported.

Clinical Findings

A. Symptoms and Signs: The pathognomonic feature of the disease is the massive hyperkeratosis of the nail bed, which leads to a distorted tubular, tunnel-like yellowed nail plate of normal thickness. Focal or diffuse hyperkeratosis of the skin occurs in childhood, as do milia and follicular hyperkeratotic lesions on the knees, elbows, abdomen, and buttocks. Blistering of palms and soles and hyperhidrosis often accompany hyperkeratosis of these sites.

In slightly more than half of cases, oral hyperkeratosis occurs early in childhood. The tongue is most frequently involved, but the buccal mucosa and, rarely, the gingivae can be affected. Posterior commissure involvement causes hoarseness. Opaque spots, striations, or large white plaques may be present on mucous membranes. The oral lesions are not premalignant. In type II, in addition to the cutaneous features, there are natal teeth and multiple skin cysts that may involve most parts of the body, including the face and scrotum. Oral lesions do not occur in type II. In type III, in addition to the features present in type I, there is leukokeratosis of the cornea.

In types I and II, hair may be twisted, unruly, and unkempt.

B. Laboratory Findings: Oral biopsy shows large epithelial cells with cytoplasmic vacuoles and a relatively small nucleus. Skin biopsy shows thickening of the spinous and granular layers and intracellular edema associated with blistering lesions. Nail biopsy shows the nail bed to be markedly thickened.

Differential Diagnosis

Massive subungual hyperkeratosis may occur with psoriasis and fungal infections. There is a separate syndrome of subungual hyperkeratosis, onycholysis, hypohidrosis, and enamel hypoplasia. In dyskeratosis congenita, there is blistering and aplasia of the nail bed, leading to scarring and absent nail plates. The presence of teeth at birth (natal teeth) is also a feature of congenital chondroectodermal dysplasia (Ellis-van Creveld syndrome) and oculomandibulodyscephaly (Hallermann-Streiff syndrome) and is found in 0.03–0.5% of normal infants.

Prevention

Prenatal diagnosis for this disease is not available. Abstaining from reproduction by affected individuals would prevent disease transmission. The risk of genetic transmission is 1:2.

Treatment

Hyperhidrosis contributes to blistering; cool footwear (especially in summer), powder (eg, Zeasorb, talc) to absorb moisture, and antiperspirants containing aluminum chlorhydrate or aluminum chlorate (eg,

Drysol, Xerac AC) to decrease sweating should be considered. Mild keratolytics (60% propylene glycol, or propylene glycol with 6% salicylic acid [Keralyt]) can decrease hyperkeratosis. Surgical removal of the nail bed and matrix can eradicate the abnormal thickness of the nail bed, but a normal nail plate is not restored by this procedure.

GENETIC DISEASES ASSOCIATED WITH PHOTOSENSITIVITY

Individuals with hypopigmentation are particularly susceptible to ultraviolet light. In the diseases to be discussed, photosensitivity occurs despite normal skin pigmentation.

BLOOM SYNDROME

Essentials of Diagnosis
- Photosensitivity.
- Dwarfism.
- Increased chromosome breaks and gaps and sister chromatid exchanges.

General Considerations
Males are affected more frequently by this rare autosomal recessive hereditary disease, which is most common in Ashkenazi Jews originally from southeastern Poland and the northwestern Ukraine. There are multiple abnormalities of chromosomal structure and DNA repair in this disease, but the basic genetic defect is unknown. Somatic recombination may be related to the increased incidence of neoplasia associated with this disorder.

Clinical Findings
A. Symptoms and Signs: Proportionate dwarfism (average birth weight, 1900 g) is present at birth. During the first month of life, exposure to sunlight causes erythema, blistering, and eventually persistent areas of erythema and telangiectatic vessels on the ears, the bridge of the nose, the cheeks, and the dorsa of the hands. Sun sensitivity is within the UVB range (sunburn spectrum, 290–320 nm). Adults are short (average 145 cm) and have normal intelligence and sexual development; males often have small testes. Respiratory and gastrointestinal infections are frequent.

B. Laboratory Findings: There is decreased DNA replication. Chromatid and isochromatid gaps, rearrangements, and breaks can be seen on karyotype analysis of phytohemagglutinin-stimulated lymphocytes. Complicated karyotypic abnormalities are

seen, including triradial and quadriradial configurations. Lymphocytes respond poorly to mitogens, and immunoglobulin deficiency may be present.

Differential Diagnosis
Erythropoietic protoporphyria causes sun sensitivity in early childhood and can be diagnosed by fluorescent microscopy of red cells and quantitative determination of red cell protoporphyrias. Erythropoietic porphyria can also be diagnosed by red cell fluorescent microscopy and urinary porphyrin determinations (see Chapter 38).

In Rothmund-Thomson syndrome, there is telangiectasia and hyperpigmentation on sun-exposed areas, dwarfism, sparse hair, and cataracts. In Cockayne's syndrome, there is facial telangiectasia early in the second year of life and a wizened appearance due to subcutaneous tissue atrophy. Neonatal lupus erythematosus may be associated with epidermal atrophy and telangiectasia and may be diagnosed by serologic tests for the Ro (SS-A) and La (SS-B) antibodies in sera from the infant and its mother or by skin biopsy. The telangiectases of patients with ataxia-telangiectasia are predominantly in the axillas, the antecubital fossae, the conjunctiva, and the ears. The photosensitivity in Hartnup disease is associated with ataxia, a pellagralike rash, and a monoacidic, monobasic aciduria. Ataxia is not seen in Bloom syndrome. Increased chromosome breaks and an increased frequency of lymphosarcoma, lymphocytic leukemia, and gastric adenocarcinoma occur in ataxia-telangiectasia.

Prevention
Sister chromatid exchange is increased in cells grown from amniotic fluid and allows prenatal diagnosis. Genetic counseling should emphasize the 1:4 risk of giving birth to an infected child in subsequent pregnancies.

Treatment
Topical sunscreens with p-aminobenzoic acid and its derivatives will prevent the sunburn reaction and decrease sun damage.

Prognosis
The incidence of cancer is markedly increased in this disease, with expected shortening of the life span. Neoplasms include acute leukemia in adolescence, lymphomas, and squamous cell carcinomas of the mouth and esophagus.

XERODERMA PIGMENTOSUM

Essentials of Diagnosis
- Photosensitivity to UVB (290–320 nm).
- Melanocyte hyperplasia in skin.
- Abnormal DNA repair.

General Considerations

This is a rare (1:250,000–1:65,000 births) group of abnormalities of DNA repair; each individual form of the disease is inherited as an autosomal recessive trait. Excision of ultraviolet-induced pyrimidine dimers is the defect in most cases. In some, excision is normal but postexcision repair is slow. Different genetic complementation groups have consistently shown different decreases in repair. In group A (repair < 2%), forms of the disease with neurologic manifestations are common.

Clinical Findings

A. Symptoms and Signs: In infancy or early childhood, sun exposure leads to prolonged erythema because the minimal erythema dose is reduced. With ordinary sun exposure and no photoprotection, increased freckling, atrophy, and telangiectasia may be seen. Exposed areas are most affected and doubly covered areas (eg, beneath underpants) least affected. Dermal sclerosis leads to distortion of the eyes, nose, and mouth. Photophobia occurs early, and blepharitis, keratitis, and corneal ulcers are common.

In patients with the more severe forms of the disease, there is frequently microcephaly, choreoathetosis, cerebellar ataxia, mental retardation, and testicular hypoplasia (De Sanctis-Cacchione syndrome).

B. Laboratory Findings: Studies of DNA repair on cultured fibroblasts, lymphocytes, and epidermal cells are abnormal and show decreased DNA repair.

Differential Diagnosis

The various causes of photosensitivity discussed under Bloom syndrome should be considered. Hyperpigmentation would suggest progeria, Peutz-Jeghers disease, LEOPARD syndrome, and familial melanoma (these are discussed in detail in other chapters).

Prevention

Prenatal diagnosis in families at risk is advised, because DNA repair studies can be detected in affected individuals in utero.

Treatment

Avoidance of UVB light and use of sunblocks and sunscreens with an SPF of 15 are mandatory. Tumors are treated by surgical excision.

Prognosis

Basal cell carcinomas, squamous cell carcinomas, keratoacanthomas, and melanomas occur frequently and may lead to death. Squamous cell carcinoma of the tip of the tongue is common.

DYSKERATOSIS CONGENITA

Essentials of Diagnosis

- Hyperpigmentation of chest and neck.
- Diffuse thickening of palms and soles and loss of dermatoglyphics.
- Blistering of nail beds and loss of nail plates.
- White oral plaques.

General Considerations

Almost all cases of this rare syndrome have been seen in males, and X-linked inheritance is assumed because the trait is lethal in females. Sister chromatid exchange is increased after treatment of cells from patients with psoralens and ultraviolet light, and there is delayed excision of the DNA-psoralen cross-links.

Clinical Findings

A. Symptoms and Signs: In early childhood, epiphora develops from obstructed lacrimal ducts. In the middle of the first decade, blistering of the palms, nail beds, and matrix occurs. This leads to loss of the nail plates and bulbous atrophy at the ends of the digits, which sometimes contain only small amounts of nail plate. Irregular persistent intraoral buccal plaques appear. On the palms and soles, diffuse atrophic hyperkeratotic areas are devoid of dermatoglyphics.

In adolescence, on the trunk and neck, a finely reticulated hyperpigmentation surrounds central hypopigmented areas.

B. Laboratory Findings: DNA repair and excision studies establish the diagnosis (see above). Pancytopenia is present (see below).

Differential Diagnosis

Pachyonychia congenita is associated with hyperkeratosis and blistering of the soles and oral lesions, but the nail beds are hypertrophic rather than atrophic. In epidermolysis bullosa and tyrosinemia, the blistering starts earlier in life.

In Fanconi's syndrome, a more uniform hyperpigmentation may occur in childhood. Digital, carpal, and renal abnormalities occur. An aplastic anemia completes the syndrome.

In the Naegeli syndrome, there is a fine reticulated hyperpigmentation on the neck that begins in childhood. Hyperkeratotic palms and soles are also accompanied by a loss of dermatoglyphics. The inheritance is autosomal dominant.

Treatment

There is no treatment other than symptomatic relief for various cutaneous signs. Avoid known occupational carcinogens and mutagens, including UV light and tobacco.

Prognosis

Aplastic anemia and an increased incidence of cancer are the main complications of this disease. Adenocarcinoma of the rectum and squamous cell carcinomas of the oral, esophageal, nasopharyngeal, and cervical epithelial areas and the tongue occur.

Pancytopenia presages a downhill course and death within a few years.

DISORDERS ASSOCIATED WITH URTICARIA & EDEMA

Persistent or intermittent edema and swelling occur in a number of diseases that are tabulated in Table 20–3.

CONNECTIVE TISSUE DEFECTS

The collagen and elastin of the dermis are abnormal in several inherited disorders. Some of the diseases in this group are related to sclerosis or premature aging of connective tissue; others present as abnormal elasticity or papule formation. Fig 20–3 outlines the differential diagnosis of this group of diseases.

DISEASES ASSOCIATED WITH PREMATURE AGING & SCLEROSIS

1. WERNER'S SYNDROME

Affected individuals of both sexes are short and have premature graying and loss of scalp hair, sclerodermatous changes on the extremities, diabetes mellitus, hypogonadism, calcification of blood vessels and myocardial infarction at young ages, and leg ulcers. The disease is manifested in the second and third decades of life and is transmitted in an autosomal recessive pattern. Cells undergo premature aging in vitro and cannot be passed in culture for as long as cells from age-matched controls. The mottled pig-

Table 20–3. Genetic disorders with urticaria or edema.

Disease	Age at Onset and Genetics	Clinical Features and Treatment
Amyloidosis with urticaria and deafness	Adolescence, dominant	Chills and fever accompany urticaria. Limb pain in some kindreds. Absent organ of Corti. Kidney involvement present.
Cold urticaria	Childhood, autosomal dominant	Generalized chilling (eg, walking in the cold, swimming in cold water, not local chilling or ice cubes) precipitates chills, fever, headache, arthralgia, and edema. Avoid cold exposure.
Familial angioedema	Childhood, autosomal dominant	Nonpruritic, nonpitting edema lasting up to 72 hours. Symptomatic upper respiratory and gastrointestinal involvement common. Inhibitor of activated first component of complement (C1INH) defective or absent. **Emergency treatment** may require tracheostomy and epinephrine. Replacement with plasma or C1INH helpful. Danazol (a nonandrogenic steroid) increases plasma level of C1INH in most patients and is used for chronic preventive therapy (not useful in acute attacks).
Familial localized heat urticaria	Childhood, autosomal dominant	Wheals after 1½–2 hours in heat; last up to 1 day. Avoid heating; antihistamines may help.
Familial lymphedema	Birth to adulthood, dominant	Initially reversible with rest and pittable. Fibrosis and infection contribute to persistence. Some late-onset forms associated with distichiasis (2 rows of eyelashes) or ptosis.
Familial Meterranean fever	First 2 decades, dominant, most frequent in Armenians and Sephardic Jews	Urticaria and erysipelaslike erythema accompany attacks of serositis, abdominal pain, and arthritis. Colchicine may prevent attacks. Amyloidosis in some patients.
Sickle cell anemia	Infancy and childhood, autosomal	Hands and feet affected. Other signs of sickle cell disease, eg, anemia, crisis, are present.
Turner's syndrome	Infancy, sporadic, females affected	Hand and foot edema resolves with age. Other features such as webbed neck, broad chest, and low hairline suggest diagnosis. Karyotype most commonly shows missing X (45/XO) and establishes the diagnosis.

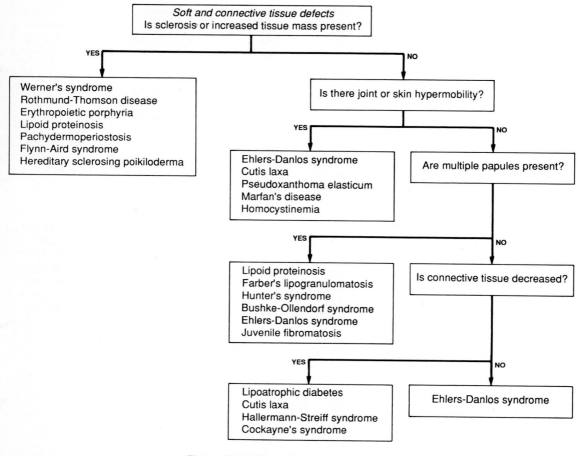

Figure 20–3. Soft and connective tissue defects.

mentation, telangiectasia, and sclerosis require differentiation from dyskeratosis congenita. The incidence of internal malignancy is increased.

There is no known treatment. Death usually is from accelerated atherosclerosis.

2. PROGERIA

Alopecia begins in the first 18 months of life. Sclerodermatous or morphealike changes on the scalp with prominent, superficial blood vessels are often an early sign of the disease. Generalized growth is decreased, and there is facial hypoplasia with frontal bossing and micrognathia. The skin is sclerotic and atrophic. Accelerated arteriosclerosis leads to death from coronary artery disease, often in the second decade. The cells from affected individuals age rapidly in culture. The disease has autosomal recessive inheritance.

There is no effective therapy.

DISEASES ASSOCIATED WITH ABNORMAL ELASTICITY OR PAPULE FORMATION*

1. EHLERS-DANLOS SYNDROME

This is a heterogeneous group of genetic disorders in which there is a deficiency or defect of normal collagen, with resulting abnormal skin extensibility and friability and frequent soft joint laxity, bony abnormalities, or changes in collagen in other internal tissues.

Details of the classification of these diseases are presented in Chapter 24.

2. CUTIS LAXA

This is a group of genetically heterogeneous disorders of connective tissue in which skin abnormalities

*Lipoid proteinosis (hyalinosis cutis et mucosae) is discussed in Chapter 31.

often presage serious internal disease. In the first year of life, the sides of the face begin to form loose folds, leading to sagging jowls and a "sad sack" or bloodhound appearance. There is a long philtrum and inverted nostrils.

See Chapter 24.

3. OSTEOPOIKILOSIS WITH CONNECTIVE TISSUE NEVUS (Buschke-Ollendorff Syndrome)

In this autosomal dominantly inherited syndrome, there are circumscribed sclerotic areas in epiphyseal and metaphyseal bone that are asymptomatic and associated with multiple raised red-orange skin papules. Elastic tissue is markedly increased in these lesions.

No treatment is required; there are no serious sequelae.

4. FARBER'S LIPOGRANULOMATOSIS

Infants with this disease have a weak, hoarse cry and swollen joints. Multiple subcutaneous nodules are especially prominent in juxta-articular locations. Death usually occurs in the first decade. Mucosal, lung, and subcutaneous tissues are infiltrated with foam cells, histiocytes, lymphocytes, and plasma cells. Free ceramide is increased; ceramidase is decreased in white blood cells or cultured fibroblasts. The disease is transmitted as an autosomal recessive, and genetic counseling is mandatory.

5. PACHYDERMOPERIOSTOSIS

This is a rare autosomal dominant disease in which there is thickening and furrowing of the facial skin, especially on the forehead. Large, active sebaceous glands contribute to oiliness. Thickened hands and feet suggest acromegaly. Marked folding of the scalp skin (cutis verticis gyrata) is often present. Bony changes include periosteal proliferation and hypertrophic osteoarthropathy with clinical clubbing of the nails.

MULTIPLE NEW SKIN GROWTHS

Papules and nodules occur in a variety of genetic diseases. In Fig 20–4, a logical scheme for distinguishing some of them is presented. The nature of these disorders is outlined in Tables 20–4 and 20–5. A few of them are discussed in more detail below.

EPIDERMODYSPLASIA VERRUCIFORMIS

In this disease with autosomal recessive inheritance, red, fibrous papules resembling flat warts or tinea versicolor appear in childhood. The lesions can be generalized and contain human papillomavirus (HPV). Specific types of wart viruses are associated with these lesions, especially HPV-5 and HPV-8. Patients usually have deficient cell-mediated immune function. Lesions may become malignant.

Treatment with transfer factor has been successful in restoring host immunity in some patients.

GARDNER'S SYNDROME

In Gardner's syndrome, benign soft tissue tumors occur during the first decade of life and include epidermal inclusion cysts, fibromas, and desmoids. Osteomas occur as well. Later in life, large intestinal polyps frequently become malignant. Jaw cysts and supernumerary teeth (detected by x-rays) may be an early sign of the disease. Close follow-up for intestinal malignancy is warranted.

Because the disorder is inherited as an autosomal dominant, relatives should be investigated for stigmas of the disease.

GENETIC DISORDERS ASSOCIATED WITH SKIN ULCERATION

These diseases are listed in Table 20–6, and some are discussed elsewhere in this chapter or in the text.

In the Flynn-Aird syndrome, transmitted as an autosomal dominant, subcutaneous tissue atrophy and ulceration similar to that of Werner's syndrome or scleroderma are seen. There is deafness, retardation, convulsions, baldness, and stiff joints, which begin the first and second decade of life.

In prolidase deficiency, transmitted as an autosomal recessive, leg ulcers with thickening of surrounding skin appear in the early decades of life. Associated abnormalities include atrophic scars on the face, extremities, and buttocks; premature poliosis and alopecia; facial defects, including saddle nose, hypertelorism, and jaw hypoplasia; and bilateral deafness. Hyperkeratosis over the elbows and knees is also present. Increased urinary excretion of proline-containing dipeptides is seen.

Lesch-Nyhan syndrome is characterized by severe mental retardation, self-mutilation, choreoathetosis, hyperuricemia, and uricosuria. The disease is X-linked; only males are affected.

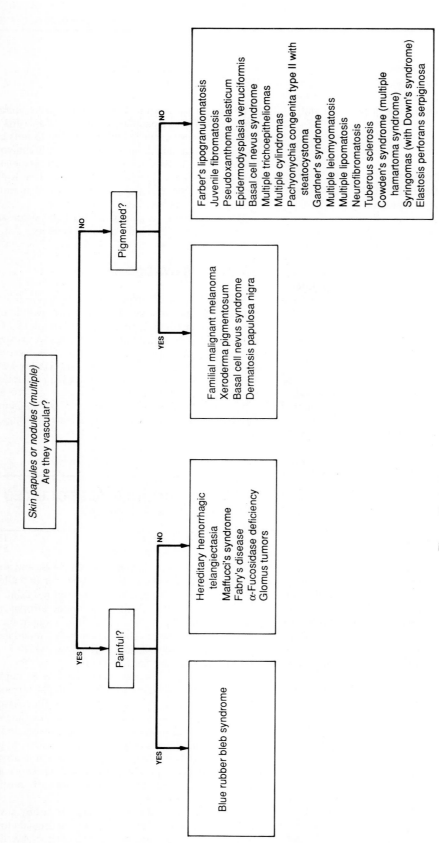

Figure 20–4. Skin papules or nodules (multiple).

Table 20–4. Dominantly inherited skin diseases with multiple skin papules and nodules.

Disease	Age at Onset	Basic Lesions	Characteristic Location	Complications and Associations	Histology
Adenoma sebaceum	First or second decade.	Flesh-colored papules with telangiectasia.	Face.	Tuberous sclerosis with convulsions, retardation, hypopigmented macules.	Angiofibromas.
Basal cell nevus syndrome	Second or third decade.	Flesh-colored papules.	Face.	Jaw cysts, rib defects, calcified falx, frontal bossing, short fourth metacarpal bone.	Basal cell proliferation often with calcification.
Cowden's disease	Childhood, puberty.	Shiny or slightly hyperkeratotic papules.	Face, palms, tongue, oral mucosa.	Fibrocystic disease, internal cancer.	Facial lesions, tricholemmomas on biopsy.
Cylindromas	Early adulthood.	Papule to nodule; may be pedunculated.	Scalp.	Frequently, patients have trichoepitheliomas.	Two cell types streaked with hyalinized material; lumina of glands within lesions.
Dermatosis papulosa nigra	First or second decade.	Small brown or black individual papules.	Face.	In about one-third of US blacks.	Hyperkeratosis and acanthosis as in seborrheic keratoses.
Familial melanoma	First and second decades.	Reddish-brown papules with some splay of pigment.	Sun-exposed skin; scalp.	Melanomas at early ages; may be multiple.	Atypical melanocytic hyperplasia with new vessel proliferation.
Leiomyomas	Third decade.	Multiple discrete or grouped pink papules and nodules.	Anywhere.	Painful, especially with pressure or cold.	Bundle of smooth muscle cells.
Lipomas	Puberty to fourth decade.	Subcutaneous.	Arms.	Sometimes painful (Dercum syndrome).	Multiple fat lobules in a fibrous capsule.
Multiple glomus tumors	First or second decade.	Flesh-colored or blue discrete or grouped papules.	Anywhere.	Painful (rarely).	Nonencapsulated with glomus cells surrounding endothelial cells.
Steatocytoma multiplex	First or second decade.	Flesh-colored nodules.	Anywhere; extremities, scrotum common.	May rupture and become infected; oily fluid may be discharged.	Cyst with sebaceous lobules and eosinophilic cuticle.
Trichoepitheliomas	First and second decades.	Small flesh-colored papules with telangiectasia.	Face, periorbitally and in the nasolabial folds.	Frequently have cylindromas; important to distinguish from the adenoma sebaceum of tuberous sclerosis and from acne.	Sharply delimited basal proliferation with immature follicular features.

Table 20–5. Genetic skin disorders with prominent vascular features.

Disease	Age at Onset	Genetics	Clinical features	Diagnostic Tests
Blue rubber-bleb nevus syndrome	Birth, infancy.	Dominant (or sporadic).	Nipplelike little hemangiomas on limbs or trunk; millimeters to centimeters in diameter; gastrointestinal bleeding from similar lesions.	
Fabry's disease	Late first decade to second decade.	X-linked.	Purple papules from 1 to a few mm in diameter with hyperkeratosis, especially on lower trunk, buttocks, thigh, and genitals; corneal opacities, neuropathy, heart intolerance.	α-Galactosidase A deficiency leading to ceramide trihexoside deposition.
α-Fucosidosis	First decade.	Autosomal recessive.	Similar skin lesions to Fabry's disease, frequent mental retardation.	Decreased α-fucosidase levels in cells.
Hereditary hemorrhagic telangiectasia	Childhood.	Dominant.	Sharply delimited telangiectatic mats on face, ears, oral and nasal mucosa, gastrointestinal tract, and lungs; epistaxis, gastrointestinal bleeding, pulmonary arteriovenous fistulas common.	
Maffuci's syndrome (dyschondroplasia with cavernous angiomas)	Early in first decade.	?	On fingers and toes there are raised hemangiomas; multiple enchondromas and pathologic fractures are common; bone or vascular neoplasia occurs.	X-rays of long bones show enchondromas and are diagnostic.

CHROMOSOMAL DEFECTS & SKIN DISEASE

Table 20–6. Ulceration and mutilation associated with genetic skin diseases.

Aplasia cutis
Flynn-Aird syndrome
Hemoglobinopathies (sickle cell, thalassemia)
Klinefelter's disease
Lesch-Nyhan syndrome
Prolidase deficiency
Werner's syndrome

Chromosomal abnormalities are often associated with defects in many organ systems. Some of the chromosomal abnormalities have prominent skin manifestations which, in connection with other phenotypic features of the syndrome (or multiorgan involvement suggesting a chromosomal defect), warrant karyotyping. Such disorders and their features are listed in Table 20–7.

REFERENCES

Alper JC: The genodermatoses. Dermatol Clin 1987;5:1.

Beauregard S, Gilchrest BA: Syndromes of premature aging. Dermatol Clin 1987;5:109.

Bergsma D (editor): *Birth Defects Compendium,* 2nd ed. Alan R. Liss, 1979.

Birnbaum PS, Baden HP: Heritable disorders of hair. Dermatol Clin 1987;5:137.

Carney RG: Incontinentia pigmenti: A world statistical analysis. Arch Dermatol 1976;112:535.

Cowan MJ et al: Multiple biotin-dependent carboxylase deficiencies associated with defects in T-cell and B-cell immunity. Lancet 1979;2:115.

Demmel U: Clinical aspects of congenital skin defects. 1. Congenital skin defects on the head of the newborn. Eur J Pediatr 1975;121:21.

Der Kaloustian VM, Kurban AK: *Genetic Diseases of the Skin.* Springer-Verlag, 1979.

Eil C et al: A cellular defect in hereditary vitamin D-dependent rickets type II: Defective nuclear uptake of 1,25-dihydroxyvitamin D in cultured skin fibroblasts. N Engl J Med 1981;304:1588.

Goldsmith LA, McKusick VA: Genetics in relation to the skin. Pages 1619–1633 in: *Dermatology in General Medicine,* 3rd ed. Fitzpatrick TB, Freedberg IM (editors). McGraw-Hill, 1987.

Goldsmith LA: Molecular biology and molecular pathology of a newly described molecular disease: Tyrosinemia II (the Richner-Hanhart syndrome). Exp Cell Biol 1978; 46:96.

Gonzalez JJ et al: Acquired hypertrichosis lanuginosa: Rare

Table 20–7. Skin manifestations associated with chromosomal abnormalities.

Disease	Defect	Skin Manifestation
4P–	Deletion of the short arm of chromosome 4.	Central scalp defects.
Trisomy 8	Extra autosome.	Short nails; redundant skin on posterior neck. No patella. (Important to distinguish trisomy 8 from the nail-patella syndrome.)
Inversion 9	Pericentric inversion of chromosome 9.	Inversion of 9 usually a harmless polymorphism. Features of anhidrotic ectodermal dysplasia in obligate females with inversion; obligate females without inversion normal. One family.
Trisomy 10	Extra autosome.	Congenital scalp defect.
Trisomy 13	Trisomy 13 (D group). Extra autosome.	Scalp defects (parietal-occipital). Low posterior hairline. Redundant skin on neck. Nails narrow and hyperconvex. Scrotal-type skin extending to tip of penis.
Ring 13	Deletion of portions of 13 associated with ring formation.	Epicanthal fold. Alopecia and (?) scalp defect. Symmetrical hypopigmentation (arciform).
Ring 14	Ring of chromosome 14.	Epicanthal folds. Café au lait spots (some linear). Redundant neck skin. Multiple depigmented macules. Seizures (myotonic). (Need to consider in differential diagnosis of tuberous sclerosis.)
Ring 17	Ring of chromosome.	Multiple café au lait spots.
18p–	Deletion of the short arm of chromosome 18.	Congenital alopecia.
Monosomy 21 (mosaic)		EEC syndrome (ectrodactyly, ectodermal dysplasia, cleft lip and palate). Sparse scalp hair.
Down's syndrome	Trisomy 21 (as an additional autosome or due to a translocation).	Elastosis perforans serpiginosa. Vasculature instability (acrocyanosis, cutis marmorata). Premature wrinkling of the skin. Frequent syringomas. Frequent alopecia areata. Hyperkeratotic palms, skin, and ichthyosislike changes. Fissured and furrowed skin (xerosis).
Turner's syndrome	XO (deficiency of one X chromosome or presence of an abnormal X chromosome, XX₁(iso-X).	Congenital and persistent lymphedema. Hypoplastic nails. Increased number of nevi. Redundant skin on neck; cystic hygromas. Low posterior hairline. Increased aging of skin.
XYY	Extra Y chromosome.	Cystic acne. Frequent port wine stains (?). Varicose veins and ulceration increased.
Klinefelter's syndrome	XXY (XXY mosaics, XXXY, XXYY).	Thirteen percent with leg ulcers.

manifestation of urinary bladder carcinoma. Arch Intern Med 1980;140:969.

Gorlin RJ, Pinborg JJ, Cohen MM Jr: *Syndromes of the Head and Neck,* 2nd ed. McGraw-Hill, 1976.

Hazen PG et al: Premature cataracts in a family with hidrotic ectodermal dysplasia. Arch Dermatol 1980;116:1385.

Kraemer KH: Xeroderma pigmentosum: A prototype disease of environmental-genetic interaction. Arch Dermatol 1980;116:541.

Lambert WC: Genetic diseases associated with DNA and chromosomal instability. Dermatol Clin 1987;5:85.

Lutzner MA: Epidermodysplasia verruciformis: An autosomal recessive disease characterized by viral warts and skin cancer. A model for viral oncogenesis. Bull Cancer 1978;65:169.

McKusick VA: *Mendelian Inheritance in Man: Catalogs of Autosomal Dominant, Autosomal Recessive, and X-Linked Phenotypes,* 8th ed. Johns Hopkins Press, 1988.

Neldner KH, Hambidge KM, Walravens PA: Acrodermatitis enteropathica. Int J Dermatol 1978;17:380.

Ogata A et al: Autosomal recessive prolidase deficiency: Three patients with recalcitrant ulcers. Arch Dermatol 1981;117:689.

Oorthuys JW, Beemer FA: The Langer-Giedion syndrome (trichorhino-phalangeal syndrome, type II). Eur J Pediatr 1979;132:55.

Polani PE: DNA repair defects and chromosomal disorders. Page 81, in: *Symposium on Genetics and Human Biology: Possibilities and Realities.* Porter R, O'Connor M (editors). Ciba Foundation Excerpta Medica, 1979.

Schonfeld PHIR: The pachyonychia congenita syndrome. Acta Dermatovener (Stockholm) 1980;60:45.

Sirinavin C, Trowbridge AA: Dyskeratosis congenita: Clinical features and genetic aspects. Report of a family and review of the literature. J Med Genet 1975;12:339.

Solomon LM, Cook B, Klipfel W: The ectodermal dysplasias. Dermatol Clin 1987;5:231.

Solomon LM, Keuer EJ: The ectodermal dysplasias: Problems of classification and some newer syndromes. Arch Dermatol 1980;116:1295.

Stanbury JB et al: *The Metabolic Basis of Inherited Disease,* 5th ed. McGraw-Hill, 1983.

Trojak JE et al: Immunologic studies of cartilage-hair hypoplasia in the Amish. Johns Hopkins Med J 1981;148:157.

21 Disorders of Keratinization

Mark V. Dahl, MD

Disorders of keratinization are generally characterized by obvious epidermal disruptions such as fissures, scales, or thickening of the stratum corneum. Inflammatory changes, if present, are presumed to be secondary to the disordered epidermis.

DARIER'S DISEASE (Keratosis Follicularis)

Essentials of Diagnosis

- Waxy, keratotic papules in "seborrheic" distribution.
- Macerated intertriginous papules and plaques.
- Nails: distal fragility, longitudinal ridges, red and white linear subungual bands.
- Cobblestonelike white papules on mucosa.
- Histopathology: Epidermal suprabasilar lacunae with acantholytic and dyskeratotic cells.

General Considerations

Darier's disease, an uncommon autosomal dominant disorder, usually begins in childhood or adolescence. Sporadic cases are not unusual and presumably represent new mutations. The disorder affects the skin, mucosa, and nails, producing a characteristic clinical picture and diagnostic histopathologic features. Histologically, a severe defect in cornification is seen; however, the biochemical abnormality is unknown.

Clinical Findings

A. Symptoms and Signs: Pruritic, greasy brown, keratotic papules coalesce to form plaques in the seborrheic areas (scalp, ears, face, neck, upper trunk). Intertriginous involvement results in eroded or macerated papules and plaques. Rarely, thick keratotic plaques cover much of the body surface (cornifying variant). Sunlight frequently induces lesions. Distinctive nail changes consist of fragile, short, relatively widened nails with distal notching, wedge-shaped subungual hyperkeratosis, longitudinal ridging, and red and white linear streaks in the nail bed. Asymptomatic involvement of the oral mucosa is characterized by white cobblestoned confluent papules, most prominent on the gingiva. Punctate keratoses of the palms and soles are characteristic, as are dorsal acral keratoses (clinically identical to acrokeratosis verruciformis of Hopf; see below). The skin disease is frequently worsened by exposure to ultraviolet radiation.

B. Laboratory Findings: Skin biopsy is diagnostic. Foci of suprabasilar clefts and lacunae contain characteristic acantholytic keratinocytes and dyskeratotic cells (the so-called *corp ronds* and grains). A thickened, parakeratotic stratum corneum develops over these lacunae.

Patients with Darier's disease may have decreased numbers of T cells in their peripheral blood and mild cell-mediated immunodeficiency.

Differential Diagnosis

Darier's disease must be differentiated from seborrheic dermatitis and benign familial pemphigus (Hailey-Hailey disease). Biopsy usually helps. A similar histologic picture is seen in transient acantholytic dermatosis (Grover's disease), some epidermal nevi, and warty dyskeratomas, but these differ clinically. Since the disorder consists of follicular papules in the seborrheic areas, it may be misdiagnosed as acne, although comedones, pustules, and nodules are absent.

Complications

Secondary bacterial infection is common. Patients are at risk for serious, widespread cutaneous viral infections (Kaposi's varicelliform eruption), most commonly due to herpes simplex virus.

Treatment

Patients should assiduously avoid sun exposure and routinely use an effective sunscreen (SPF 15). Secondary infection should be treated with topical and oral antibiotics—eg, dicloxacillin, for 2 weeks—after appropriate culture samples have been collected. Topical tretinoin (Retin-A) 0.05% cream may be applied 1–2 times daily; however, irritation frequently limits its effectiveness. Intermittent wet compresses (eg, Burow's solution 1:40) or tap water soaks help decrease odor and crusts. Oral vitamin A should not be used because of its toxicity and limited efficacy. Treatment with synthetic retinoids—etretinate (Tegison) or isotretinoin (Accutane)—often induces remission, but chronic administration is often required to prevent recurrences. Many patients who have received these retinoids for several years have developed diffuse idiopathic skeletal hypertrophy, so chronic continuous therapy is rarely justified. Deep dermabrasion followed by split-thickness skin grafting has been advocated for some patients with the severe cornifying variant.

Prognosis

Although the disorder waxes and wanes, there is a tendency for the disease to become progressively more severe with time.

ICHTHYOSIS

Ichthyosis (from Gk *ichthys* "fish") denotes a group of acquired and hereditary disorders characterized by excessive scaling. The genetic forms are classified by their clinical characteristics and mode of inheritance. At least 5 major types of hereditary ichthyosis are recognized (Table 21–1). In 3 (lamellar ichthyosis, congenital ichthyosiform erythroderma, and epidermolytic hyperkeratosis), clinical scaling is accompanied by—and perhaps due to—a markedly increased rate of epidermal proliferation, similar to psoriasis. In contrast, in the 2 most common forms (ichthyosis vulgaris and recessive X-linked ichthyosis), epidermal turnover is normal and clinical scaling is apparently due to abnormal retention of stratum corneum. There are several minor forms, as well as a number of syndromes in which ichthyosis occurs as part of a multisystem disorder. A new classification system has been proposed and is being revised as the biochemical bases for these disorders are clarified (Table 21–1).

ACQUIRED ICHTHYOSIS

The distinction between overly dry skin (xerosis) from environmental causes (excessive bathing, harsh soaps, low humidity) and acquired ichthyosis is sometimes difficult. The sudden onset of generalized pronounced scaling in adulthood demands explanation. Internal malignant tumors—particularly lymphoma—may first present as scaling with a clinical

pattern similar to ichthyosis vulgaris (see below). Hypothyroidism can be manifested as acquired ichthyosis and must be ruled out by thyroid function tests. Dry, ichthyotic skin may be a feature of chronic renal insufficiency, perhaps due to mild hypervitaminosis A, and—in severe malabsorption or following prolonged total parenteral nutrition—possibly a manifestation of essential fatty acid deficiency. Ichthyosis may be a cutaneous feature of lepromatous leprosy. Certain drugs that interfere with cholesterol metabolism may produce ichthyosis, acanthosis nigricans, or palmar-plantar keratoderma as a side effect. Clofazimine, used in treatment of leprosy and pyoderma gangrenosum, produces ichthyosis, but its mechanism is not known.

ICHTHYOSIS VULGARIS

Essentials of Diagnosis

- Scaling on extensor extremities more than trunk; flexural sparing.
- Increased palmar markings to frankly thickened palms and soles.
- Onset after 3 months of age.
- Association with atopy.

General Considerations

Ichthyosis vulgaris is a common autosomal dominant disorder affecting about one of every 300 people. When mild, it may be indistinguishable from severe xerosis (dry skin). Atopic dermatitis is a frequent accompaniment. The fundamental abnormality is unknown; however, a defect in keratohyalin formation is suspected on morphologic grounds.

Clinical Findings

A. Symptoms and Signs: The skin is normal at birth but becomes rough and scaly during the first year of life. Fine, white branny scales over the trunk and larger, more adherent scales over the extensor surfaces of the extremities are characteristic. Flexures and the face are spared, and scaling is less pronounced on the trunk than on the extremities. The palms and soles are thickened, but this thickening may be mild and manifested as increased palmar markings.

B. Laboratory Findings: A skin biopsy is usually not necessary for diagnosis but demonstrates a thickened stratum corneum with a diminished or absent granular cell layer. On electron microscopy, keratohyalin granules are poorly developed.

Differential Diagnosis

There is a continuum between dry skin and ichthyosis vulgaris. The latter term is usually used if almost all skin is affected and the disorder has been present since childhood. The following features of ichthyosis vul-

Table 21–1. Classification of generalized genetically transmitted disorders of cornification.[1]

Type	Name	Inheritance[2]
1. Vulgaris	Ichthyosis vulgaris	AD
2. Steroid sulfatase deficiency	Recessive X-linked ichthyosis	XR
3. Bullous	Epidermolytic hyperkeratosis; bullous congenital ichthyosiform erythroderma	AD
4. Lamellar-recessive	Lamellar ichthyosis	AR
5. Congenital erythrodermic	Lamellar ichthyosis; congenital ichthyosiform erythroderma	AR
6. Lamellar-dominant	Autosomal dominant lamellar ichthyosis	AD
7. Harlequin	Harlequin fetus	AR
8. Curth-Maklin	Ichthyosis hystrix type Curth-Maklin	AD
9. Netherton	Netherton's syndrome; icthyosis linearis circumflexa	AR
10. Sjögren-Larsson	Sjögren-Larsson syndrome	AR
11. Phytanic acid storage	Refsum's disease; heredopathia atactica polyneuritiformis	AR
12. Neutral lipid storage	Neutral lipid storage disease; Chanarin-Dorfman syndrome	AR
13. Multiple sulfatase deficiency	Multiple sulfatase deficiency syndrome	AR
14. Trichothiodystrophy	Tay's syndrome; trichothiodystrophy; BIDS syndrome	AR
15. Keratitis-deafness	KID syndrome; atypical ichthyosiform erythroderma with deafness	AR?
16. Unilateral hemidysplasia	CHILD syndrome	XD?
17. Chondrodysplasia punctata syndromes	Conradi-Hünermann syndrome; chondrodysplasia punctata	AR; XD?
18. Erythrokeratodermia variabilis	Erythrokeratodermia variabilis	AD
19. Erythrokeratolysis heimalis	Erythrokeratolysis heimalis	AD
20. Erythrokeratodermia progressiva symmetrica	Erythrokeratodermia progressiva symmetrica	AD
21. Peeling skin	Peeling skin syndrome; familial continuous skin peeling	AR
22. Darier	Darier's disease; keratosis follicularis	AD
23. Giroux-Barbeau	Giroux-Barbeau syndrome	AD
24. Keratosis follicularis spinulosa decalvans	Keratosis follicularis spinulosa decalvans	XD?

[1]Modified and reproduced, with permission, from Williams ML, Elias PM: Genetically transmitted, generalized disorders of cornification: The ichthyoses. Dermatol Clin 1987;5:155.
[2]AD = autosomal dominant; AR = autosomal recessive; XD = X-linked dominant; XR = X-linked recessive.

garis permit distinction from other forms:

(1) From acquired ichthyosis: Onset in childhood, affected family members.

(2) From recessive X-linked ichthyosis: Complete flexural sparing, absence of corneal opacities, palmar-plantar involvement, smaller and whiter scales, normal steroid sulfatase activity, normal serum lipoprotein electrophoresis.

(3) From lamellar ichthyosis: Not present at birth, flexural sparing, no ectropion, no erythroderma.

(4) From epidermolytic hyperkeratosis: Flexural sparing, no blistering, histopathologic features.

Treatment

In mild cases, use of an emollient such as hydrophilic petrolatum (eg, Eucerin) cream or a 10–20% urea cream (Nutraplus, Aquacare/HP, Carmol 10 or 20) may suffice. Forty to 60 percent propylene glycol in water with occlusion by plastic occlusive suit at bedtime is effective. Five percent lactic acid in hydrophilic ointment or 12% ammonium lactate lotion (Lac-Hydrin) applied twice daily usually works well. Coexisting atopic dermatitis may complicate therapy because of increased sensitivity to irritant reactions from keratolytic agents.

Prognosis

The disorder improves with age. Residence in a mild moist climate may help.

RECESSIVE X-LINKED ICHTHYOSIS

Essentials of Diagnosis

- Skin normal at birth but peels and scales within the first few months.
- Adherent brown scales on trunk and extremities.
- Posterior neck always involved; other flexures are usually spared.
- Males only.
- Corneal opacities in adults.
- Steroid sulfatase deficiency.
- Abnormal mobility of β-lipoproteins on lipoprotein electrophoresis.
- Increased serum levels of cholesterol sulfate.

General Considerations

Recessive X-linked ichthyosis affects 1:6000 males. Absence of activity of the enzyme steroid sulfatase leads to accumulation of the enzyme's substrate, cholesterol sulfate (readily detected by abnormal lipoprotein electrophoretic mobility), within scale and serum. Failure to cleave cholesterol sulfate in the epidermis leads to faulty desquamation. In utero, placental insufficiency of the enzyme may lead to failure to initiate labor. Characteristic comma-shaped corneal opacities in affected men assist in the diagnosis but are asymptomatic.

Clinical Findings

A. Symptoms and Signs: The scales in this form are frequently browner than those of ichthyosis vulgaris and have a characteristic tacked-on appearance. There is generalized involvement of the trunk and extremities, with sparing of the face, palms, and soles. The flexures and face are relatively spared. The posterior neck, however, is always involved. Unlike ichthyosis vulgaris, the disorder begins during the first month of life. The skin is usually normal at birth.

B. Laboratory Findings: Biochemical diagnosis of this disorder is possible by assaying steroid sulfatase activity in cultured fibroblasts, scale, leukocytes, and amniocytes (permitting prenatal diagnosis). Abnormal mobility of the β-lipoproteins on lipoprotein electrophoresis is a readily available alternative to enzymatic assay. High levels of cholesterol sulfate confirm the diagnosis. Slit-lamp examination for corneal opacities may be useful in affected adults and, in some instances, carrier females.

Treatment

Lactic acid (5–10%) in petrolatum or hydrophilic petrolatum 1–2 times a day is effective, as is 40–60% propylene glycol in water under occlusion overnight. A lotion containing 12% ammonium lactate (Lac-Hydrin) may also help if applied twice daily.

Prognosis

Like ichthyosis vulgaris, this disorder improves with residence in warmer climates and in warmer seasons. There is no tendency to amelioration with age. Prenatal diagnosis in early pregnancy is possible by assaying sterol sulfatase in amniocytes.

LAMELLAR ICHTHYOSIS

Essentials of Diagnosis

- Erythema and scaling at birth ("collodion baby").
- Large, thick, dark, platelike scales.
- Generalized scaling disorder involving flexures, face, palms, and soles.
- Ectropion or facial tautness.

General Considerations

Lamellar ichthyosis is a rare autosomal recessive disease of unknown cause. The disorder is always present at birth and is frequently complicated by prematurity and encasement in a taut, inelastic membrane ("collodion baby"). Although clinical variability exists, this is usually a severe form producing considerable disability and deformity.

Clinical Findings

A. Symptoms and Signs: Babies may be born encased in a membrane that is eventually shed. Lamellar ichthyosis is characterized by generalized scaling. In some patients, large, platelike, dark scales (lamellae) dominate. All body surfaces, including all flexures, are involved. Facial involvement often results in ectropion and, in newborns, eclabium. Erythroderma is prominent in infancy, usually persisting to a greater or lesser degree through life. Alopecia occurs in some patients. Nails may be normal or dystrophic. Dentition is normal.

B. Laboratory Findings: Histologic findings of acanthosis and marked hyperkeratosis are characteristic but nondiagnostic. Epidermal proliferative activity is somewhat increased. There are increased amounts of free sterols and ceramides in the stratum corneum.

Treatment

At birth, collodion babies should be kept in a humid environment; the membrane should not be manually debrided.

Topical preparations containing 3–6% salicylic acid (eg, Keralyt gel) should be used with caution since systemic salicylism may occur. Topical tretinoin 0.05% or 0.1% cream (Retin-A) or one of the topicals outlined in the preceding sections may be helpful.

The need for continuous widespread applications and unsatisfactory responses to topical therapies have led to a search for alternatives. Experimental studies using the oral synthetic retinoids isotretinoin (Accutane) and etretinate (Tegison) have been promising. However, because continuous therapy at relatively high doses is required, further knowledge of long-term toxicity is needed before these agents can be generally recommended, particularly for children.

Complications

In addition to the problems of prematurity, collodion babies are at risk for sepsis, because cutaneous fissures provide a portal of entry, and for water and electrolyte imbalance.

CONGENITAL ICHTHYOSIFORM ERYTHRODERMA

Essentials of Diagnosis

- Born in a "collodion membrane."
- Generalized nonbullous erythroderma.
- Scales are fine and white but may be thick and dark on the legs.
- Flexures are involved.

General Considerations

Many still consider this to be a form of lamellar ichthyosis inherited as an autosomal recessive trait. The biochemical basis is unknown.

Clinical Findings

A. Symptoms and Signs: Most babies are born encased in a "collodion membrane" that is promptly shed. The skin then is erythrodermic and covered with fine white rough scale. Later, scales may be thicker and darker (lamellar), particularly on the legs. The face, palms and soles, and flexures are all affected. Ectropions, diffuse nonscarring alopecia, and nail plate thickening and ridging may occur. Obstruction of sweating may lead to heat intolerance. Mild growth retardation is not unusual.

B. Laboratory Findings: Epidermal turnover rates are increased, and there are increased levels of alkanes in the scales. Histologically, there is acanthosis, hyperkeratosis, and at least occasional parakeratosis. The stratum corneum may stain pink with periodic acid-Schiff (PAS) reagent.

Differential Diagnosis

The disorder mimics lamellar ichthyosis. About two-thirds of all "collodion babies" have congenital ichthyosiform erythroderma. The absence of bullae and characteristic histologic features distinguish the disorder from epidermolytic hyperkeratosis.

Treatment

The disorder responds to treatment with emol-lients, alpha-hydroxy acids such as lactic acid ointment, and keratolytics (see above).

Prognosis

Collodion babies may die from sepsis or electrolyte imbalance. Ectropion and eclabium may occur. Development of the cartilage in the nose and ear may be impaired and cause deformity. The scaling persists for life.

EPIDERMOLYTIC HYPERKERATOSIS (Bullous Congenital Ichthyosiform Erythroderma)

Essentials of Diagnosis

- Blistering and erosions at birth.
- Generalized scaling with accentuation in flexures.
- Warty or spiny ridges of thickened stratum corneum, usually in flexures.
- No ectropion.

General Considerations

Epidermolytic hyperkeratosis is a rare, autosomal dominant form of ichthyosis of unknown cause. Although its histopathologic features are distinctive, they are not specific since the same histologic pattern is seen in some patients with palmar-plantar keratodermas or epidermal nevi. Extensive bilateral epidermal nevi (ichthyosis hystrix) with this histologic picture may represent a forme fruste of generalized epidermolytic hyperkeratosis; the 2 forms have occurred in the same kindred. Many cases are sporadic, presumably new mutations. As in other forms, clinical severity varies; however, in most instances, epidermolytic hyperkeratosis is severe, chronic, and disabling.

Clinical Findings

A. Symptoms and Signs: Extensive denudation of skin in areas of trauma—more than scaling—characterize the newborn with epidermolytic hyperkeratosis. Blistering decreases with age, usually ceasing to be important after childhood. Similarly, erythroderma is intense in newborns but improves with age. Scaling is generalized and often most pronounced in flexures, where heaped-up keratotic spines form ridges. A foul odor from macerated scales and secondary infection is common. Palms and soles are usually affected, as is the scalp.

B. Laboratory Findings: Skin biopsy is diagnostic and permits prenatal diagnosis through fetoscopy and fetal skin biopsy. Upper spinous and granular cells have indistinct cell borders, vacuoles, and an increased number of irregular keratohyalin granules (granular degeneration). Pronounced hyperkeratosis overlies an acanthotic epidermis.

Treatment

Therapy is difficult. Topical therapy used in other forms of ichthyosis is frequently too irritating for the fragile skin of this disorder. Moreover, the stratum corneum forms an imperfect barrier, placing patients at risk for salicylism or hyperadrenocorticism, when salicylic acid or topical corticosteroids are employed. Because oral synthetic retinoids produce epidermal fragility, their usefulness in this disorder may be limited.

Secondary infection may play a significant role in blister formation; blisters and erosions should be cultured and oral antibiotics effective against anticipated pathogens (usually *Staphylococcus aureus*) utilized. The foul odor emanating from bacterial colonization of macerated scales may improve with antibacterial soap (eg, povidone-iodine or chlorhexidine) and sometimes with oral antibiotics (eg, erythromycin, 500–1000 mg/d).

ERYTHROKERATODERMA VARIABILIS (Mendes da Costa Syndrome)

Erythrokeratoderma variabilis, a rare autosomal dominant disorder with variable expressivity, is characterized by 2 types of lesions: (1) fixed hyperkeratotic plaques, most frequent on the face, extremities, and buttocks; and (2) shifting rings or arcs of erythema induced by wind or temperature change fading within hours to days.

SJÖGREN-LARSSON SYNDROME

Sjögren-Larsson syndrome is a rare autosomal recessive disorder characterized by ichthyosis plus central nervous system manifestations. The scaling abnormalities most closely resemble lamellar ichthyosis, and the patient may present at birth as a collodion baby. Flexural accentuation is characteristic. All patients exhibit spasticity and mental retardation by 5 years of age; retinitis pigmentosa, ocular hypertelorism, "glistening dot" retinopathy, seizures, and dental and skeletal anomalies constitute variable features. An abnormal fatty acid profile suggests that an abnormality of lipid metabolism may cause the disorder. Indeed, there are reports of dramatic response to a diet in which all of the lipid is in the form of medium-chain triglycerides.

ICHTHYOSIS LINEARIS CIRCUMFLEXA (Netherton's Syndrome)

Ichthyosis linearis circumflexa is a clinically distinctive scaling disorder in which migratory circinate, erythematous plaques exhibit a pathognomonic, double-edged train track-like scale at the margins. At birth there is generalized erythroderma. Sometimes the ichthyosis mimics lamellar ichthyosis, and occasional infants are collodion babies. The histologic picture is nondiagnostic and may include features of eczematous dermatitis. **Netherton's syndrome** denotes the triad of ichthyosis linearis circumflexa, atopic dermatitis, and a hair shaft anomaly called trichorrhexis invaginata (bamboo hair). The hair shaft abnormality is due to intussusception of the distal portion of the hair shaft into the proximal portion. Netherton's syndrome is a rare autosomal recessive disorder of unknown cause.

KERATITIS-ICHTHYOSIS-DEAFNESS (KID) SYNDROME

In this rare syndrome, progressive keratitis leads to corneal neovascularization and blindness associated with neurosensory deafness and an unusual scaling disorder. All cases have been sporadic. Distinctive cutaneous features include fixed hyperkeratotic plaques—particularly periorally—a generalized hyperkeratosis imparting a leathery quality to the skin, follicular hyperkeratosis, a diffuse, pebbly palmarplantar keratoderma, leukonychia, and sparse hair. Other reported associations include mental retardation, tight heel cords, leukoplakia, dental dysplasia, and cryptorchidism. Recurrent infections—particularly severe granulomatous dermatophyte infections—occur in about half of patients. The biochemical basis for this disorder is unknown.

BIDS SYNDROME (Trichothiodystrophy)

Ichthyosis is a frequent feature of a syndrome characterized by *b*rittle hair, *i*ntellectual impairment, *d*eafness, and *s*hort stature (BIDS syndrome). The alternative name, trichothiodystrophy, has been proposed because the structural hair defect, characterized by alternating bands of birefringence on polarizing light microscopy, is accompanied by a marked decrease in sulfur content. The ichthyosis most closely resembles lamellar ichthyosis, though scaling may be mild and focal. Other associations include palmar-plantar keratoderma, nail dystrophy, dental dysplasia, and cataracts. Tay syndrome (ichthyosis, hair shaft anomalies, mental and growth retardation) and Marinesco-Sjögren syndrome (sulfur-deficient hair, mental and growth retardation, cerebellar ataxia, cataracts) may be variants.

REFSUM'S DISEASE (Heredopathia Atactica Polyneuritiformis)

Inability to metabolize dietary phytanic acid leads to progressive neurologic deterioration, wasting, and generalized scaling, resembling ichthyosis vulgaris.

CHONDRODYSPLASIA PUNCTATA
(Conradi-Hünermann Syndrome)

A peculiar form of ichthyosis occurs in some patients with chondrodysplasia punctata, characterized by whorls of yellow-white scales in a nevoid pattern on the trunk and limbs. The underlying skin is erythematous and rough, corresponding to the marked follicular hyperkeratosis seen on skin biopsy. The skin disorder spontaneously resolves within the first 6 months of life, although cicatricial alopecia and follicular atrophoderma may persist. Skeletal involvement ranges from mild (radiographic evidence of stippled epiphyses) to severe (proximal-limbed dwarfism).

Two distinct forms are recognized: (1) The rhizometric type (severe dwarfism, lethal in infancy), which occurs by autosomal recessive inheritance; and (2) Conradi-Hünermann disease, characterized by milder to asymptomatic bone involvement. Cataracts and skin involvement occur in both groups. Mental retardation is more common in the rhizomelic type. Cardiovascular and renal anomalies occur.

HARLEQUIN FETUS

The harlequin fetus is a rare form of ichthyosis. Infants are born encased in extremely thick plaques of scales that produce severe soft tissue deformity and a grotesque appearance. Most affected infants are born dead or have died shortly after birth from restrictive respiratory failure and inability to feed. Inheritance appears to be autosomal recessive; more than one genetic defect may produce this phenotype. Some infants have shown an underlying defect in lipid metabolism; others, an abnormality in protein metabolism (keratin synthesis). The condition can be diagnosed prenatally.

NEUTRAL LIPID STORAGE DISEASE

Essentials of Diagnosis
- Generalized ichthyosis with erythroderma, present at birth.
- Lipid vacuoles in polymorphonuclear leukocytes and monocytes.

General Considerations
Neutral lipid storage disease is inherited as an autosomal recessive trait and is rare. The metabolic basis for the disorder is unknown, but the neutral lipids that accumulate are triglycerides.

Clinical Findings
A. Symptoms and Signs: Ichthyosis is present at birth and suggests congenital ichthyosiform erythroderma. Myopathy may be present. Growth retarda-

tion, sensorineural deafness, and cataracts may be part of this syndrome.

B. Laboratory Findings: Polymorphonuclear leukocytes and monocytes contain round, clear, lipid-laden vacuoles that can be seen by carefully inspecting a peripheral blood smear. Occasionally, lipid droplets are also present in some cells of the lower epidermis and appendages. Serum muscle enzyme levels are often elevated, even when the degree of clinical myopathy is small. In contrast, liver function studies may be normal even though biopsy almost always reveals severe fatty change.

Differential Diagnosis
The ichthyosis suggests congenital ichthyosiform erythroderma, but the finding of lipid droplets in phagocytes identifies the disease.

Treatment
No specific treatment is available. Applications of emollients, keratolytic agents, and alpha-hydroxy acid ointments (see above) are helpful.

OTHER SYNDROMES WITH ICHTHYOSIS

Ichthyosis occurs in multiple sulfatase deficiency, which probably shares a common pathogenesis with recessive X-linked ichthyosis.

Rud's syndrome is an ill-defined complex of ichthyosis, mental retardation, seizures, and hypogonadism. A rare syndrome of unilateral congenital ichthyosiform erythroderma and skeletal, visceral, and central nervous system anomalies is also reported, and there are isolated reports of individuals or kindreds with ichthyosis and a wide variety of other abnormalities (immunodeficiency, renal disease, mental or growth retardation, etc). The type of ichthyosis and its relationship to the other observed abnormalities remain to be determined in many instances.

FOLLICULAR HYPERKERATOSES

KERATOSIS PILARIS

Essentials of Diagnosis
- Discrete follicular keratotic plugs on extensor extremities.
- Common in childhood.
- More severe in winter.
- Associated with atopy and ichthyosis vulgaris.

General Considerations
This common asymptomatic condition gives the skin a sandpaperlike texture. A variant form is associ-

ated with a red halo around each plugged follicle (keratosis pilaris rubra).

Clinical Findings

A. Symptoms and Signs: Discrete follicular asymptomatic keratotic papules on the extensor extremities are extremely common in children, in individuals living in cold climate, and in patients with ichthyosis vulgaris.

B. Laboratory Findings: On skin biopsy, dilated follicles contain a keratotic plug and entrapped hairs. However, the diagnosis is usually made clinically without biopsy.

Differential Diagnosis

Phrynoderma is a similar disorder associated with vitamin (A, B complex) and nutritional (essential fatty acid) deficiencies. Sometimes each follicle is surrounded by a halo of erythema. When generalized, this suggests pityriasis rubra pilaris. Some of these patients have a confluent erythema of the cheeks that is particularly resistant to treatment.

Treatment

Treatment with an emollient, such as hydrophilic petrolatum (eg, Eucerin cream), or a 10–20% urea cream may be of some value. Tretinoin (Retin-A), 0.05% cream twice daily, is an alternative. Most patients improve following exposure to ultraviolet radiation.

Prognosis

The disorder is chronic but improves in summer months.

DISSEMINATED & RECURRENT INFUNDIBULOFOLLICULITIS

Essentials of Diagnosis

- Flesh-colored follicular papules on neck, trunk, and proximal extremities resemble gooseflesh.
- Limited to blacks.

General Considerations

This is a recurrent or persistent dermatosis of unknown cause occurring almost exclusively in blacks.

Clinical Findings

A. Symptoms and Signs: Mildly pruritic follicular papules, without scale or pustulation, are seen over the trunk, neck, and proximal extremities.

B. Laboratory Findings: Skin biopsy demonstrates spongiosis and hyperkeratosis of the upper portion of the hair follicle.

Differential Diagnosis

Disorders to be distinguished include keratosis pilaris, lichen planus, secondary syphilis, pityriasis

rosea, psoriasis, tinea versicolor, drug eruptions, and viral exanthems, but the disease is usually clinically diagnosable.

Treatment

The disorder is best treated with low-potency topical corticosteroids (eg, 1% hydrocortisone cream) and emollients (eg, alpha-hydroxy acid [Lacticare] lotion, hydrophilic petrolatum [Eucerin, others]) if symptomatic.

HYPERKERATOSIS FOLLICULARIS ET PARAFOLLICULARIS (Kyrle's Disease)

Essentials of Diagnosis

- Horny filled craters with a surrounding rim of erythema.
- Most common on extremities.

General Considerations

The criteria for diagnosis of Kyrle's disease are controversial. If strictly defined histologically, the disorder is uncommon. A similar disorder appears more frequently in patients undergoing chronic hemodialysis.

Clinical Findings

A. Symptoms and Signs: Small keratotic plugs with a surrounding rim of erythema may enlarge to 1–2 cm in size and coalesce to form plaques. Lesions are most numerous on the extremities but may occur anywhere.

B. Laboratory Findings: Marked hyperkeratosis, epidermal atrophy, and a superficial infiltrate of lymphocytes are seen in early lesions. Later, an invaginating plug of keratin penetrates the epidermis.

Treatment

Use of a keratolytic agent (eg, Keralyt gel) or application of liquid nitrogen may be helpful.

OTHER FOCAL HYPERKERATOSES

ACRAL HYPERKERATOSIS

Table 21–2 compares the features of 3 disorders of acral hyperkeratoses: stucco keratoses, acrokeratosis verruciformis (Hopf's disease), and hyperkeratosis lenticularis perstans (Flegel's disease).

Table 21–2. Disorders of focal hyperkeratosis.

	Clinical Feature	Age at Onset (years)	Histopathology	Inheritance
Stucco keratoses	Keratotic papules on distal extremities, especially dorsal feet and ankles. Easily removed without bleeding by curet or even fingernail.	>40	Hyperkeratosis with papillomatosis	Acquired
Acrokeratosis verruciformis	Keratotic papules on dorsal hands, feet, elbows, and knees. May have diffuse palmar-plantar keratoderma.	0–50	Hyperkeratosis with papillomatosis	Autosomal dominant
Hyperkeratosis lenticularis	Keratotic papules on dorsal feet and lower legs. Removal of scale results in bleeding base.	>30	Hyperparakeratosis with epidermal atrophy and superficial dermal lymphocytic infiltrate	?Autosomal dominant

TRANSIENT ACANTHOLYTIC DERMATOSIS (Grover's Disease)

Essentials of Diagnosis

- Scattered erythematous papules over neck and upper chest, trunk, and back.
- Histopathologic features: acantholysis with varying degrees of dyskeratosis.

General Considerations

Grover's disease is fairly common, particularly in men over age of 40. Although of unknown cause, sunlight may play a role in its pathogenesis. The term "transient" is misleading, since the disorder frequently persists.

Clinical Findings

A. Symptoms and Signs: Discrete erythematous papules or papulovesicles with crusting are scattered over the upper trunk and extremities. Pruritus is variable.

B. Laboratory Findings: Histopathologically, varying degrees of acantholysis and dyskeratosis are seen, mimicking Darier's disease.

Differential Diagnosis

Although the histopathologic picture may suggest Darier's disease, Hailey-Hailey disease, or pemphigus vulgaris, the clinical pattern does not. Clinically, the disorder most commonly suggests insect bites. Drug eruptions must be differentiated.

Treatment

Treatment is frustrating. Topical corticosteroids (eg, triamcinolone 0.1% cream), retinoids (eg, Retin-A 0.1% cream daily) or alpha-hydroxy acid creams (eg, Lac-Hydrin or Lacticare twice daily) may help.

DERMATOSIS PAPULOSA NIGRA

See Chapter 52.

ACANTHOSIS NIGRICANS

Essentials of Diagnosis

- Velvety brown, poorly marginated plaques with accentuation of skin markings.
- Characteristic distribution: (1) flexures, especially axillas and neck; and (2) acral prominences: elbows, knuckles, occasionally palms and soles.

General Considerations

Acanthosis nigricans occurs in varied clinical settings (Table 21–3). It may be expressed in childhood as a benign autosomal dominant trait. In adults, it is frequently seen in obese and darker skinned individuals. It is also associated with visceral cancer (see Chapter 47), particularly gastrointestinal adenocarcinomas. This dermatosis precedes or presents simultaneously with the cancer. Therefore, the sudden onset of acanthosis nigricans in an adult demands prompt evaluation.

Acanthosis nigricans occurs also in association with a number of endocrinopathies and metabolic disorders, including Cushing's syndrome and insulin-resistant diabetes. Nicotinic acid is at least one drug that can cause acanthosis nigricans.

Clinical Findings

A. Symptoms and Signs: Velvety brown plaques with accentuation of skin markings are found in flexural (axillas, neck) and acral (knuckles, elbows) distribution. When associated with an internal malignancy, the disorder may be pruritic and widespread, including palmar-plantar keratoses, mucous membrane papillomatosis, and seborrheic keratosis-like growths (sign of Leser-Trélat).

B. Laboratory Findings: The benign- and malignant-associated forms do not differ histopathologically, since both demonstrate papillomatosis with a thickened stratum corneum (orthohyperkeratosis). Clinical pigmentation is due to hyperkeratosis rather than increased melanin.

Treatment

Therapy is directed toward recognition and treatment of the underlying disorder, eg, obesity, endocrinopathy, or cancer. In severe cases, bacterial overgrowth causes an offensive odor. Topical antibiotics such as 2% erythromycin solution may help in such cases.

Prognosis

Familial and obesity-related acanthosis nigricans is stable and nonprogressive. The course of cancer-associated acanthosis nigricans parallels the course of the neoplasm. In most instances, these have been highly malignant adenocarcinomas.

POROKERATOSIS

Essentials of Diagnosis

- One or more nummular plaques with raised, hyperkeratotic, furrowed borders.
- Central scaling or atrophy.
- Characteristic histopathologic features ("coronoid lamellae").

General Considerations

Three autosomal dominant clinical syndromes have been associated with porokeratosis (see Table 21–4). The histopathologic picture is distinctive because of an invaginating parakeratotic column, the "coronoid lamella." The coronoid lamella may be due to an abnormal clone of keratinocytes exhibiting accelerated proliferation or premature keratinization (or both).

Clinical Findings

A. Symptoms and Signs: The clinical lesion of porokeratosis is unique. An annular, raised keratotic border may have a central furrow or depression. The center this border surrounds is scaly or atrophic.

In porokeratosis of Mibelli, the lesions occur anywhere on the body and are usually well developed, ie, possess a sharp, elevated border and central atrophy. There may be a single annular plaque of varying size or multiple plaques arranged in linear or segmental "nevoid" distribution. The onset is in childhood, usually before age 10.

The lesions of disseminated superficial actinic porokeratosis (porokeratosis of Chernowsky) are smaller, more numerous, and symmetrically distributed, especially over sun-exposed areas of the body, including the legs. The palms and soles are spared. Most patients are fair-skinned adults. Sunlight elicits these lesions. Unlike the Mibelli form, the keratotic border is less distinct, there is less central atrophy, and the lesions are often pruritic.

The lesions of porokeratosis plantaris, palmaris, et disseminata (porokeratosis of Guss) are clinically most similar to disseminated superficial actinic porokeratosis. These patients differ because the porokeratosis plaques occur at an earlier age (in the second decade), and initial localization to palms and soles is followed later by generalization.

B. Laboratory Findings: The skin biopsy is

Table 21–3. Acanthosis nigricans.

Type	Features
Familial	Autosomal dominant. Onset in infancy or childhood.
Obesity-associated ("pseudo-acanthosis nigricans")	More apparent in dark-skinned obese individuals.
Endocrine-associated	Reported endocrine associates include diabetes mellitus, insulin-resistant syndromes, diabetes insipidus, acromegaly, Addison's disease, Cushing's disease, Stein-Leventhal syndrome.
Metabolic-associated	Reported metabolic associations include Bloom syndrome, Down syndrome, congenital lipodystrophy, phenylketonuria, Wilson's disease, cirrhosis, chronic hepatitis.
Malignancy-associated	Vast majority are adenocarcinoma; 60% gastric. Other sites include lung, bronchus, pancreas, esophagus, breast, ovary, and prostate. Other reported malignancies include squamous cell carcinomas of various sites, lymphoma, osteosarcoma, testicular carcinoma, malignant pinealoma.
Drug-related	Nicotinic acid, "street drugs?"

pathognomonic. Histologically, the furrow or depression represents an invaginating parakeratotic column ("coronoid lamella") arising from a focus of dyskeratosis.

Differential Diagnosis

Lesions on the palms and soles must be distinguished from verrucae, arsenical keratoses, and other focal palmar-plantar keratodermas. Linear or nevoid plaques should be differentiated from epidermal nevi, lichen striatus, and linear lichen planus. The superficial plaques of disseminated superficial actinic porokeratosis may be confused with a variety of dermatoses: lentigines, nummular or asteatotic eczema, actinic or seborrheic keratoses, psoriasis, lichen sclerosus et atrophicus, stucco keratoses, and other papulosquamous disorders.

Complications

Because squamous cell carcinomas may develop, careful follow-up is warranted, especially in porokeratosis of the Mibelli type.

Treatment

In the Mibelli form, surgical removal should be considered for small lesions, particularly on the extremities or in sites of previous radiation. Patients with the disseminated superficial actinic form should be advised to avoid sunlight and to use effective sunscreens or sunblocks. Liquid nitrogen sufficient to produce a blister may be effective—but impractical if lesions are too numerous. Fluorouracil 2% solution or 5% cream applied twice daily for 3 weeks may be useful in some patients.

Prognosis

In the Mibelli form, lesions slowly enlarge. In the other 2 forms, the number of lesions increases with time.

PALMAR-PLANTAR KERATOSIS

Palmar-plantar keratosis is a descriptive term for thickening of the horny layer of the palms and soles. A wide variety of acquired and hereditary disorders may affect the palms and soles primarily or as part of a more generalized defect in cornification; an extensive differential diagnosis must be considered (see Table 21–5). The age at onset, the family history, the clinical pattern of palmar-plantar involvement—eg, focal (keratoses) versus diffuse (keratoderma)—and the presence of skin lesions elsewhere or involvement of other ectodermal structures (hair, nails, teeth, etc) must be considered to arrive at an accurate diagnosis.

Secondary forms of palmar-plantar keratosis are discussed elsewhere (see chapters on psoriasis, genetic diseases, atopic disorders, contact dermatitis, and other sections of this chapter; see Table 21–5).

FOCAL KERATOSES

1. CORNS, CALLOSITIES, & WARTS

These punctate (corns) or more diffuse (callosities) keratoses occur over pressure points in response to trauma. They are often painful and interfere with walking. Treatment is directed toward relief of pressure foci, usually produced by ill-fitting shoes. Regular paring and the use of doughnut-shaped pads to redistribute pressure are useful when change in footgear is impractical.

2. ARSENICAL KERATOSES

Punctate, cornlike keratoses of the palms and soles occur as a manifestation of chronic arsenic intoxication. Lesions may be numerous and involve the dorsum of the hands and proximal extremities. These lesions may become invasive carcinomas. Patients with arsenical keratoses should be followed carefully for the development of Bowen's disease elsewhere on the body and for visceral carcinoma. Preliminary cancer chemopreventive studies utilizing the new oral synthetic retinoids (isotretinoin and etretinate) suggest that they may prove useful for the management of patients with widespread premalignant keratoses.

3. KERATODERMA CLIMACTERICUM

Round or oval hyperkeratotic plaques involving the palms and soles may progress to generalized keratoderma, usually in postmenopausal obese women.

Treatment is symptomatic. Hormonal replacement is not useful.

4. HEREDITARY FORMS

Punctate palmar-plantar keratosis is an autosomal dominant disorder in which numerous hard horny papules are randomly distributed over the palms and soles. Painful over pressure points, the central corn may be lost, leaving a pit with a keratotic wall. In blacks, a common variant is seen in which punctate keratoses align themselves along palmar-plantar creases. The presentation of tyrosinemia (type II) in infancy as painful, tender palmar-plantar keratoses must not be overlooked, since the sequelae—mental retardation and blindness—can be prevented by early institution of a low-phenylalanine, low-tyrosine diet (see Chapter 20).

Table 21–4. Porokeratosis: Clinical classification.[1]

	Mibelli	Disseminated Superficial Actinic Porokeratosis	Porokeratosis Plantaris, Palmaris, et Disseminata
Age at onset	1st Decade	3rd–4th Decade	2nd Decade
Sex predominance M : F	2–3 : 1	1 : 1	2 : 1
Size of lesion (cm)	Variable, up to 20	Most < 1	Most < 1
Height of border	>1 mm	<1 mm	<1 mm
Furrow in border	Yes	No	No
Number of lesions	Single or few	Numerous	Numerous
Distribution	Usually single or unilateral	Bilateral, symmetrical	Bilateral, symmetrical
Palmar-plantar lesions	Occasional	Never	Always
Pruritus	Usually not	Often	Often
Sunlight-induced	No	Yes	Maybe
Squamous cell carcinoma	Uncommon	Rare	Uncommon

[1]Adapted from Guss SB, Osbourn RA, Lutzner MA: Porokeratosis plantaris, palmaris, et disseminata: A third type of porokeratosis. Arch Dermatol 1971;104:366.

DIFFUSE KERATOSES
(Keratoderma)

The hereditary palmar-plantar keratoses are the major consideration in this group; their clinical features are summarized in Table 21–6. With the exception of the Unna-Thost type, most are rare. When the onset is delayed until childhood or adolescence, the clinician should consider Howel-Evans' syndrome. Most patients with this rare syndrome eventually develop esophageal carcinoma.

Clinical Findings

The diagnostic features are listed in Table 21–6.

Pain on walking, fissuring, and hyperhidrosis may produce considerable occupational or functional disability.

Treatment

Regular use of a topical keratolytic (eg, Keralyt gel plus occlusion at bedtime) followed by paring help maintain function. Painful fissures may be sealed with Castellani's paint or flexible collodion. The oral synthetic retinoids may prove useful, but they should be reserved for severely disabled patients. Etretinate usually is more effective than isotretinoin, and doses as low as 25 mg/d may be quite effective.

Table 21–5. Classification of palmar-plantar keratoses (PPK).

	Acquired	Hereditary
Primary (hyperkeratosis confined mostly to palms and soles)		
Focal (keratoses)	Calluses, corns, verrucae, arsenical, keratoderma climactericum, hand eczemas, tinea, porokeratosis plantaris discreta, scabies	PPK-striata, PPK-punctata, tyrosinemia (II) (Richner-Hanhart syndrome), PPK with corneal dystrophy, keratosis circumscripta
Diffuse (keratoderma)	PPK-manual labor, tinea (2 foot-1 hand disease), hand eczemas, keratoderma climactericum	Unna-Thost PPK, Howel-Evans syndrome, mal de Meleda, progressive PPK (Greither), PPK mutilans (Vohwinkel), Papillon-Lefèvre syndrome.
Secondary (part of generalized disorder of cornification)		
Focal (keratoses)	Lichen planus, atopic or contact eczema, syphilis, yaws	Psoriasis, Reiter's syndrome, incontinentia pigmenti, basal cell nevus syndrome, Darier's disease; porokeratosis palmaris, plantaris et disseminata; pachyonychia congenita, epidermodysplasia verruciformis, acrokeratoelastoides
Diffuse (keratoderma)	Pityriasis rubra pilaris, atopic or contact eczema, Sézary's syndrome	Ichthyosis vulgaris, lamellar ichthyosis, epidermolytic hyperkeratosis; some ectodermal dysplasias; keratitis-ichthyosis-deafness syndrome, Franceschetti-Jadassohn syndrome, dyskeratosis congenita, erythrokeratoderma variabilis

Table 21–6. Primary, diffuse palmar-plantar keratoderma: Hereditary forms.

Disorder	Eponym	Inheritance[1]	Age at Onset	Cutaneous Features	Extracutaneous Features
Tylosis	Unna-Thost	AD	Infancy	Strict limitation to palms and soles with band of erythema at margin. Histopathologically 2 groups: orthohyperkeratosis and epidermolytic hyperkeratosis.	None
Keratoderma with esophageal carcinoma	Howel-Evans	AD	5–15 yr	Resembles Unna-Thost type.	70% develop esophageal carcinoma in 4th–5th decade
Mal de Meleda		AR	Infancy	Erythema followed by keratoderma. Progressive glovelike extension onto dorsum. Distant acral, flexural, and perioral psoriasiform plaques. Nail abnormalities.	Shortened digits
Progressive keratoderma	Greither	AD	Infancy	Similar to mal de Meleda.	
Mutilating keratoderma	Vohwinkel	AD	Infancy	Honeycombed, diffuse keratoderma. Digital constricting fibrous bands producing auto-amputation. Progressive stellate keratoses on dorsal hands, knees, elbows. Occasionally cicatricial alopecia.	
Papillon-Lefèvre		AR	Infancy	Similar to mal de Meleda.	Severe periodontitis with shedding of teeth

[1]AD = autosomal dominant; AR = autosomal recessive.

REFERENCES

Baden HP et al: Keratinization in the harlequin fetus. Arch Dermatol 1982;118:14.

Brown BE, Williams ML, Elias PM: Stratum corneum lipid abnormalities in ichthyosis: Detection by a new lipid microanalytical method. Arch Dermatol 1984;120:204.

Caver CV: Clofazimine-induced ichthyosis and its treatment. Cutis 1982;29:341.

Davies MG et al: The epidermis in Refsum's disease (heredopathia atactica polyneuritiformis). Page 51 in: *The Ichthyoses.* Marks R, Dykes PJ (editors). Spectrum, 1978.

Dicken CH et al: Isotretinoin treatment of Darier's disease. J Am Acad Dermatol 1982;6:721.

Dykes PJ, Marks R: Acquired ichthyosis: Multiple causes for an acquired generalized disturbance in desquamation. Br J Dermatol 1977;97:327.

Elias PM: Epidermal lipids, membranes, and keratinization. Int J Dermatol 1981;20:1.

El-Ramly M, Zachariae H: Long-term oral treatment of two pronounced ichthyotic conditions: Lamellar ichthyosis and epidermolytic hyperkeratosis with the aromatic retinoid, Tegison (Ro 10-9359). Acta Derm Venereol 1983; 63:452.

Epstein EH Jr, Krauss RM, Shackleton CH: X-linked ichthyosis: Increased blood cholesterol sulfate and electrophoretic mobility of low-density lipoprotein. Science 1981;214:659.

Epstein EH Jr, Williams ML, Elias PM: Steroid sulfatase, X-linked ichthyosis, and stratum corneum cell cohesion. Arch Dermatol 1981;117:761.

Frost P, Van Scott EJ: Ichthyosiform dermatoses. Arch Dermatol 1966;94:113.

Golbus MS et al: Prenatal diagnosis of congenital bullous ichthyosiform erythroderma (epidermolytic hyperkerato-sis) by fetal skin biopsy. N Engl J Med 1980;302:93.

Jöbsis AC et al: A new method for the determination of steroid sulphatase activity in leukocytes in X-linked recessive ichthyosis. Br J Dermatol 1983;108:567.

Jorizzo JL, Crouse RG, Wheeler CE Jr: Lamellar ichthyosis, dwarfism, mental retardation, and hair shaft abnormalities: A link between the ichthyosis-associated and BIDS syndromes. J Am Acad Dermatol 1980;2:309.

Lidén S, Jagell S: The Sjögren-Larsson syndrome. Int J Dermatol 1984;23:247.

Rand RE, Baden HP: The ichthyoses: A review. J Am Acad Dermatol 1983;8:285.

Skinner BA, Greist MC, Norins AL: The keratitis, ichthyosis, and deafness (KID) syndrome. Arch Dermatol 1981;117:285.

Toole JW, Hofstader SL, Ramsay CA: Darier's disease and Kaposi's varicelliform eruption. J Am Acad Dermatol 1979;1:321.

Weiss RM, Rasmussen JE: Keratosis punctata of the palmar creases. Arch Dermatol 1980;116:669.

Williams ML: The ichthyoses—pathogenesis and prenatal diagnosis: A review of recent advances. Pediatr Dermatol 1983;1:1.

Williams ML, Elias PM: Genetically transmitted, generalized disorders of cornification: The ichthyoses. Dermatol Clin 1987;5:155.

Williams ML, Elias PM: Heterogeneity in autosomal recessive ichthyosis: Clinical and biochemical differentiation of lamellar ichthyosis and nonbullous congenital ichthyosiform erythroderma. Arch Dermatol 1985;121:477.

Zaias N, Ackerman AB: The nail in Darier-White disease. Arch Dermatol 1973;107:193.

Disorders of Pigmentation

22

James J. Nordlund, MD & Christy A. Lorton, MD

NORMAL PIGMENT CELLS

The principal pigment determining skin color is melanin. The chemistry, quantity, character, aggregation, and distribution of melanin are the major factors that determine color and hue of cutaneous pigmentation. Three other pigments that contribute to normal skin color are oxygenated hemoglobin, reduced hemoglobin, and carotenoids.

The variety of colors conferred by the composite of these pigments in the skin, hair, and eyes is remarkable. Skin color may range from ghostly white to deep brown-black. Hair color can be white, gray, blond, light or dark brown, black, or red. The eyes can be any shade from sky blue to jet black.

EMBRYOGENESIS

All pigment cells arise from the neural crest except those of retinal pigment epithelium, which are derivatives of the primitive forebrain. Formation of the neural crest in human embryos is completed by the sixth week of gestation. The precursors of pigment cells probably begin their migration to the skin, eyes, ears, and other organs before the neural crest (Fig 22–1) is completed. By the eighth week of embryogenesis, pigment cells can be identified in the dermis.

DISTRIBUTION OF PIGMENT CELLS IN THE BODY

Skin

Most melanocytes are located in the basal layer of the epidermis (Figs 22–1, 22–2, and 22–3). They also reside within the papilla and matrix of the hair bulb. In black and Oriental infants, the skin overlying

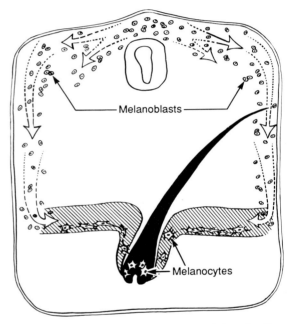

Figure 22–1. Schematic representation of the migration of melanoblasts from the neural crest to the skin and the hair bulbs. The migration begins early in embryogenesis, within 6 weeks after fertilization. The melanoblasts differentiate into mature pigment cells, called melanocytes, within the epidermis and hair bulbs. Any factors inhibiting the development of melanoblasts in the neural crest, their migration, or their differentiation within the skin or hair bulbs cause a disorder of pigmentation, eg, piebaldism.

the sacrum frequently has a bluish discoloration, ie, the mongolian or sacral blue spot, caused by dendritic melanin-containing cells in the reticular dermis.

Mucous Membranes & Respiratory Tract

Melanocytes are a normal cellular component of the mucous membranes. The oral epithelium cover-

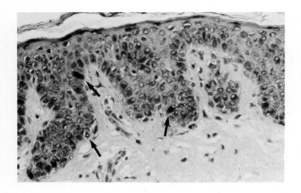

Figure 22–2. The microscopic appearance of the epidermis in cross section. Pigment cells (arrows) are darkly stained and are located within the epidermis at the dermal-epidermal junction. ×200.

ing the gingiva, buccal mucosa, and palate of all individuals contains numerous pigment cells. In dark-skinned individuals, these pigment cells normally produce large amounts of melanin, and oral mucous membranes are therefore deeply pigmented. In Caucasians, pigmentation may not be visible normally. In disease, pigment cells can be stimulated to produce more melanin, possibly by melanocyte-stimulating hormone (MSH).

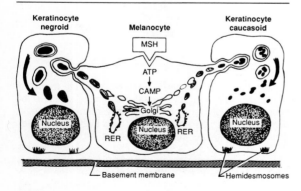

Figure 22–3. The schematic representation of the effect of the melanocyte-stimulating hormone (MSH) on melanocyte function. MSH attaches to a receptor on the cell surface and activates the enzyme adenylate cyclase (not shown), which converts ATP to cAMP, an intracellular messenger that stimulates melanin formation. The enzyme tyrosinase is produced within the Golgi apparatus. The melanosomal substructures are formed in the rough endoplasmic reticulum (RER). Vesicles from the RER and the Golgi apparatus fuse, and melanin synthesis begins. Small melanosomes, found in whites, are transported in groups into the cytoplasm of keratinocytes; large melanosomes, found in blacks, are transported individually.

A few pigment cells can be found in the mucosa of the nasal septum and respiratory tract, in the turbinates, and in the mucosa of the larynx and esophagus. Occasional bluish macules (melanosis) are found in these sites, especially the esophagus. Melanosis in these sites probably is a normal variant. Mucosal pigment cells may be the origin of primary melanomas arising in these organs.

The epidermis overlying the male and female genitalia is deeply pigmented and has a greater density of pigment cells than epidermis of other parts of the body. The mucosa of the vagina and uterine cervix has a few pigment cells along the basement membrane and may rarely exhibit melanosis or primary melanoma.

Eyes

The uvea is composed of the choroid, ciliary body, and iris. The uvea contains dendritic pigment cells similar in morphology to melanocytes in the skin. One function of melanin in the uvea is to prevent penetration of light through the sclera.

Pigment is manufactured also in the cells of the retinal pigment epithelium, which synthesize melanin almost entirely during embryogenesis. This melanin may be an essential embryologic signal. The melanin in the retinal pigment epithelium may be critical for normal formation of the uvea and for proper routing of dendrites of the ganglion cells from the neuroretinal rods and cones through the optic chiasm to the central nervous system.

In albinism, the retinal pigment epithelium lacks melanin. The fovea fails to form, and optic nerves are abnormally arranged. Such individuals are affected with a variety of anatomic and thus physiologic defects that permanently impair visual acuity not correctable with deeply tinted glasses.

Ears

The ear also contains pigment cells. The cells are components of 2 parts of the cochlea—the modiolus and Reissner's membrane—and are necessary for proper formation of the stria vascularis. Patients with genetic disorders of the pigment system often have associated disorders of hearing. For example, patients with Waardenburg's syndrome lack pigment cells in discrete areas of the facial skin, hair, and eyes. They suffer from congenital sensorineural deafness thought to be due to lack of pigment cells in the ear.

Leptomeninges

The cells that form the leptomeninges and its pigment cells arise from the cephalic portion of the neural crest. Many pigment cells are concentrated within the pia mater overlying the medulla oblongata and the proximal portion of the cervical spinal cord. The role of the pigment cells and the melanin in leptomeninges is not known. Some primary meningeal melanomas probably arise from these cells.

Other Organs; Pleura & Peritoneum

Dendritic pigment-containing cells resembling melanocytes occur in the muscles of the eyes, gastrointestinal tract, and prostate; in teratomas of the ovary; and, on rare occasion, in the pleura or the peritoneum. The origin, ultrastructure, and function of these cells are unknown.

FUNCTIONS OF THE PIGMENT SYSTEM

In humans, pigment in the skin and hair protects against the harmful effects of sunlight; in some lower animals, pigment may provide camouflage protection against predators or act as an attractant for sexual mates. Humans who lack pigment (albinos) are very sensitive to sunlight. They sunburn easily and are susceptible to developing skin cancers at a young age. The pigment system may be an alternative type of protection for animals and humans with little body hair.

Short wave ultraviolet light (290–320 nm) alters some immunologic functions. Ultraviolet light, chemical carcinogens, and phenols cause the formation of free oxygen radicals within the epidermis and perhaps the dermis. It seems likely that a primary function of melanocytes is to remove free radicals formed in the skin during a variety of inflammatory conditions. Melanocytes protect other cells of the epidermis from damage caused by release of radical oxygens. Large quantities of melanin are an indicator of an efficient and effective protective mechanism for elimination of detrimental effects of many chemical and physical toxins.

HISTOLOGY OF THE EPIDERMAL PIGMENT CELLS

The population density of epidermal pigment cells varies significantly in different parts of the body. The skin of the genitalia has the highest density of melanocytes, a mean of $2400/mm^2$; that of the trunk has the lowest population, a mean of $900/mm^2$. The number of cells per unit area (Fig 22–4) is similar for people of all races—ie, skin color does not depend on the number of pigment cells but rather on the quantity of melanin formed.

The number of epidermal melanocytes begins to decrease at age 40. Clinically, this loss of epidermal pigment cells is manifested by a lighter complexion typically observed in healthy older people. The hair bulbs also lose pigment cells. A few gray hairs can be found in 25% of Caucasians over the age of 25 years, 66% of those over the 35 years, and 90% of those over 45 years.

Melanocytes reside in the basal layer of the epider-

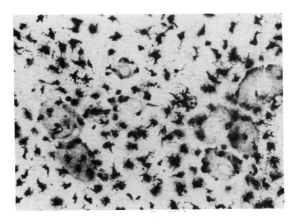

Figure 22–4. The distribution of dopa-positive melanocytes within the epidermis. For this preparation, the epidermis has been separated from the dermis. The cells are stained by incubation of the epidermal sheet in a solution of L-dopa. Note that the pigment cell extends dendrites from the cell body. ×200.

mis and abut the basement membrane (Figs 22–1 to 22–4). Pigment cells have no hemidesmosomes necessary for the attachment of keratinocytes to the basement membrane (Fig 22–3) but do have an analogous structure: the melanocyte dense plate. One in every 6 or 7 basal cells of the epidermis is a melanocyte, and each melanocyte interdigitates with an average of 36 keratinocytes and possibly some Langerhans cells. This dendritic association establishes the epidermal melanin unit as a group of integrated keratinocytes, melanocytes, and Langerhans cells.

CYTOLOGY OF CUTANEOUS MELANOCYTES

Melanocytes are oval and have a smooth cytoplasmic membrane and a round nucleus. Dendrites extend outward from the cell body (Fig 22–4). The cytoplasm is filled with many organelles and a characteristic granule, the melanosome (Fig 22–5). The Golgi apparatus is prominent (Fig 22–3). Intermediate filaments (10 nm in diameter) and microtubules (25–27 nm in diameter) are involved in the transfer of melanosomes from the pigment cell into adjacent keratinocytes (Fig 22–3).

Melanosomes formed within the cytoplasm can be transferred into the cytoplasm of other cells, usually keratinocytes (Fig 22–3), though on occasion melanosomes are obscured in Langerhans cells or macrophages. Melanosomes are formed by the fusion of several cytoplasmic suborganelles. Vesicles with lamellae called premelanosomes are formed by the rough endoplasmic reticulum. Other vesicles contain-

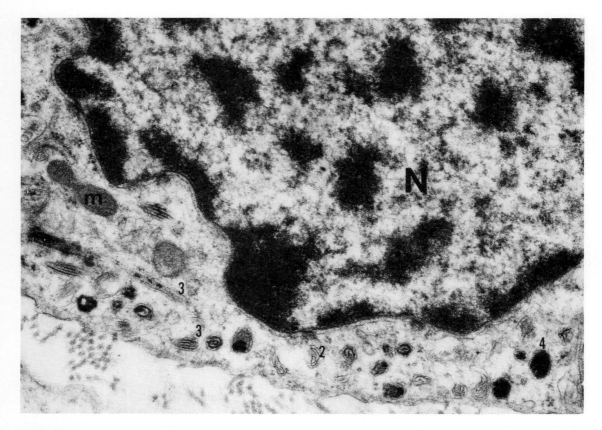

Figure 22–5. Electron micrograph of a melanocyte. The nucleus (N) is surrounded by a membrane. Mitochondria (M) are present in the cytoplasm. Melanosomes in many stages of development (2, stage II; 3, stage III; 4, stage IV) are visible. ×44,200. (Courtesy of DM Bell.)

ing tyrosinase pinch off from the Golgi apparatus and fuse with the premelanosome to initiate the synthesis of melanin.

The formation of the melanosome has been arbitrarily divided into 4 stages (Fig 22–6A, 22–6B, and 22–6C). Stage I melanosomes are oval or spherical and contain a few filaments with a characteristic periodic banding and the enzyme tyrosinase in an inactive form (Fig 22–6A); stage II melanosomes are oval organelles with numerous filaments organized into a lamellar substructure in which melanin is not present (Fig 22–6A); stage III melanosomes are partially filled with melanin (Fig 22–6B); and stage IV melanosomes are completely filled with melanin (Fig 22–6C). The immature stage I and stage II melanosomes are usually found around the nucleus; the more mature stages III and IV melanosomes are distributed into the dendrites.

The skin color of peoples of different races is determined genetically by 3 or 4 pairs of alleles. Skin color is determined to a large degree by the number and size of melanosomes, ie, the quantity of melanin produced by the melanocyte and transferred into the surrounding keratinocytes. The melanocytes of light-skinned individuals form and transfer to keratinocytes fewer and smaller (< 0.7 μm in diameter) stage II and III melanosomes; the pigment cells of dark individuals form many large (> 1 μm) stage III and IV melanosomes. Melanocytes of some individuals form small melanosomes in a basal state but larger ones when stimulated by sunlight or other melanocyte-stimulating agents (MSH). Another important determinant of skin color is the type of melanin synthesized, ie, brown or black eumelanin or red or yellow phaeomelanin (see below).

MELANIN SYNTHESIS

Human melanocytes are now known to produce 2 types of melanin: eumelanin and phaeomelanin. Eumelanin is black or brown, and phaeomelanin is red. The ratio of the 2 types of pigment largely determines the hue of human hair and skin.

Eumelanin

Eumelanin chemically is a polymer of indoles and

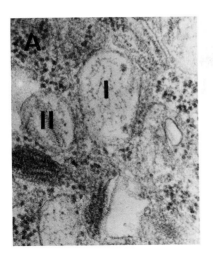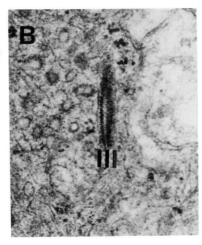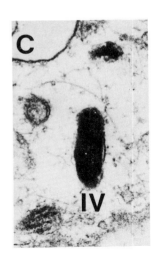

Figure 22–6. Melanosomes. **A:** Electron micrograph of stage I and stage II melanosomes. **B:** Stage III melanosome. **C:** Stage IV melanosome. ×55,000.

quinones formed by the oxidation of the amino acid tyrosine (Fig 22–7). These quinones and indoles, highly reactive chemically, are toxic to most cells. Melanin synthesis probably is restricted to the internal milieu of the melanosome to prevent these compounds from injuring the cell.

A single enzyme, tyrosinase, performs 3 different catalytic functions in the melanin pathway. This enzyme catalyzes the oxidation of tyrosine to dopa, the dehydrogenation of dopa to dopaquinone, and the conversion of dihydroxyindole to melanochrome (Fig 22–7). Tyrosinase is the best-characterized enzyme involved in melanin synthesis. Two other factors—dopachrome conversion factor and indole blocking factor—seem to be involved in regulating the rate of melanin formation. Dopachrome conversion factor is

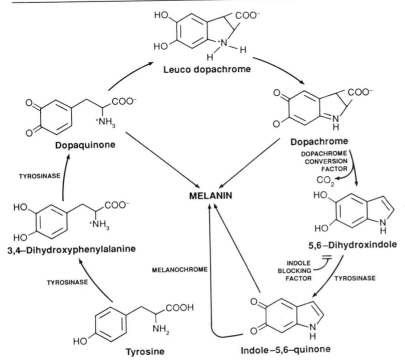

Figure 22–7. Biochemical pathway for synthesis of melanin. Tyrosine is oxidized first to 3,4-dihydroxyphenyl-alanine (L-dopa) and then to dopaquinone by the enzyme tyrosinase. The same enzyme is involved in a third oxidative step, the conversion of 5, 6-dihydroxyindole into indole-5, 6-quinone. Two other factors—dopachrome conversion factor (probably also an enzyme) and indole-blocking factor—are involved in the regulation of melanin formation. Melanin itself is a polymer composed of the many different oxidized derivatives of dopaquinone.

now well characterized as the enzyme dopachrome oxidoreductase.

Phaeomelanin

Phaeomelanin is formed from 2 amino acids: tyrosine and cysteine. In the formation of phaeomelanin, dopaquinone condenses with the amino acid cysteine to form cysteinyl dopa. Cysteinyl dopa is oxidized into cysteinyl indoles, which condense to form a red polymer, phaeomelanin. The melanosome in which phaeomelanin is formed is structurally different from that of the eumelanosome. The phaeomelanosome is round, not oval, and lacks the organized lamellar substructures characteristic of eumelanosomes.

FACTORS THAT STIMULATE MELANIN FORMATION

Many physical and chemical agents stimulate pigment formation (Table 22–1). Short wave ultraviolet light (UVB; 290–320 nm), abundant in sunlight, causes epidermal pigment cells to increase melanin formation. This process takes several days to a week to be noticeable chemically. Long wave ultraviolet light (UVA; 320–400 nm) rapidly alters the melanin polymer, causing it to become darker (immediate pigment darkening, IPD). IPD is responsible for the rapid bronze tanning observable immediately after sunbathing.

Table 22–1. Systemic causes of hyperpigmentation (increase in epidermal melanin).

Metabolic
Porphyria cutanea tarda
Advanced liver cirrhosis
Hemochromatosis
Chronic renal failure
Gaucher's disease
Niemann-Pick disease
Endocrine
Addison's disease
ACTH and MSH producing tumors
Pregnancy
Oral estrogen therapy
Acromegaly
Nutritional
Pellagra (niacin deficiency)
Pernicious anemia (vitamin B_{12} deficiency)
Kwashiorkor
Miscellaneous
Scleroderma
Inflammatory bowel disease
Cronkhite-Canada syndrome
Bleomycin therapy
Fluorouracil therapy
Busulfan therapy
Arsenical ingestion
Fixed drug reaction

Prostaglandin E_2, estrogens, and other hormones also increase the amount of pigment produced by pigment cells. Some chemotherapeutic drugs, eg, bleomycin, darken the skin by inducing melanin formation. Ingested metals such as arsenic and silver also darken the skin by depositing in the dermis.

Psoralens are tricyclic organic compounds found in many plants such as limes, celery, and parsnips. In combination with UVA, psoralens stimulate formation of melanin. Psoralens are also mutagens and form covalent bonds with the nucleic acids present in chromosomal DNA. The mechanism by which psoralens and UVA (PUVA) may stimulate pigment formation is not known.

Melanocyte-stimulating hormones (MSH) are the best-characterized stimulants of melanin formation. Four different MSH peptides have been identified, each formed in the pars intermedia of the pituitary gland. These different MSH peptides probably have a variety of functions other than causing an increase in skin color. α-MSH affects many cognitive functions, enhancing memory and visual discrimination and altering behavior. In the neonate, α-MSH may control ACTH released from the pituitary. α-MSH has a variety of anti-inflammatory properties. γ-MSH may regulate heat loss from the skin. All of these melanotropic peptides seem to have important bioregulatory effects besides merely stimulating pigmentation.

Specific receptors for MSH are present on the surface of the pigment cell (Fig 22–3). When attached to a receptor, MSH activates the enzyme adenylate cyclase to form cAMP, which is one intracellular messenger involved in activating a protein kinase and initiating formation of tyrosinase in the Golgi apparatus. The other factors needed for formation of tyrosinase are not well described. The active enzyme is transported from the Golgi to the premelanosome and synthesizes melanin. cAMP (Fig 22–3)—by itself or with inhibitors of phosphodiesterase (the enzyme that degrades cAMP)—can mimic the effects of MSH. MSH also accelerates the movement of melanosomes through the dendrites and their transfer into keratinocytes.

TRANSFER OF MELANOSOMES; MELANOSOMAL DEGRADATION

Melanosomes are transported by intermediate filaments to the tips of the dendrites (Figs 22–3 and 22–5). The tips of the dendrites are pinched off and phagocytosed by the keratinocyte. The interaction between keratinocytes and melanocytes is not well worked out. Mediators possibly by the keratinocyte may stimulate an increase in the proliferation of melanocytes as well as their melanization and dendricity. Within keratinocytes, large melanosomes (1 μm in length) characteristically found in dark skin are packaged individually; small melanosomes are packaged in groups (Fig 22–3).

The melanosome becomes a permanent granule within the keratinocyte. As the keratinocytes undergo mitoses, progeny cells containing melanosomes migrate out of the basal layer into the stratum spinosum. As the cell traverses the epidermis, it carries the melanosomes in its cytoplasm. The proteinaceous substructure of the melanosome is degraded enzymatically, but the melanin polymer persists as "melanin dust." The melanin polymer is extremely stable.

Melanin, deposited in the dermis in a variety of diseases, can be removed only by macrophages (melanophages) that ingest the polymer and transport it to lymph nodes and spleen, where, presumably, it persists throughout life.

PROLIFERATION OF MELANOCYTES

Although highly differentiated, melanocytes do divide even in normal skin. The factors regulating pigment cell growth are not well defined. Wounding or injury to the skin causes vigorous proliferation. The sunburning spectrum of sunlight (290–320 nm) is the best-known stimulant. Sunlight causes pigment cells to proliferate. It has been suggested that light releases a circulating factor. In contrast, psoralens and long wave UV light (320–400 nm; PUVA) cause only a small proliferation of pigment cells but marked increase in the amount of melanin production. MSH causes increased production of pigment without proliferation. The carcinogen dimethylbenzanthracene (DMBA) and the cancer chemotherapeutic agent bleomycin may cause pigment cell proliferation.

ABNORMALITIES OF PIGMENTATION

Abnormalities of hyperpigmentation and hypopigmentation can be subdivided into abnormalities of (1) melanocyte population densities (increased or decreased); (2) melanin production (enhanced or diminished); (3) melanosomal packaging and distribution; and (4) miscellaneous abnormalities (usually nonmelanotic). The depth of pigment deposition in the skin, whether in the epidermis or abnormally in the dermis, also affects the overall perceived color. These broad groups of clinicopathologic disorders are further divided into (1) congenital or genetic and (2) acquired diseases.

DISORDERS OF HYPERPIGMENTATION

Since melanocytes are derived from the neural crest, infants with a congenital or genetic pigmentary abnormality may have associated dysfunction of the central nervous system. Other neuroectodermal derivatives such as the teeth, hair, nails, eyes, ears, or facial features may also be defective.

Hyperpigmentation is a common problem, especially in patients with dark skin. Most cutaneous irritants cause an increase in pigmentation. However, patients of any race can suffer significant cosmetic disfigurement from localized or generalized hyperpigmentation. Hyperpigmentation may be a cutaneous sign of a serious metabolic or nutritional disorder. Fortunately, most types of hyperpigmented lesions are benign. Some are malignant, eg, melanomas. Usually one thinks of hyperpigmentation as affecting only the skin. However, it can also affect the nails or mucous membranes.

CONGENITAL OR GENETIC HYPERPIGMENTATION DUE TO AN EXCESS NUMBER OF MELANOCYTES

1. LENTIGO SIMPLEX

Essentials of Diagnosis
- Onset during infancy or early childhood.
- Small brown macules.
- Not limited to sun-exposed areas.
- Low malignant potential.

General Considerations
The lesions of lentigo simplex are small brown macules that form during infancy or, in many cases, by 6 months of age. They continue to appear throughout childhood and adult life on any part of the integument. Large numbers of lentigines have been observed to develop suddenly following sunburn; however, unlike freckles, they are not limited to sun-exposed surfaces. Lentigo simplex may have a familial occurrence and, if numerous, may be a sign of the multiple lentigines syndromes or a variant described in the following section.

Clinical Findings
A. Symptoms and Signs: (Fig 22–8.) Lentigines are flat, dark brown to black spots, usually 2 or 3 mm in diameter and rarely more than 5 mm. In young people, they are most commonly found on the trunk or proximal extremities. Lentigines do not darken with exposure to ultraviolet light, nor do they fade in the winter months.

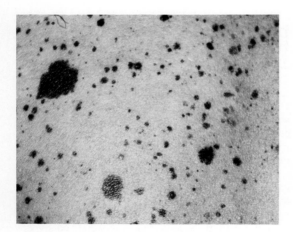

Figure 22–8. Close-up of lentigines. The patient has multiple lentigines syndrome. Note that lentigines are darkly colored (dark brown) and macular. They have normal or slightly thickened skin markings.

B. Laboratory Findings: The histologic features are an increased number of melanocytes along the basal layer and a slight and regular elongation of the rete ridges (in contrast to solar lentigines, which have marked and irregular elongation of the rete ridges). Increased melanin production is also evident in basal melanocytes and basal and suprabasilar keratinocytes and stained by Fontana-Masson silver stain.

Differential Diagnosis

Lentigo simplex differs from solar lentigo by the occurrence of the latter in later life on sun-exposed skin sites and by their larger size. Freckles are confined to sun-exposed areas and tend to show seasonal color variation. Junctional nevi often can be differentiated on a histologic basis.

Treatment

No treatment is necessary. If cosmetic lightening of the lentigines is desired, refer to Treatment of Epidermal Hyperpigmentation, below.

Course

Lentigo simplex have a low or minuscule malignant potential. They continue to increase in number until adulthood.

2. MULTIPLE LENTIGINES SYNDROME
(Moynahan's Syndrome,
LEOPARD Syndrome,
& Probable Variations:
Centrofacial Lentiginosis,
NAME Syndrome, & LAMB Syndrome)

Essentials of Diagnosis
- *L*-entigines.

- *E*-lectrocardiographic abnormalities.
- *O*-cular hypertelorism.
- *P*-ulmonary stenosis.
- *A*-bnormalities of the genitalia.
- *R*-etardation of growth.
- *D*-eafness.

General Considerations

The multiple lentigines syndrome was initially presented as the progressive cardiomyopathic lentiginosis syndrome by Moynahan. The acronym LEOPARD syndrome was derived later not only to describe the unusual clinical appearance of innumerable lentigines but also as an acronym for the major developmental defects (see Essentials of Diagnosis, above) (Fig 22–8). The inheritance is autosomal dominant, with variable expressivity. The basis for the pleiotropic effects of the defective gene are unknown. The NAME (nevi, atrial myxoma, myxoid neurofibromas, and ephelides), LAMB (lentigines, atrial myxoma, mucocutaneous myxomas, and blue nevi), and centrofacial lentiginosis syndromes are probably variants of the multiple lentigines syndrome. The latter are also inherited in an autosomal dominant mode.

Clinical Findings
A. Symptoms and Signs:
1. Skin– The patients may have just a few lentigines at birth; the number increases markedly with age. Often the adult patient has many hundreds or more brown spots distributed over all parts of the integument, including the palms, soles, lips, and genitalia. The mucous membranes are spared. They even occur in the axillas (axillary freckling), and some patients may have other pigmentary abnormalities such as café-au-lait spots. Patients with centrofacial lentiginosis have lentigines in a "butterfly" distribution across the cheeks and nose.

Lentigines differ from freckles (ephelides) and from pigment cell nevi. Freckles are flat spots confined to sun-exposed skin; they are reddish tan in color. Following sun exposure, they darken. In contrast, lentigines are dark brown spots. They are flat, but the skin lines coursing through them are thickened.

2. Electrocardiographic and other cardiac abnormalities– Electrocardiographic abnormalities and anatomic cardiac defects may occur with the various lentigines syndromes. Anatomic defects include stenosis or insufficiency of the pulmonary, mitral, or aortic valves and obstructive cardiomyopathy. The electrocardiographic abnormalities include right and left bundle branch block, left axis deviation, ventricular hypertrophy, and arrhythmias. Patients with multiple lentigines must be evaluated for the presence of atrial myxoma.

3. Ocular hypertelorism– Patients with lentigines syndrome may exhibit one or more different cephalofacial dysmorphic features. Hypertelorism (abnormally increased distance between the eyes), high-arched palate, low-set ears, a short neck, strabismus, and prognathism have all been observed.

4. Abnormalities of genitalia– Genital infantilism, cryptorchidism, delayed puberty, hypospadias, and cystic ovaries have been found.

5. Retardation of growth– Patients often have short stature and may exhibit a multitude of bony abnormalities, including bifid ribs, pectus excavatum, pectus carinatum, kyphoscoliosis, and hypoplastic digits.

6. Deafness– Most patients exhibit congenital neurosensory deafness. This defect limits significantly the ability of the child to develop mentally at a normal rate.

7. Other– Many patients are mentally retarded. They may have abnormal EEGs and slow nerve conduction rates. These more subtle abnormalities suggest that all tissues within the central and peripheral nervous system are affected. Mental retardation may be in part related to congenital deafness, a very serious sensory deficit.

B. Laboratory Findings: The histologic features of the lentigines are identical to those of simple lentigines. Characteristically, the epidermis is hyperplastic (acanthosis; Fig 22–2), with elongation of the rete ridges. There are increased numbers of melanocytes in the basal layer and increased melanization. The melanosomal content is expanded, and giant melanosomal complexes are noted.

Differential Diagnosis

Patients with any variant of the lentigines syndrome should not be difficult to distinguish from patients who have only freckles, multiple nevi, or neurofibromatosis. Freckles and nevi appear at 6 months to 1 year of age and have a characteristic clinical and histologic appearance. Patients with neurofibromatosis may have café-au-lait spots and axillary freckles but do not have lentigines. The presence of neurofibromas and Lisch nodules in the iris distinguishes neurofibromatosis from the lentigines syndrome.

Generalized lentiginosis (lentiginosis profusa) is the occurrence of multiple lentigines without other associated developmental abnormalities. It is also an autosomal dominant disorder.

Prevention

The patient's family should be counseled that all varieties of the multiple lentigines syndrome are transmitted as autosomal dominant disorders.

Treatment

Most abnormalities manifested by patients with the multiple lentigines syndrome are not treatable. Patients should be carefully examined by a pediatric cardiologist, endocrinologist, and otologist at the earliest possible time. The most immediate concerns are for early detection of atrial myxomas or deafness. Other cutaneous findings can be improved as the child matures. Improvement in the patient's appearance has been achieved by superficial dermabrasion of lentigines on the face. Refer to the section below on treatment of epidermal hyperpigmentation for more specific therapeutic details.

3. NEVUS SPILUS

Essentials of Diagnosis

- Present at birth or occasionally early infancy.
- Light brown patch speckled with dark brown macules.

General Considerations

A nevus spilus usually is a congenital light-brown patch speckled with dark brown macules. It is essentially a café-au-lait spot (light brown patch) associated with junctional or compound nevi (dark brown macules). In occasional cases, nevus spilus is first noted later during infancy or childhood.

Clinical Findings

A. Symptoms and Signs: The overall size of the café-au-lait spot varies but is generally several centimeters. Junctional or compound nevi are 2–4 mm in size and are localized within the light brown patch in a speckled pattern. The usual location is the trunk or proximal extremity. The underlying café-au-lait coloration is more easily appreciated when viewed with Wood's fluorescent lamp, which accentuates the epidermal pigment.

B. Laboratory Findings: The histologic features of the light-brown patch are identical to those of a café-au-lait spot. The brown macules have theques of nevus cells either confined to the epidermis (junctional nevus) or distributed on both sides of the dermal-epidermal junction (compound nevus).

Differential Diagnosis

Nevus spilus is clinically distinct once both components are appreciated.

Treatment

No treatment is necessary or effective.

4. MONGOLIAN SPOT

Essentials of Diagnosis

- Blue-black pigmentation of the sacrogluteal region.
- Present at birth
- Spontaneous resolution

General Considerations

Mongolian spots (congenital dermal melanocytosis) are common blue-black pigmented patches, present at birth in over 90% of Asian and black infants, 46% of Hispanic neonates, and 10% of Caucasians. The lesions are characterized by melanin-producing cells in the papillary and reticular dermis. Although the melanin is black or brown, the spot appears blue because of the physical properties of the skin, i.e, blue light is refracted within the epidermis and reflected back to the observer. Incomplete migration of melanocytes from the neural crest during fetal development may account for the dermal location.

The color of the spot is most intense at birth or soon thereafter, and the lesion tends to enlarge until 2 years of age. The pigment cells in the dermis have active tyrosinase until around age 2 years. Thereafter, the cells disappear or the tyrosinase becomes inactive. Only 5% of Japanese males entering military service had a persisting spot. In the remaining group (95%), the spots disappeared spontaneously.

Clinical Findings

A. Symptoms and Signs: The mongolian spot is a flat blue-black patch with indistinct borders usually present over the sacrum or lumbar area of newborn infants. The size can be small, 4–5 cm², or very large, over 30 cm². In contrast to large congenital nevi (nevus pigmentosus), the mongolian spot always spares the perianal area and perineum.

Aberrant mongolian spots in an extrasacral location are much less common. They may be observed within the defect of a cleft lip, on the face, or on the extremities. It is uncommon for aberrant spots to regress spontaneously. Many of them first appear around puberty. Extensive mongolian spots covering much of the trunk or an extremity fade slowly, if at all.

Mongolian spots can occur in association with several other congenital defects. Infants with multiple or an unusually large mongolian spot may also have numerous cutaneous vascular abnormalities such as nevus flammeus.

B. Laboratory Findings: The epidermis is normal. Scattered in the papillary and reticular dermis are bipolar melanocytes filled with melanin. The pigment is contained entirely within intracellular melanosomes, thereby avoiding incorporation into melanophages that can persist indefinitely. The involution and disappearance of melanocytes in the dermis is observed as lesions regress. The mechanism for regression is not known.

Differential Diagnosis

The presence of a blue-black spot over the sacrum is diagnostic. Mongolian spots must be distinguished from café-au-lait spots and congenital pigmented nevi. Extrasacral mongolian spots are differentiated from other dermal melanocytic processes such as dermal melanosis. The nevi of Ota and of Ito are always located on the face or shoulder, respectively.

Treatment

No therapy is effective in eradicating dermal pigment. Parents should be reassured that most sacral lesions regress spontaneously. Those in extrasacral areas can be camouflaged by cosmetics.

Course & Prognosis

The common type of mongolian spot regresses within months to years. Factors that portend a more persistent or even permanent course are extensive distribution and extrasacral location.

5. NEVI OF OTA & OF ITO

Essentials of Diagnosis

- Blue to gray-brown pigmented patches.
- Nevus of Ota: facial location.
- Nevus of Ito: unilateral shoulder location.
- Permanent.

General Considerations

Nevus of Ota (nevus fusocaeruleus ophthalmomaxillaris) is a blue to gray-brown pigmented patch located on the face, usually within the distribution of the ophthalmic and maxillary branches of the trigeminal nerve. The nevus of Ito is located unilaterally on the shoulder and neck (Fig 22–9). Half of these lesions are present at birth or soon thereafter. The other half become apparent around puberty. The nevus of Ota is more common in Orientals and affects 0.5% of all Japanese people and darkly pigmented races. Females are affected 5 times more commonly than males. A defect in the migration along nerves of neural crest derived melanoblasts could account for the dermatomal distribution seen at birth. There is no explanation for the onset of nearly half of the lesions at puberty.

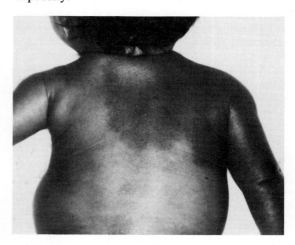

Figure 22–9. Nevus of Ito. The large blue nevus is located over the shoulder of an infant. There were many other similar lesions scattered over its integument.

Clinical Findings

A. Symptoms and Signs: The blue-brown discoloration of nevus of Ota on the face may be limited to the zygomatic arch or forehead or may cover half the face. The abnormal pigmentation can involve the bulbar and palpebral conjunctivas, the sclera, the iris, the retina, and even the optic cup. The mucous membranes of the nose and mouth are often discolored. Although the lesion rarely is bilateral, it may involve the nose but always spares the nasolabial fold.

Nevus of Ito is probably a variant of nevus of Ota. It has a similar clinical appearance except that it occurs unilaterally along the distribution of the supraclavicular and brachial nerves. The 2 lesions can occur together.

Unlike the mongolian spot, nevi of Ota and Ito do not fade with age. The coloration is less uniform, with mottled or densely spotted blue-gray to dark brown pigmentation. The tendency to become malignant is minimal. Women often report that the color intensifies during menses.

B. Laboratory Findings: The histologic features are identical to those of the mongolian spot except that the melanocytes are more numerous and distributed more superficially in the upper reticular dermis.

Differential Diagnosis

The lesion should not be confused with lentigo maligna. The latter occurs in patients in their seventh or eighth decade of life. Lentigo maligna exhibits a variety of shades of brown and black, without shades of blue. Melanosis of the eye also occurs late in life but is brown, not blue.

Treatment

There is no satisfactory treatment. Applications of dry ice or liquid nitrogen decrease the intensity of discoloration but must be applied cautiously to prevent scarring. Cosmetic cover-ups (eg, Covermark) are safe and effectively disguise the nevus.

ACQUIRED HYPERPIGMENTATION DUE TO AN EXCESS NUMBER OF MELANOCYTES

1. SOLAR LENTIGO (Senile Lentigo)

Essentials of Diagnosis

- Onset after puberty and usually after age 40 years.
- History of chronic exposure to solar radiation.
- Lesions confined to sun-exposed areas.

General Considerations

Patients with fair skin who have a history of chronic sun exposure develop solar or senile lentigines in the fifth and sixth decades of life. Patients call these liver spots or old-age spots.

Clinical Findings

A. Symptoms and Signs: Solar lentigines are moderately dark brown and large, often 1 cm or more in diameter, with irregular borders. The epidermis is atrophic, and thus their surface has fine, cigarette paperlike wrinkles. They occur on chronically sun-exposed surfaces, especially the dorsum of the hands and forearm or on the face. Like lentigo simplex, they do not darken in the summer or fade in the winter.

B. Laboratory Findings: Solar lentigines have certain histologic features that differ from those of lentigo simplex. There is marked and irregular elongation of the epidermal rete ridges with budding bulblike configurations and anastomoses of the lower ends. The number of melanocytes in the basal cell layer is increased, and an occasional melanocyte can be seen above the basal layer. The melanocytes and keratinocytes are laden with melanosome complexes that are frequently larger than in the surrounding normal epidermis. In the upper dermis, a mild perivascular infiltrate is often present.

Differential Diagnosis

Other pigmented lesions that commonly occur on the hands and face are freckles, melasma, and seborrheic keratoses. In contrast to freckles and melasma, solar lentigines do not fade in the winter but persist throughout the calendar year. Seborrheic keratoses occur additionally in nonexposed sites and can be papillomatous or have a verrucous surface.

Solar lentigines must be distinguished from lentigo maligna (Hutchinson's freckle). This distinction can be very difficult. It has been proposed that lentigo maligna can arise from a solar lentigo. The lentigo maligna tends to enlarge slowly and darken in color over a period of years. If any doubt exists, skin biopsy should be submitted for histologic diagnosis.

Treatment of Epidermal Hyperpigmentation

The treatment described in this section can apply to any of the localized processes of epidermal hyperpigmentation such as simple or solar lentigines, freckles, melasma, or postinflammatory melanosis. Epidermal forms of hyperpigmentation usually respond to treatment. In contrast, dermal hyperpigmentation (mongolian spots or nevus of Ito or Ota) and dermal melanosis do not respond to any medical treatments and usually is permanent. It is important, therefore, to determine whether the pigmentation has mainly an epidermal or dermal component. Examination of the patient with Wood's lamp ("black light") in a totally dark room can facilitate this evaluation. Epidermal melanin turns almost black when viewed with Wood's lamp. In contrast, dermal pigmentation, when observed with Wood's lamp, will not be visible to the examiner, and the blemishes on the patient's skin will disappear.

Prevention of further hyperpigmentation is paramount. Patients with sun-induced pigmentary disorders must avoid habitual sun exposure. Sunscreens or sun blocks should be applied prior to any outdoor activities. These and additional sun prevention techniques are discussed further under ultraviolet-induced hyperpigmentation (suntan).

Various bleaching medications are listed in Table 22–2. Most must be applied conscientiously 2 or 3 times every day, often for periods of 6–12 months, to achieve optimal results. There is considerable individual variation in the response to treatment, but in general most patients respond to one of the combination preparations.

Hydroquinone suppresses pigmentation probably by blocking the activity of tyrosinase, the enzyme that is primarily involved in melanin synthesis. Side effects from hydroquinone are rare but include mild skin irritation. At higher concentrations, colloid milia or dermal pigmentation has been reported. The addition of a corticosteroid cream increases the effectiveness of the hydroquinone and perhaps reduces the frequency of skin irritation. Caution must be exercised when prescribing corticosteroids for prolonged periods. On the face, steroids can cause telangiectases, atrophy, or acneiform lesions. The more potent fluorinated corticosteroids should not be used on the face except under special circumstances. On the arms and trunk, potent topical steroids can cause irreversible striae.

Tretinoin cream (Retin-A) can also be used in conjunction with hydroquinone or mild corticosteroids (or both) to decrease epidermal hyperpigmentation. There has been great interest in the use of tretinoin alone to remove pigmentation associated with photoaging. Tretinoin can be very irritating to the skin and cause erythema, desquamation, and soreness. To minimize the side effects, the following approach is suggested. Therapy should be initiated with 0.025% or 0.05% tretinoin cream applied at bedtime twice weekly for 1 month, then 3 times weekly for the second month, followed by nightly applications. Thereafter, the concentration of the cream can be increased to 0.1% if tolerated by the patient.

Monobenzyl ether of hydroquinone (Benoquin) should never be used to treat disorders of hyperpigmentation. It is always contraindicated because in some individuals it causes destruction of melanocytes and leaves permanent disfiguring white spots. Its only indication is depigmentation of patients with extensive vitiligo.

Other physical and chemical modalities for treating localized pigmented spots are available. Gentle freezing with liquid nitrogen can decrease the amount of color. Melanocytes are particularly susceptible to destruction by this treatment. One must avoid causing necrosis of the skin or blistering. Dark-skinned patients should not have lesions frozen except in special

Table 22–2. Some bleaching agents for hyperpigmentation. Apply twice or 3 times daily

Over-the-counter preparations (2% hydroquinone)
Eldopaque Cream with opaque base
Eldoquin
Esoterica Cream
Atra

Prescription preparations
Eldopaque Forte with opaque base (4% hydroquinone)
Solaquin Forte (4% Hydroquinone, PABA ester, benzophene)
HCQ Kit (4% Hydroquinone, 1% Hydrocortisone)
Ambi (2% Hydroquinone, PABA ester)
Melanex (3% Hydroquinone)

Combination of medications (to be prescribed as separate medications)
Hydroquinone 4% and salicyclic acid 2% cream
Hydroquinone 2% or 4%; hydrocortisone 2%; and tretinoin cream 0.05% applied sequentially
Hydroquinone 4%; tretinoin 0.1%; and dexamethasone 0.1% applied sequentially

circumstances because of the risk of permanent depigmentation.

Trichloroacetic acid, while effective in light-skinned patients, is generally not useful in dark-skinned individuals. It must be used with great caution, as it is extremely reactive chemically, and higher concentrations can cause instantaneous necrosis of the epidermis that can leave severe scarring. One cautious approach is to begin with a single application of 15% or 25% trichloroacetic acid on one or 2 test areas in cosmetically less critical locations. The area should be cleansed first with alcohol to remove surface lipids. A cotton-tipped applicator is used to evenly paint the acid directly on the lesion. Caution must be taken not to drip solution onto uninvolved areas. If the patient notes burning, the field is washed with soap and water. Generally, 25% trichloracetic acid produces only a mild effect and moderate results. If necessary, areas can be treated with 35% or 50% acid but only by a physician familiar with its properties. The optimal concentration of trichloroacetic acid is one that produces desquamation and disappearance of the lesion without excessive injury.

2. ULTRAVIOLET-INDUCED HYPERPIGMENTATION (Suntan)

Essentials of Diagnosis

- Light brown or golden brown coloration of exposed skin.
- Sharp demarcation lines between exposed and normal skin.

General Considerations

The constitutive or baseline skin color is genetically determined by 3 or perhaps 4 sets of alleles independently of extrinsic factors such as sun exposure. Facultative skin color is the inducible darkening of the skin which most often follows exposure to ultraviolet radiation. Suntan results from 2 different mechanisms. Long wave ultraviolet light (type A, 320–400 nm) causes pigment darkening within 15–30 minutes following exposure that disappears within hours. It is probably caused by an oxidative change in the preexisting melanin molecules. It is responsible for the golden bronze color observed immediately after sunbathing.

Short wave ultraviolet light (type B, 290–320 nm) produces both sunburn as well as delayed tanning. Delayed tanning is often much darker than the immediate type and is caused by proliferation of melanocytes as well as enhanced production of melanin. It takes 3–4 days to develop and lasts for many weeks. Both long and short wave ultraviolet light also contribute to photoaging, and both increase the risk for development of skin cancer.

Clinical Findings

A. Symptoms and Signs: Ultraviolet radiation of light-skinned individuals results in a tan ranging in color from light golden brown to bronze to grayish brown-black. There is a sharp contrast in the skin color of exposed and nonexposed sites, with typical "tan lines" demarcating the garments worn for sun bathing. Sun-exposed areas are usually evenly pigmented. After many years of prolonged exposure, the skin develops a mottled appearance characterized by spots of hypo- and hyperpigmentation. The texture may become leathery and excessively wrinkled, especially on heavily exposed areas of the face, the neck, and the dorsum of the hands.

B. Laboratory Findings: Histologic examination of sun-exposed skin shows, in addition to proliferation of melanocytes and enhanced production of melanin, features of photoaging such as basophilic degeneration of the collagen in the upper dermis and a thinned, atrophic epidermis.

Differential Diagnosis

The hyperpigmentation of Addison's disease, while more pronounced in areas of the skin exposed to the sun, can easily be distinguished by the increase in pigmentation seen in nonexposed sites, especially the genitalia, areolae, oral mucosa, scars, and palmar creases.

Treatment

The patient must recognize that reversal of sun-induced pigmentation can occur only by avoidance of exposure of the skin to all forms of ultraviolet light. There are many physical sun blocks that reflect ultraviolet light and protect the skin very well. Clothing such as beachwear and hats are excellent protectants. Other opaque chemical sun blocks such as zinc oxide, calamine, talc, titanium dioxide, and kaolin are effective sun shields. These products must be applied in a thick coat. Some preparations available commercially in spectacular colors are now cosmetically and socially acceptable. For individuals who are unusually sensitive to sunlight and who desire to enjoy outdoor activities, these sun blocks are essential.

Chemical sunscreens function in a different way. They absorb ultraviolet light especially in the short wave range (UVB, 290–320 nm). The most common chemical sunscreens contain p-aminobenzoic acid (PABA), esters of PABA, and salicylates. Other chemicals such as the benzophenone derivatives, anthranilates, and cinnamates absorb UVB and offer additional absorption in the UVA (290- to 350-nm) range.

Two factors should be considered when choosing a sunscreen: the sun protection factor (SPF) and the substantivity. The SPF is the ratio of the minimal sunburn (UVB) dose of sunlight on chemically protected skin compared to that on unprotected skin. An SPF of 15–20 (which requires 15–20 times more UVB to burn the skin) is considered to be adequate protection against UVB irradiation.

The substantivity of the sunscreen is its ability to withstand sweating and water immersion. Commercially available sunscreens with SPFs ≥ 15 that also have good to excellent water and sweat resistance include (among others) Sundown, PreSun, Super-Shade, Total Eclipse, and Photoplex. Ideally, all sunscreens should be reapplied after prolonged swimming or heavy sweating.

CONGENITAL HYPERPIGMENTATION DUE TO MELANOSOMAL DEFECTS: NEUROFIBROMATOSIS (Recklinghausen's Disease)

Essentials of Diagnosis

- Neurofibromas: usually soft, pedunculated, flesh-colored papules and nodules, "buttonhole" deformity.
- Café-au-lait macules.
- Axillary freckles (café-au-lait spots).
- Lisch nodules: yellow or brown papules on the iris.

General Considerations

Neurofibromatosis is one of a group of disorders of neural crest-derived cells, the neurocristopathies. They include pheochromocytoma, neuroblastoma, and medullary carcinoma of the thyroid (Sipple's syndrome, the neuroectodermal melanotic tumor of infancy), Hirschsprung's disease, and other syndromes. Neurofibromatosis affects one in 3000 infants and has an equal predilection for males and females, consistent with an autosomal dominant mode of transmission. Half of patients have no family history of the disorder, ie, they have the disease as a result of a

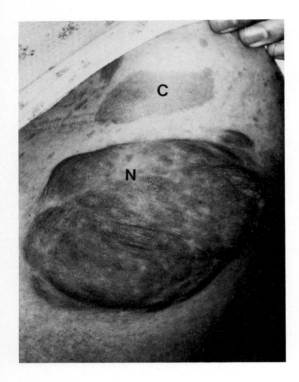

Figure 22–10. Patient with neurofibromatosis. A large plexiform neuroma (N) is present on the thigh. Several café-au-lait spots (C) are also visible.

spontaneous mutation. Clinically, neurofibromatosis has been separated into at least 6 varieties. We shall discuss Recklinghausen's neurofibromatosis in this section.

Clinical Findings

A. Symptoms and Signs: The two most important cutaneous signs of neurofibromatosis are multiple café-au-lait spots (distinctive light brown in color, like "coffee with milk") and neurofibromas (Fig 22–10). Many normal individuals have one or more café-au-lait spots. The presence of 6 or more spots larger than 1.5 cm in diameter during infancy or childhood strongly suggests the diagnosis of neurofibromatosis even in the absence of neurofibromas. The tumors may not form until late childhood or around puberty. Patients with neurofibromas have small guttate café-au-lait spots in the axilla (axillary freckling, or Crowe's sign) and on the perineum.

Neurofibromas are derived from neuroid supportive cells within the central, peripheral, or autonomic nervous system. The tumors may be of several types: neurofibromas, schwannomas, or combined forms. Clinically, they are pedunculated soft, fleshy, skin-colored tumors that seem to rise up out of a hole ("buttonhole" deformity) within the dermis, easily perceived by palpation. They may be few in number or innumerable. Many are small (1–2 cm in diameter), but occasionally a neurofibroma is 10–20 cm or more in diameter (Fig 22–10). These large tumors are called plexiform neurofibromas. The presence of café-au-lait spots (1.5 cm in diameter), axillary freckles, and cutaneous neurofibromas is diagnostic.

Neurofibromas can arise from peripheral nerves as they pass through the vertebral foramina and cause bony deformities of the spine (kyphoscoliosis). They may form virtually in any organ, including the mesentery, prostate, colon, bladder, and central nervous system. Those that arise within the spinal canal or the cranial vault—eg, acoustic or optic neuromas—usually cause severe neurologic problems. Neurofibromas on the iris are called Lisch nodules and are raised, gelatinous papules of yellow or brown color. By the age of 6 years, 92% of patients have one or more Lisch nodules.

B. Laboratory Findings: Skin from a café-au-lait spot exhibits an increased number of melanocytes in the basal layer and increased pigment in the melanocytes. As a consequence, there are a greater number of melanosomes within the melanocytes and keratinocytes. Giant melanosomes, usually varying in size from 1 to 10 μm but occasionally up to as large as 50 μm, may be seen on electron microscopy (Fig 22–5). These macromelanosomes result from aggregation of normal-sized melanosomes into a single giant organelle. Giant melanosomes are found frequently in neurofibromatosis; however, they have been observed in many other pigmentary disorders, including lentigo simplex, nevus spilus, tinea versicolor, Becker's nevus, and most nevocellular nevi. The darker color of the café-au-lait spot is caused by an increase in the amount of melanin transported into the keratinocytes.

Differential Diagnosis

The diagnosis of neurofibromatosis usually is not difficult. The constellation of 6 large café-au-lait spots, axillary freckles, and neurofibromas is diagnostic. Adult patients with only café-au-lait spots and axillary freckling are considered to have a benign variant of neurofibromatosis. Isolated neurofibromas or tumors restricted to one segment of the body should not be considered pathognomonic of neurofibromatosis.

Isolated café-au-lait spots occur in 10–20% of normal individuals. The spots are generally less than 1.5 cm in size and usually do not contain giant melanosomes. Café-au-lait spots are also seen in Albright's syndrome, a triad consisting of polyostotic fibrous dysplasia, precocious puberty, and hyperpigmented macules and patches. A few other syndromes in which café-au-lait spots are seen include Watson's syndrome (mental retardation and pulmonary stenosis), Russell-Silver dwarfism, tuberous sclerosis, and ataxia telangiectasia.

Treatment

Some neurofibromas may be removed surgically for cosmetic purposes or to prevent mechanical problems. The patients must be observed for development of tumors within the central nervous system or other life threatening disorders such as pheochromocytoma.

Prognosis

The number of pigmented spots and neurofibromas increases with age. Cosmetic disfigurement may be mild to severe. Probably for this reason, many patients do not marry or have children. Some neurofibromas become neurofibrosarcomas that can metastasize. Others are lethal because they develop within the cranial vault. Other tumors (eg, pheochromocytoma and melanoma) and endocrine abnormalities (acromegaly or thyroid dysfunction) may occur. The MEN II (Sipple) syndrome consists of medullary thyroid cancer, bilateral pheochromocytomas, hypothyroidism, and neurofibromatosis.

CONGENITAL HYPERPIGMENTATION DUE TO ABNORMALITIES OF TYROSINASE

Although there are no disorders in humans or other mammals unequivocally attributed to increased melanin formation from excessive tyrosinase activity, there are several in which the amount of melanin synthesized and transported into the keratinocyte is excessive. The hyperpigmentation may be mild or may be severe enough to be considered moderately disfiguring.

1. FAMILIAL PROGRESSIVE HYPERPIGMENTATION

Essentials of Diagnosis

- Dark-skinned individuals only.
- Reticulated, deeply pigmented patches.

General Considerations

This uncommon disorder is characterized by mottled or reticulated hyperpigmented patches on the skin present at birth. As the child ages, both the intensity of color and the number of patches on the skin and mucous membranes increase. The disorder probably is transmitted as an autosomal or X-linked dominant disorder.

Clinical Findings

A. Symptoms and Signs: The patients—always black—have darker areas of skin that increase in number and darken with age. The quantity of melanin in the stratum corneum is so great that rubbing the skin with a white towel or wearing white clothing discolors the fabrics. The hyperpigmentation has a reticulated pattern and can affect any area of the integument, the oral mucosa, or the bulbar and palpebral conjunctiva. The nails, retina, and vaginal mucosa are not affected, and the patients have no associated disorders.

B. Laboratory Findings: The population density of the epidermal pigment cells is normal. The amount of melanin visible on routine sections of skin stained by hematoxylin and eosin or by silver methenamine is markedly increased in all skin layers.

Treatment

No treatment is available.

2. HEREDITARY HYPERPIGMENTATION IN BLACKS

General Considerations

Several inherited types of hyperpigmentation are so common in blacks that they should not be considered abnormalities.

Futcher's line is a sharply demarcated line of pigmentation visible on the anterolateral side of the deltoid and the upper part of the arm. The outer arm is darkly colored; the inner part is lighter. Futcher's line is present bilaterally in 18% of blacks and unilaterally in 2%.

A thin line running down the mid trunk has been observed in 22 members of 4 generations of one kinship. Other members of the same family had a transverse hyperpigmented line extending across the nose from one nasolabial fold to the other. Both the vertical thoracic line and the horizontal nasal line were transmitted as an autosomal dominant trait. The patients were healthy in all respects.

Treatment & Prognosis

No treatment is necessary. Mild bleaching of the nasal line with 2–4% hydroquinone applied daily only to the dark area might be attempted if the patient is concerned about the cosmetic disfigurement.

3. PERIORBITAL HYPERPIGMENTATION

Darkened rings around the eyes are of concern to many patients. In many cases the darkening seems to vary with stress or lack of sleep. This observation suggests that the common dark rings are due in part to vascular changes.

Kinships have been shown to have excessive melanin in the epidermis of the upper and lower eyelids. The trait is transmitted as an autosomal dominant defect. It may be that in many people vascular alterations caused by stress or lack of sleep accentuate melanin deposition in the eyelids due to genetic traits.

4. PEUTZ-JEGHERS SYNDROME

Essentials of Diagnosis
- Brown or black macules, especially on the lips and buccal mucosa.
- Polyps of the intestines.
- Autosomal dominant inheritance.

General Considerations
Patients with Peutz-Jeghers syndrome have intestinal polyps associated with a distinctive pigmentation of the skin around the mouth and in the oral cavity.

Clinical Findings
A. Symptoms and Signs: Polyps are scattered throughout the gastrointestinal tract—occasionally in the stomach or duodenum and invariably in the jejunum, ileum, colon, or rectum. Polyps develop singly or in groups from early infancy and continue to form throughout life. Removal of polyps at any age does not prevent formation of new lesions.

The most common complication of intestinal polyposis is intussusception or rectal prolapse. Bleeding and iron deficiency anemia are also frequent. Although the polyps in the small intestine show no tendency to undergo malignant transformation, patients with the syndrome have an increased incidence of carcinoma in various other sites.

From birth or early infancy, pigmented spots develop that look like freckles—brown or black macules with sharply demarcated borders. Most are scattered around the mouth and on the lips, but some are on the hands, arms, and abdomen. They do not darken following exposure to sunlight. A diffuse light brown pigmentation of the tongue, buccal mucosa, gums, and palate may persist throughout life.

B. Laboratory Findings: Routine sections of the skin are unremarkable. Increased quantities of melanin are present, compared to the unpigmented skin and mucous membrane.

Complications
Polyposis may cause intestinal obstruction, rectal prolapse, or anemia from bleeding.

Treatment
No treatment is necessary for pigmentation. Patients should be counseled that the disease is genetic, and they should be under the care of a gastroenterologist to minimize the complications of the intestinal polyposis.

5. INCONTINENTIA PIGMENTI (Bloch-Sulzberger Syndrome)

Essentials of Diagnosis
- Female predominance (X-linked dominant).

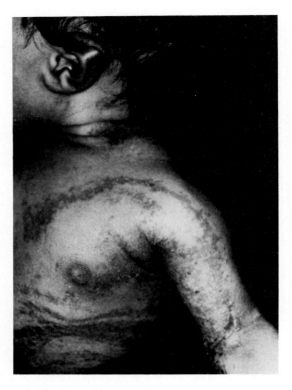

Figure 22–11. Swirls of hyperpigmentation remaining on the skin after clearing of the earlier vesicles and papules caused by incontinentia pigmenti. The hyperpigmentation spontaneously disappears, usually by the time the patient has reached adolescence or early adulthood.

- First stage: streaks of vesicles.
- Second stage: streaks of verrucous papules.
- Third stage: streaks of whorled hyperpigmentation,

General Considerations
This disorder, transmitted probably as an X-linked dominant disorder, is usually lethal to male fetuses. It occurs in female infants of all races. Incontinentia pigmenti is associated with multiple defects of the central nervous system (see Chapter 51).

Clinical Findings
A. Symptoms and Signs: At birth or within the first month of life, 95% of affected individuals manifest the characteristic skin signs. Streaks of red papules or vesicles develop most commonly over the extremities and trunk. The streaks, distributed in a swirled or marbled pattern, evolve over a period of weeks into verrucous, keratotic papules that heal and leave a brown-gray hyperpigmented discoloration

(Fig 22–11). The pigment has the same marbled appearance and distribution as the papules. Much of a child's integument may be covered by these brown-gray swirls. Most often, the verrucous pigmented lesions form after 6–12 months of age.

B. Laboratory Findings: The first stage consists of intraepidermal vesicles, eosinophilic spongiosis, and intense dermal infiltrate. In the second stage, acanthosis, hyperkeratosis, and basal cell layer vaculopathy are seen. In the third pigmented stage, the epidermis appears normal. There is a moderate deposition of melanin within the superficial papillary dermis, often within melanophages.

Differential Diagnosis

In the infant with vesicles, viral sepsis is often suspected, but the arrangement of lesions, histologic appearance, and the presence of verrucous papules should lead to the correct diagnosis. Verrucous lesions resemble viral warts. The swirling brown ("like marble cake") pigmentation of the third stage is unmistakable.

Treatment

The skin disorder requires no treatment.

Prognosis

The evolution through the 3 stages is usually rapid. Verrucous lesions are usually gone within 2 years, and the pigmentation usually disappears by age 20 years (see Chapter 51).

ACQUIRED HYPERPIGMENTATION DUE TO ABNORMALITIES OF TYROSINASE

1. FRECKLES

Essentials of Diagnosis

- Tan or red macules 1–5 mm in diameter in sun-exposed areas.
- Especially in fair-skinned people.

General Considerations

Freckles (ephelides) are pigmented macules, usually tan or reddish tan, observed in sun-exposed skin of people most often of Celtic origin.

Clinical Findings

A. Symptoms and Signs: Many children have a few freckles scattered across their cheeks and nose. Occasionally, an individual may have thousands of these macules that coalesce, covering the skin. Freckling of the skin is usually observed in patients with red or auburn hair and blue eyes. The freckles darken following exposure to ultraviolet light, a property not observed in lentigines or nevi. Both long wave (320–400 nm) and short wave (290–320 nm) ultraviolet light cause increased pigmentation. Short wave ultraviolet light stimulates melanin formation. Long wave ultraviolet light causes photo-oxidation of preexisting melanin within the keratinocyte and pigment cell.

B. Laboratory Findings: The skin on routine examination appears normal. A Fontana-Masson stain for melanin demonstrates increased melanin within the freckles. Electron microscopy confirms that the melanocyte in a freckle produces larger quantities of stage IV melanosomes than do melanocytes in the surrounding skin.

Complications

Freckles mark patients who are unusually susceptible to sunburn, actinic keratoses, and skin cancers. Freckled individuals should be instructed to avoid sunlight and to apply sunscreens daily (more often during sun exposure). They should wear protective clothing at the beach, golf course, etc.

Treatment

Freckles are not readily treated. Application of creams containing hydroquinone usually does not improve the appearance.

2. MELASMA; CHLOASMA

Essentials of Diagnosis

- Mottled macular pigmentation, usually on the face.
- Most commonly during pregnancy ("mask of pregnancy").

General Considerations

Melasma develops on the faces of some women who are pregnant or taking birth control pills. Estrogens may cause melasma by accelerating the formation of melanin and also cause darkening of the nipples and areolas and the linea nigra on the abdomen, a darkened line extending from the pubis to the umbilicus.

Melasma is not restricted to pregnant women. Many women who have neither been pregnant nor received estrogen-containing medications have melasma, as do some men.

Clinical Findings

A. Symptoms and Signs: Melasma is a brown-gray mottled discoloration most prominent on the forehead, malar eminences, and cheeks anterior to the ears. Sometimes it affects the upper lip and the chin.

B. Laboratory Findings: The epidermis appears normal. The amount of melanin in the darkened skin is increased compared to the normal skin. The number of pigment cells is normal. Melanin may also be present in dermal macrophages (pigment incontinence) and causes the gray-brown discoloration observed in some patients.

Complications

Although there are no biologic complications from melasma, some patients are markedly distressed emotionally by the cosmetic defects.

Treatment

The goal of therapy is to decrease the production of melanin without killing melanocytes. Cream containing hydroquinone in 3–4% concentration—applied twice daily to the dark areas—may decrease the production of melanin. However, the response to therapy takes months, and most patients do not respond adequately to hydroquinone alone. Fluorinated corticosteroids also decrease melanin formation, but they must be used with caution to avoid epidermal atrophy or dilatation of the superficial dermal capillaries. Hydroquinone (2% or 4%) combined with retinoic acid (0.05%) and hydrocortisone (1%) in a cream or lotion base can be applied twice daily if creams containing hydroquinone alone do not work. The melanin in the dermal melanophages cannot be bleached away with any of these preparations. It is important for the pa-

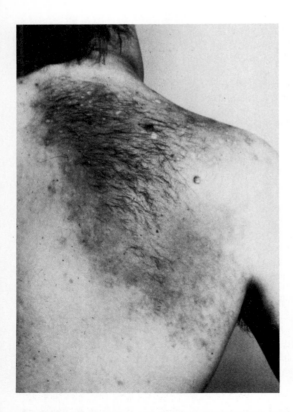

Figure 22–12. Becker's nevus on the shoulder. The skin is hyperpigmented and the hairs coarse and darkly pigmented. The lesion is a type of epidermal nevus.

tient to use sunscreens during the summer months and to avoid direct exposure to sunlight whenever possible.

Additional treatment details are given in the section on treatment of epidermal hyperpigmentation.

3. BECKER'S NEVUS

Essentials of Diagnosis
- Light brown patch usually on the unilateral shoulder and back.
- Male predominance.
- Hypertrichosis within the pigmented patch.

General Considerations

Becker's nevus (Fig 22–12) is an epidermal nevus, a benign proliferation of keratinocytes and epidermal appendages. It usually appears around puberty or in the second to third decade, sometimes after a severe sunburn. The male:female ratio is 5:1.

Clinical Findings

A. Symptoms and Signs: A light brown pigmented patch most commonly covers the shoulder or a large portion of the upper back. Most are single, but they can be multiple. Lesions may be located on the abdomen, buttocks, or distal extremities. After puberty, the area is usually covered with many dark, coarse hairs.

B. Laboratory Findings: The number of melanocytes is normal, but there is increased melanin deposition in the basal layer melanocytes and suprabasal keratinocytes. Features of an epidermal nevus are present, including acanthosis, hyperkeratosis, and papillomatosis.

Differential Diagnosis

The late onset distinguishes this nevus from the congenital black hairy (bathing trunk) nevus, which may also be large and may contain prominent hairs. In prepubertal children, Becker's nevus may be indistinguishable from a large café-au-lait spot.

Treatment

The lesions persist throughout life and are sometimes disfiguring. They do not become malignant. Attempts to bleach the skin are usually not successful. Shaving the hair may minimize the cosmetic disfigurement.

4. POSTINFLAMMATORY HYPERPIGMENTATION

Essentials of Diagnosis
- Patchy distribution following pattern of original dermatoses.
- Very common in dark-skinned patients.

General Considerations

A variety of inflammatory conditions and infections cause postinflammatory hyperpigmentation of the skin. Common inflammatory dermatoses include psoriasis, acne, cutaneous lupus, lichen simplex chronicus, lichen planus, atopic dermatitis, and trauma. Examples of infections of the skin leaving residual hyperpigmentation are herpes zoster, tinea versicolor, and chickenpox. Postinflammatory hyperpigmentation is common and rather persistent in dark-skinned people.

Clinical Findings

A. Symptoms and Signs: The dyschromia follows the pattern and distribution of the original dermatoses, but its intensity is not necessarily related to the degree of previous inflammation. The patches can be a black-brown or gray-brown color.

B. Laboratory Findings: The number of melanocytes remains the same, but the amount of melanin is increased. Often the preceding inflammation is associated with disruption of the dermal-epidermal barrier. Melanin is then deposited in the upper dermis, usually within melanophages.

Differential Diagnosis

A distribution mimicking a known cutaneous disorder, often with the original disease process ongoing, helps to make the diagnosis.

Treatment

See section on treatment of epidermal hyperpigmentation. If the pigment is primarily localized in the dermis, none of the topical therapies will be effective.

5. SYSTEMIC CAUSES OF HYPERPIGMENTATION

Generalized hyperpigmentation is associated with many systemic disorders. A few of the disorders will be discussed separately. Table 22–1 offers a partial list of metabolic, endocrine, nutritional, or miscellaneous disorders often associated with widespread or diffuse hyperpigmentation.

6. ADRENAL INSUFFICIENCY (Addison's Disease)

Essentials of Diagnosis

- Generalized brown hyperpigmentation.
- Accentuation in creases, sun-exposed sites, and genitalia.
- Excessive ACTH and MSH production.

General Considerations

Secretion of cortisone from the adrenal gland causes repression of ACTH and MSH released from the pituitary. If the adrenal gland cannot synthesize adequate cortisone to shut off pituitary release of MSH, the patient will develop hyperpigmentation. Pigment cells in all parts of the body—the mucous membranes as well as the skin—are stimulated by MSH to produce melanin.

Clinical Findings

A. Symptoms and Signs: The patient often feels well but may be less energetic than usual. However, the entire skin is darker, especially the sun-exposed areas. Hyperpigmentation of certain parts of the integument are highly suggestive of excessive MSH secretion. The gums (particularly along the alveolar ridge), the buccal mucosa, and the tongue may be minimally or deeply pigmented. The nipples, areolas, and genitalia often are especially dark. Scars and the palmar and plantar creases are darkly pigmented. The patient may note longitudinal pigmented bands on the nails. The scalp hair may darken.

B. Laboratory Findings: Serum cortisol levels obtained at 8:00 AM will be lower than normal. The response of the adrenal gland to stimulation by ACTH (the corticotropin [Cortrosyn] stimulation test) will be subnormal. Twenty-four-hour urine 17-hydroxycorticosteroid levels fail to rise.

Treatment

The medical aspects of adrenal insufficiency are not discussed here. The pigmentation disappears slowly when the patient receives adequate glucocorticosteroid replacement therapy. However, most patients retain a slight tan color for life.

7. DRUG-INDUCED HYPERPIGMENTATION

Many chemicals cause hyperpigmentation. Melanocyte-stimulating hormone is the best-characterized example and may be responsible for the hyperpigmentation associated with Addison's disease. Many other chemicals—eg, psoralens or cyclophosphamide—may also cause hyperpigmentation. A few elements such as the heavy metals can be deposited within the skin and discolor it.

Heavy Metals

Silver at one time was used as an antiseptic for the treatment of infections of mucous membranes. It is absorbed through the mucous membranes and deposited in the skin, especially around the eccrine glands. The skin and the lunulae of the nails acquire a characteristic silver or blue-gray color called argyria.

Bismuth and arsenic—also used as medications in the past—cause brown hyperpigmentation. Some patients may ingest arsenic by drinking water from contaminated wells. Others are exposed to insecticide sprays containing arsenic that are used in fruit orchards. Chronic arsenic ingestion stimulates melanin formation within the epidermis, and the hyperpigmentation is not due to deposition of arsenic within the dermis.

Tetracycline

Tetracycline itself rarely causes hyperpigmentation, but it may discolor teeth if taken during childhood. Minocycline and methacycline, both long-acting tetracyclines, can cause a striking blue-gray hyperpigmentation of the skin. The pigment is deposited in the dermis of inflamed or injured skin and in the thyroid gland. Although melanin may be present in the epidermis of the hyperpigmented areas, most of the discoloration is due to iron in perivascular histiocytes.

Cytotoxic Agents

Patients receiving cytotoxic drugs for the treatment of malignant disorders may develop hyperpigmentation. Bleomycin causes the skin to become deeply tanned. It probably stimulates proliferation of pigment cells as well as increased formation of melanin. Cyclophosphamide, melphalan, and other alkylating agents can cause longitudinal or horizontal bands of hyperpigmentation in the nails (melanonychia).

Miscellaneous Drugs

Antimalarial drugs such as quinacrine or chloroquine produce blue discoloration of the mucous membranes, especially the palate. The discoloration commonly is observed also on the nail beds, over the surface of the tibia, and on the face.

Chlorpromazine, especially if taken in large doses for prolonged periods, causes bluish discoloration of sun-exposed skin, including the hands, forearms, and cheeks. Characteristically, patients taking chlorpromazine have a yellow horizontal band on exposed portions of the sclera. Clofazimine, used in the treatment of leprosy, gives the skin a reddish-brown hue.

Fixed Drug Eruptions

Some drugs such as tetracycline, phenolphthalein (the active ingredient in many laxatives), and griseofulvin may cause localized hyperpigmentation. Patients first note a discrete red, pruritic papule, nodule, or bulla, frequently on the genitalia, the face, or the trunk. Sometimes more than one area may be affected. During healing, a hyperpigmented macule is formed. Each time the patient ingests the offending drug, the same spots become inflamed and the pigmentation becomes more intense. The mechanism by which a drug can cause a fixed or localized reaction is not known.

HYPERPIGMENTATION OF THE NAILS

The nails may exhibit abnormal pigmentation or hyperpigmentation bands. Brown longitudinal bands are normally seen in black patients. They can be observed in patients with benign lentigo or malignant melanoma of the nail matrix, Addison's disease, or malignant disorders being treated with alkylating agents (cyclophosphamide, melphalan, or bleomycin). Chlorpromazine, antimalarials, and silver cause azure discoloration of the lunula. Radiation therapy directed to the thorax—eg, in the treatment of breast cancer—may cause horizontal pigmented banding of the nails. Workers in certain chemical industries may have discolored nails due to staining. Patients using hydroquinone as a bleach may develop horizontal pigmented bands in their nails. Zidovudine (AZT), used to treat patients with HIV infections, can cause hyperpigmented brown or blue-gray longitudinal streaks of the nails.

DISORDERS OF HYPOPIGMENTATION; DEPIGMENTATION

For each type of functional or anatomic abnormality of pigment cells producing hyperpigmentation, there is an opposite abnormality resulting in hypopigmentation or depigmentation. For example, pigment cells may be absent from an area of skin, may make too few melanosomes, or may be incapable of synthesizing normal amounts of melanin.

CONGENITAL DEPIGMENTATION DUE TO ABSENCE OF MELANOCYTES

1. PIEBALDISM

Essentials of Diagnosis
- Present at birth.
- White forelock (poliosis).
- Depigmented cutaneous patches on ventral surfaces.

General Considerations

The word "piebald" is derived from "pied," meaning "having 2 or more colors." The term "partial albinism" has been used synonymously with piebaldism in medical literature. Piebaldism or white spotting of the skin and hair is a common phenomenon in mammals. Dogs, cats, horses, and mice often are bred for these patterns of white spots. Zebras have an organized and patterned form of spotting. The white spots are devoid of mature melanocytes. Absence of functional pigment cells may be due to failure of melanoblasts to form within the neural crest; to migrate into the skin or hair bulb; or to differentiate into mature functioning melanocytes after reaching the integument. The skin and hair are white because they lack melanocytes. Most genes coding for piebaldism are transmitted in an autosomal dominant fashion. Not uncommonly, the genetic defect also interferes with the pigment cells in other organs such as the eye and ear. For example, spotting in animals commonly is associated with heterochromia iridum or deafness.

Genetic traits cause piebaldism or white spotting in human subjects also.

Classic piebaldism is transmitted in an autosomal dominant fashion, and the incidence is estimated to be 1 in 20,000 births. Piebaldism probably is caused by many different genes. Most kinships affected by the piebald trait seem to exhibit a unique variant with a special pattern of spotting in combination with defects of hearing, central nervous system dysfunction, or abnormalities of growth.

Clinical Findings

A. Symptoms and Signs: White spots on the skin and a white forelock (poliosis; Fig 22–13) are present at birth. They may not be apparent for several months in infants with fair skin and blond hair. Examination of the infant's skin with Wood's lamp will detect these depigmented areas. The largest areas of depigmentation are distributed symmetrically over the ventral skin, ie, the forehead, chest, mid thigh to mid calf, and mid arm. The hands, feet, upper thigh, upper arm, and shoulders are usually spared. The hairs

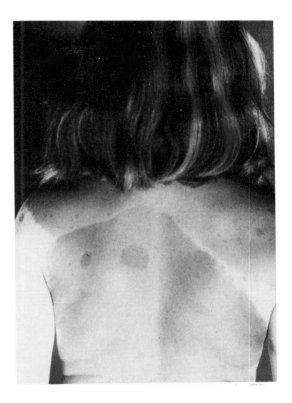

Figure 22–14. The back of a child with piebaldism. The left arm is depigmented. The skin shows multiple shades of pigmentation. Islands of deeply pigmented skin are also visible.

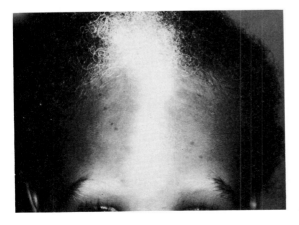

Figure 22–13. White forelock on a patient with piebaldism. Poliosis usually is a permanent feature of this disorder.

within the depigmented patches are white and remain depigmented throughout the patient's life. The central frontal portion of the scalp may exhibit the classic white forelock associated with a white triangular or diamond-shaped area of depigmentation in the middle of the forehead. Scattered within the depigmented and normally colored skin are hyperpigmented macules (piebaldism; Fig 22–14). Although the areas of depigmentation and poliosis tend to be permanent, some spots enlarge or decrease in size, and a few hairs may become pigmented.

In some families, piebaldism is associated with mental retardation; in others, with deafness; and in still others, with cerebellar ataxia and incoordination.

B. Laboratory Findings: The depigmented skin appears normal under light microscopy except for the complete absence of identifiable melanocytes. An occasional melanocyte, often morphologically abnormal, has been recognized utilizing electron microscopy. A possible explanation for this observation is the occurrence of melanocytes in transitional zones between depigmented and hyperpigmented islands of skin.

Differential Diagnosis

Piebaldism can be differentiated from vitiligo without difficulty. Vitiligo is an acquired (usually nonfamilial) cutaneous depigmentation with a distribution different from that of piebaldism. Vitiligo tends to change over time with or without treatment, whereas piebaldism is stable.

Features of piebaldism (white forelock and leukoderma) can be associated with abnormalities of other neural crest derivatives. Woolf's syndrome consists of congenital sensorineural deafness and depigmentation of the entire head and scalp hair. The inheritance is thought to be autosomal recessive. Ziprowski-Margolis syndrome also consists of congenital deafness and hypopigmented skin with hyperpigmented patches. However, histologic specimens reveal the presence of melanocytes in the hypopigmented skin. This syndrome has been reported to occur only in males and has an X-linked recessive genetic transmission.

Treatment

Successful repigmentation of leukodermic skin depends upon the stimulation of preexisting melanocytes to proliferate and migrate into depigmented skin. Attempts to repigment the white areas of piebaldism with conventional methods such as ultraviolet light and psoralens have generally been unsuccessful. This is predictable because of the absence of melanocytes in the epidermis and hair bulbs of piebald skin.

Surgical correction is possible with punch autografts, epidermal suction grafts, and thin split-thickness grafts. Repigmentation does occur, and the appearance is most often satisfactory. Covermark and Dermablend are special opaque cosmetics that can be used to conceal the more obvious depigmented areas with acceptable results.

2. WAARDENBURG'S SYNDROME

Essentials of Diagnosis

- Dystopia canthorum.
- Congenital sensorineural deafness.
- White forelock (poliosis)
- Synophrys (hypertrichosis of medial eyebrows).
- Broad nasal root.
- Heterochromia iridum.

General Considerations

Waardenburg's syndrome, like piebaldism, is an inherited defect of neural crest-derived elements. There are at least 3 genetic variants: (1) classic Waardenburg's type I, (2) Waardenburg's type II, and (3) Klein-Waardenburg syndrome (type III). An autosomal dominant mode of transmission is suggested for all 3 types, with considerable heterogeneity in phenotypic expression. Pseudo-Waardenburg syndrome and other less well described subtypes have also been described.

Clinical Findings

Waardenburg's type I is the classic syndrome described by Waardenburg in 1951. Dystopia canthorum occurs in 99% of cases and is almost invariable in the type I syndrome.

A. Symptoms and Signs: The patients show lateral displacement of the medial canthi and lacrimal puncta without widening of the interpupillary distance.

Waardenburg's syndrome is the cause of deafness in 1% of infants born with sensorineural hearing loss. The frequency of deafness in Waardenburg's syndrome ranges from 9% to 40%. The incidence is lower in type I than in type II syndrome. About 60% have a white forelock with a triangular white area of skin on the forehead. Five to 10% also have piebald spots on the extremities or trunk. The broad nasal root and synophrys are observed in two-thirds of affected individuals. Heterochromia iridum affects one-fourth of these patients. Another 25% have a peculiar bilateral whitish blue hypochromia of both irides. Visual acuity is normal. However, the fundus may exhibit decreased quantities of pigment within the retinal pigment epithelium. A distinctive facial appearance is seen with closely set nasal nares, small alar wings, a broad mandible, and an arched upper lip.

Waardenburg's syndrome type II is distinguished from type I by the absence of dystopia canthorum. The incidence of congenital sensorineural deafness is greater in type II than in type I cases. Hirschsprung's disease, or aganglionic megacolon, occurs more often in type II than in type I Waardenburg's syndrome. Intestinal bowel obstruction can occur in the neonatal period secondary to an abnormally dilated segment of bowel that has absent parasympathetic ganglion cells in the submucosal and myenteric plexuses. A common faulty embryologic event of neural crest-derived melanocytes and myenteric ganglion cells is probably responsible for both cutaneous and intestinal abnormalities.

Features that distinguish Klein-Waardenburg syndrome (type III) are musculoskeletal defects of the upper limb. These include hypoplasia of the upper arm and pectoral muscles, axillary webs, rigid joints, and camptodactyly of all fingers.

B. Laboratory Findings: The histology of the white skin from patients with Waardenburg's syndrome is unremarkable by light microscopy. Silver stains for melanin and the dopa technique for detection of active tyrosinase enzyme confirm the absence of melanin and functional melanocytes within the epidermis and hair bulbs. The lack of pigment cells has been confirmed by electron microscopy.

Treatment

The therapy for the cutaneous depigmentation is

the same as for patients with piebaldism. Conventional modalities of repigmentation are not effective.

A family history should be investigated thoroughly. If possible, family members should be examined with Wood's lamp to determine if a parent of the affected child carries the gene. If not, one must assume that the child represents a spontaneous mutation. Genetic counseling is important.

ACQUIRED DEPIGMENTATION DUE TO ABSENCE OF MELANOCYTES

1. VITILIGO

Essentials of Diagnosis
- Paper-white macules and patches.
- Symmetric or segmental distribution.
- Typically affects skin over bony prominences.
- No melanocytes in affected skin.

General Considerations

Patients with vitiligo, born with normal skin and hair color, develop white spots later in life (Fig 22–15). The white spots on the skin are caused by destruction of epidermal pigment cells. The causes and mechanisms of pigment cell destruction are unknown. Genetic factors probably predispose the pigment cells of some individuals to destruction. Eight percent of individuals with vitiligo have one or more children with vitiligo. The prevalence of vitiligo in children of parents with vitiligo is about 5%, compared to 1% in the general population. Only occasionally do 2 children within one family have vitiligo. In an occasional kinship, vitiligo will affect several individuals in 3 or 4 successive generations. The pattern of inheritance suggests that vitiligo is a polygenic disorder or that genetic predisposition requires special conditions for expression. Patients can develop vitiligo at any age, though half acquire vitiligo before the age of 19 years and most are affected before the age of 50 years.

Vitiligo is a disorder classically characterized by cutaneous depigmentation. The destruction of pigment cells, however, is not limited to the skin but also affects melanocytes within the choroid and retinal pigment epithelium of the eye and possibly within the leptomeninges. A few patients develop neurosensory hearing loss (Vogt-Koyanagi-Harada syndrome and Alezzandrini's syndrome).

Three theories have been proposed to explain the mechanisms by which pigment cells are destroyed: the autocytotoxic, immunologic, and neural theories. No compelling data are available to indicate which one (if any) is correct. The autocytotoxic theory is based on the observations that certain hydroquinones (derivatives of phenol) are selectively toxic in vitro to pigment cells. The structures of some hydroquinones such as monobenzyl ether of hydroquinone are similar to dopaquinone or the indoles formed within a melanocyte during melanin synthesis. The autocytotoxic theory suggests that vitiligo may be a form of cellular suicide in which intermediary metabolites of melanin selectively destroy pigment cells.

The second hypothesis postulates an autoimmune mechanism. Vitiligo is associated with several autoimmune endocrinopathies. About 20% of patients have Hashimoto's thyroiditis, 5% have insulin-dependent diabetes mellitus, and a few individuals have pernicious anemia or idiopathic adrenal insufficiency. Two-thirds of patients have circulating autoantibodies to nucleoproteins, microsomes, parietal cells, or thyroglobulin. Vitiligo is commonly observed in patients with other disorders of the immune system, eg, Down's syndrome. About one-third of patients with familial endocrinopathies and mucocutaneous candidiasis have complement-fixing antibodies directed against the cytoplasm of epidermal pigment cells. This antibody probably is not cytotoxic; it can be found in the serum of patients with mucocutaneous candidiasis without vitiligo. Also, many patients with vitiligo have antibodies directed against melanocyte surface antigens. These melanocyte-associated antibodies are found in other disturbances of melanocytes, such as melanoma, but are not seen in nonpigmentary conditions. Patients who develop lymphoproliferative neoplastic disorders—especially mycosis fungoides, multiple myeloma, or Hodgkin's disease—may develop vitiligo.

The neural theory for the cause of vitiligo is based on the observation that in some patients vitiligo is confined to a portion of one side of the body. Segmental vitiligo may affect one side of the face, part of the trunk, or one extremity. It stops at the midline.

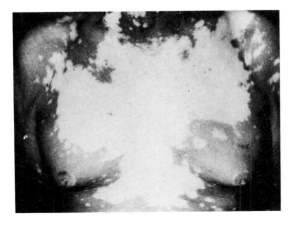

Figure 22–15. The chest of a patient with widespread vitiligo. The white areas are totally depigmented. The depigmentation is caused by destruction of pigment cells within the epidermis.

The distribution of depigmentation does not conform to known dermatomal patterns. However, because of the localized pattern of depigmentation, it is difficult not to implicate some neural or developmental influence.

Vitiligo may be associated with melanomas. Although patients with vitiligo do not have an increased probability for developing a melanoma, about 10% of patients with metastatic melanomas develop vitiligo.

Typically, patients have a high-risk primary melanoma, ie, usually more than 1.5 mm in thickness. Vitiligo in patients with melanoma suggests a high probability of metastatic disease, though it also portends a reasonable possibility that the individual will survive longer than expected. Whether the melanoma causes the vitiligo or the vitiligo delays the spread of the melanoma is not known.

Clinical Findings
A. Symptoms and Signs:
1. Skin– The hallmark of vitiligo is the development of hypopigmented and, later, completely depigmented spots. Depigmentation most often begins on the fingers (Fig 22–16), hands, and wrists but soon spreads to the face and feet. Depigmentation is progressive. The individual lesions progress from hypopigmentation to depigmentation. The spots progressively enlarge, and new lesions appear on the trunk and genitalia. The skin and mucous membranes are involved. In the mouths of black individuals, the mucous membranes, which are normally pigmented, show a loss of pigment. Patients with minimal cutaneous depigmentation often have extensive depigmentation of the oral mucosa. Many patients spontaneously regain some or most of their pigment.

2. Eyes– The pigment cells in the eyes are probably destroyed by the same pathophysiologic mechanisms active in the skin. Seven percent of patients with vitiligo have active but asymptomatic (subclinical) forms of uveitis (Fig 22–17). About 30–40% have asymptomatic but discrete areas of pigment loss visible upon funduscopic examination. Occasionally, these areas of retinal damage are located in the macula, with significant loss of visual acuity. Five percent of patients attending eye clinics for the treatment of idiopathic forms of iritis and uveitis have vitiligo, a prevalence significantly greater than the 1% in the general population. Patients with vitiligo, bilateral uveitis or iritis, poliosis, and hearing impairment are categorized as having Vogt-Koyanagi-Harada syndrome. Alezzandrini's syndrome seems to be a unilateral variant of Vogt-Koyanagi-Harada syndrome. Some patients with Vogt-Koyanagi-Harada syndrome have aseptic meningitis. The meningitis may be due to inflammatory destruction of the meningeal melanocytes by the vitiliginous process.

B. Laboratory Findings: A routinely processed biopsy specimen taken from an area of spreading vitiligo shows few abnormalities. A minimal lymphocytic infiltrate may be visible. Silver or dopa stains for melanin and tyrosinase document the lack of pigment and pigment cells in the white skin.

Under the electron microscope, pigment cells are absent. In the surrounding pigmented skin, the pigment cells exhibit fibrillar degeneration. The keratinocytes exhibit a vacuolar type of degeneration. Extracellular debris—probably microsomes from degenerated keratinocytes—is clumped between keratinocytes. The cell membranes of the keratinocytes and Langerhans cells are excessively ruffled.

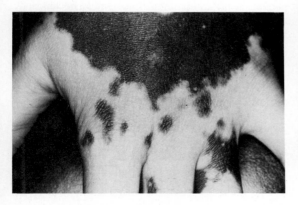

Figure 22–16. Hand of a patient with spreading vitiligo. The fingers (a common site for vitiligo to begin) are totally depigmented. At the leading edge, the skin is a lighter brown than the normally pigmented skin.

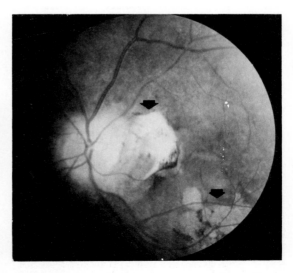

Figure 22–17. Chorioretinal scars affecting the eyes of a patient with vitiligo (Vogt-Koyanagi-Harada syndrome). The patient was legally blind. About one-third of patients with vitiligo have similar but smaller areas of retinal depigmentation usually located in the periphery of the retina. The peripheral lesions do not affect visual acuity.

Complications

The most obvious complication is the severe psychosocial impact. Relationships with spouses, friends, and relatives are affected. The white spots on the face and hands significantly impair the patient's ability to interact with others. Laymen are often suspicious that vitiligo may be contagious. Patients in occupations that require an attractive appearance, eg, receptionists and sales people, have been dismissed from their positions because of vitiligo. The white skin is susceptible to sunburn.

Occasional patients have active uveitis. Appropriate physical examination and laboratory workup for thyroid, adrenal, or pancreatic disease should be undertaken if the patient exhibits signs or symptoms of endocrine dysfunction. Routine laboratory studies for patients with vitiligo are probably not indicated.

Treatment

All patients with vitiligo should be instructed in the proper use of sunscreens. Sunscreens are recommended for 3 reasons: (1) areas of vitiligo are more susceptible to sunburn, (2) sunburn injury can extend the depigmentation (Koebner response), and (3) sun-induced darkening of the surrounding normal skin causes accentuation of the cosmetic disfigurement. They should apply a potent sunscreen (SPF > 15) daily to all affected areas that might be sun-exposed. They should reapply it frequently if actually in the sun or after swimming, bathing, or heavy exercise. The physician should be empathetic and provide emotional support. Some patients require referral for psychologic counseling.

Two medical treatments are available: repigmentation and depigmentation. Patients attempting to regain pigment may be treated with topically applied (methoxsalen) or orally administered psoralens (methoxsalen, trioxsalen). The physician should be thoroughly acquainted with the use of these potent compounds, and in general such patients should be referred to dermatologists. Use of topically applied psoralens will not even be discussed here because the treatments are complicated and the risk of phototoxic bullae is high.

Patients should be treated with psoralens every 2–3 days. Two hours after ingesting an appropriate dose of either drug, the patient is exposed to controlled doses of sunlight or ultraviolet A (320–400 nm) lamps. A standard UVB sunlamp cannot be used to treat patients with vitiligo. The optimal dose of psoralen must be tailored to the duration of light exposure.

Patients exposed to sunlight for short periods—30 minutes to 1 hour—will require about 0.25–0.3 mg/kg of trioxsalen or 0.4–0.5 mg/kg of methoxsalen. Patients exposed to 3 or 4 hours of sunlight will require less drug: 0.1–0.2 mg/kg of trioxsalen or 0.2–0.3 mg/kg of methoxsalen. Adult patients should begin therapy with 10 mg trioxsalen (20 mg

methoxsalen) and 15–30 minutes' exposure to light and gradually increase the amount of drug and the period of exposure. The amount of sun exposure must be modified by ambient intensity of sun. Intensity varies with latitude, time of day, humidity, smog and other factors.

The proper dose of psoralen and UVA (PUVA) produces modest pinking of the vitiliginous skin 24 hours after exposure to light. Ideally, PUVA should be administered every 2–3 days. Appropriate UVA opaque eyeglasses must be worn during treatment and for the rest of the day. Overexposure to UVA is associated with very painful toxic burns and bullae. Because the dosimetry of UVA from sunlight is difficult to gauge, treatment in special UVA phototherapy units is often preferred.

Depigmented areas of the skin devoid of hair, ie, the fingers and toes, or depigmented skin on which the terminal hairs are white cannot repigment. The hair bulb is the source of new pigment cells (Fig 22–18). Because pigment cells must divide repeatedly

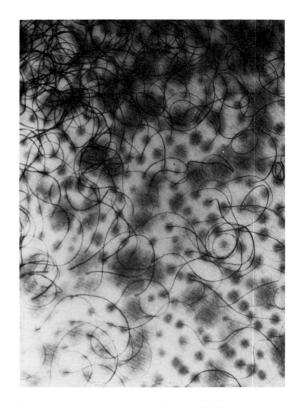

Figure 22–18. Patient with vitiligo exhibiting repigmentation. The pigment cells proliferate in the base of the hair bulb, then migrate and spread out into the surrounding depigmented skin. This manner of spread causes the freckled appearance of a patient successfully responding to PUVA therapy. Skin devoid of hair follicles or in which the terminal hairs are depigmented cannot repigment in response to PUVA therapy.

and migrate into the depigmented areas, successful repigmentation requires many months of treatment. Often 50–100 or more PUVA treatments are required.

About 50% of patients will exhibit partial or total repigmentation of vitiligo, especially on the knees and legs, from nightly applications of corticosteroid creams (triamcinolone acetonide 0.1%). The treatment requires 4 months or longer.

Patients with extensive depigmentation do not repigment with psoralens and UVA even after long periods of treatment. These patients may elect to remove their remaining pigment. Their skin becomes albinoid, but the cosmetic appearance is excellent. Depigmentation is produced by one or 2 daily applications of monobenzone (monobenzyl ether of hydroquinone; Benoquin 20% cream). Depigmentation of patients with extensive vitiligo is the only proper indication for the use of this medication, because the depigmentation produced by monobenzone is irreversible. The drug destroys epidermal pigment cells. Depigmentation for patients with vitiligo should not be prescribed without appropriate consideration by both the patient and the physician. Patients who are totally depigmented must protect their skin from sun exposure with hats, clothing, and sunscreens for the remainder of their lives.

Operative treatment is available when conventional medical therapies fail. The goal of surgical correction is to introduce a new reservoir of melanocytes into depigmented skin sites that do not have a source of pigment cells in the hair bulbs. The surgical candidate preferably has nonprogressive, localized vitiligo.

Punch minigrafting using autologous pigmented donor sites is the simplest, least invasive surgical approach. Several sessions can be scheduled for large areas, and 100 minigrafts or more can be done per session. Suction cup blisters are another source of autologous pigmented epidermis for grafting onto achromic recipient sites. Epidermal grafting does not produce scarring, but the overall procedure is more time-consuming and requires specialized equipment. Thin split-thickness grafts can be harvested with a dermatome from autologous noncosmetic areas and placed on denuded vitiligo sites. The potential for scarring is greater with this technique.

A newer investigational technique involves transplantation of in vitro cultured melanocytes or in vitro cultured epidermal sheets containing melanocytes onto denuded vitiligo skin. Small autologous donor specimens can be expanded in culture to provide pigment cells for larger depigmented areas.

2. POSTTRAUMATIC DEPIGMENTATION; COLD-INDUCED DEPIGMENTATION

Any physical, chemical, or infectious agent that destroys the epidermis will destroy the pigment cells located along the basal layer. Normally, skin repigments by proliferation and migration of pigment cells from hair bulbs, other appendages, and adjacent uninvolved skin. If the injury extends deep into the dermis and involves the hair bulbs and the other appendages, the normal reservoir of new pigment cells is destroyed, and that skin will probably remain permanently white. Thermal burns, radiation, deep lacerations, or deep abrasions may cause permanent depigmentation. Infections that leave deep scars, eg, herpes zoster or chickenpox, typically leave depigmented areas. Lupus erythematosus causes liquefaction degeneration of the basal layer of the epidermis and the hair bulb; many lesions of discoid lupus are permanently depigmented.

Pigment cells seem particularly susceptible to cold injury. Freezing of the epidermis by applications of liquid nitrogen with cotton-tipped swabs or cryotherapy units may cause temporary depigmentation. After a period of time, new pigment cells migrate into the area from the hair bulbs and adjacent skin. Minor lesions such as seborrheic keratoses or epidermal nevi in dark-skinned individuals should be treated with cryotherapy only with great caution. Deep freezing used for the destruction of basal cell epithelioma or squamous cell carcinoma may leave an area of permanent depigmentation because of the destruction of the pigment cells in the hair bulbs. This side effect should be considered when the physician chooses a method treatment for this type of skin cancer.

Numerous other inflammatory and infectious dermatoses that result in postinflammatory hypopigmentation as opposed to complete depigmentation are listed in Table 22–3.

3. CHEMICALLY INDUCED DEPIGMENTATION

Essentials of Diagnosis
- History of exposure to industrial cleaning solutions, germicidal agents, rubber products, depigmenting medications.
- Irregular white patches beginning on exposed surfaces.

General Considerations
A variety of chemicals—mostly derivatives of

Table 22–3. Postinflammatory hypopigmentation.

Psoriasis	Syphilis
Eczematous dermatitis	Lichen planus
Atopic dermatitis	Pityriasis rosea
Seborrheic dermatitis	Pityriasis lichen-
Diaper dermatitis	oides chronica
Tinea versicolor	Lichen striatus
Varicella	

phenols—can produce depigmentation of the skin mimicking vitiligo in most respects. Catechol is *o*-hydroxyphenol; hydroquinone is parahydroxyphenol. Each inhibits melanin formation. In contrast, phenols, catechols, and the hydroquinones that have a side chain at the para- position—monobenzyl ether of hydroquinone, *p*-tert-butylcatechol, and 4-hydroxyanisol—are cytotoxic to pigment cells. Several germicidal agents also contain parasubstituted phenols and may produce a vitiligolike depigmentation. Workers in the rubber and plastic industries are exposed to agents such as monobenzyl ether of hydroquinone and *p*-tert-butylcatechol and sometimes develop depigmentation of the hands that may also involve other parts of the body. Whether the depigmentation on nonexposed skin is due to inadvertent contamination of the area, circulation of the compound through the blood, or a self-perpetuating cytotoxic process is not known.

All patients who have a progressive vitiligolike depigmentation beginning on the hands and spreading to other parts of the body should be questioned about exposure to phenolic compounds, employment in the rubber and plastics industries, or the use of germicidal agents. Another common cause is inappropriate prescription of monobenzyl ether of hydroquinone (monobenzone; Benoquin) for treatment of cutaneous hyperpigmentation. All topical medications used by a patient with leukoderma should be checked for the presence of monobenzyl ether of hydroquinone.

Sulfhydryl compounds (mercaptoamines) are also known to cause depigmentation. They are probably cytotoxic to melanocytes.

Clinical Findings

Confettilike white macules or small irregularly shaped white patches are seen on exposed surfaces, typically the dorsal hands. The depigmentation usually begins 2–6 months after continual exposure. In time, depigmented patches can develop in remote areas. The distribution is often asymmetric. Examination with Wood's light reveals milk-white accentuation suggesting complete depigmentation. Some patients develop a bluish-gray discoloration indicating dermal melanosis. This is permanent and very disfiguring.

Differential Diagnosis

It may be difficult or even impossible to clinically and histologically differentiate chemical leukoderma from vitiligo. A high index of suspicion is necessary to make the historical correlation with known depigmenting agents that can exist in diverse sources.

Treatment

If a chemical origin for the depigmentation has been identified, the patient should be protected from further exposure. Repigmentation of hair-bearing skin can be achieved with PUVA, as with vitiligo.

CONGENITAL HYPOPIGMENTATION DUE TO ABNORMAL FORMATION OF MELANOSOMES

1. TUBEROUS SCLEROSIS

Essentials of Diagnosis

- Ash-leaf hypopigmented macules.
- Epilepsy.
- Mental retardation.
- Multiple hamartomas.

General Considerations

Tuberous sclerosis belongs to the group of disorders called phakomatoses, ie, diseases characterized by the presence of multiple disseminated hamartomas involving eyes, skin, and brain. Hamartomas are anomalous benign proliferations of tissue. These tumors arise from several cell types. The multiple cellular origin distinguishes a hamartoma from cancer and benign adenoma, both of which are derived from a single type of cell.

The incidence of tuberous sclerosis is 1:100,000–1:30,000 live births and accounts for 0.1% of patients hospitalized for mental retardation. The disorder is transmitted by an autosomal dominant gene. About 25% of patients have an affected parent. For the other 75% of affected individuals, the defect arises by spontaneous mutation. Patients with tuberous sclerosis form astrocytomas in the brain, glial tumors in the retina, and fibromas in the mucous membranes and along the fingernails and toenails. Classically, angiofibromas begin to form on the skin around the nose and across the cheeks between the ages of 2 and 8 years. A Shagreen patch—a yellowish, bumpy patch caused by proliferation of capillaries, fibroblasts, and deposition of collagen—appears usually on the back and is highly suggestive of tuberous sclerosis.

Clinical Findings

A. Symptoms and Signs: One of the earliest signs is the presence of hypopigmented macules, found in 65–85% of individuals with tuberous sclerosis. They are visible at birth or soon after. The hypopigmented macules can have one of many shapes. The classic shape is the ash-leaf or lanceolate macule. It is round at one end and tapered at the other. The more common shape is polygonal or thumbprint. Less common shapes are confettilike or dermatomal. They are most easily observed by examining the skin with Wood's lamp, which makes the macules more visible but does not cause stark white accentuation as in vitiligo.

Other cutaneous manifestations of tuberous sclerosis are café-au-lait spots, poliosis, gingival and ungual fibromas, and fibrous plaques on the forehead. Periventricular brain calcifications (with or without history of seizures) associated with cutaneous white macules is pathognomonic of tuberous sclerosis.

B. Laboratory Findings: Routine histologic methods reveal no abnormalities in the hypopigmented macules. However, electron microscopic examination shows that the number of melanosomes in the hypopigmented macules is fewer and their size smaller than those of melanosomes in the surrounding, normally pigmented skin.

Differential Diagnosis

Other congenital localized leukodermas such as nevus depigmentosus and nevus anemicus must be considered in the differential diagnosis. Vitiligo is not difficult to differentiate because of its onset in childhood or later, its tendency to progress, and its characteristic distribution. Chemical or postinflammatory hypopigmentation is differentiated by their history.

Treatment

No treatment for the pigmentary abnormalities is needed. A child with ash-leaf spots should be carefully followed by his family physician or pediatrician in order to detect the development of fibromatous tumors in the skin, mucous membranes, brain, kidneys, or other organs. The patient and the parents should be counseled that the disorder is transmitted in an autosomal dominant fashion.

HYPOMELANOSIS OF ITO (Incontinentia Pigmenti Achromicans)

Essentials of Diagnosis
- Present at birth.
- Bizarre hypopigmented macules in linear whorls and streaks.

General Considerations

Hypomelanosis of Ito is also referred to as incontinentia pigmenti achromicans because the pattern of hypopigmentation appears as a negative image of the hyperpigmentation seen in the third stage of incontinentia pigmenti. Incontinentia pigmenti remains a separate and distinct disorder, however, with a different pattern of inheritance and clinical manifestations.

Hypomelanosis of Ito has an autosomal dominant mode of transmission, is invariably present at birth, and has a male:female ratio of 2.5:1. The cutaneous leukoderma is commonly associated with disorders of the central nervous system, eyes, hair, nails, teeth, musculoskeletal system, or internal organs. A defect of neural crest-derived tissues might explain these associations.

Extracutaneous manifestations occur in up to 75% of patients. The most severe associations are mental retardation and seizures (40%). The eyes may exhibit nystagmus. The retina may have a tessellated appearance. Ptosis and strabismus caused by muscular weakness have been observed in a few patients; others exhibit generalized hypotonia of all skeletal muscles. The breasts may be hypoplastic and asymmetric. Some patients have dysplastic teeth, thickened lips, saddle nose, and a high-arched palate.

Clinical Findings

A. Symptoms and Signs: On the skin of the trunk and extremities are bizarre patterns of hypopigmented macules. There are linear, mottled, or whorled streaks and splashes. The patterns of pigmentary changes observed in hypomelanosis of Ito follow the lines of Blaschko (developmental zones of skin surface areas). The number of hypopigmented streaks may be few or multiple. The pigmentary changes are present at birth and are often the first sign that the infant is not normal. The hypopigmented areas tend to be hypohidrotic, and the sweat glands respond subnormally to injections of pilocarpine. Hair on the scalp may be thin.

B. Laboratory Findings: The hypopigmented skin has either a normal or fewer number of melanocytes. Electron microscopy reveals that the number of melanosomes in keratinocytes is markedly decreased.

Differential Diagnosis

Incontinentia pigmenti (can have hypo- and hyperpigmentation in whorls and streaks), dermatomal tuberous sclerosis, nevus depigmentosus (especially the systematized variant), and segmental vitiligo must be considered in the differential diagnosis.

Treatment

As with the other congenital hypopigmentation disorders, there is no definitive treatment for the cutaneous manifestations. A combination of methoxsalen applied topically to hypopigmented areas and exposure to ultraviolet A radiation may lessen the degree of hypopigmentation and minimize the cosmetic disfigurement, but such treatments should be given only by dermatologists. Patients with hypomelanosis of Ito may have multiple incapacitating anomalies often requiring institutional care. For these patients, the complex treatments are not desirable.

3. NEVUS DEPIGMENTOSUS

Essentials of Diagnosis
- Present at birth or acquired in adult life.
- Localized irregular patch of cutaneous leukoderma.

General Considerations

Nevus depigmentosus is an uncommon, localized cutaneous leukoderma that can be present at birth or acquired during adult life. The defect is developmental, not inherited. It is not hamartomatous, as the name implies, but patterned and thus is misnamed. Generally, nevus depigmentosus occurs without any associated abnormality, but it has been rarely reported with mental retardation, seizures, or unilateral limb hypertrophy. It might more properly by called a variant of hypomelanosis of Ito when associated with these latter defects.

Clinical Findings

A. Symptoms and Signs: Cutaneous pale-white macules and patches with irregular borders occur on the trunk or proximal extremities. These are often better observed with illumination from Wood's light in a darkened room. The most common clinical pattern is an isolated unilateral circular or polygonal patch that is stable in size. The macule enlarges in proportion to the growing child. Dermatomal or systematized unilateral whorled patterns have been observed.

B. Laboratory Findings: The light microscopic examination is normal, with the normal number of melanocytes. Electron microscopy reveals melanosomes that are smaller in size, shape, and number or are abnormally aggregated within phagolysosomes in poorly developed melanocyte dendrites. Keratinocytes have markedly reduced melanosomes.

Differential Diagnosis

Segmental vitiligo (acquired, amelanotic), tuberous sclerosis, nevus anemicus (disappears with Wood's lamp illumination), and hypomelanosis of Ito must be considered in the differential diagnosis.

Treatment

There is no effective method of repigmentation for the leukoderma. Concealment with cosmetics (Covermark, Dermablend) is available if desired.

4. CHÉDIAK-HIGASHI SYNDROME

Essentials of Diagnosis

- White or fair skin and hair (albinoid appearance).
- Defect of membrane bound organelles.
- Recurrent bacterial infections.

General Considerations

Chédiak-Higashi syndrome, a disorder of membrane-bound cytoplasmic organelles—ie, lysosomes and melanosomes—has been observed in many mammalian species, including felines, Aleutian minks, beige mice, and even killer whales. The defect affects many cytoplasmic organelles in many cell types. It is transmitted as an autosomal recessive trait.

Patients have an increased susceptibility to infections. Neutrophils, after phagocytosing bacteria, normally release the bactericidal contents of lysosomes into the phagocytic vacuoles. Neutrophils from patients with Chédiak-Higashi syndrome do not release sufficient bactericidal products to kill bacteria. Thus, patients with this syndrome suffer from recurrent and often fatal bacterial infections.

Melanosomes are membrane-bound organelles. Pigment cells in patients (or animals) with Chédiak-Higashi syndrome produce deformed and abnormally large melanosomes that are apparently readily transferred into the keratinocyte of skin and hair.

Clinical Findings

A few patients with Chédiak-Higashi syndrome have an albinoid appearance, ie, their skin and hair are white and resemble those of an albino. Some patients have nystagmus. Most patients with Chédiak-Higashi syndrome have blond or gray hair, blue eyes, and fair skin.

Complications

The most serious complication is recurrent infection. Some patients have inadequate quantities of melanin in the choroid and the retinal pigment epithelium of the eyes and suffer from photophobia and decreased visual acuity.

Treatment

There is no therapy for this pigment defect. The use of vitamin C, 500 mg 3 times daily, to aid neutrophil function is controversial. Parents and patients with Chédiak-Higashi syndrome should be counseled regarding the transmission of this disease. Patients should be protected against infection and should be instructed in the use of sunscreens and sunglasses.

CONGENITAL HYPOPIGMENTATION DUE TO DECREASED SYNTHESIS OF MELANIN: OCULOCUTANEOUS ALBINISM

Essentials of Diagnosis

- Abnormally white skin.
- Light-colored hair.
- Nystagmus.
- Poor visual acuity.
- Lack of normal amounts of melanin in melanosomes.

General Considerations

Albinism comprises a heterogeneous group of congenital, universal, hypomelanotic disorders. Oculocutaneous albinism is characterized by disturbed melanogenesis of the skin, hair, and eyes, whereas ocular albinism is associated with primarily eye manifestations. There are at least 10 different phenotypes of oculocutaneous albinism: (1) tyrosinase-positive, (2) yellow mutant, (3) tyrosinase-negative, (4) minimal pigment, (5) brown, (6) rufous, (7) Hermansky-Pudlak syndrome, (8) autosomal dominant, (9) platinum, and (10) Cross syndrome.

Albinos have normal numbers of cutaneous and ocular pigment cells that form melanosomes in abundance. However, melanin synthesis is defective, and the melanosomes are incompletely melanized. The melanocytes in some albinos lack active tyrosinase. In others, the enzyme functions at a low rate. Patients with tyrosinase-positive albinism have an active tyrosinase enzyme, but other factors may severely limit the rate of formation of melanin.

The presence of melanin in the retinal pigment epithelium during embryogenesis seems critical for proper development of the optic tracts between the neuroretina and the occipital lobes. Normally, the optic tracts from the neuroretina pass through the optic chiasm and divide into 2 bundles. Half the fibers go to each of the 2 areas of visual cortex in the ipsilateral and contralateral brain. In the absence of melanin during embryogenesis, excessive numbers of the optic tracts cross to the contralateral occipital cortex. In addition, the fovea forms poorly. These anatomic abnormalities may cause the poor visual acuity and the nystagmus that afflict all albinos.

The overall incidence of oculocutaneous albinism is 1:20,000. All but one type are genetically transmissible as an autosomal recessive gene. Some are caused by genes at different loci on different chromosomes; ie, the offspring of parents with 2 different forms of albinism may be normal.

There are 4 common types of albinism in the USA: tyrosinase-positive, tyrosinase-negative, yellow mutant, and the Hermansky-Pudlak varieties. The clinical features of each of these will be discussed separately

Clinical Findings
A. Symptoms and Signs:
1. Tyrosinase-negative– The tyrosinase-negative variety of albinism is the most severe variant and affects about one in every 33,000 individuals. The skin, eyes, and hair of these patients are almost completely devoid of melanin. The hair is white at birth and remains so throughout life. The skin is pink-white. Nevi form on the skin but are amelanotic. The irides of these children are grayish in a dimly illuminated room; in bright light, they are pinkish. On funduscopic examination, no pigment is visible in the iris, the retinal pigment epithelium, or the choroid, and the choroidal capillaries are easily observed. The patients suffer from severe photophobia, nystagmus, and poor visual acuity. Most are legally blind. Dark glasses help minimize the photophobia but do not improve vision. Patients with albinism are very susceptible to sunburn. A small percentage are severely retarded.

2. Tyrosinase-positive– The genes that cause the tyrosinase-positive and tyrosinase-negative forms of albinism occupy different loci. Children born of one tyrosinase-positive and one tyrosinase-negative parent will have normal skin color; however, they will be carriers for both types of albinism. The biochemical abnormality that causes tyrosinase-positive albinism has not been identified. Pigment cells do contain active tyrosinase enzyme. The deficiency of pigment can be explained in several ways. The quantity or activity of the enzyme may be very low. It is equally possible, however, that factors which regulate melanin synthesis are defective and may retard the normal rate of pigment synthesis.

Tyrosinase-positive albinism affects about one in 37,000 infants. At birth and during early childhood, these children phenotypically may be indistinguishable from individuals with the tyrosinase-negative disorder. They lack pigment in the skin, retinal pigment epithelium, and choroid and have white hair and severe photophobia. As these children grow older, their hair becomes yellow-blond or reddish. Their irides become blue. Nevi become lightly pigmented, and numerous freckles form in the sun-exposed areas of the skin. Photophobia ameliorates. The nystagmus, which may be most prominent during childhood, persists throughout life but decreases in severity as visual acuity improves.

3. Yellow mutant– The yellow mutant type of albinism is rare and affects only one in 100,000 individuals. The gene for this variant may occupy the same chromosomal locus as the gene for the tyrosinase-positive form of albinism. The hair of these children is white at birth but acquires a yellow-red hue during early childhood. The nevi acquire pigment, and freckles appear on the sun-exposed skin. The children may have poor visual acuity, severe photophobia, and nystagmus. However, these ocular problems ameliorate as the child grows older. The irides of adults with the yellow mutant are blue.

4. Hermansky-Pudlak syndrome– Hermansky-Pudlak syndrome is a tyrosinase-positive form of albinism associated with a hemorrhagic diathesis caused by a platelet defect. About one in 2000 Puerto Ricans has this syndrome. In Lencois Island, Brazil, as many as one in every 30 individuals may be affected. Consanguineous marriages are frequent within communities where such high rates of Hermansky-Pudlak syndrome are found. Some affected individuals have severe mental retardation.

Affected infants have white or pale yellow hair. The hair may remain yellow or acquire a red-brown color. The skin of children and adults may have many freckles and deeply pigmented nevi. Nystagmus, photophobia, and poor visual acuity all are severe during infancy but ameliorate with age.

Patients with Hermansky-Pudlak syndrome bleed and bruise easily. Epistaxis, postpartum and postsurgical bleeding, and heavy menses are common problems. Platelet counts are normal. Clotting time, prothrombin time, partial thromboplastin time, and the plasma content of clotting factors (fibrinogen, prothrombin, factors V and VII–XIII) are normal. The platelets of patients with Hermansky-Pudlak syndrome contain abnormally low quantities of ADP and serotonin; thus, they cannot undergo secondary aggregation. The impaired release of ADP and serotonin seems responsible for the bleeding diathesis.

Patients with Hermansky-Pudlak syndrome also have a disorder of lipid storage. Clumps of fatty acids, cholesterol, cholesteryl esters, and ceroid are present in macrophages of the bone marrow; in the circulating white blood cells; in cells within the urinary sediment, the oral epithelium, and the intestinal mucosa; and possibly in the epidermal Langerhans cells.

The accumulation of ceroid may cause complications. Patients develop pulmonary fibrosis and pulmonary insufficiency. They have restrictive lung disease, reduced lung volume, and poor oxygen diffusion. Histologic examination of the lung shows peribronchial fibrosis and macrophages filled with ceroid.

B. Laboratory Findings:

1. Tyrosinase-negative– By light microscopy, the skin looks normal. Melanin cannot be detected by histochemical stains. Pigment cells do not stain when the skin is incubated in solutions of levodopa, a histochemical technique for the detection of the tyrosinase enzyme—ie, the cells are tyrosinase-negative, and hair bulbs are also tyrosinase-negative. As seen by electron microscopy, pigment cells contain stage I premelanosomes and stage II melanosomes but few if any melanosomes that contain melanin (stage III and stage IV).

2. Tyrosinase-positive– The skin, nevi, and hair contain small amounts of melanin visible by histochemical stains (Fontana-Masson melanin stain). The pigment cells in the skin and hair have active tyrosinase enzyme (tyrosinase-positive). By electron microscopy, melanosomes with small amounts of melanin (stage III) are typically found in pigment cells and in keratinocytes.

3. Yellow mutant– A biopsy of skin stained by the Fontana-Masson technique resembles that from patients with the tyrosinase-positive variety of albinism. Small amounts of melanin are present in the skin, but cells are tyrosinase-negative. However, if cysteine is added to the solution of levodopa, the pigment cells in the skin and hair stain a yellow-red color. This biochemical characteristic suggests that the cells are capable of forming only phaeomelanin. This unique feature is confirmed by electron microscopy, which demonstrates the presence of many stage III phaeomelanosomes in the skin and hair.

4. Hermansky-Pudlak syndrome– The hair bulbs are tyrosinase-positive. As seen by electron microscopy, stage III melanosomes are predominant. Many melanosomes are larger than normal, ie, macromelanosomes.

Differential Diagnosis

Oculocutaneous albinism, common throughout the animal kingdom, must be distinguished from other disorders that may have an albinoid appearance, ie, the Chédiak-Higashi syndrome, piebaldism, or total vitiligo. Patients with Chédiak-Higashi syndrome have an abnormality of melanosomes; those with piebaldism or total vitiligo lack pigment cells in their skin.

Oculocutaneous albinism must also be distinguished from known inborn errors of metabolism that result in pigmentary dilution of the skin, eyes, and hair. Phenylketonuria is the most common of these disorders, with a frequency of 1:20,000 births. Phenylalanine hydroxylase, which is absent, normally converts phenylalanine to tyrosine. Tyrosine is a melanin precursor; therefore, a decrease in tyrosine will result in less substrate for melanin production. Also, there is inhibition by accumulated phenylalanine and its metabolites. Phenylketonuria is diagnosed by elevated urinary and serum phenylalanine. Patients with phenylketonuria also have mental and growth retardation, skeletal and cardiac defects, and sclerodermoid and eczematous dermatitis.

Other congenital universal hypomelanoses to be differentiated because of pale skin, light blue eyes, and fair hair are histidinemia (deficient histidase activity), homocystinuria (deficient cystathionine synthetase activity), and Menkes' kinky hair syndrome (deficient copper levels).

Complications

Patients with albinism suffer most from sensitivity to sunlight. Their skin burns very easily. Actinic keratoses, basal cell epitheliomas, and squamous cell carcinomas are common. Occasionally, albinos will develop melanomas. Albinos have difficulties with photophobia and poor visual acuity. Most are legally blind; a few are mentally retarded.

Treatment

Albinism is a genetic disorder transmitted in an autosomal recessive mode. Genetic counseling is important for patients and for the parents of albino infants. Avoidance of sun exposure may prevent formation of skin cancers.

ACQUIRED HYPOPIGMENTATION DUE TO DECREASED SYNTHESIS OF MELANIN: TINEA VERSICOLOR

Tinea versicolor is so named because it can manifest with various colors, though the most common presentation is hypopigmented macules on the chest and back. It is a superficial infection of the stratum corneum caused by the lipophilic yeast *Pityrosporum orbiculare*. A fungal enzyme converts unsaturated fatty acids in the skin to azelaic acid, a dicarboxylic acid that inhibits tyrosinase activity. It has been suggested that penetration of the epidermis by the acid is responsible for the hypopigmentation. The hypopigmentation often persists for many months after the infection is eradicated.

Further details about the diagnosis and treatment of tinea versicolor are reviewed in Chapter 16.

ACQUIRED HYPOPIGMENTATION DUE TO DECREASED TRANSFER OF MELANOSOMES: PITYRIASIS ALBA

Essentials of Diagnosis

- Hypopigmented macules on the face.
- Very fine scale.
- Associated dermatitis.

General Considerations

Pityriasis alba is mild dermatitis in which there appears to be a block in the transfer of the melanosomes from the pigment cell to the keratinocyte. The cause of this disruption of melanin synthesis and melanosomal transfer is not known.

Pityriasis alba begins in childhood or adolescence. It occurs in all races but is more evident in darker-skinned people. There is often an associated dermatitis, especially atopic dermatitis. Spontaneous resolution usually occurs by adulthood.

Clinical Findings

A. Symptoms and Signs: The patient complains of hypopigmented macules on the cheeks, the backs of the upper portions of the arms, over the triceps, and on the thighs. The skin has poorly defined hypopigmented macules, often with a slight scale.

B. Laboratory Findings: The epidermis, by light microscopy, shows a mild spongiosis and exocytosis. The number of pigment cells and melanosomes in the keratinocytes is less than that in unaffected skin.

Treatment

Pityriasis alba is accompanied by a mild inflammation of the epidermis. Therapy is directed at suppressing the inflammatory process. High-potency fluorinated steroids may suppress pigment formation, so their use in the treatment of pityriasis alba is ineffective. Application of weak, nonfluorinated steroids such as hydrocortisone 1% or 2.5%, twice daily for 3–4 weeks, often is more successful.

ACQUIRED HYPOPIGMENTATION DUE TO MISCELLANEOUS CAUSES

1. POSTINFLAMMATORY HYPOPIGMENTATION

There are numerous infectious and inflammatory cutaneous disorders that resolve with hypopigmented macules and patches in the distribution and pattern of the original dermatosis. The more common disorders causing postinflammatory hypopigmentation are listed in Table 22–3. Several mechanisms may explain the hypopigmentation. Edema and spongiosis (secondary to inflammatory mediators) may physically block the transfer of melanosomes to keratinocytes. In hyperproliferative disorders, the transition rate of keratinocytes through the epidermis is increased out of proportion to the rate of melanin synthesis. In disorders characterized by hydropic degeneration of the basal cell layer, there is destruction of melanocytes.

Several other cutaneous and systemic disorders occasionally present with localized hypopigmentation. In all of these cases, hypopigmentation is not the primary disorder but an occasional manifestation of the underlying disease process. In a few of the disorders, hypopigmentation may be partially postinflammatory; in others, it may precede the development of atrophy. These disorders are listed in Table 22–4.

2. DRUG-INDUCED HYPOPIGMENTATION

Drugs can cause hypopigmentation or depigmentation of the skin. Chloroquine may cause hypopigmentation of the skin and bleaching of the hair.

Cosmetics and skin bleaches often available without prescription may contain hydroquinone. Hydroquinone blocks tyrosinase function and may cause mild hypopigmentation. Cosmetic agents available outside the USA often contain parasubstituted phenols. These are melanocytotoxins and cause a permanent depigmentation that resembles vitiligo (see above).

3. LEUKONYCHIA

Leukonychia may involve the entire nail, a portion of the nail, or a horizontal or longitudinal band. The

Table 22–4. Cutaneous or systemic disorders occasionally presenting with hypopigmentation.

Granulomatous	Atrophic/Fibrotic
Sarcoidosis	Scleroderma
Infectious	Morphea
Tuberculoid leprosy	Lichen sclerosus et atrophicus
Indeterminant leprosy	Balanitis xerotica obliterans
Syphilis	Dego's disease
Pinta	**Inflammatory**
Yaws	Pityriasis lichenoides chronica
Onchocerciasis	Alopecia Mucinosa
Miscellaneous	Cutaneous lupus
Arsenic ingestion	erythematosus
Hypothyroid	**Neoplastic**
	Cutaneous T cell lymphoma

causes are protean. Some patients have an inherited variety. Arsenic and antimetabolites used for the treatment of leukemia may cause white banding of the nails. Patients with liver disease have total leuk-

onychia. Azotemia is associated with the half-and-half nail, ie, leukonychia of the proximal half of the nail.

No therapy is available for these conditions.

REFERENCES

Bolognia JL, Pawelek JM: Biology of hypopigmentation. J Am Acad Dermatol 1988;19:217.

Falabella R et al: On the pathogenesis of idiopathic guttate hypomelanosis. J Am Acad Dermatol 1987;16:55.

Falabella R: Grafting and transplantation of melanocytes for repigmenting vitiligo and other types of leukoderma. Int J Dermatol 1989;28:363.

Ferguson J, Frain-Bell W: Pigmentary disorders and systemic drug therapy. Clin Dermatol 1989;7:44.

Fitzpatrick TB et al (editors): *Biology and Diseases of Dermal Pigmentation*. University of Tokyo Press, 1981.

Fulk CS: Primary disorders of hyperpigmentation. J Am Acad Dermatol 1984;10:1.

Granstein RD, Sober AJ: Drug and heavy metal-induced hyperpigmentation. J Am Acad Dermatol 1981;5:1.

Kaplan P, de Chanderévian J-P: Piebaldism-Waardenburg syndrome: Histologic evidence for a neural crest syndrome. Am J Med Genet 1988;31:679.

Klein LE, Nordlund JJ: Genetic basis of pigmentation and its disorders. Int Soc Trop Dermatol 1981;20:621.

Körner A, Pawelek J: Mammalian tyrosinase catalyzes three reactions in the biosynthesis of melanin. Science 1982;217:1163.

Lee EB: Metabolic diseases and skin. Pediatr Clin North Am 1983;30:597.

Logan A et al: Melanotropin-potentiating factor (MPF) potentiates MSH-induced melanogenesis in hair follicle melanocytes. Peptides 1981;2:121.

Lucky PA and Nordlund JJ: The biology of the pigmentary system and its disorders. Dermatol Clin 1985;3:197.

Montagna W, Hu F, Carlisle K: A reinvestigation of solar lentigines. Arch Dermatol 1980;116:1151.

Mosher DB et al: Disorders of pigmentation. In: *Dermatology in General Medicine*. Fitzpatrick TB et al (editors). McGraw-Hill, 1987.

Nordlund JJ (editor): *Pigmentation Disorders*. Vol 6 of: *Dermatologic Clinics*. Saunders, 1988.

Nordlund JJ: *Genetic Basis of Pigmentation*. University of Tokyo Press, 1981.

Pawelek JM, Körner AM: The biosynthesis of mammalian melanin. American Scientist 1982;70:136.

Reuter DJ et al: Hypomelanotic macules in tuberous sclerosis. Arch Dermatol Res 1981;271:171.

Riccardi VM: Cutaneous manifestations of neurofibromatosis: Cellular interaction, pigmentation, and mast cells. Birth Defects 1981;17:129.

Sanchez J, Vasquez M, Sanchez N: Vitiligolike macules in systemic scleroderma. Arch Dermatol 1983;119:129.

Sanchez NP et al: Melasma: A clinical, light microscopic, ultrastructural, and immunofluorescence study. J Am Acad Dermatol 1981;4:698.

Susong CR, Nordlund JJ: Vitiligo: Guidelines for successful therapy. Drug Ther Bull 1985;15:133.

Takematsu H et al: Incontinentia pigmenti achromicans (Ito). Arch Dermatol 1983;119:391.

Valenzuela R, Noringstar WA: The ocular pigmentary disturbance of Chédiak-Higashi syndrome: A comparative light and electron microscopic study and review of the literature. Am J Clin Pathol 1981;75:591.

Witkop C: Albinism. Clin Dermatol 1989;7:80.

Zaias N: *The Nail in Health and Disease*. Spectrum, 1980.

Zaynoan ST et al: Extensive pityriasis alba: A histological, histochemical and ultrastructural study. Br J Dermatol 1983;108:83.

23

Circulatory Disorders

Edward E. Krull, MD & Joseph Beninson, MD

Diseases of the peripheral vasculature include diseases of the arteries, veins, and lymphatics of the 4 extremities and the skin (Table 23–1). Some benign and malignant tumors may involve blood vessels or lymphatics; these are described in Chapter 43. Other diseases with a significant vascular component, such as collagen diseases, are described in Chapter 50. Diseases associated with vasculitis and necrosis of blood vessel walls are discussed in Chapter 37. There remain, then, the more classic diseases of the peripheral arteries, veins, and lymphatics; the vasculitides, purpuras, telangiectases or diseases with significant telangiectasia; and a collection of miscellaneous and heterogeneous diseases in which the vasculature plays a prominent etiologic role. Many disorders that affect even deep, large arteries and veins cause changes in the skin.

EMBRYOLOGY & ANATOMY OF THE CIRCULATORY SYSTEM

The circulatory system, with all of its complex arborizations and varied functional activities, is essential for survival of multicellular organisms. In humans, the vascular system begins on the yolk sac as compact clusters of mesenchymal cells that develop into capillary plexuses. These spread out from primary vascular centers and unite to form the closed circuit of the circulation.

The arteries terminate in their arteriolar beds, which comprise 75% of the entire arterial tree. Arterial flow can circumvent the blood capillary bed by flowing through arteriovenous shunts that may be physiologic or pathologic. When the veins of the lower extremities are dilated by peripheral venous insufficiency or for other reasons, residual pressure from the arteriolar bed is of no help in lifting the venous load against gravity in the standing position. Under these circumstances, an arteriolar-venous reflex causes the arteriolar bed to contract. When the veins later empty, there is a compensatory maximal arterial dilation.

Muscular action of the extremities is the main

Table 23–1. Peripheral vascular disease.

Arterial
 Organic
  Occlusive
   Arteriosclerosis
   Buerger's disease (thromboangiitis obliterans)
   Arteritides
   Collagen diseases
   Thrombosis
   Embolism
   Cold injuries
   Ainhum
  Nonocclusive
   Aneurysm
   Arteriovenous fistulas
 Functional
  Vasoconstrictive
   Raynaud's phenomenon-disease
   Acrocyanosis
   Methysergide ingestion
   Ergotism
   Shoulder girdle syndrome
   Posttraumatic syndrome
  Vasodilatory
   Erythromelalgia (erythermalgia)
Venous
 Organic
  Occlusive
   Thrombophlebitis
   Thrombophlebitis migrans
   Phlebothrombosis
   Postthrombophlebitic syndrome
   Vasculitis
  Nonocclusive
   Phlebosclerosis
   Phlebofibrosis
   Phlebectasia
 Functional
   Phlebospasm
Lymphatic
 Lymphedema
  Primary
   Lymphatic dysplasia
    Milroy's disease
    Letessier's disease
  Secondary
   Lymphangitis
   Lymphadenitis
   Malignancy
    Direct pressure
    Invasion
   Nonmalignant masses
    Direct pressure

pumping force for venous return to the heart. Pressure gradient stockings and leotards improve the efficiency of this action, especially in venous insufficiency. Venous valves partition the gravitational pressure in the distal extremities by dividing the veins into smaller individual segments, each absorbing a proportionate part of the total pressure. If the valves are incompetent, venous pressure at the ankle is the total weight of the column of blood from the heart to the ankle.

The lymphatic system is a closed efferent one that exists only in the higher vertebrates and serves to return essentially all of the circulating plasma proteins that enter the extravascular space from the postarteriolar capillary bed. From 50% to 100% of this protein mass leaves and returns every 24 hours in healthy human adults. Of the 20 L of plasma water that accompany this protein mass to the extravascular space, about 16–17 L are resorbed by the venous capillaries; the other 2–4 L accompany the protein into the lymphatic channels. Because of the absence of valves of the superficial lymphatic arcade and because the lymphatics traverse the midline, cancerous tissue, particulate matter, and fluids can spread to any area, as can infection. For example, streptococcal infections spread through the superficial lymphatic arcade to cause erysipelas. Red streaks are seen clinically when the infection empties into the deep lymphatic collecting vessels.

Lymphatics, unlike veins, do not have communicating channels between the superficial and deep vessels; they meet at the regional lymph nodes. The regional lymph nodes have more afferent than efferent lymphatic channels.

ARTERIAL DISEASES

Intermittent claudication, pain with elevation partially or totally relieved by dependence, and paroxysmal neuropathic pain—especially at night—are important symptoms of significant arterial disease. Associated signs may include thin, shiny, pale skin; coolness of the skin; dependent rubor and pallor with elevation; absence of hair on the toes; dystrophy of nails (especially ridging); atrophy of muscle tissues; and dry, nongranulating painful ulcers. Peripheral pulses must be carefully assessed and may be diminished or absent.

Various noninvasive and invasive studies may help in the diagnosis and treatment of arterial and other peripheral vascular diseases. These include venography, arteriography, ultrasound, Doppler flow measurements, and plethysmography.

The organic arterial diseases are more common than the functional ones (Table 23–1). Functional diseases are characterized by alterations of circulation caused by a transient and reversible changes in the diameter of the vessel. Organic diseases are associated with structural changes in vessels that affect circulation. An overlapping or combined process may be present. For example, in Raynaud's phenomenon—considered functional—organic, structural changes can frequently be demonstrated in the vessels. Thus, classification of vascular disease is imperfect and oversimplified.

ARTERIOSCLEROSIS

The term "arteriosclerosis" denotes hardening and induration of the arteries and includes atherosclerosis, Mönckeberg's calcification, and arteriolosclerosis. The term "arteriosclerosis" and "atherosclerosis" are sometimes used interchangeably, but the latter term more specifically, denotes the patchy, irregular lipid deposits that form plaquelike intimal elevations within the larger vessels. Occlusion and emboli may result. Surgical procedures are far more successful in treating this disease than disease of the smaller vessels (arteriolosclerosis). Mönckeberg's medial calcification does not produce signs or symptoms of occlusive disease. Arteriosclerosis obliterans is a chronic atherosclerotic occlusive disease of the aorta and its main branches to the extremities.

Arteriosclerosis occurs primarily in men 40 years of age or older. It is more common in diabetics. The arteries of the distal legs and feet are most frequently affected.

Clinical Findings
The decreased blood flow produces cool, pale lower extremities and, in advanced stages, atrophy of musculature, loss of normal hair distribution, and nail abnormalities. In still later stages, reddish-blue cyanosis and ischemic pain are present. Pain is increased when the leg is elevated, so many patients sleep sitting up with the legs dangling down to relieve pain. Over bony prominences, stubborn acral ulcerations resist healing until new arterioles invade the area. Gangrene results from severe or complete occlusion.

Treatment
Patients should stop smoking and protect the skin from injury and cold. If circulation is significantly impaired, surgical bypass of the occlusion, balloon dilatation, laser surgery, or transposition of a vein from the axillary-subclavian area may help bring blood into the ischemic limb. Vasodilators are not especially beneficial. Pentoxifylline may be helpful by reducing blood viscosity.

THROMBOANGIITIS OBLITERANS
(Buerger's Disease)

Thromboangiitis obliterans is characterized by thromboses of the medium and small arteries of the extremities. It is frequently a panarteritis affecting adjacent veins and nerves as well. The cause is unknown; smoking is deleterious to the vessels and may be the most important causal factor.

Clinical Findings
Peripheral ischemia leads to trophic changes (ulcers, gangrene, loss of digits), coldness, rubor, and pain. Mottling discoloration with blanching and cyanosis and hyperhidrosis occur, the latter partly related to the associated neural involvement. Superficial migratory phlebitis may be present.

Treatment
Early discontinuation of smoking prevents further progression and is the most critical feature of management. Analgesics, care of ulcers, sympathectomy, and amputation of gangrenous parts are other forms of treatment.

ARTERIAL EMBOLI

Acute arterial emboli come from various sources, including atheromatous plaques, cardiac mural thrombi, and fat as a result of trauma. Signs are blue toes, infarctive ulcers, and gangrene, depending on the size and location of the embolus and the involved vessel. Treatment may include administration of low-molecular-weight dextran, anticoagulants, vasodilators, and surgical procedures such as endarterectomy and various bypass procedures.

ERYTHROMELALGIA
(Erythermalgia)

Erythromelalgia is a paroxysmal bilateral vasodilation of the feet and sometimes the hands, associated with burning pain and erythema relieved by exposure to cool soaks. The cause is unknown. A primary (idiopathic) and a secondary form exist. The secondary type may be related to neurologic disorders, hypertension, polycythemia vera, and gout.

Clinical Findings
Initially, the palms, soles, or both develop burning sensations bilaterally that may last minutes to hours. Sweating may be increased. The patient may have headaches, vertigo, and palpitations. Redness, heat, and edema are present, and symptoms may be triggered by warmth or exercise. Raising the skin temperature to 35 °C will reproduce the symptoms; this occurs more rapidly with dry rather than humid heat.

Treatment
Relief is frequently produced by cool soaks or by walking on cool surfaces. Elevation of the extremities reduces swelling. Other treatments include avoidance of warm environment, aspirin to relieve pain, and antihistamines and prednisone for the swelling. Vasoconstrictors (ephedrine and methysergide) occasionally have been helpful. Sympathectomy is not usually successful. Treatment of secondary erythromelalgia is directed at the underlying disease.

RAYNAUD'S PHENOMENON
& DISEASE

Raynaud's phenomenon, a bilateral paroxysmal vasospastic disease produced by cold and emotional stimuli, is characterized by ischemic episodes involving usually a few digits of both hands or feet rather than the entire part. During an attack, the digits become white and then cyanotic. During recovery, before the normal color returns, there is reflex vasodilatation producing a bright red color. Other skin changes include sclerodermoid changes of the digits, necrosis, scarring, and loss of the pulp of the fingertips of the palmar aspects of the hand. Raynaud's phenomenon may be a primary process or secondary to many diseases (see Chapters 47 and 50).

ACROCYANOSIS

Acrocyanosis is benign symmetric cyanosis of the hands—occasionally the feet, and rarely the forearms and legs—with few if any symptoms. Young women are especially susceptible to the disorder. Arteriolar vasospasm in conjunction with venular and capillary dilatation allows extensive deoxygenation of the blood, and the cyanosis produces the bluish color. Abnormal cold sensitivity, induced even by the coolness of room temperature, seems to be the inciting process. Blue or bluish-red discoloration of the hands and feet, coldness and swelling (especially of the digits), and hyperhidrosis (especially of the palms and soles) are the usual skin manifestations. No trophic changes occur.

Treatment is frequently unnecessary. The patient should avoid cold and tobacco use. Vasodilators and sympathectomy are not usually needed.

OTHER VASCULAR DISEASES
RELATED TO COLD

Some vascular diseases result from hypersensitivity to cold and may present with urticaria (cold urticaria), vasculitis and vascular occlusion (cryoglobulinemia and cryofibrinogenemia), and vasoconstrictive phenomena (Raynaud's phenomenon, acrocyanosis). Others reflect a normal adverse response to cold, including immersion foot, chilblain, and frostbite.

Immersion foot results from prolonged exposure to cold or warm water. Chilblain (erythrocyanosis) is a mild cold injury, usually appearing in cold, damp climates. In frostbite, the tissue actually freezes and the tissue injury is a consequence of both vasoconstriction and the freezing effect. All of these disorders and their treatments are discussed in Chapter 45.

ERGOTISM

Marked vasoconstriction can be produced by the ingestion of ergot; the source may be drugs or wheat or rye infected with ergot-producing fungi. Methysergide occasionally produces peripheral vasospasm similar to that of ergot. In addition to vasoconstriction, there may be thickening of the media of the arteries, which undergo hyaline changes, intimal infolding, and thrombosis.

Clinical Findings

Vasoconstriction causes coolness, mottling, pallor, muscle cramps, and intermittent claudication of the acral areas. Raynaud's phenomenon may occur. When the disease is severe, gangrene may affect the digits and possibly the ears and nose. All of these tend to be more frequent in the chronic form of ergotism.

In the more acute form, headaches, paresthesias, seizures, vertigo, nausea, vomiting, and diarrhea may be prominent complaints, as well as vasospastic phenomena that may lead to gangrene.

Treatment

Administration of ergot or methysergide, vasodilators, and anticoagulant drugs should be stopped. The end results are significantly better if gangrene has not occurred.

ARTERIAL OCCLUSION

Arterial occlusion may be caused by an embolus or thrombosis. The usual source of a pulmonary embolus is phlebothrombosis or as a result of thrombophlebitis. Arterial emboli affecting the skin usually come from the heart (valvular or mural disease or arrhythmias leading to clots in the heart), from atheromatous plaques, or from fat mobilized by trauma. Arterial occlusion also results from many other diseases, including thromboangiitis obliterans, arteriosclerosis obliterans, polyarteritis nodosa, polycythemia, thrombotic thrombocytopenic purpura, and various infections, including mycotic arteritis. Leriche's syndrome is progressive occlusion at the bifurcation of the abdominal aorta that produces ischemic pain in the hips and thighs, especially when walking.

Clinical Findings

Progressive occlusion of the anterior tibial artery leads to the anterior tibial compartment syndrome. Paresthesias, pain, tenderness, and swelling of the anterior surface of the leg develop in the early stages. Later, patients may develop fever, foot drop, absent pulses in the tibial artery, and gangrenous changes, including ulcers of the involved skin.

Treatment

Treatment is related to the areas involved. The occlusion may be bypassed by surgically implanting a new vessel to carry the blood. Embolectomy may be successful if performed early. Low-molecular-weight dextrans have been given to aid circulation through peripheral arteriolar areas. Anticoagulants, vascular dilators, and sympathectomy may be indicated. The involved extremity should not be elevated or subjected to heat above room temperature.

VENOUS DISEASES

The venous system consists of the superficial, deep, and communicating (perforating) veins of the 4 extremities and the other veins of the head, neck, and trunk. The veins in the limbs resemble a ladder with rungs, one side of the ladder being the superficial veins, the other side the deep veins, and the rungs the communicating veins.

Blood flows from the superficial to the deep veins through the communicating veins. All of these vessels have bicuspid (bucket) valves that minimize backflow. The calf muscles are the peripheral pumps that force blood through the veins to the heart.

Varicose veins are irregular dilatations of veins, primarily seen in the lower extremities, caused by valvular incompetence and variations in the components of the vessel wall.

THROMBOPHLEBITIS & PHLEBOTHROMBOSIS

A clot in an inflamed vein constitutes thrombophlebitis. The portion of the clot that extends proximally beyond the area of thrombosis may break off and travel through the veins as an embolus. Phlebothrombosis represents a venous clot in a vein that is not inflamed. These blood clots are especially prone to embolize.

Clinical Findings

Deep thrombophlebitis usually causes venous obstruction and edema distal to the thrombosis. Pain is variable but may be severe and may occur at rest or only with activity such as walking. Increased heat and a tender cordlike induration may be palpable over the affected vein.

With phlebothrombosis, pain may be mild or absent because of the lack of inflammation. Other signs may also be less evident or absent.

When the thromboses extend into or involve both the femoral and the iliac veins, the swelling is marked and rapid in onset and involves the entire leg. Rarely, ischemic changes—pallor, cyanosis, and gangrene—may occur with extensive iliofemoral venous thrombosis.

Superficial thrombophlebitis is usually tender over the site. A cordlike, reddish-brown band delineates the involved segment of vein that is painful. If the lesion is within 8 cm above or below the knee, the phlebitis may extend to involve deep vessels because of the special intercommunications of the superficial veins with the deep venous system at this site.

A special type of superficial thrombophlebitis is **Mondor's disease,** which involves the superficial veins of the chest wall from the axilla to the lower costal margin. Superficial migratory thrombophlebitis, which can involve large or small vessels, recurs at various sites over a period of months to years. It usually occurs in superficial vessels of the extremities, abdominal wall, and flanks. It is frequently idiopathic but may be caused by infections, malignant disease (especially of the pancreas), Buerger's disease, or Behçet's disease.

Treatment

Treatment varies to some extent depending on which component of the venous system is involved (superficial or deep) and the extent and site of involvement.

For thrombosis or phlebitis of the deep veins, bed rest, heat, and anticoagulants such as heparin or dicumarol are important. Occasionally, heat may exacerbate pain owing to increased metabolic requirements that cannot be met because of the venous occlusion. Various surgical procedures can be used to prevent or treat emboli.

Because of the infrequency of associated thromboembolic disease, superficial thrombophlebitis does not usually require anticoagulation, except perhaps near the knee and the proximal part of the thigh. Heat and rest help, and ibuprofen or indomethacin can be given to reduce inflammation and pain.

PHLEGMASIA CERULEA DOLENS

Venous gangrene (phlegmasia cerulea dolens) is extremely rare. Severe thrombotic disease of the deep veins is associated with arterial spasm. The limb is bluish-violet and acutely painful. In the later stages, there may be bullae, necrosis, and paresthesias that may progress to motor paralysis.

VENA CAVAL OBSTRUCTIONS

Obstruction of the superior vena cava leads to edema and a dusky cyanosis of the face, neck, thorax, and upper extremities. Obstruction of the superior vena cava is in most instances produced by bronchogenic carcinoma, but other metastatic cancers, lymphomas, tuberculosis, histoplasmosis, thrombophlebitis, aortic aneurysms, fibrous mediastinitis, and injury to the veins of the upper extremity can cause the obstruction.

The skin may be painful. Dyspnea may be present, and all symptoms are aggravated when the patient is lying down. This resultant increased pressure can cause headaches, drowsiness, stupor, loss of consciousness, and convulsions.

Obstruction of the inferior vena cava causes edema, plethora, and caput medusae (distended veins radiating from the umbilicus or from the inguinal region).

LYMPHATIC DISEASES

The lymphatics drain the extravascular space of proteinaceous and particulate matter through regional lymph nodes to the thoracic duct or the right lymphatic duct, depending upon the areas involved. Both empty into the jugular vein. There are deep and superficial lymphatics; they do not have communicators, as do veins, and they contain more valves than the veins. Lymphatics of the skin may cross the midline and have 2 or 3 lymphatic capillary arcades. Whereas edema tends to compress veins and arteries, the lymphatic walls are drawn farther apart by edema, because connective tissue fibrils that anchor them to the surrounding tissue are stretched. The greater the edema, the wider the diameter of the lymphatics, which in turn increases removal of proteinaceous and particulate matter from the extravascular space.

LYMPHEDEMA

Lymphedema occurs when the lymphatics of the region are not capable of removing proteins and particulate matter from the extravascular space of that part. Lymphedema is usually firm, nonpitting, and painless (unless infection occurs)—features that tend to differentiate it from edema due to other causes (Fig 23–1). Ulcers rarely occur.

Lymphedema may be primary or secondary. The primary lymphedemas result from hypoplasia, hyperplasia, or aplasia of lymphatic vessels. Primary lymphedema can be subdivided into 2 groups: **Milroy's lymphatic dysplasia,** which is congenital, familial, and present at birth; and **Letessier's lymphatic dysplasia,** which is familial but not congenital. Lymphedema praecox usually appears in the teens and as late as the early 30s. A tardive form has been seen with onset as late as 49 years of age. Secondary lymphedemas are mostly due to trauma, ablative surgery, and infections, especially streptococcal cellulitis, filariasis, and lymphogranuloma venereum.

Repeated streptococcal infections presenting as lymphangitis are common in lymphedema of the lower extremities as well as in postmastectomy lymphedema. Fissures between the toes caused by tinea pedis are frequent entry points for infection. These repeated infections lead to destruction of the remaining lymphatics.

Streptococcal infection should be treated with more than the usual dosage of penicillin because of the diluting effect of the edema.

MOSSY FOOT

Mossy foot is usually seen in a postthrombophlebitic limb that has had many superimposed streptococcal infections causing lymphangiosclerosis and excrescences of the superficial lymphatics (Fig 23–2). This can be successfully treated by employing a pumping device (eg, Jobst pump), pressure-gradient supports, and prophylactic oral penicillin. When the mossy foot involves the toes, one sometimes must resort to individual wrapping with strips of elastic bandage.

An uncommon complication of chronic lymphedema is lymphangiosarcoma, referred to as the Stewart-Treves syndrome. The most common clinical setting is postmastectomy lymphedema, but lymphangiosarcoma has also occurred in other forms of chronic lymphedema including congenital lymphedema. It is not observed in postvenous thrombophlebitis. Clinical manifestations of lymphangiosarcoma are reddish-purple macules, papules, nodules, and tumors.

Body areas affected by lymphedema can be compressed with special inflatable pressure devices. Once edema is reduced by decompression, an appropriate pressure gradient garment is fitted to the area. Pa-

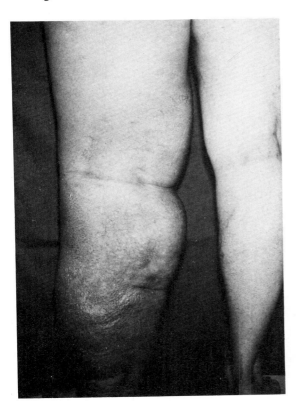

Figure 23–1. Lymphedema of entire left leg.

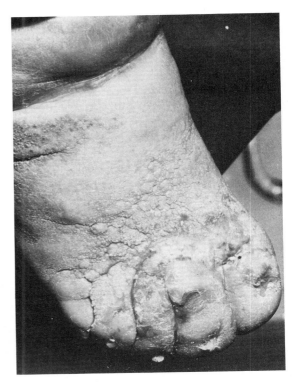

Figure 23–2. Mossy foot with lymphatic excrescences.

tients with repeated streptococcal infections should be treated with prophylactic oral penicillin or erythromycin to prevent recurrence of infection and further damage to lymphatics. Many surgical techniques for lymphedema have been explored, but no successful therapy has been developed.

OTHER LYMPHATIC DISEASES

Two major types of lymphangiomas are (1) cavernous lymphangioma—called cystic hygroma when situated in the neck; and (2) lymphangioma circumscriptum. Both are usually present at birth or appear in the first or second years of life.

Cavernous lymphangiomas are soft cystic tumors. The lesions may be located entirely in the subcutaneous tissues or may have a surface component of lymphangioma circumscriptum. Treatment is surgical.

Lymphangioma circumscriptum presents as patches or clusters of translucent vesicles suggestive of frog eggs. Occasionally they may have a reddish color from admixture of blood. The surface lesions are frequently associated with deep lesions that appear as soft swellings. The cause is unknown. However, there are, on rare occasions, similar lesions that appear as a result of scarring and lymphatic obstruction that represent true lymphangiectases.

Treatment of the surface lesions with destructive methods is usually not successful because of the deep underlying component. Excision of the deeper lesions require some method of study to determine the extent of tumor.

PYODERMA GANGRENOSUM

Pyoderma gangrenosum is a clinically characteristic ulcerative skin disease without diagnostic laboratory or histopathologic findings. This disease is often associated with internal disorders primarily involving the gastrointestinal, hematologic, and musculoskeletal systems. It is idiopathic in 20% of cases.

Inflammatory bowel disease is the most commonly associated disease, with ulcerative colitis much more frequent than regional enteritis. Usually the colitis precedes the appearance of pyoderma gangrenosum.

Hematologic disorders, especially myelogenous leukemia and myeloproliferative disease, may be related to pyoderma gangrenosum. In these situations—and contrary to what is experienced with ulcerative colitis—pyoderma gangrenosum may precede the appearance of hematologic disease. In leukemia, the skin lesions may be bullae; in fact, bullous

pyoderma gangrenosum should raise a suspicion of underlying leukemia. Paraproteinemias—especially elevation of IgA—are also associated with pyoderma gangrenosum, but true multiple myeloma is uncommon.

Musculoskeletal disease, serologically positive rheumatoid arthritis, and serologically negative inflammatory arthritis (especially with peculiar progressive erosive arthritis) also occur with pyoderma gangrenosum. Chronic active hepatitis has also been associated with pyoderma gangrenosum.

Clinically, the lesions may start as pustules that often develop rapidly into progressive necrotic ulcers with a characteristic undermining of the edge, which is a deep reddish-blue color (Fig 23–3). The lesions enlarge, often several centimeters each day. Trauma to the site precedes the onset of the lesion in about one-third of cases (pathergy).

Diagnosis is based on the typical clinical lesions; the nonspecific biopsy; failure to recover fungi, bacteria, and acid-fast organisms; the presence of associated diseases; and exclusion of other conditions, especially the vasculitides.

Treatment successes have been achieved with topical, intralesional, and systemic corticosteroids and

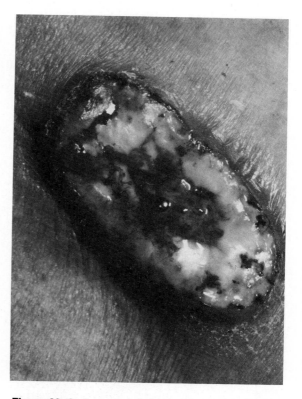

Figure 23–3. A characteristic ulcer of pyoderma gangrenosum with necrotic center and reddish-blue undermined borders.

with dapsone, sulfapyridine, cytotoxic agents, cromolyn compresses, minocycline, clofazimine, protection, and treatment of the underlying disease.

COUMARIN CONGENER & HEPARIN NECROSIS
(Anticoagulation Syndrome)

Severe reactions to coumarin and its congeners happen infrequently, mostly in young women. The onset is usually 3–10 days after initiation of a coumarin drug (dicumarol, warfarin). Continuation or discontinuance of the drug does not alter the course.

The lesions begin as petechiae or ecchymoses. Necrosis occurs rapidly, sometimes within 24 hours after the appearance of the petechiae. Necrosis can extend into the deep subcutaneous fat, and the resulting ulcer may take months to heal. If the lesion is not necrotic, healing may be rapid.

About 80% of lesions appear on the lower body, especially in areas with significant subcutaneous fat. Biopsies reveal occlusions of dermal and subcutaneous veins with fibrin thrombi and extravasation of red cells but no significant inflammation.

Heparin necrosis without the use of coumarin drugs has also occurred. The lesions appear at the subcutaneous injection sites 4–11 days after start of treatment and progress rapidly into large necrotic areas that require excision and grafting.

No specific treatment has been considered successful.

Amputation of the breast or penis when these are severely involved has been recommended. Surgical debridement and skin grafts have been necessary at other sites. Coumarin necrosis has been associated with protein C deficiency.

PURPURA

Purpura is the extravasation of blood into the skin or mucosa, causing a purple macule or papule. Usually the initial lesions are bluish or reddish-blue. With time and absorption, the color develops shades of yellowish or reddish brown. Purpura does not blanch with diascopy. Lesions a few millimeters in diameter are referred to as petechiae (small spot); lesions larger than 3 cm are called ecchymoses. These latter lesions constitute what is commonly referred to as "black-and-blue" discolorations, or bruising. Deeper accumulations of blood are hematomas.

A variety of adjectives are used to qualify purpura. The word "vibex" (pl "vibices") is used to denote a linear hemorrhage that might result from the lash of a whip. Other terms may reflect prevalence in the aged (senile purpura), etiologic mechanisms (thrombocytopenic purpura), or course of disease (purpura fulminans).

A classification of purpuras may be based on a number of factors, such as the quantity of platelets, the presence or absence of inflammation, defects in the coagulation system, the palpability of the lesions, and the presence of an immunologic reaction. No one classification system is entirely satisfactory; flexibility is needed, because more than one process may be occurring simultaneously.

A classification that assists in the recall of the various types of purpura is based on whether the reason for the purpura is within the vessel, in the vessel wall itself, or in the supporting tissue (Table 23–2).

THROMBOCYTOPENIC PURPURA
(Immune Types)

Hemorrhagic tendencies increase with diminishing platelet count. Bleeding diatheses generally do not

---

Table 23–2. Classification of purpura.

Intravascular-vascular contents
  Thrombocytopenia
    Immune
      Autoimmune thrombocytopenic purpura (idiopathic thrombocytopenic purpura)
      Other immune, including some drug reactions
    Nonimmune
      Some drug reactions
      Disseminated intravascular coagulation
      Purpura fulminans
      Thrombotic thrombocytopenic purpura
      Kasabach-Merritt syndrome
      Wiskott-Aldrich syndrome
      Hematologic disorders
  Nonthrombocytopenic
    Coagulation defects
    Functional platelet disorders (thrombocytopathies)
    Psychogenic purpura
    Thrombocytoses: thrombocythemia
    Drug reactions
    Dysproteinemias (may also be vasculitic)
Vascular wall
  Vasculitis
  Nonvasculitis
    Hereditary hemorrhagic telangiectasia
    Amyloid
    Pseudoxanthoma elasticum
Supporting tissues
  Senile purpura
  Corticosteroid purpura
  Scurvy
  Ehlers-Danlos syndrome

occur until the platelet counts reach 50,000 or less. Counts below 20,000 are usually associated with cutaneous and mucosal hemorrhage. Trauma and surgery may result in abnormal bleeding with platelet counts as high as 100,000.

Thrombocytopenia may be separated into immune and nonimmune types (Table 23–2).

1. AUTOIMMUNE THROMBOCYTOPENIC PURPURA (Idiopathic Thrombocytopenic Purpura)

In autoimmune thrombocytopenic purpura, platelets are destroyed but the numbers of platelets and megakaryocytes in the bone marrow are normal or increased. The spleen is not enlarged. Antiplatelet antibodies are diagnostic of immune thrombocytopenic purpura.

The acute form of autoimmune thrombocytopenic purpura is most common and usually occurs in children 2–6 years of age. An acute systemic illness precedes appearance of the purpura by 3 weeks. Ecchymoses or petechiae of the skin suddenly appear (Fig 23–4), and bleeding of the mucous membranes may result in epistaxis, melena, and gingival and conjunctival hemorrhage. Menorrhagia may appear in menstruating young women. Platelet counts are usually below 20,000/μL. The course is usually self-limiting, but a few children may develop a more chronic and serious form. Systemic corticosteroids usually shorten the course of the initial episode and

lessen the severity of the disease but do not seem to prevent development of chronic forms. Intravenous gamma globulin has also caused an increase in platelet count. Splenectomy has been only variably helpful and usually is withheld for use only in management of chronic forms.

The chronic form of autoimmune thrombocytopenic purpura occurs more often in the third and fourth decades of life, especially in women. In contrast to the acute form, antecedent infection is not apparent. The course is more subtle and insidious, with bruising, heavy or long menstrual periods, or other evidence of a moderate bleeding diathesis.

The gradual onset and the less dramatic skin and oral purpuric lesions reflect the less significant decrease in platelets, which may range between 25,000 and 90,000/μL. The risk of intracranial bleeding is significant, and death may be a consequence.

Corticosteroids and splenectomy have been used successfully.

2. NEONATAL IMMUNE THROMBOCYTOPENIC PURPURA

Neonatal immune thrombocytopenic purpura may result from transplacental passage of persistent maternal antiplatelet antibodies. In the mother, there is a high incidence of bruising and bleeding from episiotomy incisions. Purpura occurs in about 70% of these infants. The risk to the mother and the fetus is much less in previously splenectomized mothers. Physician awareness, prenatal corticosteroids, corticosteroids administered to the fetus, possible cesarean section, and neonatal plasma exchange to lower platelet antibodies may be important for treatment.

3. ISOIMMUNE NEONATAL PURPURA

Isoantibodies to platelets (an antibody developed against an antigen not present on one's own platelets) causes congenital thrombocytopenia in about 0.02% of births because of maternal absence of the PL^1 antigen. The PL^1-negative mother is sensitized to these antigens by fetal platelets that cross the placental barrier. The firstborn is affected half the time, and antibodies to paternal and fetal platelets are readily detected in the mother's serum. Petechiae and ecchymoses occur in the fetus (not the mother) within a few hours after birth, especially over bony prominences and presenting parts. Neither the spleen nor the liver is enlarged, and treatment options are the same as for maternal autoimmune thrombocytopenic purpura.

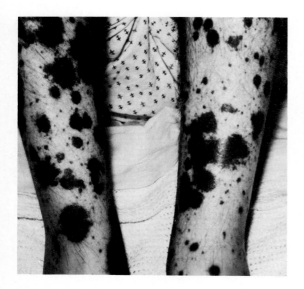

Figure 23–4. Marked petechiae and ecchymotic lesions in a patient with thrombocytopenia who developed a superimposed drug vasculitis. (Courtesy of Ruth Hanno, MD.)

4. POSTTRANSFUSION PURPURA

Potentially fatal thrombocytopenic purpura can occur within 1 week of blood transfusions. Over 50% of the reactions are related to the PL^1 antigens; other platelet antigens are involved in the other cases. PL^1 antigens are present on platelets of 98% of the population. When transfused into a patient who does not have these common platelet antigens, the antigens elicit antibodies to the transfused platelets. A significant thrombocytopenia results. The platelet counts may be 10,000/μL or less. Heavy bleeding into tissues appears suddenly, and the risks of intracranial hemorrhage are significant. Plasmapheresis will remove antibodies and is probably the treatment of choice.

5. DRUG-INDUCED PURPURA

Drugs may induce purpura by toxic mechanisms, vasculitis, and immune thrombocytopenia. Drugs more commonly implicated are quinidine, quinine, sulfonamides, thiazides (sulfonamide derivatives), digitoxin, and antimalarials. All drugs—both prescribed and over-the-counter medications—should be suspected and eliminated or replaced by another chemically unrelated medication. Once sensitization has developed, lifelong reactivity probably persists. The patient should know which drug caused the problem and should be cautioned to avoid medications with similar chemical composition. Disappearance of the purpura within a few days after stopping the drug strongly suggests a drug etiology. Rechallenge carries a high risk and is not indicated. Corticosteroids may be useful in the acute phase.

Cutaneous petechiae and ecchymoses, hemorrhagic bullae of the mucosa, and bleeding of the gastrointestinal or genitourinary system may occur within 6–24 hours. Platelet counts may be less than 10,000. Antibodies to most drugs except quinine derivatives are difficult to detect.

NONIMMUNE PURPURAS

1. NONIMMUNE DRUG-INDUCED THROMBOCYTOPENIA

All cytotoxic drugs are capable of causing thrombocytopenia if given in high enough doses. Clinical findings may be similar to those of immune drug thrombocytopenia and may reflect the damage to other cell systems affected by the toxic reaction. Treatment consists of stopping administration of the drug and administering specific antagonists if available.

2. DISSEMINATED INTRAVASCULAR COAGULATION

Disseminated intravascular coagulation results from inappropriate activation of the coagulation cascade, usually caused by an underlying disease. Widespread excessive activation of thrombin, overactivation of the fibrinolytic system, an increase in fibrin and fibrinogen degradation products, hypofibrinogenemia, and thrombocytopenia result in 2 main cutaneous skin changes: (1) widespread thrombosis of both larger and smaller vessels and (2) hemorrhage. Thrombosis results from excessive activation of thrombin and may cause loss of function, pulmonary embolus, acral cyanosis, and gangrene. Hemorrhage from depletion of platelet and coagulation factors and activation of the fibrinolytic system cause petechiae and purpura, resulting in palpable petechiae, ecchymoses, hematomas, and hemorrhagic bullae. Bleeding may also occur at surgical sites and at sites of venipunctures, indwelling tubes, and catheters.

Disseminated intravascular coagulation may follow a fulminant course, with coma, fever, and shock with significant neurologic, cardiopulmonary, hepatic, and renal involvement. Milder disease may be of little clinical significance. This great variability explains some inconsistencies in establishing criteria for diagnosis.

Disseminated intravascular coagulation is caused by many underlying diseases and disorders, including incompatible blood transfusions, intrauterine death, abruptio placentae and other obstetric conditions, leukemia (especially during lysis with chemotherapy), surgical or other extensive trauma, sepsis, viral infections, polycythemia vera, cyanotic heart disease, large or multiple cavernous and capillary hemangiomas, and arterial aneurysms. Diagnosis is a clinical and laboratory correlation: inappropriate coagulation, widespread bleeding, and the presence of thrombosis. Fibrin degradation products in the blood confirm the diagnosis but are not themselves diagnostic of disseminated intravascular coagulation. Prolonged prothrombin and thrombin times, hypofibrinogenemia, and thrombocytopenia strongly suggest disseminated intravascular coagulation.

To treat disseminated intravascular coagulation, the underlying disease or condition must be treated—eg, with appropriate antibiotics for sepsis. Replacement of hemolytic factors, especially if surgery is necessary, may be indicated, though the procedure is controversial. Heparin is probably helpful in some patients.

3. PURPURA FULMINANS

Purpura fulminans is a severe form of disseminated intravascular coagulation that usually occurs in children. The appearance of the disease is usually preceded by infection up to 4 weeks previously. Disseminated intravascular coagulation and purpura in the acute phase of meningococcemia with septic emboli are not considered part of purpura fulminans by some because of the absence of a latent period and the presence of microorganisms in the lesions.

The most common antecedent infections are bacterial and include streptococcal pharyngitis, scarlet fever, group A streptococcal bacterial infections, meningococcemia, and staphylococcal bacteremia. Varicella is the most common viral cause.

A patient suddenly develops extensive ecchymoses, hemorrhagic bullae and necrosis, acral cyanosis, and peripheral focal gangrene. Lesions are usually symmetric and more frequently on the lower extremities. The skin lesions are purplish-black, swollen, and hard. Systemic symptoms are severe, with hypotension, shock, and rapidly progressive anemia.

Adequate blood volume must be maintained. Exchange transfusions and heparin are useful, especially early in the course of the disease. Corticosteroids have not been especially effective and may be contraindicated as sole therapy. Corticosteroids in conjunction with heparin have been recommended by some. Persistence of inciting infection should be excluded; if present, appropriate treatment should be devised.

4. NONIMMUNE THROMBOTIC THROMBOCYTOPENIC PURPURA

This uncommon disease has 5 major elements: thrombocytopenic purpura, microangiopathic hemolytic anemia, central nervous system symptoms, renal disease, and fever. Thrombotic lesions in the cardiac conduction system are a fairly common feature.

Microvascular hyaline thrombi of platelets, fibrin, and immunoglobulins occlude segments of arterioles and capillaries. Fibrinolysis is limited, and levels of fibrinogen-fibrin degradation products are normal or slightly elevated in most patients, tending to distinguish thrombotic thrombocytopenic purpura from other diseases that cause thrombi, such as disseminated intravascular coagulation.

Three of the 5 symptoms and signs (anemia, purpura, and neurologic disease) appear together in 75% of cases. Petechiae and ecchymoses are common. Bleeding of the mucous membranes or conjunctiva, epistaxis, retinal hemorrhage, gross hematuria, and gynecologic and gastrointestinal bleeding also occur. Differential diagnosis should include lupus erythematosus (which may be associated with thrombotic thrombocytopenic purpura), disseminated intravascular coagulation, immune thrombocytopenic purpura, and subacute bacterial as well as nonbacterial thrombotic endocarditis.

Diagnosis is made on the basis of the multisystem involvement, clinical findings, microangiopathic Coombs-negative hemolytic anemia, thrombocytopenia, and normal or mildly altered coagulation studies. Tissue biopsies, especially of mucous membrane,

are often nonspecific. The great majority of cases develop without apparent cause. Pregnancy, drugs, and infectious agents have precipitated the disease in some patients. There is evidence that a platelet-aggregating factor or large multimers of factor VIII:von Willebrand factor may be the cause of thrombosis.

Without appropriate treatment, patients may die in less than 2 weeks, though the prognosis has improved significantly in recent years because of rapid diagnosis and aggressive treatment. Corticosteroids have been of limited benefit. Of the cytotoxic agents, vincristine has been perhaps the most successful. Hemodialysis (renal failure), platelet suppressant drugs (dextran 70, combinations of aspirin and dipyridamole), and plasmapheresis have helped.

Fresh frozen plasma, which may replace immunoglobulins and inhibit platelet-agglutinating factor and factor VIII:von Willebrand factor, has been successful in some cases.

5. KASABACH-MERRITT SYNDROME

Large hemangiomas of the cavernous and strawberry type may cause thrombocytopenia. Although trapping of platelets has been the most accepted theory for the thrombocytopenia, studies have not consistently supported this explanation. A localized form of disseminated intravascular coagulation may produce fibrin degradation products and a microangiopathic hemolytic anemia.

Except for the rare internal organ hemangioma, large or multiple hemangiomas are visible in the skin. Hemorrhage into the skin and mucous membranes and gray cyanosis of the acral areas are the usual clinical signs.

Treatment may include surgical or radiation treatment of the hemangioma. Systemic corticosteroids are usually preferable.

6. WISKOTT-ALDRICH SYNDROME

Wiskott-Aldrich syndrome is an X-linked recessive disease characterized by thrombocytopenia, recurrent infection, and a dermatitis that resembles atopic dermatitis. The thrombocytopenia is probably related to an inherent defect in the platelets that makes them small and decreases platelet survival time. Cell-mediated and humoral immunologic abnormalities explain the recurrent infections.

The initial sign is often a hemorrhagic eczematous dermatitis. By the end of the first year, infection with the polysaccharide-containing organisms (pneumococcus, meningococcus) appear. Lymphoreticular cancers develop then or later. Death usually occurs early in life from infection, bleeding, or the lymphoreticular tumors. Treatment has been directed toward intercurrent infections. Replacement of immunoglobulins and platelets has been used, and bone marrow transplantation has been beneficial in some patients.

7. HEMATOLOGIC DISORDERS

Petechiae, purpura, ecchymoses, and hemorrhagic necrosis may be the result of leukemia and myeloproliferative disorders. Monocytic leukemia and granulocytic leukemia are especially apt to be associated with skin lesions. Thrombocytopenia causes hemorrhage from the gums and nasal mucosa. Marked hypertrophy of the gingiva from leukemic infiltrates may also appear. Other skin manifestations include marked pruritus (especially in Hodgkin's disease and myeloproliferative disorders), plum-colored nodules and tumors of specific infiltrates, pyoderma gangrenosum, and severe disseminated, necrotic herpes zoster.

Treatment is aimed at the underlying diseases.

8. COAGULATION DISORDERS

Congenital bleeding disorders can usually be elicited by the history, especially of bleeding in association with trauma, tooth extractions, tonsillectomies, menorrhagia, hemarthrosis, and cutaneous hematomas.

Von Willebrand's disease can be more subtle and may cause excessive bleeding in procedures—such as hair transplantation—that stress the coagulation system. Other causes of acquired bleeding disorders relate to change in platelet function or numbers; these changes may be caused by drugs, especially aspirin.

Four simple tests identify the most common important bleeding problems and thus are especially helpful in routine evaluation of patients undergoing hair transplant or other surgery. These include the prothrombin time (assesses the extrinsic system), partial thromboplastin time (assesses the intrinsic system), the number of circulating platelets, and bleeding time.

Clinically, the patient with a coagulation disorder bleeds severely, especially in some of the congenital types such as hemophilia. Prolonged and severe bleeding following trauma and therapeutic injections, hemarthrosis, and mucosal bleeding are common.

Treatment is directed toward specific causes, replacement of missing factors, avoidance of offending drugs (especially aspirin), and protection from trauma. Appropriate history taking and basic testing before skin surgery may avoid serious bleeding problems or adverse effects on wound healing as a result of hematoma.

9. THROMBOCYTOPATHIES

Defects of platelet function may be hereditary or acquired. Some hereditary forms are the Wiskott-Aldrich syndrome, some cases of albinism, Hermansky-Pudlak syndrome (albinism and ceroidlike pigment in marrow macrophages), thrombasthenia (Glanzmann's disease), long bleeding times, abnormal clot retraction, failure of platelet aggregation with ADP, and Chédiak-Higashi syndrome (partial oculocutaneous albinism, abnormally large neutrophilic granules, and susceptibility to infection).

Acquired defects in platelet function have occurred with drugs (especially aspirin), liver disease, uremia, scurvy, and alcoholism.

Clinical signs of defects in platelet function include petechiae, easy bruising, ecchymoses, epistaxis, and bleeding and hematomas in conjunction with surgery. In addition, signs of the related disease, such as albinism, may be striking.

10. PSYCHOGENIC PURPURAS, INCLUDING GARDNER-DIAMOND SYNDROME

The patients (95% are female) may first note redness, tenderness, and burning or stabbing pains of the lower extremities. The skin lesions become bluish in a matter of a few hours or as late as 3 days and later resemble bruises. Recurrence of lesions, sometimes in groups, is typical. Trauma may induce a typical lesion. Biopsies of lesions sometimes suggest an inflammatory process. The disease may be due to some sort of hypersensitivity to red blood cell stroma. Accordingly, skin tests help establish the diagnosis. About 0.1 mL of autologous venous blood is injected into the skin of each anterior thigh with a 27-gauge needle; control injections with 0.1 mL of saline are administered in adjacent areas.

Somatic manifestations include nervousness, headaches, syncope, diplopia, abdominal complaints, chest pain, dysuria, and arthralgias. Psychologic components include hysteria, masochism, depression, anxiety, and inability to deal with one's own hostility. Therapy has been relatively ineffective; psychiatric therapy has had mixed results.

Self-induced (factitial) bleeding problems are not uncommon. The ecchymoses may be difficult to distinguish from those associated with autoerythrocyte sensitization and autosensitization to DNA (which can produce an analogous syndrome).

Lesions may disappear if occluded under appropriate protective devices such as plaster casts.

11. THROMBOCYTOSIS

The term "thrombocytosis" refers to an increase in the number of platelets, sometimes secondary to some other disease. Hemorrhage and thrombosis cause purpura and extensive bleeding into the skin or other deeper tissues.

12. WALDENSTRÖM'S MACROGLOBULINEMIA

Waldenström's macroglobulinemia is characterized by the excessive production of a monoclonal macroglobulin IgM. Hallmarks of Waldenström's macroglobulinemia include anemia, bleeding diathesis, pleomorphic marrow involvement, increase of high-molecular-weight globulins, and serum hyperviscosity. This disease must be distinguished from purpuric hyperglobulinemia of Waldenström, a polyclonal hyperglobulinemia that affects only the skin (petechiae of the lower legs) and usually occurs in young women.

In Waldenström's macroglobulinemia, most of the symptoms are derived from the macroglobulinemia and the induced hyperviscosity syndrome. This produces retinal lesions and failing vision, various neurologic symptoms, and hemorrhage. Cryoglobulins may cause Raynaud's syndrome and cold urticaria. Cellular proliferation resembles a lymphoma with lymphadenopathy, hepatosplenomegaly, and infiltration of the marrow. Peculiar firm translucent papules and nodules containing IgM may develop on the extremities.

Treatment includes cytotoxic agents such as chlorambucil, cyclophosphamide, and melphalan and plasmapheresis for the hyperviscosity syndrome.

13. PURPURA HYPERGLOBULINEMICA OF WALDENSTRÖM (Benign Hypergammaglobulinemic Purpura of Waldenström)

Patients with purpura hyperglobulinemia of Waldenström have purpura, polyclonal hypergammaglobulinemia, mild anemia, and an elevated sedimentation rate. Petechiae, predominantly on the lower extremities, occur in crops at 4-week intervals. No mucosal lesions or coagulation defects are present. The polyclonal gammopathy consists primarily of IgG; IgA may be elevated in some, but IgM is low or normal. A few patients have circulating cryoglobulins, and some biopsies in both types show necrotizing vasculitis. Rheumatoid factor is common. Patients with polyclonal gammopathy apparently do not develop multiple myeloma.

In the secondary type, other diseases such as Sjögren's syndrome, lupus erythematosus, and chronic lymphatic leukemia cause the hyperglobulinemia. In the primary type, no underlying disease is present.

Treatment includes support stockings. Treatment with chlorambucil improves the purpura but does not affect the immunoglobulin abnormalities. Corticosteroids have not been beneficial.

14. CRYOGLOBULINEMIA

Cryoglobulins are immunoglobulins that precipitate reversibly from serum at temperatures below 37 °C. The greater the number of cryoglobulins, the higher the temperature at which precipitation occurs.

The cryoglobulins are divided into 3 types. Type I cryoglobulins are monoclonal immunoglobulins, most frequently an IgM, less commonly IgG, IgA, or Bence Jones proteins. Type II cryoglobulins consist of a monoclonal immunoglobulin and at least one other type. Usually it is a combination of 2 immunoglobulins, most frequently IgM and IgG. Type III cryoglobulins are usually polyclonal immunoglobulins in small amounts. Types II and III are frequently referred to as mixed cryoglobulins.

About one-fourth of type I cases have Waldenström's macroglobulinemia—not to be confused with Waldenstroöm's hypergammaglobulinemic purpura. Some patients present with hyperviscosity syndrome. Cold exposure may cause precipitation of globulins in the blood vessels, resulting in purpura, edema, urticaria, stasis, necrosis, and gangrene.

In the mixed types, IgG and IgM may be approximately equal in amounts. Women are most commonly affected, developing arthralgia, severe recurrent purpura of the legs, and symptoms of malaise and weakness. Hepatosplenomegaly is frequently present. Renal disease may be rapidly progressive.

In about one-third of cases, the cause of cryoglobulinemia is unknown. The remainder may be associated with a variety of diseases, including Waldenström's macroglobulinemia; multiple myeloma, lymphomas, and other malignant neoplasms; connective tissue disorders (especially lupus erythematosus), rheumatoid arthritis, and Sjögren's syndrome; chronic infections, including subacute infective endocarditis, malaria, leprosy, and kala-azar; and chronic liver disease, especially cirrhosis and hepatobiliary disease.

Detection of cryoglobulins requires a special regard for temperatures at the time of collection and testing. Blood must be drawn with a warm syringe, and the sample must be immediately placed in a 37 °C water bath to clot. The serum is removed and kept at 0 °C for 72 hours. It is then centrifuged under refrigeration, and the separated cryocrit is tested.

Cutaneous lesions commonly include petechiae and ecchymoses, especially on the legs. Only about 30% of patients note purpura after cold exposure. Ulcers and gangrene may occur, especially in association with high levels of cryoglobulins or severe cold exposure (or both). Other skin findings include

Raynaud's phenomenon, leukocytoclastic vasculitis, acrocyanosis, cold urticaria, and livedo reticularis.

Patients with cryoglobulinemia should protect themselves against cold exposure. Plasmapheresis has been used to reduce the quantity of cryoglobulins. Underlying diseases, if any, should be treated.

15. CRYOFIBRINOGENEMIA

Cryofibrinogens are proteins precipitated from the plasma rather than the serum. Cryofibrinogenemia is much less common than cryoglobulinemia. Idiopathic and secondary types occur. Associated diseases include nonlymphomatous cancers—especially metastatic prostatic carcinoma—and leukemias.

Skin findings include petechiae, ecchymoses, cold intolerance with acrocyanosis, Raynaud's phenomenon, ulcers, and gangrene. Cryofibrinogenemia is found with collagen vascular disease, pregnancy, excessive smoking, myocardial infarction, diabetes mellitus, and ingestion of oral contraceptive agents. The disease may be transitory.

16. SENILE PURPURA

Ecchymoses commonly occur on the dorsa of the arms and hands in elderly patients. Shearing forces and other trauma damage vessels that are poorly supported by connective tissues.

Ecchymoses of variable sizes and shapes, solitary and multiple, develop on the dorsa of the arms and hands. Actual tears of the skin may be present. Occasionally, hematomas may form. Corticosteroids and rheumatoid arthritis seem to significantly aggravate senile purpura.

There is no known way to develop connective tissue support for vessels or to make vessels more sturdy. If corticosteroids are being used they should be discontinued, if feasible, and the skin should be protected from trauma (eg, by heavy clothing).

17. PIGMENTED PURPURIC ERUPTIONS (Benign Hemosiderosis; Peculiar Progressive Pigmentary Diseases of the Skin)

A group of diseases having in common rustcolored macules and papules, especially on the lower extremities, have been grouped together in what is termed pigmented purpuric eruptions, or benign hemosideroses. There are 3 clinical subtypes that may be variations of the same process. Capillaritis causes the rust-colored pigmentary changes by leaking blood into tissues and causing endogenous hemosiderin tattoos. Although the eruptions tend to predominate on the lower extremities, the capillaries are usually involved in a more generalized fashion. The Rumpel-

Leede tourniquet test is usually positive in all 3 subgroups. Histopathologic study reveals a lymphocytic vasculitis of the upper dermis.

The 3 subtypes are as follows:

(1) Progressive pigmentary dermatosis (Schamberg's disease): The lesions are located on the distal part of the lower extremities and are small macular petechiae and brown pinhead-sized macules that enlarge and coalesce. The rust color and pinhead size account for its familiar name, "cayenne pepper spot." Pruritus is not common.

(2) Purpura annularis telangiectodes (Majocchi's disease): The lesions are usually rust-colored macules and papules with perifollicular telangiectasia. Early lesions may be more erythematous and tend to form rings or even concentric rings. Sites of predilection are the lower extremities and lower abdomen. Pruritus is usually absent.

(3) Pigmented purpuric lichenoid dermatitis (Gougerot-Blum syndrome): Lesions tend to be more exclusively papular initially and coalesce into generally pruritic plaques. Although the sites of predilection are the lower extremities, the lower trunk and abdomen and even the arms may be involved. Other forms of pigmented purpuric eruptions have been described related to the presence of pruritus and other changes.

Treatment is unsatisfactory. Fortunately, the disorder is primarily a cosmetic problem, since internal organs are not involved and the lesions do not usually itch. Suspected drugs should be eliminated and other causes of purpura excluded, though most other diseases do not have rust-colored lesions as a prominent feature. Support stockings may be beneficial. Systemic corticosteroids are usually effective, but the risk:benefit ratio usually weighs against their use. Topical corticosteroids, especially under wet dressings or plastic occlusion, may be effective.

18. LICHEN AUREUS

In lichen aureus, unique golden-brown patches are asymmetrically located, usually on the distal lower extremities. A segmental distribution is rarer.

The primary lesions may resemble those of the pigmented purpuric eruptions—ie, punctate reddish tending to become rust-colored—or may appear more like a bruise that subsequently assumes the golden-brown color. Histopathologic changes are similar to those of the pigmented purpuric eruptions. Mild pruritus and chronicity are usual. Treatment with topical corticosteroids is not effective.

19. OTHER CAUSES OF PURPURA

In scurvy, hemorrhages into the follicles and surrounding tissues and perifollicular telangiectasia are characteristic lesions. Patients with primary amyloidosis have amyloid in vessel walls and may develop petechiae and ecchymoses, especially in scratch marks. Periocular and perianal ecchymoses are suggestive of amyloid. Ehlers-Danlos syndrome and pseudoxanthoma elasticum are also associated with purpura.

Various infectious diseases causing purpura include Rocky Mountain spotted fever (purpuric lesions of the palms and soles), typhus, sepsis, and subacute infective endocarditis (petechiae of the skin, conjunctiva, and nail beds [splinter hemorrhages]). Purpura has also been caused by food and drug additives.

TELANGIECTASES

Telangiectases are dilated capillaries, small veins, and arteries. Some of the configurations include linear, spiderlike, matted, or punctate forms.

GENERALIZED ESSENTIAL TELANGIECTASIA

In generalized essential telangiectasia, blood vessels become dilated over extensive areas of the body. No underlying disease is apparent. Women in the fourth and fifth decades of life usually are affected. The initial telangiectases are usually on the legs, but new telangiectases may eventually cover much of the body.

Clinical patterns may vary; the dilated vessels may be linear, retiform, confluent macules and patches, or generalized. There is no spontaneous bleeding in the skin, mucous membranes, or internal organs. The absence of alkaline phosphatase in histologic studies of the involved vessels suggests that the dilated vessels are venules.

Tetracycline has been used with some reported successes. The mechanism of action is not known.

UNILATERAL NEVOID TELANGIECTASIA

Telangiectasia may occur in one extremity or on one side of the face or body. Uncommonly, unilateral nevoid telangiectasia is a congenital disease; far more often, it is acquired. The disease may result from acquired stress on a congenitally altered vasculature. Estrogens (especially at menarche or with pregnancy), alcohol, and liver disease have a major role.

Clinically, the telangiectases are scattered in a uni-

lateral distribution. About two-thirds of cases have been reported in females.

Unilateral nevoid telangiectasias associated with pregnancy may fade and disappear in the postpartum period, but other types tend to be chronic.

Lasers—especially tunable dye micropulse lasers—may be helpful in therapy.

HEREDITARY HEMORRHAGIC TELANGIECTASIA (Rendu-Weber-Osler Syndrome)

Hereditary hemorrhagic telangiectasia is a dominantly inherited disease, with telangiectases of the skin, mucous membranes, and other organ systems, and is associated with significant episodic hemorrhage. Lesions may be present at birth but more often become noticeable after puberty and progress with age.

The clinical lesions may be red 1- to 4-mm puncta or linear, spiderlike angiomas. Common locations are the lips, oral and nasal mucosa, face, ears, fingers and toes, and nail beds. Lesions of the gastrointestinal and genitourinary systems, liver, larynx, and bronchi occur. Arteriovenous aneurysms may lead to severe pulmonary symptoms and clubbing. Central nervous system vascular abnormalities may also appear. Plasminogen activator may be increased in blood, implicating fibrinolysis in the bleeding diathesis.

Hemorrhage is common and often serious. Epistaxis may be progressively more difficult to control. Hemorrhage of other organ systems (ie, gastrointestinal bleeding, hematuria, and hemoptysis) may also occur. Anemia and death may result from hemorrhages and may be a consequence of the severe repeated epistaxis alone.

Treatment is difficult. Epistaxis may be controlled by electrocautery, but in time this modality of treatment becomes less effective. Surgical grafts may be necessary. Embolization therapy to occlude the telangiectases has been useful, as has administration of estrogen. Laser destruction of blood vessels has been helpful.

ANGIOMA SERPIGINOSUM

Angioma serpiginosum is a vascular nevus usually appearing in young females. The disease usually begins by the age of 14 years. The lesions are pinhead-sized capillary puncta that blanch partly with compression. Hemorrhage or rust-colored pigmentation is not seen. Although usually on the extremities, the lesions may occur on any part of the skin but spare mucous membranes. Lesions enlarge, usually reaching and persisting at some fixed size. The lesions rarely regress. No systemic findings or symptoms occur. A few familial cases have been reported. Angioma serpiginosum is probably a capillary nevus rather than simple ectasia.

ATAXIA TELANGIECTASIA

Ataxia telangiectasia (Louis-Bar syndrome) is a recessively inherited disease characterized by ataxia, oculocutaneous telangiectasia, and a high incidence of sinopulmonary infection.

Ataxia and choreoathetosis are important aspects of this syndrome. The ataxia is noted by 2 years of age and is usually progressive. Intellectual deterioration is not prominent.

Telangiectases are usually noted on the bulbar conjunctiva (bloodshot eyes) but may not appear until the end of the first decade. Other sites include sunexposed areas, especially the butterfly area of the face, the center of the anterior neck, the tops of the ears, and the popliteal and antecubital fossae. Other skin findings include graying of the hair and loss of skin elasticity and subcutaneous fat.

Sinopulmonary infection may lead to bronchiectasis and death.

Immunologic deficiencies include diminished or absent IgA and IgE (not always) and a flawed response to bacterial antigens. Cutaneous anergy and reduced lymphocytic responsiveness to mitogens have been found. Levels of alpha-fetoprotein are often elevated.

Neoplastic disease—especially lymphoma—is common and is second only to infection as the cause of death. Death usually occurs by the fifth decade.

Patients are sensitive to therapeutic x-ray radiation but not to ultraviolet light. A defect in DNA repair has been suggested. Immobile cilia syndrome has been suggested as a possible mechanism for the sinopulmonary infections.

COCKAYNE'S SYNDROME

Cockayne's syndrome is a recessively inherited form of dwarfism with a diagnostic habitus and associated central nervous system symptoms and photosensitivity. The patients are dwarfs with long arms, large ears, and sunken eyes. Joint contractures are progressive. Microcephaly and mental retardation are present, as are deafness, retinitis pigmentosa, optic atrophy, and cataracts.

Photosensitivity is associated with erythema and telangiectasia, loss of subcutaneous fat, and cold, blue extremities. The hypersensitivity to sunlight is probably not related to DNA repair defects. Association with internal cancer or skin cancer does not occur. In Cockayne's syndrome, the cells do not seem to be sensitive to x-ray radiation.

ROTHMUND-THOMSON SYNDROME (Poikiloderma Congenitale)

Rothmund-Thomson syndrome is a recessive disorder characterized by skin changes, short stature, small hands, photosensitivity, juvenile cataracts, hypotrichosis, and hypogonadism. Intelligence is not affected. Erythematous patches develop on the cheeks, forehead, extensor surfaces of arms and legs, and buttocks. Vesiculation may occur. Reticular telangiectases with atrophy and hypopigmentation (poikiloderma) follow. One-third of patients are photosensitive. No DNA repair defects have been detected.

Differentiation must be made from other congenital poikilodermas, such as Werner's syndrome (poliosis, atrophied fat, beaked nose, and pinched face in Werner's versus saddle nose, wide forehead, and normal subcutaneous fat in Rothmund-Thomson syndrome) and progeria (absent fat, beaked nose, micrognathia, normal stature, sparing of the face except for the eyelids, and sclerosis of the palms and soles). Linear and reticulated hyperkeratotic and sclerotic bands occur in the axillae and the antecubital and popliteal fossae in hereditary sclerosing poikiloderma.

CUTIS MARMORATA TELANGIECTATICA CONGENITA

Cutis marmorata telangiectatica congenita (van Lohuizen's disease) is present at birth as an exaggerated network-type marbling of the skin referred to by some as livedo reticularis and by others as cutis marmorata. Telangiectases and superficial ulcerations occur but improve with age. The extremities, trunk, face, and scalp are most frequently involved, but the whole body may be affected.

Various abnormalities may be associated with this syndrome. Inheritance is unclear; sporadic appearance in siblings suggests possible dominant inheritance with low penetrance and great intrafamilial variability.

OTHER TELANGIECTASES

Spider angiomas are a characteristic vascular lesion with a central pulsating body and radiating legs. They are frequently associated with pregnancy and cirrhosis. Children and some normal adults may also develop the lesions, which may disappear spontaneously but also may be persistent. The usual sites are the face, neck, upper thorax, and arms. Atypically distributed and unilateral lesions may be seen. The central feeder vessel can often be successfully destroyed by electrosurgery, a special electrosurgical technique using a very fine wire electrode called a "cat's whisker" threaded down the vessel before cauterizing. Laser ablation has also been used.

Venous lakes are bluish cystic ectasias, most commonly seen on the ears, face, and lips. They represent dilated veins and probably are not related to other gastrointestinal disease. The best treatment, if desired, is to electrosurgically or cryosurgically destroy the vein or to surgically excise it. Laser destruction has also been used successfully.

Cherry or senile angiomas are common 1- to 5-mm bright red dome-shaped papules most prominent on the trunk. Lesions may first appear in adolescence, but most older patients have them. They are not associated with internal disease. Tiny lesions may resemble petechiae. No treatment is necessary, but they can be destroyed with electrosurgery, cryotherapy, or laser therapy.

Venous stasis and superficial venous ectasias (venous stars) are related to venous insufficiency and chronic increased venous pressure. They are more common in women and are located on both the upper and lower parts of the leg. Treatment with electrosurgery has not been successful. Injection of sclerosing solutions, including hypertonic saline, has produced good results. Repeated treatment is usually necessary because the underlying venous insufficiency is not changed by this treatment.

LEG ULCERS

There are many causes of leg ulcers, but the most common is venous disease and the second most common is arteriosclerosis. Ulcers may be caused by more than one process. Smoking aggravates vasospastic ulcers. Trauma—even minor trauma—may trigger lesions in many of these diseases and is a special problem in venous ulcers. Cancer may occur in chronic ulcers, especially those associated with burns and x-radiation.

Determining the cause of leg ulcers may be difficult and confusing if the typical changes and sites of the 2 most common lesions—venous and arterial—are not present. Some of the causes of leg ulcers are listed in Table 23–3.

To arrive at a diagnosis, a detailed medical history is required, including details about the onset and course of the disease, review of systems, family history, travel history, occupation, medications taken, and treatments attempted. A careful general physical examination must be performed. Particular attention should be paid to the ulcer edges, walls, floor and base, and surrounding tissues.

Some clues suggesting the appropriate diagnosis are given below:

(1) Arterial ulcers: Dry, pale ulcers without granulation tissue; necrosis especially of the heels and toes. Pain with elevation; some relief with dependence. Insufficient pulses.

(2) Venous ulcers: Located near medial malleoli; venous insufficiency; hemosiderin pigmentation with edema, granulation tissue in ulcer base.

(3) Hypertensive vasculitis: Small painful ulcers located on the mid leg or ankle, especially in hypertensive females.

(4) Vasculitis: Palpable purpura; necrotic ulcers; black central eschars.

(5) Hemoglobinopathy ulcers: Family or racial history of spherocytosis, thalassemia, and sickle cell anemia; abnormal red blood morphology or hemoglobin electrophoresis.

(6) Cold reaction: Purpura, cold urticaria in cryopathies.

(7) Ulcerative necrobiosis lipoidica diabeticorum: Yellow or brown patches with prominent telangiectases surrounding the ulcer. Usual location on anterior tibia. Usually diabetic patient.

(8) Sporotrichosis: Ulcers develop proximally along the lymphatic drainage.

(9) Blastomycosis: Pustular vertical outer edge; gradual sloping toward center ("stadiumlike").

(10) Neoplastic ulcers: Persistent, continue to enlarge; failure to respond to treatment; occur especially in ulcers due to thermal burns, physical burns, chemical irritation, or x-ray radiation; chronic.

(11) Trophic ulcers: Develop over pressure sites, in skin that has markedly decreased or no sensation.

(12) Panniculitis: Develops in areas with abundant fatty tissue; causes include systemic lupus erythematosus, pancreatic disease, and tuberculosis.

(13) Pyoderma gangrenosum: Reddish-blue edges, necrosis centrally with undermined edges; associated with underlying diseases, especially inflammatory bowel disease, myeloproliferative disorders, and rheumatoid arthritis (Fig 23–3).

VENOUS LEG ULCERS

Essentials of Diagnosis

- Ulcer near medial malleolus.
- Presence of stasis dermatitis.
- Presence of hemosiderin pigmentation and edema.
- Venous incompetence.

General Considerations

The postthrombophlebitic syndrome may account for over 50% of venous leg ulcers. Stasis dermatitis, as a reflection of the postthrombophlebitic state or

Table 23–3. Classification of leg ulcers.

Vascular	**Metabolic diseases (continued)**
Arterial (large vessel)	Gout
Arteriosclerosis	Gauchers' disease
Thromboangiitis obliterans	Porphyria cutanea tarda
Periarteritis nodosa	**Infections**
Venous (large vessel)	Bacterial
Stasis dermatitis	Ecthyma
Postphlebitic syndrome	Furunculosis
Lymphatics	Sepsis
Chronic inflammation	Anaerobic: Meleney's synergistic ulcer
Vasculitis and small vessel disease	Acid-fast bacterial
Necrotizing vasculitis	Tuberculosis
Nodular vasculitis	Leprosy
Degos's disease	Atypical mycobacterial infections
Hypertensive leg ulcers	Swimming pool granuloma
Livedo reticularis with ulcerations	Fungal: superficial, intermediate, and deep
Livedo vasculitis (atrophie blanche)	Majocchi's granuloma
Cutaneous periarteritis	Blastomycosis
Pernio	Coccidioidomycosis
Raynaud's phenomenon and disease	Histoplasmosis
Connective tissue disease	Sporotrichosis
Hematologic	Nocardiosis
Red cell disease	Actinomycosis
Sickle cell anemia	Chromoblastomycosis
Thalassemia	Madura foot
Hereditary spherocytosis	Cryptococcosis
Polycythemia	Spirochetal
White cell disease	Syphilis, especially tertiary
Leukemia	Yaws
Dysproteinemia	Protozoan
Cryopathies	Leishmaniasis
Cryoglobulinemia	**Neoplasms**
Cryofibrinogenemia	Epithelioma
Macroglobulinemia	Squamous cell carcinoma
Platelets	Basal cell carcinoma
Coagulation defects, platelet disorders, thrombocytosis	Sarcoma
Metabolic diseases	Kaposi's hemorrhagic sarcoma
Diabetes	Lymphangiosarcoma
Necrobiosis lipoidica diabeticorum	Other
Neuropathy	Mycosis fungoides
Associated with atherosclerosis	

other causes of venous insufficiency, frequently precedes ulcer formation. Occupations and activities that require prolonged standing and sitting without opportunities for moving around contribute to venous stasis, edema, and venous insufficiency. Trauma of even minor nature may initiate an ulcer. Treatment of the ulcer or dermatitis with over-the-counter and prescribed medications may cause irritation or allergic dermatitis that further contributes to worsening of the lesions. These dermatitic lesions may then be a source of distant dermatitis (autoeczematization).

Clinical Findings

Edema, erythema, scaling, oozing, and crusting are skin changes associated with venous insufficiency. A combination of hemosiderin and melanin produces a reddish-brown pigmentation. Varicosities may be prominent. Ulcers usually form on or near the medial malleolus. Rarely do venous ulcers involve the feet. If stasis is persistent and chronic, brawny induration and fibrosis may lead to chronic and disabling ulcers.

The ulcers are red and shallow, and granulation tissue is usually evident within them. Size may vary from small lesions to ulcers involving much of the lower leg.

Complications

Bacterial infections may contribute to enlargement or persistence of the ulcer. The diagnosis of an infection is a combination of the clinical and bacteriologic findings, because bacteria are usually recovered from cultures whether or not true infection is present. Venous leg ulcers are particularly prone to allergic contact dermatitis from topical medicaments. The resulting dermatitis compounds the discomfort of the stasis dermatitis and can cause ulcer enlargement or produce dermatitis at remote sites.

Treatment

Many topical treatments have been recommended, including enzymes, hydrophilic beads of dextranomer (Debrisan), benzoyl peroxide, aloe vera, gold leaf, hyperbaric oxygenation, cromolyn sodium (Intal), biosynthetic dressings, and antibiotics. None have been satisfactory unless combined with treatment to decrease venous stasis.

The foundation of successful treatment is to restore systemic and local factors to as normal a state as possible. Every effort must be made to increase circulation and decrease venous stasis. The leg should be elevated, if possible, and prolonged standing should be discouraged. A form-fitted elastic stocking may be used to maintain fluid dynamics and minimize stasis dermatitis. Usually the thigh-high or pantyhose types provide the best support. Open-crotch styles are available for men. Modified Unna dressings as soft casts can be applied to the leg with greater pressure at the ankle and decreasing pressure as the dressing is applied proximally to encourage venous return and decrease edema. Additionally, biologic dressing may be beneficial. Antibiotics topically or systemically are used for infected lesions. Topical corticosteroids may be used to suppress surrounding dermatitis and local pruritus. Trauma should be avoided or devices added to protect the healed ulcer from injury. Surgical procedures such as split-thickness grafts may be beneficial and decrease healing time. Some of these basic principles may be equally beneficial for many of the other types of ulcers as well.

ARTERIOSCLEROTIC ULCERS OF THE LOWER EXTREMITIES

Associated findings with arteriosclerotic ulcers of the legs are hair loss, especially on the dorsal toes, atrophy of the skin, and nail dystrophy of the involved extremity. Peripheral pulses may be of poor quality or absent. Dependent rubor and pallor with elevation may be prominent. A peculiar reddish-blue discoloration may occur on the toes. Intermittent claudication is common.

The ulcers are usually on the heels and toes or other sites of trauma and bony prominences. They are pale and without granulation tissue. The base may be gangrenous or covered with a yellowish, gray, or black membrane. The ulcer is usually more painful with elevation and more comfortable with dependence.

The legs should be protected from trauma and cold. Patients should stop smoking. Vascular surgery, balloon angioplasty, or laser recanalization may be indicated if a large vessel is blocked. Vasodilators are not especially helpful. Pentoxifylline may be helpful by reducing blood viscosity. Biologic dressings may be useful. Amputation is indicated for significant gangrene.

REFERENCES

Auletta MJ, Headington JT: Purpura fulminans: A cutaneous manifestation of severe protein C deficiency. Arch Dermatol 1988;124:1387.

Baker WF Jr: Clinical aspects of disseminated intravascular coagulation: A clinician's point of view. Semin Thromb Hemost 1989;15:1.

Berg E et al: Rothmund-Thomson syndrome: A case report, phototesting, and literature review. J Am Acad Dermatol 1987;17:332.

Berndt MC et al: Drug-mediated thrombocytopenia. Blood Rev 1987;1(2):111.

Bolton-Maggs PH et al: Diffuse angiomalike changes associated with DIC. Clin Exp Dermatol 1988;13:180.

Callen JP et al: Pyoderma gangrenosum and related disorders. Med Clin North Am 1989;73:1247.

Carbonari M et al: Relative increase of T-cells expressing the gamma/delta rather than the alpha/beta receptor in ataxia telangiectasia. N Engl J Med 1989;332(2):73.

Carr ME Jr: Disseminated intravascular coagulation: Pathogenesis, diagnosis, and therapy. J Emerg Med 1987; 5:311.

Chenaille PJ et al: Purpura fulminans: A case for heparin therapy. Clin Pediatr (Phila) 1989;28:95.

Clancy JM et al: Treatment of leg ulcers with cultured epithelial graft. (Letter.) J Am Acad Dermatol 1988; 18:1356.

Colver GB et al: Unilateral dermatomal superficial telangiectasia. Clin Exp Dermatol 1985;10:445.

Comerota AJ et al: The diagnosis of acute deep venous thrombosis: Noninvasive and radioisotopic techniques. Ann Vasc Surg 1988;2:406.

Cruces MJ et al: Multiple eruptive verrucous hemangiomas: A variant of multiple hemangiomatosis. Dermatologica 1985;171:106.

El-Dessouky M et al: Kasabach-Merritt syndrome. J Pediatr Surg 1988;23:109.

Falanga V, Eaglstein WH: A therapeutic approach to venous ulcers. J Am Acad Dermatol 1986;14:777.

Ferreiro JE et al: Benign hypergammaglobulinemic purpura of Waldenström associated with Sjögren's syndrome: Case report and review of immunologic aspects. Am J Med 1986;81:734.

Flint SR et al: Hereditary hemorrhagic telangiectasia: Family study and review. Oral Surg Oral Med Oral Pathol 1988;66:440.

Gilliland EL et al: Bacterial colonization of leg ulcers and its effect on the success rate of skin grafting. Ann R Coll Surg Engl 1988;70:105.

Goldman MP, Bennett RG: Treatment of telangiectasia: A review. J Am Acad Dermatol 1987;17:167.

Golitz LE et al: Diffuse neonatal hemangiomatosis. Pediatr Dermatol 1986;3:145.

Haboubi NY et al: Zinc deficiency in senile purpura. J Clin Pathol 1985;38:1189.

Hansson C: Studies on leg and foot ulcers. Acta Derm Venereol Supp (Stockh) 1988;136:1.

Harrison PV: Split-skin grafting of varicose leg ulcers: A survey and the importance of assessment of risk factors in predicting outcome from the procedure. Clin Exp Dermatol 1988;13:4.

Heng MC: Venous leg ulcers: The post-phlebetic syndrome. Int J Dermatol 1987;26:14.

Invernizzi F et al: Hypergammaglobulinemic purpura of Waldenström: A report of serologic and immunogenetic studies and long-term follow-up in 18 patients. Ric Clin Lab 1988;18:23.

Jimenez-Acosta F et al: Response to tetracycline of telangiectasias in a male hemophiliac with human immunodeficiency virus infection. (Letter.) J Am Acad Dermatol 1988;19(2 pt 1):369.

Knupp CL et al: Thrombotic thrombocytopenic purpura in older patients. J Am Geriatr Soc 1988;36:331.

Lewis M: Leg ulcers: Getting skin to grow. Cutis 1989;44:123.

Oranje AP: Blue rubber bleb nevus. Pediatr Dermatol 1986;3:304.

Peery WH: Clinical spectrum of hereditary hemorrhagic telangiectasia (Osler-Weber-Rendu disease). Am J Med 1987;82:989.

Picascia DD, Esterly NB: Cutis marmorata telangiectatica congenita: Report of 22 cases. J Am Acad Dermatol 1989;20:1098.

Poon MC et al: Epsilon-aminocaproic acid in the reversal of consumptive coagulopathy with platelet sequestration in a vascular malformation of Klippel-Trenaunay syndrome. Am J Med 1989;87:211.

Prystowsky JH et al: Present status of pyoderma gangrenosum: Review of 21 cases. Arch Dermatol 1989;125:57.

Rossignol M et al: Skin telangiectases and ischemic disorders in primary aluminum production workers. Br J Ind Med 1988;45:198.

Ryan T: Management of leg ulcers. Practioner 1988;232(1454 pt 2): 1014, 1016, 1021.

Saleem S, Saleem A: Thrombotic thrombocytopenic purpura: A brief review of recent literature. Tex Med 1989;85:46.

Sato Y: Embolization therapy in the management of infantile hemangioma with Kasabach-Merritt syndrome. Pediatr Radiol 1987;17:503.

Schlesinger I: Ataxia telangiectasia: A familial multisystem disorder. Conn Med 1989;53:135.

Seagle MB, Bingham HG: Purpura fulminans. Ann Plast Surg 1988;20:576.

Seiden AM: Postoperative deep venous thrombosis and pulmonary embolism: Diagnosis, management, and prevention. Am J Otol 1986;7:377.

Settle EC Jr: Autoerythrocyte sensitization successfully treated with antidepressants. JAMA 1983;250:1749.

Sierakowski SJ et al: Thrombocytopenic purpura: A review. Cor Vasa 1988;30:60.

Sorensen RU et al: Psychogenic purpura in adolescent patients. Clin Pediatr (Phila) 1985;24:700.

Standen GR: Wiskott-Aldrich syndrome: New perspectives in pathogenesis and management. J R Coll Physicians Lond 1988;22:80.

Steinberg D et al: Lipoproteins and the pathogenesis of atherosclerosis. Circulation 1989;80:719.

Watzke H, Linkesch W, Hay U: Giant hemangioma of the liver (Kasabach-Merritt syndrome): Successful suppression of intravascular coagulation permitting surgical removal. J Clin Gastroenterol 1989;11:347.

Wilkin JK et al: Unilateral dermatol superficial telangiectasia: Nine new cases and a review of unilateral dermatomal superficial telangiectasia. J Am Acad Dermatol 1983;8:468.

Wong HY: Hypothesis: Senile purpura is a prognostic feature in elderly patients. Age Ageing 1988;17:422.

Yatsu F, Fisher M: Atherosclerosis: Current concepts on pathogenesis and interventional therapies. Ann Neurol 1989;26:3.

24   Diseases of the Dermis

Robert W. Goltz, MD

The dermis is composed of a complex mixture of collagen, elastin, ground substance, vascular tissues, nerve endings, and fat. While usually considered separately, no clear line can be drawn between the dermis and the underlying subcutaneous tissue (hypoderm) in certain disease states or normal hypoderm at some sites. Adipose cells are sometimes found high in the dermis and are particularly frequent in certain nevi such as involuting moles and nevus lipomatosus.

The dermis varies in thickness and density from layer to layer and from one area of the body to another. Its structure is adapted to its function; the reticular dermis supports and affords mechanical protection to the underlying organs, while the papillary dermis provides a nutrient bed for the overlying epidermis.

Any system of classification of diseases of the dermis is artificial. Disorders of collagen, elastin, fat, ground substance, blood vessels, or other components of the dermal connective tissue blend together. Diseases of the dermis are not always distinct from those of the underlying hypoderm; tumors or inflammatory processes frequently involve both. It is even difficult to make a sharp distinction between hereditary and acquired disorders. An example of this is neurofibromatosis, which is clearly of genetic origin, yet affected individuals may develop new lesions throughout life. Elastosis perforans serpiginosa, a disorder associated with several genetic diseases such as osteogenesis imperfecta, Marfan's syndrome, and pseudoxanthoma elasticum, does not appear until many years after birth. In cutis laxa, various members of the same family may have lesions at birth or may develop them many years later. Thus, any system of classification of connective tissue disorders is artificial and to that extent misleading. For additional comments, see Chapter 20.

CUTIS LAXA

Cutis laxa is a group of inherited or acquired diseases characterized by loss of normal elasticity, resulting in looseness and sagging of skin. Some laxity

is necessary for motion. In pregnancy, loosening of the connective tissue of the birth canal is an important part of parturition. The appearance of old age is largely due to increasing laxity of the skin, particularly in sun-exposed areas.

In cutis laxa, laxity may be localized or generalized and may be associated with significant connective tissue disease elsewhere in the body. Excessive laxness is generally associated with disruption and dysfunction of elastic fibers, with collagen being less clearly involved. In some cases, obvious damage to elastic fibers—and collagen to a lesser extent—can be demonstrated microscopically; in others, it has not been possible to demonstrate structural changes in elastin or collagen.

Defects of collagen such as occur in some forms of the Ehlers-Danlos syndrome may later develop areas of cutaneous laxity.

1.   GENERALIZED CUTIS LAXA
(Generalized Elastolysis)

Generalized cutis laxa has been divided into dominant, recessive, and X-linked genetic types, with concomitant variations in expression and severity.

Clinical Findings

The most severe form, probably recessive, is characterized by early onset of generalized sagging and bagging of the skin, producing a striking appearance of premature old age (Fig 24–1). Laxity of the skin is not limited to light-exposed areas but involves the entire body. Changes occur in connective tissues elsewhere in the body, resulting in pulmonary emphysema, multiple diverticula of the gastrointestinal tract and bladder, prolapse of the rectum, and multiple hernias at various sites. Severely affected individuals do not survive infancy. Others may survive to adulthood but with various disabilities. In some cases the earliest expression of the disease is evident in an internal organ. An example is tracheobronchomegaly (Maunier-Kuhn disease), in which laxity of the lids

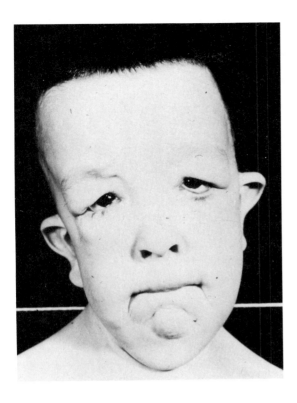

Figure 24–1. Five-year-old boy with recessive generalized form of cutis laxa (generalized elastolysis).

destroyed by too much stretching over the loose joints.

Extensive laxity of the skin may follow inflammatory diseases. A small epidemic of cutis laxa developed after an outbreak of an erythema multiforme-like skin disorder. Urticarial or erythema multiforme-like inflammatory lesions may be followed by loss of elastic tissue and laxity of the skin over extensive areas, usually on the trunk. In these cases, it is difficult to know whether the inflammatory disorder resulted in the destruction of the elastic and other connective tissue components or whether a breakdown of elastic tissue in these tissues caused the otherwise unexplained inflammatory process.

Treatment

There is no satisfactory treatment for the generalized form of cutis laxa. Attempts to tighten the skin surgically are usually followed by prompt reappearance of folds. Treatment of internal disorders such as pulmonary emphysema is symptomatic. Surgical repair of hernias and prolapsed organs may or may not be successful.

2. LOCALIZED FORMS OF CUTIS LAXA

Cutis laxa can also occur only in focal areas, either independently or as part of the syndrome of generalized elastolysis. Blepharochalasis (abnormal laxity of the lids) may occur as a result of aging or may begin early in life. Localized disease may be the only expression of cutis laxa or may be an early manifestation of a more widespread form.

Clinical Findings

A. Symptoms and Signs: The term "anetoderma" denotes loss of tissue in the skin, usually in coin-sized areas, sometimes with outpouching of underlying tissue (Fig 24–2). Loss of dermal substance results in "keyholing"––so called because there seems to be a hole in the dermis when the area is palpated. Patches of anetoderma may appear spontaneously or may occur after injury to the skin by inflammatory or infiltrative disorders such as syphilis, erythema multiforme, acne, urticaria, varicella, or lymphoreticular disorders. There may be a genetic predisposition to this condition.

B. Laboratory Findings: Histologically, lesions of anetoderma are characterized by diminution of the elastic fibers; in some lesions, there is loss of collagen as well.

Differential Diagnosis

Lesions of anetoderma need to be distinguished from neurofibromas. Localized forms of cutaneous laxity occur at sites of acne, usually on the upper back, shoulders, and chest. A form of localized cutis laxa, called perifollicular elastolysis, is caused by

and later of the entire skin appeared several years after the onset of respiratory problems.

Differential Diagnosis

The striking appearance of patients with fully developed cutis laxa is unmistakable. The sagging and bagging of the skin and the appearance of premature old age can hardly be mistaken for anything else. But cutis laxa must be distinguished from other congenital disorders in which the skin is thrown into folds, including the mucopolysaccharide disorders, the so-called Michelin tire baby, and the prune belly syndrome. Similarly, the pendulous lesions of neurofibromatosis could be mistaken for a localized form of cutis laxa.

Cutis laxa must be distinguished from cutis hyperelastica (Ehlers-Danlos syndrome). In the latter, the skin and frequently the joints are hyperextensible. However, the skin and joints return to original configuration when released from tension, whereas in cutis laxa the skin remains hanging loosely. However, after many years, patients with Ehlers-Danlos syndrome can develop skin laxity over the hyperextensible joints, perhaps because the elastic fibers were

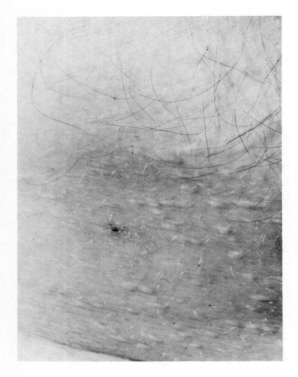

Figure 24–2. Anetoderma.

destruction of elastic fibers by elastolytic enzymes in microorganisms residing in the follicles. The distinction between perifollicular elastolysis and anetoderma following acne is blurred. Lesions of anetoderma in which there is loss of substance without significant outpouching must be distinguished from other forms of cutaneous atrophy, including morphea (localized scleroderma) and the atrophoderma of Pasini and Pierini.

Treatment

There is no way to treat this condition other than to avoid trauma that might produce inflammation and subsequently new lesions. Cosmetically objectionable lesions can be excised surgically, but this should be done with great caution because the wounds may not heal well and the scars may spread and gape.

Course & Prognosis

Lesions appear throughout life, though most arise during childhood and adolescence.

CUTANEOUS ATROPHY

"Atrophy" of the skin somewhat inaccurately denotes loss of substance of the skin. Both epidermis and dermis are usually involved. The skin is thin,

easily wrinkled, and fragile. Subcutaneous blood vessels show through. The dermal vessels, poorly supported by surrounding connective tissues, are easily ruptured at points of trauma and produce multiple bruises—so-called Bateman's purpura. Minute tears in the skin of the backs of the hands and forearms result in the development of "stellate pseudo scars."

Histologically, all components of the skin are involved. The epidermis is thinned, but the most striking changes occur in the dermal collagen fibers, which are markedly attenuated and spread apart. The elastic fibers are involved to a lesser extent.

Cutaneous atrophy is a normal result of aging. In the aged, it is particularly marked on light-exposed areas, where it is accompanied by hyper- or hypopigmentation, roughened lentigines, and keratoses. Senile atrophy is most obvious when exposure to sunlight has been excessive.

1. PROGERIA

Atrophy of skin may also be a feature of progeria, a disease in which the body ages prematurely. The causes of progeria are unknown, but the accompanying tendency toward development of cancer and immunologic deficits implies a profound disturbance of homeostatic mechanisms. Death occurs in most cases by the third or fourth decade.

2. IATROGENIC ATROPHY

Cutaneous atrophy is commonly produced by corticosteroids, either systemically or topically administered (see Chapter 53). Thinning of the skin associated with systemic corticosteroid use occurs everywhere on the body. It differs clinically from senile atrophy because it lacks epidermal changes on light-exposed areas. Corticosteroids apparently interfere with the formation of collagen. As in senile atrophy, stellate pseudo scars and Bateman's purpura may be seen; the latter is due to fragility of the poorly supported dermal blood vessels.

3. STRIAE DISTENSAE
(Striae Atrophicae)

Striae distensae ("stretch marks") are linear areas of thin skin. Their cause is unknown, but hormones influence development. Striae are particularly apt to appear at puberty, during pregnancy, during lactation, after corticosteroid therapy, or after abrupt changes in body weight. Common sites are the abdomen in pregnancy, the breasts during lactation, and at points of stretching of the skin. Striae also result from prolonged use of topical corticosteroids in occluded areas such as the inner thighs. They can appear in a bandlike pattern on the arms or legs or across the back in growing children given systemic corticosteroids. Striae frequently develop in weight lifters, apparently as a result of mechanical forces.

Histologically, striae distensae show absence of elastic fibers in the involved area and clumping and attenuation at the borders of the streak.

4. ACRODERMATITIS CHRONICA ATROPHICANS

Acrodermatitis chronica atrophicans is rare in the USA, perhaps because infection with *Borrelia* organisms appear to have only recently appeared on this side of the Atlantic. It is more common in Europe, where it occurs chiefly in middle-aged women years or even decades after inoculation of the causative organism. The initial event is a reddened, edematous thickening of the skin of acral parts such as the backs of the hands or tops of the feet, followed by pronounced thinning of the skin in these areas. This process extends proximally to the knees, elbows, or higher, sometimes as far as the trunk. In addition to thinning, wrinkling, and transparency of the skin (underlying blood vessels are visible), subcutaneous fibrous nodules occur. Ulnar bands are well circumscribed thickenings extending from the elbow to the fingers or over the tibia. The thin skin frequently ulcerates; resulting ulcers heal poorly, and carcinoma has been reported to develop in them. Frequently there is associated osteoarthritis as well as osteoporotic changes in the bones.

Acrodermatitis chronica atrophicans is probably a late sequela of *Borrelia* infection. Penicillin or tetracycline given over a long period prevents the spread of acrodermatitis chronica atrophicans, particularly if given early during the inflammatory phase.

EHLERS-DANLOS SYNDROME (Cutis Hyperelastica)

Essentials of Diagnosis
- Hyperextensible joints.
- Fragile, easily torn skin.
- Numerous widely spread scars.
- Ecchymoses and hematomas.

General Considerations
Ehlers-Danlos syndrome is of a group of hereditary disorders characterized by varying degrees of hyperextensibility of the skin, ligaments, joints, and other connective tissue structures, fragility of the skin and other organs; a bleeding tendency; and ocular defects.

The syndrome comprises a family of 10 or more separate genetic disorders with varying inheritance patterns, some dominant, some recessive, and some X-linked. Four have been linked to specific enzymatic deficiencies.

Ehlers-Danlos syndrome is primarily a disorder of collagen with lesser involvement of other components of the connective tissue. The skin is hyperextensible, resulting in the characteristic ability of the skin to be stretched far beyond its usual length, but it usually resumes its original shape after distention. The contortionists of the circus side show are frequently victims of Ehlers-Danlos syndrome. Other connective tissues are also involved, notably the supporting tissues of the joints. Involvement of blood vessels results in many of the other clinical manifestations of the disease. Until relatively late in life, many patients with Ehlers-Danlos syndrome are not obviously distorted; in late stages, laxity of the skin, scarring due to fragility of the skin, and joint changes may result in considerable cosmetic deformity.

Several types of Ehlers-Danlos syndrome show abnormalities in fibroblasts and in the synthesis or processing of collagen fibrils, with defective lateral aggregation and reduced fiber thickness. Specific enzymes or cofactors required for normal collagen synthesis may be lacking.

Clinical Findings
The skin and joints can be extended far beyond the usual limits but return to their original configuration on release. Cutaneous hyperelasticity is most marked over the major joints. Although the skin is not lax in the earlier stages of this disease, the skin of the hands and feet may be redundant from the outset, with pronounced wrinkling of the palms and changes in the dermatoglyphic pattern. Fragility of the skin results in easy tearing and bruising; gaping wounds may develop after the slightest trauma. Surgical sutures hold poorly. Characteristically, prominent scars are present over sites of frequent injury such as on the forehead, chin, knees, and shins (Fig 24–3).

There may be repeated subcutaneous hematomas; the combination of tearing and hematomas results in outbagging of skin—so-called molluscoid pseudotumors. Some of these calcify or ossify. Elsewhere, there may be loose scars containing varying amounts of fat and calcium. In the vascular type (type IV) of Ehlers-Danlos syndrome, the skin is markedly thinned and the deep blood vessels show through.

Ligament and tendon laxity result in characteristic hyperextensibility of joints in some forms. The hands are soft, and the handshake is characteristic. Hyperextensibility of the fingers allows them to be bent 90 degrees dorsally (Fig 24–4). The thumb can be opposed to the wrist; there is also hyperextensibility of elbows and knees. Patients are able to rest their hands on the floor when bending forward. A high-arched palate, long neck, and sloping shoulders are characteristic. Kyphoscoliosis and other spinal deformities are common, and there may be spondylolisthesis. Dislocations of the patella, hips, and temporal mandibular joints are common. Repeated distortion of the joints as a result of hypermotility eventually leads to degenerative arthritis of the large joints and the spine.

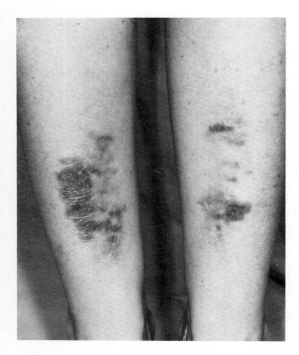

Figure 24–3. Characteristic scars on shins in type VIII Ehlers-Danlos syndrome.

There is a high incidence of hernias, diverticula, and eventration of the diaphragm. Pulmonary emphysema has been reported. Hyperextensibility can be demonstrated by Gorlin's sign, in which the tip of the tongue can be easily placed on the tip of the nose; however, a number of normal individuals can do this too.

Cardiovascular problems include cardiac valvular disturbances, aortic regurgitation, floppy prolapsed mitral valve, and tricuspid insufficiency. Aortic aneurysms and rupture are not infrequent. Excessive bleeding from the gums or after surgical operations is common, and postpartum hemorrhage is a serious risk. Microscopic or gross gastrointestinal bleeding is often present. There may be hemoptysis and hemothorax.

The bleeding tendency may be due in part to fragility of blood vessels of the soft tissues, but it is also due to biochemical factors. Various disturbances in clotting factors vary widely from kinship to kinship. Some patients have a deficiency of Christmas or Hageman factors, but other patients have a deficiency of platelet factor 3 or fibronectin.

The eyes may have blue sclerae, epicanthal lid folds, and various disturbances of the lens, including ectopia. Fragility of the eye may result in easy rupture of the globe or tears in the sclera. Glaucoma, retinal hemorrhages, and retinal tears often result in visual impairment. Angioid streaks on the retina have been reported rarely.

Patients with Ehlers-Danlos syndrome may extrude defective elastic tissue through the skin surface, giving rise to elastosis perforans serpiginosa, or Miescher's elastoma. This phenomenon and the occurrence of angioid streaks suggest that the elastic tissue may be involved as well as the collagen in at least some patients.

Treatment

Surgical treatment of the various defects may be attempted, but the tendency toward hemorrhage and poor wound healing must be considered. Avoidance of unnecessary trauma by protection of the fragile skin and joints is important. Excessive hyperextension of skin, ligaments, or joints should be avoided. Patients should be advised of the hazards of pregnancy because of the greatly increased risk of obstetric hemorrhage.

Prognosis

Recovery from Ehlers-Danlos syndrome is not to be expected. In milder forms, hyperelasticity of the joints tends to correct itself with aging. In other cases, relentless progression results in severe arthritic changes and laxity of the skin over the distorted joints. Death may occur as a result of various internal organ complications. For example, the life expectancy of patients with type IV Ehlers-Danlos syndrome is halved, since patients are prone to rupture great blood vessels, bowel, or gravid uterus.

PSEUDOXANTHOMA ELASTICUM

Essentials of Diagnosis

- Characteristic yellowish spots, papules, or plaques ("gooseflesh").

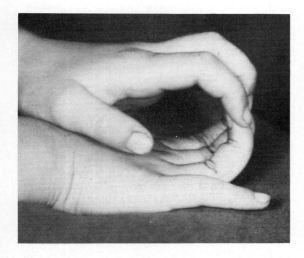

Figure 24–4. Hyperextensibility of joints of hands in Ehlers-Danlos syndrome.

- Angioid streaks of the retina and other ocular changes.
- Vascular disorders, including peripheral vessel disease, coronary artery disease, hypertension, and a hemorrhagic tendency with expression in the gastrointestinal tract or central nervous system.

General Considerations

Pseudoxanthoma elasticum is a rare multisystem disorder of elastin, and to a lesser extent, of collagen and ground substance. It is manifested by characteristic skin and eye lesions and a number of vascular disorders. In the ophthalmologic literature it is known as Groenblad-Strandberg syndrome. Most cases are transmitted genetically—some autosomal recessive and others autosomal dominant. The disorder may occur sporadically, usually in a localized form confined to the skin. It occurs chiefly in females and may be associated with Marfan's syndrome.

Clinical Findings

A. Symptoms and Signs:

1. Skin– Characteristic skin lesions generally appear after the second decade. They involve the face, neck, and axillae, the inguinal and ischial skin, the antecubital and popliteal fossae, and the periumbilical area. The skin appears relaxed, redundant, and yellowish—hence the name "pseudoxanthoma."

On the sides of the neck, the axillae, and the cubital and inguinal areas, the skin takes on the appearance of "plucked chicken skin" (Fig 24–5). It is yellowish, lax, and inelastic, with prominent follicular

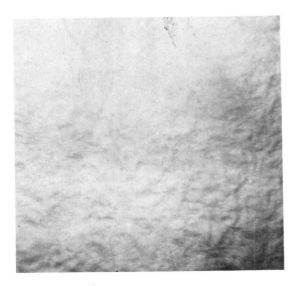

Figure 24–5. Characteristic "plucked chicken" skin on side of neck in pseudoxanthoma elasticum.

orifices. The mucous membranes of the soft and hard palate, the inside of the lips, and the vaginal and rectal mucosal may be similarly affected. Gastroscopy may demonstrate nodular or linear submucosal lesions in the lining of the stomach. Elastosis perforans serpiginosa may develop, most often on the back of the neck.

2. Eyes– The earliest ophthalmologic manifestations are mottling and pigmentary changes in the retinas. The characteristic angioid streaks are linear streaks in the fundi, wider than blood vessels and underlying them. Later, there may be scarring and hemorrhage of the retina, with loss of visual acuity. Central chorioretinitis may pose a grave threat to vision.

3. Blood vessels– The vascular system throughout the body may be involved. Damage to the elastic media of the small to medium-sized arteries leads to impingement on the lumen of involved vessels. There is endothelial and subendothelial proliferation, which may reduce the blood-carrying capacity of the involved artery to a fraction of normal. When that happens, there is intermittent claudication and easy fatigability of skeletal muscles and weakness or absence of peripheral pulses. X-ray examination of peripheral blood vessels shows medial calcification, and plethysmography demonstrates characteristic pulse wave abnormalities.

4. Gastrointestinal tract– In the gastrointestinal tract, hemorrhage is common and may be fatal. Occult blood in the stools is characteristic, but in some cases there is gross bleeding with hematemesis or melena.

5. Cardiovascular system– Patients have an increased incidence of coronary artery insufficiency, angina pectoris, and myocardial infarction. Coronary artery calcification can be demonstrated. Hypertension may result from peripheral vascular disease but especially from involvement of the renal arteries.

6. Other findings– The combination of hypertension and increased fragility of vascular walls greatly increases the risk of hemorrhage. Cerebral vascular accidents occur. Subarachnoid hemorrhage is particularly characteristic. Uterine hemorrhage may complicate the reproductive process, and hemarthrosis may result in severe joint damage.

B. Laboratory Findings: Microscopic examination shows marked disruption of the elastic fibers in the mid dermis, with calcification, and with greatly increased amounts of mucopolysaccharide ground substance nearby. In involved blood vessels, the medial elastin is disrupted. There is some alteration and fusion of collagen fibers near the altered elastin.

Treatment

Treatment is symptomatic and supportive. Patients should be advised against activities enhancing the tendency to hemorrhage and instructed as to the genetic nature of the disorder.

CONNECTIVE TISSUE NEVI

The connective tissue nevi are a group of rare conditions characterized by hamartomatous overgrowth and dysplasia of various solid components of the dermis. Solitary forms occur sporadically. A few familial cases, usually with multiple lesions, have been reported.

Clinical Findings

A. Elastomas: Nevus elasticus of Lewandowsky is characterized by overgrowth and distortion of the elastic fibers of the dermis. Clinically, a localized— usually grouped—collection of smooth skin-colored papules, sometimes perifollicular, form patches and plaques, which may be linear or zoniform. They occur most commonly on the trunk, particularly in the lumbosacral region. The diagnosis is made by biopsy.

B. Collagenomas: Connective tissue nevi of collagen are less easy to diagnose microscopically, since the dermal collagen, while increased in amount, may appear normal. Clinically, collagenomas consist of plaques measuring up to several centimeters in diameter. They usually occur on the upper trunk, sometimes the extremities. They are usually present at birth or appear shortly thereafter.

C. Adipose Nevi: Nevus lipomatosus of Hoffmann and Zurhelle is characterized by grouped yellowish nodules, forming plaques. They have a distinct predilection for the lower trunk and upper thighs. Histologically, there is proliferation of fat in the dermis so that fat cells surround the blood vessels as the vessels rise up from the subcutaneous layer and spread out to form the subpapillary plexus.

D. Shagreen Patch: Connective tissue nevi, whether of elastin, collagen, or fat, are not associated with systemic disease, but the shagreen patch is a sign of tuberous sclerosis. A shagreen patch is a large area of protruding skin resembling "shagreen leather" that usually occurs on the lower back. The diagnosis is based on the presence of the other characteristic lesions of the tuberous sclerosis syndrome, namely, fibrovascular papillomas on the face and ash leaf depigmented spots. Involvement of the central nervous system is manifested by a severe seizure disorder, varying degrees of mental deficiency, intracranial calcifications, and a distinctive "potato" deformity of the cerebral gyri.

E. Buschke-Ollendorf Syndrome: This disorder is dominantly inherited. There is an association of various connective tissue nevi of the skin with osteopoikilosis and mottling of the long bones, particularly in the regions of the epiphyses and metaphyses. The onset is usually in the second or third decade. Mostly symmetric nodules or plaques develop, chiefly on the thighs, buttocks, or abdominal wall. The connective tissue nevi are firmer than other connective tissue nevi and may resemble dermatofibromas.

Differential Diagnosis

Connective tissue nevi must be distinguished from congenital nevus cell nevi, which may have the same nodular and plaquelike configuration but are almost always heavily pigmented—in contrast to the normal or slightly yellowish skin color of connective tissue nevi. The latter also may resemble lesions of pseudoxanthoma elasticum, but they lack the characteristic multiplicity, symmetry, and predilection for the flexural surfaces. Localized lesions of neurofibromatosis may also resemble connective tissue nevi. The multiple dysplastic lesions of the focal dermal hypoplasia syndrome, in which the dermis is largely replaced by adipose tissue, have been compared with nevus lipomatosus, but the accompanying widespread dysplasia of ocular, dental, skeletal, and other tissues that characterize the focal dermal hypoplasia syndrome are not found in the Hoffmann-Zurhelle form of nevus lipomatosus.

Treatment

No treatment is needed for most connective tissue nevi, since they do not present a severe cosmetic defect. When there is a problem, surgical excision can be done.

THE FIBROMATOSES

The fibromatoses are a group of disorders in which overgrowth of fibrous connective tissue results in various degrees of dysfunction: fibrous hamartoma of infancy; infantile digital fibromatosis; juvenile palmoplantar fibromatosis; palmar and plantar fibromatosis in adults, including Dupuytren's contracture, knuckle pads, and Peyronie's disease; hypertrophic scars and keloids; and ainhum and pseudoainhum.

Fibrous Hamartoma of Infancy

Fibrous hamartoma of infancy is present at birth or soon after. Lesions usually occur in the axillae, neck, or trunk.

Infantile Digital Fibromatosis

In infantile digital fibromatosis, multiple smooth nodules on one or more fingers or toes are present at birth or develop within the first 3 years of life. Nodules are usually found on the extensor aspects of the fingers—especially the terminal phalanges—and are firmly attached to the skin.

Juvenile Palmoplantar Fibromatosis

Juvenile palmoplantar fibromatosis is characterized by nodular thickening, often over the thenar or hypothenar eminence or in the instep of the foot. Initial growth is rapid. Calcium deposits in a fine granular form may be detectable by x-ray.

Palmar & Plantar Fibromatosis in Adults

Palmar and plantar fibromatosis in adults includes **Dupuytren's contracture.** It has its onset late in life and occurs in as many as 18% of individuals over 75 years of age. It seems commoner in alcoholics and diabetics. Dupuytren's contracture is associated with an increased incidence of knuckle pads, keloids, and Peyronie's disease (see below). The earliest stage of palmar fibromatosis is an isolated nodule in the palmar fascia, generally at the base of the fourth digit. There is gradual contraction of the palmar tendon with pulling down of the fourth digit, interfering with extension of the fourth and fifth fingers.

Knuckle Pads

Knuckle pads are circumscribed thickenings, usually over the extensor portions of the finger joints. Over the course of months and years—generally in adult life—flat, smooth circumscribed nodules develop slowly. These nodules are most common over the proximal interphalangeal joints but occasionally occur over the knuckles or distal joints. Rarely, they may occur at other sites, such as the dorsum of the feet or the knees. They are sometimes familial but usually occur sporadically. Several kinships have shown an autosomal dominant inheritance pattern. An association with Dupuytren's contracture and other fibromatoses has been noted in some families.

Peyronie's Disease

Peyronie's disease—plastic induration of the penis—may occur in association with other fibromatoses, particularly palmoplantar fibromatosis, keloids, and knuckle pads, or as an isolated phenomenon. It has its highest incidence between the ages of 40 and 60 and rarely occurs in men younger than 20. It is characterized by painful erections and downward curvature (chordee) of the erect penis. There is a thickened subcutaneous plaque on the dorsal aspect in the distal third of the penis. Peyronie's disease is slowly progressive, but spontaneous regression may occur in up to half of case.

Treatment is generally unsatisfactory. Repeated intralesional injection of corticosteroids may result in improvement. Operative removal of the plaque may help in refractory cases.

Keloids & Hypertrophic Scars

There is no clear-cut difference between keloids and hypertrophic scars. Both are characterized by excessive overgrowth of dermal collagenous connective tissue. Keloids tend to grow indefinitely, whereas hypertrophic scars tend to reach a certain size, level off, and spontaneously regress. Keloids may occur in anyone but are sometimes familial; they are particularly apt to occur in blacks. They have a distinct predilection for the upper sternal area, the upper shoulders, the earlobes (from ear-piercing), and elsewhere on the face and neck. They are rare in infancy and old age. Their appearance increases in frequency throughout childhood, reaching a maximum between puberty and the age of 30. There may be endocrine factors involved, since they have been known to arise during pregnancy. Initially, there is a transient inflammatory phase with considerable redness.

Prevention of hypertrophic scars centers on avoidance of injury to the skin, especially in early adult life and in areas of predilection. Earlobe puncturing and excision of nevi and other congenital lesions on the upper sternal area or other keloid-prone areas should be done with great caution in young persons, particularly in blacks.

Treatment of keloids and hypertrophic scars is generally unsatisfactory. They tend to recur after attempts at surgical excision and can become larger and more unsightly than before. Intralesional injections of corticosteroids (eg, triamcinolone acetonide, 20 $\mu g/mL$) may be helpful, but it is difficult to obtain even distribution of the injected material, and an uneven surface thus results. Hypopigmentation is another complication of this treatment. Repeated application of flurandrenolone tape to the lesion often helps.

Surgical excision (eg, with CO_2 lasers) can be followed by x-ray radiation therapy or intralesional injection of triamcinolone acetonide, 2–5 $\mu g/mL$, to reduce the chance of recurrence. Prolonged application of pressure by special appliances after surgical removal may also prevent recurrence but is frequently impractical.

Ainhum & Pseudoainhum

Ainhum and pseudoainhum are names applied to constricting bands of fibrous connective tissue usually involving the dermis and subcutaneous areas of the fingers or toes. In Africa and other tropical areas where people go barefoot, constricting bands develop around the toes, perhaps as a result of repeated injury and infection. Progressive constriction of the proximal portions of the toes may lead to gangrene or spontaneous amputation. Constricting digital bands may also develop in hyperkeratotic disorders such as mal de Meleda and Vohwinkel's syndrome. Pseudoainhum has been reported in conditions leading to decreased blood supply such as scleroderma or Raynaud's disease, diabetes mellitus, or decreased sensation due to any cause.

On examination of constricting bands, special care should be taken to look for extraneous causes of constriction, such as hairs, rubber bands, sutures, or other foreign materials tied or entangled around the affected finger or toe. This is especially true in infants and children.

Treatment of constricting digital bands consists of surgical interruption of the band. Often this is permanently helpful, though the fibrotic constriction may sometimes recur. Occasionally, amputation of the affected digit may be the only alternative.

FOCAL DERMAL HYPOPLASIA

The rare syndrome of focal dermal hypoplasia consists of widespread dysplasia of mesodermal and ectodermal structures throughout the body. The syndrome derives its name from the obvious underdevelopment and dysplasia of the dermis with characteristic areas of thinness of the skin and outpouching of adipose tissue. It predominates in females and has been reported in several female members of the same family. There is a high frequency of miscarriages and stillbirths in affected families. The complete syndrome may be incompatible with life in males.

The occurrence of linear skin and bone lesions has led to the suggestion that this disease may represent a form of genetic mosaicism. Fibroblasts from affected skin show markedly reduced growth potential.

Affected individuals are usually small in stature and have facial or extremity asymmetry; some have mental deficiency or epileptiform seizures. Many other defects of the eyes, mouth, skeleton, and soft tissues characterize the syndrome, including small stature, oddly shaped face, skeletal asymmetry, hearing loss, and cardiac abnormalities.

Cutaneous abnormalities include the characteristic underdevelopment and thinness of areas of the skin, which may be in a reticular, vermiform, cribriform, or frequently linear distribution. In some cases there has been total absence of the skin from some sites at birth. Herniation of subcutaneous fat through the attenuated dermis gives rise to characteristic yellow nodules resembling lipomas (Fig 24–6). There may be telangiectases, and in some cases hyper- or hypopigmentation. Radial folds around the mouth are common, and papillomas around body orifices, including the lips, gums, tongue, anus, and vulva, continue to appear throughout life (Fig 24–7).

Disorders of sweating occur, including hypohidrosis and hyperhidrosis. The hair may be sparse,

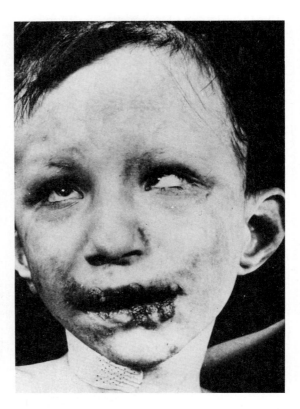

Figure 24–7. Facial hypoplasia and asymmetry, ocular defects, and labial papillomas in focal dermal hypoplasia syndrome.

brittle, or totally lacking from small areas of the scalp or pubic regions. The fingernails and toenails may be absent, poorly developed, or dystrophic.

These changes are usually present at birth, but an early inflammatory or desquamative phase, sometimes associated with blistering and crusting, has been reported in a few cases.

Surgical correction of some of the more disfiguring or disabling skeletal and soft tissue anomalies is frequently of value. Repeated removal of papillomatous lesions around the body orifices may be needed.

PERFORATING DISORDERS*

There is a family of several disorders characterized histopathologically by perforation of the dermis through the overlying epidermis as though the body were trying to extrude tissue (transepithelial elimina-

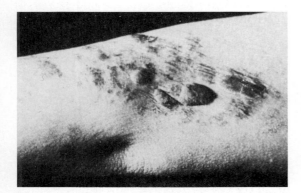

Figure 24–6. Adipose nodules due to protrusion of subcutaneous fat through attenuated dermis in focal dermal hypoplasia syndrome.

*Kyrle's disease is discussed in Chapter 21.

tion). The perforating disorders include elastosis perforans serpiginosa, perforating collagenosis, perforating folliculitis, Kyrle's disease, and perforation occurring in other connective tissue disturbances such as granuloma annulare and necrobiosis lipoidica diabeticorum and pseudoxanthoma elasticum.

1. ELASTOSIS PERFORANS SERPIGINOSA

Elastosis perforans serpiginosa results from extrusion of defective elastin through the overlying epidermis. The result is a circular or arcuate keratotic eroded lesion, often secondarily infected, with verrucous changes due to secondary epidermal hyperplasia (Fig 24–8). Elastosis perforans serpiginosa occurs as part of several connective tissue disorders such as Ehlers-Danlos syndrome, Marfan's syndrome, osteogenesis imperfecta, Down's syndrome, acrogeria, and Rothmund-Thomson syndrome. It may be familial. Men outnumber women 4:1. Some cases occur spontaneously without known association with other connective tissue disorder. It has been produced by penicillamine, usually given for the treatment of Wilson's disease or scleroderma. Penicillamine chelates copper, which prevents normal cross-linking of elastin. The disorder has also been reported to occur in association with renal disease.

Elastosis perforans serpiginosa usually appears during the second or third decade. A characteristic location is on one side of the back of the neck, but lesions on the upper extremities are not infrequent.

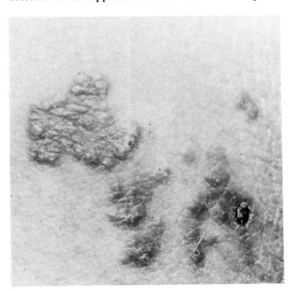

Figure 24–8. Arcuate and ringed hyperkeratotic plaques with extrusion of damaged elastin in elastosis perforans serpiginosa.

Involvement may be symmetric. Lesions have occurred on the face and lower extremities, but rarely the trunk.

Microscopically, there is epidermal hyperplasia with acanthosis and hyperkeratosis. Through the hypertrophic epidermis, abnormal elastin is extruded. The elastin in the upper dermis appears abnormal, increased in amount, and has poor staining and irregularity in outline of the fiber.

Treatment of elastosis perforans serpiginosa is generally unsatisfactory. Surgical excision may be attempted.

2. REACTIVE PERFORATING COLLAGENOSIS

This rare disease is characterized by extrusion of abnormal collagen through the overlying epidermis. It usually occurs in childhood, and a familial tendency has been reported. Sites of predilection are the backs of the hands, forearms, elbows, and knees. Small cutaneous papules (approximately 0.5 cm in diameter) have a central area of umbilication in which keratinous material is lodged.

No treatment is needed, since the lesions usually involute spontaneously. However, freezing with liquid nitrogen or electrodesiccation may speed resolution.

3. PERFORATING FOLLICULITIS

Perforating folliculitis consists of hyperkeratotic follicular papules usually on areas of friction with clothing, such as the extensor surfaces of the thighs, buttocks, or upper arms. On microscopic examination, these hyperkeratotic lesions show large keratotic plugs that have eroded through the wall of the follicle and set up a necrotizing inflammatory reaction in the nearby dermis. Necrotic connective tissue in turn enters the hair follicle and is extruded through it. The cause of this condition is unknown, but in some cases it has been related to wearing of tight clothing, especially stretch pants. Formaldehyde in synthetic fabrics has been suspected to be a cause.

4. OTHER PERFORATING DISORDERS

Perforation has also been reported to occur in diseases in which there is necrosis of connective tissue, including granuloma annulare, necrobiosis lipoidica diabeticorum, and pseudoxanthoma elasticum, and where there are hyperkeratotic plugs (Kyrle's disease).

REFERENCES

Altman LK et al: Pseudoxanthoma elasticum: An under-diagnosed genetically heterogeneous disorder with protean manifestations. Arch Intern Med 1974;134:1048.

Balus L et al: Granulomatous slack skin. Arch Dermatol 1985;121:250.

Beighton P: The dominant and recessive forms of cutis laxa. J Med Genet 1972;9:216.

Burgdorf WHC et al: Acrodermatitis chronica atrophicans. Int J Dermatol 1979;18:595.

Burgdorf WHC et al: Focal dermal hypoplasia in a father and daughter. J Am Acad Dermatol 1981;4:273.

Chan WY, Garnica AD, Rennert OM: Cell culture studies of Menkes' kinky hair disease. Clin Chim Acta 1978;88:495.

Danks DM et al: Menkes' kinky hair syndrome. Pediatrics 1972;50:188.

Duvic M, Pinnell SR: Ehlers-Danlos Syndrome. Pages 565–578 in: *Pathogenesis of Skin Disease*. Thiens BH, Dobson RL (editors). Churchill Livingstone, 1986.

Finlay AY et al: Juvenile hyaline fibromatosis. Br J Dermatol 1983;108:609.

Fitzsimmons JS et al: Variable clinical presentation of cutis laxa. Clin Genet 1985;28:284.

Fleischmajor R et al: Juvenile fibromatoses. Arch Dermatol 1973;107:574.

Goltz RW et al: Cutis laxa: A manifestation of generalized elastolysis. Arch Dermatol 1965;92:373.

Goltz RW et al: Focal dermal hypoplasia syndrome: A review of the literature and report of 2 cases. Arch Dermatol 1970;101:1.

Hammerschmidt DF et al: Maternal Ehlers-Danlos syndrome type X. JAMA 1982;248:2487.

Harris RB, Heaphy MR, Perry HO: Generalized elastolysis (cutis laxa). Am J Med 1978;65:815.

Hollister DW et al: Genetic disorders of collagen metabolism. Adv Hum Genet 1982;12:1.

Lewis PG et al: Postinflammatory elastolysis: Cutis laxa. J Am Acad Dermatol 1990;22:40.

Marchase P, Holbrook K, Pinnell SR: A familial cutis laxa syndrome with ultrastructural abnormalities of collagen and elastin. J Invest Dermatol 1980;75:399.

Mehregan AH: Perforating dermatoses: A clinicopathological review. Int J Dermatol 1977;16:19.

Neldner KH: Pseudoxanthoma elasticum. Int J Dermatol 1988;27:98.

Prockop DJ, Kivirikko KI: Heritable diseases of collagen. N Engl J Med 1984;311:376.

Scars JK et al: Papular elastorrhexis: A variant of connective tissue nevus. J Am Acad Dermatol 1988;18:409.

Uitto J et al: Focal dermal hypoplasia: Abnormal growth characteristics of skin fibroblasts in culture. J Invest Dermatol 1980;75:170.

Van Joost T et al: Elastosis perforans serpiginosa: Clinical, histomorphological, and immunological studies. J Cutan Pathol 1988;15:92.

Wilson-Jones E, Marks R, Pongsehirun D: Nevus lipomatosus: A clinicopathological report of 20 cases. Br J Dermatol 1975;93:121.

Wiswell TE et al: Infantile myofibromatosis: The most common fibrous tumor of infancy. J Pediatr Surg 1988;23:315.

Disorders of the Subcutaneous Tissue

25

José M. de Moragas, MD

The subcutaneous fat, or panniculus, lies between the lower edge of the dermis and the deeper tissues such as fascia and muscle. This layer of skin is responsible for the contour of the body and functions as a heat insulator, shock absorber, and nutritional depot, all of which are mobilized during starvation. This layer of fatty tissue is well anchored to the lower surface of the dermis but loosely bound to its underlying structures, facilitating mobility of the skin over the deep fascia.

ANATOMY OF SUBCUTANEOUS TISSUE

The fat lobules of the subcutaneous tissue are surrounded by strands of collagen, which contain the major vascular networks, lymphatics, and nerves in their path from the fascia to the dermis. The deep dermal vascular plexus, just superior to the panniculus, establishes connections with the vascular networks of the subcutis. The basic unit of the panniculus is the primary microlobule (1 μL in volume) formed by lipocytes, which manufacture fat. Each microlobule is supplied by one arteriole, 2 draining veins, and numerous minute capillaries. The secondary lobule (1 mL in volume) is made up of a collection of about 1000 primary lobules. The rich supply of blood vessels in and around the panniculus serves mainly thermoregulatory functions. As a lipid storage organ, the fat lobule is vulnerable owing to lack of vascular connections with neighboring structures, either surrounding dermis or adjacent fat lobules. Any defect in the vascular supply may cause irreversible damage to the dependent fat lobule.

REACTION TO INJURY

The subcutaneous fat is fragile. Physical, chemical, enzymatic, infectious, or immunologic processes may damage the vascular network or the lipocytes. The damaged panniculus clinically appears as a deep-seated inflammatory nodule. Fatty tissue reacts to injury in a characteristic sequence. The site of injury is first infiltrated by neutrophils, followed by lymphocytes, histiocytes, and eventually fibroblasts.

FAT ATROPHY

Fatty tissue is what gives skin its softness and contour. If fat cells are destroyed, removed, or otherwise not present, the surface of the skin appears depressed. If atrophy is generalized, the bony prominences give a gaunt appearance.

Localized or generalized atrophy of subcutaneous fatty tissue characterizes a group of uncommon disorders known as the lipodystrophies or lipoatrophies.

PARTIAL LIPODYSTROPHY (Barraquer-Simmons Disease)

Partial (progressive cephalothoracic) lipodystrophy is characterized by symmetric loss of subcutaneous fat over part of the body surface. Patients gradually (over several years) lose fat in clearly demarcated areas, often after some febrile illness. Wasting usually begins on the face and extends downward. Facial involvement produces a gaunt appearance. Females are affected 4 times as often as males. A decrease in serum C3 level was found in 70% of unselected patients with partial lipodystrophy. A circulating "nephritic factor" capable of splitting C3 was found in patients with partial lipodystrophy and membranoproliferative glomerulonephritis of the dense deposit type. This glomerulonephritis may lead to renal failure. There is complete absence of subcutaneous adipocytes in affected areas.

There is no effective treatment.

LIPOATROPHIC DIABETES
(Generalized Lipodystrophy)

Two forms of lipoatrophic diabetes are recognized: a congenital form, appearing at an early age (usually in the offspring of a consanguineous union, inherited as an autosomal recessive trait); and an acquired form, frequently developing after a serious illness with high fever, appearing in late adolescence.

The clinical patterns of both forms are similar. The loss of fat is generalized, involving subcutaneous fat and fat of the mesentery, retroperitoneum, and epicardium. The loss of facial fat pads results in the typical gaunt appearance. Mammary fat may be preserved. In the congenital form, hypertrichosis is present at birth. Curly scalp hairs grow nearly to the eyebrows. Acanthosis nigricans, hyperpigmentation, genitomegaly, and polycystic ovaries are associated features. There is accelerated skeletal growth and muscular development, with muscular hypertrophy. Cardiomegaly may be accompanied by asymmetric septal hypertrophy. These patients have insulin-resistant diabetes, with high plasma insulin levels, hyperglycemia, and absence of severe ketonemia; about 50% of patients also have complications of diabetes mellitus, such as retinopathy, neuropathy, and nodular or diffuse glomerulosclerosis. The combination of overproduction and defective removal of lipoproteins results in hyperlipoproteinemia of type IV or V, with an excess of serum chylomicrons and prebetalipoproteins. These patients have voracious appetites but gain little weight.

There is no effective treatment.

INSULIN LIPOATROPHY

Repeated injections of insulin may induce localized decreases in subcutaneous fat or, rarely, an increase in fat at the site of the injection, predominantly in female patients under 20 years of age. The atrophy appears 6 months or more after injection as an obvious depression with visible underlying vessels and fascia.

Rotating the site of injection minimizes the chances of insulin lipoatrophy. Spontaneous resolution of lipoatrophy may take as long as 10 years.

HYPERTROPHY OF SUBCUTANEOUS FAT

ADIPOSIS DOLOROSA
(Dercum's Disease)

Adiposis dolorosa is a rare condition of unknown cause characterized by localized overgrowth of subcutaneous fat that produces tender and painful tumorlike masses. It is not known why pain occurs. Middle-aged women are chiefly affected. Of slow and insidious onset, in an obese individual the fatty deposits may be diffuse or nodular, symmetric or irregular, and located on the trunk or around joints of the knee, elbow, and ankle. The pain ranges in severity from slight tenderness to agonizing. Asthenia may be incapacitating.

Surgical excision of individual tumors may sometimes be indicated.

PANNICULITIS

Inflammatory diseases of the subcutaneous fat are grouped under the general term "panniculitis." Many diseases cause panniculitis, but the clinical manifestations are often quite similar. Inflammation in the fatty tissues causes pain, tenderness, ill-defined erythematous nodules, and occasionally ulceration of the overlying skin. In the absence of ulceration, the epidermis is usually not affected. Because clinically the disorders appear similar, biopsy is often required to establish a correct diagnosis. Punch biopsy is generally inadequate because the fat will separate from the dermis at its junction, so insufficient fatty tissue will be available for histologic examination. Instead, biopsy should be excisional or incisional, utilizing a scalpel to remove a fusiform, full-thickness piece of skin including epidermis, dermis, and subcutaneous fat.

Panniculitis is conveniently classified on the basis of histologic examination into either septal or lobular types (Table 25–1). In septal panniculitis, the inflammation primarily involves the fibrous septa that separate the lobules of fat. In lobular vasculitis, the inflammation centers on the fat itself. Each type of panniculitis has been subdivided according to the presence or absence of vasculitis.

Table 25–1. Classification of panniculitis.

Lobular panniculitis
  With large-vessel vasculitis
    Nodular vasculitis
    Erythrocyanosis with nodules and pernio
  Without vasculitis
    Sclerema neonatorum
    Subcutaneous fat necrosis of the newborn
    Poststeroid panniculitis
    Weber-Christian syndrome
    Subcutaneous sarcoidosis
    Subcutaneous granuloma annulare
    Lipodystrophy
    Infections (eg, with fungi or bacteria)
    Lupus erythematosus profundus
    Pancreatic panniculitis
    Physical (thermal, mechanical, chemical) and factitial panniculitis
    Lymphomatous and leukemic "panniculitis"
Septal panniculitis
  With vasculitis
    Small-vessel
      Leukocytoclastic vasculitis
    Large-vessel
      Subcutaneous polyarteritis nodosa
      Scleroderma, acute lesions
      Thrombophlebitis
        Multiple segmental (migratory) thrombophlebitis (Trousseau's)
        Varicose thrombophlebitis
  Without vasculitis
    Erythema nodosum
    Necrobiosis lipoidica
    Scleroderma, chronic lesions
    Fasciitis with eosinophilia (Shulman's)

LOBULAR PANNICULITIS
(Nodular Vasculitis)

Essentials of Diagnosis

- Red nodules and plaques on the lower extremities.
- Usually ulcerate; heal with scarring.
- Occlusive arteriolar vasculitis and lobular panniculitis.

General Considerations

Erythema induratum is an old name for nodular vasculitis caused by tuberculosis. The disorder is a true vasculitis, and ulceration is due to ischemic necrosis.

Etiology

Nodular vasculitis is a reactive erythema with causes, course, clinical features, and histology that differ from those of erythema nodosum. Mycobacterial and streptococcal antigens have been found in the nodular lesions.

Erythrocyanotic changes develop in the lower extremities, with decreased fibrinolytic activity in the tissues. Immunoglobulins, the third component of complement and fibrin, have been found in the walls of the papillary dermal capillaries and in the perivascular tissue of the subcutis. Fibrin is usually found in the site of an antigen-antibody reaction.

Clinical Findings

A. Symptoms and Signs: The chronic recurrent, indolent, inflammatory nodules of nodular vasculitis involve the lower legs and calves. Bilateral involvement is common, but unilateral lesions may be present. The nodules, initially in the subcutaneous tissue, later involve the dermis and, in ulcerative lesions, the epidermis. The skin overlying the nodules is bluish-brown, scaly, and of almost normal temperature. The ulcerated nodules form ragged ulcers, with a bluish margin that heals by scarring. Flat subcutaneous plaques may heal with pits and scars. Perniosis, erythrocyanosis, livedo reticularis, and follicular hyperkeratosis may be present.

B. Laboratory Findings: The 2 cardinal histologic features of nodular vasculitis are occlusive arteriolar vasculitis and lobular panniculitis. The muscular arteries are involved in severe vasculitis. This produces ischemia in the fat and causes lobular panniculitis with caseation necrosis and a mixed acute and granulomatous infiltrate. Eventually, all or some of the fat lobules are replaced by fibrous tissue.

The tuberculin test is strongly reactive in some patients. The erythrocyte sedimentation rate is normal or moderately increased.

Differential Diagnosis

Nodular vasculitis is a noduloulcerative panniculitis found typically on the calves of young and middle-aged women. Some nodular eruptions of the legs are difficult to classify. They may have small nodules with or without ulcerations at various locations on the extremities or large, diffuse areas of chronic induration without ulceration. The chronic forms of erythema nodosum should be considered. Histologic examination will distinguish these disorders because nodular vasculitis is a vasculitis but inflammation is mostly lobular. The leg nodules of migratory thrombophlebitis are tender, cordlike segments that may extend to the thighs and occur in crops. The distinct linear fibrotic reaction is, however, recognizable on palpation of these tissues.

Complications & Sequelae

Chronic persistent ulceration may drain a serosanguineous exudate through single or multiple openings. Hyperpigmented, depressed scars are common residuals.

Treatment

Antituberculous therapy in nodular vasculitis is sometimes curative and may be used in patients with positive tuberculoid skin tests. Isoniazid, 5 mg/kg, and rifampin, 600 mg/d, in a single oral morning dose, should be given for at least 6 months. Other underlying causes should be sought and eliminated.

Aspirin (250 mg every 6 hours), nonsteroidal anti-inflammatory agents (eg, ibuprofen, 400 mg every 6 hours), or potassium iodide (10 drops of supersaturated solution in a glass of water 3 times daily) may reduce inflammation and pain.

SCLEREMA NEONATORUM & SUBCUTANEOUS FAT NECROSIS OF NEWBORN

Sclerema neonatorum and subcutaneous fat necrosis are 2 uncommon diseases of neonatal (first 3 months of life) subcutaneous tissue. Cold injury is felt to play an important role in both disorders. The biochemical disturbance in the subcutaneous fat may be the same for both diseases. The fat of the newborn has an increased ratio of saturated to unsaturated fatty acids, solidifying at a higher temperature than that of the adult. Histologic features are those of a granulomatous panniculitis surrounding lipocytes with multiple needle-shaped clefts within the cytoplasm. Subcutaneous fat necrosis of the newborn is discussed in Chapter 51.

Sclerema neonatorum occurs in infants seriously ill with pneumonia, gastroenteritis, or sepsis. The subcutaneous tissue of the trunk shows a rapidly spreading, diffuse hardening that feels bound to underlying structures. The skin is cold, and the face may appear masklike. Infants may die from infection shortly after onset of the skin manifestations.

Infants with subcutaneous fat necrosis develop red indurated plaques that become bluish nodules. They are usually well-marginated, firm, and immobile and typically form on the buttocks, cheeks, or extremities. They may drain, calcify, or slowly resolve but typically leave a dimple on the skin surface.

Treatment includes supportive measures and protection against exposure to cold. Fluid and electrolyte imbalance, metabolic disturbances, and underlying infection need prompt attention. Needle aspiration of fluctuant lesions may sometimes minimize scarring after subcutaneous fat necrosis.

LUPUS PANNICULITIS

The adipose tissue may be involved in both discoid and systemic lupus erythematosus (SLE). In cases associated with SLE, the systemic disease follows a benign course (see Chapter 21).

PANCREATIC NODULAR FAT NECROSIS

Essentials of Diagnosis

- Recurrent crops of tender nodules.
- Eruption accompanied by episodes of abdominal pain.

- Serum amylase and lipase levels are elevated.

General Considerations

Pancreatic nodular fat necrosis is a syndrome of recurrent crops of tender erythematosus subcutaneous nodules that appear in a patient with silent or severe pancreatitis or a pancreatic tumor of exocrine elements. Associated features are polyarthritis, fever, abdominal pain, lytic bone lesions, eosinophilia, and elevated serum lipase.

This is a rare disease occurring in adults. In patients with pancreatitis, both sexes are equally represented. In cases associated with pancreatic tumor, older males predominate.

Pancreatic lipase and colipase, escaping from the pancreas, have been incriminated as the cause of nodular fat necrosis, but the precise mechanism is not known. The vascular system, directly or via lymphatic channels, seems to play a role. In some patients, elevated levels of circulating pancreatic lipase are detected each time new lesions appear. It has been postulated that lipase hydrolyzes neutral fat to glycerol and free fatty acids, with resultant fat necrosis.

Clinical Findings

A. Symptoms and Signs: Pancreatic nodular fat necrosis has a wide distribution over the general body surface. More often in the lower extremities, a crop of raised, erythematous, tender nodules (< 2 cm in diameter) may appear over pressure points such as the tibia, epicondyles, thighs, and buttocks. In mild cases, the disease may involve only the supramalleolar area, resolving in 2–3 weeks and leaving a slightly depressed hyperpigmented scar. The skin lesions may precede overt pancreatitis by up to 3 years. In more severe cases, usually associated with a pancreatic tumor, the panniculitis forms part of a syndrome with polyarthritis, fever, fat necrosis of the bone marrow, lytic bone lesions, eosinophilia, polyserositis, low serum calcium levels, and elevated serum lipase. Occasionally, the nodules become fluctuant, break down, and drain an aseptic oily material.

B. Laboratory Findings: Serum lipase levels are elevated before the appearance of each crop of new lesions. Urine amylase levels may be normal. The white blood cell count is elevated, with 7–12% eosinophils. Calcium levels are diminished. The erythrocyte sedimentation rate is markedly elevated. Other abnormalities are secondary to the underlying pancreatic disease.

Pancreatic nodular fat necrosis is a form of lobular panniculitis involving portions of the fat lobule with adjacent portions spared. On histologic examination, the lipocytes have a fine basophilic granular material in the cytoplasm and a shadowy cell wall. They have been compared to "ghosts" of fat cells. The basophilia is due to saponification of the fatty acids by calcium salts. Peripherally to the fat necrosis, the inflammatory infiltrate is sparse (neutrophils, nuclear dust, and multinucleated histiocytes).

Differential Diagnosis

Erythema nodosum and polyarteritis nodosa have different clinical and histopathologic features. Inflammatory cordlike induration readily identifies the superficial thrombophlebitis commonly present in patients with pancreatic neoplasms. The vessel involvement in nodular vasculitis is not seen in pancreatic nodular fat necrosis.

Complications & Sequelae

Mild cases resolve, leaving a slightly depressed hyperpigmented scar. In severe forms, large fluctuant plaques are formed by coalescence of individual nodules draining through several openings. In such a fashion, large portions of the fatty tissue on the buttocks and thighs are destroyed.

Treatment

There is no specific treatment for pancreatic nodular fat necrosis. The treatment, if feasible, should be directed to the causative pancreatic disease.

WEBER-CHRISTIAN PANNICULITIS (Idiopathic Lobular Panniculitis)

Essentials of Diagnosis

- Tender, red subcutaneous nodules.
- Crops of new lesions appear recurrently.
- Symmetric distribution.
- Malaise, fever, and arthralgias.

General Considerations

The cause of this form of panniculitis is unknown, but it is a lobular panniculitis without vasculitis associated with systemic symptoms.

Clinical Findings

A. Symptoms and Signs: Crops of tender red nodules appear and resolve at intervals of weeks to months. Lesions are usually 1–2 cm in diameter but may be larger and tend to affect the extremities, especially the legs. Occasionally, the epidermis overlying the nodules breaks down and the lesion discharges a brown liquid oil (liquefying panniculitis). The development of panniculitis is accompanied by systemic symptoms of malaise, fever, and arthralgias. Objective findings of systemic involvement may include weight loss, nausea, vomiting, anemia, leukocytosis, leukopenia, and steatorrhea.

B. Laboratory Findings: The erythrocyte sedimentation rate is usually elevated. Changes in blood count, liver function tests, and other tests reflect involvement of particular internal organs, including the lungs, pleura, heart, pericardium, kidneys, adrenal glands, and spleen.

Histologic examination shows an intense infiltrate in the lobules of fat that consists of polymorphonuclear leukocytes and lymphocytes without vasculitis. Lipocytes degenerate and necrose, and fibrous tissue surrounding the necrotic cells stains slightly blue with hematoxylin and eosin stains. Later, the area may be infiltrated with macrophages and foam cells.

Complications

Ulcerations heal only slowly, and all lesions may leave scars or depressed areas of skin. Involvement of critical internal organs may cause death.

Treatment

Systemic steroids such as prednisone may be given. Doses as high as 60 mg/d may be required to suppress the disease, but lesser doses are usually adequate. Nonsteroidal anti-inflammatory agents can reduce fever, arthralgias, and other signs of malaise. Involvement of specific organs may require specific supportive drugs. Antibiotics such as tetracycline and immunosuppressive drugs such as azathioprine have helped some patients, but the results are unpredictable.

Prognosis

The course is characterized by exacerbations and remissions for at least several years before the disorder subsides. Scarring may result at sites of lesions. If inflammation involves critical organs, death may occur.

SEPTAL PANNICULITIS

In septal panniculitis, the fibrous septum is the area primarily involved with inflammation. This may occur with or without vasculitis. Septal panniculitides with vasculitis include subcutaneous polyarteritis nodosa, acute lesions of scleroderma, and thrombophlebitis. Those without vasculitis include erythema nodosum, necrobiosis lipoidica diabeticorum, scleroderma, and diffuse fasciitis with eosinophilia.

POLYARTERITIS NODOSA

Cutaneous polyarteritis nodosa is rare among the inflammatory nodular subcutaneous diseases of the legs. More prevalent in men, it appears in bilateral and asymmetric crops of pink or red nodules of small size (0.5–2 cm in diameter), usually below the knees. Livedo reticularis occurs after the nodules develop, more prominently in dependent areas or at points of pressure: legs, feet, buttocks, and scapulas. Ulceration may occur (see Chapter 37).

THROMBOPHLEBITIS

Both thrombophlebitis from varicosities and multiple segmental migratory thrombophlebitis can cause septal panniculitis and vasculitis. These diseases are discussed in Chapter 23. The diagnosis must be considered when the lesions are unilateral. Superficial migratory thrombophlebitis can mimic other forms of panniculitis, including erythema nodosum with multiple lesions, usually located on the legs. The nodules often assume a linear configuration that aids diagnosis. Superficial migratory thrombophlebitis is associated with underlying cancers, including those of the pancreas and lung. It has also been associated with hypercoagulable states, Behçet's syndrome, Hodgkin's disease, myeloma, and infections.

ERYTHEMA NODOSUM

This is the most common form of panniculitis and presents with ill-defined, tender erythematous to slightly xanthochromic nodules, usually on the legs. This disorder is discussed in detail in Chapter 35.

NECROBIOSIS LIPOIDICA DIABETICORUM

This disorder is often associated with diabetes. It is a very indolent form of panniculitis which in its earliest stages can present as a slightly violaceous patch but which usually appears as a slightly depressed, yellow, nontender patch, often with overlying telangiectases. The histologic picture is characteristic.

PANNICULITIS SECONDARY TO PHYSICAL INJURY

Pressure and cold are capable of inducing inflammatory changes in the subcutaneous tissue of unusually predisposed individuals. Pressure panniculitis appears as crops of tender erythematous nodules on the legs and arms 2–12 hours after local pressure or a blow. The subcutaneous fat is infiltrated with acute inflammatory cells.

Cold panniculitis appears in areas exposed to severe cold, such as the cheeks and chin. Inflammatory plaques appear 1–2 days after such exposure and gradually disappear over several weeks. Experimental reproduction with direct ice application has occurred in children under 6 months of age. The hypersensitivity to cold disappears as the child grows older. Pathologic changes include the formation of large cystic spaces caused by rupture of lipocytes. Later, granulomatous inflammation may occur.

FACTITIAL PANNICULITIS

Factitial panniculitis is a rare entity, self-induced by mechanical, physical, or chemical means. It has bizarre features and location, continuing for months or years with multiple acute nodules. It is more common in emotionally immature females with obsessive compulsive personalities. Many patients have some sort of medical career or training. Psychiatric studies are necessary to confirm the diagnosis. A strong degree of suspicion on the part of the physician is necessary for diagnosis. All other forms of panniculitis must be ruled out.

Self-injection of chemical substances may involve drugs such as morphine or pentazocine or organic (milk, feces), oily, or silicone materials. Histopathologic examination reveals the absence of vascular inflammation and a mixture of small foci of acute and chronic panniculitis. There are no specific findings except for the demonstration by polaroscopy of birefringent crystals or other foreign materials.

The patient who denies self-manipulation has a poor prognosis in spite of deep and continued psychotherapy.

REFERENCES

Anagnostakis D et al: Neonatal cord injury: Evidence of defective thermogenesis due to impaired norepinephrine release. Pediatrics 1974;53:24.

Blecher M, Barr RS: *Receptors and Human Disease.* Williams & Wilkins, 1981.

Chen TH et al: Subcutaneous fat necrosis of the newborn: A case report. Arch Dermatol 1981;117:36.

Conway SP, Smithells RW, Peters WM: Weber-Christian panniculitis. Ann Rheum Dis 1987;46:339.

Förström L, Hannuksela M: Antituberculous treatment of erythema induratum Bazin. Acta Derm Venereol (Stockh) 1970;50:143.

Förström L, Winkelmann RK: Factitial panniculitis. Arch Dermatol 1974;110:747.

Gilgor RS, Lazarus GS: Skin manifestations of diabetes mellitus. Page 313 in: *Diabetes Mellitus.* Vol 5. Rifkin H, Raskin P (editors). Prentice Hall, 1980.

Good AE et al: Acinar pancreatic tumor with metastatic fat necrosis: Report of a case and review of rheumatic manifestations. Am J Dig Dis 1976;21:978.

Gouterman IH, Sibrack LA: Cutaneous manifestations of diabetes. Cutis 1980;25:45.

Lynch HT, Harlan WL: Hereditary factors in adiposis dolorosa (Dercum's disease). Am J Hum Genet 1963; 15:184.

Panush RS et al: Weber-Christian disease: Analysis of 15 cases and review of the literature. Medicine 1985; 64:181.

Sarkany I, Macmillan AL: Recurrent nonscarring pressure panniculitis. Proc R Soc Med 1969;62:1279.

Winkelmann RK: Panniculitis in connective tissue disease. Arch Dermatol 1983;119:336.

26

Acne & Rosacea

John S. Strauss, MD

Inflammatory reactions in the sebaceous follicles are quite common and usually are accompanied by formation of papules, pustules, and abscesses—especially in areas where sebaceous glands are large, such as the face, chest, and upper back.

ACNE

Essentials of Diagnosis

- Pleomorphic disease with mixture of open comedones ("blackheads"), closed comedones ("whiteheads"), papules, pustules, nodules, and possibly scars.
- Onset chiefly in adolescence.
- Most commonly on the face; also on the back and chest, predominantly centrally.

General Considerations

Acne is a disease of a specific pilosebaceous structure known as the sebaceous follicle, which is characterized by a wide follicular canal (the orifice is visible on the skin surface), a short vellus hair, and large, multiacinar sebaceous glands.

Primarily a disease of teenagers, acne is not restricted to adolescence and may be seen much later, particularly in women, in whom it is common in the third decade. Acne affects 70–80% of all individuals in their second and third decades. The disease is slightly more common in males, as is severe involvement. Cosmetic disfigurement frequently results in emotional problems.

While there have been reports of greater and lesser incidence in various regions, this has not been proved; the reported differences may be related to differences in the socioeconomic acceptance of the disease. In the USA, acne is the most common skin disease and accounts for 25% of all office visits to dermatologists.

The follicular apparatus is small before puberty, when the follicle enlarges in response to androgenic stimulation. Under normal circumstances, the keratinous squamae formed from the follicular wall are easily shed.

The initial lesion of acne involves the accumulation of keratinized squamae in the follicular canal (the microcomedo). There is theoretical evidence linking the increase in sebum secretion accompanying puberty to abnormal follicular keratinization (Fig 26–1). On electron microscopic examination, these squamae are much denser, contain lipid droplets, and are adherent to one another. This adherence is probably the key factor in comedo development. Because there are no propulsive forces within the follicle, the accumulating keratinous material gradually expands the follicle and causes the epithelial lining of the follicular structure to undergo atrophic changes. The follicular mouth at this point is still narrow, and the initial lesion is not visible clinically ("microcomedo"). The initial clinically visible lesion is a closed comedo ("whitehead"). As further dilation of the follicle occurs, the follicular orifice dilates to produce the open comedo ("blackhead").

In some cases, instead of development of an open comedo, the wall of the closed comedo may rupture, spilling the follicular contents into the dermis and leading to development of inflammatory lesions. Whether a lesion becomes a pustule or a nodule depends on whether the resulting inflammatory response is superficial or deep.

Of the many important factors in the generation of the inflammatory changes in acne, foremost is the role played by the microflora, which is stratified. *Pityrosporum* species are found at the skin surface. A variety of aerobic cocci are in the superficial portions of the follicle, and *Propionibacterium acnes,* an anaerobic diphtheroid, is found deep in the sebaceous follicle. *P acnes* is important in the pathogenesis of inflammatory acne; however, acne is not a bacterial infection. Rather, inflammation probably results from the effect of extracellular products of *P acnes,* which include lipases, proteases, hyaluronidases, and chemotactic factors. Of these, probably the most important is a low-molecular-weight chemotactic factor diffusing out from the follicular canal and attracting polymorphonuclear leukocytes. When polymorphonuclear leukocytes ingest *P acnes,* they may release hydrolytic enzymes that may damage the follicular wall. Once the follicular wall has ruptured, other extracellular products of *P acnes* may augment inflam-

A

B

C

D

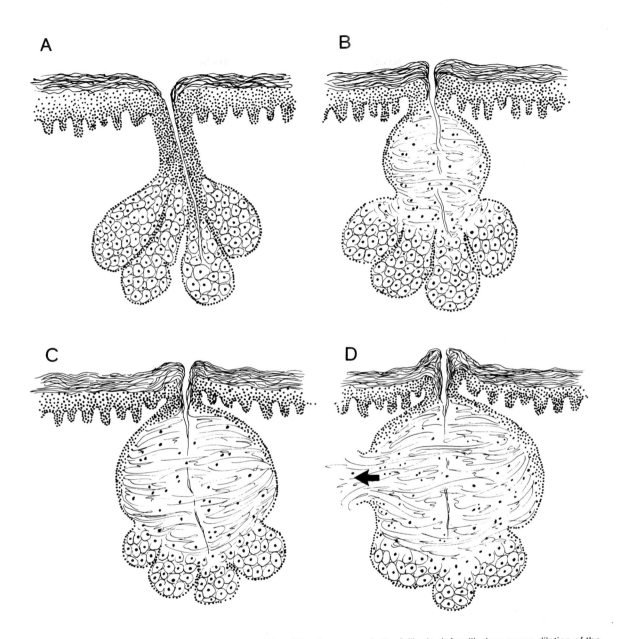

Figure 26–1. The birth of acne. Accumulation of keratinized squamae in the follicular infundibulum cases dilation of the follicular canal. Soluble products generated by extracellular enzymes and chemotactic factors from *Pityrosporum acnes* cause follicular rupture.

mation. The extruded follicular contents (lipid and keratinous components) can also induce inflammation.

Sebum is important in inflammatory acne; in its absence, acne does not develop. This is the basis for the therapeutic use of sebum-suppressive agents. There is a rough correlation between the functional capacity of the sebaceous glands and the degree of acne. Furthermore, glandular activity is greater in those with acne as compared to normal individuals. Sebum is irritating when injected into the skin; the free fatty acids generated by lipases from *P acnes* are the most irritating of the components of sebum. However, sebum's primary role may be to provide support for the growth of *P acnes,* since the number of organisms decreases greatly when the supply of sebum decreases.

Hormonal factors are important in the pathogenesis

of acne. Because acne is dependent on androgenic stimulation of the follicle, the disease is not seen in primary or secondary gonadal failure. Androgen levels may be increased in some patients with severe acne. While dietary factors were once considered of importance, there is no evidence that they have a significant role in development of acne. Instructions on dietary restrictions are not part of the current therapeutic program for the management of acne.

Clinical Findings

A. Symptoms and Signs: Lesions of acne occur most frequently on the face, chest, and back.

1. Acne vulgaris– The initial lesions are non-inflammatory closed and open comedones. Comedones are dome-shaped. In the closed comedo, the orifice is barely visible as a small central punctum. The orifice of the open comedo is much larger and has a varying amount of dark pigment at the surface. The inflammatory lesions range from small papules to pustules (Figs 26–2 and 26–3) to deep nodulocystic lesions (Figs 26–4 and 26–5). The scarring that may result from acne is usually pitted (Fig 26–6) but may be hypertrophic, particularly on the back and chest (Fig 26–7).

2. Specific types of acne– There are several types of acne; their names often reflect their pathogenesis.

a. Nodulocystic acne– This refers to presenting lesions that are primarily inflammatory nodules and fluctuant inflamed lesions often improperly called cysts.

b. Acne fulminans– This is an acute severe necrotic variety of acne accompanied by systemic symp-

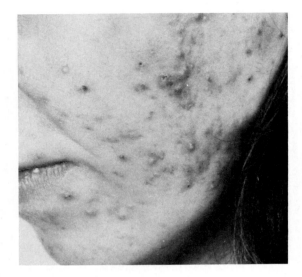

Figure 26–3. Moderate to severe acne with open comedones, pustules, and papules.

toms and signs including fever, leukocytosis, and arthralgia. It is rare and usually requires treatment with systemic corticosteroids.

c. Acne due to drugs– Certain drugs, including phenytoin, lithium, bromides, iodides, androgens, and corticosteroids, can cause acne when administered systemically. Topical and systemic corticosteroids are the most common cause of drug-induced acne. Comedones are usually absent; the disease is monomorphic, consisting of uniformly appearing papulopustular lesions.

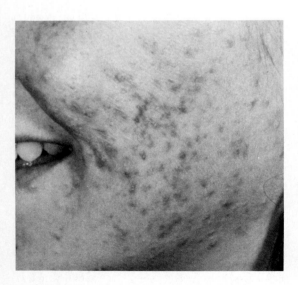

Figure 26–2. Moderate facial acne with a predominance of papular lesions.

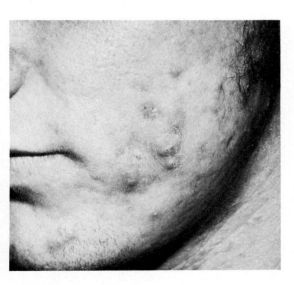

Figure 26–4. Moderate to severe acne with papules, small nodules, and scarring.

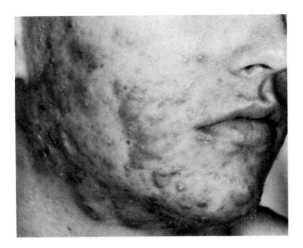

Figure 26–5. Severe acne with comedones, papules, nodulocystic lesions, and scarring.

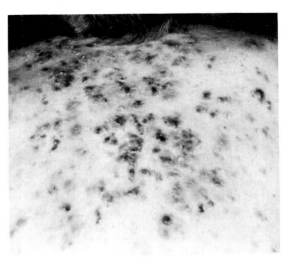

Figure 26–7. Severe nodulocystic acne of back.

d. Acne cosmetica– It is commonly believed that much of the acne seen in adult women is related to their use of cosmetics containing comedogenic materials. This assumption is probably grossly exaggerated; true acne cosmetica is probably quite rare.

e. Acne mechanica– Acne may occur from physical trauma such as rubbing. This is most common under chin straps of helmets worn by athletes.

f. Acne detergens– Whether this is a specific entity or a variety of acne mechanica remains to be determined. It occurs in some patients who are compulsive face-washers.

g. Gram-negative folliculitis– A rare result of chronic antibiotic treatment (see below) is the development of a superimposed gram-negative infection of the skin. Seeding of the gram-negative organisms probably comes from the nares. Two types of clinical lesions are seen: (1) inflammatory pustules with a large inflammatory areola, and (2) highly inflammatory fluctuant nodular lesions. Patients being treated

with antibiotics should be checked for gram-negative folliculitis if there is a sudden flare-up of previously well-controlled disease. Treatment of gram-negative folliculitis should be guided by the results of antibiotic sensitivity testing. Oral isotretinoin is the treatment of choice.

B. Laboratory Findings: Acne fulminans is accompanied by leukocytosis and an increased sedimentation rate. There may be increased androgen levels in some cases of acne, particularly treatment-resistant acne in older women.

Differential Diagnosis

The diagnosis is usually not difficult. Differentiation between ordinary acne vulgaris and acne rosacea depends on the presence of the vascular component and the absence of comedones in the latter. Differentiation of the various special forms of acne depends on an adequate history. As mentioned above, drug-induced acne is usually monomorphic.

Complications & Sequelae

Acne may have a profound psychologic effect on the teenager, especially if it is severe.

Scarring is a sequela already mentioned.

Prevention

There is no method of preventing acne vulgaris. Precipitating exogenous agents should be avoided when possible.

Treatment

A. Principles of Therapy: First one must establish whether the patient has predominant noninflammatory or inflammatory disease. The 4 principles in treating acne are listed below. The first one should

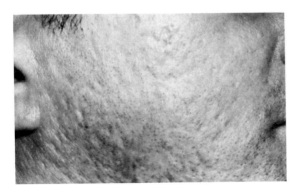

Figure 26–6. Pitted acne scarring.

dictate the primary approach in noninflammatory acne, the remaining 3 principles in treating inflammatory acne.

1. Reverse the altered pattern of keratinization within the follicle.

2. Decrease the intrafollicular *P acnes* population or the generation of extracellular inflammatory agents.

3. Decrease sebaceous gland activity.

4. Decrease inflammation.

B. Specific Agents:

1. Topical therapy–

a. Vitamin A acid (all-*trans*-retinoic acid, tretinoin)– Tretinoin is the principal drug for topical use in comedonal acne; it is a potent comedolytic agent. It is available as a gel, cream, or lotion. The lotion is potentially more irritating than either of the other forms; in general, the creams are less irritating. With either a cream or gel, therapy should be started in the lowest concentration. If there is any concern about irritation, applications should be started every other day and then increased in frequency and concentration as tolerated. Less irritation develops if vitamin A acid is applied at least one-half hour after washing. Patients should be cautioned about exposure to sunlight, because the drug can increase sun sensitivity. While vitamin A acid is indicated chiefly for comedonal acne, it also has some benefit in inflammatory acne and helps to prevent inflammatory lesions as they arise from comedones.

b. Salicylic acid– Salicylic acid is comedolytic but probably not as effective as vitamin A acid. It may be of particular use in patients intolerant of vitamin A acid.

c. Benzoyl peroxide– Benzoyl peroxide is an extremely effective topical antibacterial agent; topical application results in marked suppression of *P acnes*. It has slight comedolytic properties but is far inferior to vitamin A acid as a comedolytic agent. Therefore, benzoyl peroxide is most effective when used for inflammatory acne. By inhibiting the bacterial flora (particularly *P acnes*), it decreases the generation of inflammatory components. Most over-the-counter acne products contain benzoyl peroxide in a lotion base. The prescription items contain benzoyl peroxide in a gel base. Some irritation may follow the use of benzoyl peroxide. Allergic sensitization has occurred infrequently.

d. Sulfur and resorcinol– These agents are found in a few over-the-counter preparations. Their mechanism of action is unknown.

e. Topical antibiotics– Tetracycline, erythromycin, clindamycin, and meclocycline have been used topically for acne. Their effect, as with benzoyl peroxide, is antibacterial. They probably are not as effective as benzoyl peroxide except in mild inflammatory acne. While the literature states they are as effective as systemic tetracycline, this statement is based on trials in which full therapeutic dosages of systemic tetracyclines were not used.

A relatively new preparation that combines 3% erythromycin with 5% benzoyl peroxide in a gel base may be more effective than either component used alone.

2. Physical therapy–

a. Acne surgery– Surgery removes open comedones, closed comedones, and sometimes the very small pustules. The instrument used (comedo extractor) has a flat surface with a central orifice. When uniform pressure is exerted around the lesion, its contents are expressed through the central orifice. The orifices of closed comedones may need to be enlarged first with a small needle. The need for puncturing can usually be avoided by the use of vitamin A acid topically for 3–4 weeks, which softens the closed comedones. Removal of closed comedones is important because they are the precursors of inflammatory lesions. Open comedones are removed only for cosmetic reasons; they probably do not become inflammatory unless manipulated by the patient.

b. Intralesional therapy– The direct injection of corticosteroids intralesionally (eg, triamcinolone acetonide, 2.5–5 mg/mL) has an anti-inflammatory effect and is of great benefit in reducing inflammation in nodulocystic lesions. No more than 0.1 mL should be injected in order to avoid tissue atrophy and a depressed scar. Intralesional therapy is appropriate only for the larger cysts and should not be used for papules and pustules. Specific instruction on the use of intralesional therapy should be sought from a physician experienced in its application.

c. Ultraviolet light– This therapy has been used commonly to mask erythema. It is not very effective otherwise if it is effective at all. Acne is just as common in geographic regions where sun exposure is great as it is in more northern areas.

3. Systemic therapy–

a. Antibiotics– Ten percent of all tetracycline sold in the USA is used for acne. The major effect is probably antibacterial. Whether it has other beneficial effects remains to be seen. The initial starting dosage is 750–1000 mg/d in divided doses, with decreases governed by the clinical response. As stated previously, acne is not a bacterial disease; the activity of systemic antibiotic therapy is probably related to a decrease in the generation of extracellular inflammatory agents by *P acnes*. Treatment, then, prevents the development of additional inflammatory lesions. The response is slow because the preexisting lesions must undergo their natural course of involution. In some cases of severe resistant acne, 2–3 g/d of tetracycline may be of benefit. Laboratory parameters must be followed carefully in such patients.

Erythromycin is probably just as effective as tetracycline and is indicated for management of patients unable to comply with the requirement that tetracycline be taken at least 1 hour before or after meals. Minocycline is also effective for treatment-resistant acne in a dose of 50–100 mg twice daily;

however, at present, because of its cost it should not be used as a first-line drug in acne. Patients receiving this antibiotic should be carefully monitored for side effects such as drug deposition at sites of acne lesions, causing black macules.

b. Dapsone– This drug has been used for treatment-resistant disease with variable but in some cases excellent results. Physicians should familiarize themselves with the possible side effects of dapsone and should carefully monitor the patients. The mechanism of action is unknown.

c. Corticosteroids– Systemic corticosteroids have 2 mechanisms of action. In small dosages, they inhibit androgen production when administered to individuals with evidence of hyperadrenalism. In larger doses, corticosteroids exert an anti-inflammatory effect. However, for this purpose it is better to administer corticosteroids intralesionally; systemic administration can produce steroid acne. Systemic corticosteroid therapy is of great value in the management of patients with acne fulminans.

d. Sebum-suppressive agents– Because sebum is essential in the pathogenesis of the inflammatory disease, methods of inhibiting sebaceous gland activity have been used to control the disease, including corticosteroids. An antiandrogen, cyproterone acetate, has been used in Europe with success.

Pharmacologic dosages of estrogens inhibit the sebaceous gland. Good suppression is achieved with 0.75–1 mg of ethinyl estradiol or its equivalent given in cyclic fashion (ie, 20 days each cycle). Estrogens are indicated only in female patients with treatment-resistant acne.

e. Oral retinoids– Orally administered 13-*cis*-retinoic acid (isotretinoin) is very effective in the management of patients with severe nodulocystic acne unresponsive to other treatment regimens. Isotretinoin has produced not only remarkable clearing in patients with severe nodulocystic acne but also remissions that have persisted for years in most patients. When treated with adequate dosages of isotretinoin, 9 out of 10 patients with severe nodulocystic acne do not require any subsequent therapy or are easily controlled with more conventional agents. Isotretinoin therapy has been accompanied by many clinical side effects; the drug produces the spectrum of symptoms characteristic of chronic hypervitaminosis A. These side effects prominently involve the integumentary system and include cheilitis, dry mouth, xerosis, pruritus, epistaxis, petechiae, and conjunctivitis and eye irritation. Neuromuscular symptoms are common, and there often are dose-related elevations of serum triglyceride levels accompanied by decreases in high-density lipoproteins.

This drug, as well as other vitamin A analogues, is capable of causing pseudotumor cerebri when given in high doses, though the syndrome has not been observed very often in patients treated for acne.

Asymptomatic bony hyperostoses have also been seen in patients treated with isotretinoin.

The greatest problem related to use of the drug is that it is a potent teratogen and absolutely contraindicated in pregnancy. Retinoic acid embryopathy occurs early in pregnancy during organogenesis and involves abnormalities of the central nervous system, craniofacial tissues, the vascular system, and the thymus. Because of the potential for injury to the fetus, isotretinoin should be prescribed only by physicians who are fully trained in the diagnosis and management of severe nodulocystic acne and fully acquainted with the hazards associated with administration of this drug. Patients requiring isotretinoin therapy should be referred to such specialists.

Course & Prognosis

The course of acne varies greatly. Untreated acne probably lasts for about 7 years, but the duration can easily be influenced by environmental factors. The prognosis is excellent in most cases, but when acne is severe, considerable scarring may result.

ROSACEA & ACNE ROSACEA

Essentials of Diagnosis

- Ruddy complexion characterized by vascular dilatation with or without acneiform papules and pustules.
- Involvement of the nose often accompanied by sebaceous hyperplasia (rhinophyma).
- Preferentially affects the central face.
- Flush is often exacerbated by heat, alcohol, emotions, and other factors.

General Considerations

Rosacea is a common condition. Although it has no direct relationship to acne vulgaris, acnelike lesions are often part of the spectrum of the disease. When only the vascular lesions are present, the unmodified term "rosacea" is used. Rosacea commonly affects men and women in the age group from 20 to 50 years or older. The disease is more common in women but more severe in men. Native Americans and Caucasians seem more prone to the disorder than blacks and Asians.

The cause is not known. Patients with rosacea are prone to blushing and flushing and have ruddy complexions. Prolonged vasodilation can lead to telangiectases and probably to stimulation of the sebaceous unit, leading to acneiform papules and pustules. The sebaceous follicles are often patulous, particularly on the nose. The mite *Demodex folliculorum*, a normal inhabitant of facial follicles, has been implicated as a cause of the acneiform eruptions of rosacea, but this is unproved.

There are dilated capillaries in the superficial dermis. The acneiform papules and pustules show a perifollicular inflammation that mimics the histologic picture of acne.

Clinical Findings

A. Symptoms and Signs: Patients complain that their skin often is sensitive and easily irritated. It feels hot to them, especially during flushing episodes. Acneiform papules, if present, may be painful.

Typically, erythema is present over the cheeks, nose, and glabella. The chin and forehead are often affected, but erythema is usually mostly limited to the central face. Areas blanch on pressure. The erythema often fluctuates in intensity from minute to minute. Emotional flushing can be pronounced.

Acneiform papules and pustules mimic acne vulgaris. However, closed and open comedones are not usually seen. In severe cases, the pustular component may lead to cystic or granulomatous nodules. When acnelike lesions are present, the condition is referred to as **acne rosacea.**

A particularly distressing part of the syndrome is enlargement of the nose due to sebaceous and fibrous hyperplasia. This is known as rhinophyma, and in its ultimate expression is manifested by the "W.C. Fields" nose. Ingestion of alcohol causes facial flushing, so chronic alcoholism may predispose patients with rosacea to rhinophyma. However, not all patients with rhinophyma are alcoholics.

B. Laboratory Findings: There are no helpful laboratory findings.

Differential Diagnosis

The central facial erythema is mimicked by a ruddy complexion, mild irritant dermatitis, and seborrheic dermatitis. The butterfly erythema of systemic lupus erythematosus can occasionally lead to confusion. Flushing may suggest carcinoid syndrome or a drug reaction to vasodilators such as nicotinic acid. The papules of acne may be confused with acne vulgaris, but comedones are usually not present. Chronically persisting papules may have a granulomatous appearance and both clinically and histologically may mimic a mycobacterial infection such as cutaneous tuberculosis.

Complications & Sequelae

When the disease is present for prolonged intervals, patients with rosacea typically develop telangiectases over the affected blush areas. The nose may become huge and irregularly thickened (rhinophyma), with large follicular orifices that are usually compacted with black sebaceous material mimicking blackheads. Ocular lesions may include blepharitis, conjunctivitis, episcleritis, iritis, and keratitis (see Chapter 49). Keratitis may lead to ulceration and vision loss.

Prevention

Although rosacea cannot be prevented, the paroxysmal vascular flushing episodes can be minimized by identifying trigger factors and avoiding them. These irritants may be sunlight, heat, drugs, spicy foods, alcoholic drinks, and emotional embarrassment, although the exact relationship of these precipitating factors has not been determined. Early effective and prolonged treatment may minimize the development of telangiectases, rhinophyma, and ocular disease.

Treatment

A. Systemic Treatment: There is no good antagonist to the mediators causing the vascular blushing. However, the acneiform component of this disease typically responds to systemic antibiotics such as tetracycline or erythromycin in dosages of 250–1000 mg/d, as does acne. The dose may need to be adjusted depending upon response and patient size.

B. Topical Treatment: Topical treatments should be nonirritating to avoid exacerbating the flushing. Topical medications containing sulfur seem to be particularly helpful. Useful products include Rezamid, Liquimat, and Sulfacet-R. Topical corticosteroids are usually not recommended, and in fact the use of potent topical corticosteroids, particularly fluorinated ones, may be associated with a severe rebound phenomenon with a marked acne component when treatment is withdrawn. Furthermore, these corticosteroids are likely to increase the vascular dilatation for which the drug is being given. Topical antibiotics are also useful, particularly for the management of acneiform lesions. Recently it has been shown that rosacea can also be treated with metronidazole, 0.75% in water-base gel applied twice daily. This treatment is usually well tolerated but has no effect on telangiectasias.

C. Surgical Measures: The excessive tissue of rhinophyma can be removed by scalpel, electrosurgery, or laser. Telangiectasis can be treated with a flash-pulse tunable dye laser.

Course & Prognosis

Rosacea tends to run a long course lasting decades. If there is any indication of ocular lesions, the patient should be seen by an ophthalmologist for treatment, because ocular rosacea may lead to seriously impaired vision.

REFERENCES

Bleicher PA, Charles JH, Sober AJ: Topical metronidazole therapy for rosacea. Arch Dermatol 1987;123:609.

Downing DT et al: Essential fatty acids and acne. J Am Acad Dermatol 1986;14:221.

Ellis CN, Stawiski MA: The treatment of perioral dermatitis, acne rosacea, and seborrheic dermatitis. Med Clin North Am 1982;66:819.

Harris HH et al: Sustainable rates of sebum secretion in acne patients and matched normal control subjects. J Am Acad Dermatol 1983;8:200.

Knutson DD: Ultrastructural observations in acne vulgaris: The normal sebaceous follicle and acne lesions. J Invest Dermatol 1974;62:288.

Lavker RM, Leyden JJ, McGinley KJ: The relationship between bacteria and the abnormal follicular keratinization in acne vulgaris. J Invest Dermatol 1981; 77:325.

Leyden JJ, McGinley KJ, Kligman AM: Tetracycline and minocycline treatment: Effects of skin-surface lipid levels and *Propionibacterium acnes*. Arch Dermatol 1982; 118:19.

Leyden JJ et al: *Propionibacterium* levels in patients with and without acne vulgaris. J Invest Dermatol 1975; 65:382.

Marks R: Concepts in the pathogenesis of rosacea. Br J Dermatol 1968;80:170.

Marples RR, Downing DT, Kligman AM: Control of free fatty acids in human surface lipids by *Corynebacterium acnes*. J Invest Dermatol 1971;56:127.

Marples RR et al: The skin microflora in acne vulgaris. J Invest Dermatol 1974;62:37.

Pochi PE: Acne: Endocrinologic aspects. Cutis 1982; 30:212.

Stern RS: When a uniquely effective drug is teratogenic: The case of isotretinoin. N Engl J Med 1989;320:1007.

Strauss JS, Kligman AM: The pathologic dynamics of acne vulgaris. Arch Dermatol 1960;82:779.

Strauss JS, Pochi PE: Histologic observations following intracutaneous injection of sebum and comedones. Arch Dermatol 1965;92:443.

Strauss JS, Pochi PE, Downing DT: Acne: Perspectives. J Invest Dermatol 1974;62:321.

Tucker SB et al: Inflammation in acne vulgaris: Leukocyte attraction and cytotoxicity by comedonal material. J Invest Dermatol 1980;74:21.

Webster GF, Leyden JJ: Characterization of serum-independent polymorphonuclear leukocyte chemotactic factors produced by Propionibacterium acnes. Inflammation 1980;4:261.

Wilkin JK: Rosacea. Int J Dermatol 1983;22:393.

Wolff HH, Plewig G, Braun-Falco O: Ultrastructure of human sebaceous follicles and comedones following treatment with vitamin A acid. Acta Derm Venereol [Suppl] 1975;74:99.

27 Disorders of the Sweat Glands

Harry J. Hurley, MD, DSc(Med)

Human sweat glands are of 2 contrasting types. The eccrine glands are found in almost all parts of the body and play a vital role in thermoregulation. The vestigial apocrine glands are localized to a few areas of the skin and are of minor physiologic importance.

ECCRINE GLANDS

Heat—whether exogenous (owing to environmental causes) or endogenous (resulting from metabolic processes)—is the principal stimulus for eccrine sweating over most of the skin, but some eccrine responses to emotional or sensory stimuli may be limited to the palms and soles, the axillae, and the face. Under intense emotional stimulation, generalized eccrine sweating is possible. Physiologic and pathologic eccrine sweating is sometimes neurally stimulated by gustatory stimuli.

Eccrine glands begin functioning at birth or shortly thereafter and continue to secrete effectively through old age. They are constant morphologically from one skin region to another but are slightly larger and better developed on the palms and soles, the only areas in which sweat duct orifices are visible grossly with the aid of magnification (10×). Eccrine glands are not associated with hair follicles, in contrast to apocrine and sebaceous glands, which form apopilosebaceous or pilosebaceous units. Skin lesions of eccrine origin do not contain a hair follicle in the center as do those of apocrine or sebaceous origin.

Eccrine glands respond almost instantaneously to stimuli (eg, heat load), with a latent period of 10–30 seconds representing the time it takes sweat to travel from the secretory tubule to the opening of the duct. The glands also secrete almost without interruption, and they succumb to cellular fatigue only after hours of continuous activity.

Water is the most important component of eccrine sweat (99.5%) and is essential to its thermoregulatory function. Trace amounts of electrolytes, carbohydrates, amino acids, secretory immunoglobulin A, urea, lactate, ammonia, hormones, and ingested drugs and vitamins are also found in eccrine sweat.

Eccrine sweat is intrinsically odorless. Eccrine glands are innervated by a single set of excitatory cholinergic nerve fibers derived anatomically from the sympathetic nervous system.

APOCRINE GLANDS

Apocrine glands are a family of morphologically similar (but not identical) glands found in the axillae, anogenital skin, mammary areolae, ear canals (wax or ceruminous glands), eyelids (glands of Moll), and irregularly scattered areas on the face, anterior chest, and abdomen. Most apocrine glands function only after puberty, though those of the ear canal and the eyelid are active in infancy. Apocrine glands characteristically have ducts that open high along a hair follicle at or near its junction with the skin surface. Apocrine glands are 10 times larger than eccrine glands and in most areas are visible to the naked eye in incised, reflected skin.

The quantity of sweat produced by apocrine glands is minuscule (a fraction of a milliliter). Apocrine sweat is a viscid liquid of complex composition that forms a shiny, varnishlike residue when it dries, usually at the opening of a hair follicle. Ammonia, iron, lipid, carbohydrate, and other molecules are found in apocrine sweat. Apocrine sweat may range in color from yellow to green or blue-black but not red. Apocrine sweat droplets fluoresce to varying degrees under Wood's light (360 nm). The secretion principally responsible for "body odor" is axillary apocrine sweat, which is both sterile and odorless when it first appears on the skin surface. Within 60 minutes, however, it is degraded by aerobic diphtheroids to produce the classic acrid odor identified with underarm skin. Some individuals have unusual axillary odors (eg, musty, sour, sweet, or rancid), reflecting variations in composition of sweat. Other people apparently lack aerobic diphtheroids in their axillary microflora and develop a faint or poorly definable "acid" odor after apocrine sweat has been subjected to the action of resident micrococci. Although short-chain fatty acids have traditionally been recognized as the

340

major substances responsible for the typical acrid axillary odor, certain androgenic steroids have been identified that have distinctive odors similar to those of bacterially degraded apocrine sweat.

A distinction should be made between apocrine *secretion,* the slow, continuous formation of sweat in the apocrine secretory tubule, and apocrine *sweating,* the delivery of sweat to the surface of the skin. Apocrine sweating results from an organized myoepithelial contraction that expels preformed sweat through the apocrine duct and onto the skin. The usual stimuli for apocrine sweating are emotional or mental, but droplets can be expressed manually by "milking" the glands in a fold of skin squeezed between the fingers.

Alpha-adrenergic sympathetic neuroeffector fibers supply the apocrine glands. The most effective apocrine sudomotor drugs are epinephrine and oxytocin, which induce myoepithelial emptying of the secretory tubule. Gradual regression of apocrine function occurs with advancing years, but sweating and odor are still present in many septuagenarians.

APOCRINE SWEAT GLAND DISORDERS

APOCRINE BROMHIDROSIS

Essentials of Diagnosis
- Exaggerated intense "body odor" of an acrid character reminiscent of the underarm odor of unwashed axillary skin.
- Identification of the axillae as the regional sources of the odor. Elimination of other sites (mouth, vagina, respiratory tract, feet) and other secretions (urine, feces, discharges) as odor-producing.

General Considerations
Apocrine bromhidrosis (foul perspiration) is characterized by excessive or abnormal "body odor" derived from degraded axillary apocrine sweat. Only apocrine sweat contains the essential substrate that gives rise to the pervasive offensive odor after interaction with resident bacteria. Although the odor emanates specifically from the axillae, it results in an unpleasant general body odor. The disorder may simply reflect poor personal hygiene or failure to use axillary deodorants. Other individuals with larger, more active apocrine glands produce greater quantities of apocrine sweat that may be of varied composition and distinctive odor. Unshaved axillary hair serves to collect apocrine sweat and augments odor production. Because of a selective anosmia, some

patients are unaware of their axillary odor unless told about it and fail to adopt local preventive measures.

The onset of apocrine axillary bromhidrosis is postpubertal; axillary apocrine sweat glands are not functional earlier. The problem may persist well into later life through the 70s. Blacks with larger, more active apocrine glands tend to develop bromhidrosis more often than whites. Asians, with less well developed apocrine glands, constitute the other end of the spectrum. Women—usually more fastidious and more likely to shave axillary hair—do not have bromhidrosis as much as men do. Seasonal and climatic variations are of limited importance.

Clinical Findings
A. Symptoms and Signs: Patients with bromhidrosis may or may not be aware of their offensive body odor, though most have been apprised of the problem by other people. They have no other symptoms or local complaints and are usually in a state of general good health. Careful study of the axillary skin (which is otherwise normal) usually reveals fresh or dried apocrine sweat.

B. Laboratory Findings: No abnormal results on laboratory tests are associated with bromhidrosis.

Differential Diagnosis
Apocrine bromhidrosis must be distinguished from common eccrine bromhidrosis, which usually affects the soles of the feet in a patient with associated hyperhidrosis of the soles and palms. Intertriginous eccrine bromhidrosis of the inguinal or inframammary skin occurs most commonly in obese individuals, some of whom have diabetes. Children with unusual body odors should be examined for signs of an inherited metabolic disorder and trimethylaminuria, discussed below. Bromhidrosiphobia, seen characteristically in overly fastidious individuals in whom no odor can be detected by the examiner, may be an early delusional symptom of schizophrenia or may indicate neurologic disease, usually lesions of the temporal lobe.

Treatment
Many patients with apocrine bromhidrosis require only regular careful bathing of the axillary skin with soap and water and the routine use of a commercially available axillary deodorant containing aluminum chloride or other aluminum or zirconium salts. Topical antibiotics, such as gentamicin or neomycin creams and lotions, are often effective. Shaving of axillary hair helps reduce odor. Refractory patients may respond to treatment with aluminum chloride in anhydrous ethyl alcohol (Drysol or Xerac AC) applied at bedtime and covered with an occlusive plastic wrap. (Be sure the skin is dry before applying this; irritation is common.)

The underarm section of clothing may retain apocrine sweat and cause odor despite suppression of odor in the axillae. More frequent washing or dry cleaning of such clothing is necessary. Perfumes and ion exchange resins can be used to mask or adsorb substances causing axillary odors. Patients with marked bromhidrosis who fail to respond may (rarely) be candidates for surgical removal of the axillary apocrine sweat glands by a surgeon experienced in the procedure.

APOCRINE CHROMHIDROSIS

Apocrine chromhidrosis, or colored sweating, is a rare disorder of the apocrine glands, either of the face or axillae, that first appears during adolescence or early adulthood. The blue-black discoloration first appears on the face, usually on the cheeks, following emotional or painful stimulation. The axillary type frequently goes unnoticed except for a yellowish or green stain on undergarments.

The colored sweat may also appear after physical stimulation of the skin area (eg, stroking with a tongue depressor) or after manual squeezing of skin to empty the glands of stored sweat. The sweat droplets are tiny and viscid; they appear at the mouths of hair follicles and dry within a few minutes to a shiny, varnishlike material. Except for the darker varieties of colored sweat of the face, the colored secretion fluoresces brightly under Wood's light. Colored sweating may be induced pharmacologically by intradermal injection of epinephrine or oxytocin.

The cause is unknown, but the responsible chromogen is thought to be a lipofuscin that is excreted in larger quantities or is more highly oxidized in colored apocrine sweat.

Differential Diagnosis

Apocrine sweat colored externally by dyes, paint, or *Piedraia* or *Corynebacterium* microorganisms can produce spurious chromhidrosis. If necessary, biopsy of affected skin permits identification of chromhidrotic apocrine glands. Urinary assay for homogentisic acid helps to identify the patient with ochronosis, who may demonstrate brownish staining of axillary skin and undergarments.

Treatment

Except for surgical excision of the affected skin (impractical on the face because of the resultant scarring), there is no effective treatment. Manual or pharmacologic emptying of the glands provides a symptom-free period of 48–72 hours until the glands can form additional colored sweat. Soap and water or swabbing with organic solvents such as isopropyl alcohol removes the droplets from the skin surface.

Prognosis

Apocrine chromhidrosis is not likely to remit significantly until after menopause, when it gradually lessens.

FOX-FORDYCE DISEASE
(Apocrine Miliaria)

Essentials of Diagnosis

- Follicular papules in apocrine gland-bearing skin areas, especially the axillae, pubes, and mammary areolae.
- Diminished hair growth in affected areas.
- Apocrine anhidrosis at sites of papules.
- Reduction in or absence of apocrine odor in axillae.

General Considerations

Fox-Fordyce disease is an uncommon chronic, pruritic papular eruption of the skin in areas with apocrine glands, eg, the axillae, pubes, mammary areolae, parts of the genitalia, and occasionally the chest and abdomen. It is characterized by retention of apocrine sweat, and lesions develop following keratinous obstruction and consequent intraepidermal rupture of apocrine ducts. The disease is presumably influenced by endocrinologic factors, because (1) onset occurs only after puberty, (2) the disease is 10 times more common in women than in men, and (3) temporary improvement occurs during pregnancy. The disease may regress after menopause in some patients.

Clinical Findings

A. Symptoms and Signs: Fox-Fordyce disease is characterized by follicular papules (occasionally excoriated) in skin having apocrine glands, usually the axillae but also often the pubes, mammary areolae, and portions of the genital skin and trunk. Itching is intermittent and often occurs after evocation of apocrine sweating by emotional stimuli. Reduced hair growth or alopecia is common in affected areas and may precede the appearance of papules. Apocrine anhidrosis exists wherever the papules are found. If involvement in the axillae is extensive, apocrine odor is reduced or absent.

B. Laboratory Findings: Biopsy specimens reveal keratinous obstruction of the distal apocrine duct, intraepidermal rupture of the apocrine duct with regional acanthosis, and microvesicle formation. Dilatative and degenerative changes of the more proximal apocrine tubule and mucinous changes in the dermis occur later. Results of other laboratory studies, including hormonal assays, are normal.

Differential Diagnosis

The pruritic papular eruption limited to skin with apocrine glands is not found in any other disorder. Biopsy is definitive in equivocal cases.

Complications

Bacterial folliculitis and hidradenitis suppurativa are occasional complications.

Treatment

Topical application and intralesional injection of corticosteroids may offer symptomatic relief, and local application of vitamin A acid preparations is sometimes helpful. Topical or systemic corticosteroids occasionally may provide transient relief. Oral contraceptives or estrogens alone are often beneficial. Surgical excision of affected skin areas with grafting represents the only curative approach.

HIDRADENITIS SUPPURATIVA

Essentials of Diagnosis

- Acute, tender, cystlike abscesses in skin with apocrine glands, mainly the axillae and anogenital area.
- Fibrotic sinus tracts with intermittent drainage and periodic acute abscess formation are noted in chronic cases.

General Considerations

Hidradenitis suppurativa is a chronic suppurative disease of the apocrine glands that begins with obstruction of the ducts. Bacterial infection of the occluded ducts and retrograde spread lead to suppuration, rupture of the secretory tubules, and extension of the process, with formation of abscesses. Pointing of abscesses and eventual perforation through the skin are followed by healing and fibrosis. Repetition of the cycle results in increasing fibrosis, deep scarring, and sinus tracts.

Like other disorders of the apocrine glands, hidradenitis suppurativa does not develop before puberty, and hormonal influences are suspected. It is seen in all races and both sexes. The axillary forms develop more frequently in women and the perianal forms more often in men. Hidradenitis suppurativa is worse under hot, humid conditions as encountered in the tropics, though it has a worldwide distribution.

Obesity, acne, and follicular keratinizing disorders such as pityriasis rubra pilaris and pachyonychia congenita, in which ductal occlusion is more likely, predispose to the development of hidradenitis suppurativa.

Clinical Findings

A. Symptoms and Signs: Solitary lesions of hidradenitis are usually manifested as "blind boils" in the axilla or other apocrine areas (Fig 27–1). Recurrent disease is characterized by abscesses as well as scarring, sinus tract formation, and multiple comedones (Fig 27–2). In severe cases with multiple lesions and sinus tracts, restricted motion of the limb may be present. Apocrine sweating is markedly reduced or absent in these areas because of destruction of most of the apocrine glands. Each acute attack is marked by local pain and tenderness but minimal or absent constitutional signs unless the process is exten-

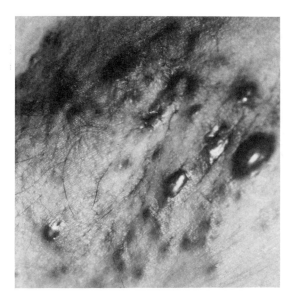

Figure 27–1. Solitary acute lesion of axillary hidradenitis suppurativa. Resemblance to "boils" or inflamed cysts is apparent.

sive and severe. Local trauma (eg, friction produced by tight-fitting clothing) often precipitates acute episodes.

B. Laboratory Findings: Microscopic examination of material from acute lesions reveals staphylococci, streptococci, and occasionally *Escherichia coli*. Chronic cases invariably demonstrate *Proteus* species that are increasingly resistant to antibiotics. Pathogenic anaerobes usually do not play a role in hidradenitis suppurativa. The results of other routine laboratory studies are usually normal except for normocytic anemia in patients with long-standing disease.

Differential Diagnosis

Hidradenitis suppurativa should be considered in any patient with abscesses in apocrine gland-bearing skin. Early lesions may be confused with infected epidermal cysts. After repeated attacks, however, fibrosis and sinus tract formation distinguish hidradenitis. Disorders such as tuberculosis, actinomycosis, tularemia, lymphogranuloma venereum, granuloma inguinale, and ulcerative colitis— which also are marked by formation of fistulas and sinus tracts—should be considered in patients with chronic disease, especially those with involvement of perianal skin.

Complications

Disseminated infection with septicemia is unusual. Marked local fibrosis with restricted limb mobility is a complication in chronic severe hidradenitis sup-

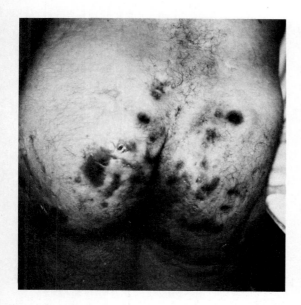

Figure 27–2. Chronic hidradenitis suppurative of buttocks and perianal skin. Scarring, sinus tracts, and abscess formation are present—all signs of chronic recurrent disease.

purativa. Urethral and rectal fistulas result from deep anogenital involvement. Squamous cell carcinomas have developed in indolent sinus tracts. Interstitial keratitis, anemia, and arthritis may occur in patients with long-standing disease. When the process is extensive and severe, amyloidosis and renal failure may be seen.

Prevention

Preventive measure seek to block development of new lesions and exacerbation of old ones. These include avoidance of frictional trauma caused by tight clothing; regular gentle local cleansing, preferably with a germicidal soap; and use of unscented talc following morning bathing to keep the skin as dry as possible. Liquid or spray antiperspirants are not contraindicated, but topical antibiotics such as clindamycin 2% lotion or neomycin cream are preferred to control axillary odor.

Treatment

Management centers around symptomatic treatment of acute infected lesions, eradication of sinus tracts, and measures designed to prevent development of new lesions. Patients with solitary or a few widely separated acute lesions can be managed conservatively with comfortably warm, wet dressings (saline, Burow's solution [1:40] in the form of compresses or soaks), topical gentamicin cream, intralesional administration of triamcinolone acetonide suspension (10 mg/mL), and systemic antibiotic

therapy. Oral erythromycin or tetracycline (1–1.5 g/d) or minocycline or doxycycline (100 mg twice daily) is recommended until resolution is complete (7–14 days). If the disease is chronic, culture of abscess or fistula material should be performed and an appropriate antibiotic selected on the basis of sensitivity studies. Hidradenitis suppurativa is due to occluded apocrine sweat ducts, however, not infection with virulent bacteria or an immunodeficient state. Cure should not be anticipated with antibiotic therapy alone.

If the disease becomes recurrent or if moderate or extensive fibrosis and sinus tract formation exist, surgery is essential for cure. In experienced hands, destruction of isolated or separated lesions by exteriorization with curettage and electrodesiccation of the interior of the tracts is effective. If surgical excision is performed, it must be wide and thorough to ensure complete removal of all sinus tract pockets. Skin grafts may be necessary for surgical closure of the resulting wound. Oral administration of 13-*cis*-retinoic acid (isotretinoin) has helped some patients, but recurrences are frequent, especially if fibrous cysts and sinus tracts remain.

Prognosis

Untreated hidradenitis may rarely resolve spontaneously, but this is exceptional. The disease is usually relentlessly progressive, with increasing discomfort and disability resulting from recurrent abscesses, sinus tracts, and scarring.

ECCRINE SWEAT GLAND DISORDERS

HYPERHIDROSIS

Hyperhidrosis denotes increased eccrine sweating. It can be classified into several clinical types on the basis of the kinds of stimuli and neural centers involved: emotional (cortical), thermoregulatory (hypothalamic), gustatory (medullary), and mass reflex (spinal) sweating. Emotional and some forms of gustatory hyperhidrosis are autosomal dominant traits. The most common causes of the various forms of hyperhidrosis are set forth in Table 27–1. The pathogenesis of most forms of hyperhidrosis remains unknown.

Sweating is generally more pronounced in warmer, humid environments where the sweat glands are conditioned to secrete more easily and in which evaporative loss is minimized. Significant racial variations in eccrine sweating are not seen. Because eccrine glands are functional from infancy onward, patients of any age can display any type of hyperhidrosis except ax-

Table 27–1. Causes of hyperhidrosis.

Neural causes
  Cortical (emotional) hyperhidrosis
    Emotion
    Axillary sweating
    Keratodermas
  Hypothalamic (thermoregulatory) hyperhidrosis
    Infectious factors
      Febrile illnesses
      Chronic illnesses (tuberculosis, lymphoma, malaria)
    Metabolic factors
      Hyperthyroidism
      Diabetes mellitus
      Gout
      Rickets
      Porphyria
      Alcoholism
    Toxic factors
      Arsenic intoxication
      Drug addiction
    Vasomotor factors
      Raynaud's phenomenon or disease
      Cold injury
      Warming erythema after exposure to cold temperatures
      Symmetric lividity of palms and soles
      Neurologic factors
        Tumors or diseases of the cerebral cortex, hypothalamus, or medulla
  Medullary hyperhidrosis
    Physiologic gustatory sweating
    Pathologic gustatory sweating
    Auriculotemporal syndrome of Frey
  Spinal (mass reflex) hyperhidrosis
    Spinal cord transection
    Syringomyelia
    Tabes dorsalis
Nonneural causes
  Local heat
  Cholinergic and adrenergic drugs
  Sudoriparous nevi

illary (emotional) hyperhidrosis, which is not seen before puberty, even though it is an eccrine response.

Clinical Findings

A. Symptoms and Signs: Patients are aware of any exaggerated sweating response and can usually identify the cause, eg, emotional stress, heat, ingestion of spicy foods or hot beverages. Appropriate stimuli to elicit sweating during clinical examination include mental arithmetic or minor pain for emotional hyperhidrosis, environmental heat (hot room, hotbox, with or without exercise) for thermoregulatory hyperhidrosis, ingestion of sour fruits or spicy foods (occasionally even mock mastication or thinking of eating) for gustatory hyperhidrosis, and various nonspecific peripheral sensory stimuli for mass reflex sweating.

Axillary (Fig 27–1) and volar (palmoplantar) are 2 of the most common forms of hyperhidrosis. Patients with these types of **emotional hyperhidrosis** are otherwise well. The excessive sweating is often embarrassing in both social and work situations. It begins when patients awake and diminishes when they fall asleep. Axillary and volar hyperhidrosis often coex-

ist. Bromhidrosis of the feet is often associated with plantar hyperhidrosis because patients wear shoes and stockings, but patients with palmar and axillary hyperhidrosis usually do not complain of bromhidrosis in those areas.

Many illnesses may induce **thermoregulatory hyperhidrosis.** Sweating occurs mainly on the trunk, which is the major site of physiologic sweating in response to heat. In febrile disorders, stimulation of the hypothalamus induces sweating, usually as the environmental temperature begins to fall. The nocturnal sweating of chronic disorders such as tuberculosis, lymphomas, and brucellosis is thermogenous. Diabetics perspire during attacks of hypoglycemia and display a characteristic compensatory hyperhidrosis of the upper half of the body with diminished or absent sweating of the lower half. Other endocrine states such as hyperthyroidism and menopause can result in thermoregulatory hyperhidrosis, as can certain metabolic and nutritional disorders, including gout, porphyria, alcoholism, and rickets. The sweating seen in parkinsonism, pheochromocytoma, and patients recovering from encephalitis results from stimulation of higher autonomic nervous centers, usually the hypothalamus.

Gustatory hyperhidrosis occurs most commonly on the face, especially the cheeks and upper lip, but may also appear on the neck, parts of the upper extremities, and (rarely) the legs. It occurs most dramatically as part of the auriculotemporal syndrome of Frey, in which regional peripheral postganglionic sympathetic and parasympathetic nerve fibers become cross-connected after recovery from surgery, trauma, or infection of the parotid area—ie, nerve fibers that originally connected to the salivary glands become connected to sweat glands, and vice versa. Thus, sweating occurs in response to salivary stimuli; and salivation occurs in response to heat. Pathologic gustatory sweating may also occur in syringomyelia and encephalitis after disruption of the brain stem nuclei governing sweating and salivation and after injury to the sympathetic trunk caused by sympathectomy, thyroidectomy, carcinoma of the lung, or subclavian aneurysm.

In **mass reflex sweating,** partial or complete transection of the spinal cord isolates lower peripheral neurons from higher hypothalamic and cortical inhibitory control. In spinal injury, tabes dorsalis, or syringomyelia, a variable pattern of segmental sweating may occur along with other autonomic, sensory, and motor changes below the level of spinal involvement.

B. Laboratory Findings: Demonstration of the various forms of hyperhidrosis does not usually depend on any laboratory determinations. Appropriate laboratory studies may be required to establish the underlying cause in sweating due to systemic disease.

Clinical confirmation of the abnormal sweating pattern and the stimuli eliciting the response is essential. A useful colorimetric test for sweating is the starch-iodine technique, in which an alcoholic solution of iodine (iodine 3%, potassium iodide 3%, in 95% ethyl alcohol) is painted on the skin and allowed to dry. Cornstarch powder dusted on treated skin turns blue-black at the pores of actively sweating glands and delineates the sweating response. Gravimetric determinations quantitate sweating by weighing gauze or cotton pads used to collect sweat from a given area both before and after the sweating response is elicited.

Differential Diagnosis

The various types of eccrine hyperhidrosis must be accurately differentiated to permit treatment (Table 27–1).

Complications

Increased eccrine sweating predisposes to development of various local bacterial, fungal, and yeast infections; to certain viral disorders (eg, warts); to miliaria, intertrigo, and acne; and to allergic and primary irritant contact dermatitis. Industrial workers with palmar hyperhidrosis are especially at risk for contact dermatitis, and their chronically wet hands may damage paper or metallic products with which they work. Social and occupational embarrassment may lead to emotional problems and thus may further aggravate hyperhidrosis.

Treatment

Sedatives, tranquilizers, and systemic anticholinergics rarely provide satisfactory control of hyperhidrosis. Biofeedback techniques and other types of behavioral and relaxation training have helped some patients with emotional hyperhidrosis. In patients whose hyperhidrosis is associated with an underlying disease, treatment of the disorder is essential. Topical control of annoying axillary and palmoplantar hyperhidrosis is generally possible using a special antiperspirant containing aluminum chloride hexahydrate, 20%, in anhydrous ethyl alcohol (Drysol, Xerac AC), applied under an occlusive plastic wrap and left on overnight. Treatment may be repeated weekly.

Scopolamine salts and other anticholinergics have been used successfully, but the risk of adverse reactions in patients with overt or incipient glaucoma, prostatic hyperplasia, and cardiovascular disorders makes them a less attractive alternative. Topical scopolamine salts, along with aluminum salts, have been used in gustatory hyperhidrosis. Other effective but less desirable topical agents for palmar hyperhidrosis are 2–10% formalin (a contact sensitizer) and 2–10% aqueous solution of glutaraldehyde (which stains the skin yellow). Tap water iontophoresis may prove adequate for some patients with emotional hyperhidrosis of the palms and soles but less so for those with axillary hyperhidrosis. These treatments require special apparatus. They should be administered daily for at least 2 weeks to achieve control and then approximately weekly thereafter to maintain it. If the above measures fail, local surgical ablation of axillary eccrine glands has been effective. Upper thoracic sympathectomy may also be used for severe palmar hyperhidrosis.

ANHIDROSIS

Anhidrosis—or abnormal deficiency of sweat—is usually partial, ie, hypohidrosis over a patchy area, a dermatomal segment, or half of the body. In central nervous system disease or congenital anhidrotic ectodermal dysplasia, total lack of sweating may occur. Disease or other interruption of the neural elements governing the sweating response—central nervous system nuclei, spinal tracts, sympathetic ganglia, or peripheral sudomotor fibers—as well as diseases of the skin (eg, psoriasis, atopic dermatitis) or eccrine glands (eg, miliaria) can cause anhidrosis (Table 27–2). Common causes of anhidrosis are drugs (anticholinergics, ganglionic blocking agents, quinacrine), dehydration, hypothyroidism, and peripheral neuropathy due to alcoholic neuritis, diabetes, amyloidosis, leprosy, or gout. Many patients with significant hypohidrosis have compensatory hyperhidrosis involving the remaining functional sweat glands. Excessive sweating in one region should alert the examiner to possible anhidrosis in another. Any variations in anhidrosis on the basis of age, sex, race, habitat, or occupation are due to the underlying cause.

Clinical Findings

A. Symptoms and Signs: Compensatory hyperhidrosis in any skin region often accompanies hypohidrosis in another area. A patient's inability to toler-

Table 27–2. Causes of anhidrosis.

Sweat gland disturbances
  Congenital defects
  Acquired defects
    Drugs
    Toxic chemicals
    Skin diseases
  Sweat duct obstruction
    Miliaria
    Inflammatory or keratotic disorders
Other disturbances
  Neuropathic
    Hysteria
    Tumors or diseases of brain, spinal cord, sympathetic
      nerves, or ganglia
  Miscellaneous or idiopathic
    Newborn
    Dehydration
    Hypothyroidism
    Toxic drugs
    Systemic disease

ate heat or to work or exercise in a hot environment should alert the physician to the possibility of widespread hypohidrosis or anhidrosis, as should the development of heat-related illnesses such as heat syncope, heat exhaustion, or heat stroke.

B. Laboratory Findings: Anhidrosis per se causes no characteristic alterations in blood or urine; however, abnormalities on laboratory tests may be associated with the underlying disease or may represent a complication of the disease, eg, fluid and electrolyte imbalance or heat exhaustion.

Anhidrotic areas must be precisely delineated with carefully conducted sweat tests using ambient heat or multiple spot sweat testing with intradermal injection of cholinergic drugs such as pilocarpine (0.01–0.1%). In patients with suspected extensive anhidrosis, general thermal stimulation or exercise to induce sweating should be performed with great care to avoid provoking a medical emergency such as hyperthermia, cardiac instability, or fluid and electrolyte imbalance. A useful examination in anhidrotic ectodermal dysplasia counts palmar epidermal ridge sweat pores, which are absent in affected males and reduced in number in heterozygous female carriers.

Complications

The major complication of extensive anhidrosis is hyperthermia. Except for compensatory hyperhidrosis of residual functional glands, no other complication can be traced to partial anhidrosis.

Treatment

The mainstay of therapy is treatment of the underlying causative disease. Patients with untreatable anhidrosis must be cautioned about the dangers of exposure to excessive heat, work, or physical activity that would normally provoke intense sweating.

MILIARIA

Essentials of Diagnosis

- Miliaria crystallina—asymptomatic transparent superficial minivesicles on uninflamed skin, often in intertriginous areas.
- Miliaria rubra—pruritic, 1–3 mm in diameter, erythematous macules, each with a tiny summit vesicle. Extrafollicular; may be pustular. Commonly on trunk and neck.
- Miliaria profunda—white papules, 1–3 mm in diameter, without erythema or pruritus. May accompany extensive chronic miliaria rubra. Commonly associated with heat stress syndrome.

General Considerations

The term "miliaria" denotes 3 disorders in which keratinous sweat duct obstruction occurs, followed by rupture of the duct and formation of a vesicle containing retained sweat. The level at which obstruction occurs and the type of vesicle that results are the differentiating features. In **miliaria crystallina,** obstruction develops superficially, within the stratum corneum. In **miliaria rubra,** or prickly heat, obstruction occurs in the epidermis and induces inflammation that produces vasodilatory erythema and itching. Ductal obstruction and rupture at the level of the dermal-epidermal junction are the hallmark of **miliaria profunda.** Bacteria may play a part in early obstructive changes in the ducts. Children are predisposed to the development of miliaria, but the tendency is frequently lost as they mature. Miliaria occurs in both sexes, in all races, and in all age groups. Prolonged exposure to heat and high humidity, as occurs in tropical climates and in certain work situations (eg, soldiers fighting in hot, humid areas for long periods) predispose to development of miliaria.

Clinical Findings

A. Symptoms and Signs: The clear crystalline vesicles of miliaria crystallina are common in the aged, debilitated bedridden patient, especially in intertriginous areas such as the axillae and the neck. Since they are asymptomatic, they may go unnoticed by the patient. Because they rupture easily, they may never be detected. The pruritic erythematous microvesicular lesions of miliaria rubra, which do not surround a hair follicle, are most common on the trunk and neck but spare the face and volar skin. Pustules—usually sterile—are seen in patients with extensive disease. Miliaria profunda develops most commonly in patients with widespread recurrent miliaria rubra and is characterized by nonpruritic whitish papules that represent sweat-retention vesicles deep in the skin. The extensive sweat gland obstruction associated with miliaria profunda commonly results in compensatory facial hyperhidrosis and inguinal and axillary adenopathy that fades when the miliaria resolves. After heat or exercise, patients with miliaria profunda are predisposed to develop thermoregulatory failure with high temperature and cardiorespiratory symptoms constituting a distinctive heat stress syndrome known as tropical anhidrotic asthenia.

B. Laboratory Findings: Miliaria is not associated with abnormal results on common laboratory tests except when a heat stress syndrome (eg, heat stroke) develops as a result of widespread sweat retention. Biopsy demonstrates sweat duct obstruction, rupture of sweat ducts, and vesicles containing retained sweat at a skin level corresponding to the type of miliaria. Inflammatory skin changes are seen in miliaria rubra.

The extent of the anhidrosis caused by miliaria can be demonstrated using a sweat test with a colorimetric technique (eg, starch-iodine).

Complications

Intolerance to heat and other heat stress syndromes

may occur in patients with widespread miliaria rubra and miliaria profunda.

Treatment

In patients with severe disease, a cool environment is essential; miliaria gradually clears over several days. Gentle cleansing and the application of a drying lotion, eg, calamine lotion or hydrocortisone 1% in a hydrophilic lotion base, may provide symptomatic relief. Experimental local application of topical gentamicin or neomycin preparations has been shown to prevent the development of miliaria in those areas.

MISCELLANEOUS DISORDERS OF ECCRINE SWEAT GLANDS

Increased concentrations of sodium and chloride in eccrine sweat are a hallmark of cystic fibrosis. An as yet unexplained defect in ductal reabsorption of electrolytes is responsible. Increased concentrations of these ions are also found in other disorders, including bronchiectasis, emphysema, diabetes mellitus, nephrogenic diabetes insipidus, Addison's disease, and myxedema, but in smaller amounts and with less predictability.

Calcium may be detected in eccrine sweat in certain types of systemic calcinosis. Uremia produces increased levels of urea in sweat; in severe cases, "uremic frost" can be seen, usually on facial skin. Large amounts of abnormal amino acids, their analogues, or metabolites are excreted in eccrine sweat in certain rare hereditary metabolic disorders such as phenylketonuria, hypermethioninemia, oasthouse urine disease, and maple syrup urine disease. The excreted compounds are generally odorous and result in specialized forms of eccrine bromhidrosis.

In trimethylaminuria, the "fish odor" syndrome, deficient trimethylamine oxidase in the liver results in the accumulation of trimethylamine, which has the odor of rotten fish, in urine and sweat. Trimethylamine is derived from bacterial degradation of eggs, fish, liver, and other choline- or lecithin-containing foods in the intestinal tract. Avoidance of these foods eliminates the odor in affected patients.

Granulosis rubra nasi is a rare inherited condition of unknown cause in which erythema, hyperhidrosis, and papulovesicular lesions are confined to the nose. Periporitis may occur in certain neonates, especially the malnourished or debilitated. Unusual multiple sweat gland abscesses may develop along with constitutional signs from infection.

REFERENCES

Giacobetti R, Caro WA, Roenigk HH Jr: Fox-Fordyce disease: Control with tretinoin cream. Arch Dermatol 1979;115:1365.

Grice K: Hidradenitis suppurativa. Pages 221–222 in: *Current Dermatologic Therapy.* Maddin S (editor). Saunders, 1982.

Hölzle E, Kligman AM: The pathogenesis of miliaria rubra: Role of the resident microflora. Br J Dermatol 1978; 99:117.

Hurley HJ: Axillary hyperhidrosis, apocrine bromhidrosis, hidradenitis suppurativa, and familial benign pemphigus: Surgical approach. Pages 717–743 in: *Dermatologic Surgery: Principles and Practice.* Roenigk RK, Roenigk HH Jr (editors). Marcel Dekker, 1989.

Hurley HJ: Diseases of the apocrine glands. Pages 704–717 in: *Dermatology in General Medicine,* 3rd ed. Fitzpatrick TB, Eisen A (editors). McGraw-Hill, 1987.

Hurley HJ: Fox-Fordyce disease. Pages 181–182 in: *Current Dermatologic Therapy.* Maddin S (editor). Saunders, 1982.

Hurley HJ: Diseases of the apocrine sweat glands. Page 1323 in: *Dermatology,* 2nd ed. Moschella SL, Hurley HJ (editors). Saunders, 1985.

Hurley HJ: Diseases of the eccrine sweat glands. Pages 1341–1365 in: *Dermatology,* 2nd ed. Moschella SL, Hurley HJ (editors). Saunders, 1985.

Hurley HJ: Local surgical management of axillary hyperhidrosis. In: *Skin Surgery,* 5th ed. Epstein E, Epstein E Jr (editors). Saunders, 1982.

Hurley HJ: Miliaria. Pages 307–308 in: *Current Dermatologic Therapy.* Maddin S (editor). Saunders, 1982.

Hurley HJ: Treatment of hyperhidrosis (emotional). Pages 232–234 in: *Current Dermatologic Therapy.* Maddin S (editor). Saunders, 1982.

Leyden JJ et al: The microbiology of the human axilla and its relationship to axillary odor. J Invest Dermatol 1981;77:413.

Quinton PM: Sweating and its disorders. Annu Rev Med 1983;34:429.

Rayner CR, Ritchie ID, Stark GP: Axillary hyperhidrosis, 20% aluminum chloride hexahydrate, and surgery. Br Med J 1980;280:1168.

Shelley WB, Shelley ED: Recalcitrant unilateral infection associated with congenital leg hypertrophy cleared by control of hyperhidrosis. Cutis 1984;33:281.

Disorders of Hair

28

Mark V. Dahl, MD

ANATOMY

The anatomy of the hair is discussed in Chapter 1 and the care of normal hair in Chapter 5. Briefly, scalp hairs are terminal hairs composed of dead, impacted keratinized cells. A central medulla is surrounded by the cortex, which in turn is shingled with cells of the cuticle. Hair is produced by the hair matrix at the tip of a dermal papilla. As cells in the matrix divide and keratinize, the hair grows. In the follicle, the hair shaft and matrix are surrounded by the inner and outer root sheaths. Anagen hairs are growing hairs with long hair bulbs, whereas telogen hairs are nongrowing hairs with keratinized "club-shaped" bulbs.

GENERAL CONSIDERATIONS

There are 2 major types of hair disorders: too much (hypertrichosis and hirsutism) or too little (alopecia). Neither is a medical problem as such, but the cosmetic impact can be devastating. In addition, there are less severe hair problems such as kinking, fraying, discoloration, tangling, curling, or straightening and breaking. Infections of the hair or scalp can cause hair loss and even permanent destruction of hair follicles. Severe inflammatory diseases such as discoid lupus erythematosus can also affect hair. Certain hair problems are associated with medical conditions requiring attention, and in such cases, having too much or too little hair serves as a marker for internal disease.

HYPERTRICHOSIS

Hypertrichosis is an increase in the amount or apparent amount of hair in nonandrogenic areas of the body. It may be generalized or localized. Ethnic backgrounds must be considered. For example, Greek men normally have very hairy chests, whereas the chests of Japanese and Chinese men are rather bare.

Classification

A. Congenital Hypertrichosis: Thin, fine, silky hair appears on the face and often also on the body during the first decade. These are the "dog boys" of circus side shows. The disorder is usually inherited as an autosomal dominant trait.

B. Congenital Localized Hypertrichosis: Long and coarse hairs develop in a specific site up to 10 cm in diameter, often related to some sort of nevus such as an epidermal nevus, linear epithelial nevus, or Becker's nevus. It is also associated with spina bifida. Circumscribed hypertrichosis over the sacrum in an infant should alert the physician to a tethered spinal cord, which could lead to spinal cord damage as the child grows.

C. Acquired Hypertrichosis Lanuginosa: This disorder is more common in females. Fine, silky hair suddenly grows all over the body, or in some cases only on the face, usually signaling an underlying malignant tumor, often of the breast, lung, gallbladder, pancreas, colon, rectum, ovary, uterus, or bladder. Coexisting lymphomas and carcinomas have been reported. Removal of the tumor may be associated with lessening of the hypertrichosis.

D. Localized Acquired Hypertrichosis: Chronic trauma or inflammation at a local site can occasionally induce hair to grow. This may result from rubbing, biting, vascular occlusion, arthritis, pretibial myxedema, or eczema.

Treatment

If possible, underlying precipitating factors should be dealt with. Removing hair by shaving is usually satisfactory, as well as use of depilatory agents, wax epilation, or electrolysis. Dark hair can be bleached with hydrogen peroxide.

HIRSUTISM

In contrast to hypertrichosis, hirsutism refers to an increased amount of terminal hair in androgen-dependent areas only. Thus, women develop male hair patterns. In general, the fine, silky, vellus hairs become coarse terminal hairs. Racial differences must be considered, because women from the Mediterranean area of Europe often have more hair on the abdomen, face, and thighs.

Classification

A. Idiopathic Hirsutism: In patients with idiopathic hirsutism, the hair follicle converts normal serum levels of androgenic hormones very efficiently. No diagnosable endocrine abnormality is found. Excessive hair growth begins in puberty and increases over the ensuing few decades. A family history of a similar disorder may be present. Pelvic examination can rule out ovarian tumors. Endocrinologic tests such as plasma levels of prolactin, dehydroepiandrosterone sulfate, testosterone, luteinizing hormone, and follicle-stimulating hormones are usually normal.

B. Polycystic Ovary (Stein-Leventhal) Syndrome: In this disorder, testosterone production by the ovaries is increased so that plasma testosterone levels are elevated. Twenty percent of patients have acne. The disorder is treated by suppression of gonadotropic hormones with estrogen or with antiandrogens such as spironolactone, cimetidine, or cyproterone acetate. Wedge resection of part of the ovary may also help some patients.

C. Ovarian Tumors: Tumors of the ovary can release hormones. Hirsutism usually develops rapidly, and virilization is also present. Androgen-secreting ovarian tumors include ovarian adenomas, arrhenoblastomas, Leydig cell tumors, hilar tumors, and granulosa-thecal cell tumors. Luteomas, which begin in pregnancy, can also cause hirsutism, especially in blacks.

D. Congenital Adrenal Hyperplasia: This adrenogenital syndrome is inherited in an autosomal recessive manner. Hirsutism occurs in about 10% of patients but is usually not present until adolescence or later. In the most common form, 21-hydroxylation of 17-hydroxyprogesterone is blocked, resulting in low levels of cortisol and elevated levels of ACTH, testosterone, and androstenedione. Hirsutism and virilization result from overactivity of the adrenal glands in an attempt to maintain normal cortisol secretion. Most patients have polycystic ovary disease. A different genetic defect in either 11-hydroxylase or 3β-hydroxysteroid dehydrogenase activity can cause a similar syndrome, as can Cushing's syndrome and various adrenal tumors.

E. Hyperprolactinemia: Excess prolactin may be produced by pituitary adenomas, hypothyroidism, stress, disorders of the hypothalamus, drugs such as phenothiazine, and hepatorenal failure. Hyperprolactinemia may be associated with galactorrhea and amenorrhea. Serum prolactin levels are elevated.

F. Acromegaly: Excessive amounts of pituitary hormones can increase both adrenal and ovarian androgen production.

G. Drug-Induced Hirsutism: Oral contraceptives and androgens may cause hirsutism and sometimes virilization as well.

Laboratory Tests for Hirsutism

Endocrinologic consultation is often recommended. Minimum tests often assess serum levels of free testosterone, dehydroepiandosterone sulfate (DHEA-S), luteinizing hormone, follicle-stimulating hormone, and prolactin. The ratio of luteinizing hormone to follicle-stimulating hormone should also be normal.

Treatment of Patients With Hirsutism

The underlying cause should be eliminated if possible. If the history, physical examination, and screening laboratory tests are normal, the patient probably has idiopathic hirsutism. Repeat examinations after several months are sometimes worthwhile. If these tests are abnormal, further evaluation by an endocrinologist is indicated. Excessive androgenic hormone can be antagonized by estrogen. Prednisone, 5 mg/d, or dexamethasone, 0.5 mg/d, may help by suppressing the pituitary-adrenal axis. In Europe, a combination of cyproterone acetate (50–100 mg/d) and ethinyl estradiol (0.05 mg/d) has been used to treat hirsutism. It is often used cyclically but has side effects, including decreased libido and depression. Spironolactone, 50–200 mg/d, and cimetidine, 300 mg 4 times daily, have antiandrogen effects.

Hair can be removed by shaving, bleaching, plucking, waxing, depilation, or electrolysis.

ALOPECIA*

Alopecia may affect localized areas of the scalp or body, the entire scalp, or even to the entire body. It can be caused by abnormalities of the hair shafts (which cause them to break off), congenital disorders of keratinization (which cause the hair shafts to be made abnormally), endocrinologic or other systemic

---

*Tinea capitis is discussed in Chapter 16.

diseases (which affect hair growth), mechanical factors such as plucking or waving the hair (which damages it), inflammatory conditions (which cause scarring of the scalp and obliteration of hair follicles), and various diseases that affect hair follicles directly.

Approach to the Patient
With Alopecia

A brief history should be followed by a brief physical examination before additional historical information is gathered. The alopecias can be conveniently grouped into 4 types that help define the differential diagnosis: generalized scarring, generalized nonscarring, localized scarring, and localized nonscarring.

Alopecia can be either diffuse or localized—ie, it can involve the entire scalp either partially or completely or only a small area of the scalp. It may be scarring or nonscarring. In scarring alopecias, no hair follicles are present, and the skin is hard and glistening and may have areas of inflammation or atrophy. In nonscarring alopecias, the scalp usually appears normal or shows inflammatory dermatoses. In doubtful cases, biopsy may be necessary to establish whether the disorder is indeed scarring or nonscarring.

The history should establish whether the patient notes primarily hair fall or hair thinning. "Hair fall" is manifested by finding excessive numbers of hairs on the pillow or clothing or in the hair brush; "hair thinning," by a decreasing density of hair over a particular body area. Hair fall usually indicates an acute process and hair thinning a more insidious one. One should also determine whether the hair is coming out "by the roots" or simply breaking off. If the patient cannot provide this information, hair should be inspected under a microscope (see below).

The physical examination should include examination of the texture and contour of the hair surface, the pattern of hair loss if it is not even, and the appearance and amounts of hair on other body areas such as the pubic fossa, axillae, and eyebrows. The skin over the entire body should be inspected for the presence of disease. Many systemic diseases affecting the hair also affect the nails, which for that reason should be examined also. Many hereditary syndromes are associated with alopecia, so congenital abnormalities and the family history should be taken into account.

Special Tests for
Assessment of Alopecia

A. Light Pull Test: The light pull test is a useful one. Here, several strands of hair are grasped lightly and pulled through the fingers. Usually only one or 2 hairs are removed by this maneuver. Excessive numbers of easily removed hairs constitute a positive light pull test.

B. Hard Pull Test: Hard pull tests are used to determine the numbers of anagen (growing) and telogen (resting) hairs on the hair-bearing areas. Thir-

ty hairs or so are grasped with a forceps fitted with rubber tubing over the jaws. A quick pull plucks these hairs from the scalp. The roots can then be examined microscopically.

C. Hair Mounts: Microscopic examination of hair shafts or bulbs is best accomplished by placing the hairs on a microscopic slide containing several drops of Permount or other sticky mounting medium. Permount has approximately the same refractive index as hair. In addition, the sticky substance anchors the hairs on the slide so they can be more easily coverslipped and examined. Low power is usually best for scanning examining hairs for the presence or absence of hair bulbs, for the type of hair bulb, and for abnormalities of the hair shaft.

D. Wood's Light Examination: Examination of the scalp under Wood's light may be useful in diagnosing certain fungal infections. In the USA, most fungal infections are due to *Trichophyton tonsurans,* which does not fluoresce. Fungi such as *Microsporum audouinii* and *Microsporum canis* fluoresce yellow under this long-wave "black" ultraviolet light.

E. KOH Examination: Hairs can be dissolved in 10–15% potassium hydroxide and examined under the microscope for spores inside or around the hair shaft. The presence of spores indicates a fungal infection. Air bubbles occasionally seen within the hair shaft may cause confusion.

F. Culture: Fungus can be isolated by culture on mycobiotic agar (Mycocel) or Dermatophyte Test Medium Agar. Because the hairs break off at the site of fungal infection, it is usually best to cut them next to the scalp margin and place the most proximal ends on the medium. If scales are present on the scalp, they can be examined directly or cultured as well.

G. Biopsy: Wedge or punch biopsy can be used to determine whether scarring is present. Specific histopathologic changes may aid diagnosis, but in general biopsies are rather nonspecific. To detect subtle changes leading to a correct diagnosis, biopsies should be interpreted by histopathologists who are experts in diagnosing hair diseases microscopically. Fungus can be observed in hair shafts on biopsy if tissue sections are stained with PAS stain.

GENERALIZED NONSCARRING
ALOPECIAS

In these disorders, hair is lost over the entire scalp. The hair loss may be complete or incomplete. The scalp skin is normal. There is neither inflammation nor scarring. Causes of generalized nonscarring alopecias are listed in Table 28–1.

1. ANDROGENETIC ALOPECIA

Essentials of Diagnosis

- Diffuse hair loss without scarring.

Table 28–1. Causes of generalized nonscarring alopecia.

Androgenetic
  Male pattern
  Female pattern
Telogen effluvium
Postpartum effluvium
Alopecia areata totalis
Anagen effluvium
Hair shaft abnormalities
  Congenital
  Acquired
Trichotillomania
Metabolic
  Sudden weight loss
  Iron deficiency
  Hypo- and hyperthyroidism
  Diabetes
  Vitamin B_{12} deficiency
  Simmonds' hypopituitarism
Systemic lupus erythematosus
Syphilis
Drugs
  Cytotoxic agents
  Anticoagulants
  Antithyroid drugs
  Triparanol
  Vitamin A
  Levodopa
  Others

- In men, recession of the frontal hairline near the temples and thinning over the vertex.
- In women, generally diffuse, unpatterned loss.
- Light pull test usually negative.
- No serum hormone abnormalities.

General Considerations

Androgenetic alopecia includes common male pattern baldness and diffuse female alopecia. These disorders are due to loss of hair from transformation of terminal follicles to vellus follicles. Increased conversion of precursors to active androgens within the hair follicle may act in conjunction with genetic predisposing factors.

Clinical Findings

A. Symptoms and Signs: Hair loss is usually insidious. Patients notice thinning of the hair rather than hair fall. In men, the hair is lost primarily over the occiput and along the frontal hairline near the temples, though some thinning over the top of the scalp is quite common. In women, thinning is much more diffuse, but the vertex of the scalp has the least hair. Pubic, axillary, eyebrow, eyelash, and other body hair growth is usually not affected.

B. Laboratory Findings: Only a few patients have elevated levels of sex hormone-binding protein or free testosterone or dehydroepiandrosterone. Menstrual irregularities or coexisting hirsutism or virilization suggest which patients should be tested.

Differential Diagnosis

Other causes of diffuse nonscarring alopecia should be considered, particularly malnutrition, drugs, and endocrine disease—especially hypothyroidism, hyperthyroidism, iron deficiency anemia, hypopituitarism, and hypoparathyroidism. The sudden appearance of male pattern hair loss in a woman may suggest an endocrine dysfunction, especially if associated with acne, hirsutism, virilization, or cessation of menstruation. Occasionally, damage to hair shafts may cause a diffuse alopecia, but more commonly this alopecia is patchy and the light pull test is positive.

Treatment

A topical solution of minoxidil 2% can be applied twice daily to selected areas to lessen hair fall and to stimulate new hair growth over the vertex of the scalp. Up to 50% of patients report moderate hair growth after 1 year. The best responses are seen in patients who have been balding for less than 5 years, have baldness of the vertex less than 10 cm in diameter, and who have more than 100 vellus or other hairs in the treatment area. One milliliter of solution is applied to affected areas of dry scalp twice daily. Hair growth may not be observed for the first few months. Pulse rate, blood pressure, and weight should be monitored after 1 month and then every 6 months, though the chances for fluid retention, weight gain, hypotension, and tachycardia seem small. The solution should ordinarily not be used if the scalp is inflamed. When treatments are stopped, the newly regrown hair falls out.

Hair transplantation can help men with male pattern alopecia. Sometimes an area of the scalp that is devoid of hair is surgically removed (scalp reduction) with or without the use of tissue expanders. Small plugs of hair are then transplanted from the occipital scalp or other dense hair-bearing areas to the frontal hairline and areas immediately posterior to it. Care must be taken to maintain a normal-appearing hairline. This technique is much more complex than it might seem and is best left to experts.

Wigs also help. Patients with mild degrees of alopecia are often benefited by a creative hair stylist who can style the hair to minimize the bald appearance.

Course & Prognosis

The disorder tends to progress in men, so that the hair thins over the entire top of the scalp to the point that few or no hairs remain. Fifty percent of women have notable thinning by age 50 years, but almost none of these go on to complete baldness such as occurs in men.

2. TELOGEN EFFLUVIUM

Essentials of Diagnosis

- Hair fall, usually generalized.
- Recent acute illness, surgery, or pregnancy.

- Positive light pull test.
- Telogen hairs on microscopic examination.

General Considerations

Humans do not have synchronous hair shedding cycles. Instead, individual hairs enter the telogen (rest) phase in an asynchronous manner. As the new hair begins to grow in a new hair cycle, the old hair is pushed out. Normally, adults lose 75–100 hairs a day in this way.

Certain events can induce follicles to enter the telogen stage. This then induces a synchronous growth of new hair follicles 6–10 weeks later such that more synchronous hair fall is seen. About 95% of women develop some degree of telogen effluvium after pregnancy or after discontinuance of birth control pills. Other causes of telogen effluvium include high fever, bulimia, excessive dieting, malnutrition, blood loss, shock, surgery, and severe psychiatric stress.

Clinical Findings

Hair fall is the only symptom. The patient usually notes increased numbers of hairs on pillows, brushes, and clothes. Usually only scalp hair is affected, but all body hair is theoretically susceptible. Light traction on the hair easily extracts more than the usual number of hair shafts from the hair follicles. Microscopic examination of these hairs discloses telogen hair (club) bulbs at the proximal end of each.

Differential Diagnosis

Cytotoxic drugs can cause anagen effluvium, in which case no bulb is usually present. Hair loss from other drugs such as vitamin A, thiouracil, propranolol, levodopa, trimethadione, mercurial diuretics, bismuth, and others may cause confusion. Alopecia areata, alopecia areata totalis, and alopecia areata universalis result in sudden hair loss (see below), in which case exclamation point hairs may be present on microscopic examination and complete hair loss may result. Excessive hair fall can be noted after chemical treatments of the hair. In this case, microscopic examination reveals no bulbs or damaged hair shafts. Systemic disorders such as syphilis and systemic lupus erythematosus should be ruled out if the history or other physical findings suggest their presence.

Treatment

Because the hair falls out as new hairs are growing, no treatment is indicated. Wigs or creative coiffures can hide severe alopecia.

3. ABNORMALITIES OF THE HAIR SHAFT

Essentials of Diagnosis

- Diffuse nonscarring alopecia.

- Incomplete hair loss with broken hairs.
- Often accompanied by other underlying congenital or epithelial defects.

General Considerations

The most common cause of hair loss from hair shaft abnormality is permanent waving or straightening procedures. During these procedures, the hair bonds are broken down. The hair is set in a different position, and the bonds are reformed. Not all bonds reform, however, so the hair is structurally weaker and prone to breakage, especially if treatments are frequent or done incorrectly. The light pull test may be positive. Broken hairs often show fraying, splitting, or other abnormalities.

Hair can also be weak because of inherited defects in keratinization. Consequently, diffuse nonscarring alopecias accompany a large number of hereditary syndromes, especially those with other epithelial defects. For example, in **anhidrotic ectodermal dysplasia,** the hair is sparse, short, and fine and associated with decreased sweating, a prominent lower lip, pointed chin, square forehead, and malformed teeth. In the autosomal dominantly inherited **tooth and nail syndrome,** sparse hair is associated with hypodontia and peg-shaped primary teeth. In **congenital poikiloderma,** the scalp hair is fine and sparse and associated with erythema of the face and ears, mottled pigmentation, atrophy, telangiectasia, and hypogonadism. In **cartilage-hair hypoplasia,** short, sparse, fine light hair is associated with dwarfism and dysostosis. Among other syndromes associated with diffuse nonscarring alopecia are hidrotic ectodermal dysplasia, XTE (xeroderma, talipes, and enamel defect) syndrome, AEC (ankyloblepharon, ectodermal defects, cleft lip and palate) syndrome, Basan's syndrome, Sensenbrenner's syndrome, onychotrichodysplasia, trichorhinophalangeal syndrome, Moynahan's syndrome, Hallermann-Streiff syndrome, progeria, Werner's syndrome, Cockayne's syndrome, bird-headed dwarfism, popliteal web syndrome, oral-facial-digital syndrome, dyskeratosis congenita, pachyonychia congenita, and Dubovitz's syndrome.

Specific Disorders

A. Trichorrhexis Nodosa: Small nodes occur along the hair shaft owing to breakage. Under the microscope, the hair appears as though 2 brooms had been shoved into each other. Trichorrhexis nodosa usually results from hair damage associated with permanent waving or other chemical treatments. It has been associated with argininosuccinicaciduria and congenital ectodermal dysplasia.

B. Trichorrhexis Invaginata: This occurs as a part of Netherton's syndrome and is inherited in an autosomal recessive manner associated with ichthyosis.

C. Monilethrix: This disorder takes its name from the beadlike appearance of the hair shafts. It is a rare disease. Onset usually occurs in late childhood. The hair breaks off at the thinned area between the beads. A defect in keratinization is responsible.

D. Pili Torti: This disorder is transmitted as an autosomal dominant trait. The hair follicles are curved, so that the hair shafts are flattened and twisted. The disorder usually appears in the first 2 years of life. The hair shaft appears to spiral when examined under the microscope.

E. Menkes' Kinky-Hair Syndrome: This X-linked recessive syndrome features twists along the hair shafts and irregularities resembling a combination of pili torti, monilethrix, and trichorrhexis nodosa. The hair abnormality is associated with mental retardation and motor dysfunction. Most untreated patients survive less than 2 years. The disorder is related to an abnormality of copper metabolism. Poor absorption leads to low serum and tissue copper levels. Copper supplementation may be helpful.

F. Trichothiodystrophy: Patients with trichothiodystrophy have brittle hair with a low sulfur content. This disease is inherited as an autosomal recessive trait. When the hair is examined under polarized light, alternating light and dark areas are seen. When associated with other signs, the disorder is often referred to as BIDS or IBIDS syndrome depending on whether ichthyosis is associated. The acronyms stand for *i*chthyosis, *b*rittle hair, *i*ntellectual impairment, *d*ecreased fertility, and *s*hort stature.

FOCAL NONSCARRING ALOPECIA

1. ALOPECIA AREATA

Essentials of Diagnosis

- Localized patch or patches of complete alopecia.
- No scarring and no scalp disease.
- May be associated with acute hair fall, especially if generalized.
- Exclamation point hairs or tapered hairs on microscopic examination.

General Considerations

Alopecia areata is common. Both sexes are equally affected, but women are more likely to seek medical care. The disorder can occur at any age but is most prevalent in the third to fifth decades. It can be localized, involving only a single patch of hair 1–2 cm in diameter, or so extensive that all body hair is lost.

The cause is unknown. Genetic factors may play a role, and autosomal dominant inheritance has occurred in certain families. Although emotional stress has been implicated as a cause, a disorder of autoimmunity seems more likely. Evidence implicating autoimmunity in the pathogenesis includes the finding of a lymphocytic infiltrate around hair follicles before the hairs are shed, the presence of coexisting autoimmune disease in certain patients, a high prevalence of

autoantibodies to various tissues, and abnormalities in the ratios of circulating helper and suppressor cells.

Clinical Findings

A. Symptoms and Signs:

1. Localized form– The patient usually discovers a small patch of hair loss. In this patch, the hair loss is complete (Fig 28–1). The patch is usually circular and ranges from 1 to 10 cm in diameter. Large patches are often associated with additional patches of hair loss elsewhere. During the active phase, the light pull test is positive at the edge of the patch but negative elsewhere unless the disorder is progressing to more generalized forms. The nails may also be affected, with ridging, pitting, or splitting of the free edge. In some cases these nail changes are extensive.

2. Alopecia totalis– In alopecia totalis, hair fall is sudden and generalized, leading to complete alopecia of the scalp. Body hair is preserved.

3. Alopecia areata universalis– In this form, all hair is lost from the body, including pubic, axillary, eyebrow, and eyelid hair.

B. Laboratory Findings: Examination of hairs removed by light pull discloses a tapering shaft with loss of pigment proximally. Frequently, a very dystrophic bulb is present at the end (exclamation point hair). If signs or symptoms of an autoimmune disease are present, laboratory tests can be directed toward detection of autoantibodies associated with them. In general, these tests are ordered only on proper indications. Among the associated disorders are thyroiditis, vitiligo, pernicious anemia, Addison's disease, and hypoparathyroidism. Many patients have antinuclear

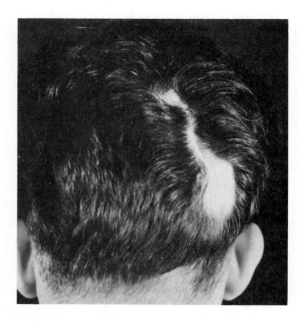

Figure 28–1. Alopecia areata. Note the well-marginated patches of complete nonscarring hair loss.

antibodies and antibodies to thyroid microsomes or thyroglobulin. Patients may also have antibodies to gastric parietal cells, adrenal tissue, or other material.

Differential Diagnosis

Alopecia areata totalis and alopecia areata universalis must be differentiated from telogen effluvium (see above). Localized alopecia areata can be differentiated from trichotillomania and tinea capitis because no hairs remain in the affected area in alopecia areata, whereas short broken hairs usually are seen in the other 2 conditions. The patch of alopecia sometimes appears scarred, in which case biopsy may be indicated to rule out causes of cicatricial alopecia.

Complications & Sequelae

Patients who have one attack of alopecia areata are liable to have another in later years. The more extensive the hair loss, the more likely the chance of recurrence and the less likely the chance for regrowth. Loss of hair over the occipital scalp is a particularly bad sign for regrowth. Patients who lose eyelash hair complain of eye irritation and frequent foreign bodies in the eye.

Treatment

There is no curative treatment. Hair can be induced to regrow with systemic corticosteroids, but their use is rarely justified. In general, high-potency corticosteroids are applied topically. Alternatively, the areas are injected with triamcinolone acetonide in a concentration of 5 mg/mL at multiple sites. Blindness has occasionally occurred following these injections. The injections must be repeated every 4–6 weeks, or hair loss will often recur. The total dose should not exceed 20 mg of triamcinolone at each treatment. Dangers from long-term systemic absorption must be considered.

Various irritants can sometimes induce regrowth of hair. Anthralin in 1–2% concentrations has been used, but pain of irritation and staining of scalp and hair have been problems.

For some reason, elicitation of allergic contact dermatitis in the areas of alopecia may induce hair growth. There is no commercially available chemical for this purpose, and this treatment must be deemed experimental.

Likewise, PUVA has been effective in some patients. However, regrowth of hair shields the scalp, so that treatments are less effective once hair starts growing.

Application of topical solutions of minoxidil can induce regrowth in some patients.

2. TRICHOTILLOMANIA

Essentials of Diagnosis

- A patch of hair loss, usually incomplete.

- History of pulling on hair.
- Scalp biopsy may show empty distorted follicles.

General Considerations

Manipulation of the hair either breaks it off or pulls it from the follicle. This may be a manifestation of psychiatric illness. A common habit resulting in trichotillomania is twirling the hair on a finger. Some patients compulsively pluck hairs, eg, on the eyebrows.

Clinical Findings

Unless hairs are being plucked with tweezers, usually some short hairs are present within the patch of alopecia. These represent broken hairs or hairs that have regrown but are still too short to grab and pull. Scarring is usually not present, nor is inflammation. Biopsy shows normally growing hair adjacent to empty hair follicles. Inflammation is absent. Empty follicles may be distorted, particularly in the intrafollicular area. The follicular epithelium may be traumatically separated from the surrounding connective tissue sheath.

Treatment

It is often difficult to convince patients to give up the habit, so the prognosis is poor. In children, trichotillomania is often simply a phase of growing up and often disappears with time. However, trichotillomania may be a presenting manifestation of severe psychiatric illness or may accompany mental retardation.

3. TRACTION ALOPECIA

Constant traction on the hair shaft can cause hair loss. Typically this is from hairstyles such as ponytails or corn rows. Traction alopecia may also occur from curlers that are applied too tightly or from vigorous hair brushing or barrettes or from attachments of hair pieces or caps. The alopecia is rarely complete, and many short hairs are seen in the area.

4. ALOPECIA MUCINOSA

In this disorder, hair follicles are infiltrated with mucin. If lesions occur on the scalp, hair loss occurs. The scalp skin may be slightly pink or hyperpigmented, and there may be scales or follicular plugs. Biopsy confirms the diagnosis. In adults, boggy plaques suggest the propensity for development of cutaneous T cell lymphomas. The relationship between alopecia mucinosa and cutaneous T cell lymphomas is not understood. A total body examination should be made to look for plaques or patches suggesting lymphoma.

No therapy is regularly effective, but topical therapy with high-potency corticosteroids may help.

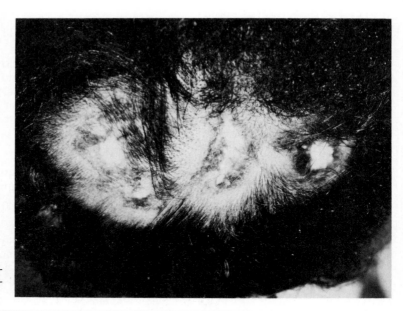

Figure 28–2. Discoid lupus erythematosus. This is an example of a focal scarring alopecia.

Intralesional injections of 0.1 mL of triamcinolone, 5–10 mg/mL in various sites, may be effective. In the absence of cutaneous T cell lymphomas, most lesions resolve within 2 years, but some leave permanent hair loss if follicles have been destroyed.

LOCALIZED SCARRING ALOPECIA

Damage to scalp skin can lead to scarring and permanent loss of hair follicles. If hair follicles are not present, the hair cannot grow. Mechanical trauma, burns, radiation, and chemicals can all cause this disorder, as can neoplasms such as basal cell carcinomas, squamous cell carcinomas, metastatic tumors, lymphomas, and adnexal tumors. Infections of the scalp—including tinea capitis—can sometimes lead to scarring and permanent hair loss. Bacterial infections, particularly staphylococcal folliculitis, are not uncommon causes. Certain dermatoses can produce permanent hair loss. These include discoid lupus erythematosus (Fig 28–2), lichen planus, sarcoidosis, lichen sclerosus et atrophicus, necrobiosis lipoidica diabeticorum, cicatricial pemphigoid, follicular mucinosis, acne keloidalis, pseudopelade of Brocq, folliculitis decalvans, and amyloidosis. The presence of skin disease on other body areas is the best clue to diagnosis. Furthermore, active (not yet scarred) lesions of these disorders may be present elsewhere on the scalp.

Developmental defects causing scarring on the scalp include aplasia cutis congenita, Darier's disease, epidermal nevi, organoid nevi, epidermolysis bullosa, and others.

REFERENCES

Alexander S: Common baldness in women. Semin Dermatol 1985;4:1.

Birnbaum PS, Baden HP: Heritable disorders of hair. Dermatol Clin 1987;5:137.

Dawber RP: Special symposium on dermatological therapy. 5. Diseases of the appendages: Alopecia and hirsutism. Clin Exp Dermatol 1982;7:177.

Mitchell AJ, Krull EA: Alopecia areata: Pathogenesis and treatment. J Am Acad Dermatol 1984;11:763.

Nelson DA, Spielvogel RL: Alopecia areata. Int J Dermatol 1985;24:26.

Whiting DA: Structural abnormalities of the hair shaft. J Am Acad Dermatol 1987;16:1.

Disorders of the Nails

29

Peter Samman, MD*

The nails have both functional and cosmetic importance. Disorders of nails can cause pain, interfere with manual dexterity, and appear ugly. Furthermore, because they may provide clues to the diagnosis of other medical problems, the fingernails and toenails should be examined routinely.

ANATOMY

The nails are formed from an invagination of epidermis on the dorsum of the distal phalanx of each digit. They are first visible in the 9-week-old embryo; the nail plate is almost complete by the 20th week. The nail fold consists of a floor, a roof, and lateral walls. The nail plate is formed from the matrix, which extends from the junction of the roof and the floor proximally to the distal edge of the lunula, or half-moon. The lunula may not be visible but can usually be seen on the thumbs (Fig 29–1, left). The matrix is well protected from injury; it is covered by the epidermis and dermis of the skin of the dorsal nail fold and below that by the dermis and epidermis of the roof of the nail fold invagination. The nail plate separates the skin of the nail fold from the matrix (Fig 29–1, right). Anterior to the matrix, the nail plate rests on the nail bed and is firmly attached to it by ridges on the undersurface of the nail plate that fit into corrugations on the nail bed in a fashion similar to that characterizing tongue-and-groove carpentry. The upper surface of the nail plate is formed from the most proximal part of the matrix; the lower surface is formed from the most distal part of the matrix.

Healthy nails are uniformly pink and bear faint longitudinal striations that become more prominent late in life. The upper surface of the nail plate is much harder than the lower, but the lower is more pliable. The space between the nail plate and the dorsal nail fold is closed by the cuticle, which is an extension of the epidermis of the dorsal nail fold onto the nail plate. A similar extension of the epidermis of the roof of the nail fold is the eponychium. The cuticle and eponychium are normally fused and appear as a single entity. At the point of separation of the nail plate from the nail bed is the hyponychium, an extension of the epidermis of the tip of the digit onto the undersurface of the nail plate.

The nail plate consists of hard keratin, a protein made up of amino acids rich in sulfur. Normally, the nail plate derives no material from the nail bed, but occasionally the nails are greatly thickened by material from the nail bed, which is not true hard keratin. The nail plate absorbs water from the environment; when a nail is saturated, 30% of its weight is due to water. The flexibility of a nail depends on its water content. A dry nail becomes brittle; a saturated nail is soft and easy to cut. Contrary to general belief, nails have little calcium.

Unlike hair, nails grow continuously. The rate varies considerably among individuals and averages from 0.5 to 1.2 mm per week; it gradually slows with age.

Nails in humans are less important than their counterparts, the claws, in other animals. The value of human nails is mainly cosmetic, but nails do contribute to the stability of the distal phalanx and assist in picking up small objects. They are also used for scratching.

DEVELOPMENTAL DISORDERS OF THE NAILS

There are 4 major developmental nail disorders and a few others of less clinical importance. No specific treatment is available for any of them, but symptomatic treatment and consultation with a podiatrist may be of benefit, especially in patients with hyperkeratoses due to pachyonychia congenita.

*The author wishes to thank the photographic departments of Westminster Hospital and St. John's Hospital for Diseases of the Skin (London) for the illustrations in this chapter.

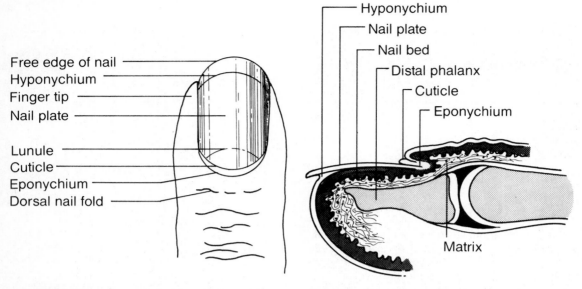

Free edge of nail
Hyponychium
Finger tip
Nail plate

Lunule
Cuticle
Eponychium
Dorsal nail fold

Hyponychium
Nail plate
Nail bed
Distal phalanx
Cuticle
Eponychium

Matrix

Figure 29–1. *Left:* Main features of the nail. *Right:* Longitudinal section through nail plate and matrix.

NAIL-PATELLA SYNDROME

Nail-patella syndrome is an uncommon congenital autosomal dominant abnormality affecting the patellas as well as the nails. The nail changes are usually the most obvious. In severe disease, the thumbnails are almost entirely missing (Fig 29–2); the other fingernails are affected to a lesser extent and in de-

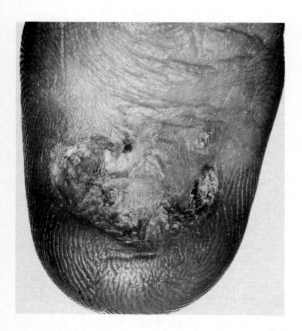

Figure 29–2. Nail-patella syndrome.

creasing severity from the index to the small finger, which is almost normal. Some nails are split into unequal parts, each of which may be spoon-shaped. In some patients whose nails are otherwise almost normal, the lunulas are triangular instead of crescent-shaped. In the mildest form of the disease, only the thumbnails are abnormal and only the ulnar half of the nail is missing.

Associated abnormalities of other parts of the body may also occur. The patellas are either small or absent. The carrying angle of the elbow is altered, so that the patient cannot totally extend the elbow to straighten the arm. A bony spur projecting from the ilium (iliac horn) is visible on x-ray. These changes cause little disability in themselves, though patients tend to develop chronic glomerulonephritis later in life.

PACHYONYCHIA CONGENITA

Pachyonychia congenita is an uncommon congenital autosomal dominant anomaly that probably comprises 3 or 4 separate conditions. The nails are typically greatly thickened, and some appear wedge-shaped, with the distal portion being the thickest (Fig 29–3). The thickening is due to addition of material from the nail bed to the true nail.

Severe painful hyperkeratoses may form on the feet, hands, and elbows after initial development of painful bullae. In some families, affected members have teeth that are fully erupted at birth; these take the place of normal milk teeth and are soft and soon shed. Other features include cysts, eg, sebocystomatosis (steatocystoma multiplex); areas of macular pigmen-

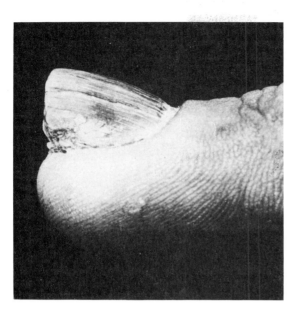

Figure 29–3. Pachyonychia congenita.

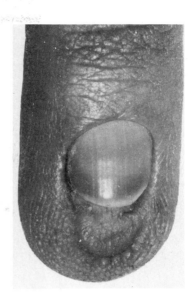

Figure 29–4. Nail in hidrotic ectodermal defect.

tation on the neck and trunk; and candidiasis and leukokeratosis of the oral mucosa.

CONGENITAL ECTODERMAL DEFECTS

Congenital ectodermal defects are classified as hidrotic or anhidrotic. The anhidrotic type is a recessive trait associated with mild nail defects in some patients, whereas the hidrotic type is an autosomal dominant condition in which all patients demonstrate nail defects and more severe involvement. The nails are small and short and fail to reach the tips of the digits. The nail bed is uncovered, and the adjacent skin of the digit has an abnormal dermatoglyphic pattern (Fig 29–4). The nails are often only loosely attached to the nail bed, and a malodorous infection may develop below the nail. Half of patients show severe alopecia of the scalp and other areas.

RACKET NAIL

Racket nail is probably the commonest (but not a major) congenital nail deformity. It is actually an abnormality of the distal phalanx of the thumb, which is shorter than normal; consequently, the nail is short and wide (Fig 29–5). It is an autosomal dominant trait and occurs more commonly in women than in men. One or both thumbs may be affected.

OTHER DEVELOPMENTAL DISORDERS

Other developmental disorders of the nails include (1) familial clubbing and koilonychia (spoon nails); (2) periodic shedding of nails; (3) abnormalities of specific digits, such as congenital malalignment of the nails of the great toes; and (4) congenital onychodysplasia of the index fingers.

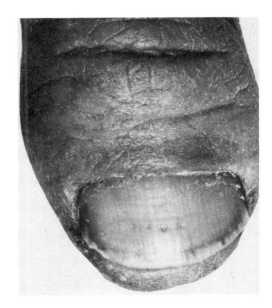

Figure 29–5. Racket nail.

INFECTIONS OF THE NAILS

ACUTE PARONYCHIA

Acute paronychia is usually caused by staphylococci. The patient presents with tender swelling of the dorsal nail fold. Superficial infection may present as a pustule, which should be incised and drained. For deeper lesions, antibiotics such as dicloxacillin, 250 mg 4 times daily for adults, are required. Less often, acute paronychia complicates chronic paronychia (see below) when various other organisms, including gram-negative bacteria, are involved. The choice of antibiotics may be based on the results of culture and sensitivity tests.

HERPES SIMPLEX INFECTION

Herpes simplex infection occurring on the distal phalanx is known as herpetic whitlow. It is manifested as grouped painful vesicles and is especially common in nurses, dental technicians, and other medical personnel who are exposed to the virus shed in the secretions of infected patients. Oral acyclovir, 200 mg every 4 hours, 5 times each day, may shorten the attack, which otherwise lasts about 10 days. Viral culture and Tzanck smears can differentiate herpetic whitlow from acute bacterial paronychia if the clinical appearance is confusing.

CANDIDIASIS

Infection with *Candida* species is the most important etiologic factor in chronic paronychia. The disorder is especially common in women who often have their hands in water. Although it is rare in men, it is seen in those who are bartenders, fishmongers, and bakers. It occurs frequently in diabetics and in persons who have cold hands. It rarely occurs on the toes.

Clinical Findings

Candidal infection of the nails is common and presents as redness and swelling of the dorsal nail fold (Fig 29–6). Typically, the cuticle is missing entirely or in part and infection enters the nail fold, from which pus may occasionally extrude. Later, the edge of the nail becomes irregular and discolored, possibly as a result of secondary infection with gram-negative organisms, especially *Pseudomonas aeruginosa*. *Candida*, usually *C albicans*, can almost always be recovered in material taken from the nail fold; it is often seen in material from the nail edge, but true

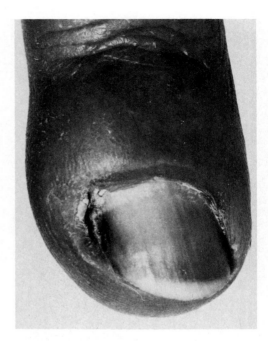

Figure 29–6. Chronic paronychia.

invasion of the nail plate is rare and is normally found only in immunodeficient patients.

Treatment

The most important feature of management is to keep the hands dry and warm. Rubber gloves may be helpful but should be worn only over cotton gloves and not directly next to the skin.

Nystatin ointment, frequently applied, provides relief. Clotrimazole cream (1%) or miconazole cream (2%) may also be used. Candidiasis should not be considered cured until all swelling has subsided and the cuticle has regrown; this may take 3 months or more.

DERMATOPHYTE INFECTIONS
(Onychomycosis)

Essentials of Diagnosis

- Yellow, thick, crumbly nail plate.
- Distal onycholysis.
- Fungi seen in nail plate (KOH preparation).
- Superficial chalky-white color.

General Considerations

True fungal invasion of the nail commonly occurs on the feet in association with tinea pedis; it is much less common on the hands. The infection spreads to the nail plate from the nail bed and is usually due to

Trichophyton rubrum or *Trichophyton mentagrophytes.*

Clinical Findings

A. Symptoms and Signs: Infection initially appears as discoloration of the nail edge and progresses proximally until the entire nail plate is discolored and ragged. Less often, there is only a superficial infection of the upper surface of the nail plate, which gives the nail a chalky appearance (Fig 29–7). The nail sometimes separates from the nail bed (onycholysis).

B. Laboratory Findings: The diagnosis is confirmed by finding fungal filaments and spores in potassium hydroxide preparations of the nail plate. (Full-thickness clippings of the affected nail are soaked in a few drops of potassium hydroxide 5% for 24 hours. The clippings soften and can be easily prepared for microscopic examination.) Culture is useful but not essential, because negative cultures occur even when abundant filaments are seen microscopically.

Treatment

Fungal infections of the fingernails are conspicuous, and the resulting dystrophy may interfere with normal activities such as paper handling. Most cases should be treated.

A. Griseofulvin: Griseofulvin microsize, 750–1000 mg/d orally, is the drug of choice. Treatment is continued until the affected nail grows out; this takes as long as 6 months. The drug is well tolerated by most patients, but a few develop headaches or photosensitivity, in which case treatment should be discontinued. The effectiveness of treatment depends largely on patient compliance. Cure can be obtained in most cases if the patient has not undergone previous treatment with griseofulvin; second or third courses of treatment are much less satisfactory, because the dermatophyte develops relative resistance.

Toenail infections are less important than fingernail infections and are difficult to treat, partly because it takes 12–18 months for a toenail to grow from matrix to tip. Except in young children, griseofulvin is usually *not* prescribed unless fingernails are also infected. In children, the dosage is griseofulvin microsize, 10 mg/kg/d orally. If only one or 2 nails are affected, they may be surgically removed and griseofulvin given for a few weeks.

B. Ketoconazole: Ketoconazole, a wide-spectrum antifungal antibiotic effective against dermatophytes and *Candida*, should be used only in patients with severe infections that have failed to respond to griseofulvin or in patients who are unable to take griseofulvin. The dosage is 200 mg orally once daily with food. Liver function tests must be monitored (see Chapters 16 and 53).

C. Other Drugs: Topical applications of antifungal preparations play little part in the treatment of most dermatophytic infections of the nails, but superficial infections (chalky appearance) may respond to ciclopirox, clotrimazole, or miconazole creams. Coexisting tinea pedis must be treated with a standard regimen.

TRAUMA TO THE NAILS

SUBUNGUAL HEMATOMA

Subungual hematoma commonly occurs after trauma to the nail, eg, from a direct blow, trapping the finger in a door or drawer. Pain is reduced if the blood is released by puncturing the nail plate with a cautery, drill, or fine scalpel blade. Without treatment, the nail may be shed. If the injury involves the matrix, an unsightly permanent ridge or split may develop.

NAIL BITING & CUTICLE TRAUMA

Self-inflicted injury in the form of nail biting is common and results in a short, ragged nail bitten back to the hyponychium. Biting is one of the causes of recurrent acute paronychia. Viral warts around bitten nails are common (see below).

The habit of pulling back the cuticle of the thumb

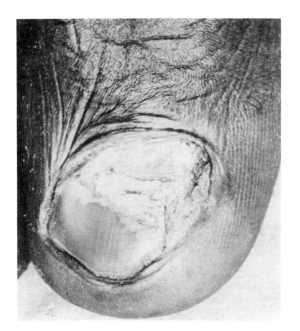

Figure 29–7. Superficial fungal infection of nail.

with the index finger of the same hand produces a ridge down the center of the nail with numerous cross ridges extending from it to the edge of the nail (Fig 29–8).

MEDIAN NAIL DYSTROPHY

Median nail dystrophy is an uncommon disorder that is similar to self-inflicted cuticle injury. The cause is unknown but is probably associated with trauma; all patients with this condition have large lunulas, so that more of the nail matrix is exposed than usual. Median nail dystrophy is characterized by a true split through the nail (Fig 29–9) that first appears at the cuticle and progresses until the entire nail is split. It usually affects one or both thumbs, but other nails may be affected. The split may clear spontaneously only to reappear later. A ridge on the nail may replace the split.

CHEMICAL TRAUMA

Continuous Wetting
Lamellar dystrophy (splitting of nails into layers) occurs commonly in homemakers and others who have their hands frequently in water. The cause is thought to be the often repeated absorption and evaporation of water from the nail plate, with resulting loss of adhesion between nail cells.

Cosmetics
Cosmetics may produce minor disorders. In some

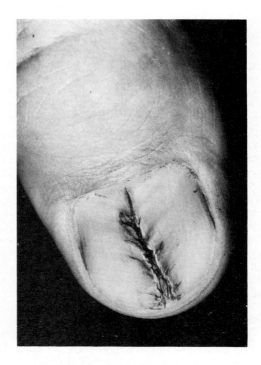

Figure 29–9. Median dystrophy.

nail polishes, pigments may leak into the nail plate and cause staining of the nail. The nail may be stained a color different from that of the polish, because only one of the mixture of several pigments may enter the nail plate.

Nail Hardeners
Nail hardeners—especially those containing formaldehyde—may produce onycholysis of one or several nails. Artificial nails may produce roughness of the nail surface or local infection resulting from a reaction to materials in the false nail.

DRUG REACTIONS AFFECTING THE NAILS

Bullous lesions affecting the tips of the digits may disturb the nail matrix and result in temporary or permanent loss of the nail. The bullae may be caused by drugs such as sulfonamides that provoke a reaction resembling the lesions of erythema multiforme.

Discoloration of the nails may be caused by various drugs, eg, a blue-gray color due to mepacrine or chloroquine, a yellow color from prolonged use of

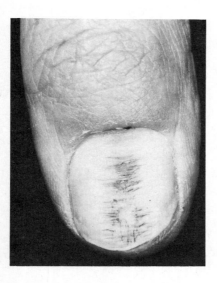

Figure 29–8. Deformity of nail due to habitual self-inflicted trauma to cuticle.

tetracycline, or darkening of the nail due to hydroxy-urea.

DERMATOLOGIC DISORDERS INVOLVING THE NAILS

Many nail abnormalities are due to primary dermatologic disorders. In most cases, the nail changes constitute a minor manifestation of the disease, but in a few conditions the nail changes are characteristic and important.

PSORIASIS

Essentials of Diagnosis
- Pitting or onycholysis, often irregularly proximal to the hyponychium, and yellow-colored (oil spot) nails; or
- Grossly thick, friable nail plates with subungual hyperkeratosis.
- Presence of psoriasis on the skin.

General Considerations
Most patients with psoriasis are likely to experience nail changes at some point during the disease. Toenails are affected less often than fingernails.

Clinical Findings
A. Pitting: Pitting (often called "thimble pitting") is the most common change in psoriatic nails. The pits are usually small (≤ 1 mm) and scattered over one or more nails (Fig 29–10). Sometimes they are closely packed and cover all nails. Pits are due to psoriasis of the nail matrix.

B. Onycholysis: Onycholysis is the second most common change in psoriatic nails; it is often associated with a change in color (salmon patch or oil spot) over a small area adjacent to the site of onycholysis (Fig 29–11). The onset of separation may be abrupt and affect several nails, and it is often associated with some discomfort.

C. Roughening and Loss of Luster: The nails may become dull, rough, and discolored. No fungal elements are found in nail clippings. Less often, the nail is greatly thickened—best seen on the toes. The shape of the nail plate may be distorted and the edge lifted up by subungual hyperkeratosis from psoriasis of the nail bed.

Differential Diagnosis
The diagnosis of psoriatic nails is usually obvious from the associated skin lesions but may be difficult if these are lacking. Pitting is not limited to psoriasis; it

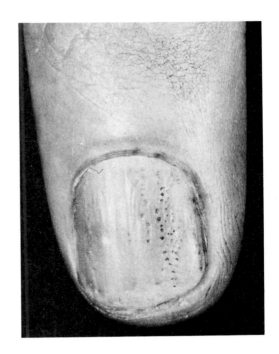

Figure 29–10. Pitting psoriasis.

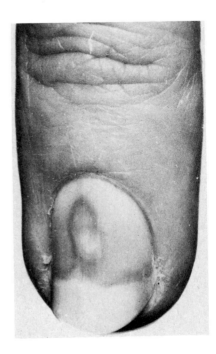

Figure 29–11. Onycholysis and salmon patch associated with psoriasis.

occurs also in alopecia areata and eczema, and a few isolated pits may be found in the nails of healthy individuals. In alopecia areata, the pits are usually smaller and fewer than those in psoriasis. In eczema, they are usually larger than those in psoriasis and they are irregularly shaped.

Onycholysis may be due to many causes, eg, fungal infections, some drug eruptions, and impaired circulation; in a few patients, onycholysis is idiopathic. The associated salmon patches are seen only in psoriasis and closely related conditions. The only important differential diagnosis with regard to changes in gross appearance is fungal infection, which is easily ruled out on the basis of microscopic examination of nail cuttings. Arthritis of the distal interphalangeal joints is commonly associated with psoriasis and is helpful in confirming the diagnosis. The same changes can also be produced by conditions closely related to psoriasis, eg, pustular psoriasis (Fig 29–12), pityriasis rubra pilaris, and Reiter's syndrome.

Treatment

There is no specific treatment for nail psoriasis. Spontaneous improvement occurs in many cases. Application of one of the more potent topical corticosteroids (eg, fluocinonide solution) to the dorsal nail fold may bring about improvement in lesions resulting from a matrix disorder. When corticosteroids are applied under loosened nails, however, they may encourage infection.

ECZEMATOUS DERMATITIS

Atopic eczema and constitutional hand eczema (pompholyx, or dyshidrosis) are the types of eczema most likely to involve the nails. Eczema affecting the nails is usually on the hands, particularly the dorsum of the fingers, but it may have resolved before nail changes appear.

Eczema affecting the nails is usually manifested as coarse pitting or irregular cross-ridging (Fig 29–13) of one or several nails. Occasionally, the nail is greatly thickened. The diagnosis is usually obvious when the patient presents with eczema of the hands or a recent history of eczema; however, many patients are referred with an initial diagnosis of fungal infection.

Treatment of the associated eczema will bring about slow resolution of the nail changes.

LICHEN PLANUS

Nail changes occur in up to 10% of patients with lichen planus. The most common change is an increased number of the normal longitudinal striations of the nail plate. This change is usually seen in association with widespread lichen planus and is a transi-

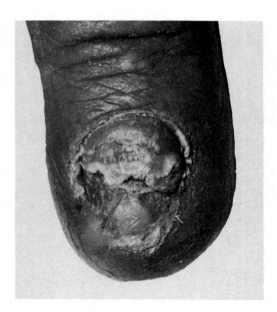

Figure 29–12. Pustular psoriasis.

tory condition that clears spontaneously. Occasionally, nail changes occur with no other evidence of lichen planus. A more serious change in the nail matrix occurs less frequently, when the dorsal nail fold fuses with the matrix to form a pterygium (Fig 29–14). Sometimes the entire matrix is destroyed, resulting in permanent nail loss with scarring (Fig 29–14, little finger).

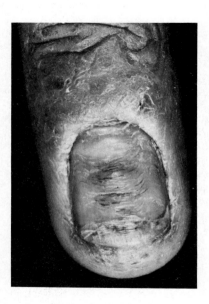

Figure 29–13. Eczema causing distortion of nail.

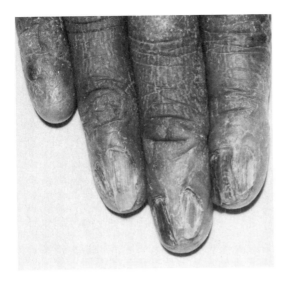

Figure 29–14. Lichen planus.

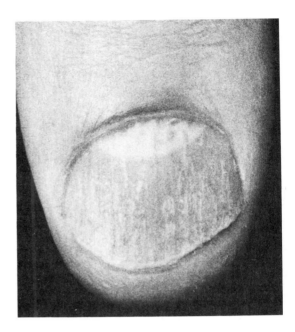

Figure 29–15. Nail dystrophy in alopecia areata. Note mottling in lunula.

More serious changes are usually heralded by erythema and discomfort around the dorsal nail fold, and it is these that are most likely to affect the nails of the great toe and to be associated with ulceration of the soles.

When severe changes are thought to be imminent, administration of oral corticosteroids may lessen the damage. A standard regimen is prednisone, 30 mg/d orally for 6 weeks, followed by a gradual reduction in dosage so that treatment can be discontinued after 3 months. Lichen planus is uncommon in childhood, but severe nail changes are seen more frequently in children than in adults.

ALOPECIA AREATA

Alopecia areata is usually a disorder of childhood that gradually clears spontaneously. As in the case of lichen planus, alopecia areata is associated with nail changes in about 10% of patients; the changes are more likely to occur when alopecia is widespread. The usual change is fine pitting of one or several nails that must be distinguished from psoriasis. Rarely, all fingernails and toenails roughen, lose their luster, and demonstrate koilonychia. There may be mottling of the lunulas (Fig 29–15). Some nails are thinner and some thicker than normal.

There is no known treatment.

DARIER'S DISEASE

Darier's disease is a rare skin condition in which nail changes are present in most patients. The disease is characterized by a linear white streak that extends from the tip of the fingernail to the cuticle and passes through the lunula (Fig 29–16). Less characteristic is a similar brown streak. A triangular niche is often found where the streaks meet the free edge of the nail. The nails are usually ragged and broken.

There is no known treatment.

TUMORS INVOLVING THE NAILS

VIRAL WARTS

Viral warts are the only common tumors that usually grow near the nails. They are frequently seen in children and are often associated with nail biting. They arise in the lateral or dorsal nail fold and may almost encircle the nail. They occasionally grow under the tip of the nail, which may then be displaced upward.

The conventional treatment regimen for warts is satisfactory if it is followed conscientiously (see Chapter 14).

PERIUNGUAL FIBROMA

Periungual fibroma is a benign tumor most often seen in patients with tuberous sclerosis; multiple le-

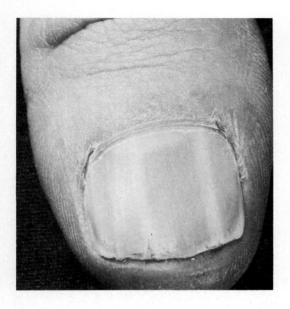

Figure 29–16. Darier's disease.

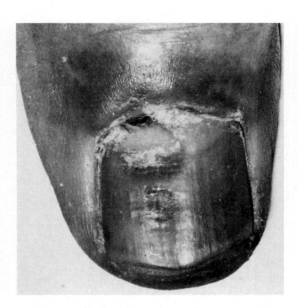

Figure 29–17. Mucous cyst distorting the nail.

sions are common. They grow beneath the nail fold and may cause depressions of the nail plate but are otherwise harmless.

GLOMUS TUMORS

Glomus tumors occasionally develop beneath the nail, where they give rise to a painful bluish mark visible through the nail.

Surgical removal is required.

MUCOUS CYSTS

Mucous cysts are not true tumors. They present as a swelling of the dorsal nail fold, often in association with osteoarthritis of the distal interphalangeal joints. If they cause pressure on the matrix, they give rise to a linear depression on the nail surface. They may discharge their contents periodically (Fig 29–17) and therefore fluctuate in size.

Surgical removal or intralesional injection of triamcinolone acetonide suspension, 5 mg/mL, is not always successful.

LONGITUDINAL PIGMENTED BANDS ON THE NAIL SURFACE

In dark-skinned individuals, longitudinal pigmented bands on the nails are of little significance.

When they occur in a Caucasian, however, they are often due to a junctional (melanocytic) nevus in the nail matrix. Such nevi occasionally become malignant, and any enlargement is an occasion for biopsy.

MALIGNANT MELANOMA

Subungual malignant melanoma is a tumor occurring below the nail and is usually classified as an acral lentiginous melanoma. It has both radial and vertical growth phases and frequently metastasizes. It may present as a pigmented band, as a warty lesion on the nail bed, as a pyogenic granuloma, or as chronic paronychia. Chronic paronychia that affects a single nail and is refractory to treatment should be regarded with suspicion, and a biopsy should be obtained.

If treatment is started during the radial growth phase, the prognosis is good. If treatment begins during the vertical phase—and the growth pattern may change swiftly from lateral spread to vertical development—the outlook is more uncertain. Surgical removal of the lesion is required, and amputation of the digit may be necessary.

EPITHELIAL TUMORS

Epithelial tumors are rarely encountered below the nail but may present as chronic paronychia. Local removal is advised.

NAIL DISORDERS ASSOCIATED WITH SYSTEMIC DISEASE

Numerous nail changes are associated with medical disorders, but because the same nail changes may also occur in the absence of these disorders, undue emphasis must not be placed on the association between the two.

KOILONYCHIA

Koilonychia (spoon-shaped nails) is characteristic of iron deficiency anemia, and this possibility should be considered whenever koilonychia is present. However, spoon-shaped nails may also occur as a developmental anomaly and may occasionally result from thinning of the nail due to other causes. In nail-patella syndrome, the nail may be split into 2 parts, and each part may be spoon-shaped.

FINGER CLUBBING

Clubbed fingers are associated with pulmonary and congenital heart diseases with cyanosis. The most severe manifestations are found in association with bronchial carcinoma, though clubbed fingers may also occur as a congenital anomaly without underlying disease.

BEAU'S LINES

Beau's lines are transverse depressions across the nails (Fig 29–18) that may occur in association with coronary thrombosis and certain infections such as measles or mumps. The depression is first visible at the cuticle a few weeks after onset of the underlying disease. When Beau's lines occur with systemic disease, all the fingernails and toenails are likely to be affected. If only one or 2 nails are involved, trauma or exposure to severe cold should be suspected as the cause.

YELLOW NAIL SYNDROME

Yellow nail syndrome is an uncommon condition in which nail growth slows or ceases and the nail plates turn yellow. The cuticles are usually missing. The nails are overcurved. Onycholysis may be severe; some nails are shed but are slowly replaced (Fig 29–19). Edema of the ankles is common and is due to abnormalities of the lymphatic system. Yellow nail syndrome often occurs in association with chronic bronchitis, bronchiectasis, or pleural effusion; sinusitis is also common.

There is no specific treatment. Some nails return to normal spontaneously. Associated underlying conditions should be treated.

OTHER COLORED NAILS

White nails occur in association with renal and liver diseases (Fig 29–20). The color change is in the

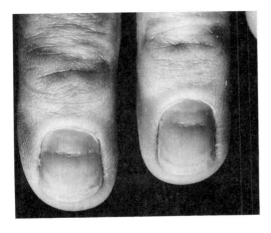

Figure 29–18. Beau's lines.

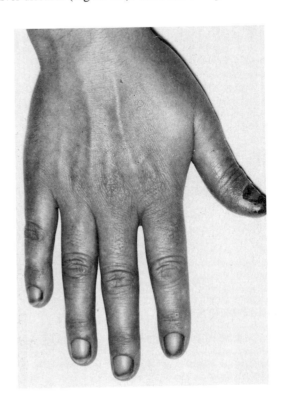

Figure 29–19. Yellow nail syndrome.

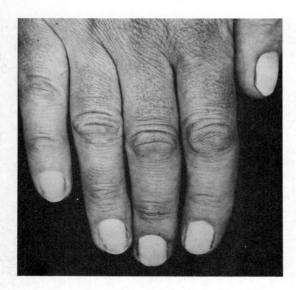

Figure 29–20. White nails in liver disease.

nail bed, not in the nail itself. In chronic heart failure, the lunulas may be red, whereas in Wilson's disease (hepatolenticular degeneration), they may be blue.

ONYCHOLYSIS

Onycholysis (discussed above) is a common symptom for which no cause can be found in some patients (idiopathic), though in many instances it is associated with thyroid disorders, including hypothyroidism and hyperthyroidism.

SPLINTER HEMORRHAGES

Splinter hemorrhages were once thought to be associated with subacute infective endocarditis, but they are now known to occur in many other general systemic and dermatologic diseases as well. These hemorrhages also occur after minor injury to the digits.

SYSTEMIC LUPUS ERYTHEMATOSUS & DERMATOMYOSITIS

Although the nails themselves are usually not affected in systemic lupus erythematosus and dermatomyositis, tortuous capillaries are visible in the dorsal nail folds, and the folds themselves appear red.

RIDGING, THINNING, & SPLITTING OF NAILS

Impaired peripheral circulation due either to spasm (Raynaud's phenomenon) or to physical obstruction of the digital vessels may cause nail changes. There is increased ridging, the nails are thinned and split (Fig 29–21), and they lose their even, pink color. Parts of the nail are darker than usual, and the tips tend to be white owing to associated onycholysis.

Some improvement may be obtained by treating with vasodilator drugs such as nifedipine, 10 mg orally 3 times daily.

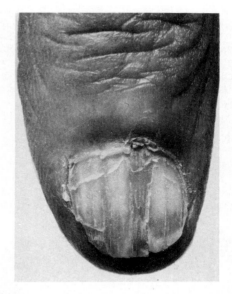

Figure 29–21. Nails in patients with impaired circulation.

REFERENCES

Baran R, Dawber RP (editors): *Diseases of the Nails and Their Management.* Mosby, 1984.
Beaven DW: *Color Atlas of the Nails in Clinical Diagnosis.* Year Book , 1984.
Daniel CR III: The nail. (Symposium.) Dermatol Clin 1985;3:371. [Entire issue.]
Daniel CR III, Scher RK: Nail changes secondary to sys-

temic drugs or ingestants. J Am Acad Dermatol 1984; 10:250.
Gunnoe RE: Diseases of the nails: How to recognize and treat them. Postgrad Med (Sept) 1983;74:357.
Jeanmougin M, Civatte J: Nail dyschromia. Int J Dermatol 1983;22:279.
Kechijian P: Onycholysis of the fingernails: Evaluation and

management. J Am Acad Dermatol 1985;12:552.

Norton LA: Diseases of the nails. In: *Dermatology,* 2nd ed. Moschella SL, Hurley HJ (editors). Saunders, 1985.

Salasche SJ, Peters VJ: Tips on nail surgery. Cutis 1985; 35:428, 435.

Samman PD, Fenton DA: *The Nails in Disease,* 4th ed. Heinemann, 1986.

Scher RK: Diseases of the nails. In: *Conn's Current Therapy.* Rakel RE (editor). Saunders, 1984.

Scher RK: Onychomycosis: Examining, diagnosis and treatment. Mycol Observ 1984;4:1.

Scher RK: Toenail disorders . In: *Clinics in Dermatology.* Parish LC (editor). Lippincott, 1983.

Scher RK, Daniel CR III: Surgery of the nails. In: *Clinical Dermatology.* Vol 1. Demis DJ (editor). Lippincott, 1985.

Zaias N: *The Nails in Health and Disease.* Spectrum, 1980.

30

Mast Cell Diseases*

D. Joseph Demis, MD, PhD

Mast cell disease (mastocytosis) includes a wide spectrum of clinical entities characterized by infiltration of tissue with mast cells. The clinical spectrum ranges from an innocuous single small cutaneous nodule, most common in children (**mastocytoma**)—to diffuse distribution of benign hyperpigmented macules or papules (**urticaria pigmentosa**)—to urticaria pigmentosa lesions with systemic involvement principally of the liver, spleen, and bone—to malignant **mast cell leukemia** and other rare variants. Symptoms occur in a minority of patients and include flushing, nausea, vomiting, upper gastrointestinal tract pain, tachycardia, syncope, and shock. This symptom complex gives rise to **mastocytosis syndrome**.

The course of the disease varies with the age at onset and the clinical form, but for most patients the prognosis is excellent and the course uncomplicated. In children, the skin lesions are often self-limited and frequently clear spontaneously. In adults, the skin lesions seldom disappear; although most adults experience a benign course, a few with systemic involvement have a progressively downhill lymphoma-like course. Rare cases terminate in cancer.

Classification & Clinical Picture

Mast cell disease can be classified on the basis of the clinical and pathologic findings (Table 30–1). Although many stimuli apparently can lead to deposition of an increased number of mast cells in the skin, this response is not related to the pathogenesis of mastocytosis. Healing wounds—especially burns—often contain increased numbers of mast cells, as do many chronic inflammatory dermatoses, including atopic dermatitis and lichen planus. Speculation about the cause of this disease has continued for years, but to date the cause has not been determined.

Mast cells can be found in all normal human tissue

Table 30–1. Classification of mastocytosis.

Benign
Cutaneous
Generalized (urticaria pigmentosa)
Isolated (mastocytoma)
Systemic
Skin, bone, liver, spleen, and gastrointestinal tract involvement
Malignant
Leukemia

except the brain and appear to be particularly numerous in developing connective tissue. Human mast cells are known to contain histamine and heparin, which are stored in their metachromatic granules. Both are synthesized in mast cells. There is no evidence of the presence of serotonin.

Mast cell disease is most common in Caucasians, though it also has been reported in blacks and Orientals. Hereditary factors seem to be operative only in rare cases.

MASTOCYTOMAS

Essentials of Diagnosis

- Usually solitary brown or tan plaque.
- Surface may resemble orange peels.
- Urticate or vesiculate when stroked.

General Considerations

Mastocytomas represent approximately 10% of the reported cases of mast cell disease and occur almost exclusively in children.

Clinical Findings

A. Symptoms and Signs: Mastocytomas usually appear at birth or within the first few weeks of life. Most are noted before 1 month of age. The lesions are usually solitary, but 3 or 4 may be present; they are most common on the trunk, neck, and arm, especially near the wrist.

*Modified and reprinted, with permission, from Demis DJ: Mast cell disease (urticaria pigmentosa). Curr Concepts Skin Dis 1985;6:11.

Typical lesions are raised brown or tan plaques 2–5 cm in diameter, often essentially linear though they may be annular. Their surfaces usually have the appearance of orange peel (peau d'orange). Isolated mastocytomas frequently swell or urticate, and bullae often develop; hemorrhagic bullae have been noted occasionally. Attacks of flushing, either facial or generalized, may occur and sometimes have been related to trauma to the lesion. In some infants, colic also has been attributed to lesion trauma.

B. Laboratory Findings: Biopsy specimens show large numbers of mast cells (see below).

Differential Diagnosis

Lesions may be confused with xanthomas and juvenile xanthogranulomas. The history of urtication after rubbing is virtually pathognomonic.

Treatment

Isolated mastocytomas may be excised, particularly if flushing and colicky symptoms are severe in infants. However, excision often is deferred in infants because spontaneous disappearance is the almost invariable rule. Adults do not seem to develop symptoms from mastocytomas.

Prognosis

Isolated mastocytomas occurring in childhood usually regress in a few years and generally are gone by 10 years of age, though some have persisted into adult life and a few have been followed by widespread skin lesions.

URTICARIA PIGMENTOSA

Essentials of Diagnosis

- Usual onset in childhood.
- Red to brown slightly elevated papules or nodules.
- Lesions urticate when stroked (Darier's sign).

General Considerations

The age at onset of mast cell disease is usually before 2 years; children are most commonly affected. In one series of 112 patients, 75% had onset before age 2 years (usually as urticaria pigmentosa) and most of the others between ages 15 and 40 years. Skin lesions often appear within 1 or 2 months after birth but may appear at any age; a few infants are born with the skin lesions. In general, these babies are well nourished, and growth and development are not affected.

Pathology & Pathogenesis

A. Childhood Disease: Children most often have multiple small red-brown hyperpigmented macules

(urticaria pigmentosa) or slightly elevated papules scattered principally over the trunk in symmetric distribution. The classic lesion becomes definitely erythematous and urticated in response to mild trauma (Darier's sign). Rubbing the lesion with a tongue blade is a useful office test.

Individual lesions usually are oval and do not have well-defined borders. Involvement of the neck, scalp, and extremities is common, and as a rule there are few lesions on the palms, soles, or face and only occasional lesions in the mouth or on other mucous membranes. Generally there are fewer of the larger macular lesions; most children have from 25 to 100. These larger macules are more common on the face, especially the forehead. Many patients have both the numerous small macules and several larger ones. At times the lesions may become virtually confluent.

Papules, plaques, and even nodules occur in association with macular lesions. After urtication by trauma, these larger lesions may produce local discomfort that at times may become extreme.

Vesiculation of preexisting skin lesions is common before age 2 years; as many as 70% of infants develop vesicles. Vesicles and bullae are usually clear, though lesions may appear as pustules that can resemble impetigo. New vesicles rarely develop after the age of 2 years. Bullous lesions may appear in the neonatal period and may be associated with systemic involvement and a poorer prognosis, while bullae of later onset appear to be associated with a better prognosis. Children with systemic involvement, including hepatosplenomegaly and ascites, may be stunted in growth and of strikingly short stature. A few children die.

B. Urticaria Pigmentosa in Adults: Adult patients with urticaria pigmentosa usually are said to have acquired their lesions in adult life.

1. Skin involvement– The skin lesions often start out as discrete, scattered macules similar to the characteristic childhood lesions; however, a distinctly adult form of urticaria pigmentosa begins to develop. With time, the lesions multiply and become virtually confluent—an uncommon occurrence in children. As in children, individual lesions urticate with trauma. Pruritus occurs in the majority of patients; yet for most it is surprisingly mild and inconstant. Often it takes a hot shower to induce itching or vigorous rubbing with a towel to urticate the lesions. Dermographism is present in about 50% of patients.

2. Liver and spleen– Hepatomegaly has been reported in 10–15% of patients. Liver biopsy often reveals mast cells, and fibrosis of the liver may develop. Hepatic involvement appears to predominate in adult men and is usually asymptomatic. Splenomegaly usually is associated with hepatomegaly and occurs about as frequently. The spleen contains increased numbers of mast cells and may reach a very large size, yet rupturing has not been reported.

3. Gastrointestinal tract– The gastrointestinal

tract often is involved, with lesions in the small intestine. Biopsy specimens taken from the small bowel show mast cell infiltration. A radiologic study with barium sometimes reveals characteristic rugal thickening and multiple mucosal outgrowths in the small intestine. Malabsorption of a variable but usually mild degree occurs in some patients; however, steatorrhea, gross malabsorption, and even tetany have been reported.

4. Bone– Bone lesions are frequent, occurring in 10–15% of patients. The incidence of bone lesions in children seems to be about 2%, whereas it approaches 30% in adults. The radiologic changes are variable and represent both osteoporosis and osteosclerosis. They are more frequent in adults and may be diffuse or localized.

5. Other sites– Mast cell infiltrates of lymph nodes, kidneys, periadrenal fat, and peripheral blood have been demonstrated. In fact, mast cell infiltrates may occur in any tissue with the apparent exception of the musculature and the central nervous system. Mast cells can also be found in the choroid plexus and around the blood vessels in general.

Bone marrow infiltration deserves special comment. In patients with other evidence of systemic mastocytosis, bone marrow biopsy (as opposed to aspiration) frequently reveals a moderate to large number of mast cells. Conversely, few patients in whom large numbers of mast cells are found in the bone marrow during hematologic investigation prove to have systemic mastocytosis. Tissue mast cells in peripheral blood have been reported; most patients with this manifestation have died.

Clinical Findings

Diagnosis of a typical case usually is made easily. Urtication of a hyperpigmented skin lesion (Darier's sign) is diagnostic when performed correctly. Dermographism also may be a helpful finding. Skin biopsy usually is required primarily for confirmation but may be diagnostic in atypical cases. Roentgenologic studies, bone marrow examination, and biopsies of other organs aid in establishing systemic involvement. Urinary histamine and metabolite (1,4-MIAA) determination may be helpful in the diagnosis, particularly in cases with systemic involvement.

A. Symptoms and Signs: Most patients with mastocytosis have few or no symptoms, and even symptoms that appear to be related to the disease tend to be mild. Yet a number of symptoms have been associated most commonly with systemic involvement. Mastocytosis syndrome may involve a symptom complex including skin lesions, bone lesions, and hepatosplenomegaly, as well as pruritus, headache, nausea, vomiting, diarrhea, and other gastrointestinal complaints.

Analysis of symptoms in all patients (adults and children) indicates that less than 15% have major symptoms of vomiting, syncope, or shock. Symptoms are often banal, chronic in nature, and frequently difficult to evaluate. There may be weakness, aching bones, tender ribs and vertebrae, fatigue, and malaise. Weight loss of up to 40 lb has been seen exclusively in adults with long-standing disease. Gastrointestinal symptoms (often of the peptic ulcer type), including anorexia, nausea, vague epigastric distress, hypermotility, vomiting, and diarrhea, most often are chronic. Malabsorption and occasionally frank steatorrhea may occur.

Flushing occurs most often in infants and children and seems to be of several types. A few infants with evidence only of skin lesions experience transient erythematous blotches of the trunk, neck, and face. These are usually bright-red circular macules, 10–30 cm in diameter, which disappear in 15 minutes or more and are not associated with edema. Clinically, these macules appear to be histamine-induced, and measurements of urinary histamine excretion have been correlated.

Flushes most often involve the face, neck, and upper area of the chest (blush areas). They tend to be episodic, are bright-red, and generally last 20–30 minutes. Edema is rare. Gastrointestinal symptoms may accompany flushes, and increased urinary excretion of histamine can occasionally be correlated. Chronic erythematous flushing of the upper trunk, neck, and face sometimes occurs in adult patients; generalized chronic flushing sometimes occurs in children.

Episodes of flushing most commonly develop with no discernible precipitating cause. However, some patients attribute flushing to exercise, hot baths, and food (especially cheese, alcohol, and spicy foods). Certain drugs regularly induce attacks of flushing and other symptoms in some patients; codeine and aspirin have been reported often, and other drugs (including morphine and its derivatives and atropine derivatives) known to be capable of degranulating mast cells also have been implicated.

Severe acute attacks rarely occur but tend to affect adult patients. These attacks may be dramatic but tend to be transient, usually lasting for only a few hours. Often they occur with enough regularity to be relatively predictable, suggesting the release of a mediator from mast cells followed by a refractory period during which degranulated mast cells have time to resynthesize their mediator stores. In a typical acute attack, the patient experiences a feeling of fullness of the face and head, followed by bright-red flushing of the face and a pounding headache. The patient notices tachycardia and a pounding heart. Nausea rapidly develops, and within a few minutes vomiting occurs and is followed by defecation. Syncope is the rule, and hypotension may be striking; some of the author's patients have sustained a blood pressure of 30/0 mm Hg for more than 1 hour. Sweating and chills develop, and right upper quadrant tenderness often appears.

B. Laboratory Findings:

1. Biopsy– Skin biopsy specimens from patients with mastocytosis show a characteristic infiltrate of mast cells. Specimens should be handled gently to avoid loss of granules. Typical cases show many mast cells resembling fibroblasts with spindle-shaped nuclei, though some are cuboidal with abundant eosinophilic cytoplasm. Ordinarily the cytoplasmic granules can be seen on routine stains, but special stains (Giemsa's, toluidine blue, Luna-Ishak, and methylene blue) may be required. Nodular lesions and isolated mastocytomas tend to have massive tumor-like mast cell infiltrates. The densely packed cells may fill the entire corium, extending from the epidermis to the subcutaneous fat.

2. Other laboratory findings– Laboratory studies may be helpful in diagnosing systemic mastocytosis. However, liver function test results are usually normal, even in the face of marked liver enlargement. Bone marrow examination may be indicated but requires careful interpretation. Urinary excretion of free histamine and metabolites, especially 1,4-methylimidazoleacetic acid (1,4-MIAA), may be increased markedly. Abnormal metabolism of prostaglandin D_2 by patients with mastocytosis also has been reported, but its specificity remains to be confirmed.

C. Imaging Studies: Roentgenographic studies of bone may reveal localized or generalized lesions; hepatosplenomegaly may be seen on a flat-plate x-ray film of the abdomen.

Differential Diagnosis

A number of conditions may be confused clinically with urticaria pigmentosa. The hyperpigmented macules may be mistaken for nevi or ephelides, and the xanthomas and nevoxanthoendotheliomas may be mistaken for the papular and nodular lesions. Drug eruptions often are considered.

In the bullous types of mast cell disease, bullous insect bites and bullous urticaria must be ruled out. Leukemia frequently is suggested in infants with extensive bullous lesions. Erythema multiforme with vesicles may also mimic the disease.

In patients with acute attacks, particularly with a history of recurrence, the carcinoid syndrome often is part of the differential diagnosis.

Complications

Known complications in addition to systemic involvement and possible sudden death in infants include cancer of the reticuloendothelial system. Some cases (especially in adults) have shown progression of systemic mastocytosis to lymphoma or leukemia, particularly mast cell leukemia.

Treatment

Treatment is of no proved value in the generalized types of mast cell disease. Antihistamines, steroids, antimitotic drugs, and radiation have been tried repeatedly with poor results. Antihistamines, especially the combination of H_1 (diphenhydramine) and H_2 (cimetidine) inhibitors, may be helpful in the relief of pruritus; occasionally, these agents may initiate flushing or other symptoms associated with mastocytosis syndrome, but they are usually ineffective. Use of histamine liberators for treatment of symptoms is of dubious rationale and has not proved effective. Cromolyn seems to relieve gastrointestinal symptoms in some patients.

Prognosis

The prognosis and course depend largely on the age at onset and the type of mastocytosis.

Urticaria pigmentosa with widespread skin lesions appearing in early childhood has an excellent prognosis. More than half of cases clear by late adolescence. Prognosis is less favorable with adult onset. A few patients with onset either in infancy or childhood develop systemic lesions, but only a few fatal cases have been recorded. Sudden death has occurred in several infants with widespread skin lesions.

Urticaria pigmentosa with onset in adult life tends to persist unchanged. Lesions improve in a number of cases and disappear entirely in a few, but about 10% of adult patients develop systemic lesions. Systemic involvement is much more common in adults than in children; several hundred cases are known, with approximately 50 related deaths.

REFERENCES

Caplan RM: The natural course of urticaria pigmentosa: Analysis and following of 112 cases. Arch Dermatol 1963;87:146.

Demis DJ: Mast cell disease. Page 1 in: *Clinical Dermatology.* Demis DJ (editor). Lippincott, 1989.

Demis DJ: The mastocytosis syndrome: Clinical and biological studies. Ann Intern Med 1963;59:194.

Demis DJ, Walton MD, Higdon RS: Histaminuria in urticaria pigmentosa. Arch Dermatol 1961;83:127.

Roberts LJ II, Fields JP, Oates JA: Mastocytosis without urticaria pigmentosa: A frequently unrecognized cause of recurrent syncope. Trans Assoc Am Physicians 1982; 95:36.

31

Diseases of Nutrition & Metabolism

Jo-David Fine, MD, Paul Brooke, MD, & Samuel L. Moschella, MD

Abnormalities of the skin reflect not only localized skin disease but aberrations in nutrition and metabolism as well. In some systemic disorders, subtle skin changes provide the first clue to diagnosis of the underlying disease. In others, even in the absence of skin abnormalities, one may obtain diagnostic information from evaluation of normal-appearing skin by electron microscopy or enzymatic assays of skin biopsy-derived fibroblast cultures. In this chapter, we discuss systemic diseases and nutritional disorders with cutaneous manifestations.

I. DISORDERS OF NUTRITION

Abnormal nutrition may result from inadequate dietary intake, maldigestion, malabsorption, or increased nutrient metabolism. Diseases and drugs can interfere with nutrition as well. Such patients may exhibit protein-energy malnutrition with or without one or more vitamin or mineral deficiencies.

PROTEIN-ENERGY MALNUTRITION

The 2 classic types of protein energy malnutrition are marasmus and kwashiorkor. Both are caused by inadequate food intake. Marasmus results from starvation due to complete food deprivation and kwashiorkor chiefly from inadequate protein intake. Other conditions leading to protein energy malnutrition include diseases associated with maldigestion or malabsorption, those resulting in excessive protein loss by the gut, and diseases such as metastatic cancer and chronic renal failure resulting in prolonged catabolic states. Patients with protein energy malnutrition commonly also suffer from multiple deficiencies of other nutrients, including vitamins and trace minerals.

MARASMUS

Marasmus is due to insufficient food intake and occurs chiefly in infants. Patients exhibit marked weight loss with atrophy of subcutaneous tissues, muscles, and internal organs. The children are emaciated but mentally alert. The skin is usually normal in appearance but may be thin, dry, or wrinkled; the hair is usually unaffected. Diarrhea may occur, but edema and hepatosplenomegaly are absent. Hypoalbuminemia is less frequent than in kwashiorkor.

KWASHIORKOR

Kwashiorkor is due to dietary protein deficiency. It is most common in impoverished inhabitants of the Third World; it also occurs in elderly persons and in some patients with systemic diseases characterized by protein malabsorption or maldigestion.

The first skin finding is blanchable erythema, followed by macules and petechiae over the legs, buttocks, abdomen, arms, and upper back. These lesions may coalesce and become darker and raised. The skin may appear dry and scaly and look like "flaky paint." The hair may be brittle, have less texture or curliness, and have smaller diameter or tensile strength with a reduced rate of growth. Color changes of hair are not infrequent; relapse may be evident by the presence of horizontally striped hair ("flag sign"). The nails tend to be soft and thin.

The liver characteristically becomes infiltrated with fat, may become fibrosed, and is often enlarged. Fibrosis and atrophy of endocrine and exocrine glands, atrophy of intestinal mucosa, and renal and cardiac manifestations can also occur.

The mainstay of treatment is adequate dietary replacement with protein-rich sources. Other nutritional abnormalities including vitamin deficiencies and deficiencies of iron or zinc must also be corrected. Severe untreated kwashiorkor may result in death. Septicemia kills about 30% of patients with kwashiorkor.

VITAMIN ABNORMALITIES

VITAMIN A DEFICIENCY

Essentials of Diagnosis
- Bitot's spots (stratified epithelium along the scleral conjunctiva), night blindness, xerophthalmia.
- Phrynoderma (hyperkeratotic follicular papules).
- Xerotic, ichthyotic skin.

General Considerations
Vitamin A, a fat-soluble vitamin, is in the diet either as such or as a precursor, β-carotene. Most ingested vitamin A is stored in the liver, where 1 year's supply may be found. Development of vitamin A deficiency therefore requires a protracted period of inadequate dietary intake.

This vitamin is involved in production of retinal protein, carbohydrate metabolism, and glycoprotein synthesis. Vitamin A deficiency results in squamous metaplasia of the mucous membranes. Major sites of involvement in vitamin A deficiency are eye and skin. Deficiency due to inadequate intake is rare in industrialized countries. Deficiency also may be induced by abnormal gastrointestinal absorption resulting from a variety of acquired or inherited diseases of the small intestine, biliary tract, or extensive gastrointestinal tract surgery. In addition, hepatic storage of vitamin A may be affected by the presence of liver injury (viral, alcohol, other toxins), diabetes, and thyrotoxicosis.

Clinical Findings
A. Symptoms and Signs: Eye findings include punctate keratopathy, periocular gland metaplasia, Bitot's spots (stratified epithelium along the conjunctival sclera), and xerophthalmia. Diminished retinal levels of rhodopsin and opsin result in night blindness. Untreated xerophthalmia results in blindness.

Skin findings include inflammation secondary to generalized dryness (asteatosis), hyperkeratotic follicular papules on the arms and thighs (phrynoderma), and cracking of the skin. Acneiform eruptions may occur.

Eye examination reveals abnormal dark adaptation.

B. Laboratory Findings: Serum levels of vitamin A or carotene are depressed. Anemia and an increased basal metabolic rate may be present.

Differential Diagnosis
The skin findings must be differentiated from asteatotic eczema, xerosis, keratosis pilaris, and acquired ichthyosis.

Complications
Untreated xerophthalmia may result in blindness. This is the most common cause of blindness in underdeveloped nations.

Treatment
Treatment consists of replacement of vitamin A in the diet. Supplemental vitamin A can be given to adults in tablet or capsule form (eg, 25,000 units twice daily) to replenish vitamin A storage sites. Higher doses and longer therapy may be needed if there is corneal injury. Several months may be required for return of eye findings to normal.

VITAMIN A TOXICITY

Acute vitamin A toxicity after excessive intake is characterized within the first few hours by nausea, vomiting, and headache. Bulging fontanelles may be seen in affected infants due to increased intracranial pressure. The skin may develop exfoliative dermatitis. Soft tissue calcification, with associated hypercalcemia and hypophosphatemia, may occur.

Chronic vitamin A toxicity is more common and results from prolonged ingestion of lower doses. The skin appears dry and feels rough. There is pruritus, scaling, localized or generalized hyperpigmentation, hair loss, brittle nails, fissuring of the lips, and glossodynia. Other findings may include anorexia, lethargy, weight loss, insomnia, altered mentation, nausea, and abdominal pain. Exophthalmos, menorrhagia, finger clubbing, arthralgias, fever, hepatomegaly, and cirrhosis may also be seen. Chronic vitamin A toxicity is one cause of benign intracranial hypertension. Anemia, leukopenia, hypoplasia of the bone marrow, and characteristic radiographic findings may be seen.

As might be expected, many of these findings are also side effects of treatment with other retinoids such as isotretinoin (Accutane) and etretinate (Tegason).

The treatment for hypervitaminosis A is to decrease ingestion of the retinoid.

RIBOFLAVIN DEFICIENCY

Riboflavin (vitamin B_2) forms part of the flavoprotein coenzyme critical in intracellular oxidation-reduction reactions. Tissue stores may be rapidly depleted so that deficiency states occur in patients consuming diets high in carbohydrates or alcohol—as well as in pregnancy, hyperthyroidism, cancer, fever, gastrointestinal diseases, and chronic debilitating diseases. Some drugs also interact with riboflavin. Phototherapy for neonatal icterus may cause vitamin B_2 deficiency.

The first sign of riboflavin deficiency is cheilitis. Other findings include purplish-red discoloration and fissuring of the tongue, flattening or atrophy of the surface of the tongue, superficial keratitis and ulcerations of the eye, and a seborrheic dermatitis-like eruption on the earlobes, ala nasi, bilateral malar areas, and canthi of the eyes. Hyperpigmentation of the vulva or scrotum may occur, resembling zinc deficiency. Normocytic normochromic anemia is common.

The cheilitis must be differentiated from that due to candidiasis or of malocclusion. The glossitis may be difficult to differentiate from deficiencies of niacin, folic acid, and vitamin B_{12}.

Riboflavin deficiency is treated with riboflavin supplementation, 5–20 mg/d.

PYRIDOXINE DEFICIENCY

Pyridoxine (vitamin B_6) serves as an important coenzyme in amino acid (tryptophan) metabolism, heme synthesis, and neural tissue biochemistry (aminobutyric acid synthesis); deficiency may result in peripheral neuritis, seizures, cheilitis, glossitis, and a seborrheic dermatitis-like skin eruption. Symptoms include weakness, nausea, vomiting, and dizziness.

Treatment is with pyridoxine, 100 mg/d.

NIACIN DEFICIENCY
(Pellagra)

Essentials of Diagnosis
- Dermatitis, diarrhea, dementia ("the three D's").
- Multiple neurologic findings in chronic cases.

General Considerations
Niacin (nicotinic acid; nicotinamide) is part of the vitamin B complex and may be synthesized from tryptophan; alterations in tryptophan intake or metabolism may result in pellagra-like states. Pellagra occurs most frequently in the spring and in populations whose major dietary intake is maize or millet. Carcinoid syndrome can cause pellagra because dietary tryptophan is shunted into synthesis of serotonin and away from synthesis of niacin. Niacin deficiency has also been seen in patients with chronic malabsorption, alcoholism, and Hartnup disease, and has been associated with use of the following drugs: isoniazid, sulfonamides, anticonvulsants, antidepressants, fluorouracil, and mercaptopurine.

Clinical Findings
A. Symptoms and Signs: In the earliest cases, weakness and fatigue are common. The diagnosis is made by the presence of the three D's: dermatitis, diarrhea, and dementia. The symmetric skin eruption—most often on the face, the neck ("Casal's necklace"), the backs of the hands, the wrists, the elbows and knees, and the inframammary and perianal areas—consists of erythema with development of vesicles or blisters. The eruption may be triggered by sunlight. The epidermis becomes reddish-brown, scaly, and thickened, as though it were not desquamating properly. Oral cavity findings include dryness and fissuring of the lips, dryness, erythema, smoothness, and aphthous-like ulcerations of the buccal mucosa and swelling and purplish discoloration of the tongue. The patient may have pruritus or a burning sensation. All parts of the gastrointestinal tract may be involved; achlorhydria may develop. Gastrointestinal symptoms include anorexia, dyspepsia, and abdominal pain. Neurologic signs and symptoms are protean, including insomnia or irritability and, later, tremor, numbness, rigidity, paralysis, psychosis, or encephalopathy.

B. Laboratory Findings: When pellagra is secondary to the carcinoid syndrome, elevated urinary levels of 5-hydroxyindoleacetic acid may be detected. Laboratory findings consistent with Hartnup disease may also be seen in those cases.

Treatment
Several weeks' supplementation with nicotinic acid or nicotinamide, 500 mg/d, is necessary to reverse the signs and symptoms of this disease. Most patients prefer the use of nicotinamide to nicotinic acid, since the former does not produce facial flushing.

ASCORBIC ACID DEFICIENCY
(Scurvy)

Essentials of Diagnosis
- Hemorrhage in tissues (skin, gingiva, subperiosteal, genitourinary, gastrointestinal, central nervous system).
- "Scorbutic rosary" (enlarged costochondral junctions in the chest wall).
- Perifollicular hyperkeratotic papules with central curled hair and surrounding erythema and purpura.

General Considerations
Ascorbic acid (vitamin C), a water-soluble vitamin, is found in fresh fruits and vegetables and is necessary for proline hydroxylation during biosynthesis of collagen. Cytochrome P-450 is influenced by vitamin C. Other effects include enhanced iron metabolism and alterations of phagocytic and immunologic function. Vitamin C maintains tetrahy-

drofolic acid in its reduced form; its deficiency further worsens anemia due to folate deficiency. This vitamin also contributes to the normal growth and mechanical stability of hair, since it reduces disulfide links.

Vitamin C deficiency is seen in underdeveloped countries, geriatric populations, alcoholics, and patients with extensive small intestine disease or advanced malignancies.

Clinical Findings

A. Symptoms and Signs: Infantile scurvy is seen particularly in children fed unsupplemented cow's milk or formula and results in irritability, anorexia, and weight loss. Sites of hemorrhage include the gingivae, long bone periosteum, gastrointestinal and genitourinary tracts, skin, and central nervous system. Enlargement of the costochondral junctions of the chest wall results in the characteristic "scorbutic rosary."

Scurvy in adults often presents as perifollicular hyperkeratotic papules, especially over the buttocks, thighs, and legs. Each papule has a corkscrew hair centrally, surrounded by erythema and purpura. Other findings include splinter hemorrhages of the nails, leg ulcers, and swelling, bleeding, and ulceration of the gums. Rarely, scleroderma-like induration of the skin may occur. Symptoms include anorexia, weakness, lassitude, fatigue, irritability, and arthralgias and myalgias, particularly of the legs—the latter a reflection of hemorrhage into joints and muscles.

B. Laboratory Findings: Normocytic normochromic anemia may be present. Characteristic radiologic features include the presence of dark bands within bone metaphyses and "champagne cork"-like changes in the distal portions of the ribs.

Differential Diagnosis

When widespread hemorrhagic signs are seen, other causes of coagulopathy must be considered, though in the infantile form the characteristic chest wall findings support this diagnosis.

Treatment

Treatment consists of addition of vitamin C to the diet or replacement with 100–500 mg (adult dose) once or twice daily. Response may be rapid, especially in infants.

Prognosis

If untreated, especially in children, adrenal insufficiency, shock, convulsions, and death may occur.

VITAMIN D EXCESS

Vitamin D is important in normal calcium metabolism. Although vitamin D deficiency leads to no cutaneous lesions, excessive intake may produce widespread metastatic calcification. Such lesions appear yellow and feel hard. They commonly occur beneath the fingernails, along the lips, in the conjunctiva, and anywhere on the skin.

Treatment is directed at the cause, eg, removal of parathyroid adenoma.

BIOTIN DEFICIENCY

Biotin is a slightly water-soluble vitamin that serves as a coenzyme for enzymes (cocarboxylase) involved in the metabolism of amino acids and pyruvic acid. Although biotin deficiency is rare in humans, when it occurs it is usually associated either with ingestion of raw egg whites (due to the binding of biotin by avidin) or with total parenteral nutrition in the absence of adequate biotin supplementation.

Clinical features of biotin deficiency vary with the age of the patient. In adults, findings are usually confined to the lips (fissuring) and oral cavity (erythema and tenderness of the tongue; erythema and dryness of mucosal surfaces). In infants, 2 forms have been reported. In the first form—often lethal—associated with a cocarboxylase defect, skin findings are similar to those of generalized seborrheic dermatitis or ichthyosis. In the second form, diffuse erythema, scaling, and crusting are noted, particularly at junctions of skin and mucosal surfaces, in association with alopecia (scalp, eyebrows, eyelashes), similar to the findings that occur in essential fatty acid deficiency and in acrodermatitis enteropathica. Photophobia and blurred vision may occur, secondary to the development of keratitis and keratoconjunctivitis, respectively. Infrequently, paresthesias, tremors, ataxia, or depression may also occur.

Treatment consists of intravenous supplementation of biotin.

II. DISORDERS OF METABOLISM

DISORDERS OF AMINO ACID METABOLISM

PHENYLKETONURIA

Essentials of Diagnosis

- Fair complexion, blue eyes, and light-colored hair.

- Atopic-like eczema commonly seen.
- Progressive neurologic deterioration.
- Multiple skeletal abnormalities.
- Elevated serum phenylalanine and urinary phenylpyruvic acid levels.

General Considerations

Phenylketonuria is a rare autosomal recessive disease not infrequently associated with consanguinity. Most cases are due to phenylalanine hydroxylase deficiency, impairing conversion of phenylalanine to tyrosine. Less frequently, "variant" phenylketonuria patients have normal phenylalanine hydroxylase levels but abnormal dihydrobiopterin synthesis or deficient dihydrobiopterin reductase.

Clinical Findings

A. Symptoms and Signs: Children with phenylketonuria are normal at birth. They have fair complexions and light or blond-colored hair and blue eyes. With time, half of phenylketonuria patients develop an eczematous dermatitis; rarely, sclerodermatous changes or atrophoderma may occur. Within the first 6 months—if untreated—there is progressive neurologic deterioration manifested by delayed physical and mental development and later by seizures, tremors, abnormal posturing, bizarre behavior, and hyperactivity. Pyloric stenosis is associated. Skeletal changes include microcephaly, syndactyly, pes planus, and shortened stature.

B. Laboratory Findings: After the first few months of life, phenylketonuria patients have consistently elevated serum phenylalanine levels by bacteriologic assay (Guthrie test); false-negative results may occur in younger children. As a screening test, addition of ferric chloride to the urine turns it a bluish-green color. Carriers for this disease tend to have abnormal phenylalanine tolerance tests. Prenatal diagnosis is now feasible for all known forms of phenylketonuria.

Complications

If treatment is not begun by age 4 months, neurologic deterioration occurs. Without treatment, the average IQ is approximately 50. Even with treatment, some patients may still experience significant deficits in IQ by the age therapy is conventionally terminated, evidence of behavioral disorders, and even reemergence of hyperphenylalaninemia after treatment has been withdrawn.

Treatment

The patient with classic phenylketonuria is maintained on a low phenylalanine diet. Unfortunately, patients with variant forms of phenylketonuria do not respond to dietary therapy. In certain disease variants, carbidopa, levodopa, and 5-hydroxytryptophan can be used. Resumption of the phenylketonuria diet

is particularly critical for phenylketonuric women who become pregnant; in the absence of such a restrictive diet, there is approximately an 80% chance of severe irreversible brain damage in the fetus.

HOMOCYSTINURIA

Essentials of Diagnosis

- Fair complexion, light hair.
- Malar blush, livedo reticularis.
- Variable eye and skeletal abnormalities.
- In older patients, accelerated atherosclerosis.
- Increased homocystine and methionine blood levels and elevated homocystine urinary levels.

General Considerations

Homocystinuria is an autosomal recessive disorder of methionine metabolism. Cystathionine synthetase levels are diminished, allowing accumulation of homocystine within blood and tissue. Methionine levels also become elevated. Less frequent variants are associated with abnormal folate or vitamin B_{12} metabolism or vitamin B_{12} deficiency.

Clinical Findings

A. Symptoms and Signs: Children with homocystinuria appear normal at birth. They tend to have fair complexions, light-colored hair, blushing of the malar eminences, and livedo reticularis. Eye findings include glaucoma, posterior dislocation of the lens, myopia, proptosis, and retinal detachment. Neurologic abnormalities include strokes, seizures, and progressive mental retardation. Multiple skeletal abnormalities are due to excessive growth and structural weakness of the long bones, resulting in skeletal disproportion, abnormal vertebrae, high-arched palate, sternal deformities, scoliosis, and genu valgum. Patients may develop hepatomegaly and accelerated atherosclerosis, the latter manifested by myocardial infarction or stroke. Infrequent findings include cardiac murmurs, cardiomegaly, aortic aneurysms, and hypertension.

B. Laboratory Findings: The disease is suggested by a positive nitroprusside cyanide test on urine and confirmed by demonstration of increased homocystine and methionine blood levels and elevated homocystine urinary levels. Anemia secondary to folate deficiency is common. Platelets have diminished life spans.

Differential Diagnosis

Homocystinuria is most frequently confused with Marfan's syndrome.

Complications

These patients tend to experience thromboembolic phenomena and accelerated atherosclerosis, manifested by pulmonary emboli, myocardial infarction, and stroke. Homocystinuric patients are especially at risk during surgery, anesthesia, and angiography because they are prone to thromboembolism.

Treatment

Patients with homocystinuria are treated with low-methionine diet, pyridoxine supplementation, and folic acid supplementation.

Prognosis

Most patients die at an early age due to thromboembolic events, especially pulmonary emboli. Other causes of morbidity include myocardial infarction and stroke.

ALKAPTONURIA
(Ochronosis)

Essentials of Diagnosis

- Grayish or bluish-gray discoloration of the conjunctiva, cornea, eyelids, sclerae, and pinnae.
- Degenerative arthritis.
- Abnormal spine x-ray.
- Elevated levels of homogentisic acid in urine and blood.

General Considerations

Alkaptonuria is an autosomal recessive disorder due to the absence of the enzyme homogentisic acid oxidase. Homogentisic acid accumulates in excessive amounts and may polymerize in connective tissue, resulting in a brownish-black pigment; the disease is then referred to as ochronosis.

Clinical Findings

A. Symptoms and Signs: In the second decade of life, the sclerae and axillary regions become discolored. Pigment deposition in the eyes discolors gray the bulbar conjunctiva, tarsal plates, cornea, sclerae, and eyelids. The cutaneous pigmentation occurs in areas rich in sweat glands such as the malar eminences and the axillary folds. Discoloration is also prominent in areas where cartilage or tendons have a thin covering of skin, including the ears, nasal tip, and hands. Other findings include prostatic nodularity, a result of ochronotic stones, renal stone formation, and aortic valve murmurs.

B. Laboratory Findings: The laboratory hallmark is the demonstration of elevated amounts of homogentisic acid in blood and urine. Ochronotic pigment may be demonstrated within affected tissues by special stains. Serum and urinary uric acid levels also may be elevated.

C. Imaging Studies: Skeletal abnormalities include lumbosacral spondylosis, abnormalities within the intervertebral disk spaces (narrowing, calcification [a pathognomonic finding], herniation), and loss of curvature of the spine. Severe degenerative arthritis may be seen.

Differential Diagnosis

Ochronosis must be differentiated from pseudo-ochronosis due to exposure to one or more drugs or chemicals including quinacrine, phenol, carbolic acid, resorcinol, benzene derivatives, and hydroquinone. The latter agent, applied topically, may result in striking ochronosis-like hyperpigmentation, perhaps due to the inhibition of homogentisic acid oxidase in the skin, leading to polymerization of homogentisic acid into ochronotic pigment.

Other disorders that must be considered include argyria, hemochromatosis, Addison's disease, porphyria, and pellagra.

Complications

Although at autopsy one can detect diffuse bluish pigmentation in all cartilaginous structures, usually there are no cardiac valvular complications. Occasional cases of hemodynamically significant aortic stenosis are presumed to be secondary to deposition of this material within the valve.

Treatment

Patients with alkaptonuria are placed on low tyrosine-low phenylalanine diets. Ascorbic acid has been suggested as a means of decreasing pigment formation, but the efficacy of this measure is unproved. Attempts at treatment of pseudo-ochronosis secondary to topical hydroquinone may include trials of topical corticosteroids, chronic use of sunscreens, avoidance of excessive sunlight, and discontinuing further use of hydroquinone—though even a partial beneficial response, if any, may be measured in years.

ARGINOSUCCINICACIDURIA

Arginosuccinicaciduria is a rare autosomal recessive disorder due to deficiency of arginosuccinase. Arginosuccinic acid levels are elevated in blood, urine and cerebrospinal fluid.

The hair is sparse, dull, short, fragile, and longitudinally grooved; abnormally rotated; and has focal areas of fraying that look like 2 brooms pushed together (trichorrhexis nodosa).

Patients develop seizures and coma and subsequently die. Some patients benefit from diets low in protein and supplemented with arginine or keto analogues of essential amino acids.

HARTNUP DISEASE

Hartnup disease is a rare autosomal recessive metabolic disorder due to defective intestinal and renal tubular transport of neutral amino acids. Laboratory screening reveals urinary excretion of amino acids and indole derivatives of tryptophan. The earliest clinical feature is a pellagra-like photoeruption, most commonly in patients between 3 and 9 years of age (infrequently earlier). Neurologic findings include ataxia, progressive dementia, and spasticity. Other physical findings may include short stature, abnormal hair, glossitis or stomatitis, and diarrhea. Patients are treated with nicotinamide supplementation.

TYROSINEMIA TYPE II
(Richner-Hanhart Syndrome)

Tyrosinemia type II is an autosomal recessive disorder due to the absence of the enzyme tyrosine aminotransferase. Patients have tyrosinemia, tyrosinuria, phenolic aciduria, and elevated urinary levels of tyrosine metabolites.

Characteristic skin findings are symmetrically distributed linear erosions, which become crusted and hyperkeratotic, over the distal fingers, palms, and soles. These lesions may become so painful as to prevent ambulation. Ocular findings include dendritic ulcerations and corneal clouding. Photophobia, excessive lacrimation, and erythema may be present (at times mimicking herpetic keratitis). Mental retardation may occur.

Treatment consists of diets low in tyrosine and phenylalanine.

PROLIDASE DEFICIENCY

Prolidase deficiency is a rare, probably autosomal recessive disorder seen in infancy. The enzyme prolidase is absent.

Skin findings are protean: chronic recurrent ulcerations of the lower extremities, diffuse telangiectasia, and shallow atrophic scarring over the face and buttocks. Hyperpigmentation may be seen in scarred areas and lymphedema in sites of chronic ulceration. Other cutaneous findings include generalized skin fragility, purpura, premature graying of hair, fissuring and erythema of the palmoplantar surfaces, papular eruptions of the face and extremities, and dry crusted areas on the face and buttocks. Facial findings include saddle nose, hypertelorism, jaw hypoplasia, and the development of multiple dental caries. Extracutaneous features include mental retardation, splenomegaly, partial deafness, eye abnormalities, and hyperextensible or dislocated joints. Recurrent otitis media and sinusitis are frequent findings. There is no treatment.

SYSTEMIC AMYLOIDOSIS

Amyloidosis is the general term for a group of entities that lead to deposition of the fibrillar protein amyloid in tissues. Ultrastructurally, amyloid fibrils are arranged in anti-parallel, twisted β-pleated sheets. On routine histologic staining, they appear amorphous and eosinophilic. Amyloid exhibits apple-green birefringence when stained with Congo red and examined with the polarizing microscope. Amyloid fibrils are insoluble and resistant to proteolytic enzymes.

There are 2 methods of classifying amyloidosis. The older method distinguishes groups of patients with primary (idiopathic) or secondary disease; in the latter classification, amyloidosis develops in conjunction with one of several inflammatory or neoplastic diseases. A more recent classification divides patients according to whether they have immunocyte-derived or reactive systemic amyloidosis. The distinction is important because treatment depends upon whether amyloidosis is immunocyte-derived or reactive. Selected patients with immunocyte-derived amyloidosis benefit from cytotoxic drugs. In contrast, treatment of the underlying infectious, inflammatory, or neoplastic disease sometimes beneficially affects the course of secondary amyloidosis. In patients with secondary amyloidosis and familial Mediterranean fever, colchicine may prove beneficial.

Pruritus can be treated symptomatically with oral antihistamines.

IMMUNOCYTE-DERIVED AMYLOIDOSIS

Essentials of Diagnosis
- Pinch purpura (purpura occurs where skin is pinched or stroked).
- Yellow discrete and confluent papules.
- Induration of skin and tongue.
- Abnormal serum protein electrophoresis or immunoelectrophoresis or presence of light chains in urine.
- Amyloid in biopsied skin.

General Considerations
Several immunocyte or plasma cell-related diseases may be accompanied by amyloid deposition, including multiple myeloma, Waldenström's macroglobulinemia, benign monoclonal gammopathy, heavy chain disease, immunoblastic lymphadenopathy, nodular malignant lymphoma, and agammaglobulinemia. In all of these and in primary idiopathic

amyloidosis, the amyloid fibril is similar or identical to the immunoglobulin light chain (most commonly the lambda type). This suggests that these disorders are related. A globular glycoprotein known as amyloid P-component, the exact role of which is unknown, may be present in serum and tissue.

Clinical Findings

A. Symptoms and Signs: Male Caucasians, most frequently in the fifth and sixth decades, are the usual patients who develop primary amyloidosis or amyloidosis associated with multiple myeloma. Organs involved include the skin, heart, tongue, carpal ligaments, peripheral nerves, and gastrointestinal tract.

Skin manifestations may be seen in 40% of patients with primary systemic (immunocytic) amyloidosis. The most common sign is pinch purpura (purpura develops easily when the skin is pinched or stroked). Amyloid infiltration of the skin may appear as asymptomatic, translucent waxy or amber-colored papules, plaques, or nodules. Less frequently, the skin may develop a xanthomatous yellow, indurated appearance, or there may be diffuse facial infiltration mimicking myxedema or the leonine facies of leprosy. Although the skin in general appears pale, redness or hyperpigmentation may also be seen. If induration of the fingertips is prominent, immobility of the joints and contractures may result. There may be thickening or hyperkeratosis of the palms and thickening and enlargement of the ears, lips, and eyelids if amyloid deposition is marked. Similarly, the scalp may develop deep folds resembling cutis verticis gyrata. Alopecia may occur. Some patients develop blisters. Sclerodermoid changes, bullae, subcutaneous nodules, and tumefactions have been noted. The nails may appear brittle, crumbling, longitudinally ridged, or longitudinally streaked. On some fingers there may be no nails.

Infiltration of nerves may cause autonomic nervous system involvement or peripheral neuropathy (stocking glove, carpal tunnel syndrome). Cardiac manifestations include restrictive cardiomyopathy, "sick sinus syndrome," arrhythmias, and enhanced sensitivity to digitalis; approximately 40% of all deaths may result from intractable congestive heart failure or arrhythmias. Hepatomegaly and lymphadenopathy may occur in as many as 50% and 10% of patients, respectively. Renal disease, in the form of nephrotic syndrome, may occur in up to 30% of cases and is another leading cause of death. Amyloid infiltrates within the gastrointestinal tract may lead to hemorrhage or malabsorption. Lung involvement may be characterized by nodular or diffuse parenchymal infiltrates. Musculoskeletal findings include polyarthropathy of large joints, shoulder-pad sign (accumulation of amyloid material in the glenohumeral joint space), osteolytic lesions, pathologic fractures, pseudohypertrophy of muscle, and myopathy. Associated hematologic complications include factor X deficiency and disseminated intravascular coagulation.

Roughly 20% of patients with primary amyloidosis develop macroglossia that may interfere with eating and breathing. The tongue is smooth, dry, diffusely enlarged, and immobile. Less frequently, localized amyloid papules may be seen along the surface of the tongue. Rare findings include eye manifestations, panhypopituitarism, thyromegaly, sicca syndrome, and splenomegaly.

B. Laboratory Findings: Lesional skin biopsies confirm the presence of amorphous eosinophilic material within the upper dermis. Even biopsies of normal-appearing skin may be positive for amyloid in up to 50% of cases. Serum concentrations of IgG are often increased, and serum protein electrophoresis or immunoelectrophoresis may disclose monoclonal spikes. Urine may contain immunoglobulin light chains (Bence Jones protein)—best evaluated by immunoelectrophoresis—and bone marrow may be abnormal.

Treatment

Treatment considerations are discussed above.

REACTIVE SYSTEMIC AMYLOIDOSIS

As opposed to immunocyte-derived amyloidosis, the amyloid fibrils are not homologous with light-chain immunoglobulin (AL fibril) but instead are composed of a distinct nonimmunoglobulin protein, AA protein. Amyloid P-component and tissue and serum proteins may be seen in reactive systemic amyloidosis. The most prominent findings are hepatosplenomegaly and nephrotic syndrome. Only rarely is there cutaneous involvement in secondary systemic amyloidosis.

Diseases resulting in secondary amyloid deposition include rheumatologic disorders (adult and juvenile rheumatoid arthritis, ankylosing spondylitis, Behçet's syndrome, Reiter's syndrome, psoriatic arthritis, scleroderma, dermatomyositis, systemic lupus erythematosus), infectious diseases (tuberculosis, leprosy, syphilis, chronic pyelonephritis, malaria, bronchiectasis, osteomyelitis, chronic skin wounds), gastrointestinal diseases (ulcerative colitis, regional enteritis), and several tumors (hypernephroma, Hodgkin's disease).

LOCALIZED CUTANEOUS AMYLOIDOSIS

1. LICHEN AMYLOIDOSIS

Lichen amyloidosis, the most common localized cutaneous amyloidosis, is not associated with systemic disease and is usually seen in middle-aged and frequently in Oriental patients. These often intensely pruritic lesions appear as translucent or yellowish-brown dome-shaped papules, some covered with scales, distributed symmetrically over the extensor lower extremities, thighs, feet, and lower back. Other areas may be infrequently involved. These lesions are not purpuric as opposed to those in primary amyloidosis. Examination of a biopsy specimen reveals amyloid deposition within the papillary dermis. As compared with primary or secondary amyloidosis, there is no amyloid deposition around dermal blood vessels, appendages, or within the subcutaneous tissue.

2. MACULAR AMYLOIDOSIS

Grayish-brown reticulated macules are noted on the upper back, breasts, buttocks, arms, ankles, and thighs. These lesions may be pruritic but are not associated with systemic amyloidosis. At times, both macular and papular forms of localized cutaneous amyloidosis may be observed in the same individual.

3. OTHER FORMS OF LOCALIZED CUTANEOUS AMYLOIDOSIS

Primary nodular or tumor-like amyloid lesions may occur anywhere on the skin surface without evidence of systemic amyloidosis. No satisfactory treatment is available, though variable responses have been noted anecdotally with topical corticosteroids, UVB irradiation, topical DMSO, and even surgical manipulations such as dermabrasion. In addition, focal amyloid may be seen within many skin lesions, including both benign and malignant tumors.

4. HEREDOFAMILIAL AMYLOIDOSIS

There are several familial forms of amyloidosis, which may be transmitted in autosomal dominant (Muckle-Wells syndrome) or autosomal recessive (familial Mediterranean fever) fashion. In the latter syndrome, which is treatable with colchicine, patients develop intermittent fever, serositis (peritonitis, pleuritis, synovitis), renal amyloidosis, and a variety of skin findings ranging from urticaria-like and erysipelas-like lesions to vasculitis. Other types of heredofamilial amyloidosis may be primarily of neurologic or cardiac origin. As opposed to immunocyte-derived or reactive systemic amyloidosis, the amyloid fibrils are not all biochemically the same.

CUTANEOUS MUCINOSES

Mucins are highly polymerized carbohydrates. Mucins containing protein are referred to as proteoglycans. These substances comprise a substantial portion of the noncellular ground substance of the dermis. Mucin may be deposited primarily or secondarily in several dermatologic and systemic disorders. For example, local secondary deposition occurs in mucocysts, lesions of fibrocytic and histiocytic proliferation, tumors (neural origin, adnexal, basal cell carcinoma, dermatofibroma), lupus erythematosus, and Degos' disease (malignant atrophic papulosis).

FOLLICULAR MUCINOSA (Alopecia Mucinosis)

Grouped follicular papules or plaques containing excessive dermal mucin may be associated with localized loss of hair. In the primary (idiopathic) form, children are most commonly involved. Patients develop pink or flesh-colored lesions, with scale and follicular plugging, on the face, neck, and scalp. These lesions may spontaneously resolve, often after years.

In the adult, similar lesions may become nodular or plaque-like. Such lesions may herald the onset of cutaneous T cell lymphoma (mycosis fungoides). In the adult form, lesions tend not to occur on the head or neck. There is no effective therapy for either the adult or childhood form, though radiation therapy and topical and intralesional corticosteroids have been tried.

CUTANEOUS FOCAL MUCINOSIS

A single flesh-colored or white papule or nodule develops on the face, neck, trunk, or extremity. Such lesions contain excessive amounts of mucin. These lesions have no increased risk of systemic disease, and are readily amenable to surgical excision.

CUTANEOUS MUCINOSIS OF INFANCY

In such infants, small, densely grouped papules develop symmetrically on the elbows, the arms, and the backs of the hands.

RETICULAR ERYTHEMATOUS MUCINOSIS SYNDROME

Patients with this disorder develop a persistent palpable reticular erythema over sun-exposed sites on the chest, back, face, and arms. The eruption can be made worse or reproduced with natural or artificial sunlight and may be benefited by treatment with oral antimalarial drugs.

PRETIBIAL MYXEDEMA

Pretibial myxedema comprises one part of the triad of Graves' disease (nonnodular goitrous hyperthyroidism, ophthalmopathy, dermopathy), occurring in up to 10% of such patients. It often develops following acute surgical or radioactive iodine treatment of thyrotoxicosis. However, pretibial myxedema may rarely occur also in the absence of hyperthyroidism. Patients with pretibial myxedema contain within their serum a circulating factor which in vitro enhances polysaccharide biosynthesis by fibroblasts from the pretibial areas.

Lesions of pretibial myxedema are sharply marginated, flesh-colored, pink, or violaceous plaques or nodules most common over the anterolateral lower extremities. They characteristically are symmetric, nonpitting, may be waxy to feel, and may become yellowish-brown and develop increased hair within their margins. The lesions may also be found over the backs of the hands, the arms, the face, or the trunk.

There is no satisfactory treatment, although some patients improve following intralesional injection of corticosteroids or application of potent topical corticosteroids under plastic occlusion with or without overlying compression bandages. Attempts at excision and subsequent split-thickness skin grafting have proved unsuccessful; lesions tend to recur within donor graft sites.

LICHEN MYXEDEMATOSUS (Papular Mucinosis; Scleromyxedema)

Essentials of Diagnosis

- Discrete or generalized lichenoid papules with or without sclerodermatous changes.
- Diffuse or nodular infiltration of other skin areas.
- Large amounts of acid mucopolysaccharides within the dermis.
- Presence of a circulating paraprotein, usually IgG.

General Considerations

Lichen myxedematosus often develops in the third to fifth decades of life. Patient's serum often contains a factor that causes fibroblast proliferation in vitro.

Clinical Findings

A. Symptoms and Signs: There are several different cutaneous presentations. In the most dramatic forms, patients develop diffuse or nodular infiltration of many skin sites, including the ears, neck, scrotum, and perianal areas. Facial features may become exaggerated, with extensive deep rolling furrows. Affected skin is markedly indurated. In some patients, acral areas become diffusely thickened. Other patients have pink wheal-like plaques coexisting with nodules or with asymmetric red or flesh-colored soft small papules, densely grouped. Other patients have generalized or localized violaceous (lichenoid) plaques suggestive of lichen planus. In most cases, only dermatologic findings are seen; occasional patients have associated myopathies, polyarthritis, or evidence of accelerated coronary or cerebrovascular disease.

B. Laboratory Findings: Serum electrophoresis reveals a paraprotein, usually IgG but occasionally IgM or IgA, most commonly of the lambda variety. However, there is no correlation between the level of paraprotein present and the extent or course of disease activity. Bone marrow biopsy may reveal increased numbers of plasma cells. Skin biopsy demonstrates increased mucin and frequently fibroblast proliferation within the dermis.

Complications

Infrequently, patients eventually develop multiple myeloma.

Treatment

Some patients have been partially responsive to cyclophosphamide. Other treatments which in selected patients may be beneficial include radiotherapy, dermabrasion, systemic corticosteroids, and other parenteral chemotherapeutic agents.

LIPOID PROTEINOSIS (Hyalinosis Cutis et Mucosae; Urbach-Wiethe Disease)

Lipoid proteinosis is a rare autosomal recessive disorder involving the skin, oropharynx, larynx, and other mucosal surfaces.

The earliest clinical finding in an infant is progressive hoarseness due to hyaline infiltration of the vocal cords. With time, as more areas of the pharynx and larynx become involved, significant dyspnea may occur and tracheostomy may be necessary.

In the first 2 years of life, pustules or blisters appear on the face and exposed areas of the arms and legs. These lesions heal with white scars. Later skin lesions are papules, nodules, and verrucous plaques. The papules appear waxy, yellow, or ivory in color and are located on the face, posterior neck, hands, and fingers. A linear array of such lesions on the free edges of the eyelids—the "string of beads" sign—is characteristic. The verrucoid plaques are red and scaly and may be noted over the elbows, knees, fingers, buttocks, and face. The extensor surfaces of the forearms may become diffusely indurated; some patients develop generalized waxy thickened yellow skin. Alopecia may occur of the scalp, beard, eyebrows, and eyelashes.

The tongue, vagina, rectum, and conjunctiva may also be involved, as may the lung, kidney, bladder, gastrointestinal tract, striated muscle, lymph nodes, and parotid glands. Symmetric intracranial calcifications of the hippocampal gyri occur in one-half of patients.

There is no known treatment. Patients developing upper airway obstruction due to increasing luminal lesions may require tracheostomy. There is an increased incidence of diabetes mellitus.

MUCOPOLYSACCHARIDOSES

Seven major types of mucopolysaccharidoses—comprising at least 14 clinical subtypes—have been described, each the result of a specific lysosomal enzyme deficiency within the mucopolysaccharide biosynthetic pathway. One or more tissues becomes infiltrated with at least one glycosoaminoglycan. All except Hunter's syndrome are transmitted by an autosomal recessive inheritance pattern. These different entities may be differentiated from one another by the relative distribution of organ involvement as well as by demonstration of the specific enzyme defect. Although none of these disorders can as yet be treated specifically, therapeutic replacement of the missing enzymes may some day be possible.

Hunter's syndrome (MPS II) is an X-linked recessive disorder due to deficiency of iduronate sulfatase. Although seen in only 20% of cases, skin findings are pathognomonic. Characteristic lesions are white or flesh-colored papules or nodules that may coalesce to form ridges or reticulate patterns symmetrically between the scapulas and posterior axillary lines, the nape of the neck, the pectoral chest, and the lateral aspects of the upper arms and legs. These lesions may be seen in patients before age 10 and may later resolve spontaneously.

Other clinical findings include dwarfism, deafness, coarse facies, mental retardation, cardiomegaly, hepatomegaly, and clawlike contractures of the hands. In the more severe form, patients are mentally retarded and die at an early age. There are milder forms in which patients survive into adulthood with normal mentation.

DISEASES OF LIPID METABOLISM

HYPERLIPOPROTEINEMIA

The Fredrickson classification utilizes variations in electrophoretic banding patterns to separate 5 different patient groups. Extensive biochemical studies have revealed considerable complexity in the nature of each of the diseases characterized by elevated plasma lipids. Simplistically, however, they can be grouped into disorders characterized by excessive levels of chylomicrons (types I and V), beta VLDLs (type III), VLDLs (type IV), and LDLs (type II).

Type I hyperlipoproteinemia is transmitted by an autosomal recessive pattern and manifested by eruptive xanthomas, hepatosplenomegaly, recurrent abdominal pain, and lipemia retinalis.

Type II hyperlipoproteinemia may be an autosomal dominant trait or, more commonly, a polygenically transmitted disorder. Clinical findings include tendinous xanthomas, xanthelasmas, arcus senilis, and accelerated atherosclerosis.

Type III lipoproteinemia is an autosomal recessive disorder. Clinical findings include obesity, atherosclerosis, and xanthoma formation (tuberous, eruptive, tendinous, and xanthoma striatum palmare).

Type IV hyperlipidemia is an autosomal dominant disorder characterized by hepatomegaly, recurrent pancreatitis, obesity, hyperinsulinemia, glucose intolerance, lipemia retinalis, and xanthomas (eruptive, xanthoma striatum palmare).

Type V hyperlipoproteinemia is autosomal dominant or recessive and is characterized by diabetes mellitus, pancreatitis, hyperuricemia, hepatosplenomegaly, and eruptive xanthomas.

CUTANEOUS XANTHOMATOSES

1. XANTHOMA TUBEROSUM

Tuberous xanthomas are yellow to deep orange, firm papules or large firm nodules, which may become pedunculated. They tend to arise over the extensor surfaces and areas subjected to physical trauma (elbows, knees, knuckles, heels, and buttocks). These lesions are seen in type II and type III hyperlipoproteinemia as well as hyperthyroidism and primary liver disease. They rarely resolve even after correction of the abnormal lipid disorder.

2. XANTHOMA PLANUM

Planar xanthomas are soft yellowish to tan macules, papules, or plaques occurring locally or generalized on any body site. They are frequently seen in patients with type III or type IV hyperlipoproteinemia as well as in some normolipemic patients. They may also occur in patients with lymphoma or multiple myeloma. When the lesions are flat and appear along the creases of the palm and volar finger joints, the condition is referred to as xanthochromia striata palmaris; if the lesions become papular, it is called xanthoma striatum palmare.

3. XANTHOMA TENDINOSUM

The lesions of xanthoma tendinosum are non-tender, firm nodules that may grow to several centimeters in diameter. They appear along the tendons, ligaments, fascia, or periosteum, most often on the hands, fingers, elbows, knees, and heels. These lesions are characteristically seen in type II and type III hyperlipoproteinemia and occasionally in normolipemic patients. Several cases have also been reported in association with tissue accumulation of 3 specific plant sterols. Infrequently, tendinous xanthomas may be clinically confused with rheumatoid nodules or gouty tophi.

Xanthoma tendinosum may also appear in normolipemic patients in association with cerebrotendinous xanthomatosis, in which xanthomas arise not only in tendons but also in the cerebellum and lungs. Cataracts also develop. Because of cerebellar involvement, progressive mental deficiency and ataxia are seen. This disorder is believed to be due to abnormal cholesterol storage.

4. XANTHOMA ERUPTIVUM

Eruptive xanthomas are small yellowish to red papules arising on an erythematous base. They are intensely pruritic, develop suddenly, and may later disappear as serum lipid levels drop toward normal. The most common sites are the extensor surfaces of the extremities, the buttocks, the back, the abdomen, and the chest. Facial and oral lesions may also arise rarely. Eruptive xanthomas are seen in patients with type I, III, IV, or V hyperlipoproteinemia as well as some patients treated with the retinoid isotretinoin. These lesions may arise in response to elevated serum triglyceride levels. New lesions may arise in areas of direct skin trauma (Koebner's phenomenon).

Treatment of the underlying hypertriglyceridemia should be started quickly, since these patients may develop pancreatic or myocardial infarction from atherosclerosis. Treatment may also cause xanthomas to disappear.

5. XANTHOMA DISSEMINATUM

Xanthoma disseminatum is a rare disease in which reddish-yellow to brown papules and nodules arise on flexural surfaces, mucous membranes, the eye (cornea, sclerae), the central nervous system, and bone. Diabetes insipidus is seen in one-third of patients as a result of pituitary gland involvement. Patients tend to be normolipemic.

6. XANTHELASMA

Xanthelasmas are flat to slightly elevated orange to yellowish-gray lesions seen on the upper and lower eyelids, especially near the inner canthus. Hypercholesterolemia is detected in one fourth of patients, especially in those developing xanthelasmas during young adulthood.

Xanthelasmas can be removed surgically or by local treatment (by a dermatologist) with trichloroacetic acid.

7. NECROBIOTIC XANTHOGRANULOMA

Patients have multiple xanthomatous plaques and subcutaneous nodules, especially over the flexural areas, trunk, and periorbital areas. These lesions tend to ulcerate and may be large, violaceous, centrally depressed, telangiectatic, and scarred. All patients have had monoclonal IgG paraproteinemia; other less frequent findings include hyperlipidemia, hypocomplementemia, cryoglobulinemia, elevated sedimentation rate, positive rheumatoid factor, and leukopenia. Some patients have had underlying cancer (lymphoma, multiple myeloma). Early favorable responses have been reported with prednisone or antimetabolites, either alone or in combination.

8. REFSUM'S DISEASE

Refsum's disease is a rare autosomal recessive disorder resulting from deficiency of the enzyme phytanic acid oxidase. Recently, a subset of infants have been identified with general impairment of peroxisomal functions. Phytanic acid, a compound chiefly of dietary origin, accumulates in multiple organs.

The characteristic cutaneous finding is acquired ichthyosis of the trunk and extremities, clinically similar to lamellar ichthyosis. Neurologic abnormalities include cerebellar findings, polyneuropathy, paresis, and anosmia. Increased protein may be detected in cerebrospinal fluid. The patient may complain of night blindness and on eye examination may have abnormal visual fields, cataracts, and retinitis pigmentosa. Multiple abnormalities may be seen in the skeletal system. Abnormalities within the renal mesangium as well as cardiomyopathy and impaired hearing may be seen in some patients.

The hallmark of the disease is the demonstration in serum and tissue of elevated phytanic acid levels.

Involvement of the kidney may result in lipiduria, glycosuria, cylindruria, proteinuria, and mild azotemia.

The treatment of choice is adherence to a low phytol-low phytanic acid diet. Some patients benefit from plasmapheresis.

SPHINGOLIPIDOSES

1. GAUCHER'S DISEASE

Gaucher's disease is an autosomal recessive disorder most frequent in Ashkenazi Jews. It results from deficiency of the lysosomal enzyme β-glucocerebrosidase. As a result, glucocerebrosides accumulate in one or more tissues. Involved tissue may contain Gaucher cells, large histiocytes filled with glucocerebroside deposits.

The most common skin finding is a yellowish-brown discoloration developing initially over exposed skin surfaces, later becoming generalized. It may mimic melasma when present on the face. Other secondary skin findings—ecchymoses, purpura, pallor, and, rarely, jaundice—reflect bone marrow and liver involvement.

Affected tissue contains large histiocytes filled with glucocerebroside deposits (Gaucher cells). Patients have elevated serum levels of non-tartrate inhibitable acid phosphatase activity, elevated serum levels of angiotensin-converting enzyme, and hypergammaglobulinemia. A biochemical assay is now available for the detection of carriers.

Splenomegaly or uncontrollable thrombocytopenia may be an indication for splenectomy. Bony abnormalities may require orthopedic correction. Studies are under way to determine the feasibility of exogenous enzyme replacement.

2. FABRY'S DISEASE
(Angiokeratoma Corporis Diffusum)

Essentials of Diagnosis
- Widespread angiokeratomas, especially in the umbilical and knee regions.
- Oral and conjunctival vascular lesions.
- Acral paresthesias and excruciatingly painful peripheral neuralgias.
- Extensive atherosclerosis.
- Renal disease with birefringent "Maltese crosses"—lipid inclusions in the urinary sediment.

General Considerations
Fabry's disease is an X-linked recessive disorder

due to defective activity of the lysosomal enzyme α-galactosidase A; the major accumulated substrate, trihexoside globotriaosylceramide, is found in plasma, many organs, and particularly in vascular endothelium. In addition, another accumulated material, galabiosylceramide, is deposited primarily within renal lysosomes.

Clinical Findings
A. Symptoms and Signs: The characteristic finding is the angiokeratoma, a 1- to 3-mm dark red to purplish papule with a hyperkeratotic surface. The lesions have widespread distribution but tend to be in greatest density around the umbilicus and superficially resemble petechiae. The conjunctiva and oral mucosa may be involved. Other skin findings include truncal and axillary telangiectasia, erythema nodosum-like lesions, and turtleback deformities of the fingernails. Sweating may be diminished in some patients.

Patients complain of recurrent excruciatingly painful peripheral neuralgias of the hands and feet, often worse in hot weather. There may be acral paresthesias, recurrent unexplained fever, and distal interphalangeal arthropathy of the fingers. Ocular abnormalities include an opacity of the cornea resembling a spoked wheel, vascular tortuosity, aneurysm formation, and, rarely, retinal occlusion. Vascular disease may also occur in the kidneys, heart, and brain and in most cases eventually results in death.

B. Laboratory Findings: The diagnosis is made by demonstrating elevated plasma concentrations of trihexoside globotriaosylceramide. Progressive kidney involvement may result in azotemia and secondary anemia. Methods are now available for prenatal diagnosis of affected individuals as well as postnatal diagnosis of carriers.

Complications
As a result of renal involvement, hypertension and renal failure may result. Because of extensive atherosclerosis secondary to this disorder, infarctions of brain and heart are frequent.

Treatment
There is no specific treatment, though exogenous enzyme replacement is being investigated. Renal transplant has supplied the missing enzyme and has transiently helped pain, sweating, and arthropathy. Unfortunately, continued deposition of material in the renal allograft may eventually destroy it too. The angiokeratomas can be destroyed by electrodesiccation, but this is rarely done since they are small and of only minor cosmetic significance.

Prognosis
Patients frequently die from myocardial or cerebral infarction.

3. FARBER'S LIPOGRANULOMATOSIS

Farber's lipogranulomatosis is a rare autosomal recessive disorder believed to be due to deficiency of a lysosomal acid ceramidase. Free ceramides accumulate in multiple tissues. The child develops a hoarse, weak cry and later tender, swollen joints as well as multiple subcutaneous articular and periarticular nodules. There is no known treatment, and patients usually die by age 2 years.

FUCOSIDOSIS

Fucosidosis is an autosomal recessive disease due to deficiency of the lysosomal enzyme α-L-fucosidase; fucose accumulates in excessive amounts intracellularly. Of the 3 types of fucosidosis, the one of dermatologic interest is type III disease, in which angiokeratomas, tortuous conjunctival vessels, pigmentary retinopathy, and, less frequently, hypohidrosis and purple nail bands have been reported. These patients have neurologic abnormalities including seizure disorders as well as recurrent pulmonary infections. There is no treatment.

THE GLYCOGEN STORAGE DISEASES

At least 12 distinct entities result from defective glycogen metabolism. Most are autosomal recessive in transmission and associated with hepatomegaly. Many organs may be involved; mental development is usually normal. Type I (von Gierke's) disease is the only glycogen storage disease with skin manifestations; eruptive xanthomas may occur in association with hyperlipoproteinemia.

DISORDERS OF PURINE METABOLISM

GOUT

Essentials of Diagnosis
- Recurrent painful monarticular or polyarticular ar-

thritis, especially of the lower extremities or great toe.
- Tophi (deposits of urate crystals).
- Elevated serum uric acid level.

General Considerations
Gout is characterized by hyperuricemia and urate crystal deposition within articular and periarticular tissue in the clinical setting of recurrent painful monarticular or polyarticular arthritis. The basic biochemical defect in most cases is unknown. Almost all patients are males. Although hyperuricemia may be detected asymptomatically by the time of puberty, the most frequent onset of symptoms usually is in the fifth decade of life. Acute attacks of gout may be precipitated by many factors, including drugs (especially diuretics and chemotherapy) and alcohol ingestion.

Clinical Findings
A. Symptoms and Signs: An acute gouty attack is characterized by the sudden onset of pain, redness, swelling, and warmth, usually in a single joint, most commonly the great toe (podagra). Other patients develop polyarticular arthritis. Deposits of urates occur not only in the skin but also in various tissues including the ears, bursae (olecranon, prepatellar), and tendons. These lesions are hard dermal nodules that may ulcerate and discharge a thick white material (urate crystals).

B. Laboratory Findings: The hallmark is hyperuricemia. Urate deposits may be demonstrated in biopsy specimens of tophi.

Complications
Some patients develop interstitial nephropathy, nephrolithiasis, or obstructive uropathy as a result of chronic urate deposition or excretion. Rarely, progressive renal failure occurs.

Prevention
Patients may be treated with colchicine, probenecid, sulfinpyrazone, and urine alkalinizing agents in an effort to prevent the development of acute episodes as well as reduce the possibility of urate precipitation in the urinary tract. Allopurinol, an inhibitor of xanthine oxidase, may be useful in patients with excessive uric acid production.

LESCH-NYHAN SYNDROME

Lesch-Nyhan syndrome is a rare X-linked recessive disorder resulting from deficiency or absence of the enzyme hypoxanthine-guanine phosphoribosyltransferase (HGPRT); such a defect has been recently demonstrated even within the basal ganglion. The skin is affected because these patients uncontrollably mutilate themselves by biting and digging at their skin. Patients characteristically develop hyperuricemia, progressive mental retardation, spasticity, and choreoathetosis.

Some biochemical improvement may result with uricosuric agents and allopurinol. Unfortunately, there is no therapy that has a positive effect on the patient's mentation or mutilatory behavior. Prenatal diagnosis and heterozygote detection are possible. Recent laboratory studies suggest the possibility of eventual gene therapy for this disorder.

DISEASES OF METAL METABOLISM

ABNORMALITIES OF ZINC METABOLISM*

1. ACQUIRED ZINC DEFICIENCY

Essentials of Diagnosis
- Periorificial and acral skin eruption.
- Alopecia.
- Diarrhea.
- Low serum zinc levels.

General Considerations
Skin, scalp, and gastrointestinal findings are reminiscent of acrodermatitis enteropathica (see Chapter 20). Altered mentation may also be associated. A common cause is total parenteral hyperalimentation without adequate zinc replacement; the findings have been noted usually within the second or third month of hyperalimentation, though earlier onsets have been reported. Serum zinc levels are low. The symptoms and findings have been rapidly reversible with the addition of adequate amounts of zinc to total parenteral hyperalimentation formulas or oral zinc supplements.

DISORDERS OF IRON METABOLISM

1. HEMOCHROMATOSIS

Essentials of Diagnosis
- Adult-onset diabetes mellitus.
- Hypogonadism.
- Hepatomegaly or cirrhosis.
- Bronze or bluish-gray discoloration of the skin.

*Acrodermatitis enteropathica is discussed in Chapter 20.

General Considerations
Hemochromatosis is an autosomal recessive disorder of iron metabolism in which total body iron stores are markedly increased so that many organs (including liver, heart, pancreas, other glands, synovium, and skin) develop iron deposition and overload. Hemochromatosis may be secondary to excessive exogenous iron intake or a result of several unrelated diseases (including cirrhosis, porphyria cutanea tarda, and certain forms of anemia). Primary hemochromatosis is a disorder of unknown cause with physical findings and biochemical abnormalities similar to those of secondary hemochromatosis. There is increased frequency of HLA-A3 and HLA-B14 in patients with primary hemochromatosis.

Clinical Findings
A. Symptoms and Signs: Patients with primary hemochromatosis first manifest symptoms in the fourth to sixth decades of life and may have diverse complaints, including weight loss, lethargy, arthralgias, abdominal pain, loss of libido, or diabetes mellitus-related symptoms. Hepatomegaly is found in nearly every patient; some later develop cirrhosis. Physical findings related to liver dysfunction include gynecomastia, spider angiomas, and palmar erythema. Signs and symptoms of congestive heart failure or arrhythmias may be present as a result of significant cardiac involvement. Some patients develop progressive degenerative arthritis similar to seronegative rheumatoid arthritis or pseudogout; increased stainable iron is detectable within affected synovium. Symptoms of poorly controlled diabetes mellitus may be prominent. Hypogonadism with associated testicular atrophy is common. Iron storage disease patients are susceptible to overwhelming septicemia, particularly yersiniosis.

Dermatologic findings include hair loss in the axillae, suprapubic, and chest areas; skin manifestations of liver disease; and bronze or bluish-gray discoloration of the skin. The bronze (or brownish) discoloration is first seen over exposed skin sites but later may become generalized. There may also be bluish-gray discoloration due to iron deposition in sweat glands.

B. Laboratory Findings: Patients have elevated serum iron and ferritin levels as well as increased plasma transferrin saturation. The presence of increased liver iron content may be confirmed by quantitative analysis of liver biopsy tissue. As a rule, there are only moderate elevations of serum transaminase concentrations.

Complications
A. Hepatic: As a result of progressive iron deposition in the liver, cirrhosis and subsequently portal hypertension may develop in untreated patients. In those developing cirrhosis, 30% later develop hepatocellular carcinoma.

B. Cardiac: Because of progressive iron deposition in the heart in untreated patients, congestive failure and arrhythmias may be seen.

C. Endocrine: Uncontrolled hyperglycemia, a result of progressive pancreatic involvement, may lead to the known chronic end-organ effects seen in other forms of diabetes mellitus. Hypogonadotropic hypogonadism is also a frequent finding.

Treatment

In the past, standard treatment was frequent phlebotomy as a means of slowly depleting excess body iron stores. Recently, some patients have benefited from the chelating agent deferoxamine.

Prognosis

With adequate therapy, patients with hemochromatosis have symptomatic improvement as well as enhanced long-term survival rates. In particular, a normal life expectancy, without risk of hepatocellular carcinoma, may be anticipated in precirrhotic patients who are successfully depleted of excessive iron by venesection. Without treatment, there is significant risk of developing hepatocellular carcinoma once cirrhosis is present.

ABNORMALITIES OF COPPER METABOLISM:* HEPATOLENTICULAR DEGENERATION (Wilson's Disease)

Hepatolenticular degeneration is an autosomal recessive disorder characterized by abnormal copper levels in tissue, serum, and urine.

Clinical findings reflect multi-organ involvement. Neurologic findings may be initially characterized by fine movement incoordination and later by action tremor (parkinsonian), ataxia, dysarthria, and abnormal personality or psychiatric presentations. Hepatitis or cirrhosis may occur. Almost all patients have a characteristic brown or greenish discoloration of Descemet's membrane of the cornea, referred to as the Kayser-Fleischer ring. Skin findings include hyperpigmentation along the anterior aspects of the legs and, infrequently, azure-colored lunulae of the nails. If significant hepatic decompensation occurs, spider angiomas and jaundice may be noted. Bony abnormalities are not uncommon.

Patients exhibit hypocupremia, hypoceruloplasminemia, hypercuprinuria, and elevated hepatic copper levels. Some investigators suggest that liver biopsy with assay of copper content by atomic absorption spectrometry is the most reliable test for this disease.

Treatment is with penicillamine for life. Trientine is a safe alternative for patients intolerant of penicillamine. There is no indication for prophylactic treatment of heterozygotes.

Prognosis

Untreated patients develop progressive multi-organ involvement and eventually die. If treated early, patients may expect normal life expectancy. In addition to neurologic and hepatic dysfunction, other poor prognostic indicators include hematologic involvement and renal tubular acidosis.

CUTANEOUS CALCIFICATION & OSSIFICATION

Dystrophic calcification occurs when calcium salts become deposited in previously injured or degenerating tissue in the setting of normal serum levels of calcium and phosphorus. Examples include dermatomyositis and CREST syndrome of scleroderma and pseudokanthoma elasticum.

When the serum calcium-serum phosphorus product is elevated, precipitation is referred to as **metastatic calcification** and may be due to elevated serum levels of calcium, phosphorus, or both. Metastatic calcification may occur within skin and subcutaneous tissue, as well as kidney, lung, stomach, and blood vessels. Cutaneous calcification is uncommon in chronic dialysis patients, despite the high frequency of extracutaneous metastatic calcification. Cutaneous lesions of metastatic calcification present as papules or nodules, usually overlying large joints, and may involve the dermis, subcutaneous tissue, or sweat ducts. Some lesions may become fluctuant and suppurative, extruding a chalky white material to the surface of the skin.

Some patients with secondary or tertiary hyperparathyroidism may develop arterial insufficiency and ischemic tissue necrosis following successful kidney transplantation. This phenomenon is referred to as **calciphylaxis** and may be manifested cutaneously by the development of painful ischemic ulcers on the extremities as well as painful livedo reticularis, which may progress to gangrene. Associated laboratory findings include marked hyperphosphatemia and, less frequently, hypercalcemia.

In some patients, calcification may occur in localized (calcinosis circumscripta) or widespread (calcinosis universalis) areas without prior tissue injury or evidence of concurrent metabolic abnormalities. These lesions may be papular, nodular, or plaque-like; may become tender, ulcerate, and discharge a

---

*Menkes's kinky hair syndrome is discussed in Chapter 20.

chalky white material; and usually occur over the extremities. This type of calcification is seen most frequently in children.

Tumoral calcinosis occurs early in life, is familial, and presents as large subcutaneous masses of calcium usually overlying joints or sites of pressure. Serum calcium levels are usually normal, though phosphate levels may be increased in occasional patients. Treatment includes the use of phosphorus-depleted diets where indicated as well as local excision of the lesions.

Cutaneous ossification is the occurrence of bone within skin and subcutaneous tissue. It may occur in conjunction with calcinosis cutis and in association with many localized skin conditions, including infections, nevoid lesions, and tumors.

CAROTENEMIA

Patients having excess serum carotenoid levels may develop yellowish discoloration of the skin. This is most common in the palms, soles, and central third of the face, though if uncorrected other areas of the skin may also be involved. Sweat may appear yellowish. The sclerae are usually uninvolved, which helps differentiate the disorder from jaundice. Hypercarotenemia may result from excessive ingestion of certain vegetables and fruits rich in carotene or as a result of therapy with beta-carotene for conditions such as erythropoietic protoporphyria. In addition, hypercarotenemia may be seen in association with some cases of hypothyroidism, diabetes mellitus, nephrotic syndrome, hypopituitarism, hyperlipoproteinemia, hypothalamic amenorrhea, and anorexia nervosa. When hypercarotenemia is a result of exogenous beta-carotene therapy or excessive dietary ingestion, the skin will return to its normal appearance several months after the offending diet or therapy is stopped.

LYCOPENEMIA

Lycopene is an isomer of carotene and is present in large amounts in such foods as tomatoes and certain berries. When these substances are ingested in large amounts, an orangish-yellow discoloration may appear in a distribution similar to that seen in hypercarotenemia. Serum lycopene levels will be elevated,

and there may be chemical evidence of mild liver dysfunction.

HYPERBILIRUBINEMIA

Hyperbilirubinemia may result from any of several causes of excessive serum levels of unconjugated or conjugated bilirubin. As a result, a yellowish discoloration may be seen affecting the skin, sclerae, and mucous and tympanic membranes. Hyperbilirubinemia can be easily differentiated from hypercarotenemia or lycopenemia by the presence of scleral discoloration and elevated serum bilirubin levels in the former.

CUTANEOUS MANIFESTATIONS & DISEASES OF PREGNANCY

During pregnancy, hyperpigmentation usually occurs in the genital and perianal areas, areolae, umbilicus, and linea nigra. Increased numbers and sizes of skin tags may also occur. Other symptoms and signs reported in increased frequency include melasma, guttate leukoderma, vitiligo, pruritus, urticaria, dermatographism, edema, cutaneous flushing, hyperhidrosis, hypertrichosis, palmar erythema, palmoplantar telangiectasia, spider angiomas, scalp alopecia, and nail changes.

HERPES GESTATIONIS

Herpes gestationis is an uncommon autoimmune bullous disorder that may occur at any time during pregnancy and is characterized by subepidermal blisters and pruritus. Direct immunofluorescence shows a linear band of complement C3 along the basement membrane zone. This disease is discussed in Chapter 42.

PRURITIC URTICARIAL PAPULES & PLAQUES OF PREGNANCY (PUPPP)

This common disorder, occurring during the third trimester, is characterized by the onset of pruritus and the development of red urticarial papules and plaques. Lesions may initially begin in the stria cutis distensae of the abdomen and later spread onto the thighs, buttocks, and arms. As opposed to herpes gestationis, routine histology does not reveal subepidermal blister formation. Direct immunofluorescence testing of the skin is negative.

There is no significant increase in fetal morbidity or mortality rates. Patients usually respond to antihistamines and topical corticosteroid preparations, though some may require brief courses of systemic corticosteroids for control. There is no resurgence of this disease postpartum, nor is there recurrence with oral contraceptives or subsequent pregnancies.

PAPULAR DERMATITIS OF PREGNANCY

Papular (Spangler's) dermatitis of pregnancy is a rare severely pruritic disorder that may occur at any time during pregnancy and reportedly is an associated finding in 30% of cases of stillbirth or spontaneous abortion. The disorder recurs during subsequent pregnancies. Such patients develop uniform red papules with crusting and excoriation in generalized or grouped distribution that resemble excoriated wheals. With the resolution of individual lesions, postinflammatory hyperpigmentation may be seen. Abnormal laboratory findings include elevated urinary levels of human chorionic gonadotropin, decreased plasma hydrocortisone levels, a shortened plasma hydrocortisone half-life, and normal or diminished 24-hour urinary estrogen levels.

Treatment is with systemic corticosteroids. Diethylstilbestrol is no longer used because of its proved association with vaginal carcinoma.

IMMUNE PROGESTERONE DERMATITIS OF PREGNANCY

Immune progesterone dermatitis of pregnancy is a rare disorder of the first trimester of pregnancy, characterized by a papulopustular eruption; at times the eruption may appear acneiform or psoriasiform. The lesions develop especially over the extremities and buttocks. Associated spontaneous abortions have been reported. Recurrences have been noted with subsequent pregnancies. Laboratory findings include peripheral eosinophilia, hyperglobulinemia, elevated sedimentation rate, elevated serum histamine, elevated plasma β-estradiol, and slightly diminished urinary levels of 17-hydroxysteroids and 17-ketosteroids. Direct immunofluorescence of lesions fails to demonstrate immunoglobulin deposits. Lesions have been reproduced with intradermal progesterone challenge. Symptoms are made worse by the administration of progesterone-containing oral contraceptives and suppressed by administration of estrogens.

PRURIGO GESTATIONIS OF BESNIER

This disorder, occurring during the third trimester and not associated with increased fetal or maternal mortality rates, clears during the postpartum period but may recur during subsequent pregnancies. It is characterized by small papules with excoriations and crusts, especially over the extensor aspects of the arms and forearms, the backs of the hands and the tops of the feet, and the thighs, legs, and later the trunk. In contrast to some other dermatologic disorders of pregnancy, vesicles and bullae have not been reported. Some have suggested that this entity may represent a variant of pruritus gravidarum in women with underlying atopy, though this is as yet unproved.

IMPETIGO HERPETIFORMIS

Impetigo herpetiformis, believed to be a form of pustular psoriasis seen during pregnancy, occurs chiefly during the last trimester and may be associated with significant increase in maternal or fetal mortality rates. It may recur with future pregnancies. It is associated with hypoparathyroidism. Systemic symptoms include fever, chills, prostration, vomiting, diarrhea, tetany, convulsions, weight loss, or arthralgias. Erythematous macules develop initially; later, sterile pustules may appear at the edges of lesions. With extension and coalescence of lesions, vegetative areas may occur. Characteristic sites for lesions include body folds (inguinal, mammary, axillary) and mucous membranes (oral, esophageal). Individual lesions may be pruritic or burning. Treatment is similar to that of pustular psoriasis, though antimetabolites and etretinate are preferably avoided.

PRURITUS GRAVIDARUM

Pruritus gravidarum—also known as intrahepatic cholestasis of pregnancy—is seen especially in the last trimester, clears during the postpartum period, and tends to recur with subsequent pregnancies or with administration of oral contraceptives. Symptoms include generalized pruritus, anorexia, nausea, and vomiting. Patients may appear jaundiced and may have enlarged and tender livers. Associated laboratory findings are consistent with cholestatic rather than hepatocellular injury.

REFERENCES

Adams PC, Halliday JW, Powell LW: Early diagnosis and treatment of hemochromatosis. Adv Intern Med 1989; 34:111.

Balato N et al: Tyrosinemia type II in two cases previously reported as Richner-Hanhart syndrome. Dermatologica 1986;173:66.

Barthelemy H, Chouvet B, Cambazard F: Skin and mucosal manifestations in vitamin deficiency. J Am Acad Dermatol 1986;15:1263.

Brady RO: Heritable catabolic and anabolic disorders of lipid metabolism. Metabolism 1977;26:329.

Breathnach SM: Amyloid and amyloidosis. J Am Acad Dermatol 1988;18:1.

Caro I: Lipoid proteinosis. Int J Dermatol 1978;17:388.

Cosky RJ, Mehregan A: Papular mucinosis. Int J Dermatol 1977;16:741.

Cox T, Lord D: Hereditary hemochromatosis. Eur J Haematol 1989;42:113.

Desnick RJ, Astrin KH, Bishop DF: Fabry disease: Molecular genetics of the inherited nephropathy. Adv Nephrol 1989;18:113.

Dobyns WB, Goldstein NP, Gordan H: Clinical spectrum of Wilson's disease (hepatolenticular degeneration). Mayo Clin Proc 1979;54:35.

Finan MC, Winkelmann RK: Necrobiotic xanthogranuloma with paraproteinemia. Medicine 1986;65:376.

Fine JD, Wise TG, Falchuk KH: Zinc in cutaneous disease and dermatologic therapeutics. In: *Dermatology Update: Reviews for Physicians*. Moschella SL (editor). Elsevier, 1982.

Glenner GG: Amyloid deposits and amyloidosis: The beta-fibrilloses. (Two parts.) New Engl J Med 1980; 302:1283, 1333.

Goldblatt J, Beighton P: Cutaneous manifestations of Gaucher disease. Br J Dermatol 1984;111:331.

Holmes RC, Black MM: The specific dermatoses of pregnancy. J Am Acad Dermatol 1983;8:405.

Hug G: Glycogen storage diseases. Birth Defects 1976; 12:145.

Lawrence N et al: Exogenous ochronosis in the United States. J Am Acad Dermatol 1988;18:1207.

Mam MK, Sethi TS: Alkaptonuria and ochronotic arthropathy. J Indian Med Assoc 1986;84:218.

Matsuoka LY et al: Pretibial myxedema. Arch Dermatol 1981;117:250.

Mehregan DA, Winkelmann RK: Cutaneous gangrene, vascular calcification, and hyperparathyroidism. Mayo Clin Proc 1989;64:211.

Muenzer J: Mucopolysaccharidoses. Adv Pediatr 1986; 33:269.

Parker F: Hyperlipidemia and xanthomatosis. In: *Dermatology Update: Reviews for Physicians*. Moschella SL (editor). Elsevier, 1979.

Parker F: Xanthomas and hyperlipidemias. J Am Acad Dermatol 1985;13:1.

Raimer SS, Archer ME, Jorizzo JL: Metastatic calcinosis cutis. Cutis 1983;32:463.

Ramsey ML et al: Lipoid proteinosis. Int J Dermatol 1985;27:230.

Sasseville D, Wilkinson RD, Schnader JY: Dermatoses of pregnancy. Int J Dermatol 1981;20:223.

Schaefer EJ, Levy RI: Pathogenesis and management of lipoprotein disorders. N Engl J Med 1985;312:1300.

Scriver CR et al: The Hartnup phenotype: Mendelian transport disorder, multifactorial disease. J Hum Genet 1987; 40:401.

Truhan AP, Roenigk HH Jr: The cutaneous mucinoses. J Am Acad Dermatol 1986;14:1.

Walshe JM: Wilson's disease: Yesterday, today, and tomorrow. Movement Disorders 1988;3:10.

Wanders RJA et al: Peroxisomal functions in classical Refsum's disease: Comparison with the infantile form of Refsum's disease. J Neurol Sci 1988;84:147.

Wappner RS: Mucopolysaccharide storage disorders. J Indiana State Med Assoc 1981;74:81.

Wilson JM, Young AB, Kelley WN: Hypoxanthine-guanine phosphoribosyltransferase deficiency: The molecular basis of the clinical syndromes. N Engl J Med 1983;309:900.

Immunodeficiency & Immunosuppression

32

Paul G. Quie, MD, Sigfrid A. Muller, MD, & Robert W. Goltz, MD

I. IMMUNODEFICIENCY

Paul G. Quie, MD

The skin is often the portal of entry for disease-causing pathogenic organisms in patients with immunodeficiency diseases, who are susceptible to severe life-threatening infections. Physicians should therefore know about possible associated immunodeficiency syndromes in patients with skin lesions and, conversely, about the skin manifestations of immunodeficiency disorders. Patients may have an inherited primary immunodeficiency or an acquired immunodeficiency due to atopy, malnutrition, cancer, HIV infection, immunosuppressive therapy, etc. Patients with eczema, for example, may be predisposed to development of deep-seated staphylococcal abscesses; when serum IgE levels are greatly elevated, signaling immune "dysregulation," the threat is even more ominous. Other examples of skin lesions heralding immunodeficiency include lupuslike lesions in patients with hereditary abnormalities of the complement system and purpuric lesions in patients with Wiskott-Aldrich syndrome. The characteristic skin and mucous membrane lesions due to *Candida albicans* in patients with chronic mucocutaneous candidiasis are another example of a systemic immunologic disorder resulting in skin disease due to a resident microorganism. A dramatic example of acquired immunodeficiency with prominent skin manifestations is AIDS (acquired immune deficiency syndrome; see Chapter 15), in which cutaneous lesions due to herpesvirus, opportunistic infections, and Kaposi's sarcoma are prominent manifestations.

This chapter will discuss skin disorders associated with primary and acquired immunodeficiencies involving the phagocyte, complement, antibody, and cell-mediated immune systems.

PHAGOCYTE IMMUNE SYSTEM

The body's capacity to protect the skin from infection after trauma depends on the prompt migration of normally functioning granulocytes to the wound site. Clinical evidence confirming this protective phagocytic function has been derived from patients with granulocytopenia (< 200 cells/μL) and patients with defective microbicidal function or disordered chemotaxis of granulocytes.

Patients with granulocytopenia are susceptible to infection caused by organisms resident on the skin and by enteric microorganisms on mucous membranes. Minor trauma or indwelling catheters may be associated with the development of septicemia and other life-threatening infections in patients who, because of hereditary defects or cytotoxic therapy, have few circulating granulocytes. *Staphylococcus aureus* is the most common causative bacterial species, and together with the enteric organisms *Klebsiella, Escherichia coli,* and *Pseudomonas* (most likely invasive from the gut) it accounts for nearly 50% of systemic infections in patients with granulocytopenia. Prophylaxis with broad-spectrum antibiotics may be useful in patients with severe granulocytopenia.

CHRONIC GRANULOMATOUS DISEASE

Essentials of Diagnosis

- Recurrent cutaneous and systemic bacterial infections.
- Absence of nitroblue tetrazolium reduction by stimulated neutrophils.

- Abnormal (flat) chemiluminescence response of neutrophils activated by soluble or particulate stimuli.

General Considerations

Chronic granulomatous disease is usually inherited in X-linked fashion. The disorder is usually due to defective cytochrome b function. Granulocytes normally respond to the stimulus of phagocytosis with an oxidative respiratory burst; in patients with chronic granulomatous disease, this response fails to occur, and as a result reactive oxygen radicals—eg, superoxide, hydrogen peroxide, and hydroxyl—are not formed. Abnormal cellular metabolism in these patients can be detected by the nitroblue tetrazolium dye reduction test, a highly useful screening device. Nitroblue tetrazolium turns blue on reduction; normal phagocytes contain blue-black deposits, whereas those of patients with chronic granulomatous disease do not, since the cells fail to reduce the dye. If neutrophils are incubated with opsonized zymosan, they also fail to show enhanced chemiluminescence.

Clinical Findings

A. Symptoms and Signs: Patients with chronic granulomatous disease have recurrent bacterial infections of the skin, lymph nodes, and reticuloendothelial organs. Eczematous lesions of the scalp and periorbital, nasal, and postauricular regions are typical, and they are often complicated by infection with staphylococci or other bacteria. Minor abrasions frequently lead to furunculosis and subcutaneous abscesses. Suppurative lymphadenopathy is frequent; skin manifestations in older patients include healed scars of old lesions in the cervical or inguinal areas or scars secondary to multiple surgical procedures performed to drain abscesses. Recurrent ulcerative stomatitis is present at some time in nearly all patients with chronic granulomatous disease. Abscesses characteristically heal slowly and leave prominent scars.

B. Laboratory Findings: Histopathologic findings are granulomas consisting of neutrophils and macrophages that contain yellow inclusions. Bacteria recovered from the lesions of patients with chronic granulomatous disease are usually catalase-positive. Catalase-negative hydrogen peroxide-producing species such as *Streptococcus pneumoniae, Streptococcus pyogenes,* and *Haemophilus influenzae* are not recovered from patients with chronic granulomatous disease with any more frequency than from normal individuals; however, *S aureus* and *Serratia marcescens* are commonly recovered from lesions such as liver abscesses, abscesses of the oviduct, and lymphadenitis. The recovery of *S marcescens* or *Klebsiella* from a skin infection or a suppurative lymph node of a young patient strongly points toward a diagnosis of chronic granulomatous disease.

Because chronic granulomatous disease is primarily an X-linked disease, mothers and sisters of most male patients with chronic granulomatous disease may be carriers. Carriers are not more susceptible to development of severe bacterial infections than normal individuals, but they do have characteristic skin lesions, which are slowly developing red-brown plaques that become erythematous and may be painful. The lesions are characterized by aggregates of lymphocytes in the mid and deep dermis, especially around blood vessels and adnexa.

Treatment

All infectious lesions should be cultured, and all infections should be treated with broad-spectrum systemic antibiotics after culture materials are obtained. Aggressive treatment should be instituted at the first signs of infection. Prolonged treatment may be required, since infections respond poorly to antibiotics in the absence of normal phagocyte function. A search for occult abscesses (eg, retroperitoneal) should be considered if the site of infection is not obvious. Administration of human recombinant gamma interferon has helped some patients experimentally and is a promising adjunct for prevention of serious infections. Healing eventually occurs over several months. Lesions may recur.

Prognosis

Infections are less common in adulthood, but the propensity for severe, life-threatening bacterial infections persists throughout life.

CHÉDIAK-HIGASHI SYNDROME

Chédiak-Higashi syndrome is a disorder of phagocytic cells characterized by susceptibility to infection, partial albinism, and silvery hair. Ocular albinism is prominent and together with photophobia and silvery hair is helpful in early recognition of the disease. Large pigment inclusions are present throughout the hair shafts, and giant cytoplasmic inclusions are found in most cell types that have cytoplasmic granules, including melanocytes.

The diagnosis is simple, since peripheral blood smears show the typical granulocytes with large inclusions.

Skin infections occur frequently in patients with Chédiak-Higashi syndrome and range from superficial pyoderma to deep subcutaneous abscesses and ulcers that heal slowly and result in atrophic scars. *S aureus* is the most common causative agent. Granulocytes of patients with Chédiak-Higashi syndrome display defective chemotaxis and intracellular killing of catalase-negative as well as catalase-positive organisms. The intracellular killing defect in Chédiak-Higashi syndrome is not as severe as in chronic granulomatous disease, and patients are far less susceptible to development of serious bacterial infections (see Chapter 12).

ABNORMALITIES OF PHAGOCYTE CHEMOTAXIS

Phagocytic cells have the capacity for rapid locomotion that enables them to localize and rapidly kill organisms invading the surface of the skin. It is therefore not surprising that host defenses are impaired in patients with chemotactic disorders of phagocytic cells. The skin and mucous membranes are particularly vulnerable to diseases arising from defective phagocyte chemotaxis. Excessively high levels of serum IgE may be found in certain patients with eczematous skin lesions associated with serious infections, eg, lung abscesses, life-threatening peritonsillar abscesses, and deep muscle abscesses. Patients with hyper-IgE (Job's) syndrome have depressed granulocyte chemotaxis on some occasions and normal chemotaxis at other times. More patients demonstrate depressed monocyte chemotaxis than granulocyte chemotaxis. Abnormal phagocytic cell locomotion in patients with this syndrome may not be a primary defect but rather a result of the underlying infectious disease. Patients with hyper-IgE syndrome have "cold" abscesses due to *S aureus* and may benefit from continuous antistaphylococcal therapy.

Patients with Job's syndrome who have defective granulocyte chemotaxis are especially susceptible to infections due to *S aureus,* and many have mouth lesions or vaginal lesions caused by *C albicans.* One study found that a group of patients with allergic rhinitis also had depressed granulocyte chemotaxis. Staphylococcal furunculosis frequently followed the rhinitis, and chemotaxis was normal when the furunculosis was active. It is tempting to speculate that depressed chemotaxis may have made these patients more susceptible to development of staphylococcal lesions.

Patients with ichthyosis or with acrodermatitis enteropathica have also been found to have defective phagocyte chemotaxis. Infections in patients wi these diseases include diarrhea and frequent stomatitis caused by *C albicans,* and skin lesions may be infected with bacteria or *Trichophyton rubrum.*

Patients with atopic dermatitis may also have elevated levels of serum IgE but not the excessively high levels found in patients with hyper-IgE syndrome. Patients with atopic dermatitis are less apt to have depressed granulocyte chemotaxis or recurrent severe infections. Not all patients with atopic dermatitis have immune defects, however, and appropriate immunologic tests in those few patients with recurrent invasive infections may be clinically valuable. Dermatologic manifestations in patients with deficient immunologic responsiveness are listed in Table 32–1.

Table 32–1. Dermatologic manifestations in patients with abnormalities of various immune system components.

Immune System Abnormality	Possible Manifestations
Phagocyte deficiency	Pyoderma, granuloma, furunculosis, abscesses, suppurative lymphadenitis, ichthyosis, incontinentia pigmenti, albinism, delayed wound healing.
Complement abnormality	Angioedema, lupus erythematosus, vasculitis, anaphylactoid purpura, seborrheic dermatitis.
Antibody (B cell) deficiency	Pyoderma, granuloma, furunculosis, eczema, telangiectases, purpura, subcutaneous nodules.
Cell-mediated (T cell) deficiency	Skin cancer, opportunistic infections, candidiasis, granulomas, cartilage-hair hypoplasia, graft-versus-host disease, widespread warts or molluscum.

COMPLEMENT IMMUNE SYSTEM

Patients with abnormalities of the complement system have significant clinical manifestations, many reflected in skin and mucous membrane lesions. Some of the syndromes associated with complement abnormalities are listed in Table 32–2. The proteins of the complement system circulate in an inactive state, but when activated by various nonspecific stimuli, they assume important biologic activities as mediators such as opsonins and chemotactic factors.

As might be imagined in such a biologically active system, exquisite regulatory systems may be abnormal. For example, an inhibitor of the activated first component of complement is missing in patients with hereditary angioedema (see Chapter 34). Patients lacking C1 inhibitor have bouts of subepithelial edema of the skin and mucous membranes, including

Table 32–2. Clinical syndromes associated with abnormalities of the complement system.

Angioneurotic edema
Systemic lupus erythematosus
Dermatomyositis
Chronic vasculitis
Anaphylactoid purpura
Leiner's disease
Raynaud's phenomenon
Membranoproliferative glomerulonephritis
Partial lipodystrophy

the gastrointestinal and upper respiratory tracts. Since its inhibitor is missing, activated C1 circulates as a protease, and complement-related peptides are formed, some of which increase capillary permeability and cause angioedema. Edema may affect many parts of the body, but when the larynx is involved, air exchange is compromised and the disease is life-threatening.

Patients with other hereditary abnormalities of the complement system also have characteristic skin lesions. Patients with C1q deficiency, for example, may have atrophic skin and joint symptoms, and patients with C4 and C2 deficiency may have lupus erythematosus.

Patients with C3 deficiency are highly susceptible to development of serious infection, and the clinical presentation of skin symptoms and other severe infections resembles that of patients with phagocytic abnormalities. Patients with C5 deficiency have a striking abnormality in serum opsonic activity. In the newborn, C5 dysfunction may be associated with severe dermatitis of the scalp that becomes secondarily infected with staphylococci (Leiner's syndrome). Patients with deficiency of a terminal complement component, eg, C6, C7, C8, or C9, are susceptible to systemic infections caused by *Neisseria*. These patients may also have Raynaud's phenomenon, which may progress to gangrene of the fingertips and toes. Strains of *Neisseria gonorrhoeae* that normally cause only mucous membrane lesions in patients with normal complement may produce fever, septic arthritis, and pustules in patients with hereditary complement deficiency.

Circulating immune complexes in certain diseases such as Henoch-Schönlein purpura and cryoglobulinemia may activate the complement system and produce cutaneous vasculitis. Dermatologic manifestations in patients with abnormalities of the complement system are set forth in Table 32–1.

ANTIBODY (B CELL) IMMUNE SYSTEM

X-LINKED HYPOGAMMAGLOBULINEMIA

X-linked hypogammaglobulinemia, described by Bruton in 1952, was the first primary immunodeficiency described in humans. Patients with this disease are born without lymph nodes, plasma cells, or the capacity to produce antibodies. Bacterial infections of

the skin, otitis media, and bacteremia with *S pneumoniae* or *H influenzae* occur after the antibodies passively transferred from mother to fetus have all been metabolized, ie, after patients are about 6 months of age. The diagnosis is confirmed by measurement of serum immunoglobulin levels. Accurate quantitation of IgG, IgM, and IgA levels is a standard procedure in most laboratories. IgG replacement therapy has been highly successful in protecting patients with immunoglobulin deficiency against life-threatening infections.

COMBINED IMMUNODEFICIENCY

Patients with combined immunodeficiency have abnormalities of both the antibody (B cell) immune system and cell-mediated (T cell) immune system and are highly susceptible to infection due to *Pneumocystis carinii,* cytomegalovirus, and bacterial pathogens; skin infections are common. Therapy in these patients includes transplantation of cultured human thymic tissue or bone marrow.

Common variable immunodeficiency denotes a syndrome noted in patients who acquire immunodeficiency after the first 2 years of life. Such patients demonstrate nonspecific skin reactions such as warts, molluscum contagiosum, and eczema. A relationship between immunodeficiency and ectodermal function (ie, hair growth and bone development) is suggested by the association of immunodeficiency with short-limbed dwarfism and cartilage-hair hypoplasia.

Isolated absence of IgA may be the most common immunodeficiency. Its incidence has been reported to be as high as 1:400 in some populations and 1:3000 in others. IgA is present on the surface of the respiratory and gastrointestinal tracts. Its absence is associated with allergies and autoimmune processes. When IgE antibodies are produced in the normal manner in patients lacking IgA, prominent allergic symptoms, including eczema and asthma, result. Patients with Wiskott-Aldrich syndrome have low levels of IgM and severe eczema as well as thrombocytopenic purpura. Some of these patients develop widespread herpes simplex lesions of the skin. Many are also plagued with chronic fungal infections, evidence that they suffer a deficiency of cell-mediated as well as humoral immunity. Both IgA and IgE are frequently absent in patients with ataxia-telangiectasia, and the incidence of telangiectasia increases in these patients as they become older. Dermatologic manifestations in patients with antibody deficiency are listed in Table 32–1.

CELL-MEDIATED (T CELL) IMMUNE SYSTEM

Cell-mediated immunity involves complex cooperation between lymphocytes and macrophages. Regulatory proteins, termed lymphokines, are produced by activated lymphocytes and are responsible for "activating" macrophages, which constitute a defense against viruses and fungi. Cell-mediated immunity is an essential part of the immunologic system, and any abnormalities are associated with increased susceptibility to disease caused by all microbial forms. The skin is convenient for clinical evaluation of the capacity for cell-mediated immunity in humans. The complex interaction between the reaction of "informed" lymphocytes to antigens, the production of lymphokines, the activation of macrophages, chemotactic stimulation, and migration of mononuclear cells to the site of greatest antigen concentration are necessary to mount a delayed-type hypersensitivity skin reaction. Erythema and induration of the skin after 24 hours (delayed-type hypersensitivity) occur only when all elements of the cell-mediated immune system are functioning effectively. The inability of patients to mount a delayed-type hypersensitivity reaction to intradermal skin tests with common antigens that most people are exposed to, eg, antigens from *Candida, Trichophyton,* streptokinase-streptodornase, or mumps, is strong clinical evidence for dysfunction of the cell-mediated immune system.

CHRONIC MUCOCUTANEOUS CANDIDIASIS

Candida albicans is an ubiquitous saprophyte in the gastrointestinal tract of most humans and causes persistent infections of the skin, nails, and mucous membranes in certain patients with abnormal cell-mediated immunity. This organism uses keratin as a source of nitrogen and therefore thrives and multiplies on superficial structures such as the nails and the surfaces of the skin. Patients with persistent lesions of the mucous membranes due to *C albicans* may develop esophagitis and granulomas of the skin. Cutaneous lesions due to *Candida* usually develop between the ages of 1 and 3 years. Some patients, however, are healthy until the teenage years.

Patients with superficial lesions due to *Candida* may have endocrine disorders, including hypothyroidism, diabetes, or hypoadrenalism. Genetic studies of patients with mucocutaneous candidiasis suggest that the defect in cell-mediated immunity may be transmitted as an autosomal recessive trait. More than one sibling in a family may be affected. Some pa-

tients with mucocutaneous candidiasis have abnormal granulocyte or monocyte chemotaxis, and because of this phagocytic cell defect or as a consequence of defective cutaneous defenses they have increased susceptibility to bacterial infections.

Patients with mucocutaneous candidiasis have depressed numbers of circulating T cells, and those that are present fail to respond to antigens, including *C albicans*. The T cells may demonstrate a normal response to mitogens such as phytohemagglutinin or concanavalin A. Intradermal skin tests with common antigens such as candidin and trichophytin are negative. Dermatologic manifestations in patients with cell-mediated immune deficiency are listed in Table 32–1.

IMMUNODEFICIENCY & CANCER

Increased susceptibility to cancer, especially that of the hematopoietic system or skin, is present in patients with either primary or acquired immunodeficiency. For example, a much higher incidence of lymphomas has been reported in patients with primary hypogammaglobulinemia than in normal subjects, and Kaposi's sarcoma is a common neoplasm in patients with AIDS.

II. IMMUNOSUPPRESSION

Sigfrid A. Muller, MD

The incidence and severity of bacterial, fungal, viral, and parasitic infections involving the skin and mucous membranes are significantly increased in immunosuppressed patients. Such patients are increasingly encountered in dermatologic practice and include those who have undergone organ transplantation, renal dialysis, parenteral alimentation, or therapeutic procedures such as suctioning or assisted ventilation. Patients receiving immunosuppressive drugs for neoplastic or inflammatory disorders may also present with dermatologic symptoms, especially if intensive multidrug regimens have been used.

In addition to iatrogenic suppression, other more conventional predisposing factors that increase susceptibility to infection include malignant disorders, especially lymphoma; chronic illness and debility; drug addiction; diabetes mellitus; extensive trauma; splenectomy; burns; certain parasitic infections (eg, leishmaniasis, schistosomiasis); and special genetic, nutritional, and occupational considerations. Individuals with acquired immunodeficiency syndrome (AIDS) present with a broad range of microbial infections and also frequently develop aggressive Kaposi's sarcoma and, less commonly, lymphoma (see also Chapter 15).

The term opportunistic infection has been used to describe many infections that occur in particularly vulnerable patients, though it is best reserved for infections due to pathogens not ordinarily causing disease in a healthy host. However, the term is also used appropriately to describe infections caused by common pathogens, eg, *Staphylococcus aureus,* in immunocompromised patients. Such patients may show evidence of an increased frequency of reactivation of latent or persistent viral infections (eg, herpes simplex, varicella zoster, cytomegalovirus). These patients may also demonstrate decreased resistance to primary infection with the same viruses.

The diagnosis of microbial infections is often difficult in immunocompromised patients because clinical signs and symptoms may be mild or may be confused with reactions to drugs and blood transfusions or to the underlying disease itself. Infections in immunocompromised patients are associated with a high mortality rate, and the condition of such patients often deteriorates rapidly, so that it is frequently necessary to begin empirical treatment before the diagnosis or causative organism is known. Culture of blood, body fluids, exudates, and affected tissues and examination of appropriately stained smears of material from pustules, wounds, and sinus tracts should be performed promptly. Occasionally, histopathologic examination of biopsies and smears of skin lesions may permit tentative identification of the causative organism while culture results are pending. In vitro susceptibility tests are essential for bacterial infections, especially gram-negative bacilli that vary in their susceptibility to the antibiotics of first choice.

In seriously ill septic patients, careful examination of the skin and mucous membranes may reveal subtle, small, or banal-appearing lesions that can be tested. Techniques for the detection of occult infections and localization of abscesses, particularly in soft tissues, include ultrasonography, CT scan, and gallium scintigraphy used alone or in combination with other methods. Specific and sensitive monoclonal antibody-staining methods have been developed that permit more rapid identification of many infectious organisms.

BACTERIAL INFECTIONS

Bacterial infection is manifested on the skin either as a primary infection or as a secondary manifestation of infection in other organs. Most of these cutaneous lesions are caused by *Staphylococcus aureus* and β-hemolytic streptococci. However, the widespread use of antibiotics and induced profound immunosup-

pression have been responsible for a greatly increased incidence of infection caused by other organisms, particularly gram-negative bacteria. The most important predisposing factor is granulocytopenia, which is a significant factor when the neutrophil count is less than $1000/\mu L$.

One study of the most common bacterial infections in granulocytopenic cancer patients showed that *S aureus, Pseudomonas aeruginosa, Escherichia coli,* and *Klebsiella* accounted for more than 50% of infections. The most common sites of infection were the mouth, skin and soft tissues, the anorectal area, the lungs, and the urinary tract—note that of the 5 most common sites, 3 are of special interest to the dermatologist.

Sepsis remains the principal cause of death in many immunosuppressed patients. The incidence of sepsis depends on many factors, including the underlying disease, the patient's age, the severity and duration of immunosuppression, the presence or absence of granulocytopenia, and the number of invasive therapeutic procedures performed.

Perhaps the most clinically distinctive cutaneous manifestation of bacterial sepsis is ecthyma gangrenosum, which accompanies *Pseudomonas* septicemia (Fig 32–1). *Pseudomonas* septicemia is frequently the last stage in a complex illness in a patient

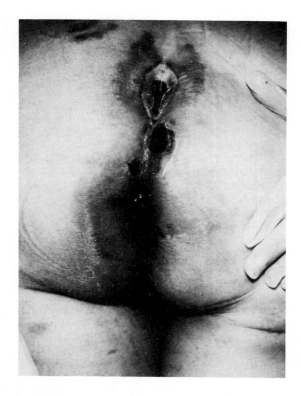

Figure 32–1. Ecthyma gangrenosum. Note the "punched out" ulcers and surrounding erythema.

with cancer or marked immunosuppression. In ecthyma gangrenosum, solitary or grouped (usually only a few) tense hemorrhagic vesicles become necrotic and form punched-out ulcers with surrounding erythema. The patient is often moribund. Disseminated intravascular coagulation may be a major complication. Other gram-negative organisms such as *Escherichia coli, Klebsiella, Proteus, Serratia marcescens, Haemophilus influenzae, Bacteroides,* and other anaerobes also cause fulminating sepsis. Sometimes sepsis is due to 2 or more of these organisms.

The mortality rate is higher and treatment more difficult in polymicrobial infection.

Treatment

Combination antibiotic therapy is often necessary in the initial treatment of many immunosuppressed patients. The object is to provide broad-spectrum antibiotic coverage until the organism or organisms causing the infection are identified. For specific doses and drug combinations, consultation with experts in infectious disease is often needed.

If bacterial cultures are negative or if the patient fails to respond to therapy, other possibilities should be considered—eg, fungal or viral infection—and further examination and cultures should be performed.

If the patient responds to treatment, antibiotics should be continued for at least 7 days and preferably for 5 days after fever has subsided. The risk of relapse must be weighed carefully against the increasing chance of superinfection if antibiotics are continued for a long time.

Special Considerations
With Mycobacterial Organisms

A. Mycobacterium tuberculosis: Reactivation of pulmonary tuberculosis and dissemination of disease are problems in immunosuppressed patients treated with large doses of corticosteroids. Tuberculin skin tests and a chest x-ray should be obtained in all of these patients before treatment is started; if results are positive, these patients should receive antituberculosis therapy and regular clinical and x-ray review.

B. Atypical Mycobacterial Infections: Infections of the skin due to atypical mycobacteria have also been reported with increasing frequency. Infections with *Mycobacterium avium* or *Mycobacterium intracellulare* have been noted to be more common in patients with AIDS. Atypical mycobacterial organisms are often resistant to a variety of drugs, including those used for tuberculosis.

FUNGAL INFECTIONS

Fungal infections of the skin and mucous membranes in immunosuppressed or debilitated patients are usually not distinguishable from bacterial infections on the basis of the appearance of lesions. Fungal infections are often even more severe and harder to treat. Fungal superinfections commonly occur in neutropenic patients being treated with broad-spectrum antibiotics and are particularly dangerous in patients receiving bone marrow transplants, in whom they are a common cause of death. Fungal superinfections have played an important role in limiting the success of marrow transplantation.

Fungal infections due to *Candida albicans* are by far the most common, but infections due to *Candida tropicalis* have definitely increased in frequency (Fig 32–2). Other fungi causing infection in immunosuppressed patients include *Aspergillus, Alternaria, Cryptococcus neoformans, Mucor, Rhizopus, Nocardia, Histoplasma capsulatum, Coccidioides immitis, Blastomyces dermatitidis, Sporothrix schenckii, Actinomyces,* and *Trichosporon cutaneum.*

Infection due to *Candida* is characterized by numerous maculopapular or erythematous nodular lesions in the initial phases of septicemia; these are frequently associated with diffuse myalgias. This syndrome typically occurs in hematologic cancers such as leukemia. Florid but benign *Pityrosporum* folliculitis involving the truncal skin may occur, mainly in severely ill patients, and may be mistaken for a

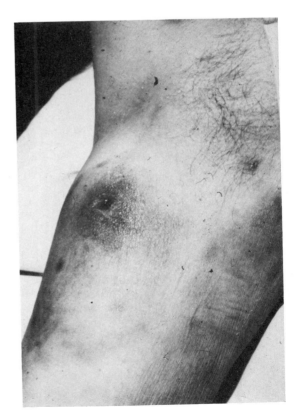

Figure 32–2. Abscess caused by Candida albicans.

systemic yeast infection. The diagnosis of invasive fungal infections of the skin should be based on biopsy specimens demonstrating dermal invasion; ideally, it should be confirmed with positive results on cultures.

Generalized superficial dermatophyte involvement of the skin has been described in immunosuppressed patients, most commonly in patients with exogenous or endogenous Cushing's syndrome. In a few patients, dermatophytes have invaded the skin and caused abscesses and sepsis with bony visceral lesions. Most of these patients have had profound neutropenia.

Blood studies for detection of fungal antibodies are not often helpful for diagnosis because of the patient's immunosuppression and the acuteness and severity of infections and because the immune response eliciting antibodies is blunted. A modified immunodiffusion test has been used for the diagnosis of *Aspergillus* infections. Testing for fungal antigens in blood is more successful, eg, detection of cryptococcal polysaccharide and other fungal antigens through latex agglutination and other methods.

VIRAL INFECTIONS

Although primary virus infections do occur, secondary infections and reactivation of previous viral infections are more common and usually result from cell-mediated immunodeficiency rather than from defects in humoral immunity. The most common and important viral infections seen in immunosuppressed patients include those caused by herpesviruses (cytomegalovirus, herpes simplex virus, varicella-zoster, and Epstein-Barr virus), papovaviruses (wart virus, BK virus), and hepatitis B virus. Multiple virus infections are common.

1. CYTOMEGALOVIRUS

Cytomegalovirus infections are often asymptomatic. Primary infection is associated with more clinical manifestations than is reactivation of previous infection, including a mononucleosis-like syndrome, hepatitis, pneumonitis, arthralgias and myalgias, cutaneous vasculitis, leukopenia, lymphocytosis, and an unusual retinitis. Dermatologic manifestations include maculopapular and purpuric rashes, chronic ulceration, and tumorlike lesions.

Cytomegalovirus also infects many normal people in childhood, especially in economically disadvantaged groups, and the virus is thought to remain latent in the host—as is true also of other members of the herpesvirus group. Flaring of latent cytomegalovirus infection in a patient with systemic lupus erythematosus or other connective tissue disease may be confused with resurgence of the underlying disease. Oc-

casionally, cytomegalovirus infection may produce pustules or papules in immunosuppressed patients or nuclear inclusions in cells observed in skin biopsies.

2. HERPES SIMPLEX VIRUS

Herpes simplex virus is a common cause of severe and persistent mucocutaneous infections in immunocompromised patients. Primary infections are particularly severe, with the development of disseminated herpes simplex virus infection in other organs, especially the central nervous system, liver, and adrenal glands.

Localized recurrent infections around the nose, mouth, and anogenital areas are the most common. Superficial large ulcerated lesions may persist for weeks to months in patients with hematologic malignancies (Fig 32–3), particularly chronic lymphatic leukemia and Hodgkin's disease; the lesions are also common in patients with AIDS or those who have undergone transplant operations. Either herpes simplex virus type 1 or type 2 may be involved, and there may be concurrent infections with bacteria or fungi. Esophageal and respiratory tract infections often occur in patients with orolabial infections.

Inapparent and asymptomatic shedding of herpes simplex virus is also common, and it is important for medical personnel—particularly those handling ventilation and suction equipment—to protect themselves against contact with respiratory secretions.

3. VARICELLA-ZOSTER VIRUS

Varicella (chickenpox) is a highly contagious primary infection usually acquired in childhood, so most

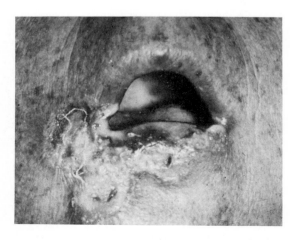

Figure 32–3. Herpes simplex labialis. Note the extensive necrotizing ulcers in this immunosuppressed patient.

adults are immune. Varicella is a potentially serious problem in children with cancer who have not already had the disease. In severely immunocompromised patients, the lesions are extensive and widespread. Many anticancer and immunosuppressing drugs adversely affect the course of varicella-zoster infections by prolonging them or increasing the risk of lethal viremias.

Zoster (shingles) occurs frequently in immunosuppressed patients and can be severe. The incidence of zoster in immunosuppressed patients with Hodgkin's disease is 11–25%. The disease is less common in non-Hodgkin's lymphoma. The risk of zoster is perhaps not increased at all in patients with solid tumors except as a result of chemotherapy and irradiation. Zoster in immunosuppressed patients is generally more severe than in immunocompetent patients but is more apt to be associated with increased morbidity than with increased mortality rates. Extensive dermatomal disease with hemorrhagic and necrotic ulcerations and dissemination of virus in the skin and viscera may occur (Fig 32–4). Postzoster neuralgia occurs more often and is more severe in immunosuppressed than in normal patients. Any dissemination of disease usually occurs within 6–10 days after the onset of lesions. Rarely, untreated zoster persists for several months as chronic ulceration.

Immunosuppressed patients without a history of chickenpox should receive zoster immune globulin (ZIG) within 72 hours after significant exposure, particularly when absence of immunity is confirmed by a negative antibody test. Zoster immune globulin is not effective once lesions have appeared. Treatment with intravenous acyclovir would then be indicated.

4. PAPOVAVIRUSES

Verrucae (warts) are caused by papovaviruses. Multiple verrucae refractory to treatment are particularly common in immunosuppressed patients; eg, in renal transplant cases, 44% of patients have developed warts, and the incidence rises with the length of time after transplantation. Warts are also more common in immunosuppressed patients with Hodgkin's disease and chronic lymphatic leukemia but not in those with multiple myeloma. Warts may improve or resolve in response to primary control of the disease or reduction or termination of immunosuppressive therapy. Rarely, warts can be more than disfiguring and may interfere with normal functioning because of their extent and involvement of the hands and feet (Fig 32–5).

Malignant transformation of warts to squamous cell carcinomas in chronically immunosuppressed patients has also been reported, particularly in skin exposed to sunlight.

The treatment of warts in immunosuppressed patients is difficult, and excessively destructive methods should be avoided since recurrences are common. It is often prudent to remove warts from family members of immunosuppressed patients.

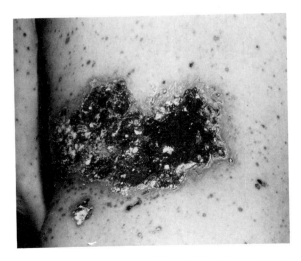

Figure 32–4. Herpes zoster. Not only has the segmental infection become necrotic, but also the virus has disseminated to produce a generalized eruption like chickenpox.

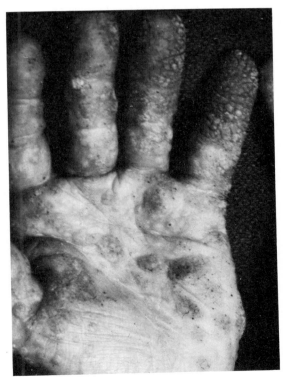

Figure 32–5. Myriad warts in a renal transplant patient.

PARASITIC DISORDERS

Parasitic infections can be atypical and severe in immunosuppressed patients. Norwegian crusted scabies and severe leishmaniasis are of special interest to dermatologists. Pulmonary infections with *Pneumocystis carinii* are common in immunosuppressed patients and have been an important presenting symptom in patients with AIDS. Unusual infections caused by *Strongyloides, Plasmodium,* and *Toxoplasma* have been noted in immunosuppressed patients. Parasitic infection, whether induced by protozoa (malaria and trypanosomiasis) or by helminths (schistosomiasis and filariasis), is characterized not only by direct deleterious effects in the host but also by impairment of the host's immune response to unrelated parasite antigens. Diffuse cutaneous leishmaniasis may in itself produce immunosuppression in which the target appears much narrower, being limited to parasite-specific antigens only. Human schistosomiasis appears to cause a similar kind of immunosuppression wherein the response is limited to a specific parasite antigen.

Repeated episodes of malaria-induced immunosuppression may contribute to the high incidence of bacterial infections in children in the tropics and may also facilitate the development of Burkitt's lymphoma.

ESSENTIALS OF MANAGEMENT

The following principles apply to infection in immunosuppressed patients:

1. Infections are common, resistant to treatment, and prone to recur.

2. Banal-appearing infections may be severe; the usual signs of inflammation may be suppressed or absent.

3. Infections often cause skin lesions that look different from those that occur in immunocompetent persons.

4. Infections are often caused by organisms that are not usual pathogens.

5. Infection is a common cause of death in immunosuppressed patients.

6. Consultation with an expert in infectious disease is often a good idea, because the drugs used and dosages required may be extraordinary, depending upon the infection and the clinical situation.

7. In general, treat early, treat long, and treat hard.

III. GRAFT-VERSUS-HOST DISEASE

Robert W. Goltz, MD

Bone marrow transplantation is being employed with growing frequency in the treatment of patients with primary immunodeficiency disorders, aplastic anemia and osteopetrosis, and especially in the management of lymphoreticular cancer. As the transplanted bone marrow repopulates the marrow of the recipient, cytotoxic cells can damage cells in the skin, liver, and gut to produce graft-versus-host disease. The new immunologically competent cells in the blood actually try to "reject" cells in the recipient organs.

Many bone marrow transplantation patients develop at least some clinical evidence of graft-versus-host disease despite careful prior matching of major histocompatibility loci and lack of reactivity in mixed leukocyte cultures. Skin involvement is usually the earliest and, in mild cases, the only obvious clinical sign of the reaction. Involvement of other epithelial organs, notably the gastrointestinal tract, may produce minor or major problems such as diarrhea. Hepatosplenomegaly and abnormalities of liver function tests are also common.

Graft-versus-host reactions also occur in patients with severe deficiencies of cell-mediated immunity, such as infants with severe combined immunodeficiency disease who receive unirradiated blood transfusions or who engraft with maternal lymphocytes transferred in utero.

ACUTE GRAFT-VERSUS-HOST REACTION

The earliest evidence of the graft-versus-host reaction appears 10–20 days after successful bone marrow implantation. Fever develops, followed in 1 or 2 days by a red maculopapular rash. There is splenomegaly and suprahepatic tenderness. Liver function tests, particularly serum AST (SGOT), alkaline phosphatase, and bilirubin, become abnormal. Diarrhea occurs. If the reaction progresses, liver function declines, high fever occurs, and the diarrhea becomes massive and bloody. Such severe reactions may end in death.

In the skin, mild graft-versus-host rashes resemble a drug eruption or viral exanthem. In more serious cases, the rash becomes bullous and resembles Stevens-Johnson syndrome or, in the most severe cases, toxic epidermal necrolysis. After several weeks, there is desquamation of the affected skin.

The rash may completely disappear or there may be gradual evolution into the chronic form of graft-versus-host disease.

CHRONIC GRAFT-VERSUS-HOST DISEASE

Chronic graft-versus-host disease may evolve directly from the acute form, may appear after months of apparent recovery from acute graft-versus-host disease, or may arise in individuals who have never been recognized to have the acute reaction. Chronic graft-versus-host disease is characterized by a wide variety of changes in the skin. Some patients have developed a lichen planus-like eruption. Depigmentation is common and may mimic vitiligo. There may be hyperpigmentation. Some cases have notable resemblances to skin manifestations of the autoimmune diseases, lupus erythematosus, scleroderma, dermatomyositis and Sjögren's syndrome (Fig 32–6). Ulceration of the skin with secondary infection has led to death. Less severe cases run a chronic course, and patients with moderate graft-versus-host disease eventually recover. The end result of skin involvement is atrophy, hair loss, nail changes, and poikiloderma.

In addition to involvement of the skin in chronic graft-versus-host disease, there may be intermittent elevation of liver enzyme levels and occasional non-bloody diarrhea, usually not as severe as in acute GVH.

DIAGNOSIS

The diagnosis of graft-versus-host reaction in the skin following bone marrow transplantation is made by the characteristic clinical and laboratory findings. Histologic confirmation may be had from biopsies of the skin or other epithelia, including the rectal mucosa. The skin shows characteristic degeneration of keratinocytes, with invasion by lymphocytes that attack the rete cells, producing the characteristic "satellite cell necrosis." Destruction of the basal layer is particularly prominent. In the connective tissue of the dermis or submucosa, there is a sparse infiltrate of mononuclear cells. Corresponding to their clinical appearance, some cases of chronic graft-versus-host

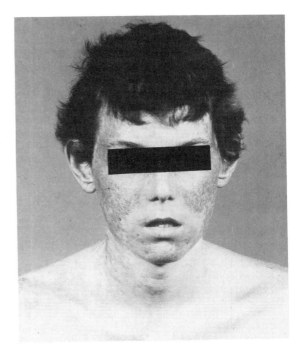

Figure 32–6. Chronic graft-versus-host disease. Scleroderma-like changes and hyperpigmentation.

disease may resemble lichen planus or scleroderma on biopsy.

PREVENTION & TREATMENT

Precise donor selection with exact tissue cross-matching is of paramount importance in prevention of the graft-versus-host reaction. Elimination from the graft material of reactive lymphocytes through prior treatment with specific monoclonal antibody or attenuation with antithymocyte sera gives promise of benefit. Treatment with immunosuppressive and cytotoxic agents, including prednisone and methotrexate, is routine. Monoclonal antibody administration after engraftment and the appearance of graft-versus-host reaction is also being tried. Irradiation of all blood products given before or after bone marrow transplantation is important in prevention or amelioration of the reaction.

REFERENCES

Araviysky AN, Araviysky RA, Eschkov GA: Deep generalized trichophytosis (endothrix in tissues of different origin). Mycopathologia 1975;56:47.

Armstrong D: Infectious complications of neoplastic disease: Their diagnosis and management. Clin Bull 1976; 6:135.

Buckley RH, Wray BB, Belmaker EZ: Extreme hyperimmunoglobulin E and undue susceptibility to infection. Pediatrics 1972;49:59.

Cao M et al: Rapid detection of cutaneous herpes simplex virus infection with the polymerase chain reaction. J Invest Derm 1989;92:391.

Chandra RK: *Primary and Secondary Immunodeficiency Disorders.* Churchill-Livingstone, 1983.

Corey L, Spear PG: Infections with herpes simplex viruses. N Engl J Med 1986;314:749.

Cyclosporine: A new immunosuppressive agent. Med Lett Drugs Ther 1983;25:77.

Dahl MV: Clinical *Immunodermatology,* 2nd ed. Year Book, 1987.

Day NK, Good RH: The complement system in human disease. Page 38 in: *Infections in the Abnormal Host.* Grieco MH (editor). Yorke, 1980.

Farmer ER, Hood A: Graft versus host disease. Pages 28-39 in: *Update: Dermatology in General Medicine.* Fitzpatrick TB et al (editors). McGraw-Hill, 1983.

Gallin JI: Recent advances in chronic granulomatous disease. Ann Intern Med 1983;99:657.

Gigli I: Comprehensive immunology. Chap 4, pp 65–100, in: *Immunodermatology.* Safai B, Good RA (editors). Plenum Pres, 1981.

Gleaves CA et al: Rapid detection of cytomegalovirus in MRC-5 cells inoculated with urine specimens by using low-speed centrifugation and monoclonal antibody to an early antigen. J Clin Microbiol 1984;19:917.

Harper JI: Cutaneous graft versus host disease. Br Med J (Clin Res) 1987;295:401.

Hermans PE, Cockerill FR III: Antiviral agents. Mayo Clin Proc 1983;58:217.

Hermans PE, Keys TF: Antifungal agents used for deep-seated mycotic infections. Mayo Clin Proc 1983;58:223.

Hill HR et al: Recurrent staphylococcal abscesses associated with defective neutrophil chemotaxis and allergic rhinitis. Ann Intern Med 1976;85:39.

Hoofnagle JH et al: Reactivation of chronic hepatitis B-virus infection by cancer chemotherapy. Ann Intern Med 1982;96:447.

Ingelfinger JR et al: Warts in a pediatric renal transplant population. Dermatologica 1977;155:7.

Johnston RB Jr, Baehner RL: Chronic granulomatous disease: Correlation between pathogenesis and clinical findings. Pediatrics 1971;48:730.

Marx JL: Human T-cell leukemia virus linked to AIDS. Science 1983;220:806.

Meunier-Carpentier F, Kiehn TE, Armstrong D: Fungemia in the immunocompromised host: Changing patterns, antigenemia, high mortality. Am J Med 1981;71:363.

Muller SA: Cutaneous infections in immunosuppressed patients. Pages 240–243 in: *Current Dermatologic Therapy.* Maddin S (editor). Saunders, 1982.

Newberger PE, Ezekowitz RAB: Phagocytic defects: II. Cellular and molecular effects of recombinant interferon gamma in chronic granulomatous disease. Hematol Clin North Am (June) 1988, page 267.

Nussenzwieg RS: Parasitic disease as a cause of immunosuppression. (Editorial.) N Engl J Med 1982;306:423.

Quie PG, Cates KL: Clinical syndromes associated with defective polymorphonuclear leukocyte chemotaxis. Am J Pathol 1977;88:711.

Rosen FS: The primary immunodeficiencies: Dermatologic manifestations. J Invest Dermatol 1976;67:457.

Rubin RH: Infection in the renal transplant patient. Pages 553–606 in: *Clinical Approach to Infection in the Compromised Host.* Rubin RH, Young LS (editors). Plenum Press, 1981.

Shulman HM: Chronic graft versus host syndrome in man: A long-term clinicopathologic study of 20 Seattle patients. Am J Med 1980;69:204.

Singer C, Kaplan MH, Armstrong D: Bacteremia and fungemia complicating neoplastic disease: A study of 364 cases. Am J Med 1977;62:731.

Van Scoy RE, Wilkowske CJ: Antituberculous agents: Isoniazid, rifampin, streptomycin, ethambutol, and pyrazinamide. Mayo Clin Proc 1983;58:233.

Vogelsang GB et al: Acute graft versus host disease: Clinical characteristics. Medicine 1988;67:163.

Wiernik PH: The management of infection in the cancer patient. JAMA 1980;244:185.

Wilkowske CJ, Hermans PE: General principles of antimicrobial therapy. Mayo Clin Proc 1983;58:6.

Winston DJ et al: Infectious complications of human bone marrow transplantation. Medicine 1979;58:1.

Wolfson JS, Sober AJ, Rubin RH: Dermatologic manifestations of infection in the compromised host. Annu Rev Med 1983;34:205.

Wood MJ, Geddes AM: Antiviral therapy. Lancet 1987;2:1189.

Youshock E, Glazer SD: Norwegian scabies in a renal transplant patient. JAMA 1981;246:2608.

Section V:
Disorders of Hypersensitivity

Contact Dermatitis

33

Klaus E. Andersen, MD, PhD & Howard I. Maibach, MD

The term "contact dermatitis" denotes an acute or chronic inflammatory skin disorder caused by chemicals or allergens. The terms "contact dermatitis" and "contact eczema" are frequently used interchangeably.

The prevalence of contact dermatitis is variously reported depending on differences in data sampling procedures. Skin diseases make up about one-half of reported occupational diseases in the USA, and contact dermatitis in the USA accounted for 4.3% of all consultations to dermatologists in 1978. In a Danish study of ambulatory care, 7% of the visitors had contact dermatitis. However, dermatologic studies sometimes underestimate the frequency of adverse reactions due to cosmetics, because most problems are solved by the patients themselves, either by discontinuing use of a product or by using other trial-and-error methods.

Dermatitis of the hands is common. Prevalence figures depend on data sampling and diagnostic variations. Surveys based on physical examination underestimate the frequency of occurrence, since dermatitis of the hand is usually episodic, with disease-free intervals of months or years. In an interview study of a stratified sample of 1961 Danish women in 1978, 22% had a history of dermatitis of the hand. The sample was representative of the general population as to age, geographic distribution, and occupational structure.

In certain occupations, the incidence of contact dermatitis is high: for women, wet work (eg, cleaning, nursing, kitchen tasks) provokes eczema; for men, building and metalworking industries constitute the major hazard, partly due to wet work, cement, and metalworking fluids. Both sexes seem equally predisposed to development of contact dermatitis; the difference in incidence in the sexes found in various studies reflects variations in exposure to causative factors.

The clinician should be at pains to distinguish between occupational and nonoccupational contact dermatitis in all patients. Contact dermatitis is a major problem in occupational medicine and has important economic and social implications. The differentiation of occupational and nonoccupational contact dermatitis may be a difficult task requiring clinical assessment and extensive experience.

Contact dermatitis can be classified into 5 types on the basis of etiology: (1) allergic contact dermatitis, (2) acute and cumulative irritant contact dermatitis, (3) contact urticaria, (4) phototoxic contact dermatitis, and (5) photoallergic contact dermatitis. Contact urticaria is characterized by wheals that develop within seconds or minutes after contact. Phototoxic reactions are generally characterized by erythema and pain resembling sunburn in skin exposed to both the contact photosensitizer and sunlight. Bullae may develop also. Clinically, eczematous contact dermatitis can be characterized as acute, subacute, or chronic. In the acute form (Fig 33–1), erythema, edema, oozing, vesicles, bullae, and crusting predominate; in the subacute or chronic forms (Fig 33–2), erythema, scaling, thickening of the skin (lichenification), and fissuring are the main manifestations.

Contact urticaria is discussed later in this chapter and in Chapter 34. Phototoxic and photoallergic contact dermatitis is discussed in Chapter 38.

IRRITANT & ALLERGIC CONTACT DERMATITIS

Essentials of Diagnosis
- Itching, burning, and erythema, often followed by edema, papules, vesicles, and bullae, in exposed areas of contact with an offending chemical irritant or allergen.

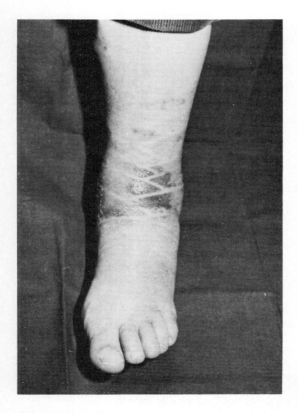

Figure 33–1. Acute vesicular allergic contact dermatitis due to colophony in an adhesive bandage.

- Later, weeping, crusting, scaling, fissuring, excoriations, and secondary infection.
- Asymmetric distribution, except when due to wearing apparel.
- Unusual configurations, such as lines, squares, perfect circles, rectilinear shapes.
- History of domestic, recreational or occupational exposure to possible offending substance; often a history of prior reaction to suspected agent.
- For allergic contact dermatitis, positive patch test results upon challenge with known allergens or suspected agents in standard test tray.

General Considerations

Irritant and allergic contact dermatitis are both eczematous dermatoses caused by chemicals coming in contact with the skin surface. Dermatitis from exposure to irritating chemicals is a result of toxic reactions, whereas dermatitis from exposure to allergens is due to immunologic reactions.

Allergic contact dermatitis is the best-studied and best-understood type of contact dermatitis, though not necessarily the most common. Irritant contact dermatitis, although more common, is an ill-defined disorder that is often a diagnosis of exclusion. In many cases, the distinction between allergy and irritation is uncertain, and both factors influence the clinical course of the disease.

Allergic contact dermatitis may be defined as a T cell-mediated immunologic cutaneous eczematous reaction characterized by a delayed onset (24–96 hours). The skin heals if further contact with the allergen is avoided, but latent hypersensitivity may be permanent and reexposure will usually elicit dermatitis.

Patch Testing

The distinction between allergic and irritant contact dermatitis is usually made by patch testing. The proper performance and interpretation of this bioassay require considerable experience. A small amount of the suspected allergen in a suitable concentration and vehicle is applied to the test site—usually the back—and covered with an occlusive dressing for 48 hours (Figs 33–3 and 33–4). The result is influenced by the skin condition; the concentration and volume of the test substance and the vehicle used; the test site; the duration of test exposure; and the number of readings. If only one reading is planned, the best time to

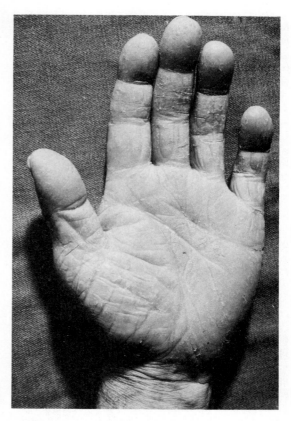

Figure 33–2. Chronic hand dermatitis with scaly, thickened, and fissured skin.

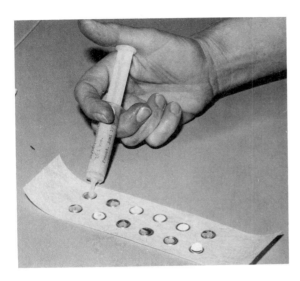

Figure 33–3. Patch tests prepared for application.

check for a reaction is 72 hours after application, but it is better to take readings at 48 hours and again at 96 hours. Because both false-positive and false-negative reactions occur frequently, patch testing is best done by dermatologists, who are also trained to advise patients about allergen substitution, relevance of the test, and prognosis. Patch tests may utilize chemicals (in proper concentrations) with which the patient has been in contact; if the possible allergen is obscure, useful information may be obtained by applying patch tests with a standardized series of the most frequently occurring contact allergens (Table 33–1).

The standard tray of allergens is regularly updated by an international and national group of experts: the International Contact Dermatitis Research Group (ICDRG) and the North American Contact Dermatitis Research Group (NACDRG).

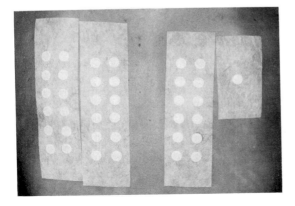

Figure 33–4. Patch tests after application.

The standard patch test series uncovers about 80% of contact sensitivities. In order to diagnose the remaining 20%, supplementary patch testing with other allergens must be done. The choice of allergens for patch testing is crucial and depends on the clinical appearance of the dermatitis, the history of domestic and occupational exposure, and the experience of the dermatologist. Frequently, potential allergens of unknown irritant or allergic capacity must be tested after the concentration and vehicle have been carefully calculated.

The hazards of false-positive and false-negative patch test reactions are obvious. A false-negative result leaves the patient with an undetected contact allergy, whereas a false-positive patch test reaction still poses the problem of interpretation. Correct interpretation can be facilitated by retesting or exaggerated provocative testing. (The supposed allergen is applied to an elbow flexure twice daily for 1 week.)

The range of individual susceptibilities to skin irritation makes it difficult to establish a "correct" recommended concentration for patch testing. To compare patch test results from different investigators, the ICDRG has standardized the terminology used to describe contact dermatitis and the recording patch test results. The use of the following symbols is recommended:

NT	=	Not tested
?+	=	Doubtful reaction
+	=	Weak reaction (nonvesicular, slightly infiltrated or edematous)
++	=	Strong reaction (edematous or vesicular)
+++	=	Extreme reaction (bullous or ulcerative).

The reading of patch test reactions is as important as performance of the test (Fig 33–5). Any reaction must be evaluated with regard to the individual patient. Some reactions may represent immunologic memory from previous attacks of dermatitis. Others cannot be explained.

Major Allergens

Table 33–2 shows the occurrence of positive reactions (in percentages) of all men and women tested in a Danish study of 2166 consecutive eczema patients patch tested with the standard series of the International Contact Dermatitis Research Group (ICDRG).

The allergens in allergic contact dermatitis are conjugates (formed in vivo) between low-molecular-weight substances (haptens) and autologous (carrier) proteins. The substances must penetrate the skin and form covalent bonds with proteins in order to cause a reaction. The ability to induce sensitization is thus related to skin penetrability and reactivity with proteins.

A. Nickel: About 10% of women in industrialized countries are sensitive to nickel; the allergy is much

Table 33–1. Patch test series of 21 substances.

Substance	Number of Tests	Some Sources of Allergens
Metals	3	
Nickel sulfate		Earrings, watchbands
Potassium dichromate		Cement, leather
Cobalt chloride		Combined with nickel and chromate
Mixtures of rubber chemicals	5	Rubber
Topical preparations	6	
Neomycin sulfate		Medicaments
Quinoline mixture		Medicaments
Local anesthetics		Medicaments
Parabens (*p*-hydroxybenzoic acid)		Medicaments, cosmetics
Benzoisothiazides (Kathon CG)		Medicaments, cosmetics
Wool alcohols (lanolin)		Medicaments, cosmetics
Balsams	2	
Peruvian balsam		Perfume, flavorings
Colophony (rosin)		Glues, coatings, cosmetics
Miscellaneous agents	5	
Formaldehyde		Resins, preservatives
Fragrance mixture		Perfumes
p-Phenylenediamine		Hair dyes
Epoxy resin		Uncured epoxy resins
p-Tertiary butylphenol formaldehyde resin		Shoe adhesive

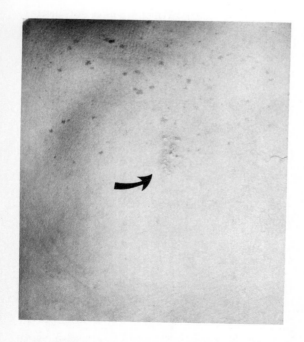

Figure 33–5. Vesicular patch test reaction at 96 hours.

less common in men. Nickel is a shiny stainless metal often used in surface plating of metal objects (eg, buttons, costume jewelry, and kitchen equipment) and as an element in many alloys.

The dimethylglyoxime spot test can be used to detect the release of nickel in significant amounts from an object. The test requires 2 solutions: 10% ammonia water and a 1% alcoholic solution of dimethylglyoxime. The test is performed by applying a few drops of each solution to the object. If a strawberry-red color appears, the object releases nickel in an amount sufficient to affect many nickel-sensitive patients. Those with strong sensitivity to nickel may develop dermatitis from objects containing very small quantities of nickel. People who are highly sensitive to nickel may even experience a flare of dermatitis from unintentional consumption of the metal, which is ubiquitous in foods as a trace element.

Nickel dermatitis often begins where metal objects such as earrings or watchbands are in prolonged contact with the skin (Fig 33–6) and is associated with an increased risk of developing dermatitis of the hand. Nickel allergy may also start with hand dermatitis, which in some cases is a chronic disabling disease

Table 33–2. Positive test results among 2166 patients tested by the Danish Contact Dermatitis Group from September 1985 to February 1986.[1] (International Contact Dermatitis Research Group Standard Series.) The percentages of positive reactions in males and females and in the totals are shown.

Substance[2]	Concentration	Males (n = 696)	Females (n = 1470)	Total (n = 2166)
Potassium dichromate	0.5%	5	3.9	4.3
Paraphenylenediamine	0.5%	0.4	0.2	0.3
Thiuram mixture	1%	2.6	2.2	2.3
Neomycin	20%	3.5	2.7	2.9
Cobalt chloride	1%	1.6	6.1	4.6
Benzocaine	5%	0.9	0.5	0.6
Nickel sulfate	5%	5.1	20.7	15.6
Quinoline mixture	6%	1.9	0.9	1.2
Colophony (rosin)	60%	2.4	4.3	3.7
Parabens	15%	1	0.6	0.7
Black rubber mixture	0.6%	1	0.6	0.7
Wool alcohols	30%	1.9	1.8	1.8
Mercapto mix	2%	1.4	1.1	1.2
Epoxy resin	1%	1.7	0.8	1.1
Balsam of Peru	25%	4	4	4
p-tert-Butylphenol formaldehyde resin	1%	0.7	1.1	1
Carba mixture	3%	4.6	3.5	3.9
Formaldehyde	1%	3.6	3.6	3.6
Fragrance mixture	8%	5.5	6.9	6.4
Ethylene diamine	1%	1.2	1.1	1.1
Quaternium 15	1%	0.1	1.7	1.2
Primin	0.01%	0.1	1.7	1.2

[1]Modified and reproduced, with permission, from Christofferson J et al: Clinical patch test data evaluated by multivariate analysis. Contact Derm 1989;21:291
[2]The vehicle for the allergens was petrolatum except for formaldehyde, which was tested in water.

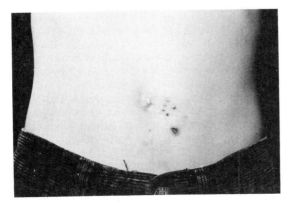

Figure 33–6. Allergic contact dermatitis due to nickel in jeans buttons.

(Fig 33–7). Workers at high risk for development of nickel allergy include hairdressers, restaurant workers, workers in metal industries, nurses, and cashiers.

Patients with nickel dermatitis should avoid nickel-skin contact and protect their hands by using moisturizing creams and polyvinylchloride gloves for wet work. The spot test is useful in identifying nickel-containing objects at home and at work.

B. Chromium: Chromium in the form of chromates is the most common allergen in men with allergic contact dermatitis. Most cases result from occupational exposure. Like nickel, chromates are common in the environment and thus difficult to avoid. The main source of chromate is cement in the building and machining industries. Leather tanned with chromates and made into shoes can cause eczema on the feet of susceptible individuals. Patients

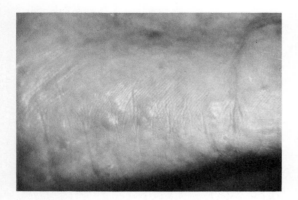

Figure 33–7. Close-up photo of vesicular hand dermatitis (dyshidrotic eczema).

tend to have persistent, often widespread dermatitis that often resembles nummular eczema in its distribution. Marked dryness and lichenification of the skin are often characteristic. Many patients fail to improve even after years of avoidance of contact with chromates. Highly motivated patients continue in their jobs if they can avoid skin contact with chromium-containing substances. Workers with mild to moderate dermatitis are sometimes encouraged to remain at their jobs, because a change in work does not guarantee that the dermatitis will not recur.

A method has recently been developed to reduce the risk of dermatitis in cement workers. The sensitizing chromates in the cement are hexavalent; if ferrous sulfate is added to the cement, these chromates are reduced to trivalent chromates, which are insoluble and therefore less sensitizing. Addition of ferrous sulfate to cement may prove to be a major breakthrough in the prevention of occupational chromate allergy.

C. Rubber: There are many allergenic rubber chemicals; most belong to the group of accelerators and antioxidants used in the vulcanization process, and they may constitute up to 5% of the finished rubber product. Tetramethylthiuram disulfide and 2-mercaptobenzothiazole and thiourea derivatives are also used as disinfectants and preservatives in other industrial processes. A problem in patch testing for rubber sensitivity is the large number of different allergenic chemicals. Cross reactions between chemically related rubber substances are common. Hypersensitivity to rubber may often be suspected from the history of direct contact between eczematous skin and a rubber product.

D. Topical preparations: Approximately one-third of patients with contact allergy in most outpatient dermatology clinics demonstrate positive results on patch tests to active or inactive ingredients in topical drugs or cosmetics. Among the most common sensitizers are lanolin, neomycin, local anesthetics,

formaldehyde, and preservatives such as the parabens (*p*-hydroxybenzoic acid) and benzoisothiazides (Kathon CG). Certain patients are at increased risk for development of topical drug allergy: those with leg ulcers and stasis dermatitis and those with disorders of the anogenital skin. Repeated applications of medications on diseased skin and bandaging or occlusion as occurs in the anogenital area because of underclothing and body folds support the development of sensitization.

When patch tests are performed on patients thought to be allergic to topical preparations, their own skin care products and drugs should be included as patch test materials and properly diluted if the original products are irritating. Note that the concentrations of individual ingredients are not necessarily the most reliable concentrations for patch testing, so that both false-positive and false-negative test results may occur.

Lanolin is derived from sheep fleece and consists of a complex variable mixture of alcohols and acids. Artificial hypoallergenic lanolin derivatives have also been developed. The frequency of lanolin sensitization ranges from 1% to 6% of dermatitis patients tested, depending on group selections and the prescription practices of the physicians.

Neomycin is a widely used antibiotic; about 5–8% of patients with eczema have become sensitive to it, though the risk of allergy is much lower when the antibiotic is applied to simple cuts or surgical wounds. The diagnosis of neomycin allergy may be difficult, because the dermatitis is not vesicular or bullous but often appears instead as an aggravation of a preexisting dermatitis, especially stasis dermatitis.

Among **local anesthetics,** benzocaine (ester group) is the most potent sensitizer, but its use has recently declined. One epidemiologic study from San Francisco in 1979 found that the benzocaine sensitization rate in a group of 1158 volunteers—which appeared representative of the population in the San Francisco Bay area—was far lower (0.15%) than for neomycin (1.1%) and nickel (5.8%). Cross reactions and concurrent reactions to related chemicals often occur, eg, *p*-aminobenzoic acid esters used as sunscreens and various dyes for hair treatment, textiles, and certain eye cosmetics. Local anesthetics of the amide group (eg, lidocaine) are weak sensitizers, so allergic reactions are only sporadically reported.

Formaldehyde is a ubiquitous potent sensitizer used in industry and medicine for its antimicrobial properties. Household products may contain formaldehyde as a preservative. Formaldehyde-releasers used as preservatives in cosmetics and industrial products are often masked by trade names or synonyms, and it is important that the physician recognize these sensitizers when tracing causes of formaldehyde allergy. Unexpected positive patch test reactions frequently occur.

E. Parabens: The most widely used preservatives

are the parabens (esters of *p*-hydroxybenzoic acid) incorporated into foods, drugs, and cosmetics. One-third of the cosmetics registered in the USA contain paraben preservatives. The incidence of paraben sensitization is low in relation to their extensive use. Most sensitized patients have been treated for leg ulcers or stasis dermatitis, and they may often paradoxically tolerate paraben-containing cosmetics on normal facial skin—the so-called "paraben paradox," since hypersensitivity is usually thought to be equally expressed in all body regions. Even in allergy states, dose-response relationships affect skin reactivity: Normal skin tolerates more and is less reactive than eczematous skin.

F. Perfumes and Fragrances: A complete perfume compound may contain 3 to more than 100 basic components, which can be classified as (1) natural products from flowers, plants, roots, herbs, woods, and gums; (2) animal products and their extracts (civet, musk); and (3) synthetic aromatic chemicals. Evaluation of perfume allergy is made more difficult because labeling of perfumes is not required. Many contain components that are identical to or cross-react with materials contained in natural resins (eg, Peruvian balsam) that are included in the standard tray of allergens to pinpoint perfume allergy. Perfume screening trays for patch testing have been developed to increase the sensitivity and specificity of perfume allergy detection. Patients thought to have perfume allergy should also be tested with their own cosmetics and fragrances.

Most patients with perfume allergy are sensitized by use of perfume products, creams, and deodorants. The small amount of fragrances in soaps and detergents rarely sensitizes or causes allergic contact dermatitis in subjects who have been sensitized to perfume.

G. Epoxy Resin: Epoxy resin is just one of the many plastics causing contact allergy. Fortunately for consumers, finished plastic products rarely sensitize, and it is working with the unpolymerized substances that involves the risk of allergic contact dermatitis. Epoxy resin is usually a condensation product of epichlorohydrin and a polyhydroxy compound. Depending on molecular size, the epoxy resin will be liquid or solid. The low-molecular-weight epoxy resins are potent allergens. The resins are cured by the addition of catalysts and hardeners and may be modified for specific applications by the use of softeners, reactive diluents, coloring materials, fillers, and preservatives. Many of these additives are themselves allergens, which makes the evaluation of allergy to plastic a difficult task requiring considerable knowledge and experience.

H. Plants: The manifestations of plant dermatitis vary with its source. Allergic contact dermatitis as well as irritant dermatitis and photodermatitis result from exposure to plants. In the USA, about 50–60% of individuals are sensitive to the allergens in poison oak or poison ivy, common members of the genus *Rhus*. Characteristic features of the plants include triple-lobed leaves with rounded borders and the "black spot" sign: When the sap from a crushed leaf is exposed to air, it turns black within a few minutes. The allergen pentadecylcatechol is present in all parts of the plant, so that not only direct but also indirect contact with plants must be avoided. Indirect contact may occur through clothing, pets, tools, or vehicles that have brushed against the plant. Smoke from burning leaves may also carry the allergen.

The severity of *Rhus* dermatitis depends on the sensitivity of the individual and the amount of allergen deposited on the skin. The dermatitis begins with erythema and swelling, which may be followed by oozing vesicles and bullae. It may be severe enough to require systemic corticosteroids, eg, prednisolone 60 mg daily for 2 weeks. *Rhus* dermatitis is a frequent occupational contact allergy in the USA. The best prophylaxis is to recognize and avoid the plant. If contact does occur, immediate washing of exposed skin and all clothing may prevent dermatitis. Hyposensitization to *Rhus* allergen through oral administration of the allergen is possible, but the results are short-lasting and the procedure is not without side effects. For these reasons it is usually not recommended.

In northern Europe, *Primula* (primrose) dermatitis is common. *Primula obconica*, which has round leaves covered with fine hair, is the usual cause; other species of *Primula* rarely cause dermatitis. The allergen is contained in the fine hairs, and the content varies with the season and the care of the plant. In *Rhus* and *Primula* dermatitis, lesions are often arranged in linear streaks and most often appear on exposed skin.

Irritant Contact Dermatitis

Irritant contact dermatitis is a nonimmunologic local inflammatory reaction following single or repeated exposures to toxic chemicals. Acute irritant dermatitis is elicited by strong irritants after a single application or sometimes a few applications. It is easily diagnosed on the basis of the history, and it often results from occupational accidents. The clinical appearance varies depending on the irritant and ranges from deep red ulcerations to dermatitis indistinguishable from acute allergic contact dermatitis.

Cumulative irritant dermatitis occurs more frequently than acute irritant contact dermatitis. Repeated insults by low-grade irritants occur over a long period. Dryness and cracking of the skin are often the initial signs. Redness, scaling, papules, vesicles, and gradual thickening of the skin may supervene.

The causative factors are complex and usually involve a combination of irritants. The initial dermatitis may be caused by a strong irritant such as a solvent or caustic agent, and the reaction is thereafter sustained by soaps and detergents. An important clinical feature is that the skin all over the body reacts as one organ: An acute irritant dermatitis of the hands lowers the threshold for irritant reactions on the back. This fact must be remembered when patch testing is performed, since false-positive reactions may occur.

Irritant contact dermatitis of the hand frequently starts in moist areas that are difficult to rinse and dry, eg, under rings and in the web spaces. Dermatitis may spread to the dorsum of the hand, where the skin is thinner and less resistant than on the palms.

Irritant contact dermatitis may be long-lasting if it is not treated early. Even when the skin appears to be healed, its protective capacity remains impaired for weeks to months. Furthermore, irritant contact dermatitis may be a precursor to the development of allergic contact dermatitis. Individuals who have had atopic dermatitis in childhood are more likely than other people to develop irritant contact dermatitis of the hand when their jobs involve wet work and dirt.

No objective test exists for diagnosing irritant contact dermatitis. Because of the clinical similarity of allergic and irritant contact dermatitis, it is important that all patients thought to have either disorder undergo patch testing.

Clinical Findings

A. Symptoms and Signs: The clinical appearance of the different types of contact dermatitis varies widely, and differentiation often cannot be achieved on the basis of history and clinical examination alone. Irritant, allergic, and photoallergic contact dermatitis are characterized by varying combinations of eczematous dermatitis, erythema, edema or induration, papules, vesicles or bullae, scaling and fissuring, and excoriations. Patients may complain of itching, burning, or pain. Rubbing and scratching frequently lead to development of secondary superficial infections with staphylococci and streptococci.

Contact urticaria is characterized by wheals that develop within seconds or minutes after contact. Phototoxic reactions are generally characterized by erythema and pain resembling sunburn in skin exposed to both the contact photosensitizer and sunlight. Bullae may develop also.

A meticulous history of the patient's daily activities and environmental exposure is required. Contact dermatitis usually first appears where there is direct contact with the allergen or irritant. In patients with widespread dermatitis, the area of onset may provide a clue to the causative agent or provide clues for further history taking. A history of previous similar dermatitis may provide important information; eg, earring dermatitis often precedes nickel dermatitis of the hands by several years. Previous dermatitis may have been complicated by allergy to topical drugs containing sensitizers the patient is now using again.

Examine the skin surface of the entire body, since the location of the lesions (sun-exposed areas, symmetric versus asymmetric distribution, etc) may point to the possible allergens, irritants, and differential diagnoses (eg, dermatophytosis, psoriasis). The morphology of the lesions may clarify the cause; eg, strong allergens such as poison oak and poison ivy may provoke a linear bullous eruption in the distribution of the original contact, whereas less potent allergens in contact with various parts of the skin cause a random pattern of distribution. For a short while after exposure, allergens may be spread to other body regions by the fingers without causing dermatitis of the hand.

B. Laboratory Findings: The histologic picture is similar for all forms of eczematous contact dermatitis: spongiotic edema, acanthosis, and parakeratosis. Vasodilatation, edema, and perivascular mononuclear cell infiltration are seen in the dermis.

Differential Diagnosis

Differential diagnosis depends on the history and the type and site of the dermatitis. Other skin disorders may be complicated by secondary sensitization to topical drugs or occupational contactants. Seborrheic dermatitis of the head and skin folds may mimic contact dermatitis. Psoriasis in the external ear or on the palms may be mistaken for contact dermatitis. Dermatophytosis of the feet may provoke vesicular dermatitis of the hand as an id reaction, and unilateral mycotic infection of the palm may resemble keratotic hand dermatitis.

Other differential diagnoses include atopic dermatitis, nummular eczema, dyshidrotic eruptions, lichen planus, polymorphic light eruptions, porphyria cutanea tarda, dermatomyositis, drug eruptions, or scabies.

Complications

Secondary bacterial or yeast infections may occur and delay healing of contact dermatitis unless the infection is treated appropriately. Depending on individual susceptibility, dermatitis may heal with hyperpigmentation or hypopigmentation that often lasts for several months.

Patients with strong sensitivity to an allergen may develop eczematous reactions when exposed to a sufficiently high concentration of the allergen by routes other than the skin. Ingestion of the allergen may cause flaring of eczema, flare of patch tests, dyshidrotic dermatitis of the hand, generalized rash, fever, and malaise. Nickel, chromate, mercury, ampicillin, and Peruvian balsam have caused systemic contact allergy.

Prevention

The best prevention is achieved in industries where physicians specializing in occupational medicine are available. Allergens in both occupational and home environments must be considered.

Allergens should be supplanted by other substances when possible—eg, phenylenediamine derivatives in hair dyes or in rubber tool handles can be replaced by other less sensitizing materials. New chemicals should be assessed for their allergenic potential before they are put into widespread use. Protective clothing and disposable gloves should be worn to reduce contact with allergens that cannot be replaced with nonallergenic substitutes. Protective devices themselves may introduce a new allergic hazard in the form of rubber in gloves, solvents in skin cleansers, etc. Automation of industrial processes may also reduce exposure of skin to potential allergens or irritants, just as dishwashing machines have diminished contact with detergents in the home.

Barrier creams are of little or no use. Neatness and cleanliness in the workplace are essential to reduce contact with potential allergens. Clean washbasins and showers should be available.

Workers must be taught to use protective clothing and to follow manufacturers' instructions. Workers should be trained to properly remove potentially hazardous substances from the skin. Paper towels, hand creams, and cleansing creams should be close at hand.

Preemployment patch testing with substances used in the occupation is without value, since a negative result does not assess the risk of future sensitization. Atopic individuals should be advised of the risk inherent in jobs with exposure to water or dirt, since repeated exposure to weak irritants imposes an increased chance of development of dermatitis. However, many atopic patients hold such jobs and suffer no ill effects.

Treatment

Treatment of acute mild to moderate exudative dermatitis consists of compresses with cool water applied for 20–30 minutes 3 times daily. Burow's solution (aluminum acetate 1:20) and potassium permanganate solution (1:16,000 to 1:4000) are astringents and germicides suitable for wet dressings, soaks, or baths. Soothing shake lotions (eg, calamine) may be used. After oozing subsides, a topical corticosteroid cream or lotion helps to reduce itching. In severe cases, systemic corticosteroids are indicated, eg, prednisolone, 40–60 mg/d tapered over a 2- to 3-week period before withdrawal. Causative allergens may cause reactions for 2–3 weeks, so patch testing should be postponed until the dermatitis has cleared and treatment with corticosteroids has been discontinued.

Chronic (nonexudative) contact dermatitis is treated with topical corticosteroids; the strength of the preparation depends on the site of the dermatitis. In the groin, low-potency hydrocortisone preparations are indicated, whereas volar hand dermatitis requires high-potency fluorinated corticosteroids applied once or twice daily. More frequent applications are not more efficient, since tolerance (tachyphylaxis) quickly develops. To avoid side effects, the patient should be instructed to apply the cream or ointment sparingly and only on involved skin. When bacterial superinfection complicates contact dermatitis, systemic antibiotics are indicated, eg, erythromycin or a semisynthetic penicillin.

The patient must be instructed to avoid irritants and to lubricate the skin with an adequately greasy, nonsensitizing, cosmetically acceptable emollient. These measures are important for both prevention and treatment and are particularly important for patients with hand dermatitis. Printed instruction sheets may prove helpful.

After patch testing, the patient should be carefully informed of alternatives to allergenic substances and irritants and provided with the exact chemical name of the allergen.

Prognosis

The prognosis for contact dermatitis depends on the cause and the possibility of avoiding reexposure. Individual factors are also important, eg, atopy, motivation, and information. Allergic contact dermatitis from easily avoidable allergens usually heals in a few weeks.

Chromium and nickel dermatitis of the hand are chronic and may last for decades. It is questionable whether a change in occupation influences the prognosis for chronic hand dermatitis. The return of a patient to the site of employment has high priority when a patient has had to stay away from work.

CONTACT URTICARIA

Contact urticaria is an immediate wheal-and-flare reaction to certain external agents. A single exposure is generally sufficient to elicit the reaction in susceptible individuals. The frequency of occurrence of this phenomenon is unknown. Patients may complain of immediate urticarial reactions to external substances and thereby make the diagnosis; but noncharacteristic itching, burning, erythema, and recurrent dermatitis are more frequent. Whether contact urticaria causes eczema or not is unproved.

Contact urticaria may be divided into 3 major groups based on the pathogenetic mechanisms: (1) nonimmunologic contact urticaria is caused by chemical compounds that release histamine and other mediators to the skin without involving immunologic processes; (2) the immunologic type is caused by immediate hypersensitivity; and (3) the third group caused by an unknown mechanism contains chemicals for which both allergic and nonallergic mechanisms can be found. Differentiation of the subtypes may be difficult: Immediate readings of skin tests (15–20 minutes) are the main diagnostic tools. Properly diluted suspected agents are applied to normal or diseased skin and left either exposed or occluded. The reactions are often seen only on diseased skin; variations in manifestations in different body regions may be impressive.

Proteinaceous material from animals, foods, and plants as well as low-molecular-weight chemicals (eg, benzoic acid used as a food preservative or cinnamic aldehyde used in fragrances) may elicit contact urticaria.

PHOTOTOXIC & PHOTOALLERGIC CONTACT DERMATITIS

Phototoxic and photoallergic contact dermatitis are counterparts to irritant and allergic contact dermatitis. A chemical on the skin is "activated" by sunlight to become an allergen or to promote erythema. Long-wave ultraviolet light (UVA; 320–400 nm) usually constitutes the action spectrum for both types of reactions; middle-wave ultraviolet light (UVB; 290–320 nm) may potentiate the effect. Phototoxic reactions are more common than photoallergic ones; they are based on a nonimmunologic mechanism and are similar to an exaggerated sunburn, whereas photoallergic reactions are uncommon and have a varied presentation that usually includes itching and extension beyond the site exposed to ultraviolet light.

Expression of photoallergic responses requires a state of acquired altered reactivity involving an antigen-antibody reaction. When evaluating patients thought to have photosensitivity related to a contactant, physicians should establish the action spectrum and reproduce the lesion on nonexposed skin by applying the chemical and exposing the area to ultraviolet radiation (photopatch test). The distinction between phototoxicity and photoallergy is often difficult to make. Many phototoxic reactions are caused by the

Table 33–3. Some photoxic and photoallergic topical substances.

Phototoxic
Coal tar derivatives
Drugs
  Phenothiazines
  Sulfonamides
Dyes
  Anthraquinone
Plant derivatives
  Bergamot oil (bergapten, 5-methoxypsoralen)
  Xanthotoxin (8-methoxypsoralen)
Sunscreens
Photoallergic
Antifungal agents
  Fentichlor
  Jadit
Fragrances
  Musk ambrette
Drugs
  Phenothiazines
  Sulfonamides
Halogenated salicylanilides
Sunscreens

same compounds that occasionally produce photoallergic reactions in sensitized individuals. Table 33–3 lists the most common phototoxic and photoallergic agents. 5-Methoxypsoralen (bergamot oil, bergapten) and 8-methoxypsoralen (xanthotoxin) are derivatives of naturally occurring furocoumarins in plants and essential oils. Phenothiazines and sulfonamides administered to patients constitute a potential occupational hazard for hospital personnel, who may become sensitized. The halogenated salicylanilides once widely used as bacteriostatic substances in toilet soap and cosmetics now rarely cause photoallergy.

REFERENCES

Adams RM: *Occupational Skin Diseases*. Grune & Stratton, 1989.
Adams RM: Patch testing: A recapitulation. J Am Acad Dermatol 1989;5:637.
Adams RM, Maibach HI: A five-year study of cosmetic reactions. J Am Acad Dermatol 1985;13:1062.
Christophersen J et al: Clinical patch test data evaluated by multivariate analysis. Contact Derm 1989;21:291.
Cronin E: *Contact Dermatitis*. Churchill Livingstone, 1980.
Epstein E: Hand dermatitis: Practical management and current concepts. J Am Acad Dermatol 1984;10:395.
Fisher AA: *Contact Dermatitis,* 3rd ed. Lea & Febiger, 1986.
Foussereau J, Benezra C, Maibach HI: *Occupational Contact Dermatitis*. Saunders, 1982.
Fregert S: *Manual of Contact Dermatitis*. Year Book, 1981.
Marzulli FN, Maibach HI (editors): *Dermatotoxicology,* 2nd ed. Hemisphere, 1983.
Menné T, Borgan O, Green A: Nickel allergy and hand dermatitis in a stratified sample of the Danish female population: An epidemiological study including a statis-

tical appendix. Acta Derm Venereol 1982;62:35.
Menné T, Christophersen J: Epidemiology of allergic contact sensitization. Curr Probl Dermatol 1985;14:1.
Menné T, Hjorth N: Reactions from systemic exposure to contact allergens. Semin Dermatol 1982;1:15.
Mitchell J, Rook A: *Botanical Dermatology*. Greengrass, 1979.
Nater JP, deGroot AC: *Unwanted Effects of Cosmetics and Drugs Used in Dermatology,* 2nd ed. Elsevier, 1985.
Prystowsky SD et al: Allergic contact hypersensitivity to nickel, neomycin, ethylenediamine and benzocaine: Relationships between age, sex, history of exposure, and reactivity to standard patch tests and use tests in a general population. Arch Dermatol 1979;115:959.
von Krogh G, Maibach HI: The contact urticaria syndrome. Semin Dermatol 1982;1:59.
Wilkinson DS et al: Terminology of contact dermatitis. Acta Derm Venereol 1970;50:287.
Wilkinson JD, Rycroft RJG: Contact dermatitis. Chap 14, pp 435–532, in: *Textbook of Dermatology,* 4th ed. Rook A et al (editors). Blackwell, 1966.

Urticaria & Anaphylaxis

34

Harold B. Kaiser, MD

ANAPHYLAXIS

Essentials of Diagnosis

- Laryngeal edema or bronchospasm (or both).
- Erythema, pruritus, urticaria, or angioedema (any or all).
- Vomiting, cramps, diarrhea.
- Hypotension, cardiac arrhythmias, or shock.

General Considerations

Anaphylaxis is an immediate and potentially life-threatening hypersensitivity reaction, usually mediated by IgE antibody, occurring within seconds to hours after exposure to some foreign material to which the patient has been previously sensitized. It is a generalized reaction involving several organ systems occurring with dramatic suddenness. *Any physician or other health professional who prescribes or administers parenteral or oral medications should be prepared to deal with anaphylaxis emergencies.*

Anaphylactic reactions (anaphylaxis) are the result of the release of chemical mediators secondary to an immunologic (antigen-antibody) reaction. **Anaphylactoid reactions** are clinically similar reactions that involve the nonimmunologic (non-antigen-antibody) release of similar mediators. The evidence is not strong that allergic individuals are more susceptible to anaphylactoid reactions.

Human anaphylaxis is usually mediated through antigen-specific IgE antibodies bound to basophils and tissue mast cells. When a specific antigen combines with specific cell-bound IgE, chemical mediators are released. These include histamine, eosinophilic chemotactic factor of anaphylaxis (ECF-A), leukotrienes, platelet-aggregating factor (PAF), kallikreins, kinins, neutrophil chemotactic factor of anaphylaxis (NCF-A), and others. These mediators bind to specific receptors on smooth muscle and blood vessels and induce vascular permeability, smooth muscle contraction, vessel dilatation, and mucous gland secretions, leading to the clinical symptoms of anaphylaxis.

Anaphylactoid reactions occur as a result of release of the same chemical mediators as in anaphylaxis, but the pathways do not involve antigen-antibody reactions. The exact mechanisms are not known, but some anaphylactoid reactions may be due to direct mediator release and activation of complement through the alternative pathway. Reactions to radiographic contrast media, aspirin, and local anesthetics are examples of common anaphylactoid reactions.

In a review of pathologic findings in 100 deaths from anaphylactic reactions to insect stings, the primary pathologic finding was in the respiratory tract of 69 cases, the vascular system of 12, and the neurologic system of 7. Anaphylactic shock accounted for 12 deaths. Most respiratory deaths showed edema or secretions of the pharynx, epiglottis, larynx, trachea, and bronchi.

Causative Agents

Any list of agents with potential to cause anaphylaxis would be incomplete. The most common causes in clinical practice (in order of frequency) are as follows:

A. Drugs: Penicillin and synthetic penicillins are the most frequent pharmacologic causes of anaphylaxis. The incidence of cephalosporin sensitivity is 4 times higher in penicillin-sensitive patients than in the general population. Other drugs often reported to cause anaphylaxis are sulfonamides, insulin, aspirin, and almost anything else.

B. Foods: Among the most common foods causing anaphylaxis are fish, shellfish, nuts, seeds, legumes (eg, peanuts, beans), milk, eggs, and citrus fruits.

C. Vaccines and Antisera: Some of these are derived from hyperimmunized animals such as horses and may contain foreign serum proteins to which the patient may be sensitive. They are used in treatment of diphtheria, rabies, and snakebite. Antilymphocytic serum used in transplantation surgery is also derived from horses. Egg-based embryo vaccines such as measles, mumps, flu, yellow fever, and rabies vaccines can induce anaphylaxis in egg-sensitive patients.

D. Hymenoptera Insects: Bees, hornets, wasps, and yellow jackets cause anaphylactic reactions in a small percentage of patients. Nonhymenoptera insects such as fire ants and deerflies may also cause anaphylaxis.

E. Allergy Injections: Anaphylaxis may occur from injections used in immunotherapy of allergic rhinitis, asthma, or stinging insect sensitivity. In very sensitive patients, even skin testing may cause anaphylaxis.

F. Other Causes: Iodinated contrast media, aspirin, and local anesthetics such as procaine are common causes of anaphylactoid reactions.

Clinical Findings

A. Symptoms and Signs: The clinical symptoms may involve the skin, the respiratory tract, the gastrointestinal tract, and the cardiovascular and neurologic systems. Respiratory distress resulting from edema of the upper airway or bronchospasm is the usual cause of death in fatal anaphylaxis, and may occur within seconds or minutes after exposure.

Advanced signs of anaphylaxis are easily recognized; early ones may be subtle and confusing. Awareness of the possibility is the first step in recognition. Even mild atypical symptoms may quickly progress and become severe, even life-threatening. The physician should be especially alert to the patient who "doesn't feel quite right," has itching of the face or the back of the throat, fright, nausea, cough, or loss of voice (from laryngeal edema). Frequently the patient has an ominous feeling of impending doom. Treatment of anaphylaxis must be prompt and vigorous even though early symptoms may be mild.

Signs, symptoms may be classified by system.

1. Skin– Erythema, pruritus, urticaria, angioedema.

2. Respiratory system– Upper airway edema including laryngeal edema, lower airway bronchospasm.

3. Gastrointestinal system– Vomiting, cramps, diarrhea, which may be bloody.

4. Cardiovascular system– Hypotension, arrhythmia, shock.

5. Neurosensory apparatus– Agitation, confusion, convulsions, coma.

B. Laboratory Findings: Because the reaction occurs so suddenly, the laboratory is of little help. Skin testing to identify patients at special risk is discussed below.

Prevention

The best treatment for anaphylactic or anaphylactoid reactions is prevention. Any patient being treated with drugs or vaccines should be asked about prior reactions to medications, especially penicillin, and egg allergy (for egg-based vaccines). Be wary of potent immunogens, including penicillin, enzymes (trypsin and chymotrypsin), horse serum and other foreign serum, and allergens for management of allergic disorders.

Anaphylaxis is often mediated by reaginic (IgE)

antibodies; skin tests have some predictive value in certain cases. Skin testing in the sensitive patient may be dangerous and should be done with very dilute solutions. The inexperienced physician should seek consultation before proceeding with skin testing. Radioallergosorbent (RAST) tests may provide information about whether the patient is sensitive to a foreign substance such as medication or food. RAST tests have the advantage of no patient risk; the disadvantages are that few laboratories are able to perform the tests, the unavailability of tests for certain agents, the possibility of false-negative test results, and delay in obtaining results.

Treatment

A. Equipment Needed: An emergency anaphylaxis kit should be readily available wherever drugs are given parenterally. A minimal kit should include syringes and needles, epinephrine 1:1000, diphenhydramine for intravenous use, an airway, a tourniquet, and a scalpel. Also desirable are oxygen, saline intravenous solution, a blood pressure cuff, vasopressor medication such as metaraminol or dopamine, corticosteroids for intravenous administration, a laryngoscope, an endotracheal airway, and a tracheostomy set. Aminophylline for intravenous injection may be helpful for patients who have acute bronchospasm without shock. The emergency equipment should be handy; physicians should rehearse the treatment of anaphylaxis in advance.

B. Procedure: (See Table 34–1.) *Call for help and start treatment immediately!*

Check the patient's airway and treat adults with epinephrine, 0.3–0.5 mL of 1:1000 aqueous solution intramuscularly as soon as anaphylaxis is recognized. The dose for children is 0.01 mg/kg. Severe reactions may be treated by slow intravenous injection of epinephrine in 10 mL of saline. If anaphylaxis has been caused by an injection, inject epinephrine into the site to provide local vasoconstriction and slow down absorption. A tourniquet should be placed proximal to the injection site. The epinephrine dose may be repeated at 15-minute intervals as needed. Diphenhydramine, 50 mg intravenously, intramuscularly, or orally, may also be given. If the patient is in respiratory distress, oxygen should be administered by mask or nasal catheter and an intravenous line with saline established. Tracheostomy may be required in cases of severe laryngeal edema. Endotracheal intubation may assist ventilation in cases of severe bronchospasm. The patient should be monitored for vascular shock. Corticosteroids are not helpful in acute anaphylaxis but may have a role in prevention of protracted anaphylaxis. Hydrocortisone intravenously or its equivalent in a dose of 100 or 200 mg every 4–6 hours for the first day is suggested for severe anaphylaxis. H_2 antihistamines such as cimetidine, 300 mg intravenously, are also useful in some cases of refractory anaphylaxis.

Table 34–1. Treatment of anaphylaxis.

1. Treatment should be started immediately. Summon help. Emergency phone numbers should be prominently displayed.
2. Check vital functions: airway, blood pressure, and circulation.
3. Establish a clear airway. If respirations have stopped, start artificial respiration (mouth-to-mouth or endotracheal).
4. Epinephrine (1 : 1000 aqueous solution), 0.3–0.5 mL SC (for adults) is the drug of first choice. The dose for children is 0.01 mg/kg. Give at the site of injection if appropriate. The dose may be repeated every 15 minutes as needed. If cardiovascular collapse and shock are present, the initial dose for adults may be 0.1 mg (0.1 mL) of 1 : 1000 dilution mixed into 10 mL of saline (resulting in a final dilution of 1 : 100,000) by IV infusion over a 5- to 10-minute period. The patient must be closely monitored for arrhythmias and severe fluctuations of blood pressure.
5. Apply a venous occlusion tourniquet proximal to the injection site (in appropriate cases).
6. Give diphenhydramine, 50 mg IV (10–25 mg IV for children) if the response to epinephrine is not rapid and sustained.
7. Give cimetidine, 300 mg IV, if the response to diphenhydramine is not rapid.
8. Give oxygen by nasal catheter or mask. A patent airway must be maintained.
9. Establish a continuous intravenous infusion of normal saline.
10. Monitor vital signs.
11. Treat hypotension as one would in other situations: Recumbent position, IV fluids, metaraminol, dopamine. Administer saline, albumin, or plasma until the central venous pressure is 15 cm H_2O. Treat acidosis.
12. If laryngeal or severe unremitting bronchospasm stridor is present, consider endotracheal tube or tracheotomy.
13. If wheezing has not responded to epinephrine, give aminophylline IV (6 mg/kg diluted in 10–25 mL of saline and infused over 10–15 minutes). Corticosteroids are not helpful in the acute situation when symptoms are prolonged but may prevent later recurrence of anaphylaxis. Administer 100–200 mg hydrocortisone or equivalent every 4–6 hours.
14. Patients with severe anaphylaxis should be hospitalized and observed overnight because symptoms sometimes recur hours later.

There is often acute loss of plasma volume, which may be primarily responsible for shock. Rapid infusion of normal saline may be helpful, but infusion of plasma or albumin intravenously is more effective. A vasopressor agent may also be necessary. Patients with anaphylactic reactions not fully responding to these measures require hospitalization, monitoring, and intensive care.

Prognosis

Anaphylaxis is rarely fatal, but deaths do occur. It is estimated that there are 500 deaths a year in the USA from anaphylactic reactions to penicillin.

Although sensitivity may disappear spontaneously over time, the patient who has had one anaphylactic reaction to a known substance should be considered at risk if he or she were to be exposed again. Emergency kits containing a syringe preloaded with epineph-rine—or an EpiPen Auto-Injector (a self-injecting epinephrine-filled syringe)—should be prescribed for such patients.

URTICARIA & ANGIOEDEMA

Essentials of Diagnosis

- Wheals: pink papules sometimes with pale centers, without epidermal changes.
- Evanescent: individual wheals disappear within 24 hours and often within minutes.
- Changing configuration: wheals enlarge rapidly and may appear annular or arcuate.

General Considerations

Urticaria and angioedema are common clinical problems that can be baffling and difficult for both the patient and physician. Chemical mediators affecting small vessels include histamine, kinins, serotonin, acetylcholine, prostaglandins, and others. Histamine produces itching and vascular permeability and is a major mediator of urticaria. The histamine wheal and flare reaction is the prototype of urticaria.

The pathogenic mechanisms may be immunologic or nonimmunologic. The most common allergic reaction causing urticaria is a type I (immediate hypersensitivity) reaction mediated by IgE. Other immunologic mechanisms may involve activation of the classic complement pathway, producing anaphylatoxins that in turn can release histamine and other permeability mediators. Nonimmunologic mechanisms include activation of the alternative complement pathway and direct release of histamine from basophils or tissue mast cells by drugs or chemicals. Other factors that may cause mediator release include fever, heat, cold, sunlight, exercise, and emotional stress.

Urticaria is common. About 25% of the population have had at least one attack of hives. Acute urticaria (persisting less than 3 months) is generally self-limited and can be controlled with antihistamines. It may be possible to identify the inciting agent by careful history.

Chronic urticaria (persisting three months or longer) may persist for years, and the cause may never be found. Some authors claim that an etiologic agent can be found in 50% of cases, while others think the cause remains obscure in over 90%. Whether or not one can arrive at a specific etiologic diagnosis, it is possible to treat most patients with chronic urticaria successfully.

Wheals are due to vasodilation and leakage of plasma into tissue.

Allergic & Metabolic Causes of Urticaria & Angioedema (Table 34–2)

A. Drugs: Common pharmacologic causes include penicillin, sulfonamides, aspirin, and diuretics. Ur-

Table 34–2. Causes of urticaria and angioedema.

Drugs
Foods
Inhalants
Infections
Noninfectious diseases
Neoplasms
Insect bites
Physical agents and dermographism
Hereditary conditions
Excessive sensitivity to endogenous acetylcholine
Vasculitis
Contactants
Psychogenic factors
Idiopathic

ticarial reactions after drug administration may occur within minutes but may be delayed for days or weeks. A thorough drug history and substitution with chemically unrelated drugs of suspected agents is central to the urticaria work-up. Ask specifically about vitamins, laxatives, aspirin, other pain pills, birth control pills, or diet pills that patients may not consider to be "drugs."

B. Foods: The offending food can often be identified by history if the reaction occurs immediately or shortly after the food is eaten; however, sometimes urticaria may not appear for hours or even days after ingestion. The most common offenders in adults are fish and shellfish, berries, eggs, nuts and peanuts, pork products, chocolate, and cola drinks. In infants, milk and milk products, eggs, wheat, and citrus fruits are common etiologic agents. Sensitivity to food additives may be a cause. About 15% of aspirin-sensitive patients are sensitive to the food coloring agent tartrazine (Yellow Dye No. 5). Certain foods, including berries, citrus fruits, and shellfish, may also act as direct histamine liberators in some patients.

The diagnosis of food allergy is best made by history. It is generally easy for the patient to identify a food that causes acute urticaria. Allergy skin testing in acute urticaria may help identify cases of food allergy mediated through IgE when the patient cannot. Skin testing is seldom helpful in the diagnosis of chronic urticaria due to food allergy. A food diary and a trial elimination diet will be more helpful here.

C. Inhalants: Pollens, molds, animal danders, organic dusts, and other air-borne substances that can cause respiratory symptoms such as allergic rhinitis and asthma will occasionally cause acute or chronic urticaria. Urticaria usually occurs during exposure concurrently with the respiratory symptoms. Avoidance is the proper treatment.

D. Infections: Parasitic infections are common causes of urticaria in tropical climates. Viral infections frequently cause acute urticaria, primarily in children. Some viruses activate the classic or alternative complement pathway to produce anaphylatoxins

and subsequent release of histamine and other mediators that cause the urticarial reaction. Infectious mononucleosis and hepatitis are sometimes associated with urticaria. Bacterial infections are rarely reported as causal agents, but occasional cases of chronic urticaria improve when bacterial infection is treated.

E. Noninfectious Disease: Many systemic diseases are sometimes associated with urticaria, including rheumatic and collagen diseases such as lupus erythematosus and polyarteritis. Hyperthyroidism and hypoparathyroidism have been associated with urticaria. Urticaria occurs also in some patients at menses, suggesting an endocrine relationship.

Urticaria and angioedema may occur in serum sickness, symptoms and signs of which are fever, malaise, arthralgias, joint swelling, lymphadenopathy, splenomegaly, and erythematous skin rashes. Serum sickness should be considered when urticaria or these other symptoms and signs occur 3 days to 3 weeks after injection or injections of a foreign protein or drug.

F. Neoplasms: Urticaria in association with neoplastic disease is unusual but has been reported in patients with lymphoma, carcinoma of the lung and colon, and other tumors.

G. Insect Bites: Some patients—especially children and fair-haired adults—develop papular urticaria in reaction to insect bites (eg, fleas, mites, mosquitoes). These are local toxic reactions. Of more significance is the patient who develops generalized urticaria or angioedema after a sting from a hymenopteran insect. These reactions in sensitive patients can be life-threatening, requiring emergency treatment for anaphylaxis, as discussed above. Patients who have had a severe generalized reaction to a stinging insect should be evaluated and carefully skin-tested with pure hymenoptera venoms for possible future hyposensitization. These sensitive patients should carry an emergency kit containing a pre-filled syringe of epinephrine when they are at risk of being stung.

Physical Causes of Urticaria

Cold, heat, sunlight, pressure, and even water may cause urticaria in some patients.

A. Dermographism: This is sometimes called "write-on-skin," because writing on the skin with a pointed object results in a few minutes in linear wheal and flare reactions along the pressure lines that may persist for 30 minutes or more. Dermographism results from increased wheal and flare reactions after mechanical stroking. It is a form of chronic urticaria, perhaps hereditary, which may persist for life. Acquired dermographism usually resolves within a year or two. Antihistamines, especially hydroxyzine, sometimes help.

B. Cold Urticaria: Cold urticaria is characterized by pruritus, hives, and swelling after exposure to cold. Lesions are confined to body parts in contact with the cold. For example, a patient outside on a cold, windy day may have erythema and urticaria limited to the face and hands. The diagnosis can be confirmed by placing an ice cube on the patient's arm for 2 minutes and observing the area for another 15 minutes. In the patient with cold urticaria, the area develops a large wheal at the site of contact. Warn the patient to avoid cold water, since deaths have been reported after diving into it. Treatment with cyproheptadine (Periactin), 4 mg 3 or 4 times a day, often increases tolerance to cold and provides significant clinical relief. Patients with cold urticaria are usually more comfortable living in a warm climate.

C. Solar Urticaria: Solar urticaria is an uncommon condition in which exposure to sunlight leads to the development of urticaria on exposed skin within a few minutes. There are 6 types of solar urticaria depending on the wavelength of light producing the condition. Prevention is the best treatment. Patients should remain indoors or cover exposed body areas with clothing or sunscreens before going out. Pretreatment with antihistamines or corticosteroids sometimes helps if this is impossible.

D. Aquagenic Urticaria: Patients uncommonly develop hives after contact with water regardless of its temperature. This condition can be tested directly by applying water to the skin. Treatment with antihistamines may be helpful.

E. Pressure Urticaria: Typically, the patient develops lesions a few hours after application of pressure in the beltline, where shoes are tied, under bra straps, or under elastic stockings. Lesions may be painful. Dermographism (immediate whealing of the skin after stroking) may or may not be present. Prolonged pressure is necessary, and whealing is delayed. Systemic corticosteroids have been used with success. Antihistamines are usually *not* effective.

F. Cholinergic Urticaria: Cholinergic urticaria is also called **heat-and-effort urticaria.** The characteristic small punctate lesions surrounded by erythematous flares are precipitated by stress, extreme heat, hot showers, exercise, and sweating. The disorder is due to excessive vascular response to acetylcholine liberated by autonomic nerves in the skin. Characteristic lesions can be reproduced by skin testing with methacholine (Mecholyl), and the condition often responds to systemic antihistamines—especially hydroxyzine—and sometimes to anticholinergic agents.

Hereditary Causes of Urticaria & Angioedema

There are several rare inherited forms of urticaria and angioedema.

A. Familial Cold Urticaria: This form is inherited as an autosomal dominant. Histologically, it is not true urticaria but edema with an intense inflammatory infiltrate.

B. Hereditary Vibratory Angioedema: Angioedema and intense itching are induced after vibratory stimulation such as a jack-hammer. Systemic antihistamines seem partially effective; these patients should be advised to avoid vibratory stimuli.

C. Other Forms: Another familial form of urticaria is seen in combination with **amyloidosis, nerve deafness,** and **limb pain.** It appears to be inherited as an autosomal dominant.

D. Hereditary Angioedema: This hereditary autosomal dominant disorder results from absence or nonfunctional inhibitor (C1INH) to the first complement component. The condition is characterized by spontaneous episodic attacks of nonpruritic angioedema of the skin and mucosa of the upper respiratory and gastrointestinal tracts. This angioedema is not usually associated with urticaria. The diagnosis is suggested by a positive family history and the presence of respiratory and gastrointestinal symptoms along with the angioedema. The most severe complication is laryngeal edema, which may be fatal. Severe attacks of abdominal pain and gastrointestinal bleeding may occur.

The serum levels of the complement substrates C4 and C2 are diminished. Serum C4 is the simplest screening test to diagnose this condition. C2 is usually normal when the patient is asymptomatic, but the serum level of C4 is diminished even when the patient is asymptomatic. If hereditary angioedema is suspected and a diminished C4 concentration is found, direct quantitative assay of serum C1INH can be performed. In 15% of cases, the C1INH is present but not functional, and so a functional or biologic assay may be required to confirm the diagnosis. A similar nonhereditary syndrome associated with low levels of C1INH is associated with lymphoreticular malignancies.

Androgenic agents such as stanozolol taken on a regular prophylactic basis reduce the frequency of attacks, and increase the concentration of C1INH and also C4. Initially, stanozolol, 2 mg daily orally, is recommended; if the patients have no attacks for 2 months or longer, the dose is gradually reduced to 1–2 mg every other day. Androgenic side effects have been a problem but are rare at this low dose. Patients with ongoing cutaneous, respiratory, or gastrointestinal attacks of hereditary angioedema may require long-term stanozolol therapy.

There are other rare hereditary complement system disorders sometimes associated with urticaria. These are usually isolated case reports of urticaria in association with a complement deficiency or abnormality, requiring a laboratory capable of determining individual complement components.

Urticarial Vasculitis

Some patients with chronic urticaria have a form of necrotizing vasculitis. The association of vasculitis and urticaria, differential diagnosis, and other considerations are discussed in Chapter 37.

Contact Urticaria

Contact of the skin with a substance to which the patient is reactive can elicit an immediate or delayed—for 1 or 2 days after contact—localized urticarial reaction. Numerous substances have been incriminated, including animal danders, wool, egg white, other foods, pollen and plants, drugs, and chemicals. Immunologic and nonimmunologic mechanisms may be responsible, depending on the patient and the contactant. Avoidance is the best treatment.

Psychogenic Causes

There is extensive literature on the role of psychologic factors in the etiology of chronic urticaria, which like other chronic diseases can be aggravated by emotional stress. In some cases, emotional factors are primary causes of urticaria. Placebo treatment may benefit some patients. The patient with chronic urticaria and significant emotional turmoil should have these factors evaluated and treated as part of total management.

Idiopathic Causes

All too often, the cause of chronic urticaria remains unknown even after extensive history taking, physical examination, laboratory studies, and environmental manipulations.

Clinical Findings

A. Symptoms and Signs: The classic abnormality is a large or small transient pink wheal. The epidermis over the wheal is normal. Lesions blanch completely with pressure and vary from a few millimeters to several centimeters in diameter. Annular wheals are not uncommon. Wheals are typically red and itchy, and individual lesions last less than 24 hours. Pruritus may be severe. Pruritus and erythema may in some cases precede wheal formation.

Hives may occur anywhere on the body but are more common in pressure areas such as the beltline or thighs and in dependent parts such as the buttocks.

Angioedema is similar in clinical presentation, but the lesions are larger and deeper (involving the subcutaneous tissues). Urticaria and angioedema often coexist, but either can occur without the other.

B. Laboratory Findings: Some patients have peripheral blood eosinophilia. The diagnosis of urticaria is a clinical one. The laboratory helps to confirm the clinical diagnosis and uncover occult causes (see below).

The major pathologic finding in urticaria is edema, intradermal in urticaria and subcutaneous in angioedema. Urticaria is associated with vasodilation and increased permeability of the small blood vessels, especially the venules in the dermis, which result in flattened rete pegs, widened dermal papillae, and separation of collagen bundles and fibers in the superficial dermis. Angioedema is similar but is located in the deeper dermis and subcutaneous tissues.

Differential Diagnosis

Other dermatologic conditions sometimes confused with urticaria include allergic contact dermatitis, erythema multiforme, multiple insect bites, bullous pemphigoid, pruritic urticarial papules and plaques of pregnancy, pityriasis rosea, scabies, and urticarial vasculitis. The specific differentiation can often be made by history and physical examination, but biopsy may be useful if the diagnosis is in doubt.

Angioedema may be confused with other types of local swelling, including local infection, cellulitis, lymphedema, Melkersson-Rosenthal syndrome, or even the superior vena cava syndrome.

Approach to the Patient With Chronic Urticaria

Since the diagnosis has often been established before the patient visits the physician and since the cause in many cases is readily apparent from the history, the common dilemma is how far to go in working up a patient with chronic urticaria of unknown cause, keeping in mind that even after sophisticated evaluation, the cause remains obscure in over three-fourths of cases.

The following guidelines are appropriate for evaluation of patients who have had episodes of urticaria daily for 3 months or more.

A. Initial Workup: First, do a complete history—unhurried and probing—and physical examination both to confirm the diagnosis and to look for underlying disease. Screening laboratory tests to eliminate the possibility of systemic disease including a complete blood count and urinalysis, blood chemistry profile, fluorescent antinuclear antibody test, and chest x-ray. Further evaluation might include tests for infectious mononucleosis and hepatitis, complement levels, stool studies for ova and parasites, heat and cold challenge tests, other specific x-rays, and skin biopsy.

B. Diet and Drug Survey: Dietary manipulation may be based on a food diary kept by the patient and elimination of specific suspected foods or commonly allergenic foods. Later, provocative food challenges can confirm the allergy. All medications should be discontinued—especially aspirin and aspirin-containing compounds. Chemically dissimilar drugs can be substituted if needed. A clinical decision must be made if the patient requires a suspected medication for other reasons (eg, propranolol for hypertension).

C. Skin Tests: Allergy skin tests are rarely helpful in determining the cause of urticaria except in stinging insect allergy; they should be reserved for patients in whom inhalant allergy or food allergy is suspected but in whom dietary manipulation has not been conclusive. Skin testing may sometimes help confirm acute urticaria due to food allergy, because these allergies are often mediated through IgE. Skin testing may help in proving penicillin allergy; if suspected, skin tests should be done with penicillin G major and minor determinants. Minor determinants are available only on a research basis. Skin tests risk anaphylactic reactions in extremely sensitive patients. Radioallergosorbent (RAST) tests are rarely of diagnostic value.

Treatment

The best treatment is elimination or avoidance of the causative agent. Since this is not always possible, drugs are needed to control urticaria. Drug treatment of urticaria is usually effective even if the cause is unknown.

Epinephrine by injection is the treatment of choice for severe acute urticaria, especially if signs or symptoms of anaphylaxis are present. An injection of 0.3 mL of 1:1000 aqueous epinephrine subcutaneously usually relieves itching, quiets the lesions, and provides temporary symptomatic relief. Epinephrine should be followed by administration of oral antihistamines on a regular basis day and night.

Antihistamines are the mainstay of urticaria treatment. They work by blocking histamine receptors on target cells and are competitive inhibitors of histamine. Diphenhydramine (Benadryl), 25–50 mg every 4 hours, and hydroxyzine (Atarax, Vistaril), 10–50 mg every 4 hours, are among the most effective antihistamines used in the treatment of urticaria. The new nonsedating antihistamines such as terfenadine (Seldane), 60 mg twice daily, and astemizole (Hismanal), 10–20 mg once daily, are also effective in many cases of urticaria and have the advantage of not making the patient tired. Cyproheptadine (Periactin), 4 mg every 4 hours, has antiserotonin and antihistamine properties and sometimes helps, usually when given in combination with other antihistamines such as hydroxyzine. Cyproheptadine is specifically used to treat cold urticaria. H_2 antihistamines such as cimetidine and doxepin may be used adjunctively if combined with conventional (H_1) antihistamines. Some patients with chronic urticaria not responding to H_1 antihistamines have done well when H_2 antihistamines were added. Oral sympathomimetics such as ephedrine are especially helpful in angioedema. Systemic corticosteroids such as prednisone may be necessary to control urticaria not responding to other therapy. Corticosteroids have significant side-effects when used on a long-term basis and should be reserved for selected patients with chronic urticaria not responsive to conventional treatment.

REFERENCES

Austen KF: Systemic anaphylaxis in the human being. N Engl J Med 1974;291:661.

Barnard JH: Studies of 400 Hymenoptera sting deaths in the United States. J Allergy Clin Immunol 1973;52:259.

Beall GN: Urticaria: A review of laboratory and clinical observations. Medicine 1964;43:131.

Burdick AE, Mathias CGJ: The contact urticaria syndrome. Dermatol Clin 1985;3:71.

Champion RH, Greaves MW, Kobla-Black A: *The Urticarias.* Churchill Livingstone, 1985.

Green GR, Koelsche GA, Kierland RR: Etiology and pathogenesis of chronic urticaria. Ann Allergy 1965;23: 30.

Harvey RP, Wegs J, Schocket AL: A controlled trial of therapy in chronic urticaria. J Allergy Clin Immunol 1981;68:262.

Jorizzo JL, Smith EB: The physical urticarias: An update and review. Arch Dermatol 1982;118:194.

Kaiser HB, Weisberg SC, Morris RJ: Cimetidine in chronic urticaria. (Letter.) Lancet 1980;2:206.

Keahy TM: The pathogenesis of urticaria. Dermatol Clin 1985;3:13.

Kohler PF: The University of Colorado chronic urticaria study. N Engl Reg Allergy Proc 1981;2:136.

Mathews KP: Management of urticaria and angioedema. J Allergy Clin Immunol 1980;66:347.

Sullivan TJ: Pharmacologic modulation of the whealing response to histamine in human skin: Identification of doxepin as a potent in vivo inhibitor. J Allergy Clin Immunol 1982;69:260.

Wasserman SI, Marquardt DL: Anaphylaxis. Pages 1365–1376 in: *Allergy Principles and Practice,* 3rd ed. Middleton E Jr et al (editors). Mosby, 1988.

Weiszer I: Allergic emergencies. Pages 374–394 in: *Allergic Diseases,* 2nd ed. Patterson R (editor). Lippincott, 1980.

Reactive Erythemas*

Mark V. Dahl, MD

A group of disorders called "reactive erythemas" or "vascular reactions" are generally characterized by pink or red wheals, papules, plaques, or nodules without alteration of the epidermis. The epidermal skin markings characteristically traverse the lesions without any disruption.

The reactive erythemas are listed in Table 35–1. Differentiation is important because different causes result in different reactive erythemas, and the treatment of choice in all cases is to eliminate the cause.

ERYTHEMA MULTIFORME

Essentials of Diagnosis

- Annular erythematous plaques, urticarial papules, or target lesions (annular plaques with central erythematous papules).
- Preservation of epidermal skin markings.
- Tendency to involve the extensor forearms, legs, palms, and soles.
- A severe clinical variant, Stevens-Johnson syndrome: erythema multiforme (often bullous), involvement of mucous membranes, fever, headache, and malaise.

General Considerations

Erythema multiforme is a reactive erythema characterized by nodular wheals and targetlike plaques, especially on acral areas including the palms and soles.

Stevens-Johnson syndrome is a serious variant associated with fever and ulcers of the mucous membranes. Its occurrence is a dermatologic emergency and may cause death due to fluid and electrolyte imbalance. When the tracheobronchial tree is affected, there is risk of death from asphyxiation. Involvement of the conjunctiva can cause blindness.

Erythema multiforme is a spectrum of reactive erythemas due to drugs, chemicals, physical agents,

*The most common reactive erythema is urticaria. It is discussed in Chapter 34.

Table 35–1. The reactive erythemas.

Urticaria (see Chapter 34)
Erythema multiforme
Toxic epidermal necrolysis
Acute graft-versus-host reaction (see Chapter 32)
Erythema annulare centrifugum
Erythema marginatum
Erythema chronicum migrans
Erythema gyratum repens
Erythema nodosum
Erythema dyschromicum perstans
Urticarial vasculitis (see Chapter 37)
Fixed drug eruption (see Chapter 36)
Erythema toxicum neonatorum
Exanthem of juvenile rheumatoid arthritis
Behçet's disease
Relapsing polychondritis

foods, or a variety of internal diseases. Often no cause is found. The eruption lasts days to weeks to years depending upon the cause. Recurrences are common, especially when the disorder has been caused by herpes simplex infection. Although erythema multiforme can occur at any age, the median age at onset is 25 years. Stevens-Johnson syndrome more often affects children.

Clinical Findings

A. Symptoms and Signs: The eruption often begins suddenly with the appearance of erythematous papules affecting any area of the body but particularly the arms, legs, palms, and soles. Pruritus may be mild or even absent. Lesions enlarge slowly and resolve centrally. After a period of time, a new crop of papules may develop, oftentimes starting in the cleared center of a previous lesion. This produces the distinctive iris "target lesion" (Fig 35–1). Coalescence may generate arcuate or serpentine plaques.

The color of plaques varies; they may be pink, red, white, or violet. In the bullous variant, bullae usually occur in the center of plaques (Fig 35–2) but may appear at the margin. Erosions and hemorrhagic crusts occur when bullae break. In the mouth and on other mucous membranes, crusts and ulcers can be found in lieu of bullae. In another variant (dermal

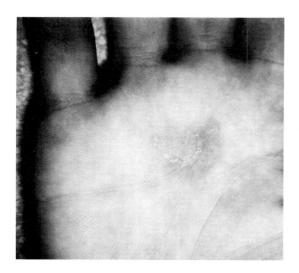

Figure 35–1. Erythema multiforme. Target lesions on the palms are frequently present.

nodular allergid), only hard, somewhat fixed dermal papules are present.

Constitutional signs such as fever, headache, and malaise are usually not present unless the eruption is severe, eg, in Stevens-Johnson syndrome.

B. Laboratory Findings: Laboratory tests are usually normal. Leukocytosis and elevated erythrocyte sedimentation rates are occasionally found. If the disorder is precipitated by an infection or other systemic disease, laboratory tests may reflect the underlying cause or organ involvement. Immune complexes have been found in the serum of patients during the acute phase, and macrophage aggregation factor may also be present.

Biopsy is helpful, especially to distinguish erythema multiforme from annular variants of urticaria. In early erythema multiforme, there is intense edema of the papillary dermis, so that the connective tissue spans across the most superficial parts of the papillary dermis in gossamerlike threads. The epidermis may show widespread necrosis or individual necrotic keratinocytes. There is a perivascular infiltrate of mononuclear cells. In other patients the necrosis is more marked, progressing to confluent basal cell necrosis and subepidermal blister formation. Acute inflammation around superficial dermal blood vessels may be associated with leukocytoclasis.

Examination of tissue from early lesions by direct immunofluorescence may demonstrate IgM, IgG, C3, or fibrinogen in these blood vessels. Herpesvirus antigens have been found in vessels, and herpesvirus DNA has been found in skin lesions using the polymerase chain reaction when herpes simplex was the cause. IgM and C3 are frequently deposited in a granular pattern at the dermal-epidermal junction, but di-

rect immunofluorescence testing is usually reserved for research purposes or to distinguish the bullous form from other bullous diseases.

Differential Diagnosis

Initially, the urticarial papules resemble urticaria or insect bites. Involvement of the palms and soles may suggest secondary syphilis, Rocky Mountain spotted fever, or atypical measles. However, erythema multiforme is rarely purpuric. As lesions become annular, the differential diagnosis includes annular urticaria, erythema annulare centrifigum, granuloma annulare, and tinea corporis, but the course of rapidly enlarging lesions usually rules out the last 2; besides, tinea corporis is a scaling disease and erythema multiforme is not.

Target lesions are nearly pathognomonic. Bullous erythema multiforme can mimic other subepidermal blistering diseases such as dermatitis herpetiformis, bullous pemphigoid, herpes gestationis, and linear IgA bullous dermatosis, and it merges clinically and histologically with toxic epidermal necrolysis. Histologic examination and direct immunofluorescence testing help to sort these out. Mouth lesions are not characteristic.

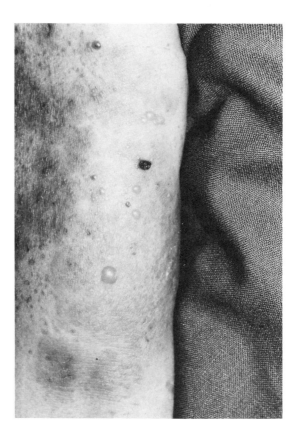

Figure 35–2. Erythema multiforme bullosum. Tense bullae arise from erythematous plaques.

Complications & Sequelae

Erythema multiforme usually resolves without scarring. Hyperpigmentation may mark the sites of lesions for some time but eventually fades. The Stevens-Johnson syndrome, however, is associated with marked morbidity. Involvement of the oral mucosa may interfere with eating, while involvement of the palpebral conjunctiva may result in photophobia and temporary or permanent loss of vision. Blindness may occur either acutely from vesicles on the cornea or later as a result of adhesions, symblepharon, ectropion, or decreased lacrimation. Involvement of the tracheobronchial tree can cause respiratory distress or may even result in asphyxiation. Scars of the urethra can result in stenosis. Other sequelae include acute glomerulonephritis, acute tubular necrosis, renal failure, myocardial arrhythmias, congestive heart failure, gastrointestinal bleeding, seizures, and coma.

Treatment

It is of first importance to identify and remove the cause (see Table 35–2). When the cause cannot be found, treatment is mostly symptomatic and suppressive. No treatment may be required in mild cases. Antihistamines are not effective.

In severely afflicted patients, systemic corticosteroids have been used. Doses in excess of 40–60 mg of prednisone are often necessary. The use of systemic corticosteroids in patients with Stevens-Johnson syndrome is controversial. If used, the dosage should be equivalent to prednisone, 1–2 mg/kg, and given for only a short period because these drugs may increase the risk of complications if given for longer periods.

Erosions may be treated with intermittent or continuous wet compresses. Patients with extensive erosions should be treated as for extensive third-degree burn.

Intravenous fluids and electrolyte replacement may be necessary, particularly when oral involvement makes feeding difficult. Treatment of mouth lesions with a topical anesthetic agent such as viscous lidocaine may provide symptomatic relief during eating. Application of petrolatum or other ointments to eroded and crusted lips often helps reduce cracking and avulsion of dry crusts. Involvement of the eye indicates a need for ophthalmologic consultation and careful lid hygiene. Systemic or local antibiotics may be necessary.

Prognosis

The eruption usually clears when the cause is removed. If the cause is a drug and that drug is readministered later, the eruption may recur. If the eruption is caused by herpes simplex, then recurrent bouts of herpes simplex may result in recurrence of erythema multiforme.

The prognosis for patients with Stevens-Johnson

Table 35–2. Some causes of erythema multiforme.

Idiopathic
Drugs
  Antipyrine
  Aspirin
  Barbiturates
  Bromides
  Chlorpropamide
  Diuretics
  Penicillin
  Phenolphthalein
  Phenylbutazone
  Phenytoin
  Quinine
  Sulfonamides
  Other
Chemicals
  9-Bromofluorene
  Others
Infections
  Adenovirus
  Coccidioidomycosis
  Coxsackievirus B5
  Echoviruses
  Herpes simplex and herpes zoster
  Histoplasmosis
  Influenza type A
  Lymphogranuloma venereum
  Milker's nodules
  Mumps
  Mycobacteria
  Mycoplasma
  Orf (ecthyma infectiosum)
  Poliomyelitis
  Pseudomonas infection
  Salmonellosis
  Staphylococcal infections
  Streptococcal infections
  Syphilis
  Trichomoniasis
  Vaccinia
  Others
Physical agents
  Sunlight
  Cold
  Therapeutic radiation
Pregnancy
Foods
  Beer hops
  Shellfish
  Other
Lupus erythematosus
Polyarteritis nodosa
Cancer
Others

syndrome is guarded. Death due to asphyxia, sepsis, or electrolyte imbalance may occur in up to 10% of severe cases. If the patient survives, major sequelae relate to scarring of the conjunctiva or other mucous membranes.

TOXIC EPIDERMAL NECROLYSIS (Drug-Induced Scalded Skin Syndrome)

Essentials of Diagnosis

• Tender skin.

- Red, scalded appearance of skin.
- Often a recent history of drug ingestion.
- Subepidermal separation of skin.
- Features of erythema multiforme major (Stevens-Johnson syndrome): stomatitis, blotchy eruption with target lesions.

General Considerations

Toxic epidermal necrolysis is a rare, serious disorder occurring mostly in adults and older children. It is a severe form of erythema multiforme major (Stevens-Johnson syndrome; Fig 35–3). The skin separates at the dermal-epidermal junction, so that the peeled skin contains all epidermal layers and the exposed raw surface is dermis.

The disorder is conceded to be a reactive erythema. Many drugs have been implicated as causes, but hazardous provocative testing is the only reliable means of showing that a given drug is responsible. This testing is not recommended. Even if done, a suspected drug may not precipitate a new attack if it has been longer than 4 months since the patient first used the drug. An additional factor may be required to trigger the reaction, eg, some inherent aspect of the infection or illness for which the drug was being used. The drugs that cause toxic epidermal necrolysis most frequently include sulfonamides (especially the long-acting preparations), barbiturates, penicillin, analgesics, anti-inflammatory agents, antirheumatics, and antiepileptics. It is difficult to obtain precise information about the relationship between the dosage of a drug and the incidence of drug-induced scalded skin syndrome; eg, phenylbutazone is frequently associated with adverse dermatologic side effects, yet many physicians regularly prescribe it for various indications and never encounter drug-induced scalded skin syndrome. The rarity of the disease and the un-predictable results of using the suspected causative agent after an attack make it difficult to know how to advise patients; the disease is a distinct though remote possibility with the use of almost all drugs.

Drugs are not the only cause, and many drugs have been falsely incriminated when in fact infection is responsible. Often a prodrome of malaise may prompt empirical drug treatment, which then is blamed as causal when toxic epidermal necrolysis appears. In some cases no cause can be found, especially in elderly women, who may be subject to repeated attacks.

Clinical Findings

A. Symptoms and Signs: A sore throat or pain on swallowing may be the first sign of impending toxic epidermal necrolysis. Malaise follows and is succeeded by a widespread blotchy eruption that becomes confluent and looks scalded in the most severely affected areas. The scalded areas may be more prominent than the blotchy eruption or may replace it altogether. Severe conjunctivitis and stomatitis are typical, and balanitis or vulvitis frequently occurs. The esophagus, trachea, and bronchi may be affected, with risk of consequent bronchopneumonia, and patients may cough up necrotic bronchial tissue. The extensive areas of raw skin are quite painful and constitute a site for the potentially lethal hazards of dehydration, electrolyte imbalance, and multiplication of bacteria. In severe disease, the hair, eyelashes, and nails are shed. Ocular involvement is common and important, because partial loss of vision or blindness may result. Renal involvement has been reported.

B. Laboratory Findings: Biopsy is recommended to confirm the diagnosis and distinguish it with certainty from staphylococcal scalded skin syndrome.

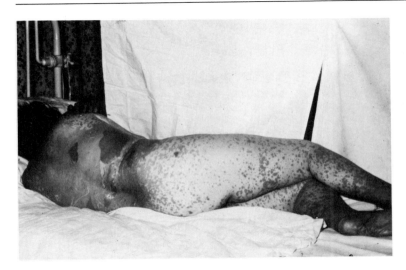

Figure 35–3. Toxic epidermal necrolysis. (Reproduced with permission from Lyell A: Toxic epidermal necrolysis: The scalded skin syndrome. J Cont Educ Dermatol 1978; 17:15.)

Shed skin consists of the entire thickness of the epidermis; cytologic microscopic examination of cells on the red, raw areas fails to reveal significant numbers of epidermal cells.

Differential Diagnosis

The distinction between toxic epidermal necrolysis and staphylococcal scalded skin syndrome is particularly important because the treatments and prognosis are so different. If physical examination is equivocal, microscopic examination of a skin biopsy or of shed skin will reveal the characteristic cleavage pattern of the epidermis. Apart from thermal burns, other causes of "scalding" must be considered, including skin contact with gasoline, kerosene, or ethylene oxide; or poisoning with carbon monoxide, barbiturates, or boric acid. Features resembling those of toxic epidermal necrolysis are present rarely in unstable psoriasis and can be distinguished by their characteristic histopathologic appearance. Toxic epidermal necrolysis is also a feature of severe acute graft-versus-host disease.

Complications & Sequelae

Corneal scarring, blindness, adhesion of the eyelids to the bulbar conjunctiva, permanent alopecia, onycholysis, and pigmentary disturbances have been reported. Eruptions of pigmented nevi may occasionally develop in affected skin after it heals.

Treatment

Treatment of severe epidermal epidermolysis represents a major challenge for both medical and nursing staff. If the patient survives the first 2 weeks, recovery is likely. The chief goals of treatment are to keep the patient as comfortable as possible, to control fluid and electrolyte balance, to discourage bacterial growth on the skin that might lead to sepsis, and to safeguard the eyes.

Hospitalization in a unit equipped to treat severe thermal burns is often desirable. A turning frame, net suspension bed, or water bed contributes to the patient's comfort by distributing weight and therefore pressure more evenly on the skin. Fluid and electrolyte metabolism should be monitored as in patients with severe burns. Topical treatment is the same as for generalized third-degree thermal burns. Many new topical regimens are being used. Topical antibiotics such as sulfadiazine or mafenide are useful but may delay epithelialization or cause leukopenia. These should *not* be used in patients allergic to sulfonamides, especially if a sulfonamide drug caused the toxic epidermal necrolysis.

Ophthalmologic consultation should be obtained early. Adhesion of the eyelids may be prevented by application of sterile petrolatum or ophthalmic ointments to the edges, and mydriatics are often instilled. Oral hygiene is particularly important to prevent acute parotitis. Because septicemia is a constant threat, it is best to avoid *intravenous* administration of drugs or other substances, if feasible. A nasogastric tube should be used as long as practicable. Antibiotics should be reserved for treatment of serious complicating infections. Prophylactic use of antibiotics is controversial.

The value of systemic corticosteroids is uncertain; they are often used but have been said to encourage bacterial toxemia. Some practitioners believe them to be lifesaving. If corticosteroids are used, they should be given in high doses for a short period rather than indefinitely at low dosages. Corticosteroids cannot be expected to save skin that has died or separated.

Heparin has been recommended if disseminated intravascular coagulation develops. Postural drainage is required for the chest, and antibiotics are necessary if bronchopneumonia develops.

Prognosis

The mortality rate from toxic epidermal necrolysis is about 25%. Death occurs from electrolyte disturbance, bacterial toxemia, or septicemia. Good nursing care is a key to survival. Eye damage may cause blindness or other visual impairments. Possible etiologic drugs should not be used again, even though it is unclear whether they would precipitate a second attack.

ERYTHEMA ANNULARE CENTRIFUGUM

Essentials of Diagnosis

- Annular erythematous plaques that enlarge centrifugally 1–3 mm daily.
- Collarette scaling on the inner edge of the red rings.
- The central cleared area may be hyperpigmented, especially near the red edge.
- Confluence of lesions or resolution of part of the circle may result in arcuate, serpiginous, or hook-like lesions.

General Considerations

Erythema annulare centrifugum is a reactive erythema with characteristic expanding ring-shaped plaques. Like erythema multiforme, this reactive erythema is characterized by annular lesions, but these lesions enlarge slowly and usually occur on the trunk. Causes include cutaneous dermatophyte infections elsewhere, cutaneous and internal infection with *Candida albicans,* ingestion of blue cheese, carcinomas, parasitic disease of the bowel, and autoimmune syndromes. Pruritus is absent. Most patients are young adults, but the disorder may occur at any time from infancy to old age and may last for years. Both sexes are affected.

Clinical Findings

A. Symptoms and Signs: The eruption begins with one to many erythematous papules without much overlying epidermal change. These enlarge while clearing centrally, so that lesions become annular erythematous plaques. The central edge of the plaque may develop an overhanging scale, pointing inward like the collar of a shirt. Complete resolution of part of an annular plaque leads to artful figured designs, crescents, and hooks. Coalescence of plaques may cause serpentine artistic patterns (Fig 35–4). Hyperpigmentation may occur centrally as a sequela of inflammation. In slowly enlarging lesions, this brown color appears more intense near the active edge than centripetal to it. Lesions can occur on almost any body site but most often on the trunk, thighs, and buttocks. The palms, soles, mucous membranes, and head are usually spared.

B. Laboratory Findings: Fungus is not present in scale as determined by KOH preparation or culture but may be present on the foot or elsewhere and actually cause the reactive erythema.

Histopathologic examination of biopsy material demonstrates an intense lymphocytic infiltrate hugging the blood vessels in the superficial dermis, giving the appearance of a "coat sleeve" around the vessels. The epidermis is usually normal except for slight hyperkeratosis.

Differential Diagnosis

Usual considerations are erythema multiforme, annular urticaria, tinea corporis, pityriasis rosea, erythema gyratum repens, erythema chronicum migrans, granuloma annulare, annular lupus erythematosus, and leprosy. Of these, tinea corporis can be ruled out by KOH examination and culture of scale. Erythema multiforme usually affects the palms, soles, and acral areas of the body, and lesions are small and may form targets. Annular urticaria is fleeting because individual lesions last less than 2 days. Pityriasis rosea characteristically has more scale and is pinker. Individual lesions of pityriasis rosea are smaller and oval and line up in a Christmas tree-like configuration on the back. Erythema chronicum migrans—typically a single lesion centered around a tick bite—could cause confusion when secondary lesions are present. Differentiation from granuloma annulare, subacute cutaneous lupus erythematosus, sarcoidosis, and leprosy is by biopsy. Most patients with annular lupus erythematosus have antibody to Ro(SSA) antigen in their sera. Erythema gyratum repens presents with more widespread swirling, pruritic lesions over the entire body, often with edema of the eyelids. Female carriers of chronic granulomatous disease may have annular erythematous plaques associated with abnormal neutrophil killing function as detected by chemiluminescence. History of an afflicted male child helps in such cases.

Complications & Sequelae

Lesions may resolve with some transient hyperpigmentation that fades slowly over months.

Treatment

If the cause is known, it should be eliminated, eg, by treatment of dermatophyte infection with topical or systemic antifungal drugs. Erythema annulare centrifugum caused by yeast infections has cleared following treatment with oral and vaginal nystatin.

Course & Prognosis

The disorder may be short-lived or persist for decades, probably depending upon the cause.

ERYTHEMA MARGINATUM

Essentials of Diagnosis

- Evanescent, rapidly changing, annular, erythematous patches or plaques.
- Confluence produces a reticulate or polycyclic pattern resembling chicken wire.
- Lesions are especially prone to appear on the trunk but may occur on the extremities. The face and hands are usually not affected.
- Crops of new lesions may recur for many weeks.
- Patients usually have signs of active rheumatic fever, including carditis, arthritis, fever, subcutaneous nodules, or chorea.

General Considerations

Erythema marginatum is a reactive erythema associated with rheumatic fever. With the decline of acute rheumatic fever, the disorder is becoming uncommon.

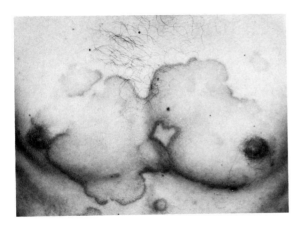

Figure 35–4. Erythema annulare centrifugum. Serpentine erythematous plaques with central clearing migrate centrifugally.

Clinical Findings

A. Symptoms and Signs: Acute rheumatic fever is associated with fever, carditis, migratory polyarthritis, Sydenham's chorea, subcutaneous nodules, and erythema marginatum. Epistaxis, abdominal pain, pneumonia, and pleurisy are associated. No single symptom, sign, or laboratory test is diagnostic; the diagnosis is based on a combination of clinical findings. Rheumatic fever may occur at any age but is most common in childhood. It usually begins 1–3 weeks after an episode of pharyngitis caused by group A beta-hemolytic streptococci.

The skin eruption consists of annular and curvilinear evanescent erythema especially on the trunk. These change size and shape rapidly and may come and go for months or even years. Sometimes an erythematous arc moves across the body in hours.

Subcutaneous nodules are a more common skin manifestation of rheumatic fever than erythema marginatum. These nodules are small, painless spheres in the skin especially grouped around extensor tendons such as those of the hands, feet, elbows, knees, back, and scalp.

A migratory arthritis usually affects the large joints of the extremities such as knees, elbows, shoulders, hips, ankles, and elbows. Often only one or 2 joints are affected at a time. The carditis is indicated by murmurs that may change pitch and character as it progresses. Pericarditis and congestive heart failure may result. Tachycardia, gallop, and arrhythmias are fairly common. The chorea is an odd, dancelike, irregular movement of muscles. Fever may be high or low and usually chronic, lasting for weeks.

B. Laboratory Findings: There is no specific laboratory test to prove the diagnosis. The antistreptolysin O test (ASO) is usually elevated over 250 Todd units. The leukocyte count, erythrocyte sedimentation rate, and C-reactive protein tests are commonly abnormal but nonspecific. Group A streptococci may be isolated from the throat. If carditis is present, the PR interval may be prolonged and other ECG changes may be present.

Differential Diagnosis

Disorders resembling erythema marginatum include erythema gyratum repens, erythema chronicum migrans (with Lyme arthritis), annular urticaria, viral exanthems, drug eruptions, and erythema multiforme. Erythema marginatum may be distinguished by its relative absence of induration and its transient, migratory character. Most patients with erythema marginatum are ill, having other signs and symptoms of acute rheumatic fever.

Complications & Sequelae

There are no complications or sequelae of erythema marginatum; however, acute rheumatic fever may permanently damage the heart. The arthritis does not cause permanent injury.

Prevention

Penicillin given in oral or parenteral doses to maintain adequate therapeutic levels for 10 days following streptococcal pharyngitis may prevent rheumatic fever. Patients who have had rheumatic fever are often treated with long-term prophylactic antibiotics to prevent recurrence of streptococcal infection.

Treatment

A. Local Measures: The skin disease is nonpruritic and does not require topical therapy.

B. Specific Measures: The streptococcal infection should be treated. The treatment of rheumatic fever and its complications is beyond the scope of this text.

Course & Prognosis

The cutaneous eruption usually subsides as the rheumatic fever becomes inactive. The overall prognosis is excellent in the absence of carditis. A recurrent attack of rheumatic fever may be associated with recurrence of erythema marginatum. Streptococcal pharyngitis may cause resurgence of rheumatic fever in up to 50% of patients.

ERYTHEMA CHRONICUM MIGRANS (Lyme Disease)

Essentials of Diagnosis

- A red macule that expands peripherally and clears centrally.
- Occasionally, multiple secondary red macules or wheals.
- Mild symptoms of headache, fever, and aching.
- May occur weeks to months later: arthritis, neurologic and cardiac abnormalities.

General Considerations

Erythema chronicum migrans is the skin manifestation of Lyme disease, which is caused by the spirochete *Borrelia burgdorferi*. The bacterium is inoculated into the skin by the tick *Ixodes ricinus* or *Ixodes dammini*. Most cases in the USA occur in the New England states; the Midwest, including Wisconsin and Minnesota; and the West Coast, chiefly California and Oregon. Cases have been reported from Europe and other countries. Most patients develop the illness between May and November.

Clinical Findings

A. Symptoms and Signs: The patient may or may not remember being bitten by a tick. After an incubation period of 3–32 days, a red macule develops at the site of the bite. This slowly enlarges and in doing so clears in the center to form an annular plaque. A central punctum may mark the bite site. The border is typically raised, and the lesion may be huge—eg, covering much of the entire back.

If treatment is not provided, secondary lesions may develop. These include blotchy erythema, annular plaques, malar rashes, or urticaria. When this occurs, systemic symptoms are often present, including malaise and fatigue, headache, fever, chills, achiness, and lymphadenopathy. More rarely, patients may have meningeal irritation, encephalopathy, splenomegaly, sore throat, cough, or testicular swelling.

B. Laboratory Findings: Until more sensitive and specific laboratory tests become available, the diagnosis depends on the clinical features. Biopsy is nonspecific and shows perivascular accumulations of mononuclear cells and edema. The spirochete has been observed rarely in biopsies from the borders of lesions using special stains and can occasionally be isolated by culture. Serologic determinations of antibodies to the infectious agent are most useful in patients who have symptoms comparable with late-stage Lyme disease. Many normal persons have antibodies to this bacterium. Most patients with only erythema chronicum migrans do not have elevated titers. A rise in antibody titer is diagnostic. The highest titers are found in patients with arthritis, often many months later. Although patients may have antibodies to other spirochetes, VDRL tests are negative.

Differential Diagnosis

Erythema chronicum migrans can be confused with tinea corporis, but the latter usually scales. Erythema annulare centrifugum and granuloma annulare may also cause confusion. The arthritis can mimic rheumatoid arthritis due to other causes.

Complications & Sequelae

The arthritis involves many joints but is often migratory and without much swelling. Tendons, bones, bursae, and muscles may also be painful. Later, the arthritis tends to attack the large joints, causing erosions of cartilage and bone.

Neurologic abnormalities include meningitis, encephalitis, and neuritis. The neuritis may be cranial, motor, or sensory. Mononeuritis multiplex or myelitis in various combinations can also occur. These manifestations usually develop weeks to months after the skin eruption.

Cardiac abnormalities also occur later and include atrioventricular block, pericarditis, myocarditis, or left ventricular dysfunction.

Prevention

Protective light-colored clothing should be worn in areas where tick exposure is likely. Pants can be tucked into the tops of socks. After potential exposure, the body should be inspected for ticks, and ticks attached to skin should be removed. Diethyltoluamide (deet) is an effective tick repellant. Permethrin 0.5% sprayed into the clothing can reduce the numbers of adhering ticks. Patients with active disease should not donate blood, because the organ-

ism may contaminate it. Treatment during the phase of erythema chronicum migrans may prevent development of late sequelae.

Treatment

Doxycycline, 100 mg twice daily for 21 (localized) to 42 (disseminated) days, is the drug of choice for children aged 9 years or older and for adults. Tetracycline is an effective alternative in a dose of 250 mg 4 times daily for 21–42 days. Amoxicillin, 1 g 3 times daily, plus probenecid, 500 mg 3 times daily, has been recommended also.

For children less than 9 years old, penicillin V, 50 mg/kg/d—but not less than 1 g/d or more than 2 g/d—can be administered in divided doses. Children allergic to penicillin and intolerant or too young to be given tetracycline or doxycycline may be given amoxicillin, 40 mg/kg/d, in divided doses. Adult patients allergic to penicillin and tetracycline may be given erythromycin, but treatment with erythromycin may be less successful than treatment with other drugs.

Patients with arthritis, neurologic abnormalities, or cardiac abnormalities may occasionally improve following treatment with intravenous ceftriaxone at a dosage of 2 g daily for 14–21 days. If this is done in the hospital, isolation is not required.

Course & Prognosis

Oral antibiotic therapy shortens the course of the rash. The skin disorder characteristically clears after treatment, but many treatment failures have been reported. Late manifestations can persist despite treatment and cause permanent damage to nerves, joints, or heart.

ERYTHEMA GYRATUM REPENS

Essentials of Diagnosis

- A bizarre generalized swirling, serpiginous, "wood grain-like" erythema.
- Usually if not always associated with malignant disease.

General Considerations

Erythema gyratum repens is a rare reactive erythema usually caused by cancer, most frequently adenocarcinoma of the breast, lung, uterus, and upper gastrointestinal tract.

Clinical Findings

A. Symptoms and Signs: This distinctive eruption is pruritic and located primarily on the trunk and proximal extremities. The individual lesion is probably an annular plaque, but lesions are so large and confluent that the overall appearance is serpentine. Adjacent lesions typically parallel one another, so that the eruption frequently resembles coils of rope or annual growth rings of a cross-sectioned tree.

B. Laboratory Findings: There are no specific laboratory abnormalities. X-rays or other tests may indicate underlying cancer. Biopsy of an affected cutaneous area shows a nonspecific perivascular lymphocytic infiltrate. Direct immunofluorescence in at least one case showed granular deposits of IgG and C3 at the dermal-epidermal junction.

Differential Diagnosis

The eruption is distinctive. The differential diagnosis includes tinea imbricata (a generalized tinea corporis), erythema annulare centrifugum, and especially the annular variant of subacute cutaneous lupus erythematosus.

Complications & Sequelae

The eruption precedes the malignancy in 60% of cases. In most of the remainder of reported cases, it has occurred concurrently or very shortly after the carcinoma was found.

Treatment

Resection or treatment of the underlying carcinoma has caused remission of pruritus and the cutaneous eruption. Topical therapy is of little help. Emollients may relieve pruritus.

ERYTHEMA NODOSUM

Essentials of Diagnosis

- Painful erythematous nodules, usually over the anterior tibial surfaces.
- Induration, warmth, and extreme tenderness.
- Lesions usually heal without scarring within 4–6 weeks.

General Considerations

Erythema nodosum is an inflammatory skin disease associated with hypersensitivity to a drug or infectious agent or associated with sarcoidosis, inflammatory bowel disease, collagen disease, lymphoma, leukemia, or some other condition (Table 35–3). In some patients, no cause is found. Most affected persons are middle-aged women, but the eruption can occur at any age in either sex. It is not uncommon and accounts for about 0.5% of new disorders of the skin in the United Kingdom. The mechanism generating inflammatory nodules is not understood but seems to involve cell-mediated immune reactions around large blood vessels in the subcutaneous fat.

Clinical Findings

A. Symptoms and Signs: Multiple erythematous painful nodules and plaques develop suddenly on the skin, especially the anterior surfaces of the lower legs (Fig 35–5). Lesions may occur on other sites such as

Table 35–3. Some causes of erythema nodosum.

Infection
Streptococcal pharyngitis
Viral infections, including viral pharyngitis
Tuberculosis
Lymphogranuloma venereum
Cat-scratch disease
Ornithosis
Milker's nodule
Orf (ecthyma infectiosum)
Glandular fever
Tularemia
Yersiniosis
Blastomycosis
Coccidioidomycosis
Salmonellosis
Leprosy
Histoplasmosis
Enteropathies
Ulcerative colitis
Regional enteritis
Cancer
Leukemia
Hodgkin's disease
Carcinoma
Sarcoidosis
Drugs
Oral contraceptives
Sulfonamides
Bromides
Others

the arms and thighs. Nodules tend to group and be oriented longitudinally along the leg. As areas age, they can become somewhat purple and later yellow-brown to resemble a bruise. They do not ulcerate but may heal with postinflammatory hyperpigmentation. Systemic signs and symptoms may be present, including fever, chills, malaise, headache, myalgia, arthralgia, or sore throat. Additional signs and symptoms may reflect underlying causal disease.

B. Laboratory Findings: There is usually mild leukocytosis. The erythrocyte sedimentation rate is usually increased. Other laboratory tests may reflect an underlying infectious disease or condition. If the cause is not obvious, initial diagnostic tests normally include an intradermal test for tuberculosis (PPD); a chest x-ray film to search for fungal infections, sarcoidosis, or tuberculosis; and a throat culture and ASO titer to uncover associated streptococcal pharyngitis. If gastrointestinal complaints are present, stool cultures should be obtained for *Yersinia* and *Salmonella*. Sometimes the intestinal tract should be investigated for inflammatory bowel disease.

Skin biopsy is best accomplished by scalpel incision or excision, including the subcutaneous fat as well as the epidermis and dermis. The epidermis is usually unaffected, and the dermis shows a scattered infiltrate. In the septa of the subcutaneous fat, areas of intense inflammation (lymphocytes, polymorphonuclear leukocytes, histiocytes, occasional plasma

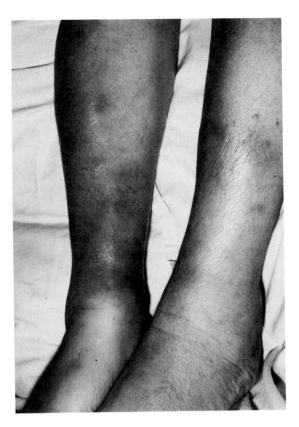

Figure 35–5. Erythema nodosum. Nodules on the legs are usually very tender.

cells and giant cells) are clustered around large blood vessels. The fat is not destroyed, and necrosis is not present. However, blood vessel walls may be thickened and damaged. Frank fibrinoid changes throughout the vessel and occlusion usually do not occur.

Differential Diagnosis

The differential diagnosis includes other forms of panniculitis (see Chapter 25). These include cellulitis, superficial migratory thrombophlebitis, Behçet's disease, meningococcemia, arthropod bites, erythema induratum, lipolytic panniculitis, Weber-Christian panniculitis, lupus profundus, nodular vasculitis, erythema nodosum leprosum, cold panniculitis, trauma, factitial disease, polyarteritis nodosa, subcutaneous nodular migratory panniculitis, abscess, poststeroid panniculitis, early herpes zoster, nodules of sarcoidosis, and metastatic neoplastic disease. If the eruption is bilateral, cellulitis, thrombophlebitis, trauma, cold panniculitis, abscess, and herpes zoster are unlikely. Lesions of Weber-Christian panniculitis may suppurate and tend to occur on the thighs and trunk rather than the lower legs. The panniculitis secondary to pancreatitis is usually associated with ab-

dominal pain and ulceration of inflamed nodules. When typical lesions of erythema nodosum persist for longer than 6 months, the diagnosis is nodular vasculitis.

Complications & Sequelae

Pain may be so severe that the patient is disabled, but permanent sequelae from erythema nodosum are unusual. Most sequelae relate to the underlying disorder, but the prognosis is good even when the cause is uncertain. Lesions usually develop for only 1 or 2 weeks and then resolve within 1 or 2 months. The disorder can recur.

Treatment

A. General Measures: Bed rest with the legs slightly elevated is important. When the patient is ambulatory, support stockings or wraps may help.

B. Systemic Therapy: If the cause of the disease is known, it should be treated or removed if feasible and medically justified. If drugs are responsible, they should be discontinued or substituted with chemically unrelated drugs if possible. Pain may be relieved with aspirin or other nonsteroidal anti-inflammatory agents. Systemic corticosteroids have been used, but they decrease host resistance if the cause is infectious and interfere with some diagnostic tests that may be necessary to establish the cause. Therefore, treatment with systemic corticosteroids should be avoided if possible. Potassium iodide given orally in divided doses of 300–900 mg/d has been effective. The mechanism of action is unknown. No carefully controlled studies have been performed to determine the efficacy and safety of potassium iodide in the treatment of erythema nodosum.

C. Topical Therapy: Warm tap water compresses are sometimes soothing. The areas are often hyperesthetic, so that rubbing against bedclothes and bed linens is uncomfortable; tenting the bedsheets to avoid skin contact helps keep the patient comfortable and in bed.

Course & Prognosis

The prognosis depends on the underlying condition. When erythema nodosum is associated with histoplasmosis, sarcoidosis, or coccidioidomycosis, the lesions are often self-limited.

ERYTHEMA DYSCHROMICUM PERSTANS

Essentials of Diagnosis

- Slate-gray persisting macules or patches of variable sizes.
- Involvement primarily of the trunk and extremities. Scalp, palm, soles, and mucous membranes are spared.
- Usually asymptomatic.
- Usually afflicts people of Hispanic origin.

General Considerations

Erythema dyschromicum perstans is a chronic, progressive pigmented disorder of unknown cause. It has also been called the ashy dermatosis (dermatosis cinecienta) because of the peculiar slatelike gray coloration in the skin. Because it is usually asymptomatic, its presence is mostly of cosmetic significance. Most cases have been in dark-skinned individuals, especially those of Latin American extraction. The cause is unknown. The possibility that the coloration represents postinflammatory hyperpigmentation is supported by the occasional appearance of slightly raised, erythematous lesions prior to development of pigmented patches and plaques.

Clinical Findings

A. Symptoms and Signs: The disorder is usually asymptomatic or only mildly pruritic. Numerous slate-gray macules and patches develop over the trunk and extremities. These are variable in size and may enlarge to cover large areas of the body. The scalp, palms, soles, and mucous membranes are usually not affected.

B. Laboratory Findings: Laboratory tests are usually normal except for biopsy findings. Edema is sometimes found within the epidermis, associated with incontinence of pigment and hydropic degeneration of the basal cell layer. A perivascular infiltrate of lymphocytes and histiocytes is sometimes present. Histiocytes are usually laden with melanin, which accounts for the ashy color of the skin.

Differential Diagnosis

Postinflammatory hyperpigmentation is the most difficult condition to distinguish from erythema dyschromicum perstans. Fixed drug reactions have a slate-gray pigmentation between episodes but are usually associated with the obvious acute appearance of urticarial-appearing patches and plaques at pigmented sites associated with ingestion of a drug. The pigmentation of argyria is similar but is usually generalized and without definable margins. Photodermatoses, chloasma, maculae ceruleae of pediculosis, hemochromatosis, Addison's disease, leprosy, and urticaria pigmentosa are other conditions that sometimes must be considered in the differential diagnosis.

Complications & Sequelae

There are no complications, but the disease tends to persist and spread.

Treatment

No effective treatment is available. Makeup can cover cosmetically unacceptable areas. In the same way, deliberate suntanning can also mask lesions.

Course & Prognosis

The disorder is chronic and tends to spread.

ERYTHEMA TOXICUM NEONATORUM

Essentials of Diagnosis

- Occurs from several hours to 5 days after birth.
- The primary lesion is a 1- to 3-mm sterile pustule on an erythematous base.
- Pink macules or patches develop, especially on the trunk.

General Considerations

Erythema toxicum neonatorum is a common but transient erythema occurring in the neonatal period in 5–50% of term infants and characterized by papules, pustules, and pink macules. It is less common in premature infants. The cause is unknown. Because it is associated with peripheral blood eosinophilia and eosinophil-laden pustules, the disorder has been attributed to an allergy. However, there is no immunologic support for this hypothesis. An eosinophilic response is the usual one to inflammation among newborn term infants during the neonatal period.

Clinical Findings

A. Symptoms and Signs: Because the condition is limited to the neonatal period, the degree of pruritus cannot be assessed. The disorder usually develops on the second to fifth day after birth. Onset as late as day 14 has been reported. A few infants have had skin disease at birth, but these may represent a different but similar disorder called transient neonatal pustular melanosis. The typical skin lesion of erythema toxicum neonatorum is a white pustule on an erythematous base. Pustules are sometimes not present, in which case papules or macules or a splotchy erythema is the hallmark. Any body area may be affected, but lesions are most notable on the trunk and rare on the palms and soles. In some infants the eruption is extensive, whereas in others only one or a few lesions are present.

B. Laboratory Findings: There is generally peripheral blood eosinophilia, often as high as 15%. The pustules also contain eosinophils. These can be demonstrated by biopsy or by smear of the pustular contents. All pustules are sterile, and Gram and PAS stains of smears and biopsies therefore do not reveal bacteria or fungi. On biopsy, pustules are often associated with hair follicles and develop in the upper parts of the epidermis, often just beneath the stratum corneum.

Differential Diagnosis

Staphylococcal folliculitis is often asymmetric; smears show gram-positive cocci in clumps, and cultures isolate *Staphylococcus aureus*. Transient neonatal pustular melanosis, often present at birth, is much more common in blacks (5%) than in whites (0.5%) and is characterized by papules and hyperpigmented macules. Acropustulosis of infancy is associated with vesicles or pustules on the hands and feet, and the palms are frequently involved, whereas lesions on the palms are rare in erythema toxicum neonatorum. Pustules can also occur from *Candida* infection, in which case KOH examination or PAS stains may demonstrate yeast forms. Miliaria pustulosa and miliaria rubra are associated with sweat ducts rather than hair follicles and often occur in areas where the skin has been occluded. Pustules can also be seen in infants with sepsis, but these patients are usually ill.

Treatment

No treatment is necessary. The eruption is self-limited, and there are no complications.

BEHÇET'S SYNDROME

Essentials of Diagnosis

- Oral ulcers, genital ulcers, and iritis or uveitis constitute the clinical triad of Behçet's syndrome.
- Tender subcutaneous nodules and pustules at sites of trauma are often present.
- The diagnosis is also suggested when 2 of the triad are present plus one of the following: other cutaneous lesions, arthritis, thrombophlebitis, lesions of arteries, involvement of the central nervous system, genitourinary tract involvement.

General Considerations

This uncommon disorder occurs throughout the world but especially in Japan and in the region around the Mediterranean Sea. It is more common in men. Onset can occur at any age, but most patients are young adults. The cause is unknown. Viruses have been implicated because the disorder has been passively transferred with cerebrospinal fluid and because inclusion bodies have been observed in smears. Histopathologic changes in tissues have mimicked those of viral infection. An abnormality in clotting has been implicated because of the prevalence of thrombophlebitis, the presence of inhibitors of plasminogen activator in plasma, and elevated levels of fibrinogen and factor VIII. An autoimmune origin has been suggested by the frequent presence of circulating antibodies to cell cytoplasm in many patients, by lymphocyte-mediated cytotoxicity to oral mucosal cells in some patients, and by sudden decrements in total hemolytic complement levels at the time of relapse. Furthermore, an association of Behçet's syndrome with HLA-A5 has been confirmed (relative risk about 5), indicating that genetic factors predispose certain persons to the syndrome.

Clinical Findings

In complete Behçet's syndrome, patients have recurrent ulcerations of the mouth, skin lesions (nodules, thrombophlebitis, or pathergy), eye lesions (hypopyon, iritis, iridocyclitis, or chorioretinitis), and ulcers of the external genitalia. In the incomplete syndrome, 3 of these 4 major criteria should be present. The diagnosis of Behçet's syndrome is strongly suggested by the presence of oral ulcers, scrotal ulcers, and iridocyclitis or uveitis.

A. Symptoms and Signs: The signs and symptoms of Behçet's syndrome depend on the particular organ involved.

1. Mouth– In the mouth, erythematous or edematous macules or papules enlarge and ulcerate. Vesicles are not seen. Ulcers may range in size from 2 to 10 mm in diameter and are frequently punched-out in appearance, surrounded by erythema, and often covered with a pseudomembrane. They often occur in crops and tend to affect the cheeks, tongue, tonsils, larynx, or gingiva. Ulcers of the pharynx, palate, and tonsils are unusual. The ulcers are painful, interfere with eating, and heal slowly, often with scarring.

2. Genitalia– Genital ulcers are common. They usually occur on the labia of females and on the scrotum of males (scrotal ulcers are highly suggestive of this disorder). Oral ulcers are usually present when genital ulcers are present. Genital ulcers also tend to occur in crops and in women are more likely to appear just prior to menses.

3. Skin– A variety of skin lesions have been associated: papules, vesicles, pustules, abscesses, subcutaneous thrombophlebitis, and nodular lesions suggesting erythema nodosum. The most distinctive cutaneous finding is called pathergy. After puncture of the skin with a needle, the puncture site becomes inflamed and develops a small sterile pustule. Pathergy is an uncommon finding among patients with Behçet's syndrome, but when present it strongly suggests the diagnosis.

4. Eyes– The eyes are frequently affected. A highly characteristic type of eye involvement is iridocyclitis with hypopyon. The pus often layers out and can be easily observed without specific optical aids. Inflammation at the back of the eye is more serious and may cause choroiditis, retinal thrombosis, retinal arteritis, or papillitis. Ocular sequelae include glaucoma, cataracts, and blindness.

5. Joints– When joints are involved, it is usually the large joints that are are affected. The knee is particularly prone to chronic arthritis. Involvement is usually asymmetric and recurrent. In most patients the arthritis, though nondestructive, may be associated at its onset with fever, leukocytosis, and erythema nodosum.

6. Arteries– Involvement of arteries is much less common. Focal inflammation can cause aneurysms to form in large arteries. Arterial occlusion can lead to gangrene. Recurrent thrombophlebitis occurs in about one-fourth of patients. The lower extremities are most commonly affected. Thrombosis of veins in the eye causes serious ocular sequelae.

7. Nervous system– Involvement of the central

nervous system is uncommon and usually occurs years after onset of the syndrome. Manifestations include meningitis, encephalitis, and inflammation of the brain, spinal cord, and nerves. Patients may become psychotic. Involvement of the central nervous system often is a poor prognostic sign, and most patients die within 1 year after onset of central nervous system signs.

8. Gastrointestinal system— Gastrointestinal involvement can lead to abdominal pain, distention, loss of appetite, nausea, diarrhea, malabsorption, and intestinal paralysis. Ulcerating esophagitis and ulcerative colitis have also been described.

9. Genitourinary system— Some patients have developed amyloidosis affecting kidney function. Epididymitis or orchitis is more common. Urethritis, cystitis, and ulceration of the bladder have also been recorded.

10. Other sites of involvement— Inflammation of the lungs, pleura, heart, and pericardium is uncommon.

B. Laboratory Findings: Biopsy of the skin often shows an ulcerated epidermis with lymphocytic perivascular infiltration; there may be occlusion and obliteration of blood vessels. The erythrocyte sedimentation rate is often elevated. Antibodies against cytoplasm can sometimes be detected by indirect immunofluorescence. Neutrophil chemotactic responses may be abnormally quick.

Differential Diagnosis

The differential diagnosis of Behçet's syndrome is vast because of the many organ systems involved. The most difficult differential diagnosis relates to chronic ulcerations of the mouth. Like Behçet's syndrome, recurrent aphthous stomatitis is characterized by one to many painful ulcerations affecting the tongue, palate, and buccal mucosa, but these patients lack genital, eye, or skin lesions. Major aphthae (periadenitis mucosa necrotica recurrens) are deeper ulcers and are more likely to scar. Herpes stomatitis can mimic Behçet's syndrome. Primary herpes infection usually affects children, and vesicles may sometimes be identified. In recurrent herpes simplex, ulcers may be grouped, and Tzanck smear or culture may help confirm the diagnosis. Chronic erythema multiforme can cause similar mouth ulcers, but skin lesions are often present simultaneously, and the disorder tends to be self-limited and infrequent. Cicatricial pemphigoid affects individuals over the age of 60 years and is associated with marked scarring and deposition of IgG and C3 along the dermal-epidermal junction of adjacent mucosal skin. Desquamative gingivitis may present with bullae and intense erythema of the gingiva. Mouth ulcers are usually present in patients with pemphigus. Patients with pemphigus almost always have antibodies to the intercellular areas of stratified squamous epithelium present in their own skin and serum. Patients with Reiter's syndrome oc-

casionally have many of the findings seen in Behçet's syndrome.

Complications & Sequelae

The disorder is associated with marked morbidity and even mortality, depending upon which organ systems are involved. It typically runs a protracted course with attacks generally lasting for several weeks and recurring frequently. Involvement of the eye and central nervous system is particularly ominous. Eye involvement can result in blindness, and central nervous system involvement can result in marked neurologic or psychiatric sequelae and death.

Treatment

Oral and genital ulcerations can usually be treated by local measures, though these measures do not prevent new ulcers from forming. Topical corticosteroids may reduce inflammation, and topical anesthetic agents may relieve pain. Individual lesions generally heal over the course of several weeks.

In severe cases or when vital organs are affected, systemic corticosteroids may be necessary. These may protect the central nervous system or eye, but there are no prospective studies that document the efficacy of systemic corticosteroids in reducing morbidity or mortality.

Immunosuppressive therapy with azathioprine, chlorambucil, or cyclophosphamide has been used, but their efficacy is still debated.

Colchicine, 0.6 mg 2 or 3 times daily, has been used with good results. The rationale relates to interference with neutrophil chemotaxis.

Treatment with levamisole or agents that augment fibrinolysis has also been effective in some patients.

RELAPSING POLYCHONDRITIS

Essentials of Diagnosis

- Usually 3 or more of the following are present: bilateral auricular chondritis, nonerosive seronegative inflammatory polyarthritis, nasal chondritis, ocular inflammation, respiratory tract chondritis, audiovestibular damage.

General Considerations

Relapsing polychondritis is a rare chronic autoimmune inflammatory disease of cartilaginous structures. Cartilage in the ear, nose, joints, eyes, blood vessels, trachea, and bronchial tree may be affected and destroyed. Deafness may occur. The frequent occurrence in patients with various rheumatic and autoimmune disorders suggests that relapsing polychondritis may be of similar origin. Using special techniques, antibodies against cartilage have been detected in sera from patients.

Clinical Findings

A. Symptoms and Signs: The chondritis on the ear is usually manifested by large, swollen, red, tender pinnae. The earlobe is characteristically spared because it contains no cartilage. The inflammation persists for 1–2 weeks and disappears but then recurs. When the joints are involved, there is migratory polyarthritis. Ocular involvement is manifested by keratitis, episcleritis, and conjunctivitis. Respiratory tract involvement is marked by a tender red nose, but hoarseness, loss of voice, dyspnea, and stridor are other signs. Occasionally, systemic signs of fever, malaise, and cutaneous vasculitis develop. Recurrent attacks lead to destruction of cartilage. Fibrous replacement of the cartilage of the ear leads to "cauliflower ears." Nasal involvement causes unusual dips of the nasal bridge and facial flattening. Destruction of cartilage in the respiratory tract leads to airway collapse. When the cardiovascular system is involved, aneurysms and cardiac valve disease may lead to death.

B. Laboratory Findings: The erythrocyte sedimentation rate is usually raised. Autoantibodies such as rheumatoid factor or antinuclear antibodies may be present. Indirect immunofluorescence may demonstrate antibodies to cartilage in serum. The sections of cartilage must first be incubated with hyaluronidase to unmask binding sites before indirect immunofluorescence is performed. The antibody present is usually IgG, but IgA has also been found.

Biopsy of cartilage characteristically shows loss of the normal basophilic staining and inflammatory infiltrate of polymorphonuclear leukocytes or histiocytic cells. As the cartilage is destroyed, it is replaced by fibrous tissue.

Differential Diagnosis

The diagnosis is usually not mimicked by other conditions. In the acute stage, cellulitis or facial erysipelas may cause confusion. Acute allergic contact dermatitis can cause swelling of the ears, but such swelling usually is not painful and may be accompanied by the presence of vesicles.

Complications & Sequelae

About 30% of patients die, usually about 4 years after onset. The most frequent cause of death is airway collapse or obstruction. However, involvement of the cardiovascular system can lead to ruptured aneurysms and cardiac failure. Even when the cardiovascular system or tracheobronchial tree is not affected, the disorder can cause marked disability. The ears and nose can become deformed, and joints may be destroyed.

Treatment

Topical therapy is ineffective. Systemic corticosteroids can control or ablate inflammation, but high doses are usually required. Therapy is difficult to evaluate because of the frequent spontaneous remissions and exacerbations. Dapsone has helped some patients, and in those patients dapsone may be safer than systemic corticosteroids. The usual starting dose is 100 mg/d. However, this drug may cause severe side effects (see Chapter 53).

Course & Prognosis

The course is unpredictable, but about one-third of patients die. Exacerbations and remissions are common. Some patients have only a few episodes and then recover. Others have many episodes leading to severe deformities.

REFERENCES

Amon RB, Dimond RL: Toxic epidermal necrolysis: Rapid differentiation between staphylococcal- and drug-induced disease. Arch Dermatol 1975;111:1433.

Arbesfeld SJ, Kurban AK: Behçet's disease. J Am Acad Dermatol 1988;19:767.

Arstikaitis MJ: Ocular aftermath of Stevens-Johnson syndrome: Review of 33 cases. Arch Ophthalmol 1973; 90:376.

Burkhart CG: Erythema multiforme. J Am Acad Dermatol 1979;1:357.

Chajek T, Fainaru M: Behçet's disease: Report of 41 cases and a review of the literature. Medicine 1975;54:179.

Foidart JM et al: Antibodies to type II collagen in relapsing polychondritis. N Engl J Med 1978;299:1203.

Goldstein SM et al: Toxic epidermal necrolysis: Unmuddying the waters. Arch Dermatol 1987;123:1153.

Hannuksela M: Erythema nodosum. Clin Dermatol 1986; 4:88.

Harrison PV: The annular erythemas. Int J Dermatol 1979;18:282.

Heimbach DM et al: Toxic epidermal necrolysis: A step forward in treatment. JAMA 1987;257:2171.

Holt PJ, Davies MG: Erythema gyratum repens: An immunologically mediated dermatosis? Br J Dermatol 1977; 96:343.

Horio T et al: Potassium iodide in the treatment of erythema nodosum and nodular vasculitis. Arch Dermatol 1981; 117:29.

Howland WW et al: Erythema multiforme: Clinical, histopathologic, and immunologic study. J Am Acad Dermatol 1984;10:438.

Huff JC: Erythema multiforme. Dermatol Clin 1985;3:141.

Huff JC, Weston WL, Tonnesen MG: Erythema multiforme: A critical review of characteristics, diagnostic criteria, and causes. J Am Acad Dermatol 1983;8:763.

Kaplan EL: Acute rheumatic fever. Pediatr Clin North Am 1978;25:817.

Leigh IM et al: Recurrent and continuous erythema multiforme: A clinical and immunological study. Clin Exp Dermatol 1985;10:58.

Lyell A: Toxic epidermal necrolysis (the scalded skin syndrome): A reappraisal. Br J Dermatol 1979;100:69.

Martin J et al: Relapsing polychondritis treated with dapsone. Arch Dermatol 1976;112:1272.

McAdam LP et al: Relapsing polychondritis: Prospective study of 23 patients and a review of the literature. Medicine 1976;55:193.

Nethercott JR, Choi BC: Erythema multiforme (Stevens-Johnson syndrome): Chart review of 123 hospitalized patient. Dermatologica 1985;171:383.

Novick NL, Phelps R, Tom C: Erythema dyschromicum perstans. Int J Dermatol 1986;25:322.

Rasmussen JE: Erythema multiforme in children: Response to treatment with systemic corticosteroids. Br J Dermatol 1976;95:181.

Shimizu T et al: Behçet disease (Behçet syndrome). Semin Arthritis Rheum 1979;8:223.

Shrestha M, Grodzicki RL, Steere AC: Diagnosing early Lyme disease. Am J Med 1985;78:235.

Skolnick M, Mainman ER: Erythema gyratum repens with metastatic adenocarcinoma. Arch Dermatol 1975;111:227.

Steere AC, Schoen RT, Taylor E: The clinical evolution of Lyme arthritis. Ann Intern Med 1987; 107:725.

Steere AC et al: The early clinical manifestations of Lyme disease. Ann Intern Med 1983;99:76.

Taylor WB, Bondurant CP: Erythema neonatorum allergicum. Arch Dermatol 1957; 76:591.

White JW: Erythema nodosum. Dermatol Clin 1985;3:119.

Drug Reactions **36**

Robert S. Stern, MD

Mucocutaneous reactions are among the most common undesired consequences of therapeutic drug use. They are important because of the associated morbidity and because they may be the first or most obvious sign of a generalized hypersensitivity or toxic reaction involving other structures and organs, including the joints, hematopoietic system, liver, and kidneys. In spite of their frequency, the precise mechanism of action for many types of drug-related cutaneous changes remains largely conjectural.

Cutaneous reactions to drugs are categorized according to the latency period between drug administration and development of the reaction, the presumed mechanism of action, and the morphologic appearance. Simultaneous consideration of each of these variables and the drugs used by the patient is essential in assessing the likelihood that a cutaneous eruption is due to a particular drug.

Immediate hypersensitivity reactions are the best-understood type of hypersensitivity reaction. They are manifested clinically as urticaria or angioedema and are IgE-mediated. Substances released from mast cells and leukocytes as part of this reaction can produce laryngospasm, bronchospasm, and hypotension and may lead to life-threatening anaphylactic shock.

Because of the delay between drug administration and development of the reaction and because of recurrence with rechallenge, a variety of common drug eruptions, including morbilliform eruptions and erythema multiforme, are generally considered manifestations of delayed hypersensitivity. Skin mechanisms, still not well defined, are also most likely keys to the etiology of drug-induced vasculitis, fixed drug eruptions, and erythema nodosum.

MECHANISMS OF DRUG REACTIONS

Altered Hormonal or Cellular Function

Some drugs alter hormonal or cellular function. Adverse cutaneous effects of corticosteroids parallel those observed in Cushing's disease. Hormonal therapy alters sebaceous gland activity and may pro-

duce acne or pigmentary changes. It is less clear how several other agents aggravate preexisting dermatologic diseases (eg, effect of lithium on acne and psoriasis).

Drug Deposition in the Skin

Deposition of drugs in the skin and appendages can be responsible for mucocutaneous reaction. A drug's adverse effects on normal tissue may limit the total therapeutic dose. Alopecia and mucous membrane ulcers, which can be caused by certain chemotherapeutic agents, are notable examples.

Enhanced Cutaneous Response to Physical Agents

Drugs can also enhance the effect of physical agents such as ionizing and nonionizing radiation. Radiation recall and photosensitivity eruptions due to drug-induced phototoxicity are 2 examples.

Unexplained Mechanisms

For some interesting and important drug eruptions, including toxic epidermal necrolysis, lichenoid eruptions, and coumarin-induced necrosis, few data are available on the mechanisms.

APPROACH TO DIAGNOSIS OF DRUG REACTIONS

To assess the likelihood that a given agent is responsible for changes in the skin or mucous membranes, the following elements should be evaluated systematically: (1) prior experience with the drug, including the frequency of eruptions associated with the drug's administration, the pattern of morphologic reactions, and the patient's experience during previous exposures; (2) alternative etiologic candidates; (3) the timing of events; (4) the drug dose; (5) dechallenge results; and (6) rechallenge results.

Obtaining the necessary information for this evaluation requires attention to selected details in the history and physical examination. For a complete drug history, the clinician must collect information about the time each drug used was administered in relation to the development of the eruption, past use of each agent, and prior reactions to any drugs. Current and past use of nonprescription, habitual, and illicit drugs should be recorded; analgesics, laxatives, sleeping pills, and "street" drugs are often overlooked. When multiple drugs have been used, a flow chart with dates of administration and doses of each drug is helpful.

The possibility of foods and beverages as causative factors should be considered, since an almost endless variety of chemical compounds used in the processing of foods and beverages adds to the difficulty in identifying an offending chemical agent.

The physician should inquire about symptoms suggesting an alternative cause. Infections—particularly viral infections—sometimes cause eruptions resembling those caused by drugs. In certain cases it may be difficult to determine whether an illness or its treatment is the cause of an eruption. For example, erythema multiforme may follow infection or may be due to drugs used to treat the infection. In such cases, the results of drug dechallenge and rechallenge aid in diagnosis. Rechallenge is risky and is usually recommended only if a precise etiologic diagnosis is very important for patient care decisions.

Drugs differ in the risk of reaction accompanying their use and in the morphology of the reaction. Based on a prospective study of hospitalized patients, allergic skin reaction rates are available for many common drugs (Table 36–1). The reaction rate associated with each drug that might be responsible for a patient's rash is helpful in determining the likelihood that a given drug is responsible. Knowledge about the distribution of lesions, the character of the individual lesions, associated symptoms, and evolution over time is crucial.

MORPHOLOGIC CLASSIFICATION OF DRUG ERUPTIONS

Urticarial and morbilliform eruptions are by far the most frequent types of drug eruptions. Table 36–1 presents the relative reaction rates of these types of reactions for classes of drugs used in hospitalized patients. Although not included in this study of hospitalized patients, phenytoin (Dilantin) is also often associated with cutaneous reactions.

Common classes of drugs associated with the less common eruptions discussed below are listed in Table 36–2.

Urticarial Reactions

Urticaria is an immediate hypersensitivity reaction characterized by pruritic red wheals in symmetric distribution. The lesions, representing dermal vasodilatation and edema, vary in size from a small point to a large area. The epidermis is usually not involved.

Table 36–1. Rates of cutaneous reactions to selected commonly used drugs.[1]

Drug	Reaction Rate[2]
Amoxicillin/ampicillin	4
Trimethoprim-sulfamethoxazole	3
Penicillins	2
Blood, blood products	2
Cephalosporins	2
Benzodiazepines	1
Barbiturates	0.4
Allopurinol	0.8
Furosemide	0.5

[1]Adapted from Bigby M et al: Drug-induced cutaneous reactions. JAMA 1986;256:3358.
[2]Reactions per 100 recipients averaged for drugs of that class, eg, penicillins include semisynthetic penicillins and penicillin G.

Dermal and subcutaneous tissues may become so swollen that they impair respiration, which may contribute to life-threatening anaphylaxis. As an IgE-mediated hypersensitivity reaction, urticaria usually occurs within 36 hours after drug administration but can occur within minutes. Individual lesions rarely last more than 24 hours. Although aspirin, penicillin, and blood products are the most frequent causes, many drugs can cause urticarial eruptions.

Morbilliform Eruptions

Morbilliform eruptions are sometimes loosely referred to as maculopapular exanthems. They are the most common of all drug-induced eruptions. Lesions are frequently symmetric, usually beginning as small erythematous macules and papules that become confluent and form red plaques. Morbilliform eruptions often start on the trunk or in areas of pressure or trauma. Involvement of mucous membranes, palms, and soles is variable. Mild fever is sometimes present; pruritus is common. In contrast to urticaria, the dermis and epidermis are involved.

Occasionally, a morbilliform eruption that has recurred on rechallenge with a particular drug will fade even if the suspected drug is continued. More often, continued administration will stimulate a more extensive and symptomatic reaction. Generally, morbilliform eruptions have a longer latency period than do urticarial eruptions, but most occur within 1 week after introduction of a drug. Penicillin may induce this reaction 2 or more weeks after its introduction, and with agents not rapidly excreted—such as thiazide diuretics—the eruption may occur days after the drug has been discontinued. Ordinarily, these eruptions and their associated symptoms fade within 2 weeks after the drug is withdrawn. It is often difficult to determine whether the eruption is caused by a virus or a drug.

Table 36–2. Commonly used drugs associated with cutaneous eruptions with distinctive morphologies.

	Type of Eruption					
	Vasculitis	Erythema Nodosum	Fixed Drug	Lichenoid	Photosensitivity	Toxic Epidermal Necrolysis
Penicillins		x	x			x
Barbiturates		x	x			x
Phenytoin	x	x				x
Sulfonamides	x	x	x		x	x
Phenothiazines		x		x	x	
Griseofulvin	x	x			x	x
Phenolphthalein		x	x			x
Tetracyclines		x	x	x	x	x
Nonsteroidal anti-inflammatory drugs	x	x	x		x	x
Cimetidine	x	x				
Benzodiazepine		x	x		x	

Erythema Multiforme

Erythema multiforme is an acute, self-limited inflammatory disorder of the skin and mucous membranes characterized by a wide variety of lesions, including distinctive iris ("bulls-eye") or target lesions (Fig 36–1). The onset is usually sudden, and malaise and sore throat are commonly present. Occasionally, erythema multiforme becomes generalized and is accompanied by fever and visceral involvement (Stevens-Johnson syndrome). The severe form occurs more frequently in children and young adults and may pose a significant threat to life.

Although the mechanism of this reaction remains obscure, it is probably immunologic. Drugs most often implicated in erythema multiforme include penicillin, sulfonamides, phenothiazines, thiazides, and phenytoin. Other causes of erythema multiforme include viral (especially herpes simplex) and *Mycoplasma* infections. When these infections are treated with drugs, it may be impossible, except by rechallenge, to determine if the eruption is due to the drug or to the infection. Because of the attendant risks, rechallenge is justified only when careful supervision is possible, when the patient is fully informed of those risks, and when the information to be obtained justifies the work and risk.

Fixed Drug Eruptions

Fixed drug eruptions—circumscribed inflammatory skin lesions recurring at the same locations—have a distinct morphology and a clear temporal relation to drug use. Initially, they present as a solitary lesions or as a few well-demarcated red stinging or pruritic papules. The genitalia and face are sites with special predilection. Although the erythema resolves in days or weeks, hyperpigmentation persists in the area, sometimes for long periods. Local factors play

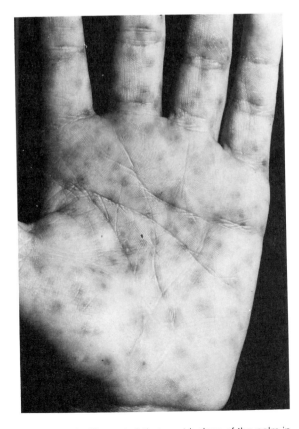

Figure 36–1. Characteristic target lesions of the palm in erythema multiforme.

an important role; rechallenge is followed by a flare only at previously affected sites. However, fixed drug eruptions are thought to be immunologically mediated.

Erythema Nodosum

Erythema nodosum presents as red, tender subcutaneous nodules on the legs. Young women are most frequently affected. The cause is usually unknown, but erythema nodosum is often associated with sarcoid or with infectious diseases such as tuberculosis and deep fungal infections. Drugs, especially oral contraceptives, appear to trigger some cases (see Chapter 35).

Toxic Epidermal Necrolysis

Drug-induced toxic epidermal necrolysis is a potentially life-threatening disorder. Initially, patients present with diffusely red, tender skin. Gentle lateral pressure on these areas later results in epidermal separation and the formation of erosions (Nikolsky's sign). Toxic epidermal necrolysis in adults is often caused by drugs. Nonsteroidal anti-inflammatory agents, phenytoin, barbiturates, sulfonamides, and penicillin-based antibiotics are especially important causes of this reaction. Large erosions cause fluid and electrolyte imbalance and increase the risk of sepsis. Treatment in a burn unit is often indicated.

Lichenoid Drug Eruptions

Lichen planus-like drug reaction is a pruritic eruption characterized by symmetrically distributed purple polygonal papules that appear most frequently on the ventral forearms and less often on the lower legs and genitalia. Mucous membranes—especially the buccal mucosa—are sometimes involved. Although the eruption suggests lichen planus, the morphology, distribution, and histology are often atypical in one or more ways. Gold, antimalarials, thiazides, and tetracyclines are the most frequent drug-related causes.

Pigmentary Changes

The inflammatory dermatoses discussed above are usually of sudden onset; in contrast, pigmentary changes induced by drugs are often insidious and slowly progressive and may be dose-related. Color changes may be a result of direct deposition of a drug or its metabolites in the skin (eg, minocycline), stimulation of melanocytes (eg, by silver in argyria), or deposition of other pigments such as iron. Sun exposure may accentuate pigmentary changes.

Photosensitivity Disorders

Ultraviolet radiation and occasionally visible light can interact with drugs or alter their effects, triggering a variety of cutaneous eruptions. The most frequent reactions caused by the interaction between a drug and ultraviolet light are phototoxic reactions.

These reactions may resemble sunburn or solar urticaria or they may present initially as stinging or burning. They are usually confined to exposed areas, and their severity is proportionate to drug dose and ultraviolet exposure.

Photoallergic eruptions occur when ultraviolet radiation alters a drug so that it serves as a foreign antigen. Such reactions are relatively infrequent but may persist even after the drug has been withdrawn, leaving patients with a reaction to the sun for extended periods.

Purpuric Eruptions

Nonblanching, raised purple papules and plaques are the clinical manifestations of vasculitis involving the skin. Drugs are one of many causes of cutaneous vasculitis; among those implicated are thiazides, sulfonamides, hydantoins, and nonsteroidal anti-inflammatory drugs. Vasculitis due to drugs may involve the kidney, central nervous system, joints, or other organs in addition to the skin. Therefore, patients with cutaneous vasculitis should be examined for involvement of these organs as well. (See Chapter 37.) In the patient with thrombocytopenia or a coagulation defect, a purpuric drug eruption is not necessarily vasculitic.

Exfoliative Erythroderma

Exfoliative erythroderma is a generalized erythematous and scaling eruption ordinarily accompanied by fever and malaise. Although usually a manifestation of an underlying dermatologic disease such as eczema, psoriasis, or mycosis fungoides, drugs such as isoniazid, phenytoin, phenylbutazone, and streptomycin have been implicated in some cases.

Other Forms

In addition to their immunologic and toxic properties, some drugs may induce or exacerbate diseases that have prominent cutaneous components. Lithium may worsen acne or psoriasis. Alcohol abuse, phenytoin, barbiturates, busulfan, estrogens, and hexachlorobenzene may induce porphyria cutanea tarda. Isoniazid may induce pellagra. Lupus erythematosus can be induced by drugs such as hydralazine and procainamide and can cause serious illness. However, cutaneous findings are less frequent when this disorder is caused by a drug.

MULTISYSTEM REACTIONS INVOLVING THE SKIN

Serum Sickness

Serum sickness is a combination of urticarial, morbilliform, or purpuric skin lesions and inflammation of other structures and organs, most often the liver, joints, and kidneys. This syndrome probably reflects immune complex deposition. In addition to cutaneous manifestations, fever, arthralgias, and lymphadenopathy are prominent. Serum sickness was first described after administration of heterologous serum; since then, a clinically indistinguishable syndrome has been noted after administration of oral as well as parenteral drugs, including penicillin, streptokinase, halothane, various vaccines, and phenytoin. Unlike urticaria and angioedema, which occur promptly after drug exposure, serum sickness usually develops 1–3 weeks after exposure.

Phenytoin Hypersensitivity Syndrome

Phenytoin hypersensitivity syndrome is an infrequent but severe reaction that can occur in the first weeks of phenytoin use. Patients develop fever, an erythematous eruption that later becomes purpuric, facial edema, generalized painful lymphadenopathy, leukocytosis, hepatitis, and occasionally nephritis. Sulfasalazine (Azulfidine) has been associated with a syndrome clinically indistinguishable from that due to phenytoin.

LABORATORY FINDINGS IN DRUG REACTIONS

Laboratory examinations are not often helpful in the diagnosis and treatment of drug-induced cutaneous reactions. Although mild leukocytosis may occur with widespread eruptions, this finding does little to help the clinician determine whether the condition is due to drugs or infection. Eosinophilia is neither a sensitive nor a specific indicator of drug allergy. In the case of purpuric eruptions, measurements of platelet and clotting factors help to determine whether purpura is caused by a defect in hemostasis or by primary vascular injury due to a drug, a hypersensitivity disorder unrelated to drug use, or an infection.

In toxic drug eruptions, measurements of the drug level in the serum or tissues may provide further evidence of the cause. Many chemotherapeutic agents that inhibit cell division produce dose-related alopecia and mucositis. Ordinarily, these findings are so striking and so clearly related to dose that it is unnecessary to determine serum levels to confirm the diagnosis.

Special Examinations

A. Biopsy: Special laboratory examinations can sometimes differentiate a drug eruption from an eruption with a different cause. In toxic epidermal necrolysis, examination of a frozen section of skin biopsy of a patient with sudden onset of generalized blistering shows the epidermal split lower in the epidermis when the reaction is caused by a drug and higher when it is caused by a staphylococcal infection. Other drug eruptions with characteristic histopathologic features include the vegetative stages of

inactive iododerma and bromoderma. In cases of pigmentary alteration, biopsy study with appropriate stains can differentiate hyperpigmentation due to the deposition of melanin, iron, or a drug. Photoallergic and phototoxic reactions also have characteristic histopathologic characteristics. Immunofluorescent examination of a skin biopsy can differentiate lupus erythematosus from a photosensitivity eruption and a primary blistering disease such as pemphigoid from a bullous drug eruption or toxic epidermal necrolysis.

Other eruptions that can be caused by drugs may have characteristic histopathologic features also. These include erythema multiforme, fixed drug eruptions, erythema nodosum, and lichen planus. While biopsy confirms or suggests the specific diagnosis of such eruptions, they can usually be diagnosed by clinical examination alone; biopsy provides little help in determining a specific cause.

B. Drug Allergy Tests: In many cases, it is impossible to identify with certainty the agent causing an eruption; in vitro and in vivo tests for immunologic reactivity to a specific drug can be useful. Antigens for immediate skin tests are available for a limited number of drugs, including penicillin. Minute amounts of the haptens of penicillin most often responsible for immediate (IgE-mediated) hypersensitivity reactions are injected into the skin. (*Caution:* The test injection may precipitate anaphylaxis in extremely allergic patients.) A local wheal-and-flare reaction is noted within 1 hour if the test is positive. Many patients with clinical histories of penicillin allergy but negative skin tests tolerate the drug without incident; a positive test with a history of penicillin allergy indicates that the patient has a high risk of developing an immediate hypersensitivity reaction such as urticaria or anaphylaxis with rechallenge.

Radioallergosorbent (RAST) tests, which measure serum IgE against specific antigens, have been used to detect immediate hypersensitivity to penicillin and other drugs. Tests for delayed hypersensitivity to drugs are less sensitive and specific than tests for immediate hypersensitivity; the former are used for investigational purposes.

TREATMENT OF DRUG REACTIONS

The first step in the treatment of a drug reaction is to identify and withdraw the responsible agents. Additional therapy depends on the type and severity of the eruption. Although simple urticaria can be treated with an oral antihistamine, patients with systemic symptoms such as bronchospasm or signs of anaphylaxis may require emergency treatment with epinephrine as well as parenteral antihistamines and corticosteroids (see Chapter 34). Morbilliform eruptions should be treated symptomatically with oral antihistamines, topical antipruritic lotions, and baths. The value of treating these eruptions with topical and systemic corticosteroids is not established, and their use is seldom justified.

Eruptions with prominent oropharyngeal mucous membrane involvement, such as erythema multiforme, may require local analgesia and a special diet or even intravenous alimentation. Systemic analgesics may be required for widespread cutaneous eruptions, especially those characterized by loss of the normal cutaneous barrier. In widespread blistering eruptions, the patient must be monitored for secondary infection and fluid and electrolyte imbalance. Such patients are often hospitalized in special units used to treat severe thermal burns. Although systemic steroids are often used to treat toxic epidermal necrolysis, erythema multiforme, bullous skin eruptions, and vasculitis due to drug hypersensitivity, their efficacy has not been documented by well-controlled studies.

COMPLICATIONS & SEQUELAE

The principal complications of cutaneous drug eruptions are secondary infection and eczematization of a pruritic eruption as a result of continued scratching. When organs besides the skin are involved (eg, kidney, liver, joints, or lungs), the affected organ's normal function is sometimes permanently impaired. In the skin, pigmentary changes—including postinflammatory hyperpigmentation—may be associated with drug-induced inflammatory dermatitis. The characteristic pigmentation seen after resolution of fixed drug eruptions often persists for years and may be a substantial cosmetic liability. In diseases exacerbated by drugs, removal of the agent may be insufficient to bring the disease under control.

COURSE & PROGNOSIS

Most cutaneous drug eruptions will remit within 2 weeks after withdrawal of the responsible agent, leaving no permanent sequelae. Some of the reactions such as anaphylaxis, toxic epidermal necrolysis, vasculitis, severe erythema multiforme, and exfoliative erythroderma may be life-threatening. In general, the more extensive an eruption, the longer the period required for resolution. Once resolved, inadvertent rechallenge and recurrence are the principal danger.

REFERENCES

Bigby M et al: Drug-induced cutaneous reactions: A report from the Boston Collaborative Drug Surveillance Program on 15,438 consecutive inpatients, 1975 to 1982. JAMA 1986;256:3358.

Bruinsma W: *A Guide to Drug Eruptions,* 4th ed. American Overseas Book Co., 1987.

Dahl MV: A guide to the guises of drug-induced skin eruptions. Mod Med 1982;50:104.

Hutchinson TA, Lane DA: Assessing methods for causality assessment of suspected adverse drug reactions. J Clin Epidemiol 1989;42:5.

Jick H: Adverse drug reactions: The magnitude of the problem. J Allergy Clin Immunol 1984;74:555.

Revuz J et al: Toxic epidermal necrolysis: Clinical findings and prognosis factors in 87 patients. Arch Dermatol 1987;123:1160.

Wintroub BU, Stern R: Cutaneous drug reactions: Pathogenesis and clinical classification. J Am Acad Dermatol 1985;13:167.

Wintroub BU, Stern RS, Arndt KA: Cutaneous reactions to drugs. In: *Dermatology in General Medicine,* 3rd ed. Fitzpatrick TB, Freedberg IM (editors). McGraw-Hill, 1987.

Vasculitis

37

Frank Taliercio, MD, John M. Pelachyk, MD, & Edward A. Krull, MD

Although the term vasculitis can be loosely applied to many diseases, including those associated with only perivascular inflammation, the term should be reserved for disorders in which there are inflammatory cells in the vessel wall accompanied by fibrinoid deposits, necrosis, or other changes. A variety of classifications can be established on the basis of factors including the predominant inflammatory cell type (polymorphonuclear leukocytes, lymphocytes, histiocytes), the presence of nuclear dust (leukocytoclastic vasculitis) or significant necrosis, the size of the vessels involved, and the significance of systemic aspects of the disease. There are 2 major vasculitic groups that will be discussed: hypersensitivity vasculitis and systemic necrotizing vasculitis (Tables 37–1, 37–2, and 37–3).

SYSTEMIC NECROTIZING VASCULITIDES (Polyarteritis Nodosa & Allergic Granulomatosis)

Essentials of Diagnosis

- Constitutional symptoms of fever, malaise, and weight loss.
- Palpable purpura, nodules, ulcers, or plaques.
- Arthritis, arthralgias, or myalgias.
- Pulmonary, renal, and central nervous system involvement may be seen.

General Considerations

The polyarteritis nodosa group includes classic and cutaneous polyarteritis nodosa, allergic granulomatous angiitis (Churg-Strauss syndrome), and the "overlap syndrome" of systemic necrotizing vasculitis.

Polyarteritis nodosa is a necrotizing vasculitis of small and medium-sized muscular arteries involving renal and visceral arteries but not pulmonary vessels. Histopathologically, the vascular lesions tend to be segmental, in various stages of development, located at bifurcations and branching points of vessels, and forming aneurysms. Polyarteritis nodosa appears to

Table 37–1. Classification of vasculitis.

Large vessel vasculitis (predominantly an arteritis; terminology: systemic necrotizing vasculitis)
  Polyarteritis nodosa
    Systemic forms
    Cutaneous venulitis
  Wegener's granulomatosis
  Allergic granulomatous angiitis of Churg-Strauss
  Lethal midline granuloma
  Temporal arteritis
  Takayasu's arteritis
  Mucocutaneous lymph nodes syndrome (Kawasaki disease)
  Lymphomatoid granulomatosis
Small vessel vasculitis (predominantly postcapillary venules; terminology: hypersensitivity vasculitis, cutaneous necrotizing venulitis, leukocytoclastic vasculitis)
  Henoch Schönlein purpura
  Cryoglobulinemia
  Connective tissue disease
  Tumor-associated vasculitis
  Exogenous antigenic exposure
    Serum sickness and drugs
    Immunization
    Injections
  Exposure to other exogenous agents such as herbicides and insecticides
  Miscellaneous syndromes associated with leukocytoclastic vasculitis
    Granuloma faciale
    Erythema elevatum diutinum
    Hypocomplementemic urticarial vasculitis
    Retroperitoneal fibrosis
    Primary biliary cirrhosis
    Chronic active hepatitis
    Goodpasture's syndrome
    Inflammatory bowel disease
    Intestinal bypass surgery
    Eosinophilic fasciitis
    Benign idiopathic vasculitis of Cupps and Fauci

be an immune complex-mediated disease; hepatitis B antigenemia is implicated as a possible cause in approximately one-third of patients. Arterial hypertension often plays an important exacerbating role and probably contributes significantly to the compromise in renal function seen with the disease. There is a male:female ratio of 3:1, and the mean age at onset is 45 years. An infantile form of polyarteritis nodosa

Table 37–2. Diagnostic features of vasculitis.

Large vessel vasculitis (systemic necrotizing vasculitis)
Constitutional symptoms of fever, malaise, and weight loss.
Nodules, ulcers, plaques predominate; palpable purpura may also be present.
Arthritis, arthralgias, and myalgias may be present.
Pulmonary, renal, and nervous system involvement may be seen.
Small vessel vasculitis (hypersensitivity vasculitis; also referred to as cutaneous necrotizing venulitis or leukocytoclastic vasculitis)
Skin manifestations include palpable purpura predominantly but also urticarial plaques, vesicles, bullae, and nodules
Arthralgias, arthritis, hematuria, gastrointestinal bleeding, and occasionally neuropathy may be seen.
Constitutional symptoms and fever are present only in a minority of patients.

may have an extremely high frequency of involvement of the coronary arteries. In the cutaneous form, lesions of necrotizing vasculitis identical to those found in classic polyarteritis nodosa are found in small to medium-sized muscular arteries of the subcutaneous tissue and muscles, with sparing of the visceral vasculature.

Clinical Findings

A. Classic Polyarteritis Nodosa: The presenting signs and symptoms in classic polyarteritis nodosa are often nonspecific and include fever, malaise, and weight loss. Less commonly, mononeuritis multiplex and joint or muscle involvement are found. Renal involvement, though characteristic of polyarteritis nodosa, rarely produces symptoms. Clinical signs and symptoms relating to other systems include nausea, vomiting, abdominal pain, congestive heart failure, myocardial infarction, hypertension, cerebral vascular accidents, and altered mental status. Characteristic cutaneous lesions include tender subcutaneous nodules, purpura, and livedo reticularis. Frequently occurring laboratory abnormalities include an increased erythrocyte sedimentation rate, leukocytosis, anemia, thrombocytosis, active urinary sediment, circulating immune complexes, elevated rheumatoid factor, and a decreased complement level. Visceral

Table 37–3. Small vessel vasculitis. Drugs associated with hypersensitivity vasculitis, cutaneous necrotizing venulitis, leukocytoclastic vasculitis

1. Potentially, any drug can induce hypersensitivity vasculitis.
2. Some drugs implicated in hypersensitivity vasculitis
   a. Penicillin
   b. Sulfonamides
   c. Amphetamines
   d. Thiazides
   e. Street drugs
   f. Quinine and its derivatives
   g. Phenytoin sodium

angiography often shows multiple vascular or fusiform aneurysms in involved vessels.

B. Cutaneous Polyarteritis Nodosa: In cutaneous polyarteritis nodosa, systemic symptoms such as fever and arthralgias occur only occasionally. The skin lesions may include ulcerations, livedo reticularis, and nodules. The nodules may be painful and often occur in the livedo pattern. Laboratory studies usually show an elevated sedimentation rate and leukocytosis, with a normal urinalysis.

C. Allergic Granulomatous Angiitis (Churg-Strauss Syndrome): Allergic granulomatous angiitis shares many features with classic polyarteritis nodosa but is distinguished from it by frequent involvement of the pulmonary vasculature, involvement of vessels of various types and sizes, intra- and extravascular granuloma formation, and association with severe asthma and peripheral eosinophilia. Histopathologically, the disorder manifests as a panarteritis of small and medium-sized vessels, often with intense eosinophilic infiltration. The lesions tend to be multistaged. The sex ratio and mean age at onset are similar to those of classic polyarteritis nodosa.

D. Both Classic Polyarteritis Nodosa and Churg-Strauss Syndrome: Patients exhibiting clinical and pathologic features of both classic polyarteritis nodosa and allergic granulomatous angiitis but not classifiable in either category comprise a group termed the "overlap syndrome" of systemic necrotizing vasculitis.

Differential Diagnosis

Diseases that may be associated with necrotizing vasculitis similar to that seen in classic polyarteritis nodosa include acute otitis media, streptococcal infection, hepatitis B antigenemia, endocarditis, collagen vascular diseases, hairy cell leukemia, amphetamine drug abuse, and enteritis.

Diseases associated with granulomas, hypereosinophilia, or pulmonary symptoms should be considered in the differential diagnosis of allergic granulomatous angiitis. These include Wegener's granulomatosis, allergic aspergillosis, Loeffler's syndrome, sarcoidosis, and idiopathic hypereosinophilic syndrome.

Complications & Sequelae

Complications of untreated polyarteritis nodosa include glomerulosclerosis with renal failure, myocardial infarction, intestinal infarction with bleeding and pain, severe hypertension, and peripheral neuropathy. Many of the complications of allergic granulomatous angiitis are similar to those of polyarteritis nodosa, except that there is a lower incidence of renal failure and the occurrence of pulmonary complications such as pneumonia and status asthmaticus in allergic granulomatous angiitis.

Treatment

Corticosteroid therapy alone often induces only

partial remission of polyarteritis nodosa or masks smoldering disease, so that acute disease activity is suppressed while insidious, relentless organ system damage continues. For that reason cyclophosphamide, alone or in combination with prednisone, is the treatment of choice. Careful control of hypertension must be maintained.

To control the manifestations of *cutaneous* polyarteritis nodosa, corticosteroids, aspirin, sulfapyridine, and dapsone have been utilized. The use of cytotoxic agents such as cyclophosphamide has met with variable success.

The mainstay of treatment of allergic granulomatous angiitis is corticosteroids with or without cytotoxic agents.

Course & Prognosis

The overall 5-year survival rate for untreated classic polyarteritis nodosa is 13%. Treatment with corticosteroids improves the outlook to 48%, while combination therapy with immunosuppressive agents and corticosteroids increases the 5-year survival rate to over 80%. Patients with cutaneous polyarteritis nodosa generally do not develop systemic signs, and the long-term prognosis in patients with this disease is good regardless of treatment. Untreated allergic granulomatous angiitis has a 5-year survival rate of only 4%, while treatment with corticosteroids or cytotoxic agents increases this figure to approximately 60%.

WEGENER'S GRANULOMATOSIS

Essentials of Diagnosis

- Sinusitis, rhinitis, nasal obstruction.
- Cough, dyspnea, chest pain.
- Glomerulonephritis.
- Palpable purpura;, or nodules, plaques, necrosis, or skin ulcers.
- Granulomatous vasculitis.
- Presence of antineutrophil cytoplasmic antibody in serum.

General Considerations

Wegener's granulomatosis is characterized by necrotizing granulomatous vasculitis of the upper and lower respiratory tracts, glomerulonephritis, and variable degrees of small vessel vasculitis. Patients may develop large skin ulcers. The mean age at onset is approximately 40 years, and there is a slight male preponderance. A "limited" form of Wegener's granulomatosis, characterized by the absence of upper respiratory tract symptoms and glomerulonephritis, has been described. The pathogenesis of this disorder is unknown.

Clinical Findings

A. Symptoms and Signs: Patients with Wegener's granulomatosis most frequently present with signs and symptoms referable to the upper respiratory tract, including sinusitis, rhinitis, and nasal obstruction. Destruction of the nasal septal cartilage may produce a "saddle nose" deformity. Cough, dyspnea, and chest pain are associated with lower respiratory tract involvement. Glomerulonephritis is often manifested as an abnormal urinary sediment. Cutaneous manifestations occur in half of patients, and these include palpable purpura, nodules, plaques, infarctive lesions, and ulcers. Acne conglobata-like cysts associated with draining otitis and rhinitis has also been described. Other organ systems involved include the eyes, ears, heart, and central nervous system.

B. Laboratory Findings: Elevations of the erythrocyte sedimentation rate to 80 mm/h or greater are frequent, as are leukocytosis, thrombocytosis, elevated rheumatoid factor, and elevated immunoglobulins. Patients typically have antibodies in serum that react with cytoplasm of normal neutrophils in vitro. Typical findings on chest x-ray include multiple bilateral nodular cavitary infiltrates.

Differential Diagnosis

The differential diagnosis includes diseases with a predominantly vasculitic picture, granulomatous diseases, or diseases with a combined vasculitic and granulomatous process.

Complications

Complications of Wegener's granulomatosis include progressive pulmonary and renal failure, cachexia, destruction of the paranasal sinuses, intractable cardiac arrhythmias, and severe episcleritis.

Treatment

Initial therapy with cyclophosphamide and prednisone, followed by cyclophosphamide maintenance therapy, is a highly effective therapeutic approach to Wegener's granulomatosis. Cyclophosphamide intravenously may be necessary initially to control rapidly progressive renal disease. Sinusitis is treated with drainage, local irrigations, and appropriate antibiotic therapy. Cyclosporine has also been used successfully in patients resistant to conventional therapy. Trimethoprim-sulfamethoxazole may be helpful ancillary treatment.

Course

Untreated Wegener's granulomatosis is a progressive, rapidly fatal disease and has a 90% mortality rate 2 years after diagnosis, with a mean survival rate of only 5 months. Use of corticosteroids alone has resulted in only a modest improvement in this figure, while cyclophosphamide therapy in combination with prednisone has induced clinical remission in a large percentage of patients.

LYMPHOMATOID GRANULOMATOSIS

Essentials of Diagnosis

- Cough, dyspnea, chest pain.
- Fever, malaise.
- Pink macules or papules, or large nodules and ulcers.
- Angiodestructive granulomatous vasculitis with atypical lymphocytes.

General Considerations

Lymphomatoid granulomatosis is an angiocentric and angiodestructive lymphoreticular proliferative and granulomatous disorder, characterized by multisystem infiltration with atypical plasmacytoid and lymphocytoid cells. Pulmonary involvement is characteristic, but the kidneys and the reticuloendothelial system are usually spared. Skin lesions are variable and range from pink macules and papules to nodules or ulcers. Lymphomatoid granulomatosis is rare, with a mean age at onset of 48 years and a male:female preponderance of 2:1. The cause is unknown. The disease represents a spectrum ranging from a benign, localized form to a frankly neoplastic lymphoproliferative disorder that may retain some of the features of the more benign disease.

Clinical Features

A. Symptoms and Signs: Most patients with lymphomatoid granulomatosis have signs and symptoms of lower respiratory tract involvement, including cough, dyspnea, and chest pain. Intranasal destruction or ulcerative lesions in the palate or nasopharynx may occur. Constitutional symptoms including fatigue, fever, weight loss, malaise, and arthralgias are common. Seizures or peripheral neuropathy may occur. Skin lesions, seen in 45% of patients, include erythematous macules, indurated plaques, or subcutaneous nodules, often present on the lower extremities.

B. Laboratory Findings: Leukocytosis is seen in 50% of patients, and a relative lymphocytosis may suggest progression to a frank neoplastic process. Leukopenia is present in 20% of patients, but the hematocrit, sedimentation rate, urinalysis, and immunoglobulin levels are usually normal. The most common chest x-ray finding consists of bilateral nodular densities of various sizes in the lower lung field.

Differential Diagnosis

The differential diagnosis of lymphomatoid granulomatosis includes the other systemic necrotizing vasculitides, as well as lymphomatoid papulosis and lymphoma.

Complications

The most severe complication of lymphomatoid granulomatosis is progressive pulmonary disease leading to respiratory insufficiency or massive pulmonary hemorrhage. Uncontrolled central nervous system disease and progression to atypical lymphoma with involvement of the reticuloendothelial system are other serious sequelae.

Treatment

Early treatment of lymphomatoid granulomatosis with the cyclophosphamide and prednisone regimen utilized in polyarteritis nodosa and Wegener's granulomatosis has been somewhat effective in producing partial remission. Its use in patients with late or widespread disease has a uniformly poor result. Adjunctive radiation therapy may be valuable in treating symptomatic localized lesions.

Course & Prognosis

In considering the entire spectrum of lymphomatoid granulomatosis, patients with untreated disease have an extremely poor prognosis, with a greater than 90% mortality rate by 3 years after diagnosis and a mean survival rate of only 11 months. Some long-term remissions in patients have been achieved with combined cyclophosphamide and prednisone therapy, especially if treatment is begun early before widespread systemic involvement is present.

MIDLINE GRANULOMA

The many causes of lethal midline granuloma have led to confusion in terminology. The disease was first called "progressive lethal granulomatous ulceration." Because of improved outcomes with current treatment methods and a better understanding of etiologic factors, the simpler term "midline granuloma" with further subclassification as occasioned by the clinical presentation is now favored. Midline granuloma may be subclassified into midline malignant reticulosis, idiopathic midline granuloma, and Wegener's granulomatosis.

The average age at onset is 45 years, with a range of 18 to 80 years. Males predominate in a ratio of 3:1.

Clinical Findings

A. Symptoms and Signs: Midline granuloma is a progressive localized, destructive, necrotizing granuloma of the nose, paranasal sinuses, and palate. It usually begins with swelling of nasal tissue and nasal or sinus drainage, followed by ulceration. Progression of ulcerations may lead to extensive destruction of the face, sinuses, hard palate, hypopharynx, and larynx. Death may result from infection, cachexia, or hemorrhage.

B. Laboratory Findings: Multiple biopsies may be required to separate midline granuloma from Wegener's granulomatosis and malignant lymphomas. Infectious causes need to be excluded by appropriate studies.

Differential Diagnosis

A number of diseases may cause destructive midline disease. These include infections such as syphilis and malignant disorders such as lymphoma and carcinoma. Differentiation from Wegener's granulomatosis may be difficult, and some consider Wegener's granulomatosis to be a form of midline granuloma. However, Wegener's granulomatosis may well be a disease distinct from midline granuloma. The vasculitis in Wegener's granulomatosis appears in nonnecrotic sites and infrequently develops only upper airway lesions. These findings are in contrast to those of idiopathic midline granuloma. Infectious causes of ulcers should be ruled out by biopsy.

Treatment

Treatment should be directed toward the underlying disease. Both the malignant reticulosis form and idiopathic midline granuloma respond to irradiation. Wegener's granulomatosis responds to cyclophosphamide and corticosteroids.

Every effort should be made to arrive at a specific diagnosis for which a specific treatment program can be developed. In the early phases of the disease, this may be difficult. Repeated studies and biopsies may be necessary, but even so the diagnosis may not be clear. Initiation of cyclophosphamide or irradiation treatment may have to depend on the clinician's best diagnostic assessment of the patient's clinical and pathologic status.

GIANT CELL ARTERITIDES

The giant cell arteritides include temporal arteritis and Takayasu's arteritis. Both are characterized by granulomatous vasculitis of medium and large arteries, with characteristic involvement of branches of the carotid artery in temporal arteritis, and of the aortic arch and its branches in Takayasu's arteritis. Cutaneous lesions are seen only rarely in temporal arteritis (nodules, ecchymosis, or necrosis in skin supplied by a temporal artery) and are absent in patients with Takayasu's arteritis.

MUCOCUTANEOUS LYMPH NODE SYNDROME
(Kawasaki Disease)

Mucocutaneous lymph node syndrome is a febrile illness that occurs predominantly in children under 5 years of age, characterized by (1) acute nonsuppurative cervical lymphadenopathy; (2) fever persisting 5 days or more; (3) changes in the peripheral extremities (initially indurating edema and redness; later, desquamation of the palms and soles); (4) bilateral conjunctival injection; (5) changes of the oral mucosa, including diffuse erythema of the oropharynx, red lips, and "strawberry tongue"; and (6) a polymorphous but frequently scarlatiniform body rash. Five of the 6 principal criteria should be present to make a diagnosis. Other signs and symptoms include diarrhea, arthritis-arthralgia, and encephalopathy. The most frequent serious feature is cardiac disease with coronary arterial involvement. Biopsies of vessels are consistent with those of polyarteritis nodosa. About 2% of the children die. The cause is unclear.

Aspirin and intravenous gamma globulin, alone or in combination, may reduce the coronary vessel complications. Systemic corticosteroids may be necessary for the acute shocklike symptoms, but the benefit in terms of long-term coronary vessel and myocardial effects is controversial.

HYPERSENSITIVITY VASCULITIS

Essentials of Diagnosis

- Palpable purpura; occasionally, urticarial plaques, vesicles, bullae, and nodules (Fig 37–1).
- Arthralgias, arthritis, hematuria, gastrointestinal bleeding, and neuropathy (variable).
- Constitutional symptoms and fever are infrequent.

General Considerations

The spectrum of hypersensitivity vasculitis can be grouped into a number of diseases (Tables 37–1 and 37–2) characterized histopathologically by intense neutrophilic infiltrations in and around skin venules. Neutrophils lyse (leukocytoclasis), so the perivascular area also contains remnants of neutrophil nuclei (nuclear dust). Accompanying the neutrophilic infiltrate are edema, fibrinoid necrosis of the blood vessel walls, and extravasation of red blood cells into the perivascular space. Specimens from early lesions tend to demonstrate a more acute inflammatory response (polymorphonuclear leukocytes and leukocytoclasis), whereas in chronic vasculitis, lymphocytic infiltrate may be dominant.

Organ systems other than skin can be involved, most frequently the kidneys (hematuria), gastrointestinal tract (melena), central nervous system (peripheral neuropathy), and joints (arthralgias).

The mechanism responsible for development of hypersensitivity vasculitis is related to the deposition of immune complexes in blood vessel walls. In several processes, specific antigens have been identified.

Classification
& Clinical Findings

A. Serum Sickness and Drugs: Serum sickness results from a reaction to foreign or heterologous serum protein. This is rare because human globulins have generally replaced animal globulins as antitoxins. Penicillin, sulfonamides, and other drugs may produce a serum sickness-like reaction. Immune complexes result in postcapillary venulitis.

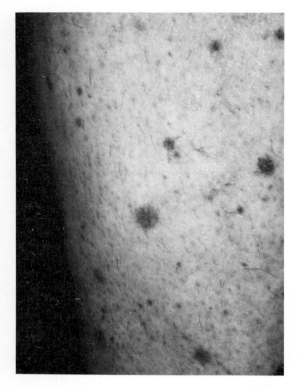

Figure 37–1. The hallmark of hypersensitivity vasculitis is palpable purpura.

The syndrome occurs within 7–10 days following initial exposure and sooner following reexposure. Skin lesions are usually in the same stage of development. Palpable purpura or urticarial plaques are seen most often. Patients with serum sickness develop a rather unique serpentine-bordered erythema of the feet with purpura. Fever, arthralgias, and lymphadenopathy are frequent. Glomerulonephritis, peripheral neuropathy, carditis, and encephalitis are rare. Recovery is generally complete within 2 weeks if the offending antigen is removed.

Laboratory findings include elevated sedimentation rate and polymorphonuclear leukocytosis. Total hemolytic complement levels may be decreased, and circulating immune complexes may be detected. IgG antibodies against heterologous serum proteins can be demonstrated occasionally in cases of true serum sickness.

Immunization and infection may cause a similar syndrome. Frequently implicated infections include hepatitis B, tuberculosis, and infections with streptococci, Epstein-Barr virus, and cytomegalovirus.

Insecticides, herbicides, and other exogenous agents can produce a hypersensitivity vasculitis by a similar mechanism.

B. Henoch-Schönlein Purpura: This process affects mainly children and young adults and occurs most often in the spring following an upper respiratory infection. The most common skin manifestation is palpable purpura, though maculopapular wheals and occasionally ulcers are seen. The lesions are fairly uniform in size and localized to dependent areas such as the legs; they may contain a small dusky center representing epidermal necrosis. Fever, joint symptoms, abdominal pain, gastrointestinal bleeding, and proliferative glomerulonephritis are common. The renal disease, characterized clinically by hematuria, is generally self-limiting.

Pathogenetically, Henoch-Schönlein purpura is a vasculitis caused by deposits of IgA immune complexes with activation of the alternate complement pathway. Mild leukocytosis, an elevated sedimentation rate, microscopic hematuria, proteinuria, red blood cell casts, and elevated serum IgA are frequent laboratory abnormalities. Immunofluorescence may disclose IgA in the blood vessel walls in about 70% of cases, but biopsies must be from new lesions or normal skin. Because blood vessels and usually immune complexes are quickly destroyed by inflammation, direct immunofluorescence examination of normal skin is often worthwhile.

C. Cryoglobulinemia: The mixed monoclonal-polyclonal type II cryoglobulinemia is associated with vasculitis due to cryoprecipitate deposition in blood vessel walls. The clinical and histologic presentation of cryoglobulin-associated vasculitis is similar to that of other forms of hypersensitivity leukocytoclastic vasculitis. This subject is discussed in more detail below.

D. Vasculitis Associated With Connective Tissue Disease: Vasculitis occurs most often with rheumatoid arthritis and systemic lupus erythematosus but may be seen with dermatomyositis, Sjögren's syndrome, scleroderma, and rheumatic fever. The offending antigen is sometimes traced to endogenous antigens such as serum proteins or DNA.

The most frequent skin lesions are urticarial vasculitic plaques and palpable purpura. In patients with rheumatoid arthritis, vasculitis is seen, especially in patients with high titers of rheumatoid factor.

E. Tumor-Associated Vasculitis: Endogenous tumor-associated antigens may be responsible for leukocytoclastic vasculitis. Patients with Hodgkin's disease, other lymphomas, multiple myeloma, malignant melanoma, breast cancer, esophageal cancer, osteogenic sarcoma, and other cancers can have associated hypersensitivity leukocytoclastic vasculitis. Circulating immune complexes have been demonstrated by the Raji cell assay. The spectrum of disease resembles other forms of hypersensitivity vasculitis.

F. Miscellaneous Syndromes: A variety of different syndromes listed previously are associated with leukocytoclastic vasculitis. In most, the offending antigen is unknown, although a hypersensitivity phenomenon is suggested.

Prevention

Removal of the offending antigens and treatment of known infections are helpful in decreasing the incidence of these disorders. Heterologous serum should not be given unless the indications seem to outweigh the risks.

Treatment

The causal antigen should be eliminated if possible. If the condition is suspected to be due to a drug, administration of the drug should be stopped. Antibiotics may remove antigens of infectious origin. Plasmapheresis may be used in severe cases with life-threatening vasculitis of internal organs.

Many patients do not require treatment, especially when the vasculitis is limited to the skin. Colchicine, 0.6 mg twice daily, may help adults, as may dapsone, 100 mg daily (see Chapter 53). Nonsteroidal anti-inflammatory agents such as aspirin may help and may also decrease the pain of arthritis and arthralgias.

If renal disease is present or if other organ systems are involved, systemic steroids (eg, prednisone) may be necessary at the lowest dosage that controls the vasculitis. Cyclophosphamide has also been used.

Course & Prognosis

The eventual outcome depends on the primary disease process. In the case of infections and drug-associated hypersensitivity, the prognosis is excellent if the offending agent is removed. Other forms of vasculitis may persist as long as the primary disease process is active. Sometimes the kidney vasculitis can persist after skin lesions are gone and eventually cause renal failure.

URTICARIAL VASCULITIS

Urticarial vasculitis is a heterogeneous symptom complex in which urticarial lesions show histopathologic evidence of leukocytoclastic vasculitis. This symptom complex may represent a spectrum extending from predominantly urticaria (with perhaps 20% of patients showing evidence of vasculitis) to hypocomplementemic vasculitis with significant systemic involvement.

The more characteristic cutaneous lesions of urticarial vasculitis include (1) individual wheals that frequently extend beyond 6 hours to as long as 24–72 hours, as compared to a few hours for most lesions of simple urticaria; (2) purpura reflecting vasculitis; and (3) in some cases, Raynaud's phenomenon, livedo vasculitis, erythema multiforme-like lesions, and angioedema. Systemic symptoms and other organ involvement may include (in descending order of frequency) arthralgias and arthritis, gastrointestinal symptoms, renal disease (especially glomerulonephritis), neurologic symptoms, lymphadenopathy, and asthma. A high percentage of cases are associated with low complement levels, and about half have circulating immune complexes. Immunoglobulin-complement deposition in vessel walls may be demonstrated by direct immunofluorescence. Sedimentation rates are elevated in most patients.

Treatment is similar to that of hypersensitivity vasculitis and has included corticosteroids, cytotoxic agents, indomethacin, sulfonamides, nicotinic acid, and plasmapheresis. The course tends to be chronic.

GRANULOMA FACIALE

Granuloma faciale is an uncommon skin disease. A single reddish or reddish-brown macule, plaque, or nodule develops almost exclusively on the face, but disseminated forms occur. The lesions are asymptomatic; the surface is smooth and intact. No systemic symptoms or signs occur. Laboratory data are not helpful. Biopsy reveals a dense infiltrate in the dermis, with a clear "Grenz" zone between the epidermis and the infiltrate. The infiltrate is polymorphous, with significant eosinophilia. Leukocytoclastic vasculitis is also present.

Treatment has not been consistently successful. Dapsone is usually preferred, but cryotherapy, intralesional corticosteroids, and x-ray have sometimes been of benefit.

ERYTHEMA ELEVATUM DIUTINUM

Erythema elevatum diutinum is a rare disease characterized by persistent, symmetric brownish red, pink, sometimes yellowish or purple papules, plaques, and nodules on the extensor surfaces of the arms and legs. Often they involve the elbows and knees, as well as the skin over the joints of the hands and feet. Extracellular cholesterosis, associated with secondary lipid deposits, is probably a variant of erythema elevatum diutinum. Although systemic involvement is uncommon, arthralgias and persisting bacterial infections are occasionally associated. The course of erythema elevatum diutinum is chronic; the disease may spontaneously involute after 5–10 years. Biopsies reveal leukocytoclastic vasculitis and fibrinoid changes in the vessel walls.

Dapsone (initial dosages of 100–250 mg) may control the process.

LIVEDO RETICULARIS

In this vascular phenomenon, a fixed reddish-blue reticular pattern gives the skin a mottled or blotchy appearance. Ulcerations may occur (Fig 37–2). Depending on the underlying cause, the distribution may be localized, diffuse, or generalized. Transient physiologic blotchy reticular patterns, seen especially in

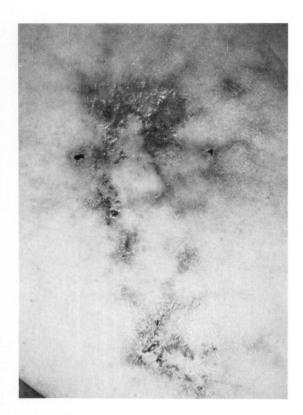

Figure 37–2. Livedo reticularis with skin ulcers.

infants, young children, and women exposed to cold, are termed cutis marmorata rather than livedo reticularis.

Livedo reticularis is a physical sign of many underlying diseases, including arteriosclerosis, the collagen-vascular diseases, and intravascular occlusive diseases (ie, cryoglobulinemias, thrombocythemias). Extensive livedo reticularis has been associated with cerebrovascular disease, including cerebral vascular accidents. Abnormal antiphospholipid activity may account for thrombotic phenomena and cerebral vascular accidents associated with livedo reticularis. When the diagnosis of livedo reticularis is made, underlying causes must be sought.

Treatment is directed toward the underlying disease.

ATROPHIE BLANCHE
(Livedo Vasculitis)

Atrophie blanche is the name given to peculiar scars which are porcelain-white and studded with pepperlike red macules and telangiectases. They are the healed result of painful vasculitic infarctive lesions that may or may not cause overt ulcers. If livedo

is also present, this syndrome is called livedo vasculitis; but atrophie blanche can also occur in polyarteritis nodosa, lupus erythematosus, and stasis dermatitis (Fig 37–3). Immunoglobulin and C3 have been noted in the vessel walls, suggesting a possible immunologic mechanism. In addition, abnormal antiphospholipid activity, ie, the anticardiolipin syndrome, may account for thrombotic symptoms of the skin, central nervous system, and other organs.

The more common sites of such lesions are the dorsa of the feet, ankles, and legs. The lesions may begin as purpuric macules and papules that progress to ulcers and characteristic white, painful scars.

The disorder is associated with a decrease in fibrinolytic activity in skin and increased platelet adhesiveness.

Phenformin and ethylestrenol in combination have been effective in the treatment of atrophie blanche, probably because of their enhancement of fibrinolytic activity. Combinations of aspirin (325 mg daily or 3 times a day) and dipyridamole (50 mg 3 times daily), which affect platelet function, are helpful. Pentoxifylline (Trental), 400 mg 3 times daily with meals, has also been used.

DIABETIC DERMOPATHY

Slightly depressed, light brown, 0.5- to 2-cm lesions occurring over the anterior tibia in diabetic patients have been termed diabetic dermopathy. Although appearing as residua of trauma, neither the

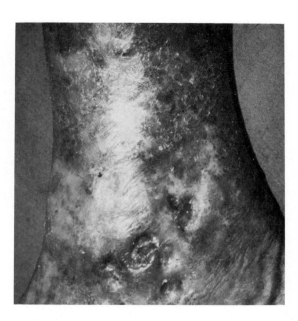

Figure 37–3. Atrophie blanche. Note the porcelain-white irregularly shaped patch studded with macules that resemble red chili peppers.

history nor attempts at duplication by trauma lend credence to this theory. Biopsies are not specific. The lesions tend to be associated with an increased incidence of retinopathy, nephropathy, and neuropathy, and so the skin lesions may be due to angiopathy.

MALIGNANT ATROPHIC PAPULOSIS
(Degos' Syndrome)

Malignant atrophic papulosis is a rare, frequently fatal disease characterized by porcelain-white skin lesions. The initial lesions are usually erythematous or flesh-colored papules about 1 cm or smaller. After a few weeks, umbilication occurs and the typical porcelain-white center appears. The number is variable, ranging from as few as 5 to as many as 100. Half the cases develop gastrointestinal involvement in weeks to years. White patches occur on the serosal surface of the intestine, and single or multiple bowel perforations ensue. Bowel involvement usually is associated with a fatal course. Central nervous system involvement is usually also fatal. Identical lesions have been reported with systemic lupus erythematosus.

Histopathologically, the early lesions show mucin accumulation. In older lesions, a wedge-shaped eosinophilic area may extend to the surface of the skin, and the vessel may be filled with fibrin. Immunoglobulin deposits in the vessel walls are infrequently demonstrated. The media and adventitia, unlike those in many of the vasculitides, are not involved. Decreased fibrinolytic activity at the local level has been noted, but phenformin and ethylestrenol (fibrinolytic enhancers) have not been successful.

No effective treatment is known. Surgical excision of bowel lesions is not feasible because of the number of lesions and the continuous course.

REFERENCES

Aboobaker J et al: Urticarial vasculitis. Clin Exp Dermatol 1986;11:436.

Bacon PA: Vasculitis: Clinical aspects and therapy. Acta Med Scand 1987;715(Suppl):157.

Bauer M, Levan NE: Diabetic dermangiopathy: A spectrum including pigmented pretibial patches and necrobiosis lipoidica diabeticorum. Br J Dermatol 1970;83:528.

Bierman FZ.: Kawasaki disease. J Pediatr 1987;111:789.

Bisaccia E et al: Urticarial vasculitis progressing to systemic lupus erythematosus. Arch Dermatol 1988;124:1088.

Borleffs JCC, Derksen RHWM, Hené R: Wegener's granulomatosis and cyclosporine. Transpl Proc 1988;20(Suppl 4):344.

Burton JL: Livedo reticularis, porcelain white scars, and cerebral thromboses. Lancet 1988;1:1263.

Callen JP: Colchicine is effective in controlling cutaneous leukocytoclastic vasculitis. J Am Acad Dermatol 1985;13:193.

Callen JP: Cutaneous vasculitis and its relationship to systemic disease. Australas J Dermatol 1989;28:49.

Camisa C: Lymphomatoid granulomatosis: Two cases with skin involvement. J Am Acad Dermatol 1989;20:571.

Case Records of the Massachusetts General Hospital: Case 17–1986: 18-year-old man with apical infiltrate and skin lesions (Wegener's granulomatosis). N Eng J Med 1986;314:1170.

Case Records of the Massachusetts General Hospital: Case 18–1987: 31-year-old woman with asthma and neurologic deficits (Churg-Strauss). N Eng J Med 1987;316:1139.

Case Records of the Massachusetts General Hospital: Case 31-1988: Fever, rash, pains in the lower legs (periarteritis nodosa). N Eng J Med 1988;319:292.

Champion RH: Livedo reticularis: A review. Br J Dermatol 1965;77:167.

Chumbley LC, Harrison EG Jr, DeRemee RA: Allergic granulomatosis and angiitis (Churg-Strauss syndrome): Report and analysis of 30 cases. Mayo Clin Proc 1977;52:477.

Drucker CR, Duncan WC: Antiplatelet therapy in atrophie blanche and livedo vasculitis. J Am Acad Dermatol 1982;7:359.

Ekenstam E, Callen JP et al: Cutaneous leukocytoclastic vasculitis: Clinical and laboratory features of 82 patients seen in private practice. Arch Dermatol 1984;120:484.

Evans GH et al: Degos' disease: A rare cause of multiple intestinal perforation. J R Coll Surg Edinb 1987;32:371.

Fauci AS et al: Midline granuloma or Wegener's granulomatosis. Ann Intern Med 1976;84:609.

Fauci AS et al: Wegener's granulomatosis: Prospective clinical and therapeutic experience with 85 patients for 21 years. Ann Intern Med 98:76-85, 1983.

Fauci AS, Haynes B, Katz P: The spectrum of vasculitis: Clinical, pathologic, immunologic, and therapeutic considerations. Ann Intern Med 1978;89:660.

Ford EG et al: Management of Henoch-Schönlein purpura and polyarteritis nodosa. Tex Med (Aug) 1987;83: 54.

Fredenberg MF et al: Sulfone therapy in the treatment of leukocytoclastic vasculitis. J Am Acad Dermatol 1987;16:772.

Friedman I: McBride and the mid-facial granuloma syndrome. J Laryngol Otol 1983;96:1.

Gammon WR: Urticarial vasculitis. Dermatol Clin 1985;3:97.

Grob JJ et al: Thrombotic skin disease as a marker of the anticardiolipin syndrome: Livedo vasculitis and distal gangrene associated with abnormal antiphospholipid activity. J Am Acad Dermatol 1989;20:1063.

Grob JJ et al: Thrombotic skin disease as a marker of the anticardiolipin syndrome: Livedo vasculitis and distal gangrene associated with abnormal antiphospholipid activity. J Am Acad Dermatol 1989;20:1063.

Guillevin L et al: Clinical findings and prognosis of polyarteritis nodosa and Churg-Strauss angiitis: A study in 165 patients. Br J Rheumatol 1988;27:258.

Hudson LD: Granuloma faciale: Treatment with topical psoralen and UVA. J Am Acad Dermatol 1983; 8:559.

Katz SI et al: Erythema elevatum diutinum: Skin and systemic manifestations, immunologic studies, and successful treatment with dapsone. Medicine 1977;56:443.

Kern AB: Atrophie blanche: Report of two patients treated with aspirin and dipyridamole. J Am Acad Dermatol 1982;6:1048.

Mackel SE, Jordon RE: Leukocytoclastic vasculitis: A cutaneous expression of immune complex disease. Arch Dermatol 1982;118:296.

O'Connor JC et al: Review of diseases presenting as "midline granuloma." Clinical implications for the appropriate workup of patients with midline granuloma syndrome with emphasis on recent diagnostic advances in lymphoid neoplasms that present as midline destructive lesions. Acta Otolaryngol 1987;(Suppl 439):1.

Pallesen RM, Rasmussen NR: Malignant atrophic papulosis: Degos' syndrome. Acta Chir Scand 1979;145:279.

Rossignol M et al: Skin telangiectases and ischaemic disorders in primary aluminum production workers. Br J Ind Med 1988;45:198.

Rowley AH et al: Kawasaki disease: New etiologic clues and advances in therapy. Pediatr Dermatol 1987;4:134.

Ruey-Bin C et al: Treatment of "idiopathic midline destructive disease" by irradiation. J Cranio-Max-Fac Surg 1988;16:375.

Rusin LJ, Dubin HV, Taylor WB: Disseminated granuloma faciale. Arch Dermatol 1976;112:1575.

Sams WM Jr: Livedo vasculitis therapy with pentoxifylline. Arch Dermatol 1988;124:684.

Sams WM Jr: Necrotizing vasculitis. J Am Acad Dermatol 1980;3:1.

Schroeter AL et al: Livedo vasculitis (the vasculitis of atrophie blanche): Immunohistopathologic study. Arch Dermatol 1975;111:188.

Stephens WP, Ferguson IT: Livedo reticularis and cerebrovascular disease. Postgrad Med J 1982;58:70.

Van Hale HM et al: Henoch-Schönlein vasculitis: Direct immunofluorescence study of uninvolved skin. J Am Acad Dermatol 15:665-670, 1986.

West BC et al: Wegener granulomatosis and trimethoprim-sulfamethoxazole: Complete remission after a 20-year course. Ann Intern Med 1987;106:840.

Photosensitivity Diseases

38

John H. Epstein, MD

The photobiologic effects of most interest to the dermatologist are those caused by the visible light portion and adjacent ultraviolet bands (UVA, UVB, UVC) of the electromagnetic spectrum: UVA: long-wave ultraviolet light (320–400 nm); UVB: middle-wave ultraviolet light (290–320 nm); UVC: short-wave ultraviolet light (200–290 nm); visible light: wavelengths of 400–760 nm.

The rays of the sun that reach the earth's surface extend from about 290 nm in the UVB range through the visible wavelengths, infrared wavelengths, and beyond. Most photobiologic events occurring in the skin are produced by UVB rays, which inhibit DNA, RNA, and protein synthesis and mitosis formation, stimulate vitamin D production, cause sunburn (acute erythema), induce new pigment formation, produce cell death, inhibit delayed hypersensitivity, and are carcinogenic. In general, UVB radiation does not pass through window glass.

In contrast, UVA radiation does penetrate through window glass and can also induce significant photobiologic effects, though in general it induces biologic changes in skin much less efficiently than UVB radiation. In human skin, UVA can darken melanin that is already present, induce new pigment formation and even erythema, inhibit delayed hypersensitivity responses, augment acute UVB injury, and aggravate certain photosensitive diseases.

In experimental animals, UVA has been shown to augment UVB-induced cancer formation and in large enough amounts can be carcinogenic in itself. UVA radiation also is extremely important to human photobiology because it is responsible for almost all exogenously photosensitized reactions in the skin, eg, those due to topical chemicals or systemic medications.

Photosensitivity denotes adverse reactions to sunlight or artificial light. Two types of reactions may occur: phototoxic or photoallergic. Phototoxic reactions can be photodynamic or nonphotodynamic; photodynamic reactions (eg, in the porphyrias) require oxygen, whereas nonphotodynamic reactions (eg, involving psoralens) do not. This chapter considers both types together.

Phototoxic reactions are commonplace and will occur in anyone given sufficient appropriate radiant energy and sufficient amounts of exogenous or endogenous photosensitizers in the skin. Reactions usually take the form of delayed erythema and edema followed by hyperpigmentation resembling sunburn. Ordinary sunburn is the most common phototoxic reaction.

In contrast, photoallergic reactions are uncommon and represent acquired altered reactivities mediated by immunologic hypersensitivity mechanisms. Lesions vary from immediate urticarial reactions to delayed papular or eczematous eruptions. In general, less radiant energy is required to produce photoallergic reactions than phototoxic reactions.

Photosensitivity reactions may be grouped into 3 categories: (1) due to loss or lack of protection against the damaging effects of sunlight, (2) due to an endogenous or exogenous photosensitizing molecule (photosensitizer) in the skin, and (3) due to unknown causes (ie, no apparent loss or lack of protection and no known photosensitizer).

PHOTOSENSITIVITY DUE TO LOSS OR LACK OF PROTECTION

Most cases of photosensitivity due to loss or lack of protection are due to deficiency or absence of melanin, the main natural protection in humans (see also Chapter 22). Such patients may have oculocutaneous albinism, in which melanocytes are present but are defective in the tyrosinase enzyme system (essential for melanin formation); vitiligo, a disease with loss of pigment cells; or Chédiak-Higashi syndrome or phenylketonuria, 2 diseases characterized by pigmentary dilution. In xeroderma pigmentosum, patients also demonstrate extreme photosensitivity, but lack of protection is not due to defects or lack of melanin. Instead, these patients lack the ability to repair DNA after it has been altered by ultraviolet radiation.

There are 8 distinct genetic variations of this autosomal recessive disorder, all characterized by defects in repair of DNA damaged by ultraviolet light. Patients with xeroderma present an elaborate inventory of effects due to chronic actinic damage compressed in the first years of life, including atrophy, telangiectasia, and all varieties of sunlight-induced premalignant and malignant cutaneous growths (actinic keratosis, basal and squamous cell carcinoma, malignant melanoma).

Photosensitivity reactions occur most commonly in light-complexioned individuals (blue eyes and blond or red hair) who sunburn easily and who with repeated injury develop chronic actinic damage (Fig 38–1) and skin cancer. The action spectrum is in the UVB range, and the response is phototoxic.

These patients must avoid exposure to UVB rays; the extent of protection required depends upon individual sensitivity. Protection can be achieved by wearing appropriate clothing, avoiding exposure to sunlight between 9 AM and 4 PM (depending on latitude and time of year), and consistently using potent sunscreens with a sun-protective rating (SPF) of 15 or greater (see Chapter 53). Lesions such as actinic keratoses or carcinomas resulting from chronic injury may need to be removed (see Chapter 43).

PHOTOSENSITIVITY DUE TO ENDOGENOUS PHOTOSENSITIZERS

Photosensitizers may be endogenous or exogenous. If exogenous, they penetrate the skin through topical applications or systemic dissemination through the bloodstream. The porphyrin molecules uroporphyrin, coproporphyrin, and protoporphyrin are the only endogenous photosensitizers synthesized by the human body. When produced in excess, they cause the porphyrias.

The porphyrias (Table 38–1) are characterized by disorders of porphyrinogen metabolism. Each type has distinct clinical, biochemical, and genetic features. Abnormal amounts of porphyrins may be produced in bone marrow only (erythropoietic porphyrias), in bone marrow and liver (erythrohepatic porphyrias), or in the liver only (hepatic porphyrias). All porphyrias except acute intermittent porphyria are associated with characteristic photocutaneous manifestations. In acute intermittent porphyria, nonphotoactive porphyrin precursors—δ-aminolevulinic acid and porphobilinogen—are produced in excess, whereas in all other porphyrias, photoactive preformed porphyrins (uroporphyrins, coproporphyrins, and protoporphyrins) are present in abnormal amounts.

Reactions are phototoxic (photodynamic), with a peak action spectrum around 400 nm; manifestations range from marked photodestruction of tissue noted in congenital erythropoietic porphyria to the fragility and blistering characteristic of hepatic porphyrias (Fig 38–2).

1. PORPHYRIA CUTANEA TARDA

Essentials of Diagnosis
- Fragility (skin shears off with slight trauma).
- Vesicles or bullae in sun-exposed areas subjected to trauma.
- Hypertrichosis with coarse hairs especially prominent over the cheekbones and periorbitally.
- Milia in areas of previous denudation or blisters, especially the dorsa of the hands.

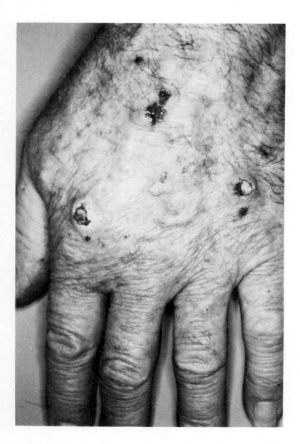

Figure 38–1. Chronic actinic damage and multiple actinic keratoses of the dorsal hand.

Table 38–1. The porphyrias.

Erythropoietic porphyrias
    Congenital erythropoietic porphyria
    Erythropoietic corpoporphyria
Erythrohepatic
    Erythropoietic protoporphyria
Hepatic porphyrias
    Acute intermittent porphyria
    Porphyria cutanea tarda
    Variegate porphyria
    Hereditary coproporphyria
    Acquired porphyria

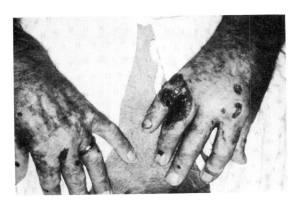

Figure 38–2. Dorsum of the hands of a patient with porphyria cutanea tarda, demonstrating crusting, scarring, and depigmentation due to sunlight-induced fragility of the skin.

- Hypo- or hyperpigmentation, especially of the face.
- Sclerodermoid changes of the face, chest, back, and at times the hands.
- Elevated 24-hour quantitative urine uroporphyrin level.

General Considerations

Porphyria cutanea tarda results from an aberration of heme synthesis, resulting in accumulation of photosensitizing porphyrins. In the case of porphyria cutanea tarda, decreased activity of uroporphyrinogen decarboxylase leads to accumulation of uroporphyrin. Although a genetic deficiency is present in at least some patients, the disease is usually not manifested until adult life. It is usually precipitated by ingestion of alcohol, estrogens, or iron.

Porphyria cutanea tarda occurs throughout the world and in both sexes.

Clinical Findings

A. Symptoms and Signs: Patients usually notice fragility of the skin on the dorsum of the hands. Bumping the hands against hard objects seems to strip the skin of the epidermis from the dermis. The skin condition may be worse in the summer and is precipitated and aggravated by exposure to sunlight. Patients usually develop frank vesicles or bullae following trauma.

In addition to fragility and blisters on the hands, most patients have hypertrichosis. The fine downy hair on the face becomes coarse and dark. In men it resembles beard hair, but it may occur on the forehead, the cheeks, and under the eyes, so that the distribution clearly suggests hypertrichosis. In women the hypertrichotic changes may be more obvious, resembling a full-face beard.

Milia usually occur in areas of blister formation.

Sclerodermatous changes may resemble progressive systemic sclerosis. Sun-exposed skin in such cases is usually indurated, yellow, and thick and may limit mobility. Calcification is unusual but may occur.

Pigmentation often involves the face and presents a mahogany to plethoric appearance.

Porphyria cutanea tarda may coexist with lupus erythematosus and has been associated with hepatitis and hepatic tumors.

B. Laboratory Findings: Patients with porphyria cutanea tarda have elevated urine levels of uroporphyrins. If the elevations are marked, the urine may be dark and may fluoresce pink when illuminated with Wood's light, particularly after acidification with acetic or hydrochloric acid. Patients also have increased amounts of isocoproporphyrin in feces and a deficiency of uroporphyrinogen decarboxylase in hepatocytes and, in familial cases, in red blood cells as well.

Histologic examination reveals a subepidermal bulla with a sparse inflammatory infiltrate. The clean line of cleavage between the epidermis and dermis is pronounced, and dermal papillae project into the blister (festooning). The chronically exposed skin shows a homogeneous pink material around the upper dermal blood vessels with H&E staining. These areas are PAS-positive and diastase-resistant with PAS staining. Direct immunofluorescence examination of the skin shows homogeneous deposits of IgG in or around the upper dermal blood vessel walls and often a band of IgG at the dermal-epidermal junction overlying these blood vessels.

Differential Diagnosis

Porphyria cutanea tarda must be differentiated from other photosensitive diseases, including other porphyrias, polymorphic light eruption, and lupus erythematosus. The sclerodermoid changes may suggest progressive systemic sclerosis, CREST syndrome, or mixed connective tissue disease. The fragility and numerous erosions may be mistaken for neurotic excoriations or epidermolysis bullosa acquisita. The differential diagnosis of bullae on the hands associated with exposure or trauma includes bullous pemphigoid, pemphigus vulgaris, epidermolysis bullosa, dermatitis herpetiformis, chemical or thermal injury bulla associated with renal dialysis, and administration of nonsteroidal anti-inflammatory agents, tetracycline, or nalidixic acid.

Complications & Sequelae

Total body iron stores may be increased. The glucose tolerance test is positive in about 25% of patients, but overt diabetes is unusual. The disease is associated with lupus erythematosus.

Prevention

Elicitation of lesions of porphyria cutanea tarda requires a second factor, usually ingestion of alcohol, estrogens, or iron. Patients with the disease may become entirely asymptomatic if these agents are avoided.

Treatment

Removal of the precipitating factor should be a mainstay of treatment. This may require total abstinence from alcohol and discontinuance of iron or estrogens used for postmenopausal symptoms or for contraception.

Phlebotomy is second-line treatment. Approximately 500 mL of blood is removed weekly or every other week until the hemoglobin decreases to 10 g/dL. Phlebotomies are resumed when hemoglobin levels rise above 12 g/dL until the urine uroporphyrin excretion is reduced to 200–300 μg/24 h. The ferrous ion inhibits uroporphyrinogen decarboxylase, so that removal of iron may increase that enzyme activity. Blistering and fragility are usually the first signs to improve, but hypertrichosis, pigmentary changes, and sclerodermoid features also remit eventually.

Chloroquine is normally contraindicated in patients with porphyria cutanea tarda. However, in minute doses the drug may help. The usual dose is about 125 mg once or twice weekly. Chemical hepatitis may be precipitated even by this low dose. Eventually this treatment will bring the patient into remission. The liver must be monitored closely.

Alkalinization of the urine increases excretion of urinary uroporphyrins but has not proved to be of much therapeutic value.

Prognosis

If the precipitating factor is identified and removed (eg, abstinence from alcohol), the disorder may become completely asymptomatic and require no ongoing therapy.

2. ERYTHROPOIETIC PROTOPORPHYRIA

Essentials of Diagnosis

- Photosensitivity characterized by pruritus, burning, and stinging of the skin almost immediately after exposure to sunlight.
- Erythema, edema, and, rarely, bullae in sun-exposed areas.
- Chronic exposure may lead to thickening of the skin and scarring in exposed areas.
- Onset in early childhood.
- Elevated red blood cell and plasma levels of protoporphyrin.
- Ferrochelatase deficiency in red blood cells and fibroblasts.

General Considerations

Patients with erythropoietic protoporphyria usually have profound photosensitivity. The exact incidence is unknown, but the disease is not rare. Decreased levels of ferrochelatase activity appear to be responsible for the biochemical and associated clinical changes.

Clinical Findings

A. Symptoms and Signs: The disease begins early in life with photosensitivity. Infants often cry when exposed to sunlight and a few hours later develop swelling in the sun-exposed areas. Bullae are unusual, but erosions may occur and leave atrophic waxy scars. These scars are prominent on sun-exposed areas, including the hands, nose, eyes, and ears. Later, the skin over the knuckles often appears thick and wrinkled, as though it had aged prematurely. The disorder is not associated with hypertrichosis, milia, sclerodermoid change, or hyperpigmentation.

B. Laboratory Findings: Fecal protoporphyrin levels are almost always elevated, and the levels of free protoporphyrin in red blood cells are characteristically increased as well. Plasma protoporphyrins may also be elevated. If red blood cells are examined under a fluorescence microscope with proper filters, about 20% of red blood cells will transiently fluoresce a red color.

Biopsy from sun-exposed skin shows homogeneous pink material around upper dermal blood vessels on H&E staining. Indeed, the vessel walls contain deposits that stain with PAS stain. On direct immunofluorescence, one sees deposition of immune globulin—primarily IgG—in or around the upper dermal blood vessel walls and at times in the basement membrane zone.

Differential Diagnosis

The profound sensitivity essentially limits the differential diagnosis to other photosensitivity diseases. Hydroa vacciniforme and other forms of porphyria are highest on the list. Contact dermatitis, angioedema, and urticaria can usually be differentiated on clinical grounds, but the diagnosis is normally made by finding elevated fecal or red blood cell protoporphyrin levels. Lipoid proteinosis is a rare genodermatosis that histologically may mimic erythropoietic protoporphyria, but the pink homogeneous material can be seen in biopsies from nonexposed areas as well as in exposed skin in lipoid proteinosis.

Prevention

Patients with erythropoietic protoporphyria should scrupulously avoid exposure to sunlight, because lesions generally result in severe scarring.

Complications

Scarring is characteristic and may be permanent. Some patients have mild hemolytic anemia, hepatic failure associated with jaundice, and hepatic cirrhosis. Many have gallstones.

Treatment

Oral administration of beta-carotene in a dosage of 60–180 mg/d may reduce photosensitivity and allow increased tolerance to light, but the drug is rarely completely effective. Serum carotene levels should be maintained above 600 pg/dL. Carotenemia is usual with this treatment. The drug appears to quench free radicals produced by the interaction of ultraviolet light and porphyrins.

Some patients have improved after treatment with iron or hematin, but in others the disease is exacerbated, suggesting that there may be 2 separate forms.

3. VARIEGATE PORPHYRIA

Essentials of Diagnosis

- Autosomal dominant inheritance.
- Fragility (skin shears off with slight trauma).
- Vesicles or bullae in sun-exposed areas.
- Hypertrichosis.
- Milia in areas of previous blisters.
- Hypo- or hyperpigmentation.
- Sclerodermoid changes of the hand.
- Decreased protoporphyrinogen oxidase in liver and fibroblasts with increased protoporphyrin, coproporphyrin in feces, and increased δ-aminolevulinic acid and porphobilinogen in urine during acute abdominal attacks.

General Considerations

Variegate porphyria is also called mixed porphyria because it has features of both porphyria cutanea tarda and acute intermittent porphyria. The disorder is apparently caused by a decreased protoporphyrinogen oxidase enzyme activity, but other enzymes involved in porphyrin metabolism may also be altered.

Clinical Findings

A. Symptoms and Signs: Clinically, this disorder precisely mimics porphyria cutanea tarda, but it has the additional features and symptoms of acute intermittent porphyria. As in porphyria cutanea tarda, fragility or blisters may occur in sun-exposed areas. Hypertrichosis, milia, and hyperpigmentation may also occur. In addition, patients with variegate porphyria may have acute abdominal attacks of pain, nausea, and vomiting, sometimes associated with behavioral disturbances, paralysis, or seizures.

B. Laboratory Findings: Urinary δ- aminolevulinic acid and porphobilinogen are elevated during acute attacks but usually normal otherwise. All patients have elevations of stool protoporphyrin and, to a lesser extent, coproporphyrin, both during and between acute attacks. Like porphyria cutanea tarda, urine uroporphyrins are usually increased, but less so than those of coproporphyrin.

If a blister is present, histologic examination shows a subepidermal festooning, noninflammatory bulla similar to what is found in porphyria cutanea tarda. PAS staining and direct immunofluorescence findings are also similar to those found in porphyria cutanea tarda.

Differential Diagnosis

The acute abdominal pain can mimic an acute abdomen such as cholecystitis or appendicitis. The skin disease otherwise mimics porphyria cutanea tarda, and the differential diagnosis is the same.

Treatment

Patients with variegate porphyria must avoid drugs that precipitate acute abdominal attacks. Treatments that seem successful for porphyria cutanea tarda usually do not help the patient with variegate porphyria. Beta-carotene, however, administered as for erythropoietic protoporphyria, may occasionally be useful.

4. ERYTHROPOIETIC PORPHYRIA

Erythropoietic porphyria is a rare disorder caused by deficiency of uroporphyrinogen III cosynthase. Patients have severe photosensitivity and pain when skin is exposed to sunlight, even in infancy. The urine is usually slightly pink to brown or burgundy. After sun exposure, the skin blisters. Phototoxic injury with or without secondary infection leads to severe mutilating scarring. Hirsutism, alopecia, ectropion, hypo- and hyperpigmentation, and increased skin fragility are often seen. Splenomegaly and hemolytic anemia may occur as complications.

The teeth fluoresce pink or brown with Wood's light. There is almost always hemolytic anemia and splenomegaly. The urine is pink and contains excessive amounts of uroporphyrin I. Coproporphyrin I levels are high in feces. Bullae are subepidermal, with usually very little inflammation but frequently with evidence of scarring.

The severe photosensitivity usually suggests a form of porphyria. Assessment of red blood cell, plasma, urine, and fecal uroporphyrins, coproporphyrins, and protoporphyrins sorts out the diagnosis.

Porphyrin binding with activated charcoal given orally has proved to be remarkably effective in reducing the circulating and urinary excreted porphyrin levels and in eliminating the acute signs and symptoms of disease. Until recently, the only treatment consisted of absolute shielding from sunlight. Topical sunscreens are not effective, but sun-blocking agents may help. Oral administration of beta-carotene may cause slight improvement in sunlight tolerance.

A partial benefit after splenectomy has been reported, but there is little evidence of specific longterm improvement.

Repeated transfusions raising the hematocrit to 37% have been shown to suppress porphyrin formation along with signs and symptoms of the disease.

PHOTOSENSITIVITY DUE TO EXOGENOUS PHOTOSENSITIZERS

Essentials of Diagnosis

- No genetic predisposition.
- Phototoxic reactions common; characterized by delayed erythema and edema followed by hyperpigmentation and desquamation limited to areas exposed to sunlight.
- Photoallergic reactions less common; usually characterized by delayed papular or eczematous lesions extending beyond exposed skin. Rarely, immediate urticarial responses.
- Action spectrum in the UVA range in most cases.

General Considerations

Exogenous photosensitizers may penetrate the skin through local application of topical preparations or through dissemination via the bloodstream.

A. Topical Photosensitizers: Topical photosensitizers are common ingredients of cosmetics, face creams, perfumes, aftershave lotions, and soaps; medications such as coal tars and psoralens that are deliberately used to induce photosensitivity to help treat various skin disorders; or phenothiazines and sulfonamides, which may produce unintended photosensitivity when applied to or accidentally spilled on the skin. Antibacterial agents such as the halogenated salicylanilides and related compounds that were once used in deodorant soaps, first aid creams, and so forth were responsible for an epidemic of photosensitivity reactions in the 1960s. Sunscreens—all potential photosensitizers—rarely cause photosensitivity.

Plants such as celery, wild carrots, gas plant, limes, and grass (meadow grass) contain photosensitizing psoralens. Industrial contaminants and air pollutants such as tars and polycyclic aromatic hydrocarbons are also potent photosensitizers.

Most reactions are phototoxic; however, halogenated salicylanilides and certain scents (musk ambrette and 6-methylcoumarin) produce mainly, if not exclusively, photoallergic reactions.

The action spectrum for these reactions, whether phototoxic or photoallergic, usually falls in the UVA range.

B. Systemic Photosensitizers: Potential systemic photosensitizing chemicals range from commonly used weak photosensitizers such as diphenhydramine to potent psoralen compounds used therapeutically to produce phototoxic reactions. Commonly used systemic photosensitizers include sulfonamides, thiazide diuretics, sulfonylureas, phenothiazines, and certain tetracycline derivatives (eg, demeclocycline and doxycycline). Of these agents, chlorpromazine, demeclocycline, and doxycycline are the most potent; clinically, however, thiazide diuretics produce the most reactions because they are used most frequently.

Most of these reactions are phototoxic, and the action spectrum, whether phototoxic or photoallergic, falls mostly in the UVA range.

C. Types of Reactions: Phototoxic reactions are far more common than photoallergic reactions and are usually characterized by painful delayed erythema with or without edema, followed by hyperpigmentation and desquamation. The reaction tends to be limited to sharply defined areas of exposure.

Photoallergic reactions usually have a delayed onset and are characterized by pruritic papular or eczematous lesions resembling contact dermatitis due to poison oak or poison ivy. The lesions usually extend beyond the areas of exposure. Immediate wheal-and-flare (urticaria) reactions occur rarely.

Treatment

Prevention is the best therapy. Patients using a known photosensitizer (whether topical or systemic) should avoid excessive exposure to sunlight.

Treatment of lesions is symptomatic and depends on the type, extent, and severity of the response. Most phototoxic reactions require little treatment, though cool compresses and an analgesic such as aspirin may sometimes be needed. If the process is severe (marked erythema and edema with or without blisters) and extensive, however, hospitalization with supportive therapy for fluid and electrolyte imbalance and (sometimes) shock may be necessary.

Photoallergic reactions are almost always of the delayed hypersensitivity type, as seen in allergic contact dermatitis. Cool tap water compresses can be applied continually or intermittently. Topical application of corticosteroid creams or lotions such as triamcinolone 0.1% cream 2–3 times daily can reduce inflammation. Systemic antihistamines such as hydroxyzine, 10 mg every 4 hours, may lessen pruritus. If the process is severe and extensive, systemic corticosteroids as used in *Rhus* contact dermatitis may be necessary.

PHOTOSENSITIVITY DUE TO UNKNOWN CAUSES

Photosensitivity sometimes occurs when there is no apparent loss or lack of melanin and no exposure to a known photosensitizer. Such photosensitivity reactions tend to fall into one of 4 subgroups: (1) allergic and autoimmune reactions, (2) pellagra and pellagra-like responses, (3) hereditary disorders, and (4) miscellaneous conditions.

1. ALLERGIC & AUTOIMMUNE DISEASES

Solar Urticaria

Solar urticaria is characterized by an immediate urticarial wheal with or without a surrounding flare upon exposure to sunlight. The lesions are transient, occur within a few minutes after exposure, and last from a few minutes to about 1 hour depending on the intensity of the stimulus. The action spectrum extends from the UVB wavelengths to the infrared wavelengths. Passive transfer of the reaction to other subjects using antibodies from patients' serum has been accomplished and confirms that allergy is the cause in some cases.

Avoiding exposure by wearing protective clothes and opaque sunblocks is effective but difficult to accomplish uniformly. Sunscreens are usually of little value. Chloroquine (250 mg per tablet) or hydroxychloroquine (200 mg per tablet) is effective in many patients. The usual dose is 2 tablets daily for 1–2 weeks, then one tablet daily for 1–2 weeks, then one tablet every other day with gradual reduction of the dose. Frequently, one tablet per week will control the disease, which may disappear after several months. Because retinopathy is the principal serious side effect of these agents, ophthalmologic examinations should be performed before therapy is started and at 3- to 4-month intervals thereafter.

Cyproheptadine, 4 mg orally 3–4 times daily, or terfenadine, 60 mg twice daily, is sometimes useful for prevention or treatment. Repeated daily exposure to slowly increasing amounts of the action spectrum radiation will control the disease in many patients but is frequently difficult to perform. PUVA therapy is useful in some cases (see below).

Solar urticaria may be chronic and persistent; remissions are not uncommon and may be either temporary or permanent.

Polymorphous Light Eruptions

Polymorphous light eruptions due to exposure to sunlight are among the most common and baffling of photosensitivity diseases, because the pathobiologic mechanisms are mostly unknown. They occur in all races but are especially common in the North and Central American Indian and Finnish populations. The disease appears at any age from infancy through late adult life, but onset is most commonly during the 30s and 40s. In Native Americans, however, it generally begins in childhood. The incidence is somewhat higher in females than in males.

The eruptions range from multiple small papules, papulovesicles, and eczematous lesions (Fig 38–3) to large papules and plaques. Usually, one type of lesion is more prevalent in a given individual; however, combinations of lesions and eruptions in various stages of transition may occur. The eruptions occur mostly at sites exposed to sunlight, though conditioned irritability (a heightened excitability of normal skin) and sensitization responses may cause spread beyond exposed areas. If spread occurs, exposed sites are still more heavily involved.

The eruption occurs a few hours to several days after exposure and usually persists for 24 hours or

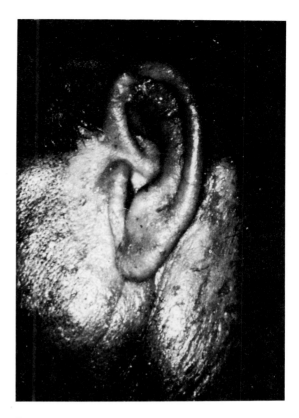

Figure 38–3. Eczematous response of the face, ear, and neck of a patient with polymorphous light eruption.

more after onset; it is not caused by a photosensitizer.

The action spectrum is within the UVB range, though certain patients respond abnormally to UVA rays as well; a subset of patients appear to respond adversely to UVA rays only.

The disease tends to be seasonal, and flare-ups are often associated with sunny weather. Many patients experience a flare-up of disease in the spring and improve as summer wears on; these patients appear to become hardened or desensitized with repeated exposure, so that moderate doses of sunlight may be tolerated normally.

The course is generally chronic once the disease begins, and exacerbations continue to occur with each exposure to sunlight; however, in some patients the disease disappears either for a few years or permanently.

Patients whose eruptions are provoked by UVB radiation should avoid the midday sun and use protective clothing and sunscreens or sunblocks. Antimalarial drugs can be used as in solar urticaria, though more prolonged high doses may be needed in polymorphous light eruption. Systemic corticosteroids are necessary for severe reactions, and topical midstrength corticosteroids help decrease inflammation and reduce pruritus in less severe reactions. Occasionally, PUVA treatment can be used for patients with chronic severe disease (see below).

Lupus Erythematosus
(See also Chapter 50.)

The role of exposure to sunlight in discoid and systemic lupus erythematosus is apparent from the characteristic distribution of lesions on the nose and malar areas. Not all lesions, however—eg, those in the ears, mouth, trunk, and palms—are related to sun exposure. About 40–80% of patients with systemic lupus erythematosus are photosensitive; others do not appear to be photosensitive at all. Even if skin lesions are not present or the patient is not photosensitive, systemic lupus erythematosus can be aggravated by exposure to sunlight, because the UVB rays constituting the action spectrum produce abnormal DNA that can induce antibodies against it.

Patients must avoid the midday sun and wear protective clothing and potent sunscreens.

Dermatomyositis

The role of sunlight in dermatomyositis has not been thoroughly examined, and the action spectrum is unknown. Certain patients are photosensitive, and exposure to sunlight may aggravate cutaneous manifestations and most probably systemic symptoms as well.

Pemphigoid & Pemphigus
(See also Chapter 42.)

The ability of UVB rays to produce lesions in pemphigoid and pemphigus—both autoimmune bullous diseases—has been established under experimental conditions. Such reactivity appears to be clinically significant only in pemphigus erythematosus and pemphigus foliaceus, in which progression of lesions follows exposure to sunlight. However, patients with all forms of both pemphigoid and pemphigus are at risk for development of lesions, and all should avoid significant exposure to UVB radiation.

2. PELLAGRA & PELLAGRA-LIKE DERMATOSES

Pellagra is characterized by a dietary deficiency of B vitamins, most notably nicotinic acid (niacin) and its metabolic precursor tryptophan. Pellagra-like reactions occur in carcinoid syndrome (carcinoid tumor appears to use tryptophan in the production of serotonin) and in the genetic aminoacidurias (Hartnup disease, hydroxykynureninuria, and tryptophanuria), which represent disturbances of tryptophan metabolism, with reduced formation of niacin.

The antituberculosis drug isoniazid has a structure similar to that of nicotinamide. Occasionally, therapy with isoniazid leads to pellagra-like cutaneous and systemic changes, especially in malnourished pa-

tients; these effects are probably due to competition between the isoniazid and nicotinamide for an unidentified enzyme or cofactor.

The photosensitivity reaction is usually characterized by symmetric erythema and edema, followed by formation of vesicles and blisters. A rough, fissured, blackish brittle scaling supervenes. The hands and forearms are most commonly involved; the tops of the feet to the ankles and at times the lower legs and the face are also affected. A necklace-like dermatitis may occur on the neck and upper chest (Casal's necklace). The action spectrum and mechanism of this photosensitivity response are unknown. The disease responds to oral niacin, 100 mg 3 times daily.

3. RECESSIVE DEGENERATIVE GENODERMATOSES

Photosensitivity occurs in several hereditary degenerative diseases transmitted as autosomal recessive traits. For most, the only preventive treatment is photoprotection. Bloom's syndrome is characterized by dwarfism and congenital telangiectatic erythema (aggravated by exposure to sunlight) involving mostly the face. Occasionally, blistering, crusting, and bleeding occur. Patients with Bloom's syndrome have an increased incidence of leukemia, and chromosomal breaks and rearrangements are prevalent in their lymphocytes.

Cockayne's syndrome resembles Bloom's syndrome and has additional features. The cutaneous changes, consisting initially of erythema involving the nose and cheeks, appear to be a photosensitivity response that disappears with time. However, mottled pigmentation, scarring, and atrophy of these sites remain.

In Rothmund-Thomson syndrome, about one-third of patients are photosensitive, though the sensitivity declines with age. The lesions may be bullous. Keratotic growths may be found in exposed areas from adolescence onward, and squamous cell carcinomas may develop in and around these lesions.

The action spectrum for Bloom's syndrome falls in the UVB range. No studies of the action spectrum have been reported in either Cockayne's syndrome or Rothmund-Thomson syndrome.

Studies of cellular repair of DNA in patients with Bloom's and Rothmund-Thomson syndromes have shown that cells repair DNA damaged by ultraviolet light in a normal manner.

4. MISCELLANEOUS DISORDERS OF UNKNOWN CAUSE

Keratosis Follicularis
(Darier-White Disease)

This is an autosomal dominant disorder characterized by hyperkeratotic papular lesions that have a specific histologic picture (see Chapter 21). Exposure to sunlight is not essential for development of lesions, though worsening of preexisting lesions and production of new lesions can be induced by sunlight. The action spectrum is in the UVB range. The mechanism of the adverse response to ultraviolet light has not been established. The most commonly accepted theory views keratosis follicularis as an isomorphic (Koebner) phenomenon; the lesions can be produced by various kinds of trauma such as thermal burn injury and application of liquid nitrogen.

Familial Benign Chronic Pemphigus (Hailey-Hailey Disease)

Although the distribution of lesions does not resemble that of a primary photosensitivity disorder, seasonal variations in the manifestations have suggested that sunlight may cause the adverse responses. Under controlled conditions, exposure to wavelengths throughout the ultraviolet spectrum may cause the characteristic acantholysis on normal skin in these patients (see Chapter 42).

Hydroa Estivale Vel Vacciniforme

This is a rare disease that may be an autosomal recessive trait. It generally begins in infancy or childhood, mainly in males, and takes the form of vesicles on areas exposed to sunlight; the lesions progress to crusting and varioliform scarring, especially of the nose, ear rims, cheeks, and backs of the hands. A mixed polymorphonuclear and lymphocytic perivascular infiltrate is seen in the dermis. The vesicles contain PMNs, lymphocytes, and fibrin. Hydropic degeneration may occur in the epidermis. The action spectrum falls in the UVA range.

Disseminated Superficial Actinic Porokeratosis

This is an autosomal dominant disorder characterized initially by multiple tiny, usually follicular, keratotic brownish-red papules with raised borders. The lesions enlarge peripherally to leave a depressed center. The lesions are found on areas exposed to sunlight and most commonly affect women in their 30s and 40s. Pruritus occurs frequently. Flaring of disease after exposure to ultraviolet light has suggested the importance of sunlight to the development of lesions; recent studies reproduced the lesions under controlled conditions. The action spectrum and mechanism of the response have not yet been clarified.

Granuloma Annulare

This is an idiopathic disease characterized by papules and nodules that frequently occur in an annular configuration. Granulomatous foci and necrobiosis are histologic hallmarks of the disease. In certain patients, exposure to sunlight causes or aggravates le-

sions. Actinic granuloma is probably a form of granuloma annulare in which actinically damaged elastic tissue is engulfed by giant cells in the granulomatous inflammation.

Herpes Simplex Virus Type I Infections & Verruca Plana (Flat Wart) of the Face

These are 2 viral disorders commonly precipitated or worsened by exposure to sunlight. Lymphogranuloma venereum and varicella are occasionally aggravated by exposure to sunlight. The action spectrum and mechanism involved in these photoresponses have not been elucidated.

Acne Rosacea

This is a common photosensitive disorder that usually begins when patients are in their 40s or 50s. Women are more commonly affected than men. Acne rosacea is characterized by a hyperactive flushing response of the head, neck, and chest and an inflammatory acneiform eruption of the face. The acneiform lesions readily respond to systemic tetracycline, 250–1000 mg/d. In contrast, the vascular component of the disease, which ranges from mild erythema to an intense flushing response with severe stinging and burning sensations, fails to respond to therapy. Antiprostaglandin medications such as naproxen, 250 mg every 12 hours, appear to effectively relieve vascular symptoms of some patients.

Psoriasis, Lichen Planus, & Sarcoidosis

These disorders are occasionally aggravated by sunlight.

PHOTOTHERAPY

Sunlight has been used therapeutically for over 3000 years. Herodotus used sunlight to restore general health to sick patients in the second century BC. Rickets was treated with sunlight in the 18th century. The importance of ultraviolet radiation as a therapeutic measure was acknowledged in 1903 when Niels Finsen was awarded the Nobel Prize in Medicine for his work on phototherapy for lupus vulgaris. Although chemotherapy has replaced ultraviolet radiation in the treatment of this form of cutaneous tuberculosis, ultraviolet radiation is still a useful treatment in many diseases..

The major sources of ultraviolet radiation currently in therapeutic use include (1) high- or medium-pressure mercury arc lamps, which have a high energy output in the UVB range, though significant amounts of UVC and UVA rays are also emitted; (2) fluorescent sunlamps, which emit mostly UVB rays; and (3) fluorescent black light (Wood's light) lamps, which emit UVA rays. Low-pressure cold quartz lamps that emit mainly UVC rays are used occasionally.

Acne vulgaris usually responds favorably to repeated mild erythema produced by sunlight, UVB, or UVC radiation. Certain papulosquamous eruptions—pityriasis rosea, psoriasis, parapsoriasis en plaque, pityriasis lichenoides et varioliformis acuta, pityriasis lichenoides chronica, and mycosis fungoides—may respond to repeated erythematous doses of UVB radiation. In some patients, phototherapy with repeated exposure to UVB radiation may inexplicably relieve the intractable pruritus associated with renal failure. The mechanism of this effect has not been established.

Photochemotherapy

The field of phototherapy has been expanded to include photochemotherapy. Photochemotherapy for vitiligo was practiced in India as early as 1400 BC and in Egypt about the 12th century AD with psoralen compounds derived from plants. Recently, certain psoralens (natural or synthetic tricyclic furocoumarins) have been used extensively as photochemotherapeutic agents. These psoralens are potent chemical photosensitizers that become activated after they absorb UVA radiation. In this excited state, the psoralens can form photoadducts to DNA and RNA, photodynamically damage cellular proteins and membranes, and stimulate melanin pigment formation.

PUVA therapy (psoralen molecules combined with UVA energy) has proved to be most effective in the treatment of psoriasis, mycosis fungoides, and vitiligo; other diseases such as polymorphous light eruption and solar urticaria may also respond well. The most commonly used agent is methoxsalen (Oxsoralen; 8-methoxypsoralen; 8-MOP), though trioxsalen (Trisoralen) has also been used extensively for its repigmenting effects in vitiligo.

The psoralens are generally administered orally, and irradiation with UVA rays is performed 2–3 hours later. Potential problems such as acute erythema, blistering responses, and possible formation of cataracts and skin cancer must be weighed against the benefits for each patient. Treatment must be individualized according to the disease being treated, the patient's body weight and skin type (susceptibility to sunburn), and the source of UVA.

Prolonged treatment lasting months is usually required, and eyeglasses that filter out UVA light are essential. Long-term effects of PUVA therapy include induction of pigmented macules and squamous cell carcinoma. Psoralens may also be applied topically to localized vitiligo or psoriatic lesions before phototherapy; the main risk is the potential for severe blistering. The use of psoralens to treat cutaneous diseases is best left to dermatologists who have the special equipment and experience needed for safe and successful treatment.

The other commonly used form of photochemotherapy is the combination of crude coal tar or its derivatives with UVB rays, UVA rays, or both. The action spectrum for coal tar and coal tar derivatives falls in the UVA range; therefore, the therapeutic effect of coal tar combined with UVB rays is a synergistic response. UVA radiation plus coal tar can produce a phototoxic effect and inhibit DNA synthesis, though the psoralens are much more effective in this regard. UVB radiation (Goeckerman technique) plus coal tar appears to be the most effective combination and has been used with great success since the 1920s. It has the additional benefit of safety: cataracts do not occur, and there is little evidence that skin cancer results from chronic therapy except under unusual circumstances.

REFERENCES

DeLeo VA (editor): Photosensitivity diseases. (Symposium.) Dermatol Clin 1986;4:253. [Entire issue.]

Epstein JH: Photocarcinogenesis and aging. In: *Aging and the Skin.* Balin HK, Kligman AM (editors). Raven Press, 1989.

Epstein JH: *Photomedicine in the Science of Photobiology,* 2nd ed. Plenum Press, 1989.

Epstein JH: Phototoxicity and photoallergy in man. J Am Acad Dermatol 1983;8:141.

Harber LC, Bickers DR: *Photosensitivity Diseases: Principles of Diagnosis and Treatment.* Saunders, 1981.

Kraemer KH, Lee MM, Scotto J: Xeroderma pigmentosum: Cutaneous, ocular, and neurologic abnormalities in 830 published cases. Arch Dermatol 1987; 123: 241.

Morison WL: *Phototherapy and Photochemotherapy of Skin Diseases.* Praeger, 1983.

Pathak MA: Sunscreens: Topical and systemic approaches for protection of human skin against harmful effects of solar radiation. J Am Acad Dermatol 1982; 7: 285.

Regan JD, Parrish JA (editors) : *The Science of Photomedicine.* Plenum Press, 1982.

Section VI:
Scaling & Bullous Disorders

Exfoliative Dermatitis

39

Harry J. Hurley, MD, DSc(Med)

The terms exfoliative dermatitis, exfoliative erythroderma, and erythroderma are interchangeable; all denote mild to severe redness of the skin and scaling, which reflects loss of stratum corneum and at times part or all of the living epidermis as well. Some writers reserve the term "exfoliative dermatitis" for disorders in which scaling is the major feature and "erythroderma" for those in which erythema is more prominent.

EXFOLIATIVE ERYTHRODERMA

Essentials of Diagnosis

- Diffuse erythema (erythroderma) over most or all of the skin.
- Extensive scaling (either fine scales or, occasionally, large sheets of skin).
- Hair loss.
- Onychodystrophy.
- Itching, malaise, weight loss.
- Low-grade fever, lymphadenopathy; occasionally gynecomastia, hypothermia, steatorrhea, and enteropathy.

General Considerations

In exfoliative dermatitis, essentially the entire skin is erythematous and scaling. In some patients, the scales are large, as in psoriasis; in others they are small, as in atopic dermatitis; and in still others the skin comes off in sheets, as in toxic epidermal necrolysis. Exfoliative dermatitis is a phenotypic expression of a variety of skin disorders of different causes, and treatment varies depending on the cause.

Clinical Findings

The best clues to the diagnosis are the signs of a previously existing skin disease. In some patients, no specific cause can be found.

A. Dermatologic Onset and Course: The onset is acute in drug-induced exfoliative dermatitis or generalized contact dermatitis. Most other types develop gradually as the primary disease becomes more extensive. Once it has appeared, untreated exfoliative dermatitis tends to persist with only slight variations in severity and extent. Clinical clues to the underlying disorder may be present in some patients and are described below.

B. Morphologic Features of Specific Types: The morphologic features of various disorders characterized by scaling and redness are listed below.

1. Psoriasis– Silvery-white lamellated scales, especially on the knees and elbows; nail abnormalities, principally pitting; and psoriasiform pustules, mainly during acute attacks.

2. Atopic dermatitis– Signs of atopy, especially epicanthal folds of the lower eyelids; white dermatographism (linear blanching in response to firm stroking of affected skin); a tendency toward lichenification in antecubital, popliteal, and neck regions; severe pruritus; and dermatopathic adenopathy, especially in children.

3. Stasis dermatitis– Edema and signs of venous insufficiency (varicosities, pigmentation, and ulcer scars on the medial and lateral ankles).

4. Pityriasis rubra pilaris– Islands of normal skin within erythrodermic areas, follicular papules on the dorsal aspects of the fingers, and thick yellow palms and soles with or without scales.

5. Pemphigus foliaceus– Erosive or crusted lesions at sites of ruptured bullae, often in an arcuate or gyrate pattern; old or healing lesions occasionally convolute to form a cauliflower-like thickening.

6. Lichen planus– Characteristic lacy, white mucosal lesions of the mouth and genitalia; anonychia or eponychial nail changes; and residual violaceous, scaling, flat-topped angular papules.

7. Norwegian (crusted) scabies– Thick crusted

lesions on the hands and feet, with nail involvement; mites abundant and easily seen in scales. Strangely, in contrast to ordinary scabies, pruritus may be minimal or absent.

8. Contact dermatitis and photodermatitis– Vesicles in early or recurrent cases; areas of skin exposed to the contactant or to light may be delineated by more pronounced inflammation.

9. Staphylococcal scalded skin syndrome– Marked erythema of medial cheeks and perioral skin, exquisitely tender skin, irritable patient, peeling exfoliative scale, and sparing of scalp. Almost all patients are children; the level of peel is beneath the stratum corneum above the viable epidermis.

10. Toxic epidermal necrolysis– The skin is diffusely red, tender, and peeling. Mucous membranes may be affected; fever is usual. Most patients are adults; the level of peel is in the epidermis.

11. Seborrheic dermatitis– An unusual cause of exfoliative dermatitis in adults. Starts on the scalp, face, and flexures. A pediatric form (Leiner's disease) is marked by generalized lymphadenopathy and severe diarrhea. A familial variant is often fatal, owing to functional opsonic defect of C5 complement.

12. Drug reactions– Typically, acute onset with symmetric lesions and pronounced erythema. Petechiae in dependent areas; often pruritic. (In all patients with exfoliative dermatitis, drugs should be considered as a possible cause.)

13. Lymphoreticular disease and visceral cancer– Cancer may appear months to years after the initial occurrence of exfoliative dermatitis. Pruritus, lymphadenopathy, and leonine facies suggest a lymphoreticular disorder, most commonly mycosis fungoides, Sézary syndrome, leukemia, lymphoma, and Hodgkin's disease. Symptoms and signs of underlying cancer, particularly of the viscera, are often present.

14. Idiopathic– The cause is not immediately demonstrable in at least 25% of patients. In such cases, spontaneous temporary remissions may occur, but permanent complete resolution is unusual.

C. Systemic Effects: Low-grade fever, a feeling of being cold, general malaise and weakness, hair loss, and postinflammatory hyper- or hypopigmentation (usually patchy) may result from the generalized inflammation. Gynecomastia may occur. Discrete nontender lymphadenopathy, often in the neck and axillae, may be pronounced. Increased heat loss and thermal dysregulation secondary to widespread erythema can occasionally result in hypothermia. The basal metabolic rate is increased. Electrolyte imbalances may occur. Loss of protein occurs as scales are shed and may cause a negative nitrogen balance in some patients. Hypoproteinemia and dependent edema also occur. Serum folate levels are decreased but rarely result in anemia. High-output cardiac failure may occur, which remits as the skin improves.

Hepatomegaly—related to cardiac decompensation in some patients and unexplained in others—occurs occasionally. Splenomegaly develops only in patients with lymphoma or leukemia. Enteropathy accompanied by steatorrhea occurs in some individuals and disappears when the dermatitis resolves.

D. Laboratory Findings: Decreased serum protein levels with hypoalbuminemia and a relative increase in serum IgE levels, lowered serum folate levels, increased levels of urinary estrogens, and steatorrhea reflect the systemic effects of exfoliative dermatitis. Eosinophilia is common, and high levels suggest hypersensitivity to drugs. Patients with psoriasis commonly have elevated serum uric acid concentrations, and those with leukemia or lymphoma have laboratory findings associated with those disorders. Skin biopsy specimens may provide clues to the underlying disorder; however, most biopsies show only nonspecific inflammatory changes.

Differential Diagnosis

See Table 39–1.

Complications

Secondary bacterial infection and septicemia occur rarely. Patients with long-standing disease often develop ectropion. Patients with exfoliative dermatitis who receive corticosteroids or cytotoxic drugs should be closely monitored for specific drug-related com-

Table 39–1. Causes of exfoliative dermatitis.

Preexisting skin disease	40%
Psoriasis	
Atopic dermatitis	
Stasis dermatitis	
Pityriasis rubra pilaris	
Pemphigus foliaceus	
Lichen planus	
Norwegian (crusted) scabies	
Staphylococcal scalded skin syndrome	
Toxic epidermal necrolysis	
Seborrheic dermatitis	
Contact dermatitis and photodermatitis	10%
Mercury	
Ragweed	
Sulfonamides	
Tar	
Others	
Drugs	10%
Arsenic	
Antimalarial drugs	
Barbiturates	
Codeine	
Iodides	
Gold	
Phenytoin	
Penicillin	
Sulfonamides	
Others	
Lymphoma, leukemia, visceral cancer	15%
Sézary's syndrome	
Idiopathic (primary)	25%

plications, because these patients often require high doses and long courses of treatment.

Treatment

Specific therapy depends upon the cause. A dermatologist should be consulted for help in diagnosis and treatment. Hospitalization may be required so that necessary diagnostic studies, nursing care, and appropriate specific and supportive treatment can be provided.

For exfoliative dermatitis due to atopic dermatitis, stasis dermatitis, pemphigus foliaceus, lichen planus, and seborrheic dermatitis, systemic corticosteroids are the mainstay of management. Give prednisone or its equivalent, 40–80 mg/d orally to start, and then add 20-mg increments every 3–4 days until exfoliation begins to stabilize, after which gradual reduction to a maintenance level, preferably on an alternate-day schedule, is made. The usual baseline clinical and laboratory evaluation and management of patients receiving long-term corticosteroid therapy should be undertaken and the patient monitored for signs of corticosteroid toxicity (see Chapter 53).

Cytotoxic drugs are useful in selected patients, including those with psoriasis and pityriasis rubra pilaris, who often benefit from methotrexate (*caution:* teratogen; see Chapter 53). Patients with lymphoma, leukemia, and visceral cancer may also benefit, but their treatment requires consultation with a radiologist, hematologist, or oncologist.

Exfoliative dermatitis in psoriasis or pityriasis rubra pilaris can be treated with etretinate. The usual dose is 0.5–1 mg/kg as a single daily dose. The dose is adjusted as the dermatitis improves, depending upon side effects. (*Caution:* teratogen.) See Chapter 53 for details.

In the familial variant of Leiner's disease, infusions of fresh plasma are often indicated and may be lifesaving.

The treatment of choice for exfoliative dermatitis occurring as a reaction to drugs is to discontinue the offending drug. The same is true for eruptions due to allergic contact dermatitis or photocontact dermatitis if the allergen is known. Lichen planus, psoriasis, and Sézary syndrome may respond to PUVA therapy (see Chapter 53).

Norwegian (crusted) scabies usually requires more intensive therapy than ordinary scabies, ie, a single application of lindane 1% lotion overnight, followed by nightly applications (for the next 5 nights) of 6% precipitated sulfur in petrolatum, followed by a second application of lindane 1% lotion overnight.

Topical therapy for exfoliative dermatitis is generally supportive. A daily 20-minute warm bath will help debride the exfoliative scales. This can be followed with applications of bland creams or ointments (eg, Aquaphor, Eucerin, Unibase) or topical corticosteroid creams or ointments (eg, triamcinolone 0.025–0.1%). Irritating compounds such as tars are best avoided.

Prognosis

In patients with a treatable underlying disease (eg, crusted scabies or drug-related eruption), the prognosis for cure or control of exfoliative dermatitis is good. In those with many of the other disorders, spontaneous remission or resolution occurs occasionally. The prognosis is poor in patients with idiopathic exfoliative dermatitis, who may die of systemic effects or complications. The course in patients with neoplastic disease varies with the type of cancer and the efficacy of treatment.

REFERENCES

Chakraborty A: Lymphoma as a cause of exfoliative dermatitis. Indian J Dermatol 1983;28:121.

Hurley HJ: Exfoliative dermatitis. Pages 543–548 in: *Dermatology,* 2nd ed. Moschella SL, Hurley HJ (editors). Saunders, 1985.

Nicolis GD, Helwig EB: Exfoliative dermatitis: A clinicopathologic study of 135 cases. Arch Dermatol 1973; 108:788.

Rosen T, Chappell R, Drucker C: Exfoliative dermatitis: Presenting sign of internal malignancy. South Med J 1979;72:652.

Tietze KJ, Gaska JA: Cefoxitin-associated exfoliative dermatitis. Clin Pharm 1983;2:582.

40

Eczematous Diseases

C.H.F. Vickers, MD

Eczematous diseases are generally characterized by scaling and pruritus. They can be differentiated from papulosquamous diseases because the lesions are not sharply marginated and because eczematous diseases tend to blister, weep, or become covered with crusts.

There are other forms of eczematous dermatitis besides those covered in this chapter. Irritant and allergic contact dermatitis are discussed in Chapter 33 and phototoxic and photoallergic eczematous dermatitis in Chapter 38. Also in the differential diagnosis are asteatotic eczema (due to overdrying of the skin), neurodermatitis—an unfortunate term—(due to habitual scratching), and polymorphic light eruption (discussed in Chapter 38).

ATOPIC ECZEMA

Essentials of Diagnosis

Major features:
- Pruritus.
- Chronic or chronically relapsing eczematous dermatitis.
- Typical morphology and distribution: facial or extensor involvement in infants and children or flexural lichenification or linearity in adults.
- Personal or family history of atopy (asthma, allergic rhinitis, atopic dermatitis).

Minor features:
- Three or more of minor features listed in Table 40–1.

General Considerations

Atopy literally means "uncommon" or "not in [the right] place." Other terms have included Besnier's prurigo and the unfortunate misnomer neurodermatitis.

Atopic eczema is common. The infantile form accounts for a significant portion of the pediatric dermatologist's clinical load. The basic abnormality is genetic, though the actual inheritance pattern is uncertain. Indeed, one member of the family may show atopic eczema, another bronchial asthma, and another hay fever. In the case of eczema, one basic defect is an inherently low threshold to pruritus. There are clear-cut pharmacologic and immunologic abnormalities in patients with atopic eczema, though none appear to be specific for the disease. Examples are the delayed blanch following intradermal injection of acetylcholine and high serum IgE levels. The incidence of the disease is around 3–4% of the population of the Western world, and it may be rising. There have been few epidemiologic studies. The disorders is most common in children.

Climatic changes influence the disease and its initial occurrence. There is a tendency for natives of one region moving to another to have either an increased or decreased incidence of the disorder. For example, Chinese-born patients living in San Francisco have an 8-fold greater incidence of atopic eczema than those who remain in China.

Microbiology & Immunology

About 80% of patients with atopic eczema develop immediate wheal reactions to various environmental allergens on scratch testing. However, these positive scratch tests may not be relevant to the disease, since it usually does not flare up when the antigens are encountered.

Elevated serum IgE levels are seen in most patients with atopic eczema, and the severity of the disease and its extent are usually reflected in the degree of elevation of IgE. However, elevations of serum IgE also occur in a number of conditions not in any way related to atopic or allergic problems (such as scabies), and the IgE levels in atopic subjects may remain high even when eczema has resolved. Furthermore, atopic eczema or an atopic-like eczema can occur in patients with low or even absent serum IgE, as in ataxia telangiectasia and X-linked hypogammaglobulinemia.

Cell-mediated immunity is disordered. Atopic children are abnormally susceptible to infection with human papillomaviruses (warts) and the viruses of molluscum contagiosum, herpes simplex, and vaccinia. Atopic subjects are less likely than others to develop cell-mediated contact sensitivity reactions superimposed on eczema. For example, sensitivity to the potent contact allergen dinitrochlorobenzene (DNCB) is

Table 40–1. Guidelines for the diagnosis of atopic dermatitis.[1]

Must have 3 or more basic features:
Pruritus
Typical morphology and distribution:
    Flexural lichenification or linearity in adults
    Facial and extensor involvement in infants and children.
Chronic or chronically-relapsing dermatitis
Personal or family history of atopy (asthma, allergic rhinitis, atopic dermatitis)

Plus 3 or more minor features:
Xerosis (uninflamed, rough, scaling skin)
Ichthyosis, palmar hyperlinearity, keratosis pilaris
Immediate (type I) skin test reactivity (especially multiple allergies)
Elevated serum IgE (especially high levels)
Early age at onset (eg, before age 5 years)
Tendency toward cutaneous infections (especially *Staphylococcus aureus* and herpes simplex) or impaired cell-mediated immunity
Nipple eczema (especially with lichenification)
Cheilitis (lick eczema, especially of upper lip)
Recurrent conjunctivitis
Dennie-Morgan infraorbital fold (especially a double fold)
Keratoconus
Anterior subcapsular cataracts (especially bilateral)
Orbital darkening ("allergic shiner")
Facial pallor or erythema
Pityriasis alba
Anterior horizontal neck folds
Itch when sweating
Intolerance to wool and lipid solvents (decreased itch threshold)
Perifollicular accentuation (pebbling)
Food intolerance
Course influenced by environmental or emotional factors
White dermographism or delayed blanch

[1] Adapted from Hanifin JM, Rajka G: Acta Derm Venereol 1980; 92(Suppl):44.

not as readily acquired by the atopic as by the nonatopic population. Many studies have shown alterations in in vitro measurements of cellular immunity, such as decreased responses of cultured lymphocytes to phytohemagglutinin. The depressed lymphocyte transformation may improve during remission and worsen with relapse of the atopic eczema. Finally, atopic subjects have a decrease in T suppressor cells that may favor increased IgE production.

Paradoxic Vascular Responses

There are subtle changes in vascular responses in the skin in atopic subjects. The facial pallor characteristic of the atopic individual is the most obvious clinical marker. White dermatographism is more frequent in the atopic individual, occurring in 80% compared to 20% of the normal population. The skin of normal people turns red after firm stroking, whereas the skin of some atopic patients turns white. Intradermal injection of acetylcholine also gives a paradoxic white reaction in 70% of atopic subjects, and this reaction is considered by some to be of diagnostic significance. This delayed blanch reaction is blocked by atropine but is not affected by procaine. Juhlin has

suggested that norepinephrine release is increased because guanethidine returns this reaction to normal. Guanethidine depletes norepinephrine deposits within the skin. Contrary to this view, Ramsey has suggested that the delayed blanch is due to dermal edema.

Clinical Findings

Patients should have at least the 3 essential features listed above. In addition, most patients have 3 or more minor features including those listed in Table 40–1.

A. Symptoms and Signs: Atopic eczema is characterized by a hereditary predisposition to a lowered threshold to itching and severe intractable itching. After repeated scratching and rubbing, the skin becomes lichenified (thick, with increased epidermal markings). Lichenification is characteristic—some say diagnostic—of atopic dermatitis. Lichenification results from chronic scratching.

The cardinal symptom of the disease is intense pruritus, characteristically worse when the patient is hot and aggravated by contact with wool or other scratchy materials and by environmental or psychologic stress. Marked changes in humidity and environmental temperatures usually also trigger itch.

Other clinical findings vary greatly at differing ages. In infants, lesions characteristically appear first on the cheeks and scalp, spreading rapidly across the whole of the face and frequently involving the antecubital and later the popliteal fossae. In severe cases, the eruption may rapidly become generalized. Weeping is common, and crusting develops rapidly on the cheeks and forehead. Other sites commonly involved are the wrists, ankles, and buttock folds (Fig 40–1). Occasionally, lesions appear on the knees and elbows, often alone or sometimes in association with the classic pattern (Fig 40–2). Many different patterns occur. Discoid lesions may occur in some sites. In patients whose dermatitis persists into the teen years or adulthood, involvement may center on the collar-

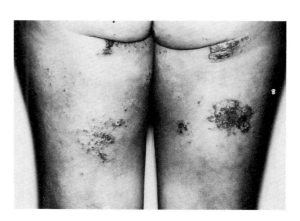

Figure 40–1. Patchy atopic dermatitis on the thighs.

ette area around the neck. The hands often become involved, and hand eczema may be a persistent problem late into the patient's lifetime.

Ichthyosis vulgaris—dry skin affecting virtually the whole body but usually sparing the popliteal and antecubital fossae—is frequently associated with atopic eczema. The dry skin (xerosis) associated with eczema usually occurs on the hands and in areas involved in the eczematous process. Keratotic plugging of hair follicles (keratosis pilaris) may occur, particularly on the upper outer arms—but since this is common in normal individuals, the relevance to atopic eczema is questionable. The eyelids are commonly involved and frequently become lichenified as a result of chronic rubbing. Excoriations may be numerous, and bleeding may occur and alarm the parents. As the lesions become more chronic, hyperpigmentation frequently occurs, especially in lichenified areas, though postinflammatory depigmentation occasionally results.

B. Laboratory Findings: Peripheral blood eosinophilia is a common nonspecific finding. High levels of eosinophils in nasal secretions may identify children who will later develop asthma. Serum levels of IgE are often elevated. Transient IgA deficiency at about 3 months of age may allow entry of allergens through the respiratory or alimentary tracts and stimulate IgE production, leading to development of the atopic state in a genetically predisposed individual.

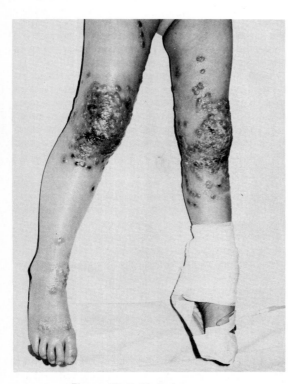

Figure 40–2. Vesicular eczema.

The histopathologic features are nonspecific, though gross hyperkeratosis and papillomatosis due to lichenification are easily recognized.

Differential Diagnosis

Cutaneous disorders that may be confused with atopic eczema include irritant dermatitis, miliaria rubra, and seborrheic dermatitis in infancy. Allergic contact dermatitis may be identified by the history or by patch testing. "Id" eruptions related to stasis dermatitis and nickel sensitivity may give rise to eruptions almost impossible to differentiate from atopic eczema except by history and patch testing.

Rare systemic disorders that mimic atopic eczema include congenital ectodermal dysplasia, ataxia telangiectasia, the Wiskott-Aldrich syndrome, X-linked agammaglobulinemia, gluten-sensitive enteropathy, ahistidinemia, phenylketonuria, and some genodermatoses associated with chromosome abnormalities. Hurler's syndrome, Hartnup disease, histiocytosis X, and acrodermatitis enteropathica may be characterized by episodes of rash with some similarity to atopic eczema. Differentiation is made easier by strict application of Rajka's criteria (Table 40–1) and by laboratory tests to rule out look-alike disorders.

Diagnosis is especially difficult (1) in early infancy, when the best approach is to await developments by naming the dermatitis "infantile eczema"; or (2) when atopic eczema arises for the first time in the age group from 20 to 30 years, in which case laboratory investigation may be helpful. Multiple positive prick, RIST, or RAST tests or very high serum IgE levels suggest atopy. The possibility of contact eczema or "id" eruption from stasis dermatitis must be carefully remembered.

Treatment

A. General Measures: The patient should avoid overheating, over-bathing, contact with wool, situations where sweating becomes excessive, and contact with irritants such soap. Do not tell the patient—child or adult—not to scratch! Doing so shows ignorance of the intensity of itching and of the irresistible urge to scratch.

The immunization program for infants should be normal. However, smallpox vaccination is best avoided, because the poxvirus may disseminate (Fig 40–3). Children of American servicemen may still be subjected to the risk of contact with vaccinia virus via smallpox vaccination, because the United States continues to vaccinate its troops. There is no credible evidence that children with atopic eczema have a higher incidence of adverse reactions to other immunization procedures than the normal population. The prospect of a child with asthma being unprotected from whooping cough, measles, and other exanthematous diseases is one that should not be considered.

At the initial interview with the parents of an atopic

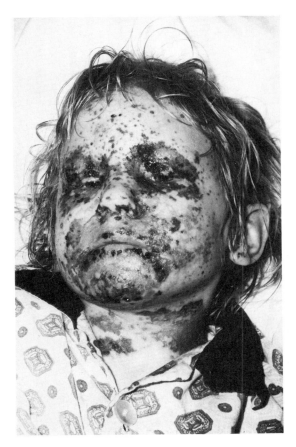

Figure 40–3. Eczema vaccinatum.

child, discussion of the problem is of great importance. Parents often have a feeling of guilt that their child is atopic, particularly if the mother has been unable to breast-feed. They need to be reassured that most patients improve as they get older. The initial discussion should also indicate that many factors exacerbate the disease and that allergy is only one possibility.

Associated asthma may require intermittent use of systemic corticosteroids. Exacerbations of the eczema may follow withdrawal of systemic steroid therapy.

A move to a dry climate may be beneficial, but some patients get worse. Humid hot climates often adversely influence the progress of the disease.

The influence of diet on the disease is still being debated. A few infants undoubtedly benefit from an egg- and milk-free diet. In most adults, the influence of diet seems to be minor. Attempts at desensitization to agents identified by RAST tests may be disastrous and frequently lead to flare-up of the eczema.

B. Local Treatment: Simple measures—especially the avoidance of irritants (soap, wool) and the addition of emollients to the bath or shower water—are of considerable importance. Occlusive nylon clothing may lead to sweat-related itching. Emollients should be applied to the skin after bathing or showering, especially in most patients with concomitant ichthyosis, and reapplied twice daily and more often as the occasion arises.

1. Lotions and compresses– In acute weeping phases, shake lotions, normal saline, 0.25% silver nitrate lotion, and tap water compresses are beneficial. These are applied for 15–60 minutes 4 times daily followed by applications of emollient ointments. Silver nitrate lotions stain skin, clothing, and other objects.

2. Corticosteroids– Topical corticosteroids usually contain the disease well. One should use the weakest preparation that gives reasonable control. Hydrocortisone 1% is best, but triamcinolone 0.025–0.1% may be necessary. It is difficult to be didactic about the corticosteroid base. In humid areas, ointments like petrolatum alba may lead to miliariasis; and in arid areas, runny or solid creams may prove too drying. Careful consideration of the risk-benefit ratio is necessary.

Minor degrees of steroid atrophy may be acceptable to the patient who is relieved of severe itching and cosmetically disabling disease. Systemic absorption of topically applied steroids may occur, especially in infants. Growth stunting is a theoretic risk but occurred in atopic children as a feature of the disease long before topical corticosteroids were discovered. Retarded growth may result from abnormal protein metabolism related to extensive skin disease.

3. Scholz regimen– Of many topical therapeutic regimens, Scholz avoids baths, ointments, and soaps and suggests application of a nonlipid emulsifying lotion and a weak steroid lotion such as 1% hydrocortisone. Results are said to be extremely good in California, but the British experience has not been favorable. It seems to work best in hot, damp climates.

4. Tar preparations– Tar preparations have a specific effect in the more chronic and lichenified lesions. Crude coal tar 1–3% in petrolatum is the preparation of choice. While cosmetically unpleasant, one can confine its use to night-time applications. More chronic lesions tend to be treated with ointments or creams containing corticosteroids or tar.

5. Occlusive dressing– Especially in infants and those with chronic lichenification, occlusive bandages are often helpful both for the therapeutic effect of the drugs used and to prevent trauma due to scratching. They increase systemic absorption of topical corticosteroids if used concomitantly. In small infants, light splinting of the arms at night only may be beneficial, but tight fixed splints are not justified.

C. Systemic Therapy:

1. Antihistamines– Antihistamines with sedative side effects (eg, hydroxyzine) are important for management of the atopic infant. They are metabolized more rapidly by infants than by adults, and relatively large doses may be indicated in very small children. Dosage for each individual child needs to be titrated, but on an average a 1-year-old baby may require 20 mg of promethazine at night to enable the child and parents to sleep. In infants, most other systemic drugs are contraindicated.

2. Corticosteroids– These agents may have value in the chronic adult atopic patient, but systemic corticosteroids or ACTH should never be used for infants and young children. For adults, ACTH injections are arguably safer than giving systemic prednisolone.

3. Sodium cromoglycate– If food allergy is suspected as a triggering cause for the attacks of eczema, it may be justifiable to administer oral sodium cromoglycate, but controlled trials have not proved this to be of real value.

4. Antibiotics– Erythromycin has been recommended in view of the frequency with which these children carry cutaneous staphylococci and the frequency of secondary infections, particularly in toddlers and young children. However, overgrowth of resistant organisms may be encouraged by the long-term administration of erythromycin, and many bacteriologists believe this to be unsatisfactory for long-term treatment.

5. Ultraviolet irradiation– Ultraviolet radiation from the sun and UVB or UVA from artificial light sources may help. PUVA is reserved for severe, refractory patients.

Complications

Before eradication of smallpox from the world, eczema vaccinatum was the most serious complication of atopic eczema. Generalization of vaccinia with viremia and severe illness lead to death in approximately 30% of affected patients (Fig 40–3).

Eczema herpeticum remains a major problem for the atopic individual. Every attempt should be made to shield the atopic child from individuals with active herpes simplex infections. The herpes virus gains access to the skin, and the resulting viremia or autoinoculation leads to the development of disseminated herpes lesions. Secondary staphylococcal infection with bacteremia and septicemia are further complications (Fig 40–4). Acyclovir, 200 mg orally every 4 hours (adult dose), should be administered to any patient with extensive eczema herpeticum. Staphylococcal superinfection occurs frequently in children, particularly toddlers and those under 10 years of age. Impetigo can become widespread over a short period owing to autoinoculation of bacteria by these children who scratch constantly.

Behavior problems occur chiefly in young children who use their disease to manipulate their parents. Parents should be warned of such possibilities, as the problem can easily be prevented. Every parent with an atopic child should be told to regard the child as

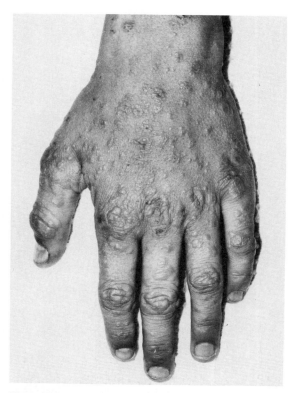

Figure 40–4. Gross secondary bacterial infection of atopic dermatitis.

normal but with a special skin. Parents should not overprotect.

Prognosis

The prognosis of infantile eczema is in general excellent; 90–95% of all cases clear during childhood. If the disorder has not cleared by age 12, persistence of eczema is likely. Adverse factors include late onset (after 2 years of age) and the reversed or inverted pattern, in which the extensor knees and elbows are affected in addition to the antecubital and popliteal fossae.

A positive family history does not worsen the prognosis, nor does the occurrence of other atopic disorders. Families do not run true to type, since parents severely affected into adult life may produce normal or minimally affected children. There is some evidence that effective treatment may improve the prognosis.

NUMMULAR (DISCOID) ECZEMA

Essentials of Diagnosis

- Well-marginated, vesiculated eczematous plaques, usually acute or subacute in intensity, covered with crust and scale.

- Extreme pruritus.
- Widespread eruption, especially on the extremities.

General Considerations

Discoid (nummular) eczema affects predominantly the older (60 and over) age groups, though it may occur at any age. It is rather common and responds poorly to topical therapy.

Clinical Findings

A. Symptoms and Signs: The lesions are characteristically vesicular, often extremely itchy, and crusted due to secondary infection. Lesions usually occur on peripheral parts of the limbs, though they may occur on the back and buttocks, rarely on the face. Lesions are clearly demarcated, oval or round, and vary in size from a few millimeters to several centimeters in diameter (Fig 40–5). They often appear suddenly and usually remain approximately the same size for the duration of the disease. There may be one or 2 small lesions, with minimal itching, or many lesions with intense itching. Crusting and secondary infection often occur at the onset; in other

cases, patients develop mostly low-grade circumscribed scaly and mildly pruritic patches.

Discoid eczema sometimes follows contact eczema or a burn. There may be a past or family history of atopic eczema. The natural history of the disease is variable, with some patients showing rapid clearing with or without therapy and others progressing to a widespread and therapeutically difficult problem. Some authors believe that bacterial infection is the basic etiologic agent, but most believe that the disorder is of totally unknown cause. Along with discoid eczema there is often an acquired (senile) ichthyosis, and this in itself may increase the intensity of pruritus.

B. Laboratory Findings: Serum IgE levels are elevated in about 25% of patients. Histopathologic examination shows spongiosis and other changes associated with eczematous dermatitis.

Differential Diagnosis

In addition to other eczemas, nummular eczema mimics papulosquamous diseases such as psoriasis because of the sharply marginated plaques. The scales of nummular eczema are smaller, the distribution is different, and the lesions are pruritic. Tinea corporis can be differentiated by KOH examination of scales.

Treatment

As in all types of eczema, avoidance of irritants such as soap, detergents, oils, and dust is important. Occasionally—especially in cases accompanied by severe exuding infection—a course of systemic antibiotics may be required.

Topical treatment consists of corticosteroids combined with antibacterials such as hydroxyquinolone used during the day and local tar preparations applied at night. Mid-strength steroids are usually necessary to control the disease. The use of emollients in the bath or shower and topical emollients after bathing has a soothing effect, especially if coincidental senile ichthyosis is present.

Systemic corticosteroid therapy may be indicated but is not very effective in low doses.

Ultraviolet light treatment may help.

LICHEN SIMPLEX

Essential of Diagnosis

- Chronic, moderately well demarcated, very thick plaque, usually somewhat violaceous in color.
- Pruritus, which is worsened by scratching.
- Commonly found on anterior shin, ankle, wrist, or nape of neck.

General Considerations

Some authors believe this condition, also called localized neurodermatitis, is a manifestation of the

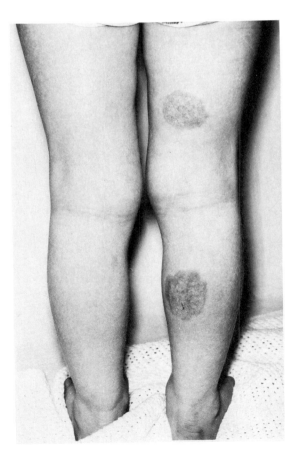

Figure 40–5. Nummular (discoid) eczema.

atopic state. The lesions appear to result purely from scratching and rubbing, usually when the patient is tense or concentrating.

Clinical Findings

The lesions characteristically consist of sharply demarcated plaques of intense lichenification. Weeping and vesiculation are absent, though excoriations may be seen. The disease is rare in children—though no age group is exempt—and more common in women than in men. Patients of Mongolian descent suffer from more severe and extreme forms of the disease. Favorite sites are those most easily accessible for scratching; the nape of the neck may be scratched when reading a book, the inner surface of the forearms may be scratched by an office worker sitting at a desk and rubbing the arm on the edge, the front of the shin may be rubbed by the opposite heel, and so on.

Differential Diagnosis

The diagnosis is usually obvious because of the singularity of lesions and intense lichenification. Mild stasis dermatitis may cause confusion or act as a trigger to scratching the ankles.

Treatment

Management is difficult, since the scratching has often become a habit not easily broken even by intelligent patients. High-potency topical corticosteroid therapy is indicated; coal tar preparations may be helpful; and in patients with lesions on the limbs occlusive bandaging is often indicated. A steroid-impregnated occlusive tape (eg, Cordran) applied at bedtime and removed in the morning may be very helpful. Most of the time the itch-scratch-itch cycle may be broken by application of potent steroids.

SEBORRHEIC DERMATITIS

Essentials of Diagnosis

- Chronic or subacute eczematous dermatitis.
- Location on scalp, ears, eyebrows, nasolabial fold, and mid chest.
- Mild pruritus.
- Scale may have a greasy quality.

General Considerations

This common type of eczema is poorly named. Although the disease occurs in seborrheic areas and there is an association with acne vulgaris and increased greasiness of the skin, this is by no means the rule. Sebaceous glands have no obvious role in causation. The disorder is probably genetically determined, though the mode of inheritance is not clear. Seborrheic dermatitis has a characteristic pattern of distribution, though it may occasionally be generalized.

Clinical Findings

The lesions of seborrheic dermatitis are often not especially pruritic and characteristically may have a yellow or orange hue. Usually there is diffuse dandruff with erythema of the scalp. Psoriasiform plaques may occur, especially if there is secondary infection secondary to scratching. Lesions occur on the face, especially the perinasal areas. Bilateral otitis externa is a common association (unilateral otitis externa being a manifestation of otitis interna). Other areas involved are the groin, the axillae, the natal cleft, the sternal area of the chest, and the back. Perineal involvement often causes pruritus ani et vulvae. This form of eczema should always be considered in such cases. Often there is a pityriasis rosea-like eruption on the trunk.

Itching is not a dominant feature, but both bacterial and candidal superinfections are difficult to manage when they occur. The condition is often most troublesome under the breasts or the pendulous abdomen of female patients. Blepharitis is common and associated with styes. Occasionally, generalization to exfoliative erythroderma results. Diffuse or localized hair loss is uncommon, and hair usually grows back after effective therapy.

Most patients with severe acne have some degree of seborrheic eczema, manifested at least by severe dandruff. The association of seborrheic eczema with psoriasis has given rise to much speculation. There are patients who appear to have both diseases; at one time, they show classic lesions of psoriasis and at another they show the lesions of seborrheic eczema. This has been referred to as "seborrhiasis" or "sebopsoriasis." Hot humid climates have a deleterious effect, as do occupations involving high humidity and temperature. Of interest is the occasional development of a mixture of seborrheic eczema and discoid eczema as a manifestation of sensitivity to methyldopa used in the treatment of hypertension. Seborrheic dermatitis is also a component of Parkinson's syndrome and is frequently seen in patients with AIDS.

Treatment

Management of seborrheic eczema is similar to that of other eczemas. Shampoos containing tar, sulfur, salicylic acid, or selenium are useful, especially if used daily. Hydrocortisone 1% cream usually controls the disease on the face and chest. Solutions of middle potency steroids (eg, fluocinolone 0.01% solution) applied to the scalp daily or twice daily help the scalp problem if shampoos alone prove ineffective. Ketoconazole 2% cream applied twice daily to affected areas is an effective alternative to topical corticosteroids. The administration of systemic antibiotics in acute exacerbations is often helpful.

POMPHOLYX

Essentials of Diagnosis
- Discrete, relatively uninflamed vesicles on the palms (cheiropompholyx) and soles (pedopompholyx).
- Intense pruritus.
- Vesicles may become confluent to form bullae.
- Tendency for periodic recurrence.

General Considerations
Whether pompholyx should be discussed separately from other eczemas is arguable, but that will be done here because therapy is different. The old name "dyshidrotic pompholyx" should no longer be used. The sweat glands play no part in causation. Pompholyx means "bubble" in Greek, and the words simply denote vesicular eczema of the palms and soles, respectively.

Clinical Features
A. Symptoms and Signs: In general, vesicles tend to be distributed on the sides of the fingers and later on the central palms and on the soles. They often become confluent and develop into large multilocular bullae. Itching is intense and secondary infection common, particularly on the feet. Often the lesions become hyperkeratotic and fissured. In some cases only the hands are involved initially, and spread to the soles occurs later; in others, the reverse is true. It is a good practice in any case of eczema to carefully examine the feet, since minor degrees of tinea pedis may result in an "id" eruption that mimics pompholyx of the palms. Precipitating factors include contact dermatitis, stress and systemic infection.

B. Laboratory Findings: The histologic picture is that of an acute eczematous dermatitis with intraepidermal spongiotic vesicles.

Differential Diagnosis
Id reactions from tinea pedis have already been discussed. A similar eczema is present on the hands of many patients allergic to nickel. Psoriasis may occasionally erupt, with vesicles appearing on the fingers.

Treatment
Therapy is based on established dermatologic principles. Low- or mid-potency topical steroids alone are often ineffective. High-potency steroids applied 3 times a day may help. Soaking the hands in 1:10,000 potassium permanganate solution, normal saline, or Burow's solution for 10–15 minutes followed by wet dressings of 0.5% silver nitrate solution or shake lotions give rapid relief. Staining of the skin and hands by silver nitrate and potassium permanganate, however, may not be acceptable.

STASIS DERMATITIS

Essentials of Diagnosis
- Poorly defined chronic eczematous dermatitis, usually near the ankles.
- Associated brown discoloration from hemosiderin deposition.
- Associated evidence of venous insufficiency, including varicose veins and pedal edema.
- Tendency for superimposed ulceration.

General Considerations
Dermatitis may complicate disorders of the venous system in the lower leg. The earliest signs may be purpura and brown discoloration due to hemosiderin deposition. Obvious varicose veins and edema are usually present as well. Neglect of stasis dermatitis may lead to the development of chronic ulcers that may be slow to heal. The disease is due to capillary venous hypertension associated with varicose veins or a deep vein thrombosis.

Clinical Findings
The legs are characteristically edematous or indurated. The initial lesion is usually over the medial malleolus, but lesions may occur over the lateral malleolus as well. Leakage of red cells into the dermis leads to marked purpura and later hemosiderin deposition. Inflammatory changes occur, and eczema develops. Ulceration often follows trauma to an area of gravitational eczema, and, once formed, the ulcer may enlarge with remarkable rapidity.

Venography may be used to assess the competence of deep and superficial veins. Patch tests can rule out superimposed contact allergy.

Differential Diagnosis
One type of gravitational disease deserves special mention, the so called atrophie blanche. White patches of atrophic skin with dilated capillaries in their centers develop over the malleoli and the dorsum of the feet. These are due to vascular insufficiency from increased intravascular pressure. When present, ulcers may follow. Although these may be small, the pain may be severe.

Stasis ulcers always show abnormal areas of skin around them (eczema, edema, brown color) whereas arterial ulcers develop in otherwise normal skin. A gravitational ulcer can occur on any part of the lower leg and even on the dorsum of the foot, though arterial ulceration is commoner in such cases. If, however, the surrounding skin is carefully examined, the differential diagnosis of the 2 types of ulceration is relatively easy.

Areas of stasis dermatitis and stasis ulcers are fertile soil for induction of allergy to topical medications. Therefore, allergic contact dermatitis may be superimposed on stasis dermatitis. Neomycin is a notorious culprit.

Treatment

The basic premise of treatment is to restore the efficiency of the "leg muscle pump" damaged by the incompetent or destroyed venous valves. This is best achieved by some form of reasonably tight elastic bandaging. Patients with sedentary occupations should be advised when sitting to raise the affected limb on blocks or a stool and to at least walk around the room once every hour. Those with occupations standing at a machine are the most disadvantaged, and again occasional moving around will allow muscular action to improve the venous circulation. Cellulitis is a frequent complication of gravitational ulceration and requires a suitable systemic antibiotic.

Since patients with gravitational eczema and ulceration seem especially prone to the development of dermatitis medicamentosa—probably due to the multiplicity of the applications because of marked chronicity of the condition—potentially sensitizing agents should be avoided. Simple applications such as Burow's solution, 2% ichthammol in zinc cream or Lassar's paste, or 0.5% silver nitrate lotion (*caution:*may stain) are often all that is required. Tight, even support with bandages or form-fit thigh-high stockings (Jobst) is the most important factor in treatment. Topical corticosteroids are of use for a limited period in the management of acute and chronic gravitational eczema but never on the ulcerated area, since vasoconstriction resulting from topical steroids may further jeopardize the cutaneous blood supply and hinder the healing process.

REFERENCES

Aly R, Maibach H: *Clinical Skin Microbiology*. Thomas, 1978.

Hanifin JM: Atopic dermatitis. J Am Acad Dermatol 6:1, 1982.

Hanifin JM, Rajka G: Diagnostic criteria for atopic dermatitis. Acta Derm Venereol 1980;92(Suppl):44.

Heskel N, Lobitz WC: Atopic dermatitis in children: Clinical features and management. Semin Hematol 1983; 2:39.

Rajka G: *Atopic Dermatitis*. Saunders, 1975.

Vickers CFH: The natural history of atopic eczema. Acta Derm Venereol 1980;92(Suppl):113.

Papulosquamous Diseases

41

Henry H. Roenigk, Jr, MD

Papulosquamous diseases are characterized by scaling papules or plaques. In contrast to the eczematous diseases, which also show scaling, the plaques of papulosquamous diseases are sharply marginated and there are rarely signs of epithelial disruption such as crusts, excoriations, or weeping. The prototypical papulosquamous disease is psoriasis.

PSORIASIS

Essentials of Diagnosis

- Well-demarcated, thick scaling erythematous plaques.
- Plaques covered with large adherent silver scales.
- Lesions typically on elbows, knees, or scalp.
- Pitted nails.
- Erythrodermatous, pustular, and guttate forms.
- Auspitz's sign: pinpoint bleeding if scale is pulled off.
- Sometimes occurs in lines at areas of trauma (Koebner's phenomenon).

General Considerations

Psoriasis is a common scaly erythematous disease of unknown cause showing wide variation in severity and distribution of skin lesions. It usually follows an irregular chronic course marked by remissions and exacerbations of unpredictable onset and duration. Factors that may lead to more lesions include drug reactions, respiratory infections, cold weather, emotional stress, surgery, and viral infections.

About 6 million people in the USA (2% of the population) have psoriasis. Psoriasis vulgaris produces stigmatizing chronic, recurrent lesions that are often emotionally and physically debilitating. Psoriasis is an expensive disease that frequently requires lifelong treatment.

The cause of psoriasis is unknown. There is a genetic predisposition, but the exact modes of inheritance are unknown. Certain HLA antigens are more common among populations of psoriatic patients, so a gene linked to or related to HLA genes may be one predisposing factor. Kinetic cell studies have shown that in psoriasis, the epidermal cells proliferate rapidly, completing a germinative cell cycle more rapidly than do the cells of normal skin. In psoriasis,

the epidermis renews itself in just 3–4 days instead of in the normal epidermal turnover time of 28–56 days. An abnormality of growth control mechanisms has been postulated.

Numerous biochemical and structural abnormalities have been found in psoriasis, but cause and effect relationships are uncertain. Immunologic abnormalities and excess production of leukotrienes and other inflammatory cells may be more important in pathogenesis than previously realized.

Clinical Findings

The diagnosis is usually obvious and is based on the typical appearance and locations of lesions. However, the many different sizes and shapes of lesions in psoriasis often mislead the general practitioner, and referral to a dermatologist or (occasionally) a skin biopsy may be needed to confirm the diagnosis. Lesions are typically round, well-demarcated, pink, scaling plaques of various sizes covered by an abundance of grayish-white imbricated scales. If these scales are traumatically removed, multiple small pinpoint bleeding sites appear (Auspitz's sign). Lesions can occur anywhere, but the elbows and knees are most commonly affected. The symmetry of plaques over both sides of the body is often remarkable. Other common sites of involvement are the scalp, sacral and perianal area, genitalia, and nails. The patient may experience a burning sensation and pruritus in acute flare-ups of the disease, but psoriatic lesions are more often asymptomatic except for the cosmetic embarrassment. Lesions may be so extensive that erythroderma covers the entire body (erythroderma psoriaticum).

A. Location of Lesions:

1. Body– Well-defined erythematous plaques (Fig 41–1) with sharp borders usually have silvery-gray scales. Plaques tend to be symmetric in distribution, with knees (Fig 41–2) and elbows most commonly affected. Active psoriatic plaques extend rapidly along the periphery and may form a ring with central clearing. Physical trauma in the active phase results in development of linear patterns of psoriasis in the injured areas (Koebner's phenomenon). Such isomorphic lesions may also be seen on the hands of factory workers in jobs requiring extensive use of the hands; they occur also in golf or tennis players. In

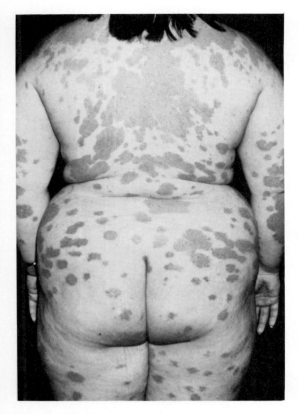

Figure 41–1. Generalized plaque-type psoriasis with symmetric distribution.

B. Types of Lesions:

1. Pustular– Generalized (von Zumbusch) pustular psoriasis may occur in a patient with classic plaque-type psoriasis or may occur de novo. There is a sudden onset of fever (to 104 °F [40 °C]), chills, and arthralgias, followed by generalized erythema studded with hundreds of small sterile pustules that resolve in 3–5 days, only to be followed by another crop.

Pustules often occur on the palmar and plantar surfaces of the hands and feet. These are routinely found in patients with the generalized (von Zumbusch) type pustular psoriasis. Some patients have pustular psoriasis limited to the palms and soles. These pustules are not associated with systemic symptoms, and the diagnosis of psoriasis is difficult because typical psoriatic plaques often are not present elsewhere.

2. Guttate– Small, erythematous droplike papules with fine scales are scattered over the entire body. The eruption may appear suddenly following upper respiratory tract infection or streptococcal pharyngitis, particularly in children and young adults.

3. Erythroderma psoriaticum– Rarely, psoriasis presents as diffuse generalized scaling (exfoliative) erythroderma with no typical demarcated plaques or

intertriginous areas (groin, axillae), erythematous plaques occur that are moist and lack the characteristic scaling and elevation above surrounding skin.

2. Hands and feet– Plaques are usually less erythematous than those on the elbows or knees but are well-demarcated and have large white scales. Pustules may occur in the plaques. Hyperkeratosis and fissures may lead to severe disability.

3. Scalp– Scalp lesions are characterized by erythema, scaling, and pruritus similar to that encountered in seborrheic dermatitis. Plaques are usually well-demarcated. Any hair loss is not permanent. There may be plaques along the forehead extending from the scalp.

4. Nails– Nail changes are common in psoriasis and may affect several or all fingernails. There may be stippling or pitting of the nail plate; yellowing or altered transparency of the nail is followed by accumulation of scales that distorts the nail plate and may lead to onycholysis. Secondary bacterial or fungal infection may result in black or green discoloration of the nail plate. Swelling, redness, and scaling of the paronychial margins occur frequently, and associated arthritis of the terminal interphalangeal joint (Fig 41–3) is often found.

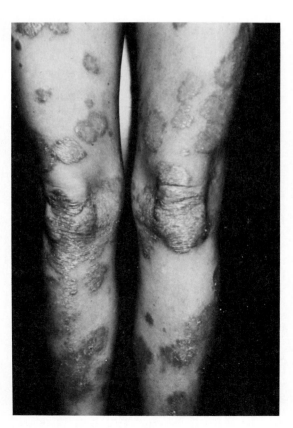

Figure 41–2. Plaque-type psoriasis of the legs with predilection for the knees.

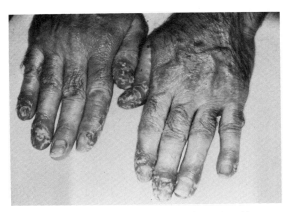

Figure 41–3. Psoriasis of nails and nail beds, with associated arthritis at the terminal interphalangeal joint.

guttate lesions. Differentiation of this form of psoriasis from pityriasis rubra pilaris or Sézary syndrome may require skin biopsy and blood tests.

C. Psoriatic Arthritis: There are 5 distinct forms of arthritis associated with psoriasis, the most common being a monarticular, nonsymmetric type affecting mainly the hand joints. Rheumatoid-type arthritis (rheumatoid factor-negative) and severe mutilating types are also seen. There is a strong correlation between HLA-B27 histocompatibility antigen and psoriatic arthritis, ankylosing spondylitis, and Reiter's disease.

Differential Diagnosis

A. Seborrheic Dermatitis: Scaling on the scalp is more diffuse than in psoriasis, and there are no individual plaques. Lesions on the face and chest are erythematous, with fine scales, and appear more eczematous than papulosquamous. Psoriasis is uncommon on the face, and seborrheic dermatitis never affects the elbows, knees, or extremities.

B. Lichen Planus: In lichen planus, plaques are small (like those of guttate psoriasis), distinctly bluish pink, and multiangled; they predominate on flexor surfaces rather than on the extensor surfaces that are more common in psoriasis. Lesions show much less scaling; only fine striae occur on the papules of lichen planus. Lesions in the mouth are common. If there is doubt, skin biopsy may confirm the diagnosis.

C. Pityriasis Rosea: The small thin, oval plaques of pityriasis rosea have fine scales at the periphery and are distributed only over the trunk; their long axes line up in a "Christmas tree" pattern.

D. Secondary Syphilis: Guttate lesions or small plaques resemble pityriasis rosea more than psoriasis. In syphilis, lesions are usually present on the palms and soles and in the mouth (mucous patches). Serologic tests for syphilis are positive in secondary syphilis.

E. Cutaneous T Cell Lymphoma: The plaques of mycosis fungoides may look identical to those of psoriasis, and only a skin biopsy can differentiate them. Plaques of mycosis fungoides are more likely to be asymmetric, nonround, and of varying thickness and tend to have little or no scaling. The erythrodermatous phase of mycosis fungoides (Sézary syndrome) and that of erythroderma psoriaticum are also similar.

F. Tinea and Onychomycosis: Fungal infections are generally localized on the feet, groin, and hands, though lesions on the trunk may resemble psoriasis. Scales are usually at the periphery of lesions, which are characterized by central clearing. Nails affected by fungal infection are thick and dystrophic but usually lack the pitting associated with psoriasis. Microscopic examination of material taken from the lesion and smeared on a slide with a drop of 10% potassium hydroxide may reveal fungal hyphae; cultures for fungus may also be diagnostic.

Complications

The major complications of psoriasis are erythroderma and generalized pustular psoriasis. Erythroderma psoriaticum may result in heat loss, pooling of fluids in skin, and high-output heart failure. Generalized pustular psoriasis may be complicated by secondary septicemia and accompanying disturbances of fluid and electrolyte balance.

Many patients with psoriasis develop arthritis that resembles rheumatoid arthritis in many ways. Patients with psoriatic arthritis do not have rheumatoid factor in their sera. The degree of arthritis does not correlate with the extent of skin involvement but usually improves when psoriasis is brought into remission. Severe psoriasis of the soles causes painful fissures that may make walking difficult.

Treatment

A. General Plan of Treatment: The goal of all therapy in psoriasis is to achieve remission in which all or almost all lesions have disappeared. Topical therapy should be used if possible. Systemic therapy is used if topical therapy fails. Exacerbations and remissions are the usual course.

If psoriasis is limited to a few plaques, topical corticosteroids or tar should be used initially. Application of topical corticosteroids under an occlusive plastic wrap (Saran Wrap; Actiderm) or intralesional injection of corticosteroids may result in rapid clearing of limited lesions.

If psoriasis is widespread and covers at least 50% of the body, an intensive course of topical corticosteroids for about 4 days, followed by treatment with tar and repeated suberythemic doses of ultraviolet light (UVB), may be used (Goeckerman regimen; see below). Treatment can be undertaken in a hospital or at a psoriasis day care center under the direction of a dermatologist and takes about 3 weeks. Remissions lasting for longer than 1 year have sometimes been achieved.

If the patient fails to respond, referral to a dermatologist is recommended. The major options then include (1) methotrexate, (2) photochemotherapy, (3) etretinate, (4) cyclosporine, and (5) combination systemic therapy. The benefits and risks of these therapies must be carefully discussed with the patient.

B. Advice to the Patient: The chronic course of psoriasis and the lack of a cure can be discouraging to both the patient and the physician if an unwarranted "nothing-can-be-done" attitude is adopted. The patient should be assured at the first visit that although there is no cure for psoriasis, the disease can be effectively controlled by one or more methods of treatment. Psoriatic lesions may disappear spontaneously or as a result of therapy, but recurrence of the disease is likely whether it occurs in a week, a month, a year, or perhaps several years.

Initially, the patient should be cautioned about factors that exacerbate psoriasis, eg, alcohol, obesity, emotional upsets, infection, trauma to the skin, and drugs (eg, lithium, beta-blockers, antimalarials, indomethacin).

Proper attention should be paid to maintaining sound nutrition and avoiding stress and fatigue, because these factors affect the patient's response to therapy. No specific dietary component seems to play a role in psoriasis, though the obese patient will benefit from losing weight. Dietary fish oil supplements may have limited benefit.

C. Topical Therapy: Most patients with psoriasis can be effectively treated with topical therapy. Even when systemic treatment becomes necessary, topical treatment should be continued so that the dosage of required systemic drugs can be reduced and excessive use of these potent agents can be avoided.

1. Topical corticosteroids– Patients with plaques limited to a few areas respond well to therapy aimed at removing scales and lubricating lesions. Topical corticosteroids are among the most useful agents for this purpose; the addition of salicylic acid 3–6%, liquor carbonis detergens 5%, or other tar bases to the corticosteroids may enhance their efficacy.

Occlusive pliable plastic dressings over topical corticosteroids increase their effectiveness, though such dressings are usually used only during sleep (6–8 hours). Plastic wrap is used on the extremities, dry cleaning bags or plastic exercise suits on the trunk, plastic food bags on the feet, and disposable plastic gloves on the hands. Whole-body reusable plastic suits can usually be purchased at department or sporting goods stores. Flurandrenolide-impregnated tape (Cordran tape) is satisfactory for occluding small areas of the body. Actiderm with or without topical steroids is effective for local areas.

Topical corticosteroids are available in several different bases. Gels are superior to ointments, which in turn are superior to creams. Prolonged use of topical corticosteroids, especially fluorinated agents or applications under occlusion, may lead to atrophy of the skin, telangiectasia, striae, and overgrowth of bacterial and fungal infections of the skin. Rapid recurrence of psoriasis (rebound phenomenon) may also occur when topical corticosteroids are used for long periods and then discontinued. Systemic absorption of corticosteroids may be sufficient to cause adrenal gland suppression and Cushing's syndrome, especially with newer "superpotent" topical steroids (eg, clobetasol propionate [Temovate]).

Intralesional injection of corticosteroids is effective for localized resistant plaques of psoriasis. Suspensions of injectable triamcinolone acetonide (Kenalog-10), 10 mg/mL (diluted to 5 mg/mL with saline), are often used. The suspension is injected with a 30-gauge disposable needle until blanching occurs. About one injection per square centimeter is sufficient.

2. Tars– Tars, crude or refined, are effective in the treatment of psoriasis when used alone or in combination with ultraviolet light therapy. The color, smell, and staining qualities of tars make them unaesthetic, however.

A bath containing 2 capfuls of Zetar Emulsion (30% coal tar) or Balnetar (2.5% coal tar) leaves a barely visible coating of tar on the skin. The traditional preparations of 1–5% coal tar in petrolatum are effective but messy. Tar is usually applied to the skin at least 2 hours before ultraviolet light therapy. Tar may not be practical for home use, because greasy black tar will stain everything the patient touches.

A more cosmetically acceptable tar-derived preparation is liquor carbonis detergens, commonly applied in concentrations of 5–10% in cold cream. If the patient's skin tends to dry out with daily bathing, bath oil may be added to the water.

Cosmetically acceptable tar preparations are available for baths or as shampoo, and some tars have been placed in a gel base (Estar, Psorigel) that makes them effective, safe, and more cosmetically acceptable to patients.

The scalp is difficult to treat, especially in patients with thick hair. Mineral oil or P&S Plus gel may be applied and left on for several hours to loosen scales before shampooing. Thick plaques on the scalp may be loosened by a preparation consisting of oil of cade (juniper tar) 20%, sulfur 10%, salicylic acid 5%, and 90 g of a nongreasy, water-removable ointment (Unibase). Most patients require at least one shampoo daily with an antiseborrheic or tar shampoo. Topical corticosteroid lotions or gels (eg, betamethasone valerate [Valisone] 0.1%, fluocinolone acetonide (Synalar), 0.01% solution) may be applied to the scalp between shampoos. Occlusion of the scalp can be obtained with a shower or bathing cap worn over the head after corticosteroids have been applied.

3. Anthralin– Anthralin paste has the potential to

irritate normal skin, so it must be applied to psoriatic plaques only—a tedious and time-consuming process; however, it does cause rapid flattening of thick psoriatic plaques. Short contact with low concentrations of anthralin may be effective without some of the side effects (eg, leaving anthralin cream on the plaques for 30 minutes and then washing it off). Dithranol 0.1, 0.2, or 0.4% paste and Drithocreme 0.1, 0.25, 0.5, and 1% cream are commercially available in the USA. All anthralin preparations stain the skin, fabrics, and other surfaces.

D. Phototherapy: Natural sunlight is effective adjunctive therapy for psoriasis, as most patients find who travel to warm, sunny climates. Psoriasis often improves in the summer for this reason also.

If natural sunlight is not reliably available, a substitute source of ultraviolet light should be found. Small portable sunlamps promoted for home use are not suitable, because only a small area of skin can be exposed to the lamp at any one time.

Artificial ultraviolet light exposure under the direction of a physician experienced in phototherapy can be best provided in a walk-in ultraviolet light booth containing 8 or more 4- to 6-foot-long UVB (290–320 nm) sunlamp bulbs. A typical "light box" allows an initial safe exposure time of 1 minute in fair-skinned individuals, 2 minutes in darker-skinned patients, and 3 minutes in black patients. Treatment time is increased by 1-minute increments with each successive treatment as tolerated or until the desired point of minimal erythema is reached. Treatment may be given every day or 2–3 times per week.

The maximum exposure tolerated without burning is usually 10–15 minutes in whites and 15–25 minutes in blacks, but maximum exposure times are dependent upon the UVB output of the box.

UVB or UVA light sources are available in many health clubs. UVB light booths are available commercially and may be purchased for home use, though they are not standardized. Home light boxes can be constructed using an empty closet lined with aluminum foil and containing 8 UVB bulbs.

During ultraviolet light therapy, special sunglasses or goggles must be worn to prevent eye damage. Long-term chronic exposure carries risks of actinic damage to skin (eg, wrinkles, freckles, lentigines) and skin cancer.

E. Goeckerman Regimen (Inpatient Treatment): When topical outpatient therapy fails or when psoriasis becomes more extensive and complications develop, hospitalization is necessary. It is helpful if the hospital has specially trained nurses to care for the many problems of psoriatic patients.

In acute, spreading psoriasis, the agents applied must be soothing; aggressive therapy should be avoided. Cool baths and petrolatum or other lubricants are safe.

The Goeckerman regimen and its variations have been a standard inpatient treatment for psoriasis for 50 years. Hospitalization usually lasts for 3–4 weeks. Clinical improvement results in remission for 6–8 months in almost all patients after discharge. Some remissions last a year or longer.

The Goeckerman procedure involves application of crude coal tar ointment 2–5% to the entire body at bedtime and left on overnight. (Application for 2 hours before exposure to ultraviolet light is an effective alternative.) In the morning, excess tar is removed with mineral oil. The patient's entire body is then exposed to ultraviolet light using a light box equipped with ordinary fluorescent bulbs (UVB range, 290–320 nm) and aluminum reflecting sides. After the ultraviolet treatment, the patient bathes to remove the remaining tar.

It is important to test the patient for the minimal erythema dose before starting ultraviolet light therapy if the patient gives a history of "light sensitivity," because in these patients such therapy will exacerbate psoriasis rather than improve it.

The amount of ultraviolet light should be gradually increased over successive treatments to a suberythema dose.

Rest and relaxation during the remainder of the day are also part of the treatment. Informal discussion between patients, nurses, and doctors helps patients understand psoriasis and the treatments they are undergoing.

A modified version of the Goeckerman routine can be used to shorten the hospital stay. Instead of applying crude coal tar at night, the patient applies topical corticosteroids with or without a plastic occlusive suit. In the morning, the remaining medication is removed, and the patient takes a tar bath before receiving ultraviolet light therapy. Topical corticosteroids should not be used for more than 4–5 days, because prolonged use may result in rebound flare of guttate psoriasis.

F. Psoriasis Day Care Center (Outpatient Treatment): Psoriasis day care centers are an outgrowth of the successes achieved by treatment during hospitalization. The same type of treatments used for hospitalized patients may be used in day care centers, where the patient stays only from 8 AM to 5 PM. This modification reduces costs and provides the same effective therapy used for inpatients.

The same combination of ultraviolet light plus tar, tar gel, or anthralin is used during daytime hours. The patient goes home or to work in the evenings and returns to the psoriasis day care center each morning.

Remissions achieved from treatment provided in psoriasis day care centers are similar to those occurring in inpatient Goeckerman therapy.

G. Systemic Therapy: Antihistamines (eg, hydroxyzine, 25 mg every 4 hours) often help relieve pruritus associated with acute flare-ups of psoriasis. Sedatives and tranquilizers (eg, diazepam, 5 mg every 6 hours) may help alleviate some of the anxiety that accompanies psoriasis. Antibiotics (eg, erythromycin, 250 mg 4 times daily) are indicated if acute guttate psoriasis follows a confirmed streptococcal infection.

1. Systemic corticosteroids– Although systemic treatment of psoriasis with corticosteroids was enthusiastically recommended 20 years ago, it quickly became obvious that corticosteroids merely controlled psoriasis and that long-term therapy caused many complications that are now well known. When corticosteroids are withdrawn, a rebound flare-up of disease occurs and the disease often becomes worse and more unstable (pustular, erythrodermic) than it was before therapy. Some recurrences take the form of generalized pustular psoriasis that is much more severe than the original psoriasis. Small doses of systemic corticosteroids may be indicated for severe, disabling psoriatic arthritis (eg, prednisone, 10–15 mg every morning).

2. Antimetabolites– Because epidermal hyperproliferation may play a part in the pathogenesis of psoriasis, antimitotic agents are a logical choice for treatment. Methotrexate is one of the oldest antimitotic drugs and has been used in treatment of psoriasis for 30 years; however, it is associated with a number of serious risks and should be administered only by a physician experienced in antimetabolite therapy. Methotrexate is the only antimetabolite currently approved by the FDA for psoriasis therapy.

The dosage of methotrexate is 15–25 mg/wk orally either in a single dose or in divided doses over 36 hours (3 doses at 12-hour intervals). Careful monitoring of laboratory parameters including especially blood counts, liver function tests, creatinine clearance, and chest x-rays (to detect methotrexate-related pulmonary fibrosis) is necessary. Because liver damage is insidious and often not detectable with serum liver function tests, periodic liver biopsies are necessary. Pregnancy is contraindicated. Specific guidelines have been published (Roenigk, 1982, 1988).

a. Indications– Because of the high risks associated with its use, methotrexate is indicated only for the symptomatic control of psoriasis that fails to respond to other forms of therapy and only when the amount of discomfort and the patient's general physical condition and degree of incapacity are felt to outweigh the risks. Some patients with the following conditions may be candidates for methotrexate therapy: psoriatic erythroderma, psoriatic arthritis, acute generalized pustular psoriasis (von Zumbusch type), localized pustular psoriasis, psoriasis that prevents employment, and extensive psoriasis. The need to discontinue systemic corticosteroids also is an indication for methotrexate therapy.

b. Contraindications– The relative contraindications to methotrexate therapy include an unreliable patient, significantly abnormal renal or liver function, pregnancy, active or recent hepatitis, fibrosis or cirrhosis of the liver, severe leukopenia or thrombocytopenia, active infectious disease (eg, tuberculosis or pyelonephritis), and anemia.

3. Photochemotherapy– Photochemotherapy (PUVA) combines the use of the photosensitivity drug methoxsalen and ultraviolet light (UVA range) administered in special ultraviolet light boxes under the supervision of physicians specially trained in phototherapy. It has proved highly effective in the treatment of severe psoriasis. Special artificial lights that have a peak irradiation of about 350 nm irradiate the skin with increasing doses (measured in J/cm^2 of light) $1\frac{1}{2}$ hours after the patient has taken oral methoxsalen (Oxsoralen-Ultra). Complete clearing of psoriasis can be achieved in over 90% of patients treated with an average of 20 PUVA treatments. Some patients experience prolonged remission and require no further treatment, but most require maintenance treatments of PUVA at 1- or 2-week intervals to remain free of symptoms. Detailed guidelines for correct use of PUVA therapy, including indications, complications, and precautions, are available. The package insert for Oxsoralen-Ultra reviews much of this information. Long-term side effects may include skin cancer, aging of the skin, and cataract formation.

PUVA is mainly an outpatient therapy. It obviates the need for topical corticosteroids, tars, anthralin, and other agents often cosmetically unacceptable to patients and also avoids the use of methotrexate and other cytotoxic drugs that require constant monitoring for hematologic, hepatic, and other potential long-term side effects. The use of PUVA is usually limited by the need for special phototherapy light sources, and thus it is normally administered only under the direction of dermatologists.

4. Etretinate– Etretinate is a retinoid drug—an analogue of vitamin A—that can be used to treat severe psoriasis. It is usually given daily in a dose of 0.5–1 mg/kg orally. Side effects are common. Most patients develop chapped lips and either a dry or sticky skin. Some lose all or most of their hair. Systemic effects include elevations of serum triglycerides or cholesterol and changes in liver function tests or blood counts. Headaches, pseudotumor cerebri, fatigue, and muscle pains are other side effects. Long-term therapy may cause diffuse idiopathic skeletal hypertrophy. Etretinate is a teratogen and must not be given to women who might become pregnant during therapy or within 1–2 years thereafter.

5. RePUVA (Retinoid-PUVA)– Etretinate can be used in combination with PUVA. About 50% of patients with psoriasis refractory to PUVA alone do improve when this retinoid is added. Combinations of etretinate with UVB, topical steroids, or other topical therapy can also be used. These combinations clear psoriasis more quickly with fewer side effects from retinoids.

6. Cyclosporine– Cyclosporine is a potent immunosuppressive drug that was developed mainly for preventing rejection of renal, heart, and liver transplants. Clinical trials have found it a highly effective systemic agent in clearing psoriasis. It has been used mainly in severe generalized psoriasis resistant to other forms of therapy. The dosage has been 5–7.5 mg/kg/d, though lower doses (2.5 mg/kg/d) may also be effective. Significant side effects can occur such as nephrotoxicity, hypertension, skin cancer, and lymphoma. Treatment of psoriasis with cyclosporine is still considered experimental. The lesions of psoriasis will return when the drug is stopped.

Prognosis

Psoriasis is often a lifelong affliction, though episodes of remission and exacerbation are common. Onset in childhood presages severe psoriasis in adult life.

PARAPSORIASIS

Essentials of Diagnosis

- Scaling plaques similar to those of psoriasis.
- Nonpruritic lesions resistant to therapy.
- Good general state of health.

General Considerations

Parapsoriasis is a confusing group of diseases characterized by superficial scaling plaques of various sizes, usually nonpruritic and resistant to therapy. Parapsoriasis looks a bit like psoriasis but is not a form of that disease and does not result from it. Some forms of parapsoriasis are chronic and cause no serious symptoms, but parapsoriasis en plaques may progress to mycosis fungoides. The initial lesion is usually a macule or maculopapule covered with a fine scale that tends to spread peripherally. Lesions usually appear first on the trunk or extremities. There are

3 main types of parapsoriasis: (1) parapsoriasis guttata, (2) parapsoriasis lichenoides chronica, and (3) parapsoriasis en plaques. Parapsoriasis varioliformis acuta is clinically and histologically different from the other 3 entities and probably should no longer be classified in this group of diseases.

Clinical Findings

A. Parapsoriasis Guttata: The lesions of parapsoriasis guttata are fine maculopapules resembling those of guttate psoriasis, with the same fine silvery scale. Unlike psoriasis, however, parapsoriasis guttata fails to respond to antipsoriatic therapy. The lesions appear mainly on the trunk, occur at any age and in both sexes, and are chronic (persisting for months to years). Pruritus does not usually occur.

B. Parapsoriasis Lichenoides: Parapsoriasis lichenoides (retiform parapsoriasis) presents with elevated, dull, red, scaly, lichenoid papules, mainly over the trunk, that tend to coalesce and create a retiform appearance. The eruption is more generalized than parapsoriasis guttata and affects the neck, trunk, and limbs. There is usually no pruritus, and the patient's general health is unaffected.

C. Parapsoriasis en Plaques: Lesions of parapsoriasis en plaques are larger than those of parapsoriasis guttata or lichenoides. The lesions are flatter than those in psoriasis and may be associated with poikiloderma elsewhere (hypo- and hyperpigmentation with subtle atrophy and telangiectasia) or be superimposed on the poikiloderma, in which case the disorder is named poikiloderma vasculare atrophicans. The plaques range from yellowish-red to brownish with a fine definite scale, and they occur mainly on the trunk (Fig 41–4), buttocks, and thighs. In contrast to the other 2 types of parapsoriasis, the lesions may be pruritic. Skin biopsies and careful

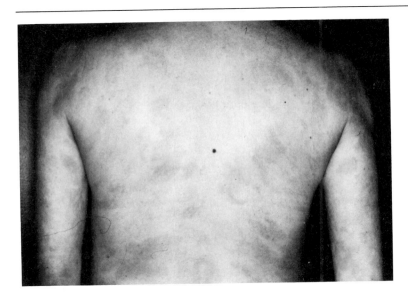

Figure 41–4. Psoriasis en plaques of the trunk.

clinical observation are essential, because in many patients the disease progresses to mycosis fungoides.

D. Parapsoriasis Varioliformis Acuta: This disease is also known as acute parapsoriasis, pityriasis lichenoides et varioliformis acuta, and Mucha-Habermann syndrome. The onset is acute, and the clinical picture resembles that of chickenpox, with crops of papules, vesicles, and pustular or crusted lesions. The lesions evolve from a papular to a pustular to a necrotic stage and leave varioliform scars. Lesions occur mainly in the second and third decades of life. The condition may last a few weeks or months and then resolve spontaneously, or it may persist for 10 years or more.

The basic lesion is the result of a lymphocytic vasculitis; skin biopsy of an early lesion will show features of the vasculitis along with destruction (necrosis) of the epidermis by hemorrhage and invasion by lymphocytes.

Differential Diagnosis

A. Psoriasis Vulgaris: Typical symmetric distribution of lesions and response to therapy distinguish psoriasis from parapsoriasis; skin biopsy is also helpful, because psoriatic lesions demonstrate more hyperkeratosis, acanthosis, and inflammation.

B. Mycosis Fungoides: Plaques and tumors have histopathologic features specific for mycosis fungoides, including atypical cells and microscopic abscesses of atypical lymphocytes in the epidermis. Asymmetry of plaques and variations in plaque thickness are clinical differentiating clues.

C. Radiation Dermatitis: A history of radiation exposure, telangiectasia, atrophy, and biopsy is helpful in distinguishing radiation dermatitis from parapsoriasis with poikiloderma.

D. Vasculitis: Skin biopsy is necessary to confirm a diagnosis of vasculitis. Small-vessel vasculitis shows necrosis of the blood vessel wall, an infiltrate of neutrophils, and a scattering of nuclear remnants near the vessels. Lesions associated with vasculitis typically occur on the lower legs.

E. Secondary Syphilis: A serologic test for syphilis should be performed to differentiate that disease from parapsoriasis.

Treatment

A. Parapsoriasis Guttata and Parapsoriasis Lichenoides: Therapy for these disorders is often not required, because lesions frequently cause no symptoms. For symptomatic patients, sunlight or topical corticosteroids may be tried, but lesions tend to be refractory to treatment.

B. Parapsoriasis en Plaques: Parapsoriasis en plaques may respond to sunlight. PUVA will cause clearing of lesions similar to that which can be achieved during the plaque stage of mycosis fungoides.

C. Parapsoriasis Varioliformis Acuta: Parapso-

riasis varioliformis acuta may respond over a month or so to large doses of antibiotics, eg, tetracycline, 1.5 g orally daily; penicillin G, 1–1.5 mg orally daily; or erythromycin, 250 mg 4 times daily—but in patients with a longer course of disease, such treatment may fail. Small doses of methotrexate, 5–7.5 mg orally daily, will control the disease, but discontinuance of the drug results in return of lesions. Close monitoring of blood counts and liver function studies are necessary if methotrexate treatment is used.

Course & Prognosis

Parapsoriasis typically has a prolonged and chronic course, though only parapsoriasis en plaques has the potential to develop into mycosis fungoides, which is potentially fatal.

LICHEN PLANUS

Essential of Diagnosis

- Flat-topped, violaceous, pruritic papules in symmetric distribution.
- Predilection for flexor surfaces, especially the ventral forearms and wrists.
- Lesions in mouth and other mucous membranes.
- Skin biopsy diagnostic.

General Considerations

Lichen planus is a papulosquamous disease that occurs at all ages and with equal frequency in both sexes. The onset is generally acute and has some features of an infectious disease, though no organisms have ever been demonstrated. The disease may be self-limiting, but a chronic form may last for years.

Many drugs may produce a skin eruption that clinically and histologically resembles lichen planus (Table 41–1).

Clinical Findings

The characteristic lesions of lichen planus are polygonal, violaceous, flat-topped papules (Fig 41–5) that tend to have a symmetric bilateral distribution. The severity of pruritus depends on the degree of involvement. A fine, whitish network covers the surface (Wickham's striae). Lesions may coalesce to

Table 41–1. Drugs causing lichenoid dermatitis.

Aminosalicylic acid	Mercury
Amiphenazole	Methyldopa
Arsenic	Phenothiazines
Chlorpropamide	Quinidine
Chloroquine	Quinine
Gold	Streptomycin
Iodides	Tetracycline
Labetalol	Thiazides
Meproquine	

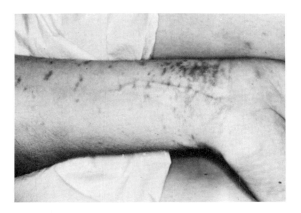

Figure 41–5. Papular lesion of lichen planus on the flexor surface of the wrist.

form groups or larger patches. Scratching or other trauma to the lesion frequently results in a linear eruption of lesions (Koebner's phenomenon). Annular patterns are common on the trunk, the mucous membranes, the dorsum of the tongue, or the penis. Distribution favors the flexor surfaces of the wrists, ankles, inner thighs, and sacral region, under the breasts, and on the buccal mucosa.

Lichen planus may involve only the mucous membranes of the vagina, mouth, or rectal areas, and the lacy white patches associated with involvement of these areas may be difficult to differentiate from dysplastic leukoplakia and other whitish plaques even with biopsy. Hypertrophic lichen planus (Fig 41–6) usually develops on the anterior aspects of the lower legs but may also occur on the backs of the hands or, rarely, may be generalized. Scalp involvement is characterized by lichen planopilaris, in which spiny follicular papules cause skin atrophy and scarring alopecia. Nails affected by acute or chronic lichen planus show pitting, parallel longitudinal grooves, or subungual keratosis. Occasionally, only the nails are involved (20-nail syndrome) and differentiation from psoriasis may be impossible. In other cases, the nail matrix may be scarred, so permanent loss of nails occurs. Lichen planus may present with erosive lesions of the feet resistant to therapy.

Histopathologic features of lichen planus, especially in the acute phase with small papular lesions, are characteristic; therefore, skin biopsy is diagnostic. There is hyperkeratosis without parakeratosis. The rete ridges are elongated and pointed like the teeth of a saw. Basal cells are degenerated, and an intense bandlike infiltrate of lymphocytes occupies the space immediately below them. Direct immunofluorescence tests of lesions show deposition of immunoglobulin below the basement membrane and may confirm the diagnosis in doubtful cases, such as in lichen planopilaris.

Differential Diagnosis

All the diseases that must be differentiated from psoriasis must also be distinguished from lichen planus. Neurodermatitis resembles lichen planus, especially the hypertrophic form, but lesions associated with neurodermatitis are much thicker than those of lichen planus and almost always excoriated. Drug-induced lichen planus may be identical to non-iatrogenic lichen planus both clinically and histologically, so that the differential diagnosis depends on the history.

Treatment

Treatment of lichen planus depends on the symptoms and extent of the disease. Topical corticosteroids of high to mid potency generally control itching and may reduce inflammation. The choice of a particular topical steroid is often based on the extent of involvement. For widespread lesions, the cost and the dangers of systemic absorption must be considered, and in such cases triamcinolone 0.1% cream is often the steroid of choice. Intralesional injection of corticosteroids is especially effective for hypertrophic lichen planus. For acute, spreading, generalized, intensely pruritic lichen planus, systemic corticosteroids are indicated, eg, prednisone, 40–60 mg/d until lesions clear (1–2 weeks), after which the dose should be slowly tapered and the drug discontinued in 4–6 weeks. Lichen planus may sometimes recur after corticosteroid treatment is stopped, but there is no rebound flare-up as occurs in psoriasis.

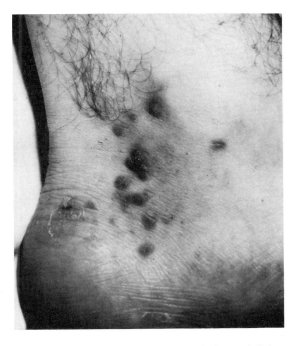

Figure 41–6. Hypertrophic papular lesions of lichen planus of the ankle.

For difficult cases, PUVA therapy can be used with the same sort of schedules as used to treat psoriasis. Griseofulvin has been effective in some forms of lichen planus, especially of the oral mucous membranes.

Course & Prognosis

The usual case of lichen planus lasts for over a year; most cases of acute lichen planus respond quickly to systemic corticosteroids, and generalized flares will frequently not recur when they are discontinued. Localized chronic lesions may persist for many years. There are no known systemic complications.

LICHEN NITIDUS

Lichen nitidus presents as skin-colored or pinkish, shiny, circinate, flat-topped papules that either remain as discrete pinhead-sized lesions or become confluent. Lichen nitidus tends to occur on the genitals, abdomen, and flexor surfaces of the forearms. Lichen nitidus is more common in blacks than in whites. There is usually no itching, and mucous membranes are seldom involved. The lesions occasionally resemble those of lichen planus. Skin biopsy is generally diagnositc and shows a focal, almost granulomatous lymphocytic infiltrate with a single dermal papilla between 2 adjacent rete ridges. The cause is unknown, and because lesions usually disappear spontaneously in a few months, no treatment is necessary. Lubrication of the skin may be helpful.

LICHEN STRIATUS

The development of small lichenoid papules resembling lichen planus in linear distribution down one extremity of a child is characteristic of lichen striatus. The lesions are asymptomatic and usually resolve spontaneously in a few months without sequelae.

No therapy is needed.

PITYRIASIS ROSEA

Essentials of Diagnosis

- Initial single plaque (herald patch).
- Generalized oval, fawn-colored eruption follows in "Christmas tree" pattern (long axes of lesions follow cleavage lines of skin).
- The major scale is often at the edge (collarette scale).
- Face, hands, and feet are usually spared.

General Considerations

Pityriasis rosea is a common self-limited disorder of unknown cause—though viral infection has been suspected—that develops abruptly, usually in the spring and fall. Both sexes and all ages are involved.

Clinical Findings

Pityriasis rosea typically presents as a generalized eruption of oval, fawn-colored plaques in symmetric distribution over the trunk and proximal portions of the extremities (Fig 41–7). A "herald patch" resembling tinea infection appears initially and is followed several days later by multiple lesions that usually appear first on the trunk. The long axis of the lesions follows the lines of cleavage of the skin ("Christmas tree" patterns). Lesions have a reddish edge and a fine peripheral collarette scale. The eruption may be extensive (Fig 41–8); itching may be severe or absent. Lesions usually clear in 6–8 weeks.

Differential Diagnosis

Secondary syphilis must always be considered in the differential diagnosis of pityriasis rosea. In syphilis, the hands and feet usually bear papular lesions. Patients with secondary syphilis may have mucous patches, condyloma lata, and patchy alopecia. A serologic test such as the rapid plasma reagin (RPR) test is positive in secondary syphilis.

A history of drug ingestion and clearing of lesions after the medication has been withdrawn differentiates pityriasis rosea from drug eruption. Intramuscularly administered gold is especially likely to cause this sort of eruption.

Tinea corporis and other fungal infections may be ruled out by microscopic examination of potassium hydroxide preparations of material from the lesions.

If lesions persist longer than 2 months, parapsoriasis guttata is a more likely diagnosis.

Treatment

Spontaneous resolution of lesions usually occurs within 6–8 weeks, so active treatment is not necessary. Antipruritic lotions and systemic antihistamines may help control generalized pruritus. Ultraviolet radiation (UVB) given daily in suberythema doses often hastens resolution. Rarely, a short course of systemic corticosteroids may be necessary for extensive lesions and severe itching. Prednisone can be given in a single morning dose of 40 mg for 2 weeks and then rapidly tapered to zero over the ensuing week.

PITYRIASIS RUBRA PILARIS

Essentials of Diagnosis

- Follicular papules with keratotic plugs.
- Generalized erythroderma that spares clear islands of normal skin.

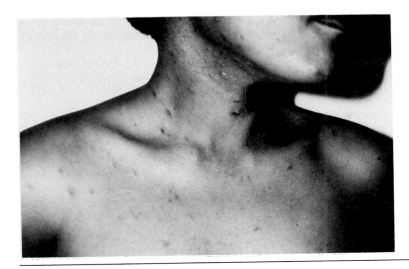

Figure 41–7. Fawn-colored papulo-squamous lesions of pityriasis rosea of the trunk.

- Yellow hooflike thickening (severe) of palms and soles.
- Chronic course; treatment-resistant.

General Considerations

Pityriasis rubra pilaris is a chronic disease with a familial and an acquired form.

A family history of the disease is often associated with the familial type, which may begin in infancy. The familial form may resemble psoriasis and last a lifetime. The acquired type usually occurs in adulthood and runs a variable course. There is no racial predilection. No infectious organism has been identified. Physical factors may play a role in onset.

Clinical Findings

The lesions of pityriasis rubra pilaris are firm, reddish-brown follicular papules that tend to coalesce

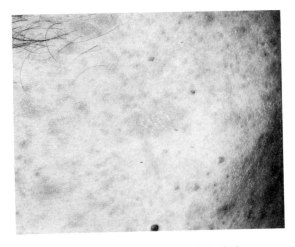

Figure 41–8. Close-up of lesions of pityriasis rosea.

and form confluent patches and groups of discrete lesions that eventually cover the entire body. Sometimes the pink plaques have a slightly orange hue. Diffuse scaling of the scalp and typical conical papules pierced by hairs occur on the dorsal surfaces of the phalanges. When the lesions become generalized and cause erythroderma, a few small clear areas of normal skin are typically spared on the trunk. Sometimes small red keratotic papules occur on each hair follicle in these spared areas. The palms and soles often show diffuse hyperkeratosis.

Skin biopsy is not diagnostic but may be helpful in ruling out other conditions.

Differential Diagnosis

In erythrodermic psoriasis there are no clear areas of normal skin and the patient gives a history of previous plaque-type psoriasis or nail changes or a family history of psoriasis.

The disease is differentiated from mycosis fungoides and Sézary syndrome because there are no plaques, tumors, or lymphadenopathy and because the lymphocyte count is usually elevated with Sézary syndrome and lymphocytes may have convoluted nuclei. Biopsy is usually helpful.

A history of ingestion of a drug and the usual onset of drug eruption as a morbilliform eruption differentiate pityriasis rubra pilaris from drug eruption.

Some keratodermas may be hereditary. Keratodermas lack the scaling and chronic course that characterize pityriasis rubra pilaris.

Treatment

Treatment of pityriasis rubra pilaris has generally been ineffective, but high doses of vitamin A (200,000–600,000 units/d orally) may produce remission. Etretinate and isotretinoin given in a dose of 0.5–1 mg/kg may be safer and produce a remission over the course of several months. Etretinate plus ultraviolet B phototherapy may have an additive effect. Topical agents such as tar and steroid creams are generally ineffective. Methotrexate in doses of 5–10 mg once weekly has been reported effective in a few cases.

Course & Prognosis

The clinical course of pityriasis rubra pilaris is variable. Familial pityriasis rubra pilaris generally pursues a prolonged course with occasional clear periods. About 80% of patients with the acquired type will experience clearing of lesions in 3 years; therapy may shorten that course.

OTHER PAPULOSQUAMOUS DISEASES

Seborrheic dermatitis is discussed in Chapter 40, fungal infection of the skin in Chapter 16, and syphilis in Chapter 13.

REFERENCES

Abel EA et al: Drugs in exacerbation of psoriasis. J Am Acad Dermatol 1986;15:1007.

Dicken CH: Isotretinoin treatment of pityriasis rubra pilaris. J Am Acad Dermatol 1987;16:297.

Ellis CN, Voorhees JJ: Etretinate therapy. J Am Acad Dermatol 1987;16:267.

Epstein JH et al: Current status of oral PUVA therapy for psoriasis. J Am Acad Dermatol 1979;1:106.

Goldsmith LA, Weinrich AE, Shupack J: Pityriasis rubra pilaris response to 13-cis-retinoic acid (isotretinoin). J Am Acad Dermatol 1982;6:710.

McMillan EM, Wasik R, Everett MA: In situ demonstration of T cell subsets in atrophic parapsoriasis. J Am Acad Dermatol 1982;6:32.

Melski JW et al: Oral methoxsalen photochemotherapy for the treatment of psoriasis: A cooperative clinical trial. J Invest Dermatol 1977;68:328.

Ortonne JP, Thivolet J, Sannwald C: Oral photochemotherapy in the treatment of lichen planus (LP): Clinical results, histological and ultrastructural observations. Br J Dermatol 1978;99:77.

Parsons JM: Pityriasis rosea update: 1986. J Am Acad Dermatol 1986;15:159.

Roenigk HH Jr et al: Methotrexate in psoriasis: Revised guidelines. J Am Acad Dermatol 1988;19:145.

Roenigk HH, Maibach HI: *Psoriasis*. Marcel Dekker, 1986.

Roenigk HH: Photochemotherapy for psoriasis: Clinical cooperative study of PUVA-48 and PUVA-64. Arch Dermatol 1979;115:576.

Sloberg K et al: Topical tretinoin therapy and oral lichen planus. Arch Dermatol 1979;115:716.

Weinstein GD, Voorhees JJ: Symposium on psoriasis. Dermatol Clin 1984;2:355.

Wilkinson JD et al: Twenty-nail dystrophy of childhood: Case report and histopathological findings. Br J Dermatol 1979;100:217.

Bullous Diseases*

42

Gerhard Tappeiner, MD & Klaus Wolff, MD

The bullous diseases, though uncommon, are a dramatic and often serious group of skin diseases. For many of the diseases discussed in this chapter, immunologic mechanisms are responsible for producing the vesicles and bullae.

PEMPHIGUS

Essentials of Diagnosis
- Flaccid blisters and weeping, painful erosions.
- Mucous membrane involvement.
- Epidermis shears off with lateral traction (Nikolsky's sign).
- Acantholysis and intraepidermal cleft formation.
- Deposition of IgG and, in lesional skin, of C3 in the intercellular spaces of the epidermis.
- Serum antibodies to epidermal cell surface antigens whose titer parallels disease activity.

General Considerations

Pemphigus is a serious autoimmune disease of skin and mucous membranes in which defective cellular cohesion leads to intraepidermal cleft formation. Clinically, it is characterized by flaccid blisters that rupture easily, producing painful, weeping, denuded lesions. According to the level of intraepidermal cleft formation, 2 major subtypes are distinguished: in pemphigus vulgaris and its rare variant pemphigus vegetans, acantholysis occurs deep in the epidermis, just above the basal cell layer, whereas in pemphigus foliaceus and its variant pemphigus erythematosus, the intraepidermal cleft forms within or just below the granular layer. Pemphigus vulgaris, when untreated, is often fatal. Pemphigus foliaceus runs a longer course, and the outlook is usually more favorable.

Pemphigus is a rare disorder; although more common in Jews and other ethnic groups of Mediterranean and Indian origin, it occurs in all races. Age at onset is between the fourth and sixth decades for pemphigus vulgaris and slightly earlier for pemphigus foliaceus, but it may also occur in children and in old age.

The cause of pemphigus is unknown. Autoantibodies directed against an antigen on epidermal cell surfaces cause acantholysis. Autoantibodies from patients with pemphigus vulgaris react with polypeptide complexes of 210, 130, and 85 kDa in pemphigus vulgaris and of 260, 160, and 85 kDa in pemphigus foliaceus and fogo selvagem. The 85-kDa protein is plakoglobin, a component of desmosomes and of adherens junctions, while the 160-kDa glycoprotein is desmoglein I, a constituent of desmosomes. These serum antibodies are detected by indirect immunofluorescence methods, and their titer often reflects disease activity; they are bound in vivo to the intercellular substance of the epidermis, where they can be visualized by direct immunofluorescence staining (see Chapter 8). Although complement is not required for acantholysis to occur, deposits of complement have been detected in lesional skin of pemphigus patients. The binding of antibodies to the keratinocyte surfaces seems to induce the keratinocytes to elaborate a proteolytic enzyme (possibly a plasminogen activator) that abolishes intercellular cohesion within the epidermis. The epidermis thus "falls apart." Acantholysis has also been induced in newborn mice as well as in human skin in organ culture by pemphigus antibodies. In vitro acantholysis in the organ culture model can be abolished by the addition of purified plasminogen activator inhibitor.

Pemphigus may be associated with other autoimmune diseases, including myasthenia gravis, lupus erythematosus, thymoma, and bullous pemphigoid. Serum samples from patients with pemphigus often have elevated levels of circulating immune complexes as assessed by C1q binding assays, but their pathogenic significance is not known. Penicillamine and captopril have induced pemphigus.

Immunogenetic factors may play a role, as suggested by the increased frequency of HLA-A10 and HLA-DR4. HLA-A10 carries a relative risk for pemphigus vulgaris of 6 and 3 in Jews and Japanese, respectively; DR4 carries a relative risk of 32 in Jews, and HLA-A10 has a relative risk of 4 for pemphigus foliaceus in Japanese.

Clinical Findings
A. Symptoms and Signs:
1. Pemphigus vulgaris— In over half of patients with pemphigus vulgaris, the earliest lesions arise on the oral mucosa, preceding skin lesions by several

---

*Transient acantholytic dermatosis (Grover's Disease) is discussed in Chapter 21.

months. Often the oral cavity remains the only site involved. Other mucous membranes may be affected.

The typical lesions on mucous membranes are erosions with a slowly advancing white edge of acantholytic epithelium; blisters are only exceptionally seen (Fig 42–1). These erosions show little or no healing tendency and are extremely painful, thus frequently impairing adequate food intake.

Skin lesions consist of flaccid bullae, usually arising on noninflammatory bases that extend peripherally and rupture easily, leading to large, denuded, weeping and often bleeding areas (Fig 42–2). Shearing pressure on seemingly uninvolved skin results in easy detachment of the superficial epidermal layers and thus in erosive lesions (Nikolsky's sign). Since blisters in pemphigus break easily, intact bullae are rarely seen and erosions and crusts may dominate the clinical presentation (Fig 42–2). The onset may be evanescent and slowly progressive or acute, with lesions spreading rapidly to involve large areas of the body. In the intertriginous areas, pemphigus vulgaris lesions tend to be vegetating; thus, there may be no clear-cut distinction between pemphigus vulgaris and pemphigus vegetans.

2. Pemphigus vegetans– Pemphigus vegetans starts like pemphigus vulgaris, but vegetating and purulent, hypertrophic granulations supervene as acantholysis progresses peripherally. Vegetating lesions often occur on epidermal-mucosal junctions, in intertriginous regions, and in the flexural areas of large joints. The course of pemphigus vegetans is slowly progressive and extremely chronic.

3. Pemphigus foliaceus– In pemphigus foliaceus, mucous membrane involvement is unusual; the disease usually begins on the scalp, face, or upper trunk and progresses slowly. Occasionally, the onset may be abrupt and the disease spreads rapidly to a generalized exfoliative erythroderma. Owing to superficial intraepidermal cleft formation, blisters are rarely seen. Lesions are erythematous, crusted patches. Normal skin is "fragile," and Nikolsky's sign is easily elicited. Burning, itching, and pain may cause considerable discomfort.

4. Pemphigus erythematosus (Senear-Usher syndrome)– Pemphigus erythematosus is a less severe variety of pemphigus foliaceus, usually confined to the face, where it may mimic the butterfly rash of lupus erythematosus; to the scalp; and to the upper and medial areas of the chest and back. Scaling and crusting are pronounced, and the eruption has a seborrheic quality.

5. Fogo selvagem– Fogo selvagem (Pg "wild fire") is clinically identical to pemphigus foliaceus, often progressing to exfoliative erythroderma and accompanied by fever. Fogo selvagem (Brazilian pemphigus) is a special form of pemphigus foliaceus endemic to certain areas in South America; isolated cases have occurred in Africa. Fogo selvagem occurs mainly in children and young adults; two-thirds of those affected are women under 30. Patients from endemic areas improve when moved to an urban environment and relapse upon return to endemic regions. The disease may be caused by an infectious agent, and there is a familial predisposition.

B. Laboratory Findings:

1. Histopathology– The histopathologic picture of pemphigus is characterized by defective cohesion of

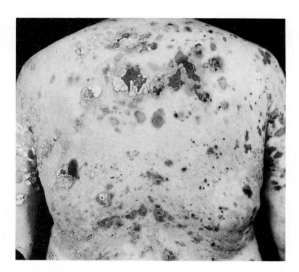

Figure 42–2. Pemphigus vulgaris. Lesions on the back. Note the typical weeping and crusted erosions with white edges of sloughed epidermis surrounded by inflammation. A few small flaccid blisters are still visible.

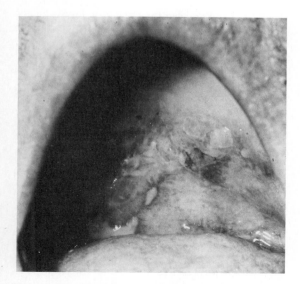

Figure 42–1. Pemphigus vulgaris. Lesions on oral mucosa. Erosions of the hard palate, partly covered by a fibrinous exudate and showing whitish edges and an inflammatory base.

epidermal cells, which lose their intercellular attachments, round up, and float off into the intraepidermal cavity thus formed (acantholysis). Acantholytic cells are initially still viable, indicating that the acantholytic factor is not cytotoxic. Electron microscopic observations show that widening of intercellular spaces (interpreted as indicative of dissolution of the intercellular substance) precedes diminution of the number of desmosomes. Desmosomes eventually split, permitting otherwise intact epidermal cells to separate. Eosinophilic spongiosis—widening of intercellular spaces and infiltration of the epidermis by eosinophils—is an early pathologic event in some patients with pemphigus and is often prominent in a clinical variant called pemphigus herpetiformis.

The intraepidermal cleft and blister formation are suprabasalar in pemphigus vulgaris and in pemphigus vegetans, where basal cells initially remain attached to the basement membrane. In pemphigus vegetans, there is downward proliferation of epidermal cells

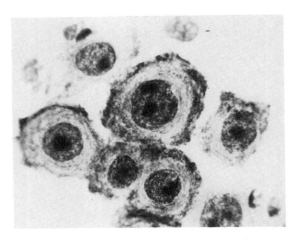

Figure 42–4. Pemphigus vulgaris. Tzanck smear from a blister, showing typical acantholytic cells.

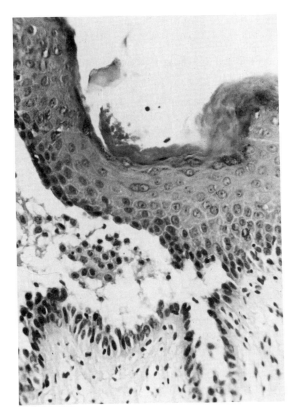

Figure 42–3. Pemphigus vulgaris. Biopsy from the edge of a blister shows suprabasal cleft formation. Epidermal cells, singly and in clusters (acantholytic cells), can be seen in the cavity. The basal cell layer, still adherent to the basement membrane zone, shows loss of intercellular adhesion. There is a scant inflammatory infiltration and discrete edema of the papillary dermis.

into the dermis, epidermal hyperplasia, and intraepidermal abscess formation by polymorphonuclear leukocytes. In pemphigus foliaceus, pemphigus erythematosus, and fogo selvagem, acantholysis occurs in the granular layer, and thus the blister is more superficial. Hyper- and parakeratosis are common in these latter disorders.

The form of the disease can be deduced by biopsy. Pemphigus vulgaris shows intraepidermal suprabasal cleft formation and acantholysis (Fig 42–3); pemphigus vegetans exhibits epithelial hypertrophy, abscesses, and granulations in addition to suprabasal acantholysis. In pemphigus foliaceus, pemphigus erythematosus, and fogo selvagem, acantholysis and cleft formation are confined to the granular layer. In all forms of pemphigus, cytologic smears obtained by scraping the base of a lesion reveal acantholytic (isolated, rounded-up) epidermal cells (Tzanck preparation) (Fig 42–4).

2. Immunologic studies– Direct immunofluorescence staining reveals IgG deposition in the intercellular spaces of the epidermis in lesional and in perilesional, normal-appearing skin of pemphigus patients; this is true for all forms of pemphigus. By immunoelectronmicroscopic techniques, pemphigus antibodies localize on the surface of epidermal cells that comprise the intercellular substance of the epidermis. Complement may be detected in the intercellular space of pemphigus epidermis but only in early acantholytic lesions.

All forms of pemphigus show intercellular deposits of IgG within the epidermis (Fig 42–5). In addition to the intercellular IgG deposits, granular bandlike deposits of immunoglobulins and complement may be found at the dermal-epidermal junction in pemphigus erythematosus similar to the immunopathologic find-

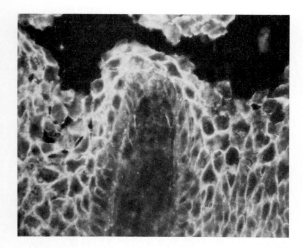

Figure 42–5. Pemphigus vulgaris. Direct immunofluorescence staining of a biopsy specimen from lesional skin with anti-IgG antiserum. Suprabasal cleft formation is apparent. Epidermal cells are outlined by the staining procedure, indicating deposition of IgG on epidermal intercellular substance. The staining is much less prominent around basal cells. The dark area in the middle of the picture is a dermal papilla.

ings in lupus erythematosus. These patients often also have circulating antinuclear antibodies.

Circulating serum antibodies directed against the intercellular substance of the epidermis are present in all forms of pemphigus. Titers of pemphigus antibodies usually reflect disease activity and are useful in the assessment of the course and therapy.

3. Routine laboratory studies– General laboratory investigations are not diagnostic but may reflect the general condition of the patient. An elevated sedimentation rate and leukocytosis are present in most patients with extensive pemphigus lesions, and in advanced cases there may be signs of derangement of fluid and electrolyte balance as well as hypoproteinemia. Eosinophilia may occur.

Differential Diagnosis

Most bullous disorders—particularly bullous pemphigoid, herpes gestationis, and blistering diseases of childhood; impetigo; and, in isolated cases, seborrheic dermatitis—must be differentiated from the pemphigus group. Bullae of pemphigus usually arise on normal-appearing skin and rupture easily, and the erosions spread peripherally. Nikolsky's sign is positive; smears reveal acantholytic cells; and histopathologic examination shows acantholytic intraepidermal cleft formation. Immunopathologic findings and the detection of circulating pemphigus antibodies confirm the diagnosis. When only erosive oral lesions are present, lichen planus, chronic discoid lupus erythematosus, bullous pemphigoid and cicatricial pemphigoid, fixed drug eruption, and erythema multiforme must be considered. The differential diagnosis of mucosal lesions can often be resolved on clinical grounds alone. A patient with a persistent painful oral erosion without skin lesions should be suspected of having pemphigus, and immunofluorescent studies should be done.

Complications & Sequelae

Patients with pemphigus become increasingly debilitated and are prone to infections to which they frequently succumb. Painful mouth ulcers may make eating painful and contribute to inadequate nutritional intake. Many complications are a result of the high doses of prednisone and immunosuppressive drugs needed to control the disease. These also predispose the pemphigus patient to systemic infection with ordinary or opportunistic pathogens. Complications of therapy may adversely affect the prognosis.

Treatment

Pemphigus is a serious disease that requires treatment with potent medications over long periods of time. Patients should be treated by dermatologists who are familiar with the disease and the drugs involved.

A. Topical Treatment: Although not sufficient in themselves, local measures can greatly increase patient comfort. Cleansing and antimicrobial baths (eg, compresses of Burow's solution, silver sulfadiazine 1% cream) will prevent superinfection, particularly in vegetating lesions. In superficial forms of pemphigus and in cases where there are only a few lesions, application of topical corticosteroids such as triamcinolone 0.1% cream 3 times daily is of value. When oral lesions are present, viscous lidocaine applied to the ulcers before meals reduces pain and helps ensure an adequate caloric and nutritional intake.

B. Systemic Corticosteroid Treatment: Systemic corticosteroids are the mainstay of treatment, and their use has completely changed the prognosis. Treatment is started with doses high enough to completely suppress formation of new blisters (up to 300 mg of prednisone equivalent per day, usually in divided doses). The dose is converted to a single morning dose and tapered carefully after complete healing. This usually takes months. An adequate maintenance dose (usually between 10 mg and 30 mg every other day) must then be found. Most patients develop side effects (see Chapter 53). Patients must be monitored frequently for side effect, including hypertension, weight gain, infection, potassium depletion, gastrointestinal bleeding, osteoporosis, and cataracts. A faster response is obtained by adding a high-dose intravenous pulse regimen (eg, 2 g methylprednisolone daily for 3 days followed by 1 g once daily for 2 days) to the treatment schedule. Except for the potentially lethal risk of shifts in serum sodium and potassium levels, this therapy is often well tolerated and can rather quickly stop the gross denudation of skin that occurs in severely affected patients.

C. Immunosuppressive Therapy: Immunosuppressive therapy, given together with corticosteroids, has a significant corticosteroid-sparing effect and improves control of disease. Azathioprine, 2–3 mg/kg body weight, or cyclophosphamide, 100–200 mg/d, are most commonly used and are also tapered to low maintenance doses. Clinical cures have been observed after long-term azathioprine-corticosteroid treatment. Azathioprine should be started early, since it requires many weeks before taking effect. Methotrexate is an alternative.

Cyclosporine has been used to treat pemphigus. While no large series nor long-term observations of such patients are yet available, preliminary studies suggest that it is ineffective when used alone but seems to have a corticosteroid-sparing effect. However, its use is fraught with severe side effects, the most serious of which is the development of "silent" renal failure. Thus, its use in pemphigus is still experimental.

D. Plasmapheresis: Although expensive, this can be a useful treatment for selected patients in the acute phase. Patients are candidates for this therapy if they have life-threatening denudations so that they cannot wait for the steroid and immunosuppressive drugs to work. Two or 3 plasma exchanges of 3 L per week are made until disease activity subsides. To avoid a rebound phenomenon after cessation of plasmapheresis, immunosuppressives and corticosteroids should be given concomitantly. This regimen results in rapid resolution of skin lesions and a considerable reduction of total corticosteroid dosage.

E. Gold Therapy (Chrysotherapy): Gold therapy can be employed concomitantly with corticosteroids, and some pemphigus patients can be managed successfully with this regimen. The response is less predictable than with azathioprine or cyclophosphamide, so these immunosuppressive agents are usually used first. A small test dose of gold sodium thiomalate is given intramuscularly; 1 week later, 25 mg, and after another week, 50 mg, are administered intramuscularly. Weekly treatment is continued until disease activity ceases, and the corticosteroid dosage can then be appreciably lowered. Maintenance therapy consists of 50 mg of gold sodium thiomalate monthly or bimonthly. Gold compounds suitable for oral administration (eg, auranofin) have been introduced recently in the therapy of rheumatoid arthritis. So far, no studies on their use in pemphigus are available, but they may prove to be of use in long-term management.

One possible side effect of gold therapy is a lichen planus-like eruption with mucosal involvement that must be distinguished from pemphigus erosions. The titer of pemphigus antibodies can help, since rising titers indicate pemphigus and falling titers favor gold toxicity.

Course & Prognosis

When untreated, pemphigus may be fatal. With the advent of systemic corticosteroids, the mortality rate was significantly reduced; with a combination of corticosteroids and azathioprine, the mortality rate was further lowered to about 5%. The disease itself runs a variable course, with exacerbations and remissions. Pemphigus foliaceus and pemphigus erythematosus are generally more benign than the deeper forms, but all patients with pemphigus need early and appropriate treatment and long-term follow-up.

THE "PEMPHIGOID GROUP"

Although clearly distinct disease entities by clinical criteria, course, prognosis, and response to therapy, several bullous disorders share an important immunopathologic feature with bullous pemphigoid, ie, the deposition of immunoglobulins and complement components at the dermal-epidermal basement membrane zone. This group of disorders, which includes herpes gestationis, cicatricial pemphigoid, epidermolysis bullosa acquisita, and "linear IgA dermatosis," is sometimes referred to as the "pemphigoid group," implying a suspected pathogenetic relationship. Our present classification of bullous diseases is tentative and incomplete.

1. BULLOUS PEMPHIGOID

Essentials of Diagnosis

- Large bullae on erythematous plaques or on normal-appearing skin; disseminated lesions.
- No or only mild involvement of mucosal surfaces.
- Cleft and blister formation at the dermal-epidermal junction.
- Deposition of IgG and C3 at the dermal-epidermal junction.
- Antibodies against basement membrane zone in patient's sera and blister fluid.

General Considerations

Bullous pemphigoid is a blistering disease, usually of the elderly, characterized by the eruption of tense bullae of variable size on erythematous or normal-appearing skin. Cleft formation is within the epidermal basement membrane zone and results in subepidermal blisters.

The disease occurs predominantly in 2 age groups: There is a small but distinct clustering of cases in prepubertal children and the much more frequent, more readily recognized occurrence in or after the sixth decade. No prevalence in sex, race, or geographic distribution has been observed.

An antibody of the IgG class directed to an antigen within the lamina lucida is usually found in the circulation. The "bullous pemphigoid antigen" is a 240-

kDa protein compound of disulfide-linked chains. It is synthesized by basal keratinocytes and is localized to only that portion of the basal cell's surface that is in opposition with the basement membrane zone. IgG and complement are bound in vivo to the basement membrane zone in lesional and perilesional skin. Occasionally, antibodies of other immunoglobulin classes (eg, IgM and IgA) may also be found. Circulating immune complexes are present in pemphigoid sera; their significance is unknown.

The pemphigoid autoantibodies may play an important role in the development of clinical disease, ie, blister formation. They activate complement; polymorphonuclear leukocytes attach to the basement membrane zone of sections of normal skin incubated with pemphigoid sera and complement, indicating a role for antibodies and complement for the recruitment and attachment of effector cells. Dermal-epidermal detachment has been experimentally produced by incubating frozen sections of skin with bullous pemphigoid antibody, complement, and leukocytes. Lesions of bullous pemphigoid have been produced on rabbit cornea by the intrastromal injection of purified IgG from bullous pemphigoid patients. Such blisters were produced by complement binding to the basement membrane zone and immigration of polymorphonuclear leukocytes.

Clinical Findings

A. Symptoms and Signs: The disease usually begins with urticarial and erythematous plaques that are often circinate and dusky, thus resembling erythema multiforme. After several days to weeks, tense blisters appear on erythematous as well as on clinically unaffected areas (Fig 42–6). Although the bullae sometimes remain localized to one area for some time, grouping of lesions is not a regular feature of bullous pemphigoid. The content of the blisters, usually intact for several days, is initially clear; later it may become turbid or hemorrhagic and, with the immigration of leukocytes, purulent. Sometimes the fluid is reabsorbed so that blisters seem to reattach to their floor. When broken, they leave an erosion that heals with hyperpigmentation but no scarring.

As a rule, the condition is initially progressive, tending to involve most or all parts of the body surface; the oral mucosa is usually spared, or involved to a much lesser degree than it would be in pemphigus. There is itching, and the oozing erosions resulting from blisters are painful, causing considerable discomfort; the patient's general health usually remains relatively good unless bacterial infection supervenes or fluid and electrolyte imbalance occurs.

B. Laboratory Findings: Routine laboratory investigations consist only of mild leukocytosis, eosinophilia, elevated IgE levels, and elevated erythrocyte sedimentation rates. In severe cases, there may be hypoproteinemia.

1. Histopathology— The histopathologic hallmark

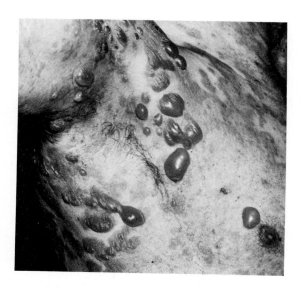

Figure 42–6. Bullous pemphigoid. Large, tense, partially coalescing blisters on erythematous bases as well as on normal-appearing skin are prominent. Red infiltrated areas without blistering but sometimes with a multiforme-like appearance can also be seen.

of bullous pemphigoid is a subepidermal blister. Electron microscopically, however, the blister is still within the epidermis as it arises between basal cells and the lamina densa. Biopsies taken from early erythematous lesions of bullous pemphigoid show neutrophilic and often predominantly eosinophilic dermal infiltration. Small aggregates of neutrophils or eosinophils may be present at the dermal-epidermal junction and are found within blisters. Biopsies taken from nonerythematous perilesional skin may be "infiltrate-poor," exhibiting only a mild mononuclear and eosinophilic perivascular infiltrate. In infiltrate-rich specimens, dermatitis herpetiformis may occasionally be impossible to distinguish on histologic grounds alone.

2. Immunopathology— The most reliable diagnostic feature of bullous pemphigoid, found in practically all patients, is deposition of IgG and complement components, particularly C3, in a linear band at the epidermal basement membrane zone of perilesional skin (Fig 42–7). Electron microscopically, these immune reactants are localized within the lamina lucida—the site where cleft formation and thus blistering occurs—and are closely associated with the plasma membrane of basal keratinocytes.

The presence of a circulating antibody to the epidermal basement membrane zone of normal skin is demonstrated in 70% of patients by indirect immunofluorescence or a variety of related techniques. This antibody fixes complement both in vivo and in vitro and allows the assembly of the membrane attack complex (C5b–9); this is thought to play a role in the

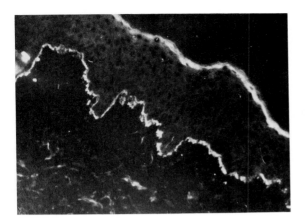

Figure 42–7. Bullous pemphigoid. Direct immunofluorescence staining of a biopsy specimen with anti-IgG antibody. The epidermal basement membrane zone is stained by the fluorescein-labeled antibody, indicating deposition of IgG-class autoantibody.

formation of pemphigoid blisters. Unlike pemphigus, however, the antibody titer found in bullous pemphigoid does not necessarily reflect disease activity.

Differential Diagnosis

The differential diagnosis of bullous pemphigoid includes all bullous diseases, erythema multiforme, bullosis diabeticorum, bullous fixed drug eruption, and porphyria cutanea tarda. The clinical diagnosis is confirmed by histopathology and immunofluorescence.

Complications & Sequelae

Complications usually result from bacterial superinfection and in severe cases from fluid and electrolyte imbalance. The formerly held belief that bullous pemphigoid is associated with internal malignancy is now considered to be statistically invalid.

Treatment

A. Topical Measures: Tepid baths, tap-water compresses, topical steroids, and antipruritic shake lotions or creams (eg, menthol 0.25% in Lubriderm) are ineffective in changing the course of the disease but are essential for relief of symptoms and prevention of bacterial superinfection. Considerations are similar to those for the treatment of pemphigoid.

B. Systemic Therapy: Treatment with systemic corticosteroids is the treatment of choice. Steroid therapy is initiated with 1–1.5 mg of prednisone per kg of body weight each day in a single morning dose. The response is usually rapid and easily observed within 3–5 days. Prednisone can be tapered as the disease process subsides. It has been suggested that immunosuppressive therapy (azathioprine, 1.5–2

mg/kg body weight) can be initiated simultaneously because of its steroid-sparing effect and maintained until all disease activity has subsided—whereupon the dose is gradually reduced. While on immunosuppressive therapy, the patient's leukocyte counts should be obtained at regular intervals.

Plasmapheresis shows considerable promise as a corticosteroid-sparing measure, but its use is still experimental. Child cases of pemphigoid may respond to sulfones.

In cases where pemphigoid occurs together with psoriasis, methotrexate treatment can be used to control both conditions.

Course & Prognosis

The course is protracted but self-limited. Disease activity may subside spontaneously but only after several months or years.

Occasionally the duration of the disease may be much shorter and the course more benign. In some elderly patients, pemphigoid may be manifested as a single episode of a few weeks' duration with no tendency to chronicity or recurrence. In these patients, the disease runs a benign course with little or no impairment of general health, so aggressive treatment is unwarranted.

2. HERPES GESTATIONIS

Essentials of Diagnosis

- Erythematous urticarial plaques, alone or with papules, vesicles, blisters, and erosions anywhere on the body but most often on the proximal extremities and the abdomen.
- Intense pruritus.
- Subepidermal blister formation.
- Deposition of C3 and, infrequently, of IgG at the dermal-epidermal basement membrane zone; "herpes gestationis factor" in patient's sera.

General Considerations

The disorder occurs in about one in 50,000 pregnancies. Tense subepidermal blisters on erythematous plaques develop during pregnancy or within a few days after delivery. Herpes gestationis shares many features with bullous pemphigoid. The disease is associated with linear deposition of C3 along the basement membrane zone of normal skin. Occasionally, deposits of IgG may be found in biopsy material.

The disease begins in the second or third trimester of pregnancy. It will usually recur in subsequent pregnancies with a tendency toward earlier onset and a more severe course.

Clinical Findings

A. Symptoms and Signs: Herpes gestationis is an extremely pruritic, generalized eruption involving the trunk and the extremities, including the palms and soles. It often begins around the umbilicus. It occurs in varying degrees of severity, ranging from urticarial papules and plaques, usually confined to the trunk, to generalized erythematous, urticarial papules and plaques covered with tense blisters and erosions. As in bullous pemphigoid, the erosions heal rapidly when not superinfected, leaving brown hyperpigmentation. Itching is pronounced and can be very distressing.

B. Laboratory Findings: Routine laboratory studies are generally noncontributory.

1. Histopathology– Histopathologic findings are characteristic but not diagnostic. There is a non-specific lymphohistiocytic and eosinophilic perivascular infiltrate of deep and superficial vessels. Dermal papillae are edematous, with an eosinophilic infiltrate that can extend into the epidermis. Focal basal cell necrosis may be seen. Blisters are subepidermal but may appear to extend into the epidermis at the edge of large blisters.

2. Immunopathology– In biopsy specimens from lesions of herpes gestationis, linear deposition of C3 along the epidermal basement membrane zone is regularly present in a linear pattern similar to that found in bullous pemphigoid. Linear deposits of IgG can be found in less than 25% of patients. Immunoelectronmicroscopy demonstrates these deposits in the lamina lucida, as in bullous pemphigoid.

Complement indirect immunofluorescence (see Chapter 8) demonstrates C3 at the dermal-epidermal junction of normal epithelial substrates. The serum factor that fixes complement is called "herpes gestationis factor" and is an IgG-antibody against an antigen in the lamina lucida that usually cannot be demonstrated by routine indirect immunofluorescence.

Differential Diagnosis

The differential diagnosis of herpes gestationis includes most acquired blistering diseases and all urticarial and papular eruptions of pregnancy, especially pruritic urticarial papules and plaques of pregnancy (PUPPP). Women with PUPPP usually do not develop bullae and do not have lesions in the umbilicus. Immunopathologic study is essential to confirm a diagnosis. The differentiation from pemphigoid may be more difficult. In those cases where circulating serum IgG can be demonstrated, the 2 conditions can be differentiated because the complement-fixing titer is much higher than the IgG antibody titer in herpes gestationis, while in bullous pemphigoid the opposite is true.

Complications & Sequelae

In patients with herpes gestationis, the concern is mainly directed toward the pregnancy outcome. Owing to the relative scarcity of reported cases, the data are preliminary. However, besides maternal morbidity, herpes gestationis is associated with increased fetal morbidity and mortality rates. Twenty-three percent of live births were premature in one study, as compared to 5–10% in the general population. Nine percent of the infants are born with lesions typical of herpes gestationis, but spontaneous remissions are the rule in these infants. Stillbirths of 7.7% in herpes gestationis contrast with 1.3% in the general population; the rate of spontaneous abortions is not increased. Another comparative study of mostly treated patients failed to confirm this greatly increased fetal risk.

Prevention

Nothing can be done to prevent a first eruption of herpes gestationis. In women who have had an episode of the disease, oral contraceptives are contraindicated since they may induce a recurrence. Patients should be advised of the high probability of recurrence of herpes gestationis in subsequent pregnancies. It is not known whether a woman who has had herpes gestationis is more prone to develop bullous pemphigoid later in life.

Treatment

Treatment with topical corticosteroids (eg, triamcinolone 0.1% cream twice daily) is worth trying, particularly in mild eruptions.

Prednisone, 0.5–1 mg/kg body weight, usually stops disease activity, relieves symptoms within 24–48 hours, and induces remissions within 10 days. However, there are exceptions to this rule. The dose should be tapered cautiously to avoid flares. Flare-ups during the perinatal and immediate postpartum periods can be controlled by temporarily increasing the steroid dosage.

No systemic treatment is necessary in infants born with lesions of herpes gestationis, as these spontaneously resolve within several days. Silver sulfadiazine 1% cream can be applied to eroded blister sites daily until healing is complete.

Course & Prognosis

Herpes gestationis is usually a self-limited disease. It may flare during the first few postpartal menstrual periods. However, it tends to recur with each successive pregnancy and upon administration of oral contraceptives. Occasionally the disease continues for months or years, but this is rare. Although the disease is bothersome for the mother, there is no increased maternal mortality.

3. CICATRICIAL PEMPHIGOID

Essentials of Diagnosis

- Tense blisters and erosions of mucous membranes, especially of the oral cavity (hard and soft palate), eyes, nose, and pharynx.
- Skin occasionally involved, rarely alone.

- Pronounced tendency to scarring, symblepharon, and strictures.
- Subepidermal blister formation.
- Deposition of IgG, IgA, and often also C3 at the basement membrane zone.

General Considerations

Cicatricial pemphigoid is a chronic blistering and scarring condition of the mucosa and the skin. Its onset is predominantly in women over age 50, but it may occasionally start in young people or in men.

Little is known about the cause of this rare condition. IgG or IgA autoantibodies are usually bound in vivo to the epidermal basement membrane zone and are sometimes demonstrable in the circulation. They are able to fix complement and are thought to play a role in the pathogenesis of cicatricial pemphigoid—analogous to the situation in bullous pemphigoid. No precipitating factors are known, but the drug practolol has rarely induced the disease. Having an HLA-B12 tissue type appears to be a risk factor.

Clinical Findings

A. Symptoms and Signs: Blisters on the mucosal surfaces of any one or all of the body orifices are the hallmark. Rarely, the skin may also be involved.

The oral mucosa is the most commonly involved site, with 2 types of lesions: desquamative gingivitis and large bullae and erosions. Involvement of the oral mucosa is found in 85–100% of patients. The roofs of oral blisters are remarkably tough and may resist rupture for several days. The erosions tend to heal slowly and leave a network of white scar tissue reminiscent of lichen planus. In contrast to erosions in pemphigus or lichen planus, the lesions of cicatricial pemphigoid are remarkably symptomless and may go unnoticed for some time.

The second most commonly affected site (two-thirds of cases)—but the one of greatest clinical significance—is the conjunctiva. Erosions tend to heal by forming adhesions that eventually lead to obliteration of the conjunctival sac and entropion (Fig 42–8). Clouding of the cornea results from keratinization and scarring. Blindness occurs in about 25% of patients and is bilateral in about 17%. Erosions, scarring, and strictures also affect the genital mucous membranes and the anus; lesions of the middle ear may result in deafness.

Two types of skin involvement are known: widespread but self-limited and transient blistering eruption reminiscent of bullous pemphigoid, and formation of a localized persistent erythematous plaque that is the site of recurrent blistering and considerable scarring. Involvement of the scalp produces permanent hair loss.

Lesions are usually on the face and neck but sometimes on the trunk and limbs. Bullae of localized pemphigoid (Brunsting-Perry type) show the characteristics of cicatricial pemphigoid but are not associ-

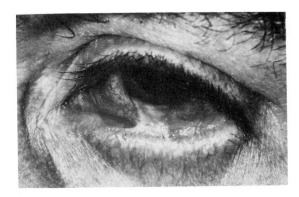

Figure 42–8. Cicatricial pemphigoid. Eye involvement. There is pronounced adhesion of the scarred lower lid to the sclera with pronounced chemosis.

ated with simultaneous or subsequent involvement of mucosal membranes.

B. Laboratory Findings: Histopathologically, subepidermal blisters contain only small numbers of inflammatory cells; in older lesions, proliferating fibroblasts and scar tissue may be seen. There is IgG and sometimes IgA in the basement membrane zone of the epidermis; circulating anti-basement membrane zone IgG may uncommonly be found. The binding site of these antibodies, as demonstrated by immunoelectronmicroscopy, is the lamina lucida of the basement membrane, as in bullous pemphigoid. The specificity of the circulating antibodies is more restricted than in bullous pemphigoid, as they do not regularly react with the skin from other mammalian species and may occasionally bind only to the patient's own skin.

Other laboratory studies are noncontributory. For a quick provisional diagnosis to distinguish pemphigoid from pemphigus, a Tzanck smear may help; acantholytic cells are found in the latter but not in the former.

Complications & Sequelae

Complications result from the slow progressive scarring that occurs on affected mucous membranes. Involvement of the oral mucosa causes little discomfort and does not impair ingestion of food, but adhesions between buccal and gingival mucosa may be bothersome. Pharyngeal, laryngeal, and esophageal strictures may necessitate operation. Ocular involvement slowly progresses to entropion, symblepharon, and ultimately blindness; scarring of the genitalia and anus may impair function. Skin lesions cause disfigurement and discomfort but rarely functional impairment; the scarring alopecia is irreversible.

Treatment

Most treatment modalities, particularly topical, have been disappointing. Intralesional injections of corticosteroids into the conjunctiva have occasionally provided temporary relief for ocular disease. While systemic treatment with corticosteroids and immunosuppressive agents has yielded poor results, a combination of corticosteroids and sulfones may halt the disease process (see dermatitis herpetiformis, below).

When functional impairment due to scarring and obliteration of mucosal surfaces occurs, operative treatment becomes necessary. Implantation of lenses may retard or prevent blindness but is frequently not tolerated well by elderly patients.

Course & Prognosis

Cicatricial pemphigoid runs a chronic but variable course in which periods of active disease may be followed by remissions lasting several months; lesions have a tendency to reappear at the same sites until mucous membranes have been replaced by scar tissue.

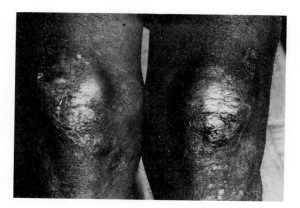

Figure 42–9. Epidermolysis bullosa acquisita. Pronounced scarring on both knees following repeated minor trauma.

4. EPIDERMOLYSIS BULLOSA ACQUISITA

Essentials of Diagnosis

- Blisters, crusts, milia, and scars, mainly on extensor surfaces of extremities.
- Oral mucosa often involved.
- Pronounced skin fragility.
- Subepidermal blister formation.
- Deposition of IgG, less frequently C3, and sometimes also other immunoglobulins at the basement membrane zone; by immunoelectronmicroscopy, these deposits occur in the dermis immediately below the basal lamina; circulating IgG-antibodies to basement membrane zone are often present.

General Considerations

Epidermolysis bullosa acquisita is rare, with onset in young to middle-aged adults; no data are available on sex, racial, or geographic distribution.

Clinical Findings

A. Symptoms and Signs: The eruption consists of blisters on the trunk and extremities, mainly at sites of minor or major trauma (Fig 42–9). The bullae eventually break, resulting in denuded areas that heal slowly, leaving hyperpigmentation and numerous milia but no scarring unless there was bacterial superinfection. Characteristically, blisters arise on normal-appearing skin.

B. Laboratory Findings: Histopathologic examination shows subepidermal blisters with little or no dermal inflammatory infiltrate. There is deposition of IgG and, less frequently, of other immunoglobulin classes and of C3 along the basement membrane zone in a pattern similar to that seen in bullous pemphigoid. By immunoelectronmicroscopy, these deposits are found below the lamina densa in the anchoring fibril zone and thus are clearly localized in the dermis below the epidermal basal lamina. Sera of patients frequently contain a circulating IgG antibody that attaches to this zone when normal human skin is used as a substrate. The antigen of epidermolysis bullosa acquisita is a 290-kDa protein that contains a collagen and a noncollagen part of 145-kDa each. It is localized at the lamina densa and at the dermal ends of anchoring fibrins but not in the banded middle part.

Treatment

Treatment consists of topical care for denuded areas, including tap water compresses (eg, 10 minutes twice daily) and topical antibiotics (eg, silver sulfadiazine 1% cream twice daily); no other established therapeutic measures are known. Dapsone has benefited some cases, but the disorder often resists treatment with systemic corticosteroids. High doses of vitamin E have also been reported to induce remission. Patients should be advised to avoid even minor trauma to help decrease the number of lesions.

Course & Prognosis

Mucosal surfaces, including the pharynx, the esophagus, and rarely even the intestinal tract, may occasionally be involved in a manner similar to that of cicatricial pemphigoid. The course is chronic with no tendency to remission.

5. LINEAR IgA DERMATOSIS

Essentials of Diagnosis

- Grouped vesicles and blisters, sometimes in rosettes.
- Subepidermal blister formation.
- Linear deposition of IgA and C3 at the dermal-

epidermal junction; circulating IgA antibodies to the basement membrane zone sometimes present.

Clinical Findings

A. Symptoms and Signs: In clinical appearance, this uncommon disease, provisionally called linear IgA dermatosis, resembles typical dermatitis herpetiformis (see below) or a mixture of dermatitis herpetiformis and bullous pemphigoid (Fig 42–10). There are tense vesicles and bullae, with a tendency to afflict flexural surfaces. Vesicles may be grouped or single. The disorder often affects children. Unlike dermatitis herpetiformis, these patients do not have gluten-sensitive enteropathy, nor do they respond to a gluten-free diet.

B. Laboratory Findings: Histopathologic examination shows neutrophils in basal vacuoles above the tips of rete ridges and generalized vacuolization and neutrophilic infiltration of the epidermal basement membrane zone—as opposed to the neutrophilic microabscesses found in dermal papillae in dermatitis herpetiformis. This is consistent with the observation that neutrophils from patients with linear IgA dermatosis or normal neutrophils preincubated with patient's serum produce active oxygen compounds that are capable of inducing tissue injury.

On direct immunofluorescence, there is a linear deposition of IgA and sometimes C3 at the epidermal basement membrane zone similar to the IgG deposits in bullous pemphigoid. At the ultrastructural level, the level of antibody binding differentiates a "lamina lucida type" and a "subbasal lamina type"; so far, no diagnostic or therapeutic consequences can be inferred from this distinction. Some patients also have circulating IgA-class antibodies to the epidermal basement membrane zone. There is preliminary evidence that the antigen in linear IgA dermatosis is a 97-kDa protein not synthesized by epidermal cells.

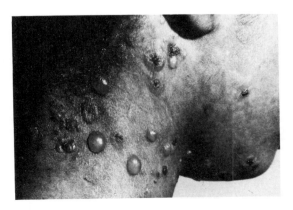

Figure 42–10. Linear IgA dermatosis. Lesions on the neck and chin. Small, tense blisters as well as infiltrated erythematous areas. Some suggestion of the typical appearance of grouping of blisters in rosettes is apparent.

No particular HLA association has been found in these patients.

Treatment

Treatment with dapsone usually works well. Its use is discussed with dermatitis herpetiformis below. Systemic corticosteroids are sometimes needed.

DERMATITIS HERPETIFORMIS (Duhring's Disease)

Essentials of Diagnosis

- Small grouped papules, vesicles, blisters, and erosions on erythematous plaques.
- Intense pruritus.
- Characteristic distribution over extensor surfaces of large joints (knees, elbows, buttocks), neck, shoulders, frontal hairline, and scalp.
- Associated with the HLA-B8 DR3/DQw2 haplotype.
- Papillary microabscesses, subepidermal split and blister formation.
- Deposition of IgA in a granular fashion subepidermally, along the basement membrane zone, frequently pronounced in the dermal papillae.
- Iodides (potassium iodide, seafood) may induce flares.

General Considerations

Dermatitis herpetiformis is a papulovesicular, intensely pruritic dermatosis associated with gluten-sensitive enteropathy and granular deposits of IgA in the dermal papillae. It may begin at any age but commonly starts between the late second and the early fourth decades. The prevalence is one in 800 dermatologic patients, though this figure varies. Males are affected twice as frequently as females; the disorder is most common in whites, particularly from Anglo-American communities; less frequent in blacks; and rare in Japanese.

The most important feature of dermatitis herpetiformis is its almost invariable association with gluten-sensitive enteropathy. This is usually an asymptomatic villous atrophy of jejunal mucosa; frank steatorrhea and malabsorption are uncommon. Gluten withdrawal in these patients not only restores normal architecture of the small intestinal mucosa but often also leads to improvement of skin lesions.

Several serologic abnormalities and diseases have been found to occur more frequently in patients with dermatitis herpetiformis: gastric hypoacidity and gastric atrophy occur in over 50% of patients, frequently associated with antigastric parietal cell antibodies; clinical or serologic evidence of thyroid disease, frequently with antithyroid antibodies, is present in 50%; glomerular deposits of IgA have been reported in several and IgA nephropathy in some patients; and, finally, there is an increased frequency of cancer, particularly of lymphomas of the gastrointestinal tract. The autoimmune disorders in patients with dermatitis herpetiformis may be explained at least partly by their common association with the HLA-B8/DR3 haplotype. The increased frequency of cancer is not readily explained but corresponds to the well-known complication of ordinary gluten-sensitive enteropathy.

Clinical Findings

A. Symptoms and Signs: The eruption of dermatitis herpetiformis is intensely pruritic and symmetric, mainly over the extensor surfaces of large joints. The sites of predilection are the elbows, buttocks, knees, hairline, neck, and shoulders (Fig 42–11A). The lesions consist of grouped papules and vesicles on an erythematous base. Because of the pruritus and scratching, the lesions tend to be excoriated (Fig 42–11B), and vesicles may be difficult to find.

B. Laboratory Findings: Routine laboratory investigations are noncontributory. Serum folate levels, xylose, and fat absorption may be reduced. There may be anemia, and jejunal biopsies usually reveal the morphologic characteristics of gluten-sensitive enteropathy. Since this tends to be multifocal and patchy, multiple biopsies may be necessary to detect jejunal lesions.

Ingestion of potassium iodide may induce a flare of the skin eruption, and patch-testing with iodine may result in the appearance of a typical lesion. These provocation tests are not usually done, since the diagnosis is confirmed by immunofluorescence.

1. Pathology– There is subepidermal blistering following a massive infiltration of dermal papillae by neutrophilic granulocytes, often so pronounced as to produce papillary microabscesses. In older lesions, eosinophils may also be present in varying numbers. The papillary dermis is edematous, and its collagen becomes basophilic. Neutrophilic infiltration may extend horizontally to form a band in the upper dermis, and there is a lymphohistiocytic and neutrophilic infiltrate around dilated blood vessels.

2. Immunopathology– The single most reliable

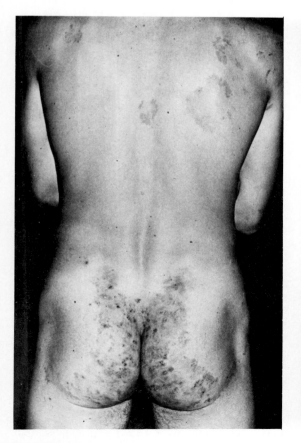
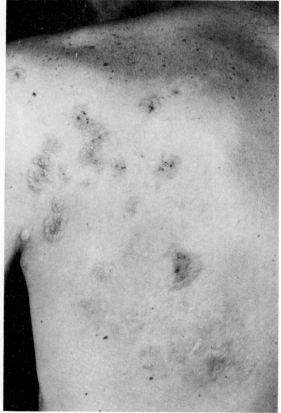

Figure 42–11. A: Dermatitis herpetiformis. Typical distribution of lesions on the buttocks, shoulders and elbows. The erythematous infiltrated nature of the lesions with small crusted erosions (scratching!) is apparent. **B:** Dermatitis herpetiformis (detail). Herpetiform grouping of vesicles on an erythematous base and small crusted erosions.

diagnostic finding in dermatitis herpetiformis is granular deposition of IgA and C3 (and sometimes other complement components) in the tips of the dermal papillae. They are invariably found in perilesional and in clinically uninvolved skin but may be absent from vesicular and bullous lesions. Granular deposits of IgA may extend and coalesce to assume a bandlike pattern, but there are no deposits in the epidermal basement membrane or in the epidermis. By immunoelectronmicroscopy, IgA is associated with dermal microfibrillar bundles and the microfibrillar components of papillary elastic fibers. The IgA, usually of the IgA_2 subclass, does not contain secretory piece or J-chain. There are no circulating antibodies to skin, but circulating antibodies to muscle endomysium may be present and reflect the degree of gluten enteropathy. Antigluten antibodies and antireticulin antibodies have sometimes—but not regularly—been found. Low levels of circulating immune complexes containing IgG and IgM have been demonstrated, probably best explained by the fact that HLA-B8 is also associated with impaired clearing of immune complexes from the circulation by the reticuloendothelial system. Immune complexes containing IgA have been detected after gluten ingestion.

Although IgA deposits cause the skin lesions, the neutrophil is the main inflammatory cell. It is not known how the disease process in skin is initiated (what mechanisms trigger an eruption).

Complications

Most complications are side effects of treatment. Patients with gluten-sensitive enteropathy may be more prone to develop intestinal lymphomas.

Treatment

Topical treatment and treatment with systemic corticosteroids are generally ineffective. The oral administration of dapsone, 50–100 mg/d, or sulfapyridine, 2–3 g/d, usually results in rapid resolution of the skin disease but has no effect on the pathologic findings in the small intestine. When either of these regimens is chosen, levels of erythrocyte glucose-6-phosphate dehydrogenase should be determined before treatment is started, since individuals with low levels are in danger of developing serious hemolytic anemia and methemoglobinemia.

A. Dapsone: Dapsone is usually given as a single daily dose. Mild hemolytic anemia always occurs but is compensated by increased rates of red blood cell synthesis reflected in high reticulocyte counts. Agranulocytosis and severe thrombocytopenia are uncommon idiosyncratic side effects, but the danger of these and severe anemia necessitate periodic assessment of hematocrit, leukocyte count, differential count, and platelet count, which should be done weekly for 1–2 months, then monthly for 1–2 months, then at least once every 6 months for the duration of therapy, which is often indefinite. Liver function should be monitored occasionally. Folate levels drop as folate is utilized to make red blood cells, and folate supplementation is often required (see Chapter 53).

Severe allergic reactions may occur, including toxic epidermal necrolysis and Stevens-Johnson syndrome. Peripheral neuropathies may develop from dapsone at any time.

The dose of dapsone may be increased if the diagnosis is certain and the response to treatment is insufficient. Very rarely, up to 400 mg/d may be necessary, but such doses require more frequent assessment for drug toxicity.

B. Sulfapyridine: Sulfapyridine is usually given as 500 mg 2–4 times daily. This drug can also cause serious severe allergic reactions, anemias, and neutropenias. Since sulfapyridine is a long-acting sulfonamide, crystallization in the kidney may occur, so all patients receiving the drug should increase their daily fluid intake.

C. Dietary Measures: A gluten-free (wheat-free) diet, if adhered to strictly, results in resolution of intestinal lesions and improvement of the eruption in most patients, but this may take a year or more, and the IgA deposits in the skin disappear even more slowly. A gluten-free diet is difficult and expensive to maintain.

Iodine ingestion (in drugs or seafood) should be avoided by these patients.

D. PUVA Treatment: Treatment with the PUVA regimen has led to fairly rapid resolution of skin lesions and thus provides an alternative to sulfone treatment, but it must be maintained continuously.

Course & Prognosis

The disease runs a long but variable course characterized by remissions and exacerbations. It tends to become less troublesome over the years, and 10–30% of patients eventually have permanent remissions.

CHRONIC BULLOUS DISEASE OF CHILDHOOD

Children can have chronic blistering diseases. The label "chronic bullous disease of childhood" is now archaic because immunofluorescence tests permit accurate classification of this previously ill-defined group of disorders. Most or all of these children suffer from bullous pemphigoid, dermatitis herpetiformis, or linear IgA dermatosis (see above). The term "chronic bullous disease of childhood" should therefore be reserved for those few patients in whom histologic, electron microscopic, and immunologic studies do not allow definitive diagnosis. An eruption not initially diagnosable may express the typical features of one or the other diseases mentioned above after several months.

BENIGN FAMILIAL PEMPHIGUS
(Hailey-Hailey Disease)

Essentials of Diagnosis

- Erosions, fissures, vesicles, and crusts on normal or erythematous skin.
- Sites of predilection: neck, axillae, groin; occasionally scalp.
- Lesions are usually superinfected with bacteria or *Candida*.
- Intraepidermal, suprabasal acantholysis.
- No immunoglobulin or complement deposition.
- No circulating antibodies.

General Considerations

Benign familial pemphigus is a rare disorder of epidermal coherence characterized by vesiculation and crusting. Acantholysis occurs spontaneously or, more frequently, as a result of physical damage or bacterial or candidal infection. Thus, the development of lesions can be triggered by inoculation into the skin of cocci or *Candida*. A hot and moist environment and sweating often are contributing factors. The disease is genetically transmitted as an autosomal dominant trait with irregular penetrance, since a positive family history can be elicited in only 70% of affected individuals. It usually manifests itself first between ages 15 and 35, and there is no predilection of sex, race, or geographic area.

The defect in cellular cohesion of the epidermis, as demonstrated by electron microscopy, seems due to a defect in the attachment of tonofilaments to desmosomes. In contrast to pemphigus, no immunologic mechanism has been implicated in the development of acantholysis.

Clinical Findings

A. Symptoms and Signs: Lesions consist of groups of tiny vesicles with an initially clear but soon turbid content. These vesicles break easily and leave eroded areas, tiny fissures, and crusts. Sites of predilection are the intertriginous areas (Fig 42–12) and the back, where chronic vegetating lesions may develop. The upper trunk, scalp, and extremities may also be involved, but mucosal lesions are exceptional. Lesions may itch or be painful on motion. They tend to enlarge, but there is a tendency to spontaneous healing without scarring. Recurrences are common. The condition can produce local discomfort but no systemic symptoms.

B. Laboratory Findings: Laboratory investigations, except histopathology, are noncontributory. The histopathologic changes consist of suprabasal cleft formation with acantholysis in the greater part of the overlying epidermis. In contrast to pemphigus, the epidermal cells have not lost their intercellular contacts completely, so that groups of cells may tenuously adhere to each other, resulting in the picture of a "dilapidated brick wall." Dermal papillae lined with

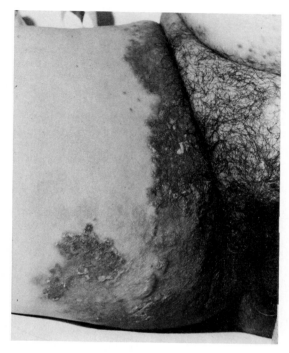

Figure 42–12. Benign familial pemphigus. Intertriginous involvement with erythema, blisters, erosions, and crusts.

basal cells protrude into the intraepidermal cavity and thus appear as "villi." In addition, there may be epidermal hyperplasia, and occasional dyskeratoses can occur. Dermal changes include papillary edema and superficial perivascular lymphohistiocytic infiltrates. Adnexal structures are usually not involved.

Differential Diagnosis

Chronic bacterial or fungal infections of intertriginous areas, pemphigus vulgaris and vegetans, and keratosis follicularis must be differentiated from benign familial pemphigus. The history and histopathologic findings rule out primary infectious disease. The absence of circulating and tissue-bound antibodies to epidermal intercellular substance, as demonstrated by immunohistologic methods, exclude pemphigus vulgaris and vegetans. Keratosis follicularis (Darier-White disease) may occasionally be more difficult to distinguish from benign familial pemphigus. The papular nature of the lesions and the distribution mainly on seborrheic areas and the extremities of Darier's disease as opposed to the vesiculation and the location in intertriginous areas of Hailey-Hailey disease should make the differential diagnosis possible.

Prevention

The only effective preventive measures are the avoidance of unnecessary exposure to heat, moisture, and physical trauma (friction) and the prevention of bacterial and candidal colonization of intertriginous regions.

Genetic counseling should be made available.

Treatment

Treatment is directed at elimination of precipitating factors, local measures for symptomatic relief, and control of infection. Topical treatment consists of cool tap water compresses and antibacterial creams and ointments. If *Candida* is present within the lesions, appropriate therapy (eg, miconazole 2% cream twice daily) should be instituted. Some patients bene-

fit from steroid creams when there is pronounced inflammation and discomfort. Systemic antibiotic treatment of infections (eg, with tetracycline or erythromycin) may also help, depending on their severity and the response to topical measures. In chronic vegetating lesions surgical removal with subsequent skin grafting may be of value.

Course & Prognosis

The disease tends to run a benign but protracted course. Periods of remission alternate with the appearance of active lesions, but in occasional cases erosions and especially vegetating lesions persist for a long time. In some patients, the condition improves with advancing age.

REFERENCES

Aberer W et al: Azathioprine in the treatment of pemphigus vulgaris: A long term follow-up. J Amer Acad Dermatol 1987;16:527.

Ahmed AR: Bullous pemphigoid. Clin Dermatol 1987;5:1.

Chorzelski TP et al: Linear IgA bullous dermatosis. In: *Immunopathology of the Skin*. Beutner EH, Chorzelski TP, Bean SF (editors). Wiley, 1979.

Hall RP: The pathogenesis of dermatitis herpetiformis: Recent advances. J Am Acad Dermatol 1987;16:1129.

Karman N: Pemphigus. J Amer Acad Dermatol 1988;18:1219.

Katz SI et al: Dermatitis herpetiformis: The skin and the gut. Ann Intern Med 1980;76:857.

Korman N: Bullous pemphigoid. J Amer Acad Dermatol 1987;16:907.

Kumar V et al: Reticulum and endomysial antibodies in bullous diseases. Arch Dermatol 1987;123:1179.

Montes LF et al: Microbial flora in familial chronic pemphigus. Arch Dermatol 1970;101:140.

Palmer DD, Perry HO: Benign familial chronic pemphigus. Arch Dermatol 1962;86:493.

Person JR, Rogers RS III: Bullous and cicatricial pemphigoid: Clinical, histopathologic, and immunopathologic correlations. Mayo Clin Proc 1977;52:54.

Rappersberger K et al: Epidermolysis bullosa acquisita: Eine klinisch-pathologische studie. Hautarzt 1988;39:355.

Richter BJ, McNutt NS: The spectrum of epidermolysis bullosa acquisita. Arch Dermatol 1979;115:1325.

Rogers RS III, Seehafer JR, Perry HO: Treatment of cicatricial (benign mucous membrane) pemphigoid with dapsone. J Amer Acad Dermatol 1982;6:215.

Savin JA: Some factors affecting prognosis in pemphigus vulgaris and pemphigoid. Br J Dermatol 1981;104:415.

Shornick JK: Herpes gestationis. J Amer Acad Dermatol 1987;17:539.

Yoshiike T, Woodley DT, Briggaman RA: Epidermolysis bullosa acquisita antigen: Relationship between the collagenase-sensitive and insensitive domains. J Invest Dermatol 1988;90:127.

Section VII:
Neoplastic Disorders

Benign & Malignant Growths

43

William A. Caro, MD

Skin tumors are common; virtually every individual has one or more at some time during the life span. The vast majority are benign, and a few are premalignant or malignant. Although only a small percentage of skin tumors can be classified as serious cancers threatening the health and life of the patient, cancers of the skin are the most common of all malignant tumors.

The skin is composed of many different kinds of cells, each of which can give rise to one or more different types of skin tumors. The skin thus produces a wider variety of tumors than any other body organ. Skin tumors also are the most common human tumors. Table 43–1 presents a classification of skin tumors based on site of origin.

Benign tumors usually can be distinguished from malignant ones clinically and microscopically, though the specific diagnosis of all tumors requires microscopic examination. Clinically, benign tumors usually are characterized by no growth or slow growth. Microscopically, such tumors have a well-organized cellular pattern. Malignant tumors tend to grow and invade adjacent tissue. Some tumors may metastasize (eg, malignant melanoma). A few skin cancers (eg, basal cell carcinomas) rarely metastasize. Others, such as squamous cell carcinomas, exhibit variable behavior—eg, those that arise in actinic keratoses metastasize with low frequency (1–3%). But those that arise on normal skin (genitalia) or in preexisting radiation scars have a high rate of metastases. Microscopically, malignant tumors show a disorganized architectural pattern and atypical cells. In addition, the pattern of tumor cells within the dermis has a malignant quality because these cells have invaded adnexa, fat, or other tissue.

Genetic and environmental factors may play an important role in the development of skin tumors. The inheritance of blue eyes and a fair complexion confers susceptibility to sun-induced tumors. Solar irradiation is important in the development of actinic ker-

atoses, basal cell and squamous cell carcinomas, and malignant melanoma. Ionizing radiations such as x-rays can produce skin cancers, as can chronic ingestion of arsenic. Contact with certain carcinogenic chemicals may induce cancers such as the scrotal skin carcinomas in chimney sweeps from contact with tars in the 18th century. Uncommonly, there may be an inherited tendency toward development of certain tumors with no relationship to environmental factors. This type of inheritance usually is autosomal dominant, and the tumors usually are multiple. Such is the case with multiple neurofibromatosis, basal cell nevus syndrome, dysplastic nevus syndrome, and Muir-Torre syndrome.

Accurate diagnosis is essential for correct treatment of skin tumors. Although many such tumors are easily diagnosed by the experienced eye, others require biopsy and microscopic examination for specific diagnosis. Small lesions may be removed in their entirety, while larger ones may be sampled and treatment determined on the basis of the biopsy of a representative area.

TUMORS ARISING FROM EPIDERMIS

BENIGN EPIDERMAL TUMORS

1. SEBORRHEIC KERATOSIS

Essentials of Diagnosis
- Domed or flat-topped verrucous papule.
- Tan, brown, or black.
- Presence of other similar lesions elsewhere.
- "Stuck on" appearance.
- Characteristic histologic features.

Table 43–1. Classification of skin tumors.

I. Tumors arising from epidermis
  A. Benign epidermal tumors
    1. Seborrheic keratosis
    2. Epidermal nevus
    3. Epidermoid cysts
    4. Keratoacanthoma
    5. Cutaneous horn
    6. Bowenoid papulosis of genitalia
  B. Premalignant epidermal tumors
    1. Actinic keratosis
    2. Leukoplakia
    3. Bowen's disease
    4. Paget's disease
  C. Malignant epidermal tumors
    1. Basal cell carcinoma
    2. Squamous cell carcinoma
    3. Carcinoma of epidermal appendages
  D. Benign tumors of epidermal appendages
    1. Trichoepithelioma
    2. Trichilemmoma
    3. Nevus sebaceus of Jadassohn
    4. Sebaceous gland hyperplasia
    5. Hidrocystoma
    6. Syringoma
    7. Cylindroma
II. Tumors of the melanocyte system
  A. Nevi (moles)
    1. Common nevus
    2. Congenital nevus
    3. Spindle and epithelioid nevus (Spitz nevus)
    4. Dysplastic nevus
    5. Halo nevus
    6. Blue nevus
  B. Lentigines
  C. Lentigo maligna
  D. Malignant melanoma
III. Tumors of mesodermal origin
  A. Tumors arising from connective tissue cells
    1. Dermatofibroma
    2. Acrochordon
    3. Dermatofibrosarcoma protuberans
    4. Atypical fibroxanthoma of skin
    5. Keloid
    6. Angiofibroma
    7. Fibromatoses
    8. Juvenile xanthogranuloma
    9. Neurofibroma
    10. Neurilemmoma
    11. Granular cell tumor
IV. Vascular tumors
  A. Benign vascular tumors
    1. Hemangioma
    2. Angiokeratoma
    3. Arterial spider
    4. Lymphangioma
    5. Glomus tumor
  B. Malignant vascular tumors
    1. Kaposi's sarcoma
    2. Angiosarcoma
    3. Lymphoangiosarcoma
V. Other mesodermal tumors
    1. Leiomyoma
    2. Lipoma
VI. Lymphoreticular tumors
  A. Benign: lymphocytoma cutis (cutaneous lymphoid hyperplasia)
  B. Malignant lymphoma
    1. Mycosis fungoides, cutaneous T cell lymphomas
    2. Other cutaneous malignant lymphomas
VII. Tumors metastatic to skin

General Considerations

Seborrheic keratoses are the most common tumors in older people and are invariably benign. They tend to increase in number with aging, and there often are more of them in seborrheic areas.

Clinical Findings

A. Symptoms and Signs: Most patients have multiple lesions, often symmetrically distributed. Seborrheic keratoses occur commonly on the face, chest, back, abdomen, and proximal extremities. The lesions themselves are usually flat, with a velvety or cobblestoned surface, and vary in color from tan to dark brown to black. With the passage of time, they tend to become more elevated and more deeply pigmented and develop a rougher contour. The lesions have sharply defined margins and frequently appear "stuck" to the skin surface. Some lesions are covered by a greasy scale.

B. Laboratory Findings: Biopsy shows acanthosis, hyperkeratosis, and papillomatosis, with keratin horn pseudocysts—small cysts of material within the epidermis.

Differential Diagnosis

Most seborrheic keratoses can be diagnosed easily from simple examination. An occasional lesion may have a less typical appearance and must be differentiate by biopsy from an ordinary nevus, a pigmented basal cell carcinoma, or a malignant melanoma.

Treatment

Because seborrheic keratoses lie on top of the skin surface, they may be easily removed with a dermal curette followed by light cautery or electrodesiccation. Liquid nitrogen application also is effective treatment. Although excisional surgery ordinarily is not indicated for seborrheic keratosis, shave excision is the treatment of choice when histologic confirmation is desired.

2. EPIDERMAL NEVUS

Although the term "nevus" usually refers to a lesion composed of nevus cells, it has also been used to denote a congenital developmental abnormality resulting in faulty production of mature or nearly mature structures. Epidermal nevi fall into this latter category, since they represent hyperplasia of surface or adnexal epithelium. These uncommon lesions may be solitary, small, and inconspicuous or may be multiple, covering large areas. They usually are present at birth but may appear during the first few months or years of life. The arrangement and distribution vary from solitary verrucous papules or plaques to multiple lesions arranged in linear distribution. Irregular configurational patterns can give lesions a striking appearance. Lesions commonly are asymmetrically distributed. Colors usually range from flesh-colored to deeply pigmented brown or black. The surface is characteristically rough and wartlike. More extensive lesions usually grow proportionately with the individual.

Large epidermal nevi may be associated with skeletal, central nervous system, and vascular abnormalities. Otherwise, except for their cosmetic importance, epidermal nevi ordinarily require no treatment. Smaller lesions may be excised, though removal of larger lesions may be technically difficult or cosmetically impractical, since the scar may look worse than the nevus.

3. EPIDERMOID CYSTS

Two major forms of epidermoid cysts occur: epidermal cysts and pilar (trichilemmal) cysts. Epidermal cysts may be single or multiple; they occur most frequently on the face, neck, upper chest, and back. Although these lesions are readily palpable, in early stages the overlying skin appears normal. As the lesion enlarges, however, the skin thins and takes on a whitish to yellowish hue. Usually the lesions are asymptomatic; but when they become infected, there may be redness and tenderness, and ultimately they may rupture and extrude purulent material.

Microscopically, epidermal cysts contain epithelial debris surrounded by an epidermal wall that resembles the normal surface epidermis.

Treatment of an epidermal cyst requires total removal or destruction of the epithelial sac; without this, the lesion may recur. Some lesions are treated by complete surgical wedge excision, though the sac sometimes may be dissected out through a small overlying incision following incision and drainage of cyst contents.

Pilar cysts, involving the hair follicles, occur much less frequently than epidermal cysts and favor the scalp. Some lesions occur on the face, neck, and trunk. They may be single or multiple and are clinically indistinguishable from epidermal cysts. Microscopically, however, the pilar cyst is lined by epithelium that more closely resembles a portion of hair follicle epithelium than it does surface epithelium. Treatment is the same as that for epidermal cysts.

4. KERATOACANTHOMA

Essentials of Diagnosis

- Rapidly enlarging nodule.
- Central keratin plug.
- Characteristic histology.

General Considerations

Keratoacanthoma is usually a benign, spontaneously regressing tumor that clinically and microscopically resembles a well-differentiated squamous cell carcinoma. Most keratoacanthomas are solitary, though occasional patients may have multiple lesions. Men are affected much more frequently than women, and most lesions begin during middle adult life or later. Sun exposure plays a major role in the development of these lesions, and most occur over sun-exposed areas, especially the face and arms.

A. Symptoms and Signs: Clinically, the typical keratoacanthoma appears as a small reddish papule that rapidly enlarges. The lesion usually reaches its full size within 1–2 months; most do not exceed 1 or 2 cm in diameter. The fully developed lesion is erythematous and firm and has a central plug of keratin material.

B. Laboratory Findings: The microscopic appearance of keratoacanthoma includes a central keratin plug with a surrounding proliferation of well-differentiated squamous epithelium extending downward into the dermis. Such lesions may be difficult to distinguish microscopically from well-differentiated squamous cell carcinoma, but keratoacanthomas do not invade deeper tissues. For this reason, the base of suspected tumors must be included in histologic sections.

Complications

After the lesion has reached its maximum size, it usually remains quiescent for a while and then slowly undergoes spontaneous regression. The end result of this regression usually will be an atrophic scar, and the entire process may take many months.

Not all keratoacanthomas regress spontaneously, and some with a typical clinical and microscopic appearance of keratoacanthoma may behave more aggressively. In such cases, the distinction between keratoacanthoma and squamous cell carcinoma is blurred.

Treatment

Treatment of keratoacanthoma usually involves simple excision, and the end cosmetic result of such excised lesions frequently will be better than the result obtained by spontaneous regression. The lesion can be excised in a surgical ellipse with primary closure. If shave excision is done, a wedge of tissue extending to fat should be excised first to provide the pathologist with adequate deep tissue to ensure that squamous cell carcinoma is not present. Biopsy across the entire depth of the lesion will give adequate material for microscopic examination, and such a procedure frequently is followed by total involution of the lesion. Aggressive keratoacanthomas may behave in a manner indistinguishable from that of squamous cell carcinoma and must be treated accordingly by wider excision. In special circumstances (where a surgical scar is particularly unacceptable, eg, the nose), intralesional injection of fluorouracil has been used. Referral to a dermatologist for this treatment is recommended.

5. CUTANEOUS HORN

The surface of cutaneous horn is composed of dense, compact keratin material. The surrounding area may be erythematous, and some bases may be indurated. Cutaneous horns tend to occur more commonly in older individuals and favor sun-exposed areas.

Cutaneous horns arise from some other underlying lesion, most commonly actinic keratosis or verruca vulgaris. Less commonly, a cutaneous horn overlies a frank squamous cell carcinoma.

Cutaneous horns may be destroyed cryosurgically or electrosurgically or excised surgically. It is advisable to have the base of the lesion examined microscopically to be sure squamous cell carcinoma is not the cause.

6. BOWENOID PAPULOSIS OF THE GENITALIA

These lesions are important because of their similarity to the premalignant dermatosis, Bowen's disease. They are produced by strains of human papillomavirus. Bowenoid papulosis occurs much more frequently in men than in women, and the shaft of the penis is the most common site. The clinical appearance suggests a small wart or seborrheic keratosis. The lesions tend to be reddish-brown to brown, average approximately 4–5 mm in diameter, protrude from the skin surface, and have a warty top.

Although the clinical appearance is benign, the microscopic appearance shows disorganization of the epidermal cellular architecture with atypical epidermal cells. Although the microscopic picture often is indistinguishable from that of Bowen's disease (see below), these lesions usually remain clinically benign and do not evolve into Bowen's disease or other premalignant or malignant conditions. Lesions of bowenoid papulosis are easily treated electrosurgically or by simple excision.

PREMALIGNANT EPIDERMAL TUMORS

These lesions can evolve into true skin cancers in a minority of cases. When such transformation does occur, the squamous cell carcinoma is the most common type.

1. ACTINIC KERATOSIS

Essentials of Diagnosis
- Red or brown rough flat-typed papule.
- Occurrence on sun-damaged skin.
- Epithelial dysplasia.

General Considerations

Actinic keratoses—also termed senile or solar keratoses—arise on sun-exposed skin, usually of older individuals.

Clinical Findings

A. Symptoms and Signs: Lesions occur most frequently on the face, the back of the hands and forearms, the neck, and exposed scalp. The lesions commonly are multiple and present as firm, sharply defined papules with a rough keratotic surface and often an erythematous base (Fig 43–1). In contrast to seborrheic keratoses, actinic keratoses usually have the feel of arising from within the skin rather than protruding from the skin surface. Most actinic keratoses are 3–6 mm in diameter, though smaller and larger lesions may occur.

The skin upon which the actinic keratosis arises frequently will show evidence of chronic sun damage, with scaling, roughness, pigment variation, wrinkling, and atrophy.

B. Laboratory Findings: Biopsy discloses disruption of normal epithelial architecture with hyperkeratosis and inflammation. The dermis also shows actinic elastosis.

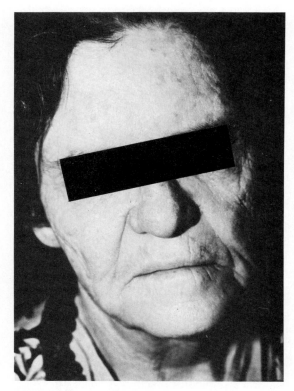

Figure 43–1. Multiple actinic keratoses of the face. The forehead and nose lesions are erythematous with some scale.

Complications

Actinic keratoses gradually enlarge. About 20–25% ultimately are transformed into squamous cell carcinomas, usually years after their first appearance. Lesions that begin to enlarge more rapidly with or without ulceration and which show increasing induration and inflammatory change may be undergoing malignant transformation.

Treatment

Actinic keratoses may be treated satisfactorily by curettage with electrodesiccation, cautery, or cryotherapy with liquid nitrogen. When there is a question of malignant transformation, the lesion should be conservatively excised or biopsied and subjected to careful microscopic examination.

Multiple lesions may be treated by the topical application of fluorouracil. A solution or cream containing 1–5% fluorouracil is applied to the entire area of involvement twice daily for approximately 3 weeks. Most actinic keratoses become intensely inflamed as they are destroyed by this drug. After the period of treatment, the area usually is treated with a topical steroid such as hydrocortisone 1% cream twice daily to speed resolution of the inflammatory process.

2. LEUKOPLAKIA

Leukoplakia is an abnormal hyperplastic response of mucosal epithelium with excessive keratinization. Clinically, the term has been used to denote whitish patches on a mucosal surface. Histologically, the term has been used to denote mucosal hyperkeratosis, often with epithelial dysplasia. It may be a premalignant disorder, since about 10% of affected patients develop squamous cell carcinomas within the area (see Chapter 48).

3. BOWEN'S DISEASE

Bowen's disease is an intraepidermal squamous cell carcinoma. It is more common in men with fair complexion, and chronic sunlight exposure may be a major inciting factor. Chronic ingestion of inorganic arsenicals has also caused Bowen's disease, though this etiologic factor is rare today.

Bowen's disease may involve any area of the skin surface but does tend to favor sun-exposed areas. In approximately one-third of patients, lesions may be multiple.

The lesion of Bowen's disease is papulosquamous and appears as a somewhat erythematous, rough-surfaced, sharply defined plaque. There may be variable scaling, and the border may be slightly elevated.

As an in-situ squamous cell carcinoma, Bowen's disease may evolve into invasive squamous cell carcinoma. Such aggressive behavior tends to be less frequent than with actinic keratoses—approximately 5% in one series. Nevertheless, squamous cell carcinomas arising from Bowen's disease usually are more aggressive than those arising from actinic keratoses. Regional lymph node metastases from these carcinomas are not uncommon.

Some studies have suggested that patients with Bowen's disease are more likely to develop other premalignant and malignant tumors. Cutaneous lesions have included actinic keratoses, basal cell carcinomas, adnexal carcinomas, and malignant melanoma, while noncutaneous cancers have included tumors of the respiratory, gastrointestinal, genitourinary, and reticuloendothelial systems.

The major lesions from which Bowen's disease must be differentiated include superficial basal cell carcinoma and inflammatory dermatoses such as psoriasis. Bowen's disease of the genitalia may resemble Paget's disease (see below), and smaller lesions may resemble actinic keratoses.

Surgical excision of lesions of Bowen's disease provides the highest cure rate. Many such lesions are treated with electrosurgical techniques such as curettage and electrodesiccation, but with these procedures there is some chance that lesions may recur.

When Bowen's disease occurs on mucosal surfaces, the clinical appearance and biologic potential change. Such lesions are termed erythroplasia of Queyrat when they occur on the glans penis, usually in uncircumcised males. They occur less frequently on the vulva. These lesions are brightly erythematous and have a somewhat velvety, glistening surface.

Although the microscopic picture of erythroplasia of Queyrat is the same as that of Bowen's disease, the rate of malignant transformation is higher in erythroplasia of Queyrat, and the resulting squamous cell carcinomas tend to be more aggressive than those arising from ordinary Bowen's disease.

4. PAGET'S DISEASE

The skin lesions of Paget's disease are produced by atypical cells lying within the epidermis, and these cells frequently arise from an underlying adenocarcinoma. Paget's disease occurs on the areola and nipple and, less commonly, in other regions such as the vulva, scrotum, and perineal and perianal areas. The typical lesion of Paget's disease is a solitary, sharply circumscribed patch that may have an eczematous surface. Paget's disease of the breast occurs almost exclusively in women; extramammary Paget's disease also occurs in men.

Paget's disease of the breast is almost always associated with an underlying carcinoma, usually of intraductal origin. Such carcinomas may vary considerably in size, and metastases may be present by the time the carcinoma is discovered.

The occurrence of an underlying carcinoma with

extramammary Paget's disease is significantly less common. Less than half of patients with extramammary Paget's disease have an identifiable carcinoma, and this usually arises from the cutaneous apocrine glands.

Clinically, Paget's disease must be differentiated from psoriasis and various forms of eczematous dermatitis. The solitary nature of the lesion, its location, its sharply marginated yet eczematous appearance, and its failure to respond to topical therapy point in the direction of Paget's disease. The diagnosis is confirmed by the specific microscopic finding of atypical Paget cells within the epidermis.

Paget's disease of the breast is treated using the accepted techniques of surgery for carcinoma of the breast, while anogenital Paget's disease is treated by wide and deep local excision with a search for an underlying carcinoma.

MALIGNANT EPIDERMAL TUMORS

BASAL CELL CARCINOMA
(Basal Cell Epithelioma)

Essentials of Diagnosis

- Translucent character and "rolled border."
- Central depression or crust.
- Telangiectasis on surface.
- Sclerosing type may look like a scar.
- Multicentric type may look like a papulosquamous dermatosis.
- Histology: basal cell proliferation and invasion of dermis.

General Considerations

Basal cell carcinoma is the most common malignant tumor affecting humans and the most easily treated and cured malignant lesion. The tumor is most common among fair-skinned individuals, particularly those with chronic exposure to sunlight, and therefore predominates on sun-exposed skin such as that of the face and adjacent areas. Men are affected somewhat more commonly than women, and the likelihood of basal cell carcinoma increases with advancing age. Nevertheless, basal cell carcinomas are not uncommon in young adults and have been seen occasionally in children.

A. Symptoms and Signs:

1. Noduloulcerative type– Clinically, the most common form of basal cell carcinoma is the noduloulcerative type. This lesion favors areas about the face and begins as a small translucent papule that may have a pale erythematous hue. As the lesion enlarges, examination often will reveal telangiectatic vessels coursing across the surface (Fig 43–2). With continuing enlargement, the central portion of the lesion may become depressed or ulcerate, with the slowly expanding border remaining relatively well defined and elevated. Although growth of the typical basal cell carcinoma is slow, such lesions enlarge progressively and ultimately may invade vital structures or vessels with resulting severe hemorrhage.

2. Sclerosing type– The sclerosing basal cell carcinoma (morphealike epithelioma) has a different appearance and presents as a yellowish-white sclerotic plaque. This lesion frequently does not have a distinct border and may resemble a small patch of scleroderma or scar. Under the microscope, such lesions show relatively fewer tumor cells, and these are in an abundant fibrous stroma. Since these lesions infiltrate the surrounding tissue, delineation of their borders is more difficult than in the case of most other basal cell carcinomas.

3. Superficial (multicentric) type– Superficial basal cell carcinoma often occurs as multiple lesions, primarily over the trunk. These lesions frequently will have an inflammatory rather than a neoplastic appearance and may resemble flat plaques of psoriasis. An irregular elevated, threadlike border is an important clue in the clinical diagnosis of such a lesion.

4. Basal cell nevus syndrome– In the rare nevoid basal cell carcinoma syndrome, multiple lesions occur throughout life. Patients with this genetically determined disorder with autosomal dominant inheritance begin developing multiple basal cell carcinomas in childhood. The lesions have widespread distribution and are not confined to the sun-exposed areas. The clinical appearance varies considerably. Many do not look like basal cell carcinomas. Although the

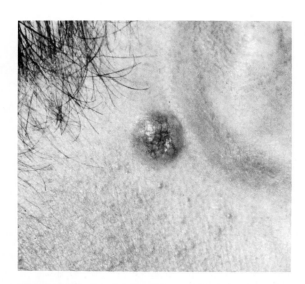

Figure 43–2. Basal cell carcinoma. Note the somewhat translucent hue and surface telangiectasia.

lesions tend to remain quiescent during childhood, most patients develop new growths at puberty, and lesions exhibit a more aggressive behavior of growth and invasion. Additional cutaneous features of the nevoid basal cell carcinoma syndrome include cysts, lipomas, and fibromas and small pits of the palms and soles. Patients with this syndrome also have characteristic bony abnormalities, including cysts of the jaw and splayed or bifid ribs. Hypertelorism, lateral displacement of the medial canthi of the eye, a broad nasal root, and frontoparietal bosselation give these patients a characteristic appearance.

B. Laboratory Findings: In all forms of basal cell carcinoma, microscopic examination reveals masses of compactly arranged basophilic cells within the dermis. These are termed basaloid cells because of their resemblance to the cells of the basal cell layer of the epidermis. Associated with these masses of cells, the dermal stroma usually shows a variable reaction of fibrosis. In the ordinary noduloulcerative type of basal cell carcinoma, the masses may be relatively large and the fibrosis mild. In the sclerosing type of basal cell carcinoma, the masses are usually small and may consist of only a few cells, while the stromal fibrotic reaction is quite pronounced. Superficial basal cell carcinoma has masses of basaloid cells extending downward from the surface epidermis, while the basal cell carcinomas of the basal cell nevus syndrome have the microscopic appearance of ordinary basal cell carcinomas,

Complications

In spite of their continuing growth, basal cell carcinomas have little tendency to metastasize. When metastasis does occur, it usually arises from a lesion that has been clinically aggressive and has had multiple recurrences following therapy. The microscopic picture of such a lesion may also be more aggressive than what is ordinarily seen. More often, basal cell carcinomas invade and destroy underlying tissues. It is this destructive, invasive tendency that makes them malignant.

Treatment

Four basic methods are used in the treatment of basal cell carcinoma, and the selection of one over another depends upon the location and nature of the lesion and the experience of the managing physician. Smaller lesions are usually treated with simple surgical excision or with destruction by curettage and electrodesiccation. Although less commonly used today, irradiation has also been an effective method of treatment, particularly for lesions around the eyelids, nose, and lips.

With recurrent basal cell carcinomas and tumors with poorly defined clinical margins, such as sclerosing basal cell carcinoma, the treatment of choice frequently will be Mohs's microscopically controlled excisional surgery (see Chapter 54). With this technique, the lesion is removed and mapped in relationship to the underlying site. Horizontally oriented frozen sections are then examined immediately, and further surgery is performed at sites where tumor cells are still present. The treatment is completed when no further tumor is found in subsequently removed tissue.

All methods for treating primary basal cell carcinomas have a high degree of success, with cure rates in the range of 95%. Those that recur are usually larger than 1–2 cm, are located over embryologic cleavage planes such as the glabella or nasolabial folds, or are of the sclerosing type. The small number of recurring lesions usually can be treated by wider excision. Some lesions will have a more aggressive course with multiple recurrences, and Mohs's surgery is the treatment of choice for such lesions.

SQUAMOUS CELL CARCINOMA

Essentials of Diagnosis
- Enlarging nodule.
- Usually arise from actinic keratosis, Bowen's disease, or leukoplakia.
- Disorganized atypical keratinocytes with invasion into dermis.

General Considerations

Although squamous cell carcinoma is quite different biologically from basal cell carcinoma, the 2 tumors share a number of characteristics. Like basal cell carcinoma, squamous cell carcinoma is much more common in fair-skinned individuals, and sun exposure is the major causal factor. Both basal cell and squamous cell carcinoma may result from other environmental carcinogens such as previous x-ray therapy of the skin. Squamous cell carcinomas are much more common in men and tend to occur at a somewhat higher average age than basal cell carcinomas. Squamous cell carcinomas are distinctly less common than basal cell carcinomas in young adults. Although both lesions occur commonly on the face, squamous cell carcinomas also occur commonly on other sun-exposed areas, such as the dorsa of the hands and forearms.

A. Symptoms and Signs: Although basal cell carcinomas ordinarily arise de novo, squamous cell carcinomas usually arise from preexisting lesions, especially actinic keratoses, Bowen's disease, or leukoplakia. Actinic keratoses evolving into squamous cell carcinoma usually show enlargement and increasing induration and inflammatory reaction. They are typically large, growing, scaling nodules.

Squamous cell carcinoma arising de novo usually appears as a small, somewhat erythematous papule or nodule with an indurated base. Such nodules enlarge somewhat more rapidly than basal cell carcinomas and ultimately ulcerate (Figs 43–3 and 43–4).

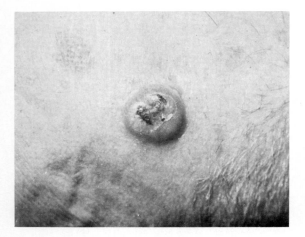

Figure 43–3. Squamous cell carcinoma with central ulceration. This was a firm lesion.

Squamous cell carcinomas usually are somewhat more firm and scaly than basal cell carcinomas.

B. Laboratory Findings: Microscopically, squamous cell carcinoma consists of a disorganized proliferation of atypical-appearing squamous cells. Groups of these tumor cells may be deeply invasive.

Complications

Squamous cell carcinomas arising from sundamaged skin usually have a relatively low rate of metastasis (0.5–3%), though this rate is higher than

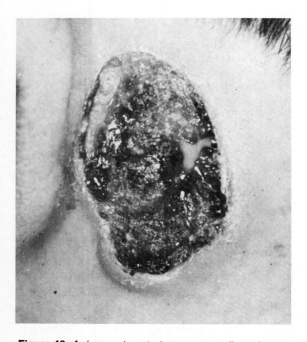

Figure 43–4. Large ulcerated squamous cell carcinoma.

that for basal cell carcinomas. Squamous cell carcinomas arising on mucocutaneous surfaces such as the lips and from areas with previous tissue alterations, such as burn scars or sinus tracts, tend to be aggressive, with more extensive invasion and a higher frequency of metastases. Squamous cell carcinomas of the lips and other mucous membranes may arise in an area of clinical leukoplakia as an indurated or ulcerated nodule.

Treatment

The treatment modalities for squamous cell carcinoma are similar to those used for basal cell carcinoma, though these lesions require somewhat more aggressive treatment (eg, wider excision) than do basal cell carcinomas. Squamous cell carcinomas on the mucous membranes should always be excised. Mohs's microsurgery may be used. Follow-up evaluation for recurrence or metastatic spread is indicated.

BENIGN TUMORS OF EPIDERMAL APPENDAGES

These tumors arise from cells with the potential for differentiation in the direction of the primary epidermal appendigeal structures: hair follicles, sebaceous glands, and eccrine and apocrine sweat glands. A large number of benign tumors fall into this category, though most are uncommon.

Trichoepitheliomas are benign tumors of the epidermis differentiating toward hair follicle structures. They may be single or multiple, and multiple lesions occur as part of an autosomal dominantly inherited trait. Solitary lesions occur primarily on the face and appear as nondescript flesh-colored papules. Multiple lesions also favor the face, and their appearance begins during the early years of life. The maximum concentration of such lesions occurs near the nasolabial folds, eyelids, and central areas of the face. The microscopic appearance of trichoepithelioma must be differentiated from that of basal cell carcinoma, which may look similar.

Trichilemmomas are benign tumors of epidermal cells with a distinctive microscopic appearance, but clinically they resemble common warts. In women with many such lesions, Cowden's syndrome must be considered. In this syndrome, multiple trichilemmomas are associated with a high incidence of breast cancer and other abnormalities.

Nevus sebaceus of Jadassohn is a benign epithelial growth that microscopically shows abnormalities of hair follicles and sebaceous and apocrine glands. The lesion frequently is present at birth or may be seen shortly thereafter as a small bald patch usually on the scalp, often slightly yellow. Following puberty, the lesion becomes a rough-surfaced plaque with a yellowish to brownish hue. These lesions vary in size and may be quite extensive. Most occur on the head. In later life, nevus sebaceus of Jadassohn may develop other benign adnexal tumors or occasionally a basal cell carcinoma. Nevus sebaceus should ordinarily be excised at or before puberty, though this may present some difficulty if the lesion is large.

Sebaceous gland hyperplasia represents a common lesion in older individuals. These lesions are usually multiple and occur almost exclusively on the face and forehead. They are yellowish, and may have a lobulated surface with a central depression. Clinically, they must be differentiated from basal cell carcinomas. They are easily treated electrosurgically, though such treatment is not required.

Hidrocystoma is a common benign sweat gland tumor that usually appears as a solitary dome-shaped flesh-colored to bluish translucent papule. Most occur near the eye. Microscopic examination reveals a large dilated cystic structure.

Syringomas occur as multiple small flesh-colored papules, primarily over the face of women. These lesions are asymptomatic but may be of cosmetic importance. They derive from proliferation of cells of the eccrine sweat duct apparatus.

Cylindromas are also benign sweat gland tumors and may occur as solitary or multiple lesions. The multiple type is autosomal dominantly inherited. Multiple lesions tend to occur primarily on the scalp. Such lesions may be large and numerous and have been referred to as "turban tumors" because of their appearance. They affect women more commonly than men.

Although some of the benign adnexal tumors have a distinctive clinical appearance, most require histopathologic examination for accurate diagnosis. An excisional biopsy will be the usual method of treatment, though with multiple benign lesions it may not be necessary or feasible to remove all of them.

TUMORS OF THE MELANOCYTE SYSTEM

NEVI
(Moles)

1. COMMON NEVI

Nevi are the most common tumors of humans. Almost all individuals have one or more nevi composed of cells that are derived from the melanocyte system. Microscopically, nevi are divided into 3 groups, depending upon the location of the nevus cells. In **junctional nevi,** the nevus cells are located within the dermal-epidermal junction. In **compound nevi,** they are within the dermal-epidermal junction and in the underlying dermis; and in **intradermal nevi,** the nevus cells are confined to the dermis.

Clinically, junctional nevi tend to be deeply pigmented, flat, and with slight elevation above the surface of the skin. They usually cannot be palpated. Compound nevi often show some elevation and may have a flat component surrounding the elevated component. Intradermal nevi tend to be nonpigmented, dome-shaped papules (Fig 43–5). In general, there is a transition from junctional through compound to intradermal nevi beginning with their appearance in childhood and progressing into adult life.

2. CONGENITAL NEVI

In contrast to the common nevi that appear after birth, congenital nevi by definition must be are present at birth. They usually remain throughout life, although a small percentage disappear spontaneously. Most congenital nevi are relatively small and may have an appearance little different from that of ordinary pigmented acquired nevi. Less commonly, congenital nevi may be quite large (giant congenital nevi) and may involve major areas of the body (Fig 43–6). These larger lesions usually favor the trunk, upper back, and shoulders. The surfaces of such lesions may be smooth or irregular. Pigmentation ranges from pale tan to brown-black is variable in intensity. Some lesions also may be associated with an overgrowth of hairs.

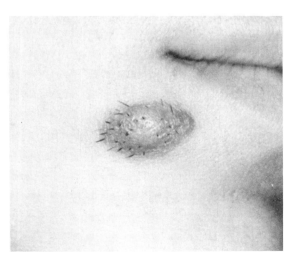

Figure 43–5. Intradermal nevus. Such an elevated pigmented lesion may or may not contain hairs.

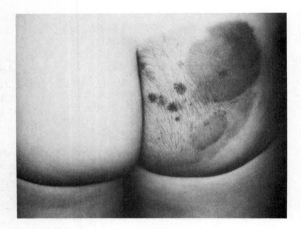

Figure 43–6. Large congenital nevus. Differing intensities of pigmentation are present, and the lesion has both flat and elevated areas.

Giant congenital nevi have a significant incidence of transformation into malignant melanoma, and this incidence averages about 5–12% in a number of reported studies. Frequently, this malignant change will occur during childhood, and such melanomas tend to be aggressive and rapidly fatal.

Congenital nevi are discussed in more detail in Chapter 51.

3. SPINDLE & EPITHELIOID CELL NEVUS (Spitz Nevus)

The spindle and epithelioid cell nevus is an important lesion because of its microscopic resemblance to malignant melanoma. Such lesions are more common in children and often present as a solitary pink to purplish-red papule or nodule. The lesions are relatively common on the face in children but tend to occur more commonly on the trunk and lower extremities of adults.

Although the microscopic features of a spindle and epithelioid cell nevus may closely resemble those of malignant melanoma, the experienced dermatopathologist will usually be able to make this distinction. Treatment of the spindle and epithelioid cell nevus is simple excision.

4. DYSPLASTIC NEVUS SYNDROME

Essentials of Diagnosis

- Usually a family history of melanoma or dysplastic nevi.
- Many large moles.
- Irregular contours.

- Irregular, variegated colors, sometimes including shades of pink.
- Atypical melanocytes seen histologically.

General Considerations

Dysplastic nevus syndrome is characterized by multiple melanocytic nevi with atypical clinical and histopathologic features. These nevi are important in that they may represent in some individuals a marker for predisposition to malignant melanoma. Melanomas may arise from such nevi or may arise de novo. The syndrome frequently is familial and usually has an autosomal dominant mode of inheritance. Many families with the syndrome have been studied and have shown an increased incidence of malignant melanoma. In an individual with dysplastic nevi who has 2 or more primary family members (parents, sibs, children) with malignant melanoma, there is a very strong likelihood that development of malignant melanoma will occur. In such an individual, this chance may approach 100%. Many previously reported cases of familial malignant melanoma have arisen in families with the familial dysplastic nevus syndrome. If a parent has dysplastic nevi without melanoma, the likelihood of the patient acquiring a melanoma is of lesser magnitude but still significantly greater than in the general population.

Patients with dysplastic nevi but no family history are said to have sporadic dysplastic nevus syndrome. Although such patients with large numbers of dysplastic nevi also appear to be at an increased risk for the development of malignant melanoma, the risk appears to be less than for patients in the familial dysplastic nevus group.

Clinical Findings

A. Symptoms and Signs: Dysplastic nevi differ clinically from ordinary acquired nevi in several respects. Dysplastic nevi tend to occur in greater numbers than ordinary nevi; patients frequently will have up to 100 or more lesions. In addition, these lesions often are larger than ordinary nevi and frequently will measure 1 cm or more. Although ordinary nevi usually have stopped appearing by early adult life, dysplastic nevi continue to develop into adult life. Thus, the syndrome often will be more easily identified in adults than in children.

Dysplastic nevi also differ from ordinary nevi in appearance. They tend to have somewhat irregular contours, and pigmentation often is also irregular. In addition to varying shades of brown, dysplastic nevi also may have some hues of red or pink, features uncommon in ordinary nevi. Where these atypical features are pronounced, it may be difficult to differentiate clinically between a dysplastic nevus and a superficial spreading malignant melanoma.

B. Laboratory Findings: Microscopically, dysplastic nevi show nests of atypical melanocytic cells at the dermal-epidermal junction. Such cells often have a spindle cell configuration. Nevus cells frequently are found within the dermis, but these usually do not show atypia. The dermis also shows a chronic perivascular lymphocytic inflammatory response and often some superficial fibrosis.

Prevention

In patients with multiple dysplastic nevi and a history of malignant melanoma in close family members, there is a strong likelihood of development of malignant melanoma. Such individuals should avoid the sun and use highly protective screening agents. They should practice self-examination of their skin and should see a dermatologist as often as every 4–6 months for continuing surveillance. Close family members should be examined to see if they are at higher risk for melanoma.

Treatment

Suspicious nevi should be excise and examined microscopically.

Prognosis

Although dysplastic nevi continue to develop as the patient grows older, the lesions generally remain stable. Only a small number of dysplastic nevi ever undergo malignant transformation.

5. HALO NEVUS

Some otherwise ordinary-appearing nevi may develop a depigmented halo around them. These lesions occur more commonly in children and young adults. The halo ranges from 1 to 5 mm in diameter, and the lesion tends to be stable. Occasionally, however, the central nevus will regress, and following this the halo may or may not repigment (see Chapter 22).

6. BLUE NEVUS

The blue nevus is usually a blue-black nodule with a relatively smooth surface. Such lesions have the same size range as ordinary nevi and usually are slightly elevated or dome-shaped. The deep pigmentation of these lesions is due to large amounts of melanin pigment within the deeper dermis. Although these lesions may be nearly black, there is no significant malignant potential. They can be easily excised.

LENTIGINES

Lentigines are small tan to dark brown macules that usually cannot be palpated. They are discussed as such in Chapter 22.

LENTIGO MALIGNA (Melanotic Freckle of Hutchinson)

Although the ordinary lentigo is a benign lesion, lentigo maligna is a premalignant lesion with the capacity to transform into malignant melanoma. It is a melanoma in situ. Such lesions may begin as small fawn-colored macules indistinguishable from benign seborrheic keratoses. In older individuals, they become larger—particularly in women, in whom they are often very large and bizarre in shape and color. Lesions occur most commonly on the face but can also occur on other sun-exposed areas. As lentigo maligna lesions evolve, they gradually enlarges to form a patch with irregular curved, jagged, and notched borders. The pigmentation frequently is irregular and may show hues of tan to dark brown or black but also erythema and whitish hues in areas of regression. After years, transformation to malignant melanoma occurs in approximately 30–50% of lentigo maligna lesions (see below).

MALIGNANT MELANOMA*

Malignant melanoma is the most important tumor of the melanocyte system. In contrast to the more common basal cell and squamous cell carcinomas, malignant melanoma is a malignant tumor with an established capacity for recurrence and metastasis. Although malignant melanoma traditionally has represented a relatively uncommon skin tumor, over the past several decades there has been a progressive increase in its frequency. At present, it is estimated that the incidence of malignant melanoma has been doubling approximately every 10 years. This increase in the incidence of malignant melanoma has not been uniform, and, as a group, young women have been developing more malignant melanomas than have other groups, often at a younger age. The lifetime risk for a Caucasian developing malignant melanoma is currently about 1:150.

Malignant melanoma shares with basal cell and squamous cell carcinomas a higher incidence among fair-skinned individuals. In addition, the incidence of malignant melanoma is higher in fair-skinned populations subjected to prolonged sun exposure. Although most malignant melanomas occur sporadically, in approximately 1–6% of melanoma patients there will be a history of malignant melanoma in a primary family member. Such melanomas may occur in association with dysplastic nevus syndrome.

Malignant melanoma may arise de novo or from a preexisting lesion such as a nevus or lentigo maligna.

---

*This section was written by James J. Nordlund, MD.

When malignant melanoma arises from a preexisting nevus, it usually appears within the melanocytic component at the dermal-epidermal junction. Malignant melanoma may also arise from the deeper components of a giant congenital nevus.

Types of Malignant Melanoma

Primary cutaneous malignant melanoma has been divided clinically into 4 major categories depending upon the clinical appearance of the lesion and its corresponding microscopic appearance. Long-term studies have established that there is no relationships between the type of malignant melanoma and the prognosis; what is important for prognosis is the thickness of the tumor, ie, the depth from the granular cell layer to the deepest tumor cell (Breslow thickness).

The 4 major forms of primary cutaneous malignant melanoma are lentigo maligna melanoma, superficial spreading melanoma, nodular melanoma, and acral-lentiginous melanoma.

A. Lentigo Maligna Melanoma: Lentigo maligna melanoma arises from the preexisting lesion of lentigo maligna (melanotic freckle of Hutchinson). Such melanomas comprise approximately 5% of all primary cutaneous melanomas and tend to occur in older individuals. Women are affected more commonly than men, and most lesions favor sun-exposed areas, especially the face.

Lentigo maligna tends to grow superficially over a prolonged period, and the onset of melanoma often will be heralded 10–15 years after the onset of the preexisting pigmented lesion. This malignant transformation occurs in approximately 30–50% of all patients with lentigo maligna.

The development of melanoma within these lesions is signaled by the appearance of a slowly enlarging nodule, which is usually deeply pigmented. In contrast to other melanomas with nodules, lentigo maligna melanoma tends to grow more slowly. Once the malignant cells have invaded the dermis, they have the same propensity for metastasis as any other melanoma.

This lesion is characterized microscopically by a proliferation of abnormal-appearing melanocytes along the dermal-epidermal junction and the ultimate invasion of such cells to produce dermal tumors.

B. Superficial Spreading Melanoma: Superficial spreading melanoma currently represents the most common clinical form of melanoma, and approximately 70% of all melanomas fall into this group. This tumor type occurs most on the lower extremities of women or the backs of men.

The lesion presents as a flat to slightly elevated pigmented papule or patch, often with a somewhat irregular contour. The earliest lesions are fawn-colored, small (1–2 cm) macules with slightly irregular borders. The enlarging lesion spreads radially, with little early tendency to form a nodule. The le-

sions vary considerably in size. Further growth typically results in an irregular surface contour with irregular borders. Superficial spreading melanoma also usually shows a variation in color, with hues ranging from black to dark brown to lighter shades of tan and also red and blue. A reddish border is common. In addition, some areas may show partial regression, and these will be hypopigmented (gray or white).

Superficial spreading melanoma usually enlarges slowly in a radial fashion prior to deep invasion and metastatic spread. This period of radial growth can be shorter, often in the range of 5–7 years, but may be as long as 20 years.

The appearance of nodules within superficial spreading melanoma is similar to that of nodules occurring within lentigo maligna melanoma, and the microscopic appearance of such nodules is the same. The distinctive microscopic features differentiating superficial spreading melanoma include the presence of discrete nests of atypical-appearing melanocytic cells within the dermal-epidermal junction and the epidermis itself. Such nests are in contrast to the proliferation of individual atypical melanocytes seen along the dermal-epidermal junction in lentigo maligna.

C. Nodular Melanoma: Nodular melanoma differs from lentigo maligna and superficial spreading melanomas in having no apparent phase of radial growth. These lesions begin clinically as nodules that enlarge both horizontally and vertically. Such lesions are much more common in men than in women and occur at an age intermediate between that common to lentigo maligna melanoma and superficial spreading melanoma. These lesions comprise approximately 15% of all primary cutaneous melanomas. Nodular melanomas occur most commonly over the head, neck, and trunk. They usually appear as deeply pigmented nodules, though amelanotic forms may occur. These lesions tend to grow more rapidly than other forms and may ulcerate.

Nodular malignant melanoma is the most common type in blacks and other dark-skinned patients.

Microscopically, nodular melanoma shows tumor cells confined to the nodule, with little melanocytic proliferation at the junction beyond the lateral extent of the nodule.

D. Acral Lentiginous Melanoma: This form of malignant melanoma accounts for less than 10% of all melanomas. It is the most common type in blacks. It is often difficult to diagnose, and late diagnosis can result in death of the patient. The lesions occur on the palms, soles, fingers, and toes. Although clinically they may closely resemble lentigo maligna with the radial irregular expansion of a deeply pigmented lesion, they tend to produce deeper nodules more readily than do lentigo maligna melanomas and thus have a much worse prognosis. In addition, features of the melanoma that might be observed on areas of thinner skin are often masked by the overlying thickness of the horny layer in these areas. Acral lentiginous melanomas may be manifested first as a pigment streak in the nail, sometimes associated with brown discoloration of the cuticle (Hutchinson's sign). Not all pigmented streaks on the nail are caused by malignant lesions.

Evaluation & Treatment

If a lesion suggests melanoma, it should be excised or biopsied. If there is reasonable clinical certainty that it is melanoma and if the lesion is small and not in a cosmetically or functionally critical area, it should be excised completely with margins that permit primary closure. If the lesion is large, incisional or punch biopsy can be done without documented increased risk of inducing metastases. If histologic examination confirms melanoma, the lesion should be excised with appropriate margins. Thin melanomas (0.75 mm or less) can be removed safely with narrow margins. Those with Breslow depth greater than 0.75 mm generally should be excised with 1- to 3-cm peripheral margins depending upon the site, thickness, and depth. Dermatologists with special training can usually provide guidance. Skin grafts or flaps may be required. The size of the margins required is under intensive study internationally, and new guidelines will be developed in the near future.

The decision to perform prophylactic lymph node dissection is controversial. If metastases are detected in regional nodes but not elsewhere, the entire nodal chain should be removed. If metastases are detected in the lung, liver, or other organs, lymph node removal is unnecessary. The decision to remove nodes prophylactically depends upon location, lymph drainage, depth of invasion, and thickness of the melanoma. The decision to perform prophylactic node dissection should be a joint decision of the melanoma treatment team.

All patients with melanomas should undergo chest x-ray and physical examination and have appropriate imaging work to detect metastases before extensive surgery. Annual follow-up chest x-rays are usually recommended as well as follow-up clinical examinations at frequencies dependent on the clinical setting. CT scans and MRI can provide better evaluation and follow-up than conventional x-rays.

Prognosis

Several methods of evaluation have been used in an attempt to accurately determine prognosis of the lesion. The microscopic parameter that appears to correlate most closely with prognosis is the thickness of the lesion (Breslow level). With increasing thickness, the likelihood of regional lymph node and distant metastases increases and the likelihood of prolonged survival decreases. If a melanoma is excised prior to onset of the nodular phase (Breslow level <0.75 mm), the prognosis usually is excellent. If the melanoma has developed a nodule greater than 1.5–2

mm in thickness, the prognosis is less good, with a likelihood of metastases.

The prognosis of nodular melanoma is worse than that for other types and is related to the usually greater Breslow thickness at the time of diagnosis.

TUMORS OF MESODERMAL ORIGIN

TUMORS ARISING FROM CONNECTIVE TISSUE CELLS

1. DERMATOFIBROMA (Histiocytoma Cutis)

Essentials of Diagnosis
- Hard brown or tan nodule.
- Usually on extremity.
- Dimples the epidermis when pinched.

General Considerations
Dermatofibroma is a common benign fibrous tissue lesion. It probably represents a reactive hyperplasia of fibrous tissue rather than a true neoplasm.

Clinical Findings
A. Symptoms and Signs: A number of patients give a history of preceding trauma such as from an insect bite, scratch, or minor skin puncture, and the common location of lesions on areas of shaving of the lower extremities of women emphasizes this etiologic possibility. Dermatofibromas also commonly occur over the upper extremities and less commonly over the trunk. They occur at any age, though most appear in early to middle adult life. Most lesions are solitary, though occasional patients may have more than one lesion. An infrequent patient may have many.

The usual dermatofibroma is less than 1 cm in diameter and presents as a round to oval, firm intracutaneous nodule. The lesion is attached to the skin surface but is freely movable. Most lesions are slightly elevated and have a dome-shaped configuration, though some actually may be somewhat depressed below the skin surface. Color ranges from dusky erythema to medium brown, and the surface may vary from smooth to somewhat rough. When the nodule is squeezed, the skin over it often dimples. Once formed, most dermatofibromas stay the same size.

B. Laboratory Findings: Microscopic examination of a dermatofibroma reveals proliferation of oval to spindle-shaped cells, usually resembling fibroblasts or histiocytes. There may also be associated overlying epithelial hyperplasia.

Treatment

These lesions ordinarily are asymptomatic and entirely benign and usually do not need treatment. If treatment is desired, the dermatofibroma can be simply excised.

2. ACROCHORDON
(Skin Tag)

Acrochordons are common papillomatous lesions usually occurring in middle age and later. These lesions occur most frequently about the neck, though the axillae and occasionally the inframammary areas may also be involved. Women tend to be affected more frequently than men. Acrochordons appear as soft, fleshy lesions ranging in size from 1–2 mm to 1 cm or greater. Larger lesions usually are pedunculated and have been termed soft fibromas. Many lesions are flesh-colored, while some may be hyperpigmented. Acrochordons ordinarily are asymptomatic, though an occasional lesion may be irritated by friction from clothing or jewelry. Treatment ordinarily is not necessary, but smaller lesions can be destroyed electrosurgically and larger lesions removed superficially with a scissors or scalpel with electrodesiccation or cautery of the base for hemostasis.

3. DERMATOFIBROSARCOMA PROTUBERANS

Dermatofibrosarcoma protuberans is an invasive fibrohistiocytic tumor that has a pronounced tendency to recur following excision. These lesions are more common in males than in females and usually have their peak incidence in the third decade of life. The upper trunk is a favored location, though the proximal surfaces of the extremities such as the shoulder are relatively common locations.

Dermatofibrosarcoma protuberans appears as a slowly enlarging firm cutaneous nodule. Because of the relatively slow growth of this lesion, medical attention frequently is not sought until the lesion has been present many years and has assumed a size of 1–2 cm or larger. Enlargement of the lesion tends to be irregular, often with a multilobular configuration. The color of dermatofibrosarcoma protuberans ranges from brownish to dusky erythema.

Although dermatofibrosarcoma protuberans is an invasive mesenchymal tumor, it has little tendency to metastasize. Nevertheless, even with what would appear to be adequate surgical excision, the lesion commonly recurs, with a frequency of 50–75% in some series. With adequate surgical excision, it often is necessary to apply a skin graft, and such patients should be followed carefully in anticipation of possible recurrence.

4. ATYPICAL FIBROXANTHOMA OF THE SKIN

Atypical fibroxanthoma is a benign histiocytic tumor clinically but histologically it may be indistinguishable from malignant fibrous histiocytoma arising in subcutaneous tissue. Atypical fibroxanthoma of the skin occurs most commonly in older individuals and usually is limited to sun-exposed areas such as the face, ears, and neck. The lesion usually appears as a small, slowly enlarging nodule, and some lesions ulcerate. They seldom exceed 2–3 cm in size. The clinical appearance does not suggest their histiocytic origin, and such lesions may be clinically mistaken for pyogenic granulomas or basal cell carcinomas.

Although the microscopic appearance of atypical fibroxanthoma is alarmingly anaplastic, the lesion has metastasized only rarely and is easily cured by simple excision.

5. KELOID

A keloid is an excessive fibrous tissue response to cutaneous injury, even though in many cases there is no history of trauma. Keloids are more likely to occur in the earlobes, the shoulders, and the sternal area of the chest. There may be a familial tendency for development of keloids, and the lesions are more common in blacks and other deeply pigmented individuals. Electrosurgical procedures are more likely to result in keloidal healing than cold steel surgical procedures. Infected wounds also have a greater tendency to be followed by keloids. In addition, susceptible individuals may develop keloids associated with acne lesions, especially on the chest and back. The most pronounced keloids frequently follow thermal burns.

A keloid usually begins as a small, firm, erythematous enlarging pruritic or tender papule (Fig 43–7). Growth may be regular or irregular, and irregular lesions may show clawlike extensions. Keloid formation may become evident within several weeks following the skin injury, and the process may continue for months or years before growth ceases. Although erythematous in their early stages, quiescent keloids usually become hyperpigmented and asymptomatic.

Management of keloids may be difficult. They should be excised only with great caution. The tendency for keloids to recur following surgical excision may be lessened by the injection of corticosteroid suspensions such as triamcinolone acetonide, 5 mg/mL, into the wound site immediately after surgery.

Keloids may be treated nonsurgically by injection of triamcinolone acetonide, 10–25 mg/mL, into the scar using a small-bore syringe with a firmly attached needle. The initial injection is typically difficult be-

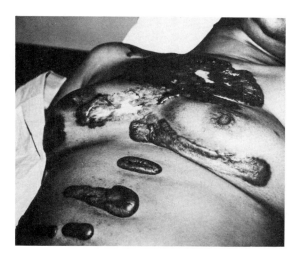

Figure 43–7. Keloids. These firm lesions are especially common over the anterior chest.

cause the dense scar prohibits adequate infiltration. Repeated injections every 2–3 months are easier.

Recently, keloids have been treated with the carbon dioxide laser with inconsistent results.

6. ANGIOFIBROMA

Several unrelated lesions can be included under the term angiofibroma. These lesions show both a proliferation of dermal connective tissue with fibroblasts and a benign proliferation of blood vessels. Although angiofibroma may occur as an inconspicuous solitary lesion of the face, multiple lesions represent an important cutaneous marker of tuberous sclerosis. The skin lesions traditionally have been called adenoma sebaceum, but they are not of sebaceous origin. In tuberous sclerosis, angiofibromas begin in childhood as small flesh-colored to erythematous papules occurring bilaterally over the nasolabial fold, cheeks, and chin. Although slowly multiplying during childhood, new lesions do not develop in adults.

Fibrous papule of the nose is a solitary lesion that frequently resembles a somewhat erythematous or flesh-colored nevus and is not related to tuberous sclerosis. Microscopically, fibrous tissue elements predominate over vascular elements. Some lesions occurring on the face show a proliferation of fibrous tissue around hair follicles, and these are termed **perifollicular fibromas.** Similar but smaller lesions around the coronal sulcus of the penis have been termed **pearly penile papules.**

Angiofibromas are benign lesions, and treatment is not required. Single lesions may be excised. Treatment of multiple skin lesions of tuberous sclerosis has not been entirely satisfactory, but excision with the

carbon dioxide laser or dermabrasion may improve appearance. Pearly penile papules are asymptomatic and ordinarily are not treated.

7. FIBROMATOSES

Fibromatoses are characterized by proliferation of fibroblasts and connective tissue. The lesions are usually numerous and frequently arise in deeper tissues in addition to the skin. Biologically, they range from relatively insignificant, clinically stable lesions to those exhibiting aggressive behavior and closely resembling fibrosarcoma. Fibromatoses frequently recur following excision, though they seldom metastasize.

The most common fibromatosis of dermatologic interest is plantar or palmar fibromatosis (Dupuytren's contracture). These lesions usually occur in adults.

Several other types of fibromatoses occur during childhood. These lesions tend to be locally aggressive, with recurrence following surgical excision.

8. JUVENILE XANTHOGRANULOMA

Essentials of Diagnosis
- Onset of lesions early in life, gradual evolution, spontaneous regression.
- Distribution favoring scalp, face, trunk.
- Small yellow to orange to tan smooth-surfaced papules.
- Characteristic histologic features.

General Considerations
Juvenile xanthogranuloma represents a benign proliferation of histiocytes that take up lipid material to give a somewhat xanthomatous appearance. It is not actually a tumor. The process usually begins early in life, develops single to multiple lesions, and usually regresses spontaneously without treatment.

Clinical Findings
A. Symptoms and Signs: The vast majority of lesions begin within the newborn period or during the first 6 months of life. Patients may have single or multiple lesions, and multiple lesions often develop rapidly, sometimes in crops. Lesions favor the scalp, face, and trunk but may also be seen on the proximal extremities and less commonly elsewhere on the cutaneous surface. Individual lesions begin as small papules that gradually enlarge and usually range from approximately 2 mm to 5 mm in diameter. These papules often are erythematous at onset but develop a yellow to orange to light-brown color often resembling a small xanthoma. The surface is usually smooth.

The lesions usually increase in number for approximately a year or somewhat longer and then gradually involute spontaneously. By the age of 5 or 6 years, all lesions usually will have regressed.

In the vast majority of cases, only the skin is affected, but in a small number there may be other associated lesions. A few patients may have café au lait spots, and in some cases these may be associated with multiple neurofibromatosis. Other rare patients may have juvenile xanthogranulomas in other areas such as the eye. Patients with juvenile xanthogranulomas should be carefully examined to rule out involvement elsewhere.

B. Laboratory Findings: Biopsy shows a proliferation of histiocytes within the dermis, and these take up lipid material to resemble xanthoma cells. In addition, such lesions have characteristic multinucleated giant cells termed Touton giant cells. Other laboratory studies are unnecessary in the usual uncomplicated cases.

Differential Diagnosis

The characteristic early childhood evolution, regression, and gross and microscopic appearance of these lesions are usually diagnostic.

Treatment

Juvenile xanthogranulomas usually regress completely without treatment and thus ordinarily require no treatment. If there is no evidence of lesions elsewhere, the patient can be observed periodically.

9. NEUROFIBROMA

Neurofibromas may occur as solitary or multiple tumors of the skin. Solitary neurofibromas frequently resemble small fleshy nevi and may be skin-colored to lightly pigmented. They have little clinical significance.

Multiple neurofibromatosis (Recklinghausen's disease) is an autosomal dominantly inherited disorder. The neurofibromas are fleshy tumors of various sizes, usually appearing in early childhood and gradually increasing in size and number throughout life. Although some lesions may be small and resemble fleshy nevi, others assume large and disfiguring proportions. In addition to a cutaneous location, neurofibromas may also occur along peripheral and cranial nerves and in subcutaneous and other soft tissues. In addition to the neurofibromas, patients with multiple neurofibromatosis have café au lait spots, axillary freckling, abnormalities of bone, neurologic signs, and endocrine abnormalities (see Chapter 20).

Solitary neurofibromas can be treated by surgical excision. The treatment of multiple neurofibromatosis is formidable. Usually only those lesions that are producing symptoms or functional problems are excised in patients with many lesions. Rare lesions may undergo malignant change to fibrosarcoma or neu-

rofibrosarcoma, and such lesions will require a more aggressive surgical approach.

10. NEURILEMMOMA

Neurilemmoma represents a benign tumor of nerve sheath derived from Schwann cells. These lesions usually occur singly along the course of cranial, peripheral, and sympathetic nerves. They have a rather widespread distribution, but approximately half of all lesions occur on the head and neck. The lesions range from several millimeters to several centimeters in size and usually enlarge slowly. Treatment of neurilemmomas involves surgical enucleation of the tumor from its adjacent nerve.

11. GRANULAR CELL TUMOR

Although the origin of the granular cell tumor has been debated, most investigators now feel it too—like neurilemmoma—is derived from Schwann cells. The lesion occurs in all age groups but is most common in the fourth to sixth decades. Although the tumor has a wide distribution, approximately one-third occur on the tongue. Lesions sometimes occur both in skin and subcutaneous tissue, and occasional ones may be identified in lung, gastrointestinal tract, and heart. In most patients, the granular cell tumor is a solitary lesion, though multiple lesions may occasionally be present. The lesion usually presents as a nondescript asymptomatic nodule that is less than 2 cm in diameter. Malignant granular cell tumors comprise approximately 3% of the entire group.

Treatment of the benign lesion is simple surgical excision.

VASCULAR TUMORS

1. HEMANGIOMAS

The hemangiomas are common benign tumors resulting from proliferation of vascular tissue in the skin and elsewhere (see Chapter 51). The most common form is the **strawberry hemangioma** (Fig 43–8). These lesions result from proliferation of immature capillary vessels. They usually appear shortly after birth and initially undergo a rapid growth phase lasting several months. Growth then slows and ceases, and the lesions begin to regress spontaneously. Most strawberry hemangiomas begin to regress by 1 year of age, and most will have regressed completely by the age of 5–7 years.

Because of the natural regression of most hemangiomas, treatment is only rarely recommended. When rapidly enlarging hemangiomas pro-

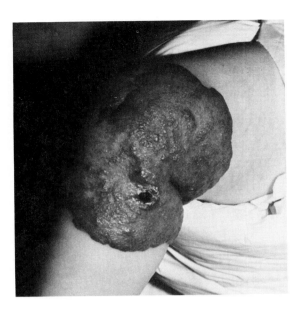

Figure 43–8. Strawberry hemangioma. This lesion enlarged rapidly and shows a dark area of ulceration.

duce functional difficulties or impinge upon vital structures, treatment is indicated. A limited course of oral corticosteroids (eg, prednisone, 1–3 mg/kg) will produce regression of these lesions in most cases.

Cherry hemangiomas occur commonly in elderly patients and usually have their onset in early adult life. The lesions are usually multiple and occur most commonly over the trunk and proximal extremities. They are bright red to somewhat purplish, smooth, dome-shaped papules approximately 1–3 mm in diameter. Although no treatment is indicated for these benign lesions, smaller ones may be electrodesiccated and larger ones removed by shave excision with electrodesiccation of the base.

Pyogenic granuloma represents an active capillary hemangioma usually arising at a site of trauma. It occurs as a solitary lesion, more commonly in areas subjected to minor trauma. Pyogenic granuloma usually has its onset as a small erythematous papule with rapid enlargement. It may have a somewhat mulberrylike surface and may become pedunculated with enlargement. Fully developed lesions usually have a yellowish or brownish hue and may be associated with a purulent exudate. Larger lesions may be quite friable and bleed easily. Pyogenic granulomas may be removed surgically, electrosurgically, or by curettage and electrodesiccation. Some recur after treatment.

Cavernous hemangiomas are derived from larger vessels than capillary hemangiomas. Many cavernous hemangiomas have a subcutaneous location and are deeper in color than capillary hemangiomas (see Chapter 51).

2. ANGIOKERATOMAS

Angiokeratomas are vascular ectasias rather than true tumors. Besides the vascular component, these lesions also have a proliferative epithelial component that makes the lesion look like a keratosis. A number of different types of angiokeratoma have been described depending upon their location and number. Individual lesions usually are soft and compressible and range from pink to red-purple. the lesions are small, seldom greater than 3 mm in diameter. Older lesions have a somewhat warty configuration. Multiple lesions have been described over the bony prominences, especially in children and young adults, while other multiple lesions are confined to the scrotum. In still other patients, angiokeratomas present as a small group of lesions frequently on a lower extremity. Rarely, a patient may develop a solitary lesion.

Angiokeratoma corporis diffusum of Fabry is inherited in an X-linked recessive fashion and results from an enzyme deficiency causing abnormal glycolipid metabolism. The angiokeratomas of this disease are a relatively minor feature, but patients develop cardiovascular and renal disease and frequently hypertension. These patients usually die prematurely from cardiac or renal failure or from a cerebrovascular accident.

3. ARTERIAL SPIDERS (Nevus Araneus)

Arterial spiders result from dilatation and proliferation of superficial cutaneous arterioles. Such lesions are more common in women than in men, and estrogens have been felt to play a role in their development. Although occasionally identified in normal individuals, such lesions are common in pregnancy and chronic liver disease. They are found commonly over the face, the anterior neck and chest, and the proximal upper extremities. Although ordinarily few in number, they may be numerous in patients with hepatic cirrhosis. The individual lesions are bright red and consist of a central punctate feeder vessel and branches radiating from the center, suggesting a spider.

Lesions associated with pregnancy ordinarily regress following delivery, and treatment is not indicated. When treatment is desired, such lesions may be electrocoagulated with a fine needle inserted into the feeding arteriole.

4. LYMPHANGIOMA

Lymphangiomas are congenital malformations of the lymphatic system. The most common form of lymphangioma of dermatologic interest is lymphangioma circumscriptum, a relatively superficial lesion. Lymphangioma circumscriptum usually presents as a group of thin-walled vesicular-appearing papules that range from flesh-colored to slightly erythematous. They occur most commonly over the proximal extremities and adjacent limb girdle areas. They are usually multiple and resemble frog spawn.

Although lymphangioma circumscriptum may appear as an isolated phenomenon, these lesions may connect with deeper lymphatic channels and thus may recur with superficial attempts at removal.

Cavernous lymphangiomas usually occur at deeper levels and are much less common than lymphangioma circumscriptum.

5. GLOMUS TUMOR

The glomus tumor is an uncommon lesion derived from smooth muscle cells of the cutaneous glomus. This structure represents a specialized arteriovenous shunt. Glomus tumors usually occur as solitary lesions and are most common over the extremities, especially within the nail beds. Less commonly, multiple glomus tumors may be inherited as an autosomal dominant trait.

The glomus tumor appears as a soft to firm, bluish to reddish papule that seldom exceeds a few millimeters in size. Solitary lesions usually are tender and may be subject to spontaneous episodic pain.

Solitary and multiple glomus tumors are benign lesions. Surgical excision is the treatment of choice and is particularly desirable in the case of solitary painful lesions.

6. ANGIOSARCOMA (Hemangiosarcoma, Malignant Hemangioendothelioma)

Angiosarcoma is a malignant tumor of endothelial cells, usually in older individuals. Dark red to purple nodules or plaques appear most commonly over the face and scalp. Although such lesions may be initially solitary, multiple lesions may be present. There may be a dusky erythema, suggesting increased vascularity about the lesion. Satellite lesions also may be present.

Angiosarcoma usually grows fairly rapidly, and lesions characteristically increase both in size and in number and may eventually involve a large area. With progression, angiosarcomas tend to ulcerate, and serious, sometimes fatal hemorrhage may result. The lesion is an aggressive invasive tumor, and metastatic spread occurs in some patients.

The prognosis of angiosarcoma is poor regardless of what form of treatment is employed. Recurrence and ultimate death of the patient usually are to be anticipated whether extensive surgery, irradiation, or chemotherapy has been employed.

7. LYMPHANGIOSARCOMA (Stewart-Treves Tumor)

Lymphangiosarcoma is closely related to angiosarcoma (hemangiosarcoma), and the microscopic pictures of these 2 tumors may be indistinguishable. Lymphangiosarcoma occurs preferentially in chronic lymphedematous extremities. Most cases have been described in lymphedematous upper extremities following radical mastectomy for breast cancer. The tumor usually develops approximately 10 years after the original surgery and many years after the onset of chronic lymphedema of the upper extremity. This lesion has no relationship to the original breast cancer.

The onset of lymphangiosarcoma normally is rapid, with development of an ecchymotic area usually over the upper arm. This change is followed by the appearance of reddish-blue to purple nodules, and the process may produce bullae. With progression there may be ulceration of larger lesions and continuing development of satellite lesions.

Lymphangiosarcoma tends to spread rapidly and metastasizes through lymphatics and blood vessels. The lungs, pleura, and thoracic wall are common sites of metastatic spread.

Treatment for lymphangiosarcoma remains unsatisfactory, and even radical surgery usually is followed by recurrence and metastasis.

OTHER MESODERMAL TUMORS

1. LEIOMYOMA

Leiomyoma is a benign tumor derived from cutaneous smooth muscle. Most such lesions are derived from the cutaneous arrector pili muscle, although smaller numbers of leiomyomas may be derived from genital or vascular smooth muscle. Leiomyomas derived from the arrector pili muscle tend to be multiple, while other forms usually are solitary. Multiple leiomyomas usually appear in late childhood or early adult life. An autosomal dominant pattern of inheritance has been identified in some kindreds. The lesions present as smooth, firm nodules that range from 2–3 mm to over 1 cm in size. Most lesions have a reddish-yellow to reddish-brown hue and may have a somewhat translucent appearance. There is a tendency for these lesions to enlarge and multiply. The most important clinical characteristic of leiomyoma is pain, which usually is spontaneous and may be paroxysmal.

The treatment is surgical excision, which is frequently requested by the patient for relief of pain.

2. LIPOMA

Lipomas are common benign mesenchymal tumors with a widespread distribution. Women are much more commonly affected than men, and the lesions usually appear in early to middle adult life. The favored locations include the posterior neck, trunk, abdomen, forearms, buttocks, and thighs. Most lipomas are several centimeters in size and are palpable as soft, movable subcutaneous masses. They are asymptomatic, and the overlying skin is unremarkable. Occasional lipomas may be massive.

Most lipomas require no treatment, though surgical excision is the treatment of choice.

LYMPHORETICULAR TUMORS

In the overall scheme of cutaneous tumors, lymphoreticular tumors of the skin are relatively rare. These tumors may be classified as benign or malignant. Lymphocytoma cutis is a benign lymphoreticular proliferation, while the malignant proliferations include mycosis fungoides, other malignant lymphomas involving skin, and leukemia cutis. This discussion will include lymphocytoma cutis, the benign lesion, while malignant lymphoreticular tumors are considered in Chapter 44.

LYMPHOCYTOMA CUTIS
(See also Chapter 44.)

Essentials of Diagnosis
- Reddish-brown papule, nodule, or plaque.
- No epidermal alterations.
- Firm consistency.
- Typical histologic picture.

General Considerations
Lymphocytoma cutis (cutaneous lymphoid hyperplasia) represents a proliferation of preexisting lymphoid tissue in the skin. Most patients have solitary lesions, and these favor sun-exposed areas, especially the face. Fewer patients have small clusters of similar lesions, and rarely the lesions may be multiple with a disseminated distribution.

Clinical Findings
A. Symptoms and Signs: The lesion usually presents as an asymptomatic smooth-surfaced papule, nodule, or plaque ranging in size from a few millimeters to several centimeters. Color ranges from dusky erythema to a reddish-brown or violaceous hue, and the lesions usually have a firm consistency. Clinically they may resemble cutaneous nodules of malignant lymphoma, and biopsy will be required for specific diagnosis. Although spontaneous regression may oc-

cur, most lesions persist. In rare instances there may be progression to malignant lymphoma, especially in patients with disseminated lesions.

B. Laboratory Findings: The pathologic changes lie within the dermis, where one sees a dense infiltration of lymphocytes and histiocytes. The cells may be arranged in a diffuse pattern or may be aggregated in lymphoid follicles. Although usually having a benign appearance, the infiltrate may show some cytologic variation and atypia. Because the histopathologic appearance may closely resemble cutaneous lesions of malignant lymphoma, these lesions require expert pathologic evaluation.

Treatment
Although lesions of lymphocytoma cutis may be excised, they also respond to intralesional injections of corticosteroid suspensions. Superficial low-dose x-ray therapy can also be employed.

VISCERAL CARCINOMA METASTATIC TO SKIN

Metastases to skin occur in 3–5% of patients with metastatic visceral cancer. In women, the most common tumor metastasizing to the skin is carcinoma of the breast, and in some instances this spread will represent direct extension rather than true metastasis. In men, carcinoma of the lung is the most common primary site, and in both men and women carcinoma of the colon also has a relatively high incidence of metastasis to the skin. Less commonly, the skin will be the site of metastases from tumors of the kidney, stomach, and ovary. The incidence of cutaneous metastases of different types reflects both the prevalence of the primary tumor in the population and the individual metastatic tendency of each tumor type.

Cutaneous metastases frequently arise close to the site of the primary tumor. Thus, metastatic carcinomas from breast and lung may be found in the chest wall, and carcinomas from the genitourinary tract may occur over the lower abdominal wall. Some tumors also tend to favor specific distant sites, and carcinoma of the breast and renal cell carcinoma metastasize to the scalp relatively frequently.

Cutaneous metastases usually appear as firm cutaneous or subcutaneous nodules. They may be single or multiple. Color varies considerably.

Cutaneous metastases usually imply dissemination of a tumor and are associated with a poor prognosis. In some instances, a metastatic lesion may be identified in the skin before symptoms of the primary tumor.

Surgical excision is usually required when treatment of a metastatic lesion is indicated, but systemic chemotherapy may cause lesions to shrink or disappear.

REFERENCES

Andrade R et al: *Cancer of the Skin.* Saunders, 1976.

Brownstein MH, Helwig EB: Metastatic tumors of the skin. Cancer 1972;29:1298.

Brownstein MH, Helwig EB: Patterns of cutaneous metastasis. Arch Dermatol 1972;105:862.

Brownstein MH, Rabinowitz AD: The precursors of cutaneous squamous cell carcinoma. Int J Dermatol 1979;18:1.

Buxton PK: ABC of Dermatology: Lumps and bumps. Br Med J 1988;296:627.

Buxton PK, Kemmet D: ABC of Dermatology: Black spots in the skin. Br Med J 1988;296:703.

Callen JP, Allegra J (editors): Cutaneous oncology. Med Clin North Am 1986;70:1.

Caro WA, Bronstein BR: Tumors of the skin. In: *Dermatology,* 2nd ed. Moschella SL, Hurley JH (editors). Saunders, 1985.

Enzinger FM, Weiss SW: *Soft Tissue Tumors,* 2nd ed. Mosby, 1988.

Fitzpatrick TB et al: *Dermatology in General Medicine,* 3rd ed. McGraw-Hill, 1987.

Graham JH: Selected precancerous skin and mucocutaneous lesions. In: *Neoplasms of the Skin and Malignant Melanoma.* Year Book, 1976.

Hashimoto K, Mehregan AH, Kumakiri M: *Tumors of Skin Appendages.* Butterworths, 1987.

Helm F: *Cancer Dermatology.* Lea & Febiger, 1979.

Hurwitz S: Epidermal nevi and tumors of epidermal origin. Pediatr Clin North Am 1983;30:483.

Jacobs AH: Vascular nevi. Pediatr Clin North Am 1983; 30:465.

Lever WF, Schaumburg-Lever G: *Histopathology of the Skin,* 7th ed. Lippincott, 1990.

MacKie RM: Skin Cancer: *An Illustrated Guide to the Aetiology, Clinical and Pathological Features, and Management of Benign and Malignant Cutaneous Tumours.* Year Book, 1989.

Rhodes AR et al: Risk factors for cutaneous melanoma: A practical method of recognizing predisposed individuals. JAMA 1987;258:3146.

Rook A et al: *Textbook of Dermatology,* 4th ed. Blackwell, 1986.

Schwartz RA: The keratoacanthoma: A review. J Surg Oncol 1979;12:305.

Schwartz RA (editor): *Skin Cancer: Recognition and Management.* Springer Verlag, 1988.

Sober AJ: Diagnosis and management of skin cancer. Cancer 1983;51:2448.

Cutaneous Lymphoma, Leukemia, & Related Diseases

44

Herschel S. Zackheim, MD

The diseases that are the subject of this chapter are divided into 3 major groups: (1) epidermotropic lymphomas, ie, having a tendency for lymphocytes to invade the epidermis; (2) nonepidermotropic lymphomas; and (3) related diseases, including the leukemias and histiocytic proliferations (Table 44–1).

The major epidermotropic diseases—mycosis fungoides and Sézary's syndrome (the leukemic variant of mycosis fungoides)—constitute about 90% of all cutaneous lymphomas in the USA. The major nonepidermotropic lymphomas are non-Hodgkin's (monomorphous) lymphomas, of either T cell or B cell lineage, which comprise the remainder.

Mycosis fungoides comprises about 85% and Sézary's syndrome about 10% of all cutaneous T cell lymphomas. The recently recognized adult T cell leukemia-lymphoma, which is caused by the retrovirus HTLV-I (human T cell lymphotropic virus), also involves the skin.

EPIDERMOTROPIC CUTANEOUS LYMPHOMAS & RELATED DISEASES

MYCOSIS FUNGOIDES

Essentials of Diagnosis

- Asymmetric, well-demarcated, thin, scaly, often atrophic patches.
- Asymmetric red or brown, scaly or lichenified infiltrated plaques.
- Nodular red or purple tumors.
- Characteristic histopathologic features.

General Considerations

The annual incidence of mycosis fungoides in the USA is about 3–4 per million and increasing. Two-thirds of cases are diagnosed between the ages of 40 and 69, though occasionally the disease is recognized in adolescence or even childhood. Male patients outnumber females by about 2:1, and the disease is about twice as frequent in blacks as in whites.

The neoplastic cell in mycosis fungoides and Sézary's syndrome is the T helper lymphocyte. Although the cause is unknown, environmental carcinogens and oncogenic viruses could be factors.

Clinical Findings

A. Cutaneous Symptoms and Signs: There are 3 principal phases in the evolution of the cutaneous lesions of mycosis fungoides: the early (patch), intermediate (plaque), and late (tumor) stages.

1. Patch stage– Lesions of the patch stage are either nonatrophic or atrophic. Nonatrophic patches are barely palpable, slightly scaly, sharply defined, usually pink lesions (Fig 44–1). They may occur on any part of the body but have a predilection for the bathing trunk area (lower abdomen, groins, hips, and buttocks).

Atrophic patches are very thin, usually wrinkled, slightly scaly, pink to dusky lesions. They commonly exhibit some degree of telangiectasia and often have a reticulated pigmentation. Superficial venules are easily seen (Fig 44–2). The combination of atrophy, telangiectasia, and pigmentation constitutes poikiloderma. Hence, atrophic patches represent the poikilodermatous form of mycosis fungoides. Atrophic patches have a strong predilection for the bathing trunk area, breasts, inner thighs, and arms.

Table 44–1. Classification of cutaneous lymphomas and related diseases.

Epidermotrophic lymphomas and related diseases
  Mycosis fungoides
  Sézary's syndrome
  Large-plaque parapsoriasis
  Poikiloderma vasculare atrophicans
  Lymphomatoid papulosis
  Follicular mucinosis
Nonepidermotropic lymphomas and related diseases
  Non-Hodgkin's (monomorphous) lymphomas
  Lymphocytic infiltrate of Jessner-Kanof
  Cutaneous pseudolymphoma
  Lymphomatoid granulomatosis
  Angioimmunoblastic lymphadenopathy
  Hodgkin's disease
Adult T cell leukemia-lymphoma
Leukemias
Multiple myeloma
Cutaneous histiocytic proliferations

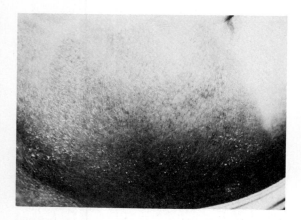

Figure 44–1. Nonatrophic form of patch-stage mycosis fungoides in a Chinese woman. There is minimal palpable infiltration, mild scaliness, and irregular pigmentation.

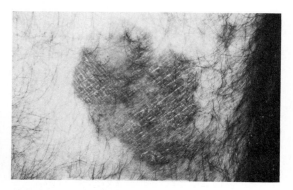

Figure 44–3. Plaque-stage mycosis fungoides. The lesion is slightly elevated, distinctly palpable, and sharply defined. The surface is irregularly lichenified.

Both forms of patch-stage mycosis fungoides vary considerably in size (commonly 2 cm to over 10 cm in diameter) and are usually only mildly pruritic or nonpruritic.

2. Plaque stage– With disease progression, moderately infiltrated plaques appear (Figs 44–3 and 44–4). These are usually asymmetric and measure several centimeters in diameter but may be much larger. Plaques may develop from preexisting patches or de novo. They are usually well-demarcated and scaly but also may be lichenified. Although some plaques are nummular, most are irregular in outline and may be arcuate. The color is most often pink or red in fair-complexioned persons and purplish or brown in those with darker complexions.

3. Tumor stage– Continued progression leads to tumors (Fig 44–5)—dome-shaped purplish or red nodules of moderate to firm consistency or deeply infiltrated plaques that ulcerate. Tumors are particularly apt to be located on the scalp and face and may arise in plaques of mycosis fungoides.

B. Systemic Disease: In the presence of extensive plaque or tumor-stage lesions, there is often palpable lymphadenopathy. Such nodes are generally freely movable and nontender. Nodal biopsies usually reveal a nonspecific "dermatopathic lymphadenopathy," but with disease progression the characteristic features of T cell lymphoma appear.

Visceral involvement may occur in late-stage disease; almost any organ can be infiltrated, but most commonly the lungs, spleen, liver, and kidney.

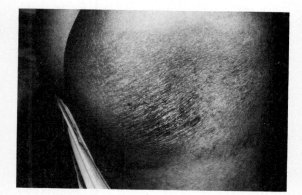

Figure 44–2. Atrophic (poikilodermatous) form of patch-stage mycosis fungoides. The skin is extremely thin and wrinkled. Telangiectasia and superficial venules can be seen.

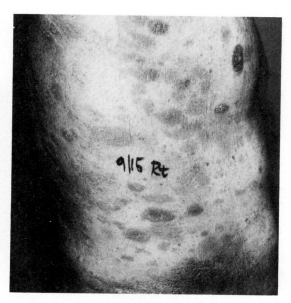

Figure 44–4. Extensive plaque-stage lesions of mycosis fungoides.

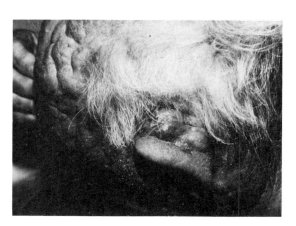

Figure 44–5. Tumor-stage nodules of mycosis fungoides on the posterior aspect of the ear and massive infiltration into the scalp.

B. Laboratory Findings:

1. Histology– The neoplastic cell in cutaneous T cell lymphomas has the appearance of a transformed or stimulated T lymphocyte. Characteristically, the nucleus is hyperconvoluted—ie, the surface is highly irregular and has deep indentations. The nuclear irregularity is best seen with the electron microscope (Fig 44–6) and less readily with the light microscope. Increases in nuclear size and staining intensity are important indications of neoplastic transformation.

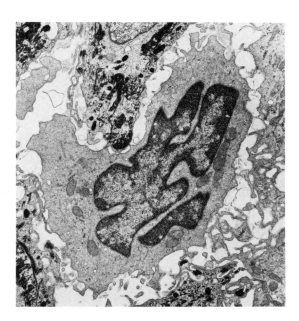

Figure 44–6. Electron micrograph of atypical lymphocyte in skin biopsy from patch-stage lesion of mycosis fungoides. The nuclear outline is highly irregular. ×11,500. (Courtesy of N. Scott McNutt, MD.)

Similar-appearing cells (but usually smaller) can occasionally be seen in benign disorders.

The important feature distinguishing mycosis fungoides from other cutaneous lymphomas is **epidermotropism,** ie, infiltration of the epidermis by lymphocytes. This infiltration consists of atypical cells or groups of cells, often forming sharply defined nests surrounded by a halo (**Pautrier's microabscesses;** Fig 44–7). Spongiosis is minimal.

In patch-stage lesions, the lymphocytes are usually mildly to moderately atypical, and there is a light, patchy infiltrate in the upper dermis. In the nonatrophic form, the epidermis is of approximately normal thickness and the rete ridges are preserved. In the atrophic form, the epidermis is thin, the rete ridges are effaced, and the dermal infiltrate hugs the basal cell layer.

In plaque-stage disease, the lymphocytic infiltrate is heavier and usually forms a bandlike pattern extending into the reticular dermis (Fig 44–8). Deeper foci may be present. The papillary dermis is com-

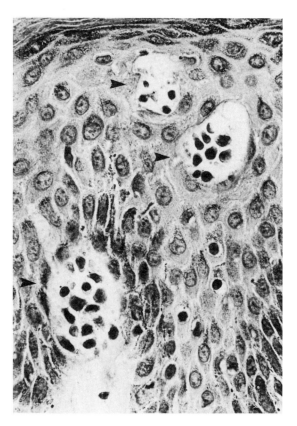

Figure 44–7. The epidermis contains 3 Pautrier microabscesses, indicated by arrowheads. These contain a number of lymphocytes with enlarged, hyperchromatic, irregularly shaped nuclei. Similar single atypical lymphocytes are also seen elsewhere in the epidermis. H&E stain, ×400.

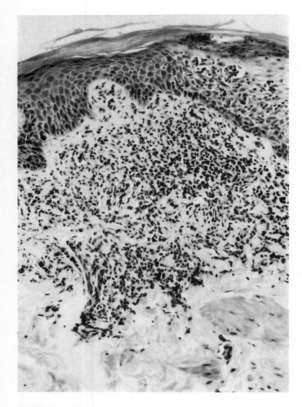

Figure 44–8. Plaque-stage mycosis fungoides. The epidermis contains single atypical lymphoid cells and Pautrier microabscesses. There is a heavy bandlike lymphocytic infiltrate in the upper dermis containing numerous atypical cells. H&E stain, ×100.

monly fibrotic. Cellular atypia is more pronounced, and varying proportions of lymphocytes with large, hyperchromatic, convoluted nuclei ("mycosis cells") are seen.

In tumor-stage disease, the infiltrate is massively deep, usually invading the subcutaneous fat and obliterating dermal appendages (Fig 44–9). The lymphoid cells are highly atypical. These may be predominantly mycosis cells or may be mostly cells with large, pale-staining nuclei and prominent nucleoli (blast forms) (Fig 44–10). The latter may be difficult to distinguish from those seen in some nonepidermotropic cutaneous lymphomas. Mitotic figures are common. The infiltrate is often polymorphic, containing histiocytes, eosinophils, and plasma cells.

2. Routine laboratory and other diagnostic studies– All patients should have a complete blood count with differential, blood chemistry panel, chest x-ray, whole body mapping of skin lesions, careful examination for peripheral adenopathy, and lymph node biopsy in the presence of adenopathy. If there is nodal involvement by lymphoma, CT scan of the abdomen and pelvis is indicated. Suspected visceral in-

volvement should be confirmed by biopsy. The most common sites are the lungs, spleen, and liver. The blood of patients with over 10% skin surface involvement, palpable adenopathy, tumors, or generalized erythroderma should be examined for Sézary cells. Following the workup, the patient should be staged according to the TNM classification.

Treatment

A. Cutaneous Therapy:

1. Patch and plaque stages– Four commonly used therapies for patch- and plaque-stage mycosis fungoides—not necessarily in order of popularity or effectiveness—are (1) oral psoralens plus ultraviolet light A (PUVA), (2) topical mechlorethamine (nitrogen mustard, HN2), (3) topical carmustine (BCNU), and (4) total body electron beam radiation.

a. Psoralens plus ultraviolet light A– PUVA therapy employs photosensitizing oral psoralens in combination with long-wave UVA radiation (320–400 nm). Treatments are given 2 or 3 times weekly for the first few months until remission is achieved and then once weekly or less often as needed. Patches and superficial plaques usually clear, but mid and

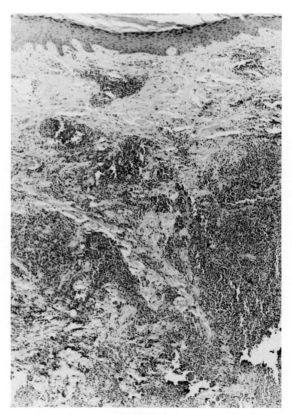

Figure 44–9. Tumor-stage mycosis fungoides. A massive, highly atypical infiltrate, obliterating dermal appendages, extends into the subcutis. H&E stain, ×40.

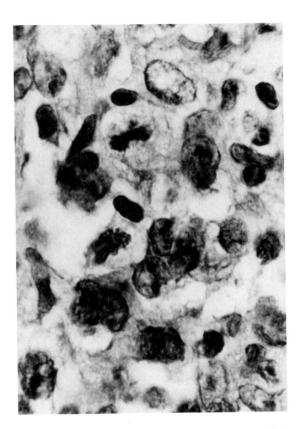

Figure 44–10. Tumor-stage mycosis fungoides. High-power view of specimen shown in Fig 44–9. The majority of the tumor cells are blast forms. These have large, pale-staining, irregular nuclei with prominent nucleoli. Some cells with large hyperchromatic nuclei are also seen. H&E stain, ×1000.

deep dermal infiltrates present in thick plaques often persist. Deeply infiltrated lesions are best treated in other ways. Prolonged use of PUVA may lead to solar keratoses and skin cancers, and patients with mycosis fungoides appear to be at greater than average risk for this complication.

b. Topical mechlorethamine– Topical applications of aqueous solutions of mechlorethamine have been used for about 30 years. The usual technique is to paint the entire body surface daily with solutions of 10 mg mechlorethamine in 60 mL of water, using a 2-inch paint brush. Complete clearing occurs in 50–75% of patients within about 2–6 months, though in some cases protracted treatment is required. Further treatment is reserved for recurrences, though some favor daily maintenance therapy for 6 months even in the absence of active lesions. The value of maintenance therapy is not established.

Topical mechlorethamine is relatively less toxic than other antineoplastic agents, though over half of patients develop irritant or allergic contact dermatitis.

Desensitization can sometimes be achieved in co-operative patients by using dilute solutions and gradually increasing the concentration. Patients receiving daily applications for prolonged periods are at increased risk for skin cancer. Mechlorethamine may also be prepared in an anhydrous ointment base. In this form, there are fewer instances of contact dermatitis.

c. Topical carmustine– Carmustine is a nitro-sourea, an antineoplastic compound that is at least as effective as mechlorethamine. It is particularly useful for treating patients allergic to mechlorethamine. It must first be dissolved in alcohol before being diluted with water.

Present schedules call for daily total body applications of 10 mg (predissolved in alcohol) in 60 mL of water for 8–12 weeks as tolerated. Substantial or complete clearing usually is achieved in lesions not in the tumor stage. Residual lesions are treated locally with more concentrated (2 mg/mL) alcoholic solutions, which may eradicate deep infiltrations. The incidence of allergic reactions is low, but carmustine tends to produce erythematous reactions that may lead to transient—or at times prolonged—telangiectasia. High-dose topical carmustine can cause bone marrow depression; this is not likely to occur with the above regimen if the total amount applied is less than 800 mg.

d. Total body electron beam therapy– This therapy gives results comparable to those achieved with topical antineoplastic agents. Electron beam therapy may be given in special radiation therapy centers. It is preferred to x-ray irradiation because of the lessened hazard of bone marrow depression and damage to underlying tissues. Daily treatments for 8–9 weeks for total doses of 3000–3600 cGy delivered at 4–6 MeV usually result in substantial or complete clearing in patch or plaque-stage disease. Electron beam therapy is particularly useful for patients with widespread deeply infiltrated plaques; however, recurrence within 6–12 months is frequent. Electron beam doses of over 3000 cGy usually cannot be repeated because of the hazard of chronic radiation dermatitis. Other complications include skin dryness, erythema, edema, bullae, and alopecia, which usually are not permanent. Local electron beam radiation is the treatment of choice for tumor-stage disease.

2. Tumor stage– The tumors of mycosis fungoides are best treated by ionizing radiation, with either local electron beam therapy or filtered x-rays. Persistent local applications or intralesional injections of carmustine or mechlorethamine may be successful for small tumors.

B. Systemic Therapy: Systemic therapy with antineoplastic agents is indicated if there are positive lymph nodes, visceral involvement, or widespread cutaneous lesions unresponsive to other therapies. Systemic chemotherapy may provide short-term palliation. Interferon alfa-2a has shown efficacy in early and advanced disease. Low-dose methotrexate (up to 50 mg orally or intramuscularly once weekly) is often of considerable value in the management of difficult patch- or plaque-stage disease.

Prognosis

Overall, mycosis fungoides is a slowly progressive lymphoma, though in a small proportion of cases disease progression is rapid. The 5-year estimated survival rate for patients with less than 10% surface involvement is over 90%, for those with over 10% involvement, 70–85%; for tumor-stage disease, 50–60%; for nodal involvement by lymphoma, approximately 20%; and for visceral involvement, approximately 10%.

The median survival, including all stages, of mycosis fungoides is approximately 10–14 years, and this is in a predominantly older age group. Ten to 20 percent of patients die from mycosis fungoides or related complications.

SÉZARY'S SYNDROME

Essentials of Diagnosis
- Generalized erythroderma.
- Generalized lymphadenopathy.
- At least 5% of circulating lymphocytes are abnormal (Sézary) cells.
- Often leukocytosis.

General Considerations

Sézary's syndrome is a rare cutaneous T cell lymphoma characterized by a generalized pruritic erythroderma and atypical circulating lymphocytes.

Clinical Findings

A. Symptoms and Signs: The erythroderma is generalized and most often universal. There is usually some scaling, though it may be purely macular (Fig 44–11). Lymphadenopathy is usually present. The palms and soles, characteristically diffusely scaly, may be fissured and painful. Pruritus is usually intense and difficult to control.

The diagnosis of Sézary's syndrome requires finding atypical lymphocytes (Sézary cells) in the blood (should constitute at least 5% of the circulating lymphocytes) identical to the hyperconvoluted cells found in mycosis fungoides skin biopsies (Fig 44–6). If suspicious-looking cells are seen in blood smears, thin (1- to 2-μm) plastic-embedded sections or electron microscopic preparations of the buffy coat are desirable. Sézary cells—usually a small percentage—may be present in some benign erythrodermas.

B. Laboratory Findings: Skin biopsies from patients with Sézary's syndrome reveal an upper dermal infiltrate of lymphoid cells, varying in degrees of atypia. Epidermotropism is usually present but is gen-

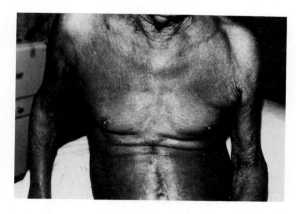

Figure 44–11. Patient with Sézary's syndrome. Almost the entire cutaneous surface is involved by a slightly scaly erythema.

erally not as pronounced as in patch- or plaque-stage mycosis fungoides.

Treatment & Clinical Course

Sézary's syndrome is relatively refractory to treatment, including topical chemotherapy, systemic therapy, electron beam radiation, and PUVA therapy. Chlorambucil is commonly given in a dosage of 2–4 mg/d, along with prednisone, 20–40 mg, every morning or less often if tolerated. However, prolonged use of chlorambucil, an alkylating agent, poses the risk of development of secondary leukemia.

Low-dose methotrexate has been recently reported to be beneficial in a majority of patients and has the advantage of not being leukemogenic.

Photopheresis has helped some patients. The procedure consists of giving the photosensitizing drug methoxsalen followed by irradiation of the blood extracorporeally. The UVA destroys abnormal cells as they pass through the photopheresis apparatus.

LARGE-PLAQUE PARAPSORIASIS

Large-plaque parapsoriasis is a rare chronic dermatitis that cannot be distinguished clinically from patch-stage mycosis fungoides. It is characterized by large, thin, scaly, red or dusky patches that may occur anywhere but which have a predilection for the bathing trunk area. Atrophy may be present but is not as marked or consistent as in the poikilodermatous type of mycosis fungoides. Pruritus is usually mild or absent.

Histologically, there is mild epidermal infiltration by single normal-appearing lymphocytes. Occasionally, small groups are seen intraepidermally but no distinct Pautrier microabscesses. There is a light perivascular infiltrate in the papillary dermis. The distinguishing feature from patch-stage mycosis fungoides is the absence of cellular atypia and Pautrier micro-abscesses.

All patients should be carefully observed for the long term. Ten to 30 percent of cases of large-plaque parapsoriasis transform into mycosis fungoides. An increase in pruritus or in size or thickness of the lesions is an ominous sign.

POIKILODERMA VASCULARE ATROPHICANS

Poikiloderma vasculare atrophicans is clinically indistinguishable from the atrophic patch-stage (poikilodermatous) form of mycosis fungoides. There are usually large, very thin, wrinkled, slightly scaly patches, chiefly in the bathing trunk area and on the breasts and inner arms. Superficial venules, telangiectases, and pigmentation are commonly evident.

Differentiation of this disorder from mycosis fungoides depends on histologic examination and is often difficult. The overall patterns are similar, but in poikiloderma vasculare atrophicans the lymphocytes appear benign, whereas in atrophic patch-stage mycosis fungoides some degree of atypia is present. The great majority of patients who present clinically with poikiloderma show some evidence of cellular atypia and are best classified as having mycosis fungoides. Patients who present with poikiloderma vasculare atrophicans should be carefully monitored for signs of malignant transformation such as itching, increased scaling, and increased lesion size.

LYMPHOMATOID PAPULOSIS

Lymphomatoid papulosis is a rare, chronic papulonodular eruption in which individual lesions heal spontaneously. The histologic picture resembles that

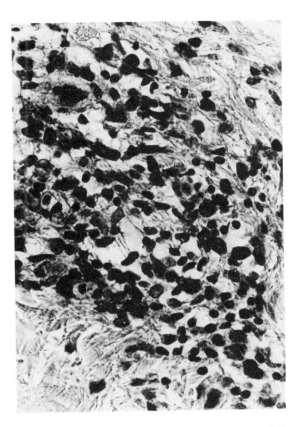

Figure 44–13. Lymphomatoid papulosis, dermal infiltrate. The infiltrate is composed of atypical lymphoid cells containing variably sized hyperchromatic, irregularly shaped nuclei, many of which are considerably enlarged.

of a highly malignant cutaneous T cell lymphoma or Hodgkin's disease. Red or purple papules, usually 20–50 in number, appear on any part of the body. They are commonly 3–5 mm in size but may be 1 cm or larger (Fig 44–12). In most patients there is crusting or even necrotic sloughing. The usual cycle from first appearance to involution is 3–6 weeks, though nodular lesions may last for 2–3 months. Simple papules involute without a trace; those with necrosis leave a depressed scar.

Histologic examination shows a perivascular and interstitial lymphoid cell infiltrate that may extend to the deep dermis. The lymphocytes are highly atypical; large, irregularly shaped hyperchromatic and pale nuclei with prominent nucleoli may be seen (Fig 44–13). Mitotic figures are common. The epidermis may be infiltrated with individual lymphoid cells or may be free of such involvement. Large Pautrier microabscesses are uncommon. There is often superficial erosion and crusting. Extravasated erythrocytes may be seen in the papillary dermis, and eosinophils may be present.

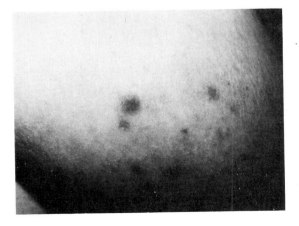

Figure 44–12. Papules of lymphomatoid papulosis on the breast. Some are mostly involuted.

The condition usually persists for years as an apparently benign disorder despite the ominous histologic picture. However, 10–20% of reported cases have been associated with or have evolved into mycosis fungoides or some other type of malignant lymphoma. Patients should be kept under careful observation, and those with particularly extensive or nodular lesions should be treated. Low-dose methotrexate, PUVA, and topical mechlorethamine and carmustine are usually helpful.

FOLLICULAR MUCINOSIS

Follicular mucinosis (alopecia mucinosa) is a rare inflammatory dermatitis of unknown cause characterized by mucinous degeneration of the pilosebaceous apparatus. The lesions present with scaly, eczematous, or infiltrated plaques on the head, neck, trunk, or extremities or as grouped follicular papules, more common on the trunk and extremities. In hair-bearing areas, there is evident hair loss. In some instances, there is gross exudation of mucin.

In several series, 9–32% of patients with follicular mucinosis either had or eventually developed mycosis fungoides. A small number developed other lymphomas, including Hodgkin's disease. Lesions of follicular mucinosis associated with mycosis fungoides are more often seen on the trunk and extremities but may also occur on the head and neck. This association is somewhat more common in older persons.

Histologic examination shows an accumulation of mucin, demonstrated by stains for acid mucopolysaccharides, in the hair follicles and sebaceous glands associated with a variable dermal infiltrate. When associated with mycosis fungoides, atypical lymphoid cells invade the pilosebaceous unit and form part of the dermal infiltrate. Histologically, follicular mucinosis is often seen in tumor-stage lesions.

Although follicular mucinosis may be associated with mycosis fungoides, it is not clear if lesions of follicular mucinosis directly evolve into those of mycosis fungoides. Nevertheless, patients with follicular mucinosis should have multiple skin biopsies to rule out the possibility of mycosis fungoides and should be kept under close observation for the possibility of development of mycosis fungoides or other lymphomatous disease.

NONEPIDERMOTROPIC CUTANEOUS LYMPHOMAS & RELATED DISEASES

Most cutaneous lymphomas other than mycosis fungoides and Sézary's syndrome are nonepidermotropic (Table 44–1).

Table 44–2. Simplified clinical evaluation scheme for non-Hodgkin's lymphomas.[1]

Cytology and Growth Pattern	Immunocytology[2]	Final Designation[2]
Small cell, nodular or diffuse	T	SnT, SdT
	B	SnB, SdB
	O	SnO, SdO
	R	SnR, SdR
Large cell, nodular or diffuse	T	LnT, LdT
	B	LnB, LdB
	O	LnO, LdO
	R	LnR, LdR
Mixed cellularity, nodular or diffuse	T	MnT, MdT
	B	MnB, MdB
	O	MnO, MdO
	R	MnR, MdR

[1] Reproduced, with permission, from Krueger GRF: Lancet 1984;1:1067.
[2] T = T cell, B = B cell, O = other (undetermined), R = reticulum cell (phagocytic, dendritic, interdigitating); S = small cell, L = large cell, M = mixed cellularity; n = nodular, d = diffuse.

Systemic lymphomas are generally classified as Hodgkin's disease and non-Hodgkin's lymphomas. Classification of non-Hodgkin's lymphoma has undergone a number of changes in the past 2 decades. The 1966 Rappaport classification is based on morphology, whereas the Lukes-Collins classification is based on the functional characterization of lymphocytes as T or B cells. Krueger has combined morphology with immunologic and cytochemical markers in a simplified classification scheme (Table 44–2).

NON-HODGKIN'S (MONOMORPHOUS) CUTANEOUS LYMPHOMAS

Most nonepidermotropic cutaneous lymphomas are non-Hodgkin's lymphomas. Cutaneous Hodgkin's disease is rare.

Non-Hodgkin's lymphomas are predominantly neoplasms of lymphocytes. The great majority of "histiocytic" lymphomas arise from transformed T or B lymphocytes and are now called "large-cell lymphomas.". However, cases of truly histiocytic lymphomas are still recognized (see also histiocytosis X, below). The non-Hodgkin cutaneous lymphomas are called "monomorphous" because they are composed mostly of lymphoma cells and lack the mixed cellularity characteristic of Hodgkin's disease and mycosis fungoides.

Cutaneous lesions of non-Hodgkin's lymphomas may appear in patients known to have systemic disease or may be the initial manifestation of lymphoma. However, in one series, further workup of patients presenting with apparent primary cutaneous lymphoma revealed extracutaneous disease, most commonly in the lymph nodes, in 60%.

Clinical Findings

A. Symptoms and Signs: The cutaneous lesions of nonepidermotropic lymphoma—nodules or infiltrated plaques having a red, blue, violaceous, or brown color—can occur on any part of the body (Fig 44–14) . The lesions are firm and usually not ulcerated. In contrast to plaques of mycosis fungoides, which are usually scaly, plaques of nonepidermotropic lymphoma have a smooth surface. However, clinical differentiation from deeply infiltrated plaques and tumors of mycosis fungoides is often difficult.

B. Laboratory Findings:

1. Histology– Infiltration of the epidermis by lymphoid cells is uncommon in non-Hodgkin's lymphoma and even then is usually limited. Characteristically, there is a grenz (border) zone of uninvolved dermis separating the lymphoma infiltrate from the epidermis (Fig 44–15). Variably sized groups of lymphoid cells are found in a perivascular, periappendageal, patchy, or diffuse distribution in the dermis and usually extend as large masses into the subcutaneous tissue. A distinct follicular (nodular) pattern is uncommon. Most cases are diffuse large-cell lymphomas (Fig 44–16).

Cell surface markers indicate that the monomorphous lymphomas are equally likely to express either B or T phenotypes. A small number are non-B, non-T.

In contrast to mycosis fungoides, the non-Hodgkin cutaneous lymphomas exhibit nonhyperconvoluted nuclei, a lack of mature helper T cell phenotype, and are Ia$^+$ rather than Ia$^-$. As a group, they display considerable immunologic, histologic, and clinical heterogeneity.

2. Routine laboratory and other diagnostic studies– If the patient is not already known to have systemic disease, a complete lymphoma workup is needed. Lymph node biopsy should be obtained in patients with clinical adenopathy. Additionally, a chest x-ray, CT abdominal scan or lymphangiogram, bone marrow biopsy, and examination of the blood for atypical cells should be ordered.

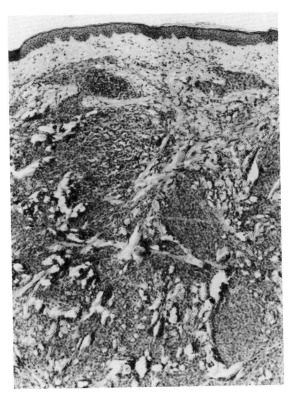

Figure 44–15. Nonepidermotropic large-cell T cell lymphoma. Biopsy specimen from lesion shown in Fig 44–14. A massive infiltrate extends into the subcutis. The infiltrate is separated from the epidermis by an uninvolved grenz (border) zone. H&E stain, ×40.

Treatment

Cutaneous lymphomas are generally highly responsive to ionizing radiation. Patients who present with disease of limited extent and who have no evidence of systemic involvement may be treated locally with either electron beam radiation or orthovoltage x-rays. Those with generalized lesions can be treated with total skin electron beam therapy. Ionizing radiation can also provide palliative relief of skin lesions in patients with systemic involvement. Chemotherapy is indicated for patients with systemic disease.

Prognosis

Inasmuch as a high proportion of patients either present with or will eventually develop evidence of systemic involvement, the prognosis for this group is guarded and is distinctly less favorable than that for the average patient with mycosis fungoides.

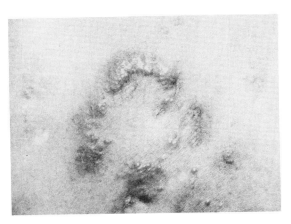

Figure 44–14. Nonepidermotropic large-cell T cell lymphoma. Shown is a hard infiltrated plaque with annular configuration.

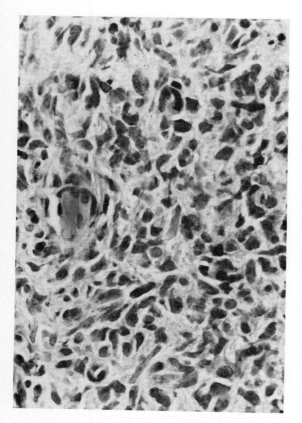

Figure 44–16. Nonepidermotropic large-cell T cell lymphoma. High-power view of specimen shown in Fig 44–15. The lymphoma cells have large, irregularly shaped nuclei and abundant cytoplasm. H&E stain, ×600.

LYMPHOCYTIC INFILTRATE OF JESSNER-KANOF

The predominant lesions are papules, small plaques, or annular infiltrations. The principal target areas are the face, back, upper chest, and arms. Age at onset is mostly between 30 and 50 years. There is no sex predominance. The disease persists for 1–10 years in most patients but is usually cyclic, with remissions and exacerbations. Itching is variable.

Histologically, the epidermis is unaffected. There are well-circumscribed superficial and deep perivascular and periappendageal aggregates of normal-appearing lymphocytes. These are predominantly T cells. Significant amounts of dermal mucin are present.

In about one-fourth of patients, lesions are aggravated by sun exposure, mostly in the early stage of the disease, and both clinical and histologic differentiation from polymorphous light eruption may be difficult.

The disorder is generally regarded as benign. Tran-

sition into malignant lymphoma has been reported, but this outcome is controversial.

Antimalarial therapy and ionizing radiation may be beneficial.

CUTANEOUS PSEUDOLYMPHOMA

The term cutaneous pseudolymphoma refers to a group of benign inflammatory dermatoses that resemble to varying degrees truly malignant lymphomas both clinically and histologically. These include lymphocytoma cutis, certain drug reactions, nodular scabies, borrelial lymphocytoma, actinic reticuloid, and lymphomatoid papulosis. Actinic reticuloid is discussed in Chapter 38, and lymphomatoid papulosis is discussed elsewhere in this chapter. It should be recognized, however, that in some situations it may be impossible to make a definite diagnosis of a benign or malignant process, and the diagnosis becomes apparent only after following the patient with repeated biopsies for some months or years.

Immunologic markers performed on frozen sections may help in the distinction of benign from malignant lymphocytic processes. In B cell proliferations, a monoclonal infiltrate, with either kappa or lambda light chains, usually indicates true lymphoma. However, polyclonality does not necessarily exclude malignancy because of admixture of accessory cells.

Lymphocytoma Cutis (Cutaneous Lymphoid Hyperplasia)

Clinically, there is usually a solitary—occasionally multiple—firm, reddish brown or purple nodule or plaque, or multiple papules. These occur most often on the face and extremities. Women are affected more often than men.

Histologically, there are dense, nodular, mixed cell infiltrates with formation of lymphoid follicles. The follicles are mostly found in early and well-developed lesions, but they may be absent in older lesions. In the follicular pattern, there are small, darkly staining, closely packed lymphocytes with scant cytoplasm surrounding aggregates of large lymphocytes. The large lymphocytes have large, irregularly shaped pale-staining nuclei and are loosely arranged because of abundant cytoplasm. The infiltrate is usually heavier in the upper than the lower dermis. Plasma cells and eosinophils are often present. The epidermis is not involved and is separated from the infiltrate by a thin zone of collagen.

In most instances the cause of lymphocytoma cutis is undetermined. In some cases, it may be induced by arthropod bites or stings, injected drugs, vaccinations, injections of antigens for hyposensitization, and acupuncture. As a rule, lesions involute within several months or a few years. However, if lesions—

particularly nodules—persist or become more numerous, repeated biopsies are mandatory to rule out the possibility of transformation to malignant lymphoma.

Phenytoin-Induced Pseudolymphoma Syndrome

A pseudolymphoma syndrome characterized by generalized adenopathy, hepatosplenomegaly, arthralgias, fever, leukocytosis, and eosinophilia may be induced by the anticonvulsant phenytoin. Cutaneous lesions may exhibit as a few erythematous plaques, as a generalized maculopapular eruption or exfoliative dermatitis, or as nodules.

Microscopically, the infiltrate is often indistinguishable from that of mycosis fungoides in that hyperconvoluted nuclei in the dermal infiltrate and Pautrier microabscesses may be seen. Sézary cells may be found in the blood. Nodular lesions suggest non-Hodgkin's lymphoma, and histologic examination of lymph node biopsy specimens may suggest lymphoma.

Nodular Scabies

Clinically, there are reddish-brown, pruritic papules and nodules, occurring most often on the elbows and genitalia and in the axillae. They may persist for many months. Fewer than 10% of patients with scabies have such nodules.

Histologically, there are dense, superficial and deep, mostly perivascular but also interstitial infiltrates of lymphocytes, histiocytes, plasma cells, and eosinophils. The infiltrate may mimic that of mycosis fungoides or Hodgkin's disease because of the presence of atypical mononuclear cells or multinuclear cells that are suggestive of Reed-Sternberg cells.

Borrelial Lymphocytoma

A solitary lymphocytoma may appear in stage I of the European form of Lyme borreliosis. It is usually the only cutaneous manifestation, though lesions of erythema chronicum migrans may be present. Spontaneous involution occurs after several months. Rarely, a borrelial lymphocytoma occurs in stage III in association with acrodermatitis chronica atrophicans. This is a blue-red nodule with predilection for soft skin areas, especially the ear lobe.

Microscopically, structures resembling lymph node follicles are often observed. Plasma cells and eosinophils may be present. Spirochetes have been demonstrated in some cases with special stains.

LYMPHOMATOID GRANULOMATOSIS

Lymphomatoid granulomatosis is a systemic disease usually involving both the skin and the lungs. Skin lesions occur in half of cases. The kidneys, lymph nodes, central nervous system, bone marrow, and other organs and tissues are often affected.

Two-thirds of patients have pulmonary symptoms; chest x-rays reveal nodular infiltrations of the lungs. Skin lesions can occur concurrently with, precede, or follow lung involvement by months to years. These may be erythematous macules, papules, or nodular lesions that tend to ulcerate. Symptoms relating to the central or peripheral nervous system are the next most common clinical manifestation.

Histologic examination shows features of inflammatory granulomatous and lymphoproliferative processes. The infiltrate is angiocentric and angiodestructive. Atypical and occasionally bizarre lymphohistiocytic cells are present, suggesting lymphoma.

Thirteen to 50 percent of patients develop frank lymphoma, and recent studies suggest that lymphomatoid granulomatosis is a form of peripheral T cell lymphoma.

Combination cyclophosphamide and prednisone therapy may produce complete remissions.

ANGIOIMMUNOBLASTIC LYMPHADENOPATHY

Angioimmunoblastic lymphadenopathy is a systemic disease characterized by generalized lymphadenopathy, severe constitutional symptoms, hepatosplenomegaly, and polyclonal gammopathy.

Typically, there is a history of rapidly enlarging, generalized lymphadenopathy for several months. A generalized morbilliform eruption may precede the adenopathy. Small erythematous nodules and acral cryoglobulinemic purpura may occur.

The lymph node architecture is altered by a pleomorphic cellular infiltrate and vascular proliferation. Immunoblasts and multinucleated cells may be present. Skin biopsies reveal a lymphocytic and plasma cell infiltrate associated with capillary proliferation.

One-third of patients develop immunoblastic lymphoma. Recent investigations suggest that the disorder is a form of peripheral T cell lymphoma.

HODGKIN'S DISEASE

Hodgkin's disease is responsible for 3200 deaths annually in the USA. There is a bimodal peak incidence affecting young adults and older age groups. The cellular origin of Hodgkin's disease is controversial.

The initial manifestation is lymph node enlargement, most frequent in the neck, usually accompanied by constitutional symptoms. Other lymph nodes may be gradually or rapidly involved. Eventually, almost any organ may be affected. With radiation and combination chemotherapy, the 5-year survival rate is over 50%.

Skin lesions in Hodgkin's disease may be non-specific or specific. Generalized pruritus is the most common nonspecific manifestation, affecting one-third of patients, and may be the presenting symptom. Papular lesions, erythema, lichenification, excoriations, localized or generalized pigmentation, and acquired ichthyosis may occur. There is a high incidence of herpes zoster among patients with Hodgkin's disease.

Specific skin lesions have been reported in 0.5–3.4% of patients. These usually present as papules or nodules that often ulcerate (Fig 44–17). Involvement of the skin results chiefly from retrograde lymphatic spread from tumor-containing lymph nodes. Direct extension into the skin from underlying lymph nodes is less common. Skin involvement usually occurs in advanced disease and implies a poor prognosis.

Four principal types of Hodgkin's disease are recognized histologically: lymphocyte predominance, mixed cellularity, lymphocyte depletion, and nodular sclerosis. A necessary but not sufficient requirement for the diagnosis of Hodgkin's disease is the finding of Reed-Sternberg giant cells in lymph nodes. This cell has several nuclei or a single multilobular nucleus and prominent nucleoli. There is usually a mixture of cell types, including atypical mononuclear cells, lymphocytes, histiocytes, eosinophils, and plasma cells.

In cutaneous Hodgkin's disease, the infiltrate often extends into the subcutaneous tissue. Patterns of the nodular sclerosing and mixed cellularity forms have

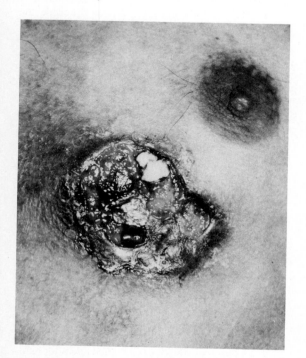

Figure 44–17. Noduloulcerative lesion in advanced Hodgkin's disease (stage IVB).

been described. Reed-Sternberg cells are usually found.

Treatment of cutaneous Hodgkin's disease is secondary to treatment of the systemic process. Ionizing radiation may provide palliation.

ADULT T-CELL LEUKEMIA-LYMPHOMA

Essentials of Diagnosis

- Adults with clinical features of an aggressive leukemia.
- Circulating malignant lymphocytes with pleomorphic nuclei.
- Mature helper T cell phenotype.
- Anti-HTLV-I antibodies.

General Considerations

Adult T cell leukemia-lymphoma (ATLL) is a recently recognized aggressive leukemia caused by the human T cell lymphotropic virus type I (HTLV-I). It is endemic in southwestern Japan, the Caribbean, central Africa, the Pacific basin, northeastern South America, and the southeastern USA. The clinical course may be chronic or acute but is usually followed by a rapidly progressive terminal outcome.

Classification & Clinical Findings

A. Symptoms and Signs: In the earliest or **pre-leukemic stage of ATLL,** patients have antibodies to HTLV-I but are asymptomatic. Typical morphologically abnormal lymphocytes are found in the blood. The only organ involved is the bone marrow. About half of all patients experience spontaneous regression; the other half have persistent lymphocytosis, and some progress to the acute phase, which is rapidly fatal.

A second group has **smoldering ATLL.** These patients present with cutaneous erythema, papules, or nodules, but otherwise have no physical abnormalities. The blood has from nil to 2% ATLL cells. Some patients progress to acute disease, usually after several years or more.

Closely related to smoldering ATLL is **chronic ATLL.** These patients have a significant number of abnormal circulating cells. They may progress to acute ATLL after some months.

The fourth group consists of patients with **subacute or acute ATLL.** They usually present with rapidly progressive localized or generalized erythroderma, nodules, nonspecific plaques, papules, or patches. About 80% have peripheral adenopathy, and about half have hepatosplenomegaly. Hilar and retroperitoneal nodes are commonly involved, but mediastinal nodes are spared. Lung and leptomeningeal involvement is also typical. These patients usually respond well to chemotherapy initially but generally relapse rapidly (see discussion of treatment).

Hypercalcemia is a prominent complication of ATLL, affecting 25–100% of all patients. Patients exhibit typical symptoms of hypercalcemia such as lethargy, constipation, confusion, dehydration, and polyuria. The hypercalcemia may be resistant to standard therapy.

B. Laboratory Findings: (In addition to those mentioned above.) Pleomorphic, medium to large lymphocytes with indented or polylobulated nuclei are consistently found in the blood. Approximately 65% of patients have leukemia at presentation. The malignant lymphocytes have a mature helper T cell phenotype, and anti-HTLV-I antibodies or HTLV-I proviral DNA sequences are present.

Skin biopsy specimens reveal dermal and subcutaneous infiltration by tumor cells. About two-thirds of patients show epidermotropism, and Pautrier microabscesses may be present. Lymph node biopsies are pleomorphic in pattern and may not be diagnostic.

Treatment & Prognosis

Patients with the preleukemic, smoldering, or chronic forms of ATLL usually need no treatment unless they progress to a more aggressive stage.

Those with subacute or acute ATLL should receive aggressive chemotherapy, radiotherapy, or both. Although most patients respond initially to treatment, remissions are short-lived. The mortality rate is about 50% in less than 5 months.

THE LEUKEMIAS

Leukemias may involve the skin either directly, by producing specific malignant infiltrates, or indirectly, by producing nonspecific eruptions sometimes called leukemids. Leukemias are classified as acute or chronic. The major acute leukemias are myelocytic (granulocytic), lymphocytic, or monocytic. The great majority of monocytic leukemias are of the myelomonocytic type. In acute leukemia, the cells are often so bizarre that classification is difficult, and cell-marker studies may be necessary to identify the malignant cell.

Myelocytic leukemia derives from multipotential stem cells in the bone marrow. Chronic myelocytic leukemia (CML) is associated with the Philadelphia (Ph[1]) chromosome. Acute myelomonocytic leukemia cells have characteristics of both myeloblasts and monoblasts and may arise from a common precursor cell. Lymphocytic leukemia arises from an abnormal type of nongranular leukocyte in the blood-forming tissues, particularly the bone marrow, spleen, and lymph nodes. Lymphocytes in chronic lymphocytic leukemia (CLL) are predominantly of the B cell type, though T cell CLL occurs also. CLL is closely related to well-differentiated lymphocytic lymphoma.

Acute lymphocytic leukemia (ALL) occurs predominantly in children. Acute myelocytic leukemia (AML), CLL, and CML are diseases of adults. Monocytic leukemia can affect all ages. CLL is the most common chronic leukemia.

Adult T cell leukemia-lymphoma (ATLL) is discussed elsewhere in this chapter.

Therapy of nonspecific or specific cutaneous lesions due to leukemia consists of systemic administration of combinations of antineoplastic drugs. For extensive or deeply infiltrating skin lesions, total body electron beam or local x-ray radiation may be of value.

CLINICAL PRESENTATIONS OF THE LEUKEMIAS

1. ACUTE LEUKEMIA

The most common nonspecific skin lesions in acute leukemia are pallor (due to anemia), hemorrhagic phenomena, oral lesions, erythema multiforme, nonspecific itching papules, pyoderma, and erythema. The hemorrhagic manifestations include petechiae, ecchymoses, bleeding from the gums, and epistaxis; these are usually due to thrombocytopenia. The oral lesions are due to bleeding, necrosis, and gingival hypertrophy.

Specific lesions are rare in acute lymphocytic and myelocytic leukemia. They are common in pure monocytic leukemia, occurring in one-third of cases and less frequently in myelomonocytic leukemia. Such lesions vary from red or brown macules to red-violet nodules (Fig 44–18). Gingival hyperplasia is also frequent in patients with monocytic leukemia.

2. CHRONIC LYMPHOCYTIC LEUKEMIA (CLL)

The most frequent nonspecific cutaneous lesions associated with CLL are prurigo-like papules, bullae, purpura, and herpes zoster. Specific lesions, occurring in 8% of patients, include papules, plaques, various types of infiltrations, nodules, and exfoliative erythroderma. The nodules may be extensive and have a predilection for the face and extremities. Erythroderma and cutaneous nodules occur in one-third of patients with T cell CLL.

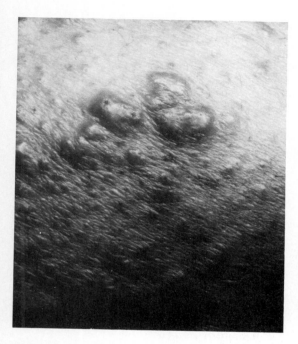

Figure 44–18. Specific nodules and papules in a patient with monocytic leukemia.

3. CHRONIC MYELOCYTIC LEUKEMIA (CML)

Nonspecific lesions are less common in CML than in CLL. Purpura, appearing as petechiae and ecchymoses, is the most frequent type, even though thrombocytopenia is rare in CML.

Specific lesions occur in 5% of cases. These are mostly papules, infiltrated plaques, or nodules, pre-

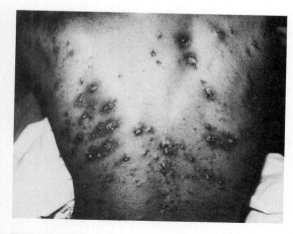

Figure 44–19. Extensive specific papulonodular and erosive lesions in a patient in terminal blast crisis of chronic myelocytic leukemia.

dominantly on the trunk—in contrast to CLL, in which the face is most often involved. Nodular lesions are termed granulocytic sarcoma. These may appear in CML shortly before transition to AML or may precede overt leukemia in the blood. Widespread cutaneous lesions may accompany a terminal blastic transformation of CML (Fig 44–19).

HISTOLOGIC FEATURES OF THE LEUKEMIAS

1. MYELOCYTIC LEUKEMIA

There is a perivascular dermal infiltrate, often extending into the subcutis. The infiltrate includes large cells with vesicular nuclei and smaller cells with clefted nuclei and granules. The chloroacetate esterase stain and the peroxidase reaction identify the myeloid nature of the infiltrate. Otherwise, differentiation from lymphoma is difficult.

2. MONOCYTIC LEUKEMIA

Monocytic leukemia is characterized by a dermal infiltrate composed chiefly of mature and immature monocytes separated from an uninvolved epidermis by a grenz (border) zone. The cells are large, with abundant cytoplasm, and may have bilobate large, notched, or oval nuclei.

3. MYELOMONOCYTIC LEUKEMIA

Specific lesions of myelomonocytic leukemia reveal an infiltrate of atypical myelocytes and monocytes that are often difficult to distinguish by light microscopy. However, they can be differentiated by the double esterase stain, in which the monocytes stain blue for α-naphthol acetate esterase (nonspecific esterase) and the myelocytes stain red for naphthol AS-D chloroacetate esterase.

4. LYMPHOCYTIC LEUKEMIA

In chronic lymphocytic leukemia, the histologic picture is similar to that of well-differentiated lymphocytic lymphoma. There are large or small masses of normal-appearing lymphocytes in the dermis. Infiltrates are commonly perivascular. Immature cells resembling lymphoblasts are infrequent. The cells are closely packed. Mitotic figures are rare. The epidermis is uninvolved. In T cell CLL, there is dermal and subcutaneous infiltration but no epidermal involvement.

In acute lymphocytic leukemia, there are diffuse

dermal and subcutaneous infiltrates of cells with large, irregular nuclei. Extensive areas of hemorrhage may be present.

MULTIPLE MYELOMA

Multiple myeloma (plasmacytoma) is a neoplasm of plasma cells arising in the bone marrow. Osteolytic lesions occur in bones with hematopoietically active marrow, such as the skull, vertebrae, ribs, pelvis, and proximal long bones. Monoclonal peaks of immunoglobulin are revealed in the serum by electrophoresis. Light-chain (Bence Jones) protein is found in the urine of 70–80% of patients.

Nonspecific skin lesions include amyloidosis, pigmentation, erythema, alopecia, and Raynaud's phenomenon. Specific skin lesions result chiefly from direct extension of the osseous plasmacytoma to the skin. Tumors arising from such extensions are usually soft and frequently ulcerated. Distant metastases to the skin are relatively uncommon.

On histologic examination, there is a dense infiltrate of atypical plasma cells with features of malignancy, such as variations in nuclear size, shape, and staining intensity; mitotic figures; and multinucleated cells. Immunoglobulins can be demonstrated by immunofluorescent techniques.

Systemic antineoplastic agents such as cyclophosphamide, melphalan, mechlorethamine, and methotrexate have benefited some patients. Topically applied mechlorethamine has cleared some cutaneous lesions. Occasionally there may be spontaneous resolution.

CUTANEOUS HISTIOCYTIC PROLIFERATION

Tissue histiocytes are part of the mononuclear phagocyte system. They derive from the blood monocyte and therefore ultimately from stem cells in the bone marrow. Van der Valk and Meijer have classified histiocytic proliferations of the skin into 4 major groups: (1) proliferation of monocytes (acute monocytic leukemia), (2) proliferations of histiocytes, (3) proliferations of Langerhans cells, and (4) proliferations of histiocytes of uncertain origin.

Monocytic leukemia has been discussed in the section on Leukemia.

MALIGNANT HISTIOCYTOSIS

Malignant histiocytosis is a rare neoplasm that may involve almost any organ system and in general has a poor prognosis. Skin lesions occur in 10–30% of patients.

Clinically, there are nodules—often ulcerated— and, less commonly, papules. Purpura and petechiae may be present. Nodules are usually multiple but may be solitary. Skin lesions may be the initial presentation in some patients, and this may indicate a more favorable prognosis, though the course is variable.

Histologically, dense nodular infiltrates are seen in the dermis or subcutis around blood vessels and appendages. There is a polymorphic proliferation of large, atypical cells with pleomorphic large nuclei and ample cytoplasm. Bi- and multinucleated cells are common. Phagocytosis is readily apparent. However, staining for histiocytic markers is necessary to distinguish the disorder from large cell lymphomas. Histiocytosis X can be differentiated with OKT6 antibody. Birbeck granules, characteristic of histiocytosis X, are rare in malignant histiocytosis.

REGRESSING ATYPICAL HISTIOCYTOSIS

Flynn et al in 1982 reported 2 patients with spontaneously regressing and recurrent noduloulcerative lesions and an apparently indolent clinical course. However, one of the patients subsequently died from the disease, and the second developed spinal metastasis.

The microscopic hallmarks of these lesions were atypical mononuclear and multinucleated giant cells with prominent nucleoli ("RAH cells"). Immunologic cell markers and enzyme cytochemical features favored an origin from histiocytes. However, some observers believe that regressing atypical histiocytosis is a form of cutaneous T cell lymphoma. Further studies are needed to clarify this issue.

FAMILIAL HISTIOCYTOSES

This is a rare group of histiocytic proliferations with clear phagocytic features. The disorder is familial, affects very young children, and is rapidly fatal. There is lymphadenopathy, hepatosplenomegaly, and thymic dysplasia. A generalized erythematous rash with papules and vesicles is seen.

Eosinophils, phagocytosing histiocytes, and lymphocytes are found at the dermal-epidermal junction with occasional epidermal invasion. Despite the relentless clinical course, there is no cytologic atypia. This syndrome thus has features of both histiocytosis X and malignant histiocytosis.

RETICULOHISTIOCYTOSIS

Lesions of reticulohistiocytosis may be limited to one or a few nodules (reticulohistiocytic granuloma), commonly on the head and neck, or may be present as multiple skin lesions associated with polyarthritis (multicentric reticulohistiocytosis).

The histology is the same in both forms. There are numerous large histiocytes containing eosinophilic homogeneous or finely granular cytoplasm, giving a "ground-glass" appearance. The cells may have a single nucleus or numerous nuclei. Early lesions show a pronounced inflammatory infiltrate composed of lymphoid and plasma cells. In older lesions, the inflammatory reaction is replaced by fibrous tissue.

In multicentric reticulohistiocytosis there are numerous flesh-colored, red, purple, or brown papules or nodules in many skin areas but with a predilection for the face and hands. In about half of all patients, papules are present on the oral and nasal mucosa. The skin lesions are associated with polyarthritis, which may be mild or severe. Mutilation of the hands due to loss of articular cartilage and subarticular bone may occur. In most instances, the disease becomes inactive after several years. Systemic therapy with methotrexate and cyclophosphamide and topical mechlorethamine may be beneficial.

LANGERHANS CELL HISTIOCYTOSIS (Histiocytosis X)

The Langerhans cell is a dendritic cell found mostly in the skin but also in lymph nodes and spleen. A prevalent concept is that it is part of the mononuclear phagocyte system and therefore derives from the bone marrow. However, the origin of this cell remains controversial. The Langerhans cell participates in the afferent limb of the immune response and is intimately involved with lymphocytes.

The term histiocytosis X has been used as a designation for 3 related clinical disorders: eosinophilic granuloma, Hand-Schüller-Christian disease, and Letterer-Siwe disease. Inasmuch as the Langerhans cell has been demonstrated as the diagnostic cell of histiocytosis X, the term Langerhans cell histiocytosis is preferred.

Langerhans cell histiocytosis affects mainly children and young adults, though older persons may also be involved. The male:female ratio is about equal. The median age at diagnosis is about 3 years.

Clinical Findings

A. Symptoms and Signs: Langerhans cell histiocytosis can involve practically any site in the body and can occur either as an isolated lesion or as a widespread systemic disease.

Bone lesions are the most common and are present in about 80% of patients. Adenopathy, skin lesions, and hepatomegaly are found in 50–60%; splenomegaly, malnutrition, otitis, and fever in about 35%; and pulmonary involvement, diabetes insipidus, short stature, exophthalmos, oral lesions, diarrhea, and jaundice in about 10–20% of patients.

Bone lesions are characteristically painful but not tender. On x-ray they appear as sharply defined areas with a "punched-out" appearance. The calvarium and other flat bones are those most frequently involved. Other common sites are the femur, scapula, rib, mandible, and vertebra.

Skin lesions are of many types (Fig 44–20). They usually begin as vesiculopustules, often with hemorrhagic crusting. Lesions may occur anywhere but are most frequent on the scalp, in the intertriginous areas, and behind the ears.

Scalp lesions are commonly scaly or exudative. Small scaly papules may appear on the trunk or scalp. The vulva is often involved in girls, and perianal involvement is common in both sexes. In disseminated Langerhans cell histiocytosis, the rash may become erythematous, maculopapular and confluent. Denuded areas may lead to sepsis. Petechiae appear with thrombocytopenia.

Brain involvement can occur from epidural extension from calvarial lesions. Cerebellar involvement has been repeatedly found in children. Diabetes insipidus is common in patients with multifocal disease. Short stature may occur in patients who have onset of diabetes insipidus prior to adolescence.

Pulmonary Langerhans cell histiocytosis is largely a disease of adults, usually men. In children, it occurs most often in those with disseminated disease. The pulmonary signs and symptoms are usually nonspecific.

Gum involvement is common in children with gen-

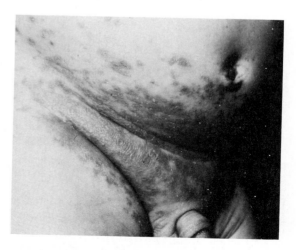

Figure 44–20. Confluent papular eruption in an infant with disseminated Langerhans cell histiocytosis. (Courtesy of Mary L. Williams, MD.)

eralized disease. Symptoms include pain and swelling of the face, loosening and premature loss of teeth, swollen gums with hemorrhage, and mucosal ulceration. There may be associated destruction of the alveolar ridge. Involvement of the ear is common and usually presents as external otitis refractory to treatment.

Hematopoietic involvement is associated with disseminated disease and occurs most often in infants. This can be secondary to splenic and bone marrow infiltration by histiocytes. Lymph node enlargement is frequently present. Commonly the nodes are regional and associated with bone or skin lesions.

B. Laboratory Findings: A *presumptive diagnosis* of Langerhans cell histiocytosis is warranted if Langerhans cells are seen in conventionally stained biopsy material and the specimen is interpreted as merely "consistent with Langerhans cell histiocytosis." A *diagnosis* is justified when these findings are supplemented by the presence of 2 or more of the following: positive stain for adenosine triphosphatase, S-100 protein, or α-D-mannosidase or characteristic binding of peanut lectin. *Definitive diagnosis* requires the finding of Birbeck granules (Fig 44–21) in lesional cells by electron microscopy or demonstration of CD2 antigenic determinants on lesional cells in a consistent clinical setting.

Treatment & Prognosis

Patients with Langerhans cell histiocytosis may be categorized into 3 groups: (1) localized disease (sin-

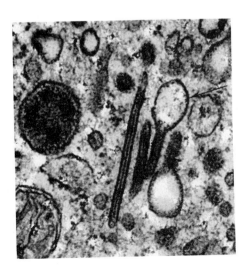

Figure 44–21. Electron micrograph of normal Langerhans cell. There are 4 Langerhans cell granules in close apposition. Arrow points to vesicle at the end of one of these granules, producing a tennis racket-like structure. ×70,000. (Reproduced, with permission, from Sagebiel RW, Reed TH: Serial reconstruction of the characteristic granule of the Langerhans cell. J Cell Biol 1968;36:595.)

gle bone lesion with or without associated soft tissue mass or regional lymphadenopathy, or skin only), (2) multifocal disease (predominantly bone and skin) without organ dysfunction, and (3) multifocal disease with organ dysfunction (most often liver, spleen, and lungs).

Solitary bone lesions are treated by surgical excision or curettage or by low-dose radiation therapy. Skin lesions are treated topically as needed. Patients with multifocal disease but without organ dysfunction are treated by surgery, chemotherapy, or local radiation. Patients with multifocal disease with organ dysfunction are usually treated with combination chemotherapy, including such drugs as vinblastine, prednisone, methotrexate, cyclophosphamide, and mercaptopurine. In a recent report, etoposide was found to have quite favorable results in this group.

The prognosis for survival for patients with localized disease is excellent. The probability of 5-year survival for patients with multifocal disease without organ dysfunction is approximately 95%, but for such patients with organ dysfunction this drops to approximately 30%. The closer the onset of disease to the neonatal period, the worse the prognosis.

SINUS HISTIOCYTOSIS WITH MASSIVE LYMPHADENOPATHY

Approximately 80% of cases of sinus histiocytosis with massive lymphadenopathy occur in the first 2 decades. Males and blacks are predisposed. The disorder is most often seen in Africa and the West Indies. The cause is unknown.

Patients typically present with cervical and commonly other adenopathy. They usually have fever, anemia, leukocytosis with neutrophilia, an elevated erythrocyte sedimentation rate, and polyclonal hypergammaglobulinemia. Extranodal involvement occurs in 8–12% of cases. The most common sites are the eyes, upper respiratory tract, skin, and bone.

Skin lesions may be the presenting sign of this syndrome even though they occur in only about 9% of cases. These include macules, papules, plaques, and nodules. In most cases the lesions are multiple.

Lymph node histology reveals expansion of the sinuses by large, foamy histiocytes and plasma cells. These collections may form nodules that focally replace the cortex. Some histiocytes may contain phagocytosed lymphocytes.

In the skin, a dermal and at times subdermal infiltrate is composed primarily of large, foamy histiocytes, plasma cells, and small lymphocytes. Phagocytosed lymphocytes may be present.

The clinical course in many patients is that of spontaneous regression over a period of months or years. However, in one large series, only about 10% actually became disease-free, and at least 7% died. Overall, intensive treatment has not been offered because there is a tendency toward spontaneous remission. Intralesional steroids have been effective for skin lesions. Systemic steroids, chemotherapy, and irradiation have helped patients with nodal enlargement.

REFERENCES

Abel EA et al: PUVA treatment of erythrodermic and plaque-type mycosis fungoides: Ten-year follow-up study. Arch Dermatol 1987;123:897.

Brodell RT, Santa Cruz DJ: Cutaneous pseudolymphomas. Dermatol Clin 1985;3:719.

Chan HL et al: Cutaneous manifestations of adult T cell leukemia/lymphoma: Report of three different forms. J Am Acad Dermatol 1985;13:213.

Coupe MO, Whittaker SJ, Thatcher N: Multicentric reticulohistiocytosis. Br J Dermatol 1987;116:245.

Dehner LP: Regressing atypical histiocytosis: The controversy continues. Arch Dermatol 1988;124:319.

Edelson R et al: Treatment of cutaneous T cell lymphoma by extracorporeal photochemotherapy: Preliminary results. N Engl J Med 1987;316:297.

Ganesan TS et al: Angioimmunoblastic lymphadenopathy: A clinical, immunological and molecular study. Br J Cancer 1987;55:437.

Gibson LE et al: Follicular mucinosis: Clinical and histopathologic study. J Am Acad Dermatol 1989;20:441.

Jambrosic J et al: Lymphomatoid granulomatosis. J Am Acad Dermatol 1987;17:621.

Lazar AP et al: Parapsoriasis and mycosis fungoides: The Northwestern University experience, 1970 to 1985. J Am Acad Dermatol 1989;21:919.

Neely SM: Adult T-cell leukemia-lymphoma. West J Med 1989;150:557.

Olsen EA, Crawford JR, Vollmer RT: Sinus histiocytosis with massive lymphadenopathy: Case report and review of a multisystem disease with cutaneous infiltrates. J Am Acad Dermatol 1988;18:1322.

Olsen EA et al: Interferon alfa-2a in the treatment of cutaneous T cell lymphoma. J Am Acad Dermatol 1989; 20:395.

Osband ME: Histiocytosis X: Langerhans' cell histiocytosis. Hematol Oncol Clin North Am 1987;1:737.

Patterson JW et al: Cutaneous involvement of multiple myeloma and extramedullary plasmacytoma. J Am Acad Dermatol 1988;19:879.

Ramsay DL, Halperin PS, Zeleniuch-Jacquotte A: Topical mechlorethamine therapy for early stage mycosis fungoides. J Am Acad Dermatol 1988;19:684.

Raney RB Jr, D'Angio GJ: Langerhans' cell histiocytosis (histiocytosis X): Experience at the Children's Hospital of Philadelphia, 1970–1984. Med Ped Oncol 1989;17:20.

Su WP, Buechner SA, Li CY: Clinicopathologic correlations in leukemia cutis. J Am Acad Dermatol 1984; 11:121.

Thomsen K, Wantzin GL: Lymphomatoid papulosis: A follow-up study of 30 patients. J Am Acad Dermatol 1987;17:632.

Toonstra J et al: Jessner's lymphocytic infiltration of the skin: A clinical study of 100 patients. Arch Dermatol 1989;125:1525.

Van Vloten WA, De Vroome H, Noordijk EM: Total skin electron beam irradiation for cutaneous T cell lymphoma (mycosis fungoides). Br J Dermatol 1985;112:697.

Vandervalk P, Meijer CJ: Cutaneous histiocytic proliferations. Dermatol Clin 1985;3:705.

White RM, Patterson JW: Cutaneous involvement in Hodgkin's disease. Cancer 1985;55:1136.

Wick MR et al: Cutaneous malignant histiocytosis: A clinical and histopathologic study of eight cases, with immunohistochemical analysis. J Am Acad Dermatol 1983; 8:50.

Wood GS et al: The immunologic and clinicopathologic heterogeneity of cutaneous lymphomas other than mycosis fungoides. Blood 1983;62:464.

Zackheim HS, Epstein EH Jr: Low-dose methotrexate for the Sézary syndrome. J Am Acad Dermatol 1989; 21:757.

Zackheim HS et al: Topical carmustine (BCNU) for mycosis fungoides and related disorders: A 10-year experience. J Am Acad Dermatol 1983;9:363.

Section VIII:
Dermatologic Trauma

Physical Injuries to the Skin

45

Robert R. Walther, MD, FACP & Leonard C. Harber, MD

INJURIES DUE TO COLD

Prolonged exposure to cold has 2 major effects on the skin: (1) Decreased skin temperature leads to localized vasoconstriction and loss of sensation associated with leakage of plasma from the vessels, hemoconcentration, and formation of small blood clots. Prolonged constriction and blockage of small vessels lead to local anoxia. (2) At freezing temperatures, small ice crystals form in the extracellular fluid. The increased tissue osmotic pressure causes direct cell damage as water is drawn out of the cell.

PERNIO
(Chilblain)

Pernio, or chilblain, is a type of injury in which the tissues are damaged by cold without being frozen. Most commonly seen in young women, pernio is a vasospastic response of acral areas (nose, pinna, fingers and toes). After an initial vasoconstrictive phase, the cooled skin undergoes a second (rewarming) phase manifested as erythematous or cyanotic doughy nodules and plaques. The bilaterally symmetric lesions may appear hours after rewarming and last for days to weeks. Burning, itching, or pain is common. Repeated episodes may lead to chronic pernio that persists throughout the winter.

Pernio may be prevented or improved by living in a warm climate or wearing adequate clothing. Acute lesions may be treated with bed rest and gentle rewarming in a 105 °F (40.6 °C) bath. The patient with chronic pernio must avoid exposure to cold. Vasodilators may provide some benefit (eg, nicotinic acid, 100 mg 3 times daily or nifedipine, 10–20 mg 3 times daily).

IMMERSION FOOT

Immersion foot is another type of cold injury in which freezing of tissue does not occur. The name is appropriate, since the disorder usually occurs in feet exposed to cold water for hours to days. Similar injury may follow prolonged exposure to tepid water (trench foot) or warm water (tropical immersion foot); the mechanism of injury is thought to be permeation of water through the stratum corneum.

Symptoms appear in 3 stages. During the wet stage, the skin gradually becomes swollen, anesthetic, and white or blue. Peripheral pulses are more difficult to palpate. As the extremity dries and becomes warm, the second, or hyperemic, stage occurs associated with intense pain, redness, bounding pulses, and anhidrosis. In severe cases, blisters and gangrene may develop. This stage may last several weeks before the third, or recovery, phase supervenes to persist for months to years. The pulses and color of the extremity return to normal, but the skin remains hyperesthetic to heat and cold. Blisters form easily, and the skin becomes atrophic. Hyperhidrosis is common, and Raynaud's phenomenon may occur.

Keeping the feet dry prevents immersion foot. During the hyperemic stage, rewarming the foot at room temperature while the skin is protected from trauma is crucial; keeping manipulation of the skin to a minimum prevents further tissue damage. Debridement is inadvisable during the early stages.

The recovery stage may be long. Physical therapy should be started, and the patient should wear shoes for protection. Surgical sympathectomy may be required if resolution of vasospasm and hyperhidrosis does not occur.

FROSTBITE

True freezing injury results from formation of ice crystals in the skin, usually associated with fatigue,

541

accident, hypoxemia (eg, at high altitudes), or alcoholic intoxication. It rarely occurs in a properly clothed acclimatized individual. Maximal tissue damage occurs if the tissue is frozen rapidly and rewarmed slowly.

Clinical Findings

Frostnip is the earliest stage of frostbite and is reversible. The skin suddenly turns white, may actually look frosty, and often has diminished sensation. Another person may recognize the early stages of frostnip more easily than the patient can, and the condition is then readily relieved by drying and rewarming, which may often be achieved by direct contact with warm skin (eg, placing the hands in the axillae or on the abdomen).

Frostnip quickly progresses to true **frostbite,** with permanent damage if exposure to cold continues. The skin becomes anesthetic, white, and increasingly hard as the depth of frozen tissue increases.

If slow rewarming or repeated freeze-thaw cycles have occurred, the affected part usually appears mottled, cyanotic, or gray. It is at this stage that most patients with frostbite first present to a physician. The skin is edematous, and blisters may form after several days. A gangrenous eschar may develop 1–2 weeks later, with sharp demarcation at the border of healthy tissue (Fig 45–1). Gangrene is usually dry unless there is secondary infection.

Rapid rewarming of patients with frostbite often lessens or prevents permanent cutaneous damage. Frozen skin becomes erythematous, with severe burning pain. Blisters develop within hours or days, and the fluid is reabsorbed over the following week. Although a black eschar is present, underlying tissue may not be gangrenous. The eschar is shed in 4–8 weeks, revealing tender, hyperesthetic, atrophic skin. Hyperhidrosis is common and may last several months. Permanent damage is often minimal.

Prevention

Frostbite can be avoided by limiting exposure to the cold and minimizing aggravating factors such as hypoxemia, fatigue, dampness, wind, smoking, and use of alcohol, phenothiazines, or tricyclic antidepressants. A buddy system in appropriate environmental circumstances is helpful not only to detect early frostnip but also to make frequent assessments of the level of sensation on the face and extremities and thereby note any alterations. The "buddy" touches the nose, fingers, and toes every 15 minutes to ascertain that touch sensation is present.

Treatment

A. Acute Measures: Rapid rewarming of patients with frostbite will often lessen or prevent cutaneous damage. The affected area should remain frozen until the patient is safe from the possibility of refreezing. Rapid rewarming may be performed with baths or

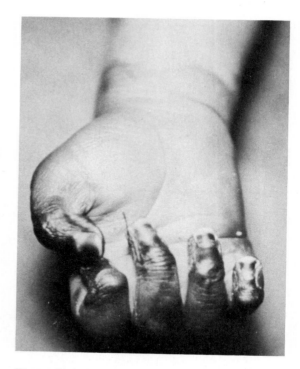

Figure 45–1. Frostbite with sharply demarcated border of the eschar at the wrist.

soaks using water heated to 105–108 °F (40.6–42.2 °C). Actual measurement of water temperature is highly desirable, since higher temperatures than these may cause increased loss of tissue. Rubbing of the skin or the use of snow, cold water, or dry heat is not recommended. A cradle over the extremities will prevent pressure, pain, and further injury.

B. General Measures: During the interval following rewarming until the eschar separates from the wound—perhaps 1 month later—minimal manipulation should be performed. Blisters should be left intact and cotton pledgets placed between affected digits. Measures to prevent infection are necessary and may include application of antibiotic creams. Analgesia, sedation, and psychologic support should be provided as necessary. Surgery is indicated only if the eschar is strangling the limb or is grossly infected. Debridement may lead to more extensive and permanent loss of tissue. Amputation should not be considered until it is definitely established that the tissues are dead.

The use of anticoagulants, arteriograms, vasodilators, and low-molecular-weight dextran early in treatment remains controversial.

Prognosis

The prognosis of any frostbite injury is in doubt during the early stages of recovery. Permanent damage is usually much less severe than suggested by the early blister and eschar, and the underlying skin may heal spontaneously even after several months. Paresthesias and cold hypersensitivity may persist indefinitely. Carcinoma developing in a frostbite scar occurs infrequently.

RAYNAUD'S PHENOMENON

Essentials of Diagnosis
- Paroxysms of pallor followed first by cyanosis and then by erythema of the digits.
- Attacks precipitated by exposure to cold and emotional stress.

General Considerations
Raynaud's phenomenon is a nonocclusive vasospastic response to cold characterized by decreased blood flow and resulting cyanosis of the digits. It is most often a clinical sign of a wide variety of underlying conditions (Table 45–1). When it is idiopathic or primary, it is called Raynaud's disease.

Clinical Findings
The initial pallor quickly gives way to cyanosis. Acrocyanosis, accompanied by pain of varying severity, lasts for a variable length of time before reactive hyperemia occurs. In some patients, the hyperemic stage is short or subtle. Pulses remain intact. Submersion of the digits in ice water may precipitate an attack. Laboratory studies may reveal abnormal blood proteins or evidence of connective tissue disease (Table 45–1).

Gangrene and loss of digits are unusual; however, small depressed pits may appear in the pulpy tips of the digits after many years of chronic involvement.

Prevention & Treatment
The patient with Raynaud's phenomenon should be evaluated for the existence of associated underlying conditions (Table 45–1), and appropriate treatment of the primary disease should be started.

Patients must avoid exposure to cold and routine handling of cold foods and beverages. They should be taught practical ways to stay warm if exposure to cold is unavoidable—eg, air is an excellent insulator, so multiple layers of thin garments are much more effective in containing natural heat than is a single thick garment. Fur, whether artificial or real, also traps layers of air when used to line garments. Battery-powered mittens with heating elements and hand-warmers are available. Moisture increases heat loss and should be avoided; synthetic materials that allow perspiration to collect should not be worn. Damp clothing should be changed. Constrictive garments compromise blood flow. There should be no exposure to the air where different garments meet, but bands and fasteners should not be so tight that they leave markings on the skin.

Table 45–1. Classification of conditions associated with Raynaud's phenomenon.

Primary
Raynaud's disease
Secondary
  Connective tissue diseases
    Progressive systemic sclerosis (scleroderma)
    Systemic lupus erythematosus
    Rheumatoid arthritis
    Dermatomyositis
    Polyarteritis
  Neurovascular compression
    Thoracic outlet syndrome
    Crutch pressure
    Carpal tunnel syndrome
  Arterial disease
    Thromboangitis obliterans
    Arteriosclerosis obliterans
    Thromboembolism
    Arteritis
  Blood abnormalities
    Cryoproteinemia
    Cold hemagglutinins
    Paraproteinemia
    Polycythemia
  Occupational
    Percussion and vibratory tool workers
    Polyvinyl chloride (acro-osteolysis)
  Drugs and toxins
    Ergot
    Methysergide
    Heavy metals
    Amphetamines
    Beta-blockers
    Bleomycin
    Clonidine
  Miscellaneous
    Causalgia
    Peripheral and central nervous system disease
    Hypothyroidism
    Pheochromocytoma
    Primary pulmonary hypertension
    Malignant disease
    Yellow nail syndrome
    Fabry's disease (angiokeratoma corporis diffusum)

Smoking causes peripheral vasoconstriction, and all patients at risk for peripheral vasospasm due to cold with or without Raynaud's disease should stop smoking.

Regional sympathectomy and vasodilators such as nifedipine, 10–20 mg 3 times daily, are useful.

INJURIES DUE TO HEAT*

THERMAL BURNS

Thermal burns are categorized by the depth of tissue damage (Fig 45–2; Table 45–2). **In superficial**

---

*Miliaria is discussed in Chapter 27.

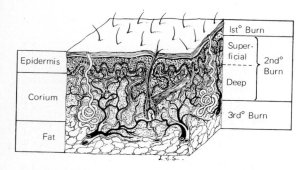

Figure 45–2. Layers of the skin showing depth of first-, second-, and third-degree burns. (Reproduced, with permission, from Way L (editor): *Current Surgical Diagnosis & Treatment,* 9th ed. Appleton & Lange, 1990.)

(first-degree) burns, the release of histamines, kinins, prostaglandins, and other mediators leads to vasodilation (redness), edema, and pain. There is no blistering, and healing usually occurs in 24–48 hours, often with desquamation. In **second-degree burns,** the epidermis and variable levels of the dermis are damaged. Pain and blister formation are common. Reepithelialization of burn ulcers occurs as keratinocytes divide and move out over the ulcer from hair follicles and the viable border. Healing usually occurs in 1–3 weeks with little or no scarring. **Third-degree burns** damage subcutaneous tissues so that there is necrosis of the epidermis, dermis, and subcutaneous structures. Muscle and bone may be involved, and the associated metabolic disturbances are profound. Considerable loss of fluids, electrolytes, and protein from the burned area occurs during the first 24 hours after injury. Third-degree burns are leathery and painless and require skin grafting to prevent contractures.

Complications

Secondary infection of a burn wound is frequent and often inevitable. Infection may result in greater necrosis with deeper tissue destruction. In severe cases, sepsis may cause death. Deep burns may heal with contractures and loss of range of motion or function. The healed skin at a burn site often remains hypersensitive to trauma and sunlight.

Treatment

A. Emergency Measures:

1. Remove the patient from the source of heat and extinguish any flames. Remove smoldering clothing.

2. Evaluate the patient's general condition, especially the airway, breathing, and circulation. Evaluate other medical problems such as possible fractures.

3. Determine whether inhalation injury has occurred, and assess the extent of all second- or third-degree burns. Estimate the age of the patient. Estimate the severity of burns using a burn severity index. When more than 5% of the body surface is burned or when vital structures are involved, the patient should be hospitalized and treated by specialists in burn management. Nonspecialist physicians in such cases should limit themselves to providing supportive emergency care (eg, maintain the airway, provide intravenous volume replacement therapy) before the patient is transferred.

4. Cool the burn; if it is small, it should be immersed in cool water to help dissipate excessive heat rapidly and prevent extension of the burn.

B. General Measures:

1. Patients with a history of tetanus immunization should receive a tetanus toxoid booster (0.5 mL). If no booster has been given during the preceding 5 years, a complete tetanus immunization regimen should be started.

2. Aspirin, acetaminophen, and codeine should be given as necessary to relieve pain.

3. Regular movement of the involved joints as well as physical therapy is helpful in preventing contractures.

4. Secondary infection should be treated appropriately. Prophylactic systemic antibiotics may lead to overgrowth of resistant organisms and should not be prescribed.

5. Patients with extensive burns should be moved to specialized burn treatment units for care and to receive needed fluid and electrolyte replacement.

Table 45–2. Characteristics of burns of different depths.

	Depth of Burn	Color and Appearance	Skin Texture	Capillary Refill	Pinprick Sensation	Healing
First-degree	First degree	Red	Normal	Yes	Yes	5–10 days; no scar
Second-degree	Superficial partial-thickness	Red; may be blistered	Edematous	Yes	Yes	10–14 days; no or minimal scar
	Deep partial-thickness	Pink to white	Thick	Possibly	Possibly	25–30 days; dense scar
Third-degree	Full thickness	White, black, or brown	Leathery	No	No	No spontaneous healing

C. Local Measures:

1. Clean small burns with a povidone-iodine or hexachlorophene solution.

2. Debride large blisters and necrotic tissue daily.

3. Apply silver sulfadiazine or other antibacterial ointment 3–4 times daily and cover with sterile gauze. Soiled dressings should be changed more often.

ERYTHROMELALGIA
(Erythermalgia)

Erythromelalgia is a rare episodic disorder characterized by paroxysmal bilateral erythema, increased skin temperature, and burning pain of the extremities. It is usually precipitated by *increased* ambient temperature. Erythromelalgia may be idiopathic or may be associated with myeloproliferative and musculoskeletal disorders. Treatment with salicylates, sedatives, methysergide, propranolol, and surgery has generally been ineffective. Staying in areas with lower room temperatures and avoiding exercise, vasodilator agents, and vasodilating stimuli may decrease the frequency of attacks.

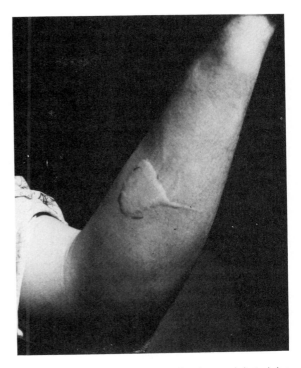

Figure 45–3. Wheal of cold urticaria precipitated by placing an ice cube on the patient's arm. Note the pattern created when ice water ran down the arm.

URTICARIA

PHYSICAL URTICARIA

Urticaria (wheals or hives) may appear in areas exposed to heat, cold, pressure, or light (Fig 45–3) (see Chapter 34). The lesions usually appear within minutes after exposure. The diagnosis is confirmed by careful history taking and provocative challenge tests using the appropriate physical stimulus. Severe episodes may result in abdominal pain, wheezing, and cardiovascular collapse.

Avoidance of known stimuli is often the only satisfactory treatment. Antihistamines and anticholinergic agents provide inconsistent relief.

CHOLINERGIC URTICARIA

Urticaria precipitated by heat, exercise, or emotional stress is known as cholinergic urticaria. Within minutes after exposure, small pruritic wheals 1–3 mm in diameter appear. Each is surrounded by a large flare of erythema that may be several centimeters wide. Unlike other forms of urticaria, the wheals do not become confluent. In severe cases, there may be nausea, wheezing, dyspnea, and abdominal pain.

Provocative exercise testing to induce sweating is the most sensitive test for cholinergic urticaria.

Oral antihistamines and avoidance of precipitating stimuli are the best treatment. Hydroxyzine, 25–50 mg 4 times daily, has been suggested as the best antihistamine. Occasionally, anticholinergic agents such as glycopyrrolate, 1–2 mg 3 times daily, seem to help.

INJURY DUE TO PRESSURE

CALLUSES & CORNS

Recurrent pressure or friction on the skin causes thickening of the stratum corneum. A callus is a circumscribed thickening of stratum corneum involving the total area of friction. A corn (clavus) is formed by pressure over a bony prominence or abnormal bony growth, eg, exostosis or spur, and is actually a cone-shaped hyperkeratosis. Corns are often surrounded by callus.

Clinical Findings

Corns are almost always tender, whereas calluses become painful only when they are very thick or fissured. The plantar surface is the most commonly affected location. However, calluses can form on any area subjected to recurrent pressure or friction. Paring the stratum corneum with a sharp scalpel aids in making the proper diagnosis, because in a callus, the thickened horn will be removed to reveal skin with normal dermatoglyphics; in a corn, the skin markings approach the core and divide to encircle it. Further paring will release the core, which can then be lifted out as a plug. **Soft corns** are found between the toes (usually the fourth and fifth toes) and lack the hard point. If thrombosed vessels (resembling black seeds) appear and are followed by multiple bleeding points, the lesion is probably a wart.

The initial thickening of the stratum corneum is a protective response. Pain and fissuring result if pressure persists and the process continues. In intertriginous areas where maceration is common (eg, soft corns between the toes), secondary bacterial or fungal infection may occur. Chronic pain may lead to changes in posture or walking with accompanying muscle strain.

Prevention & Treatment

Elimination of the friction or pressure often produces relief and permanent cure. In other cases, surgical removal of the corn and bony focus is required. Special orthoses to redistribute pressure are often of benefit.

The thickened horny layer can be removed with a sharp scalpel or file after the corn has been soaked in warm water for some time. Daily application of keratolytics such as salicylic acid plasters 40%, urea cream 20%, or salicylic acid 16.7% and lactic acid 16.7% in collodion (Duofilm) slowly removes the hyperkeratosis if the source of pressure has been eliminated.

DECUBITUS ULCERS

Decubitus ulcers, or pressure sores, form over bony prominences, especially the ischial tuberosities, heels, sacrum, and elbows, in patients who are debilitated, paralyzed, or unconscious. Decubitus ulcers result from unrelieved pressure that compromises capillary blood flow, and they may occur after only a few hours of pressure to vulnerable points. Ischemia leads to tissue death and necrosis. Nutrition, age, the patient's general physical condition, and underlying infection may affect the necrotic process. Skilled nursing care and careful observation can prevent the development of most decubitus ulcers, but in many cases inanition and less than maximal care of early lesions lead to chronic ulcers.

Clinical Findings

Early signs of impending decubitus ulcer are erythema and edema over a bony prominence that do not fade when pressure on the area is relieved. In untreated cases, blisters may form. After 24–48 hours, the epidermis sloughs, revealing a clean erosion (Fig 45–4). If damage is severe or repeated, the erosion deepens to form a yellow-gray eschar surrounded by erythema. Several days later, the dead tissue putrefies and becomes foul-smelling. Secondary bacterial infection is common and increases the extent of the ulcer. Later, the ulcer may become deep and undermined and show signs of dry gangrene.

Much of the pressure damage occurs below the surface of the skin; it is usually greater than it appears. Necrosis and infection may extend into bones (osteomyelitis), joints (septic arthritis), vessels (septicemia, hemorrhage), or body cavities such as the rectum or vagina.

Prevention

Any means of avoiding constant pressure to an area of skin is desirable. Inspection of the skin several times daily often reveals potential areas of ulcer formation. Any area showing redness or early erosion should be protected.

Bedridden patients should be turned every 2 hours so that their weight is distributed over the largest possible surface area; front-to-back turning is not necessarily required but rather a shift of weight to other bony prominences. When patients are confined to a chair, they should be moved every 10–15 minutes.

The skin should be kept clean and dry; urine and feces should be promptly removed before they irritate the skin. It is helpful to dry the skin gently. Dusting

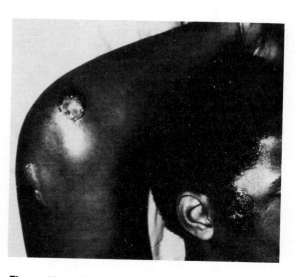

Figure 45–4. Decubitus ulcer. Blisters around the elbow and erosions on the temple in a patient found comatose 2 days previously.

powders (talc, Zeasorb) absorb remaining moisture and are helpful prophylactically.

Many mechanical devices aid in distributing pressure more effectively. Sheepskins, water and air mattresses, and foam rings can be used; however, they tend to soil easily and increase perspiration. Newer beds using air-supported glass beads (Clinitron) provide more effective distribution of weight.

Treatment

A. General Measures: It is crucial to relieve pressure as described above. In debilitated patients, wounds heal poorly even under the best nursing conditions. Dietary intake must be adequate. Hyperalimentation or total parenteral nutrition by gastric tube or intravenous catheter should be considered.

B. Surgical Measures: Necrotic tissue and eschar must be removed with a scissors or forceps or more slowly with a wet-to-dry dressing—saline-soaked gauze packed into the ulcer and allowed to dry. Necrotic tissue is extracted from the wound as the gauze is removed 3 or 4 times daily.

Formation of granulation tissue and subsequent reepithelialization may require many weeks. In some patients, primary closure, grafts, or skin flaps are warranted.

C. Topical Measures: The large number of topical preparations available for the treatment of decubitus ulcers is some indication of the difficulties of treatment. No topical preparation is a substitute for surgical debridement of the eschar or restoration of normal blood flow.

1. Elements– Zinc, gold leaf, and hyperbaric oxygen are of limited value in the treatment of decubitus ulcers and more useful in ulcers due to vascular insufficiency.

2. Antibiotics– Silver sulfadiazine may prevent overgrowth of gram-negative organisms. Other antibiotics fail to penetrate the wound and often cause secondary contact dermatitis.

3. Enzymes– Collagenase, streptokinase, and fibrinolysin (Elase) can be used to dissolve different components of necrotic tissue but are ineffective in removing thick eschar.

4. Dextran polymers– Small hydrophilic beads of dextran polymers (Debrisan) may be placed in ulcers several times daily. They absorb large amounts of serum and draw bacteria, debris, and inflammatory exudates out of the wound.

5. Synthetic dressings– Semipermeable films (Duoderm, Opsite, Tegaderm) may be used to provide the occlusive environment that favors reepithelialization. These or the nonpermeable films (Duoderm, Vigilon) are applied to the wound and usually changed after several days.

RADIODERMATITIS

Essentials of Diagnosis
- History of repeated or massive exposure to ionizing radiation.
- Diffuse atrophy, telangiectasias, pigmentary alteration, or ulceration.

General Considerations

The skin may be exposed to ionizing radiation accidentally or deliberately (eg, during radiation therapy of skin lesions and deeper tumors). In both cases, energy transmitted to individual cells leads to cell death, injury, and alteration of cellular DNA. The amount of radiation delivered to the skin depends on the type of radiation (eg, x-rays, gamma rays, neutrons). The higher-energy radiation used to treat deep tumors may actually deliver less total energy to the skin and result in fewer cutaneous reactions than the "softer" x-rays used to treat dermatologic conditions. The dermatologic reaction correlates with the total dose and rate of delivery as well as the type of radiation and amount of backscatter.

Chronic radiodermatitis and its sequelae appear years to decades after radiation exposure. While radiation therapy for cancer is often remembered by a patient, radiation treatments for acne, hirsutism, or benign dermatoses are often forgotten.

Clinical Findings

A. Radiation Erythema: Irradiation of the skin with a dose of 300–400 cGy causes transient erythema lasting 24–72 hours. A longer-lasting erythema follows in 1 week and may not fade for another week. Hyperpigmentation due to excessive melanin production then occurs. Usually no significant discomfort is present.

B. Acute Radiodermatitis: Acute radiodermatitis can be expected whenever a patient undergoes radiation therapy for cancer. It may also reflect accidental overexposure to radiation. In acute radiodermatitis, the radiation erythema described above does not regress but progresses to an acute inflammatory reaction by the second week; it is characterized by blisters, crusting, and pain (Fig 45–5). The red hue may darken and become violaceous. As inflammation decreases and healing occurs during the succeeding months, an atrophic hypopigmented scar with telangiectasias appears. Hair and sweat glands may be permanently lost.

C. Chronic Radiodermatitis: Years to decades after exposure to large amounts of therapeutic or accidental radiation, a slowly progressive chronic radiodermatitis appears. Atrophy of the skin increases, with telangiectasias and mottled hyper- and hypopigmentation (Fig 45–6). The skin is dry and easily in-

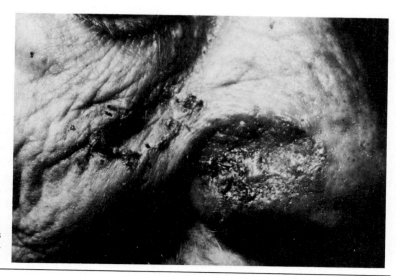

Figure 45–5. Acute radiodermatitis of the nose with erythema and crusting at the site of radiotherapy.

jured, and it heals slowly. Hair is absent, and sweat and sebaceous glands are diminished or absent in exposed areas.

Complications

Epilation and transient alopecia may follow 300–400 cGy of cutaneous superficial radiation. Larger amounts may cause permanent hair loss. Painful ulcers that do not heal may require surgical treatment, including wide excision and grafting.

An increased incidence of skin cancer is noted in areas of chronic radiodermatitis. The possibility of malignant change must be considered in any ulcer that does not heal. Basal cell carcinomas are the most common cancer. When squamous cell carcinomas develop in radiation ulcers, they are often aggressive and have a higher incidence of metastases than those

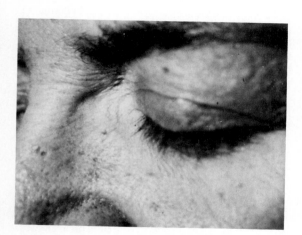

Figure 45–6. Chronic radiodermatitis of the inner canthus with telangiectasias.

induced by solar radiation. The damage due to ionizing radiation may be compounded by its synergistic action with other forms of radiation, as seen in the increased number of basal cell and squamous cell carcinomas in patients receiving psoralen and ultraviolet light therapy (PUVA) who have had previous radiation therapy.

A slightly increased incidence of benign and malignant tumors in the thyroid gland has been noted following exposure to x-ray irradiation in patients treated for dermatoses of the face and neck and more so in patients whose thymus or adenoids have been irradiated. These tumors can be avoided if the neck is properly shielded during radiation therapy.

Reactions resembling erythema multiforme have been reported during radiation therapy.

Prevention

Therapies other than radiation should be considered for treatment of nonmalignant skin disorders. Judicious use of therapeutic ionizing radiation and effective radiation safety measures can prevent unnecessary radiation damage.

Treatment

Acute radiodermatitis should be treated conservatively with cool tap water soaks and protective dressings. Bland emollients, shake lotions, or witch hazel lotions help relieve pruritus. Mild analgesics may help. Trauma to the area—especially mechanical rubbing—should be avoided. Secondary infection is treated with appropriate antibiotics. Topical corticosteroid creams are of little or no benefit.

Prognosis

Chronic radiodermatitis requires no special care. Affected sites should be protected as much as possible from physical trauma and solar radiation. The appearance of chronic radiodermatitis and associated scars usually worsens with time. Biopsy should be performed in ulcers that do not heal in order to rule out malignant degeneration.

REFERENCES

Agris J, Spira M: Pressure ulcers: Prevention and treatment. Clin Symp 1979;**31.** [Entire issue.]

Christenson C, Stewart C: Frostbite. Am Fam Physician (Dec) 1984;**30:**111.

Dressler DP, Hozid JL, Nathan P: The minor burn. Pages 177-189 in: *Thermal Injury.* Mosby, 1988.

Hirschmann JV et al: Cholinergic urticaria: A clinical and histologic study. Arch Dermatol 1987;**123:**462.

Hood IC, Young JE: Late sequelae of superficial irradiation. Head Neck Surg 1984;**7:**65.

Knight AL: Medical management of pressure sores. J Fam Pract 1988;**27:**95.

Lange RL: Current concepts in clinical therapeutics: Pressure sores. Clin Pharm 1986;**5:**69.

Porter EC, Wadsworth RC: Generalized skin eruptions during radiation therapy. J Maine Med Assoc 1976;**67:**267.

Purdue GF, Hunt JL: Cold injury: A collective review. J Burn Care Rehabil 1986;**7:**331.

Xakellis GC Jr, Garzone P: Pressure ulcers. Am Fam Physician (April) 1987;**35:**159.

46

Occupational Dermatoses

Charles Gordon Toby Mathias, MD

The skin, by virtue of its large surface area directly exposed to the environment, is particularly vulnerable to occupationally induced disease. Excluding injuries (eg, sprains, broken bones, laceration), which comprise 95% of all occupational disease, dermatoses account for nearly half of all remaining occupational illnesses. One-fourth of all workers affected by occupational skin disease lose an average of 10–12 workdays. New industrial chemicals and manufacturing processes give rise to new skin hazards and disease in the workplace. The physician can only try to keep abreast of what is going on in the work environments of his patients so that new hazards can be anticipated and dealt with appropriately.

Clues to the possibility that skin disease in a given patient may be due to occupational exposures are set forth in Table 46–1. Skin diseases in the workplace may be caused by specific occupational exposures regardless of patient factors; the age, sex, and race of the patient, environmental temperature and humidity, and personal cleanliness may be important contributing factors; and preexisting or latent skin disease may be aggravated or triggered by occupational exposures. Ultimately, the diagnosis is based not only on medical data but also on technical information about industrial processes and job performance. Because the patient may be unable to identify all exposures, it may be necessary to communicate with supervisors or safety personnel or to personally inspect the workplace. A visit is especially useful when several cases of alleged occupational skin disease have occurred. Once a list of exposures has been obtained, further technical or toxicologic information from manufacturers may be needed.

The physical examination must distinguish primarily acquired occupational skin disease from other

Table 46–1. Clues to occupational dermatoses.

1. Relevant history of occupational exposure.
2. Logical time relationship between exposure and onset of skin disease.
3. Exposure capable of producing the observed skin disease.
4. Clinical morphology and anatomic distribution compatible with skin disease caused by suspected exposure.
5. Specific diagnositc investigations, such as patch testing, show probable causal relationship.
6. Elimination of suspected causative exposure usually leads to remission or improvement of skin disease.

Table 46–2. Clinical classification of occupational skin disease

1. Systemic disease due to percutaneous absorption
2. Contact dermatitis
3. Photosensitivity disorders
4. Acne
5. Disorders of pigmentation
6. Urticaria
7. Neoplastic disorders
8. Connective tissue diseases
9. Granulomatous reactions
10. Disorders of hair and nails
11. Infections and infestations
12. Disorders caused by physical and mechanical agents

conditions that may be unrelated to or perhaps aggravated by a specific workplace exposure. A complete skin examination (Chapter 6) is usually necessary. Clinical features and diagnostic investigations should be compatible with an appropriate history of exposure before a diagnosis of occupational skin disease is made.

Although elimination of the causative exposure usually leads to improvement or remission of occupational skin diseases, this is not always the case. Severe or long-standing dermatitis may be extremely slow to resolve and may become permanent.

There are essentially 12 categories or types of occupational skin disease (Table 46–2). Each of them is discussed in the following pages.

COMMON OCCUPATIONAL DERMATOSES

SYSTEMIC DISEASE DUE TO PERCUTANEOUS ABSORPTION

Skin absorption is an important route of exposure for many substances that may produce important systemic toxicologic effects and may be the principal route of exposure for agricultural pesticides. Development of symptoms depends not only on inherent toxicity and the quantitative extent of exposure but also on the ability of the offending substance to penetrate the protective skin barrier.

Some important substances that may produce toxic systemic symptoms following percutaneous absorption from occupational exposure are listed in Table 46–3.

Pathogenesis

As a general rule, substances with molecular weights greater than 1000 are poorly absorbed through the skin. Physical alterations of the stratum corneum may increase percutaneous absorption of smaller molecules and facilitate penetration by larger ones, enhancing toxicity (see Chapter 2). Percutaneous absorption of toxic substances may be enhanced by (1) increases in stratum corneum hydration following entrapment of a substance against the skin surface by water-impermeable material (eg, protective clothing, rubber gloves); (2) damage to the stratum corneum by a local corrosive or caustic effect of the penetrating substance itself or the solvent in which it is dissolved; (3) contact with skin already "damaged" by cuts, abrasions, or preexisting dermatitis; and (4) contact with anatomic areas of skin that are most permeable (eg, genital, eyelid, and facial skin). Solvents may increase their own toxicity by damaging the stratum corneum and enhancing their percutaneous absorption. Visible inflammation (dermatitis) is not a necessary prerequisite for significant absorption. However, substances that also produce dermatitis may enhance their own toxicity.

Clinical Findings

Clinical findings depend on the systemic effects of the penetrating toxin (Table 46–3). A defective cutaneous barrier (eg, dermatitis, lacerations) may be evident at the principal site of penetration.

Table 46–3. Some important industrial chemicals with systemic toxicities following skin absorption.

Systemic Toxicity	Industrial Chemical
Methemoglobinemia, liver disease, bladder cancer	Aniline dyes
Peripheral neuritis, gastrointestinal and cardiac disturbances	Arsenic
Acute myelogenous leukemia, aplastic anemia, myelofibrosis	Benzene
Cellular asphyxia and death	Cyanide salts
Nephritis, gastroenteritis, central and peripheral nervous system abnormalities	Mercurials
Peripheral neuropathy	Methyl-*n*-butyl ketone
Liver disease, porphyria	Polyhalogenated aromatic hydrocarbons
Central nervous system abnormalities	Organic solvents
Cardiovascular, gastrointestinal, neuromuscular abnormalities	Neuromuscular insecticides

Differential Diagnosis

Symptoms of systemic toxicity must be distinguished from numerous other medical disorders. Once it has been established that symptoms are due to poisoning, the issue is whether it resulted from percutaneous absorption, inhalation, or ingestion. In clinical practice, this is a difficult determination and is usually based on circumstantial information about exposure.

Treatment

Treatment is directed primarily at reversing systemic symptoms caused by the toxin. In cases where the toxin is still on the skin, thorough washing is indicated. If the toxin may still be present in blister fluid, debridement and drainage should be performed.

Prognosis

Prognosis varies with the specific toxic exposure. Long-term effects such as carcinogenesis must be considered along with short-term effects.

CONTACT DERMATITIS

Essentials of Diagnosis

- Erythema and edema, sometimes accompanied by vesicles and bullae in area of contact with suspected agent.
- Later, weeping, crusting, or scaling.
- Sometimes a history of previous reaction to suspected contactant.
- Patch test with causal agent positive in the allergic form.

General Considerations

Approximately 90% of all occupationally acquired skin diseases are due to contact dermatitis. This is an inflammatory eczematous dermatitis induced by external contact of a substance or material with the skin surface. Most cases are due to skin irritation rather than contact allergy.

Commonly encountered industrial irritants include solvents, acids and alkalies, industrial detergents, and cleaning compounds, including abrasive soaps and waterless hand cleaners. Common occupational allergens include poison ivy or oak, metallic salts (nickel, gold, chromate, cobalt), rubber accelerators and antioxidants, epoxy resins and hardeners, acrylic resins, phenolic resins, biocidal agents used to preserve aqueous solutions and emulsifiers, and organic dyes such as *p*-phenylenediamine. Domestic sensitizers such as fragrances, cosmetic preservatives, and topical medications (eg, benzocaine, neomycin) may find their way into the workplace in the form of soaps, hand creams, and first-aid cabinet preparations.

Pathogenesis

A. Irritant Contact Dermatitis: Irritant contact dermatitis is caused by a direct local toxic effect on the skin surface and does not involve immunologic mechanisms. When effects are observed within minutes after skin contact following a brief skin exposure (eg, concentrated sulfuric acid), the injury is termed a **chemical burn.** Most industrial irritants are relatively weak and require frequent or prolonged skin contact before visible changes are induced. Factors that increase the quantitative degree of exposure and enhance percutaneous penetration (discussed above) will increase the potential for a given substance to provoke irritant contact dermatitis. Depending on the conditions under which skin exposure occurs, almost any substance encountered in the workplace may become an irritant. Workers are usually exposed to multiple potential skin irritants, and irritation may be a cumulative result of multiple exposures. Once skin inflammation has occurred, the skin barrier is compromised and the skin becomes even more susceptible to irritation.

B. Allergic Contact Dermatitis: Allergic contact dermatitis results from immunologic mechanisms involving cellular delayed hypersensitivity (see Chapter 33). Most allergens encountered in industry are relatively weak and require optimum circumstances of exposure in susceptible individuals before sensitization occurs. Months or years may pass before a reaction occurs. Thus, allergy often develops to long-standing contacts in a worker's environment rather than recently introduced substances. Once allergic sensitization has occurred, only minimal quantitative exposure may be necessary to sustain dermatitis.

Clinical Findings

Irritant contact dermatitis may be mild, the changes consisting only of dryness and chapping; or severe, with erythematous macules, papules, vesicles, bullae, and secondary exudation and crusting. The changes in allergic contact dermatitis are usually accompanied by moderate to severe inflammation. Both types may be associated with substantial itching, burning, or stinging, though burning and stinging are more characteristic of irritation.

Dermatitis usually involves areas of primary skin contact with the offending substance. Irritant contact dermatitis generally remains confined to these areas, while allergic contact dermatitis often tends to spread to areas remote from primary contact; spread may be facilitated by accidental contamination from the primary site of skin contact, indirect contact with vapors, or systemic absorption. Irritant and allergic contact dermatitis cannot usually be distinguished with confidence on morphologic grounds alone.

Patch testing should be used only for precise allergen identification. When properly performed, a positive test indicates delayed hypersensitivity (allergy) to the tested substance. Ingredients of chemical mixes may also need to be tested in order to identify the allergen precisely. (See Chapter 33 for details of patch testing and causes of false-positive and false-negative patch test results.)

The patch test is not useful in the diagnosis of irritant contact dermatitis. The conditions under which patch testing is performed (total occlusion beneath an impermeable material for 48 hours) are extreme. Many substances that produce an irritant reaction on patch testing may not produce irritant dermatitis under actual conditions of exposure, which are usually less extreme than the patch test. Thus, an irritant reaction on patch testing only indicates that under extreme conditions of actual exposure, a substance is capable of producing irritant dermatitis. A thorough understanding of the actual clinical conditions of exposure to a potential irritant is necessary before concluding that exposure actually caused the observed irritant dermatitis.

Differential Diagnosis

Occupational contact dermatitis must be distinguished from endogenous conditions (eg, atopic dermatitis, nummular eczema, seborrheic dermatitis, dyshidrosis, and psoriasis), from nonoccupational contact dermatitis, and from other exogenously acquired conditions (eg, tinea, scabies). Distribution and unusual or asymmetric patterns of skin involvement—together with an appropriate history of contact—help distinguish contact dermatitis from these other disorders; otherwise, differentiation may be difficult.

Treatment

The causative agent should be promptly identified and cutaneous exposure eliminated. Severe cases may be treated with an oral corticosteroid such as prednisone (initial dose 1 mg/kg), gradually tapering over a 2-week period. Alternatively, an injectable steroid such as triamcinolone acetonide, 40 mg once intragluteally, may be used. Topical steroids in the form of gels, creams, and ointments may be used on localized areas. High-potency topical corticosteroids are more useful when inflammation is moderate to severe. Gel and cream formulations absorb moisture and help to dry oozing, weeping vesicular dermatitis.

Prognosis

Approximately 25% of affected individuals fail to improve after developing contact dermatitis in the workplace despite protective measures and job modification. An additional 50% experience partial improvement, but only 25% experience complete healing. The reasons for this high failure rate are not known but probably reflect a combination of diagnostic failure, inadequate protection or job modification, and poorly understood endogenous factors in affected individuals.

PHOTOSENSITIVITY DISORDERS

Essentials of Diagnosis

- Erythema and edema, sometimes accompanied by vesicles and bullae, on sun-exposed surfaces.
- Later, weeping, crusting, or scaling.
- A history of sun exposure within 24 hours before onset of reaction.
- Photopatch test with causal agent positive in allergic form.

General Considerations

These disorders require for their expression activation of a chemical substance on the skin surface by ultraviolet or visible light. They usually present as acute sunburn or eczema on sun-exposed surfaces.

Polycyclic aromatic hydrocarbons, such as creosote and tar, cause immediate burning and stinging reactions following sun exposure; if severe, inflammation may follow. Severe bullous phototoxic reactions occur in celery harvesters, caused by a furocoumarin liberated from celery parasitized by a common agricultural fungus ("pink rot"). The newer polyfunctional UV-cured acrylic resins may produce phototoxic as well as photoallergic reactions. Photoallergy from vaporized epoxy resin may occur.

Pathogenesis

Chemical substances capable of producing these reactions generally have absorption spectra somewhere in the ultraviolet range and aromatic rings in their chemical formulas. Effects are produced through phototoxic or photoallergic mechanisms. Phototoxic reactions are analogous to irritant contact dermatitis and do not involve immunologic mechanisms (see Chapter 33).

Clinical Findings

Phototoxic reactions may cause stinging and burning sensations immediately upon sun exposure. Subclinical phototoxic reactions without visible inflammation or accompanying discomfort may produce striking, sometimes bizarre hyperpigmentation on sun-exposed surfaces. More severe phototoxic reactions may resemble acute sunburn and are occasionally bullous. Photoallergic reactions clinically resemble the eczematous changes of contact dermatitis. Inflammation typically affects sun-exposed cutaneous surfaces, with characteristic sparing of shielded areas such as the eyelids and inferior chin. Postinflammatory hyperpigmentation commonly follows.

Differential Diagnosis

Phototoxic and photoallergic eruptions from occupational exposure must be differentiated from endogenous photosensitive disorders (eg, porphyria, polymorphous light eruption, lupus erythematosus) and photosensitive drug eruptions. Further differentiation from other nonoccupational exogenous causes of pho-

totoxicity (eg, topical sunscreens, fragrances, halogenated salicylanilides) is necessary.

Treatment

Topical and systemic therapy is the same as for contact dermatitis. Efficient topical sunscreens containing p-aminobenzoic acid esters and benzophenones should be applied before anticipated exposure. Thick, opaque protective clothing is advisable.

Prognosis

Postinflammatory pigmentary changes may be slow to resolve following photosensitive eruptions. A state of persistent photosensitivity ("persistent light reactor") may exist in an occasional patient even after this photoallergen has been removed.

ACNE

Existing acne may be aggravated by tight-fitting masks or clothing ("acne mechanica"). Lubricating oils and greases may cause follicular irritation ("oil acne") resulting in comedonal plugging or a pustular folliculitis.

Chloracne—distinct from oil acne—is caused by specific exposure to various polyhalogenated aromatic hydrocarbons. Chloracne is a sensitive index of exposure to polyhalogenated aromatic hydrocarbons following topical exposure or ingestion and may be present in up to 95% of cases where toxic systemic symptoms (eg, hepatic disease) are present.

Oil acne is caused by heavy petroleum oils and greases. Chloracne may be caused by a variety of polyhalogenated aromatic hydrocarbons, including biphenyls (PCBs, PBBs), dibenzofurans, and 2,3,7,8-tetrachlorodibenzodioxin (dioxin).

Pathogenesis

The mechanism of induction of oil acne involves stimulation of follicular keratinization followed by ductal occlusion. In chloracne, the mechanism involves induction of squamous metaplasia of sebaceous gland ducts, followed by atrophy of the underlying sebaceous glands and subsequent formation of keratin-filled cysts. Chloracnegenic potential depends more on the stereoisomeric positioning of the halogen atoms than on the degree of halogenation. There is a correlation between chloracnegenic potential and ability to stimulate the aryl hydrocarbon hydroxylase system, with 2,3,7,8-tetrachlorodibenzodioxin being the most potent.

Clinical Findings

Oil acne is characterized by comedones and follicular papules and pustules, usually occurring in the hands and forearms, but may be severe on covered areas of the body if clothing is saturated with oil.

Chloracne is characterized by a predominance of

closed comedonal lesions, although some inflammatory pustules may be present, usually associated with the presence of almost pathognomonic noninflammatory, straw-colored cysts varying from 1 mm to 1 cm in size. The malar crescent area of the face may be first to develop lesions. In addition to usual acne areas, involvement of the ears and postauricular folds is common; covered areas outside the usual acne distribution may be involved in severe cases.

Differential Diagnosis

Oil acne and chloracne must be distinguished from acne vulgaris and bacterial folliculitis. The appearance of lesions outside the typical acne distribution is helpful in establishing the diagnosis. A history of exposure is necessary. Occurrences of chloracne have usually been associated with massive exposures, such as industrial accidents or contamination during manufacture.

Treatment

Personal hygiene measures aimed at elimination of skin and clothing contact with offending oils and greases are most effective in the management of oil acne. Topical benzoyl peroxide preparations may also be beneficial. Chloracne is more resistant to treatment and does not respond well to systemic antibiotics and topical benzoyl peroxide. Topical vitamin A analogues, such as retinoic acid creams or gels (Retin-A), may be useful. The effectiveness of oral vitamin A is sporadic; newer oral vitamin A analogues (isotretinoin) have been anecdotally effective. In some cases, acne surgery is the most effective treatment.

Prognosis

Oil acne usually resolves spontaneously when exposure to irritating oil or grease is eliminated. New chloracne lesions usually cease to form within 6 months following cessation of exposure, but existing lesions often resolve slowly and may persist indefinitely.

DISORDERS OF PIGMENTATION

Melanin synthesis may be stimulated or inhibited and the melanocytes injured or destroyed by a variety of specific or nonspecific occupational exposures.

Postinflammatory hyperpigmentation or hypopigmentation may follow any episode of contact dermatitis. Some occupational photosensitizers—particularly tar, pitch, and furocoumarins—may increase pigmentation when combined with sun exposure, even without causing overt dermatitis.

Depigmentation resembling idiopathic vitiligo ("toxic vitiligo," "chemical leukoderma") may be caused by occupational exposure to a variety of phenolic or catecholic derivatives. A partial list includes

p-tertiary butylphenol, p-tertiary butylcatechol, p-tertiary amylphenol, hydroquinone, and monobenzyl ether of hydroquinone. These chemicals function as antioxidants or germicidal disinfectants and may be encountered with exposure to rubber, photographic developing solutions, lubricating oils, plastic or adhesive resins, and hospital, institutional, or industrial cleaning solutions.

Chronic systemic intoxication from various heavy metals (eg, silver, mercury) may be associated with discoloration of the skin. Direct chemical staining of the skin may occur from a variety of external organic dyes or other substances. Explosive or abrasive forces may cause adventitious tattooing by embedding pigmented foreign material in the skin.

Pathogenesis

A. Postinflammatory Hyperpigmentation: Postinflammatory hyperpigmentation is due to the accumulation of melanin (from injured melanocytes) or hemosiderin (from extravasated red blood cells following blood vessel damage) in the dermis. Increased pigmentation from coal tar and furocoumarins is caused by enhanced melanin production by melanocyte and distribution into surrounding keratinocytes in the epidermis.

B. Postinflammatory Hypopigmentation: Postinflammatory hypopigmentation occurs when injury to the epidermis is severe enough to cause destruction and death of melanocytes. "Toxic vitiligo" secondary to phenolic or catecholic derivatives results from a structural resemblance of these substances to tyrosine, an amino acid precursor of melanin synthesis. At lower exposure levels, melanin production is simply inhibited but higher levels are cytotoxic and result in destruction of the melanocyte. The chemical structural requirement that renders a phenolic or catecholic derivative potentially cytotoxic is a nonpolar side chain in the *para* position.

Clinical Findings

Postinflammatory hypo- or hyperpigmentation is confined to areas of antecedent dermatitis and may consist of areas of irregular pigment density. Photosensitizers may increase pigmentation without obvious antecedent inflammation; bizarre patterns of pigmentation corresponding to areas of skin contact may result.

Cutaneous depigmentation resulting from exposure to specific chemical depigmenting agents occurs on surfaces where direct skin contact has occurred. Depigmentation in areas remote from direct skin contact may occur through inadvertent inoculation from the primary site of contact or systemic absorption. Chemical depigmentation may be associated with concomitant allergic contact dermatitis to the specific chemical agent but may also occur without antecedent inflammation or allergy.

Blue, slate gray, or melanotic hyperpigmentation

from heavy metal intoxication is generally diffuse but usually accentuated in sun-exposed areas. Arsenic intoxication produces a characteristic diffuse hyperpigmentation mixed with droplike areas of hypopigmentation ("raindrops on a dusty road").

Differential Diagnosis

Diffuse hyperpigmentation of sun-exposed skin caused by tar and pitch volatiles cannot be readily distinguished from melanogenesis ("tanning") stimulated by sunlight alone. It is often darker than the natural "tanning" response.

Chemical depigmentation from phenolic and catecholic substances must be distinguished from idiopathic vitiligo, which tends to occur preferentially around body orifices, knees, elbows, dorsal hands, axillas, and groin (see Chapter 22). In the absence of a history of specific exposure, this may be extremely difficult. Antecedent inflammation should raise a suspicion of chemical depigmentation and concomitant allergic contact dermatitis. A confirmative patch test may help establish the diagnosis, particularly when depigmentation occurs at the patch test site.

Treatment

Hyperpigmentary changes usually fade over time. Severe localized hyperpigmentation can be treated with twice-daily applications of topical bleaching creams containing 2% hydroquinone. Psoralens (topically or orally) followed by ultraviolet light may occasionally stimulate complete repigmentation in depigmented skin.

Prognosis

Postinflammatory hyper- or hypopigmentation may be extremely slow to resolve, particularly in pigmented individuals. Chemical depigmentation ("toxic vitiligo") sometimes resolves spontaneously but may be permanent.

URTICARIA

Essentials of Diagnosis

- Pink pruritic wheals arise suddenly.
- Individual lesions clear within 24 hours.
- No epidermal changes.
- Contact urticaria: involves skin exposed to chemical.

General Considerations

By comparison with occupational asthma, occupational urticaria is rare. Generalized allergic urticaria, when caused by occupational exposure, usually results from inhalation of antigenic material and is accompanied by other symptoms of inhalant allergy. Localized urticaria may result from exposure to a variety of substances following percutaneous absorption. This phenomenon has been dubbed "contact urticaria" (see Chapter 34).

Occupational inhalant exposures that have been associated with generalized urticaria include castor bean pomace, spices, penicillin, formaldehyde, ammonia, and sulfur dioxide. Substances that have provoked localized contact urticaria include flavorings and fragrances (eg, cinnamic aldehyde), spices, antibiotics (eg, penicillin), plant materials (eg, nettles), and various proteinaceous substances in meats and vegetables.

Pathogenesis

Urticaria may be provoked by either immunologic or nonimmunologic mechanisms. Immunologic mechanisms usually involve IgE-triggered histamine release from tissue mast cells (immediate hypersensitivity); occasionally, immunologic urticaria may be triggered by immune complexes owing to activation of C3a and C5a anaphylatoxins in the complement cascade. Nonimmunologic urticaria may be provoked by direct stimulation of blood vessels (vasodilation) or provocation of mast cell degranulation without the involvement of immunologic mechanisms (see Chapter 34).

Clinical Findings

Clinical features of urticaria consist of evanescent wheals or hives, usually erupting within 15–30 minutes following exposure. Individual lesions subside within 24 hours. Itching is usually intense. Contact urticaria occurs at the site of primary skin contact with the provocative agent. It is more common on the hands and may be superimposed on preexistent irritant dermatitis, particularly in food handlers. Presumably, antigen penetration of the skin is facilitated through continually traumatized or previously eczematized skin. Contact urticaria may become generalized if enough antigen or toxic substance is absorbed through the skin.

Prick or intradermal tests may be required to identify the causative agent, and these tests are best left to experts. RAST tests are helpful only if disks coupled with the specific allergens are commercially available; usually they are not. Contact urticaria may be diagnosed by the closed patch test procedure but with immediate readings up to 2 hours following application. Where feasible, provocative challenge testing, through inhalation or topical application on involved skin sites, confirms the diagnosis.

Differential Diagnosis

Occupational urticaria must be distinguished from a host of stimuli associated with urticaria outside the work environment (see Chapter 34).

Treatment

Topical treatment with 0.5% menthol in calamine lotion may be soothing. Systemic treatment includes antihistamines such as diphenhydramine (Benadryl) or hydroxyzine (Atarax). When severe, subcutaneous epinephrine or systemic corticosteroid treatment may be necessary (see Chapter 34).

Prognosis

Occupational urticaria resolves when the provocative exposure is eliminated.

NEOPLASTIC DISORDERS

Skin cancer became the first neoplasm with a recognized occupational etiology when Percivall Pott first suggested in 1775 that soot caused squamous cell carcinoma of the scrotum in chimney sweeps.

Ionizing and ultraviolet radiation may induce radiodermatitis, premalignant actinic keratoses, and neoplastic transformation into basal and squamous cell carcinomas and malignant melanomas following a latency period of several years. Individuals working outdoors for long periods of time in natural sunlight or occupationally exposed to ionizing radiation (eg, x-ray therapists) are at greatest risk.

Coal tar and its unrefined derivatives, such as pitch and creosote, may induce the formation of premalignant cutaneous papillomas and keratoses ("tar warts"), followed by eventual transformation into squamous cell carcinomas. Chronic intoxication with arsenic may induce the formation of both basal and squamous cell carcinomas. No chemical carcinogen has been firmly established as a cause of malignant melanoma.

Pathogenesis

Chemical induction of neoplastic disease usually requires a co-carcinogen. From an occupational standpoint, ultraviolet radiation and trauma are the most important co-carcinogens.

Clinical Findings

A. Actinic Keratoses: Actinic keratoses develop on sun-exposed surfaces of the face, neck, and arms. They characteristically appear as small, flat, red macules with superficial scales, but some degree of atrophy or hypertrophy may be present.

B. "Tar Warts": These lesions, induced by pitch, oil, or other coal tar derivatives, occur as small wartlike papillomatous growths on exposed skin surfaces, but premalignant changes are apparent on histopathologic examination.

C. Arsenical Keratoses: Arsenical keratoses characteristically arise on the palms and soles but may be present on any body surface. Clinical features of basal and squamous cell carcinomas and malignant melanoma are discussed in Chapter 43. The occurrence of basal or squamous cell carcinomas on skin surfaces that are not chronically sun-exposed should prompt a search for possible occupational exposure to chemical carcinogens.

Differential Diagnosis

Tar warts and arsenic keratoses must be distinguished from viral warts and seborrheic keratoses. Basal and squamous cell carcinomas must be differentiated from benign keratotic growths, flesh-colored nevi, and benign cutaneous appendage tumors. Malignant melanoma must be distinguished from benign pigmented cutaneous lesions (see Chapter 43).

Treatment

Premalignant actinic keratoses, arsenic keratoses, and tar warts may be treated by conservative methods of tissue destruction such as cryotherapy or electrodesiccation. Surgical excision of frank neoplasms is generally preferred to other modalities (see Chapter 43).

Prognosis

Actinic keratoses, arsenical keratoses, and tar warts may degenerate into squamous cell carcinomas. Basal cell carcinomas rarely metastasize. Squamous cell carcinomas, particularly those occurring on sun-exposed skin, have only a low potential to metastasize. The prognosis of malignant melanoma varies with type and tumor depth (see Chapter 43).

CONNECTIVE TISSUE DISEASES

Three principal types of connective tissue disorders may be induced by various occupational exposures: traumatic vasospastic disease ("vibration white finger"), scleroderma, and acro-osteolysis.

Traumatic vasospastic disease is caused by work involving the hand-held use of vibratory tools such as chain saws, pneumatic hammers, and chipping tools. **Scleroderma** may be induced by occupational exposure to silica in mining operations, an epoxy resin curing agent (*bis*-4-amino-3-cyclohexylmethane), and chlorinated organic solvents such as trichloroethylene and perchloroethylene. The scientific evidence implicating the latter exposures is mostly circumstantial. **Acro-osteolysis** has been caused only by exposure to uncured vinyl chloride monomer during the manufacture of polyvinylchloride plastics, particularly during the cleaning of reactor vessels.

Pathogenesis

Frequencies above 60 Hz are capable of inducing traumatic vasospastic disease. Because pacinian corpuscles respond to frequencies in a similar range, reflex linkage of these corpuscles to the sympathetic innervation of cutaneous blood vessels has been proposed as a possible mechanism. The mechanisms by which occupational scleroderma or acro-osteolysis is caused are not clear but may be similar to those proposed for idiopathic scleroderma (see Chapter 50).

Clinical Findings

A. Traumatic Vasospastic Disease: Traumatic vasospastic disease is characterized by paroxysmal vasospasms of the hands triggered by vibratory tools; simultaneous cold exposure may precipitate more severe attacks. Vasospasm may be unilateral, depending on the hand or arm receiving greater vibratory stimulation, but is otherwise clinically indistinguishable from Raynaud's phenomenon (see Chapter 50).

B. Scleroderma: Occupational scleroderma is clinically indistinguishable from idiopathic scleroderma (see Chapter 50).

C. Acro-osteolysis: In acro-osteolysis, lytic lesions that are apparent on x-ray examination develop in the distal and middle phalanges. These changes are associated with a peculiar papular cutaneous sclerosis, sclerodactyly, and Raynaud's phenomenon. Progressive fibrosis of the lungs, liver, and spleen has been reported. Acro-osteolysis may be complicated by the occurrence of angiosarcoma of the liver.

Differential Diagnosis

Occupationally acquired Raynaud's phenomenon and sclerodermatous skin changes must be differentiated from idiopathic scleroderma (progressive systemic sclerosis) and systemic lupus erythematosus.

Treatment

Specific medical treatment is the same as for other connective tissue diseases (see Chapter 50). Implicated chemical exposures, as well as nonspecific stimuli that trigger Raynaud's phenomenon such as cold or vibratory tools, must be avoided. Warm, protective clothing is necessary in cold climates. Special gloves that damp vibrations have been designed for use with vibratory tools.

Prognosis

Spontaneous remission is uncommon. Affected workers must usually change occupations. Change in engineering designs of some vibratory tools has improved the prognosis for traumatic vasospastic disease.

GRANULOMATOUS REACTIONS

Essentials of Diagnosis

- Firm inflammatory papules or nodules.
- Demonstration of causal agent in tissue.

General Considerations

Granulomatous reactions consist of cutaneous papules and nodules characterized histologically by aggregates of lymphoid cells, epithelial cells, and giant cells.

Foreign body granulomas may result from inoculation of particulate materials or substances into the skin. Rarely, allergic granulomas occur from inoculation of beryllium, zirconium, or silica following occupational exposure.

Pathogenesis

Foreign body granulomas result from nonallergic inflammatory reactions characterized by infiltrates of macrophages and giant cells that actively phagocytose the foreign material. **Allergic granulomas** are caused by a delayed hypersensitivity reaction characterized histologically by many epithelial cells but relatively few giant cells and resembling the granulomas of sarcoidosis.

Clinical Findings

Granulomas appear as hard, firm, violaceous or red-brown papules and nodules at the site of inoculation, with varying degrees of superficial scaling and inflammation. Beryllium granulomas may be associated with pulmonary and other systemic involvement (berylliosis). Serous or purulent exudation may be present in foreign body granulomas. Allergic granulomas are difficult to differentiate from foreign body granulomas on clinical grounds alone but usually are not associated with exudation or ulceration. Histopathologic distinction is usually easy, however. The provocative substance may be demonstrated within the granulomas by polarized microscopy or spectrographic analysis.

Differential Diagnosis

Granulomatous reactions due to occupational causes must be distinguished from granuloma annulare, cutaneous sarcoidosis, and nonoccupational infectious causes.

Treatment

Treatment of foreign body granulomas consists of removal of the foreign body. Intralesional steroids hasten resolution of allergic granulomas.

Prognosis

Foreign body granulomas resolve promptly once the foreign body has been removed. Allergic granulomas may persist for a long time.

DISORDERS OF HAIR & NAILS

Acute toxic alopecia may be caused by various toxic exposures in the work environment. **Traction alopecia** may result from acute trauma. Both hair and nails may become discolored from chemical staining. Abnormalities of nail shape and growth may result from physical or chemical injury to the nail folds and matrix. (See Chapters 28 and 29.)

Toxic alopecia may be caused by occupational exposure to thallium-containing rodenticides, boric acid, arsenic, chloroprene, and high doses of ionizing radiation.

Traction alopecia occurs when hair is caught in rapidly turning machinery and yanked from the scalp.

Nitrophenolic and other organic nitrates produce a characteristic yellowish staining of the nails as well as the skin.

Absorption of pesticides into the nail folds may cause nail plate deformation and altered growth.

Pathogenesis

Toxic alopecia is caused by acute anagen arrest of actively growing hairs, followed by rapid shedding. Nail abnormalities are caused by physical or chemical injury directly to the nail matrix, resulting in alterations of growth.

Clinical Findings

Toxic alopecia begins 1–2 weeks following acute toxic exposure. Hair loss is diffuse and patchy. Microscopic analysis of hair usually demonstrates acute tapering of hair shaft diameters near the hair bulb that are still covered by anagen root sheaths.

Traction alopecia is localized to the site of trauma, where hairs have been pulled out by the roots.

Hair and nail discoloration reflects the chromatogenous properties of the staining material.

Nail changes from physical or chemical injury are also nonspecific and include ridging, notching, thickening, and separation from the nail bed. Growth may be slowed.

Treatment

Removal from exposure is the only treatment required.

Prognosis

Once causative exposures have been eliminated, complete hair and nail regrowth usually follows, and chemical stains gradually disappear.

OCCUPATIONAL INFECTIONS & INFESTATIONS

Various infections and infestations may result from exposure to a wide range of infectious organisms encountered in the course of employment. Poor skin hygiene and minor trauma (abrasions and lacerations) are often associated etiologic factors, leading to cellulitis, deep fungal infections, or pyoderma. Intertriginous fungal infections of the groin, feet, or other body surfaces may be precipitated by hot, humid working environments. Certain occupations are associated with increased risk for specific infections from organisms to which exposure is more likely in the course of employment. Examples include anthrax in sheep and wool handlers; erysipeloid in meat and fish handlers (eg, butchers, fishermen); herpes simplex infection of fingers (herpetic whitlow) in nurses, dentists and dental assistants, physicians, and other medical personnel; orf in shepherds; milker's nodule in dairy farmers and slaughterhouse workers; sporotrichosis in gardeners and horticulturists; atypical mycobacterial infections in fishermen and aquarium keepers; and poultry and grain mite infestations in farmers.

Acquired occupational infections must be distinguished from nonoccupational cellulitis and other pyodermas, which they may resemble. Isolation of the infectious organism from both the patient and the work environment helps to establish occupational causation.

Specific types of infections and their clinical findings and treatment are discussed in Section III of this book.

DISORDERS CAUSED BY PHYSICAL & MECHANICAL AGENTS

Exposure to some physical or mechanical agents may be unique to certain occupations, resulting in a wide range of cutaneous disorders. Heat, electricity, cold, wind, vibration, and radiation may cause a variety of direct or indirect cutaneous changes, such as thermal or electrical burns, frostbite, chapping, and sunburn. Working under conditions of excessive environmental heat and humidity may result in inflammation of the sweat glands (miliaria, "prickly heat"). Warm, dry air may cause generalized pruritus. Outbreaks of nonspecific pruritus may occur in working environments where low humidity is an important quality control measure in the production process, as in semiconductor manufacturing and electronic assembly operations.

Friction and pressure may lead to blister or callus formation on the hands of laborers. Fiberglass produces pruritus from mechanical irritation, particularly in flexural areas where the fibers may be trapped beneath clothing and rubbed against the skin.

Pathogenesis

Miliaria is due to swelling and obstruction of the sweat gland duct and is more likely to occur when ambient temperatures exceed 80–85 °F and relative humidity is greater than 80%. Indoor relative humidity less than 35–40% predisposes to dryness, chapping, and pruritus. The pruritus of fiberglass dermatitis is directly related to fiber diameter and inversely proportionate to fiber length; symptoms may be particularly severe in individuals with underlying dermographism.

Clinical Findings

Thermal, solar, and electrical burns produce varying degrees of tissue damage, from simple erythema (first-degree) to blistering and superficial necrosis (second-degree) and deep tissue necrosis (third-degree). Electrical burns often produce extensive tissue damage at a much deeper level than apparent from examination of the skin alone.

Warm, dry air may produce visible skin dryness, but pruritus may be the only feature. Scratching may produce secondary transient erythema (axon flare reflex) or other secondary changes. The face and neck are affected most frequently.

Miliaria appears as intensely pruritic, small red bumps, usually over covered areas of the arms and trunk.

Blisters or callosities occur over areas of the palms where frictional forces are greatest.

Visible cutaneous changes of fiberglass dermatitis are usually secondary to rubbing and scratching, but acute erythematous papules may be present. Fiberglass spicules may be demonstrated in skin biopsies or cellulose tape strippings from inflamed papules.

Differential Diagnosis

Miliaria must be distinguished from folliculitis, scabies, and other cutaneous disorders characterized by itching red bumps. Pruritus and dermatitis caused by low humidity must be differentiated from urticaria, contact dermatitis, and atopic dermatitis. Fiberglass dermatitis may be mistaken for scabies, with which it is frequently confused.

Treatment

Miliaria responds to topical drying lotions such as calamine and prompt removal from hot, humid environments. Chapping and dermatitis from low humidity responds to topical moisturizers and low-potency corticosteroids. Correction of the responsible physical or mechanical factors in the work environment prevents recurrences.

Prognosis

These disorders usually clear promptly once environmental factors have been corrected.

PREVENTION OF OCCUPATIONAL SKIN DISORDERS

Methods to prevent occupational skin disease include protection or isolation of the worker from the harmful environment, replacement of allergenic or irritant substances with technically suitable alternatives, and removal of the worker from the workplace altogether. Removal of the worker should be considered the least desirable alternative.

Protection of the Worker

This includes protective clothing and barrier creams, good skin hygiene, good housekeeping, and process containment through appropriate engineering controls. Protective clothing (gloves, boots, sleeves, aprons, coveralls, face gear) is available in a variety of fabrics; it must fit properly, so that potentially noxious substances do not penetrate the clothing and become trapped and occluded against the skin. The physical and chemical resistance properties of protective clothing are also important in proper selection. The benefit of barrier creams against chemical substances is questionable; however, barrier creams facilitate removal of oils and greases from the skin and may be helpful when combined with a good skin hygiene program. Both protective clothing and barrier creams may aggravate dermatitis if worn or used over inflamed skin. Occasionally, workers become sensitized to allergens in these products.

Contact dermatitis may sometimes be successfully managed by replacing the offending irritant or allergenic compound with a suitable alternative. Successful substitution depends on precise identification of the actual irritant or allergen; patch testing is often necessary. Epoxy resin contact allergy may be avoided by substituting another adhesive, such as acrylic resin, when great bonding strength is unnecessary. For workers sensitized to rubber, protective clothing manufactured from nonrubber materials or without common rubber allergens may be substituted.

REFERENCES

Adams RM: Allergen replacement in industry. Cutis 1977;20:511.

Adams RM: *Occupational Skin Disease*. Grune & Stratton, 1982.

Baran RL: Occupational nail disorders. In: *Occupational Skin Disease*. Adams RM (editor). Grune & Stratton, 1982.

Birmingham DJ: Cutaneous reactions to chemicals. In: *Dermatology in General Medicine,* 2nd ed. Fitzpatrick T, Eisen A (editors). McGraw-Hill, 1979.

Birmingham DJ: Prevention of occupational skin disease. Cutis 1969;5:153.

Burdick AE, Mathias CG: The contact urticaria syndrome. Dermatol Clin 1985;3:71.

Church R: Prevention of dermatitis and its medicolegal aspects. Br J Dermatol 1981;105(Suppl 21):85.

Cronin E: *Contact Dermatitis*. Churchill Livingstone, 1980.

Ebling FJ, Rook A: Hair. In: *Textbook of Dermatology*, 3rd ed. Rook A, Wilkinson DS, Ebling FJ (editors). Blackwell, 1979.

Fisher AA: *Contact Dermatitis,* 3rd ed. Lea & Febiger, 1986.

Lim HW, Baer RL, Gange RW: Photodermatoses. J Am Acad Dermatol 1987;17:293.

Foussereau J, Benezra C, Maibach H: *Occupational Contact Dermatitis.* Munksgaard, 1982.

Gellin GA: Pigment responses: Occupational disorders of pigmentation. In: *Occupational and Industrial Dermatology,* 2nd ed. Maibach HI (editor). Year Book, 1987.

Haustein UF, Ziegler V: Environmentally induced systemic sclerosis-like disorders. Int J Dermatol 1985;24:147.

Key MM: Some unusual allergic reactions in industry. Arch Dermatol 1961;83:3.

Maibach HI (editor): *Occupational and Industrial Dermatology,* 2nd ed. Year Book, 1987.

Malkinson FD: Percutaneous absorption of toxic substances in industry. Arch Ind Health 1960;21:87.

Markowitz SS et al: Occupational acroosteolysis. Arch Dermatol 1972;106:219.

Rycroft RJ: Low-humidity occupational dermatoses. Dermatol Clin 1984;2:553.

Schwartz L, Tulipan L, Birmingham DJ: *Occupational Diseases of the Skin.* Lea & Febiger, 1957.

Taylor W, Brammer AJ: Vibration effects on the hand and arm in industry: An introduction and review. In: *Vibration Effects on the Hand and Arm in Industry.* Brammer AJ, Taylor W (editors). Wiley, 1983.

Tindall JP: Chloracne and chloracnegens. J Am Acad Dermatol 1985;13:539.

Vickers CF: Industrial carcinogenesis. Br J Dermatol 1981;105(Suppl 21):57.

Section IX:
Diseases of Special Organs & Systems

Cutaneous Manifestations of Systemic Disease

47

Jeffrey P. Callen, MD

The skin serves as a window through which the careful observer can detect internal disease. In considering the breadth of cutaneous-systemic disease, we limit discussion to the most common entities or to those with demonstrable importance. This chapter is aimed at broad disease categories that may be reflected on the skin surface, and much of the information is presented in tabular form.

There are limited ways in which the skin can behave in response to disease. Changes can occur in color, thickness, scaliness, sensation, texture, or viability. Immunologic reactions or alterations in blood flow—or both—can result in urticaria, purpura, blisters, or necrosis. These reactions are important in assessment of patient well-being.

The following tables deal not only with systemic diseases causing skin disease but also with some skin diseases causing systemic disease.

SKIN SIGNS OF INTERNAL MALIGNANCY

Certain cutaneous diseases or manifestations are commonly associated with visceral cancer. Criteria have been suggested and developed that are useful in this analysis: (1) a concurrent onset; (2) a parallel course (ie, if the tumor is removed, the dermatosis will resolve); (3) a unique tumor association (eg, acanthosis nigricans is associated mainly with adenocarcinomas of the gastrointestinal tract); (4) a genetic relationship (eg, Gardner's syndrome and colonic cancer); (5) both the dermatosis and the cancer are uncommon (eg, palmar tylosis and esophageal cancer); and (6) a statistically significant frequency of cancer occurs in association with the dermatosis. In Table 47–1, the classic relationship between cancer and associated cutaneous disorders is examined. (See also Fig 47–1.)

SKIN CLUES TO DIAGNOSIS OF GASTROINTESTINAL BLEEDING

Occasionally, a diagnosis of skin disease may be helpful in determining the cause of gastrointestinal hemorrhage. Among the common causes of gastrointestinal bleeding (peptic ulcer disease, alcoholic gastritis, and esophageal varices), skin lesions are not helpful diagnostically. If enough hemorrhage occurs, the skin may be pale. When varices are present as a complication of cirrhosis, skin findings may include palmar erythema or spider angiomas. Biliary cirrhosis may be associated with xanthomas, hyperpigmentation, and intractable pruritus.

Less common causes of gastrointestinal bleeding may have a specific cutaneous correlate. In particular, the diagnosis of Osler-Weber-Rendu disease or Peutz-Jeghers syndrome can be made by the emergency room physician. Table 47–2 details some of the more important syndromes in which gastrointestinal bleeding may occur and cutaneous disease can aid in diagnosis (Figs 47–2 and 47–3).

CUTANEOUS DISORDERS IN PATIENTS WITH MALABSORPTION SYNDROMES

Certain syndromes involving the skin include malabsorption and malnutrition. The skin can manifest abnormalities secondary to these conditions. In malnutrition, the skin becomes thinner, drier, and less elastic. It exhibits fragility as evidenced by purpura and ecchymotic lesions. Xerosis and occasionally ichthyosiform lesions are common. Alopecia and nail dystrophy may occur. Lastly, the skin often becomes hyperpigmented. Table 47–3 lists some of the disorders associated with malabsorption.

Worthy of special mention is the bowel bypass

Table 47–1. Acquired cutaneous disorders associated with internal malignancy.

Disorder	Clinical Manifestations	Tumor Type and Site	Relationship of Tumor and Skin Lesion
Acanthosis nigricans	Dark velvety discoloration in intertriginous areas. Weight loss.	Adenocarcinoma, commonly gastric or in the GI tract.	Often concurrent onset and parallel course.
Acquired ichthyosis	Rhomboidal scales on non-inflammatory base. Usually on the lower legs.	Hodgkin's disease, lymphoma; rarely, solid tumors.	Parallel course, but tumor is usually present before ichthyosis is diagnosed.
Bazex's syndrome	Paronychia, nail dysplasia, keratoderma, plum-colored acral lesions.	Squamous cell carcinoma of the upper respiratory or GI tract.	Rare occurrence. Only a handful of cases reported.
Bowen's disease	Scaly plaques with undulating borders.	Various tumors.	Different course and onset; association probably due to elevated frequency of second malignancy.
Bullous pemphigoid	Elderly patient. Tense bullae on an erythematous base. Mucosal surfaces may be involved.	Various tumors.	Classically felt related to internal malignancy but recently shown to be related to age alone. Perhaps those with mucosal involvement have a higher incidence of cancer.
Dermatitis herpetiformis	Intensely pruritic vesicles and excoriations.	Lymphoma of the intestine.	Patients have gluten-sensitive enteropathy, which has also been linked to intestinal cancer.
Dermatomyositis	Heliotrope rash: violaceous edema around the eyes. Gottron's papules: violaceous lesions over bony prominences. Myositis.	Various tumors.	May or may not have similar courses and onset. Children do not have increased risk of cancer. Cancer is not often found on nondirected search.
Diffuse plane xanthoma	Flat xanthomas often with surrounding erythema.	Multiple myeloma.	The xanthomas are often aggressive and occasionally destructive.
Erythema annulare centrifugum	Erythematous, slightly palpable annular lesions, with a fine scale inside the outer margin (trailing scale).	Various tumors.	Association is rare with tumors; more common with infections, or idiopathic.
Erythema gyratum repens (Fig 47–1)	Erythematous bands with slight scale. Appearance like "grains of wood."	Various tumors.	Similar onset, parallel course; may regress with tumor removal.
Glucagonoma syndrome (necrolytic migratory erythema)	Angular cheilitis, glossitis. Intertriginous, erythematous, slightly scaly lesions, often confused with candidiasis or seborrhea.	Alpha-cell tumor of pancreas (glucagon-secreting).	Direct relationship: removal of the tumor results in regression of the rash. Only an occasional patient with necrolytic migratory erythema does not have a glucagonoma. Diabetes, anemia, and weight loss are commonly present.
Hypertrichosis lanuginosa (malignant down) (Fig 47–3)	Fine hair growing on the face. Glossitis, weight loss are common.	Various tumors.	Similar onset and course. Over 90% of patients with "malignant down" have a tumor. Must rule out porphyria and other metabolic disorders.
Leser-Trelat sign	Acute change or appearance of multiple seborrheic keratoses. May be associated with acanthosis nigricans (see above).	GI adenocarcinomas.	Unusual occurrence; may be associated with acanthosis nigricans.
Paget's disease	Eczematous patch around the nipple or in the perineal space.	Mammary: underlying ductal carcinoma. Extramammary: apocrine, eccrine, vaginal, rectal adenocarcinoma.	Similar onset and course. When Paget's or extramammary Paget's is present, an underlying cancer is almost always found.
Pemphigus group	Blistering disease. Usually crusted lesions. Nikolsky's sign is present.	Thymoma, benign or malignant.	Combination of thymoma, pemphigus, and myasthenia gravis more than coincidental.

(continued)

Table 47–1 (Cont'd.). Acquired cutaneous disorders associated with internal malignancy.

Disorder	Clinical Manifestations	Tumor Type and Site	Relationship of Tumor and Skin Lesion
Porphyria cutanea tarda	Blisters, scars, milia on exposed skin. Darkening of the skin. Hypertrichosis.	Hepatocellular carcinoma.	Porphyria cutanea tarda is associated with cirrhosis. The association with hepatic cancer may relate to the cirrhosis.
Leukocytoclastic vasculitis	Palpable purpuric lesions, necrosis of skin, nodules, or ulcers. May be associated with systemic vasculitis.	Leukemias, particularly hairy cell. Lymphomas. Occasional solid tumor.	Malignancy in patients with cutaneous vasculitis is rare ($< 1\%$).

syndrome encountered in patients treated surgically for marked obesity. Pustular lesions and arthritis are caused by bacterial overgrowth in the blind loop of the bypassed intestine.

NEUROCUTANEOUS DISORDERS

Table 47–4 lists some important neurocutaneous syndromes. These primarily involve the skin and nervous system, both of which are of ectodermal derivation.

SKIN MANIFESTATIONS OF ENDOCRINE & METABOLIC DISORDERS

The skin is profoundly affected by hormones. Either increased or decreased hormone levels may affect the skin. For example, excess adrenal production or iatrogenic corticosteroids result in cutaneous lesions, including striae, redistribution of fat, pigmentation, ecchymoses, acneiform lesions, hirsutism, and skin fragility. Tables 47–5 and 47–6, respectively, detail the relationship of diabetes mellitus and thyroid diseases to skin disease (Fig 47–4).

Xanthomas are cutaneous tumors composed of lipid-rich (foamy) histiocytes. Several genetic hyperlipoproteinemias (primarily elevated cholesterol) are associated with plane (planar) xanthomas or xanthelasma; hyperlipoproteinemia types III, IV, and V are associated with eruptive xanthomas. In addition, xanthomas are often a prominent feature of primary biliary cirrhosis.

Amyloidosis is a metabolic disease manifested by deposition of a proteinaceous material in various body sites. The skin and mucous membranes are often involved in primary amyloidosis with "pinch purpura" (nonpalpable purpura that quickly develops when the skin is traumatized—eg, by pinching), an enlarged tongue, and a waxy-appearing skin. Alopecia and nail changes also occur. Amyloidosis can be associated with multiple myeloma.

SKIN DISEASES IN PATIENTS WITH RENAL DISEASE

Primary syndromes involving the skin and the kidneys are not common. However, because both organs have a rich vasculature that can be affected by immune complex disease, several correlates exist. Glomerulonephritis manifested by proteinuria, hema-

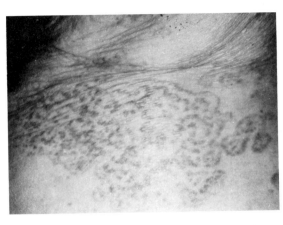

Figure 47–1. Erythema gyratum repens—a sign of internal malignancy.

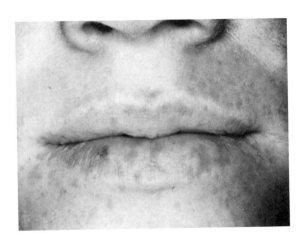

Figure 47–2. Peutz-Jeghers syndrome.

Table 47–2. Cutaneous lesions associated with gastrointestinal hemorrhage.

Disorder	Cutaneous Findings	GI Pathology	Other Manifestations
Blue rubber-bleb nevus syndrome	Blue dermal hemangiomas.	Multiple visceral hemangiomas.	Iron deficiency anemia.
Hereditary hemorrhagic telangiectasias (Osler-Weber-Rendu) (Fig 47–3)	Matlike telangiectasias on lips, acral extremities, nasal and oral mucosa.	Telangiectasias.	Autosomal dominant. Epistaxis may be severe. Pulmonary or central nervous system arteriovenous malformations.
Inflammatory bowel disease	Pyoderma gangrenosum, erythema nodosum, perirectal fistulas, aphthous stomatitis.	Ulcerative colitis, regional enteritis, or granulomatous colitis.	Arthritis, sacroiliitis, uveitis. Ulcerative colitis associated with colonic carcinoma in many cases. Regional enteritis often associated with fistulas and obstructions.
Cutaneous leukocytoclastic vasculitis (Henoch-Schönlein purpura, systemic vasculitis)	Palpable purpura (dependent areas most common). Urticaria-like lesions, nodules, ulceration, livedo reticularis.	GI vasculitis	Renal: glomerulonephritis may lead to hypertension. Arthritis. Nervous system involvement occasionally associated with hepatitis B, autoimmune disorders, or drug ingestion.
Malignant atrophic papulosis (Degos' disease)	Ivory white umbilicated papules.	Submucosal vasculitis in the GI tract with multiple infarctions.	None.
Malignant tumors	Acanthosis nigricans	Adenocarcinoma of the stomach.	Also associated with adenocarcinoma in other sites; occasionally, squamous cell carcinoma.
	Dermatomyositis (Gottron's papules, heliotrope, periungual telangiectasias).	Adenocarcinoma of colon.	Proximal muscle weakness, elevated muscle enzymes.
	Tylosis (palmar hyperkeratoses)	Esophageal carcinoma.	Autosomal dominant inheritance
	Perianal extramammary Paget's disease.	Underlying adenocarcinoma of rectum.	None.
	Multiple sebaceous adenomas and keratoacanthomas (Torres's syndrome).	Colonic carcinoma.	Variety of tumors.
	Kaposi's sarcoma	Kaposi's of small bowel or lymphoma.	Kaposi's elsewhere in body (heart, lungs, liver).
	Gardner's syndrome	Adenocarcinoma of colon.	See Table 47–1.
	Peutz-Jeghers syndrome	Adenocarcinomas	See Table 47–1.
Pseudoxanthoma elasticum	Yellow-tan papules in flexural areas.	Vascular calcification.	Autosomal dominant. Angioid streaks in eye. Claudication, angina. Genitourinary bleeding.

turia, or renal insufficiency can complicate the course of systemic vasculitis or lupus erythematosus and have prominent cutaneous features. Patients with progressive systemic sclerosis can also develop renal failure.

The most common reason for dermatologic consultation by a nephrologist is secondary changes related to therapy of chronic renal failure. In particular, patients being maintained on hemodialysis or who have received renal transplants develop a multitude of cutaneous disorders. Some are listed in Table 47–7.

SARCOIDOSIS

Essentials of Diagnosis

- Myriad of cutaneous manifestations.
- Biopsy demonstrates noncaseating granulomas.
- Pulmonary involvement; multisystem disease.
- Rule out other causes of granuloma formation.

General Considerations

Sarcoidosis is a multisystem disorder in which the skin may be affected in 20–25% of cases. The cuta-

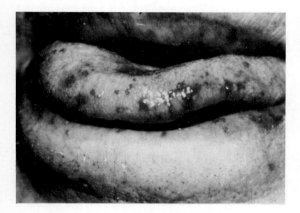

Figure 47–3. Osler-Weber-Rendu disease (hereditary).

Table 47–3. Cutaneous disorders associated with malabsorption.

Syndrome	Skin Lesions	GI Lesions	Other Manifestations	Therapy
Acrodermatitis enteropathica	Eczematous, bullous lesions around orifices; acral lesions. Alopecia.	Diarrhea, malnutrition.	Autosomal recessive. Photophobia, corneal opacities, growth retardation.	Zinc replacement.
Cronkhite-Canada syndrome	Hyperpigmentation, alopecia, onychodystrophy.	Generalized; adenomatous polyps.	Melena, malabsorption.	None known; usually progresses to death.
Dermatitis herpetiformis	Symmetric, grouped vesicles; or excoriations usually on extensor surfaces, scalp, buttocks.	Gluten-sensitive enteropathy (usually asymptomatic).	High frequency of HLA-B8; IgA in skin biopsy.	Dapsone, gluten-free diet.
Bowel bypass for morbid obesity	Pustular lesions with a purpuric base (pustular vasculitis).	Iatrogenic bypass of small intestine, forming a blind loop.	Arthritis.	Antibiotics, colchicine, NSAIDs, re-anastomoses.

neous lesions are often nonspecific, and sarcoidosis must therefore be differentiated from many skin disorders. The diagnosis is confirmed by the presence of noncaseating granulomas ("naked tubercles") in multiple organs after other causes of granuloma formation have been ruled out. Patients with cutaneous sarcoidal granulomas usually (not always) have systemic disease. Most patients with cutaneous sarcoidal granulomas follow a chronic course, while those with erythema nodosum as a manifestation of systemic sarcoidosis follow an acute resolving course.

Clinical Findings
A. Symptoms and Signs:
1. Cutaneous manifestations– Cutaneous disease in sarcoidosis can be classified as specific (gran-

Table 47–4. Neurocutaneous disorders.

Disorder	Skin Lesions	Neurologic Disease	Other Features	Therapy
Neurofibromatosis (Recklinghausen's disease)	Café-au-lait spots, axillary freckling, neurofibromas.	Intracranial tumors, seizures, acoustic neuroma, gliomas of optic nerve, peripheral nerve tumors, occasionally mental retardation.	Pheochromocytoma, bony deformities. Autosomal dominant.	Removal of any lesions causing functional or structural abnormalities, anticonvulsants, genetic counseling.
Tuberous sclerosis (epiloia)	Adenoma sebaceum: papular lesions on central face; subungual fibromas, shagreen patch (infiltrated plaque on lower back), ash leaf spots.	Epilepsy, mental retardation, gliosis of brain parenchyma (leads to calcifications ["tubers"]).	Phakomas of retina, renal hamartomas, rhabdomyomas of heart, pseudocysts of bone. Autosomal dominant.	Anticonvulsants, genetic counseling.
Sturge-Weber syndrome (encephalotrigeminal angiomatosis)	Port wine hemangioma on upper face (first and second branches of trigeminal nerve).	Contralateral seizures, and hemiparesis.	Retinal angiomas, glaucoma, buphthalmos.	Anticonvulsants, control of glaucoma.
Ataxia-telangiectasia (Louis-Bar syndrome)	Telangiectasias over bulbar conjunctiva, malar areas; late development of inelasticity.	Early onset of ataxia; oculomotor apraxia, neuronal degeneration.	Lack of serum and secretory IgA, deficient immunity, lymphoreticular malignancy, recurrent infections. Autosomal recessive.	None known.
Epidermal nevus syndrome (of Solomon)	Epidermal nevi (linear). Nevus sebaceus-like lesions, hemangiomas.	Angiomas of brain, seizures, mental retardation.	Bony defects, vascular malformations.	None known.
Behçet's disease	Aphthous stomatitis, papules, pustules, erythema nodosum-like lesions, pathergy (induction of lesions by trauma).	Headaches, hemiplegia, neuropathy, paresis, coma.	Uveitis, iritis, hypopyon, arthropathy, colon lesions (colitis), vascular lesions.	Colchicine, corticosteroids, chlorambucil or other immunosuppressive agents.

Table 47–5. Cutaneous lesions associated with diabetes mellitus.

Lesion	Clinical Appearance	Relationship to Diabetes	Therapy
Necrobiosis lipoidica diabeticorum (Fig 47–6)	Red-yellow atrophic patch with prominent telangiectasis, usually on lower leg.	Occurs in 0.3% of diabetics; 77% of patients are females. Precedes diabetes in 15%, coincides in 25%, follows in 60%. No relationship to diabetic control.	Weak topical or intralesional corticosteroids can prevent spread of lesion peripherally (need to avoid production of atrophy).
Diabetic dermopathy	Tan-brown small atrophic lesions on anterior shins.	50% of people with diabetes. Nonspecific sign. No relationship to diabetic control.	None.
Cutaneous infections	Impetigo, erythrasma, candidiasis.	Probably not specifically related to diabetes.	Specific therapy for infection.
Xanthomas	Eruptive xanthomas (yellow papules).	Poorly controlled diabetes with secondary type IV hyperlipoproteinemia.	Control of diabetes with diet, drugs or insulin, clofibrate.
Generalized lipodystrophy (Lawrence-Seip syndrome)	Subcutaneous atrophy, loss of fat, acanthosis nigricans, enlarged genitalia, hirsutism, hyperpigmentation, central nervous system disease, hepatosplenomegaly.	Insulin-resistant diabetes, congenital and acquired forms.	None.
Neurotrophic ulcer	Ulcer over pressure site.	Due to lack of pain sensation, which can occur with diabetic neuropathy.	Control of diabetes. Phenytoin may help.
Granuloma annulare	Erythematous to tan annular dermal lesions.	Usually only associated with diabetes when disseminated granuloma annulare occurs.	Antimalarials; topical corticosteroids.
Scleredema adultorum (Buschke's syndrome)	Nonpitting edema of face, neck, trunk, proximal extremities. Acute onset. Usually males. Often follows upper respiratory infection.	Patients commonly have diabetes. Infiltration of the skin with mucopolysaccharides.	Resolution usually with time.
Bullous diabeticorum	Tense bullae on noninflammatory base. Usually on lower extremities.	By definition.	Soaks, diabetic control.

Table 47–6. Cutaneous lesions associated with thyroid abnormalities.

Thyroid Function	Skin Abnormalities	Other Findings	Therapy
Hyperthyroidism	Palmar erythema, flushing of face, increased sweating, onycholysis (distal), diffuse hyperpigmentation; fine, soft hair; pruritus.	Tachycardia, fine tremor, weight loss, goiter.	Medical: propranolol, propylthiouracil, iodine. Surgical removal of thyroid. Radioactive iodine.
Hypothyroidism Congenital (cretinism)	Dryness, laxity, thick lips and tongue, fusion of eyebrows.	Hoarseness, growth retardation, constipation.	Thyroid hormone replacement.
Acquired (myxedema)	Cool skin, carotenemia, pruritus, xerosis, brittle nails.	Weight gain, fatigue, myxedema coma.	Thyroid hormone replacement.
Graves' disease (thyroid hyperplasia and hyperthyroidism)	Pretibial myxedema, clubbing (thyroid acropachy). Often these follow or worsen after treatment of hyperthyroidism.	Exophthalmos, signs of hyperthyroidism, goiter.	Treat hyperthyroidism; intralesional corticosteroids for pretibial myxedema.
Hashimoto's thyroiditis	Vitiligo, alopecia areata, dermatititis herpetiformis, pemphigoid, lupus erythematosus, scleroderma.	Eventual goiter and hypothyroidism (hyperthyroidism may be present early). Elevated TSH level even in the presence of normal T_4. Thyroid antibodies.	Treatment appropriate for thyroid function.

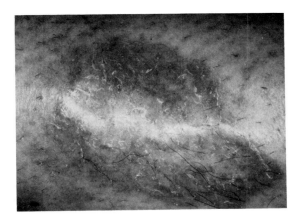

Figure 47–4. Necrobiosis lipoidica diabeticorum. These atrophic plaques frequently occur on the anterior legs of patients with insulin-dependent diabetes mellitus.

ulomatous on biopsy) or nonspecific (not granulomatous). The histologically "specific" lesions may take on multiple clinical appearances, but the usual presentation is as an infiltrated lesion such as a plaque, papule, or nodule. Facial lesions with telangiectasia, which may scar, are known as **lupus pernio** and are commonly associated with sarcoidosis in the upper respiratory tract. The most common cutaneous lesions are infiltrated papules and plaques, but alopecia, ichthyosis, and erythroderma are among the myriad of findings.

Of the histologically nonspecific lesions, erythema nodosum is the most common. Erythema nodosum occurs in acute sarcoidosis as part of **Löfgren's syndrome,** which includes a constellation of erythema nodosum, bilateral hilar adenopathy, uveitis, and arthritis. Löfgren's syndrome is a benign process, with spontaneous resolution occurring in more than 95% of cases. Other nonspecific lesions are rare.

2. Pulmonary manifestations– Intrathoracic disease is present in 80% of patients. It is radiographically staged. Stage I is bilateral hilar lymphadenopathy alone; stage II is bilateral hilar lymphadenopathy with interstitial changes; and stage III is interstitial changes alone. The stages correlate well with prognosis and abnormalities found on pulmonary function tests. Granulomas of stage I pulmonary sarcoidosis almost always resolve; patients with stage III usually develop chronic pulmonary problems.

3. Other clinical manifestations –Sarcoidosis can attack any organ but most frequently the liver, spleen, lymph nodes, and eyes. It can affect the function of the endocrine glands, the heart, or the nervous system and can cause reabsorption of tufts on bones.

Table 47–7. Skin lesions associated with renal disease.

Disorder	Skin Signs	Renal Findings	Other Features	Therapy
Nail-patella syndrome	Hypoplasia of nail plate.	Progressive renal disease (abnormal connective tissue-like material in glomerulus). Duplication of collecting system, glomerulosclerosis.	Autosomal dominant. Absent patella, iliac horns, skeletal abnormalities, ocular disorders (glaucoma).	None known.
Fabry's disease	Angiokeratomas, small blue-black papules on trunk (around umbilicus).	Renal failure secondary to glycolipid deposition.	Corneal opacities, neuropathy, cerebrovascular disease, cardiac disease (arrhythmias, hypertropy), deficiency of ceramide trihexosidase. X-linked inheritance.	Renal transplantation.
Pruritus of hemodialysis	Generalized pruritus.	Hemodialysis.	Occasionally related to secondary hyperparathyroidism.	Ultraviolet B light, activated charcoal, parathyroidectomy.
Bullous dermatosis of hemodialysis (or renal failure)	Tense bullae, usually on distal extremities (subepidermal). Occasional hyperpigmentation.	Hemodialysis; occasionally in patients with chronic renal failure not on dialysis.	Possibly related to abnormal porphyrins in some patients.	Sun avoidance, sunscreens, plasma exchange.
Skin lesions found in renal transplantation patients	Warts, chronic herpes simplex, squamous cell carcinoma, hair loss, bacterial and fungal infections.	Transplantation.	Related to the use of azathioprine and prednisone for prevention of rejection.	Specific treatment for skin lesion.

B. Laboratory Findings: Sarcoidosis is one cause of hypercalcemia and hypercalcinuria. Although there are no specific laboratory abnormalities associated with sarcoidosis, the serum angiotensin-converting enzyme (ACE) level may be raised. The ACE level may both aid in establishing the diagnosis and reflect activity of pulmonary disease. The Kveim test is also a possible diagnostic aid. Purified sarcoidal tissue is injected intracutaneously and the site biopsied after 4–6 weeks. In sarcoidosis, granulomas frequently develop.

Differential Diagnosis & Evaluation

The finding of a cutaneous sarcoidal granuloma on biopsy requires extensive evaluation. The presence of only a single skin lesion in sarcoidosis is rare, and if this is the case, foreign body granuloma should be considered. Examining the tissue under polarized light can be useful, but some foreign body granulomas require spectrophotometric analysis of tissue for diagnosis. Infectious causes must always be ruled out, so special stains and cultures for fungi and acid-fast bacteria are indicated. Granuloma annulare and granulomas from beryllium or zirconium may also produce naked tubercles.

Once the diagnosis of cutaneous sarcoidosis is made, evaluation for systemic disease should occur, including ophthalmologic examination, chest x-ray, pulmonary function tests and diffusion studies, electrocardiography, serum calcium measurements, liver function tests, and hand and foot x-ray films.

Treatment

Among the indications for systemic corticosteroids are disabling pulmonary sarcoidosis, neurosarcoidosis, cardiac sarcoidosis, hypercalcemia, and disfiguring cutaneous lesions. Cutaneous disease (plaques and lupus pernio) is usually treated with topical and intralesional corticosteroids; however, these are rarely sufficient. Some success has been reported with allopurinol or immunosuppressives.

SYSTEMIC DISEASES ASSOCIATED WITH DISORDERS CHARACTERIZED BY CUTANEOUS SCLEROSIS

Sclerotic skin is a characteristic of several systemic diseases, the most prominent of which is progressive systemic sclerosis (see Chapter 50). Table 47–8 reviews the major findings in those disorders, in which cutaneous sclerosis is related to systemic disease.

OCULOCUTANEOUS DISORDERS

Several systemic diseases have prominent ophthalmic as well as cutaneous manifestations. Most of these are discussed in Chapter 49.

The cutaneous manifestations of Reiter's disease include psoriatic lesions, circinate balanitis, and keratoderma blennorrhagica (Fig 47–5). Anterior uveitis (and occasionally conjunctivitis) is frequent. A nongonococcal urethritis, arthritis, and spondylitis complete the classic tetrad.

Erythema multiforme is a reactive dermatosis that may involve the eyes (see Chapters 35 and 49). In severe cases with systemic symptoms and involvement of multiple mucosal surfaces, the disorder is called Stevens-Johnson syndrome. Erythema multiforme and Stevens-Johnson syndrome are caused by similar processes. The most frequent associations are infections and drugs, but in about 50% of cases no cause is identified. The typical skin lesion is a "target" lesion with urticaria-like concentric rings of color. The center is dusky or bullous. The eyes, when involved, are affected by conjunctivitis, but in severe cases blistering may occur and result in corneal scarring and blindness.

Cataracts may complicate atopic dermatitis or the corticosteroid therapy used to control disease. Other characteristic disorders of the eye include keratoconus, Dennie-Morgan fold, allergic conjunctivitis, and thinning of the lateral eyebrows.

PRURITUS

Itching is a common symptom associated with many skin diseases. In the absence of a specific skin disease or skin lesions, general pruritus may be a manifestation of systemic disease. Systemic evaluation of the patient with "idiopathic" pruritus is indicated, but the diagnosis is often elusive or such studies are often unproductive. Disorders associated with pruritus include diabetes mellitus, thyroid disease, hypoparathyroidism, infections, drugs, and allergies as well as those discussed below.

Pruritus is rarely associated with malignancy other than Hodgkin's lymphoma. The pruritus of Hodgkin's lymphoma is classically severe and nocturnal.

Pruritus is a frequent feature of polycythemia rubra vera. The patient often complains of intense pruritus during or following bathing. The severity of pruritus tends to equal the severity of the polycythemia.

Generalized intractable pruritus is a feature of hepatic disease, particularly primary biliary cirrhosis. In this condition, the pruritus is believed to be related to excessive circulating bile salts, and thus the use of cholestyramine is occasionally beneficial.

Generalized pruritus can accompany pregnancy, but in the absence of skin lesions it is only of symptomatic concern. Many of these patients have mild cholestatic jaundice also.

Renal disease is frequently accompanied by pruritus. Itching is common in uremia and is also common and troublesome in hemodialysis patients. In the

Table 47–8. Syndromes associated with cutaneous sclerosis.

Syndrome	Skin Signs	Systemic Findings	Laboratory Evaluation	Therapy
Progressive systemic sclerosis (scleroderma) (CREST syndrome is a variant)	Sclerosis of skin, acrosclerosis, sclerodactyly, Raynaud's phenomenon, calcinosis cutis, matlike telangiectasias, vitiligo-like depigmentation.	Decreased esophageal motility, abnormal intestinal motility, pulmonary fibrosis, renal disease (rare, but when present usually results in death).	ANA (often speckled), pulmonary function tests, esophageal studies. CREST syndrome may be associated with anticentromere antibody.	None of proved benefit. Penicillamine may prove to be of value.
Morphea and linear scleroderma (localized scleroderma)	Localized patch of sclerotic skin	Linear scleroderma has been seen in association with thyroiditis and lupus erythematosus.	None.	Intralesional corticosteroids may help soften the lesion. Phenytoin may be of value.
Mixed connective tissue disease (Sharp's syndrome)	Acrosclerosis, telangiectasia, discoid lupus, Raynaud's phenomenon.	Myositis, arthritis, serositis, pulmonary fibrosis, renal disease (rare).	ANA (speckled pattern), high-titer ribonucleoprotein antibody (extractable nuclear antigen).	Corticosteroids.
Diffuse fasciitis with eosinophilia (Shulman's syndrome)	Sclerotic skin proximally; sclerodactyly (rare), Raynaud's phenomenon (rare).	Fasciitis on biopsy, red cell aplasia. Fatigue; occurs following exertion.	Peripheral eosinophilia, hypergammaglobulinemia	Systemic corticosteroids may be of benefit.
Carcinoid syndrome	Flushing, pruritus, sclerosis of head and neck.	Asthma-like symptoms, fatigue, weight loss.	Abnormal urinary 5-hydroxyindoleacetic acid (5-HIAA).	Removal of tumor if possible.
Porphyria cutanea tarda	Hyperpigmentation, blisters, scars on exposed surfaces, hypertrichosis. Sclerosis is a late change, usually of sun-exposed skin.	History of excessive alcohol intake is frequent. Hepatic tumors. Perhaps associated with diabetes mellitus. May occur in patients on dialysis.	Abnormal urinary uroporphyrins. In dialysis patients, abnormal serum porphyrin profile.	Phlebotomy, antimalarials, alcohol avoidance, sunscreens. Avoid certain drugs. In dialysis patients, plasma exchange.
Acro-osteolysis	Acrosclerosis, sclerosis of forearms and face, Raynaud's phenomenon.	Osteolysis of distal phalanges, history of vinyl chloride exposure.	X-ray of hands.	None known.
Scleromyxedema (papular mucinosis, lichen myxedematosus)	Sclerosis of hands, sclerotic waxy papules (may be generalized).	Abnormal serum proteins. Rare: myeloma, thyroid disease, lupus erythematosus.	Mucinous deposition on biopsy. Abnormal protein electrophoresis.	Cytotoxic agents often effective. Need for aggressive therapy weighed against benign process.
Vibratory trauma	Sclerodactyly, Raynaud's phenomenon.	None.	Rule out scleroderma.	Removal from source of trauma.
Bleomycin toxicity	Sclerosis of skin, usually the hands and arms.	Pulmonary fibrosis.	None.	Stop bleomycin.

latter, UVB phototherapy and parathyroidectomy have been the most effective treatments.

SYSTEMIC DISEASES ASSOCIATED WITH PURPURA

Purpura is not uncommon in practice but usually is not related to systemic disease. The most common form is "senile" purpura due to loss of support of capillaries in aged skin, which occurs in areas of trauma, though the injury may be mild and forgotten. Therapy consists of reassurance. Similar lesions may occur secondary to administration of systemic corticosteroids.

When purpura occurs with coagulopathies and blood dyscrasias, it is more frequently petechial. Idiopathic thrombocytopenic purpura and drug-induced thrombocytopenic purpura can be first manifested as a petechial rash. Severe thrombocytopenic purpura can be life-threatening. Dysproteinemias, including cryoglobulinemia and macroglobulinemia, may present with palpable purpuric lesions.

Leukocytoclastic vasculitis is classically manifested by palpable purpura of dependent areas. This reaction is an immune complex disorder and may be

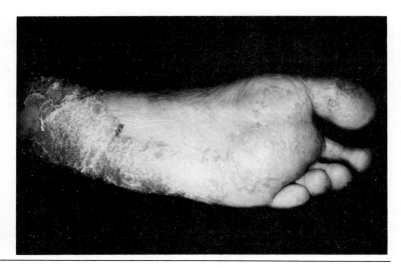

Figure 47–5. Reiter's disease. Keratoderma blennorrhagica involving the soles.

associated with arthritis, vasculitis of the gut, or glomerulonephritis. Most patients with cutaneous leukocytoclastic vasculitis have a benign course, and even if systemic disease is present it is rarely severe.

Several infections may be manifested as palpable purpuric lesions, including endocarditis, gonococcemia, meningococcemia, and Rocky Mountain spotted fever. Lastly, a left atrial myxoma embolism can produce palpable purpura.

BLISTERING DISEASE

The bullous disorders are discussed elsewhere. Internal associations are not uncommon with these chronic blistering conditions. Acute vesicles and bullae can also occur in a host of systemic diseases, but full discussion is beyond the scope of this text. Table 47–9 reviews the common internal associations seen with some chronic blistering skin diseases.

Table 47–9. Internal diseases associated with chronic blistering conditions.

Blistering Disease	Internal Association	Comment
Pemphigus	Thymoma.	May be benign or malignant.
	Myasthenia gravis	Parallel course common with thymoma.
	Red cell aplasia.	Rare.
	Lupus erythematosus.	Most often with pemphigus erythematosus.
	Malignancy other than thymoma.	Coincidental.
Bullous pemphigoid	Rheumatoid arthritis, autoimmune thyroiditis, other autoimmune disorders.	Association related to autoimmune nature of pemphigoid.
	Malignancy	Associated by age only.
Dermatitis herpetiformis	Gluten-sensitive enteropathy.	98% occurrence if carefully sought.
	Thyroiditis.	Occurs in 5–10% of patients; rarely affects dermatitis herpetiformis.
	Lymphoma of GI tract.	Associated with gluten-sensitive enteropathy.
Porphyria cutanea tarda	Cirrhosis, hepatoma.	May be related to occurrence in alcoholics.
	Diabetes mellitus.	Perhaps more common in these patients.
Epidermolysis bullosa acquisita	Dysproteinemias, myeloma	

REFERENCES

Braverman IM: *Skin Signs of Systemic Disease,* 2nd ed. Saunders, 1981.

Callen JP: Internal disorders associated with bullous disease of the skin: A critical review. J Am Acad Dermatol 1980;3:107.

Callen JP (editor): Symposium on cutaneous signs of systemic disease. Med Clin North Am 1980;64:807. [Entire issue.]

Callen JP et al: *Dermatological Signs of Internal Disease.* Saunders, 1988.

Chanda JJ: Scleroderma and other diseases associated with cutaneous sclerosis. Med Clin North Am 1980;64:969.

Curth HO: Skin lesions and internal carcinoma. Pages 1308–1344 in: *Cancer of the Skin.* Andrade R et al (editors). Saunders, 1976.

Gilchrest BA: Pruritus: Pathogenesis, therapy, and significance in systemic disease states. Arch Intern Med 1982;142:101.

Golitz LE: Heritable cutaneous disorders which affect the gastrointestinal tract. Med Clin North Am 1980;64:829.

Hanno R, Callen JP: Sarcoidosis: A disorder with prominent cutaneous features and their interrelationship with systemic disease. Med Clin North Am 1980;64:847.

48

Disorders of the Mouth

Roy S. Rogers III, MD

GENERAL PRINCIPLES OF MANAGEMENT OF DISEASES OF THE ORAL MUCOSA

Diagnosis

A disease of the oral cavity may be limited to the mouth or it may be an oral manifestation of a systemic condition. To assess the scope of the disorder, careful examination of the skin and a general medical evaluation may be needed. Treatment of the oral disease without consideration of systemic factors may yield a less than satisfactory result. Conversely, the administration of systemic therapy without controlling the periodontitis, the accumulation of calculus, or the endogenous microflora of the oral cavity may yield a treatment failure.

The oral cavity, like the skin, is readily accessible for visual inspection and palpation by the physician. A dental or ENT mirror is helpful in examining the posterior portions of the oral cavity. Most oral cancers are detectable by careful clinical examination before they become large or metastatic.

About 20,000 men and 10,000 women develop oral cancer each year, accounting for about 10,000 deaths yearly. Because most early oral cancers are mistaken for benign conditions and because they do not exhibit a specific morphologic structure, complete examination of the oral cavity and prompt biopsy of suspicious lesions are critical.

Oral Hygiene

Achieving and maintaining good oral hygiene is an excellent starting point in the prevention of oral disorders. General preventive measures include the following:

Regular tooth brushing.
Soft-bristled toothbrush.
Up-and-down strokes.
Fluoride-containing dentifrice.
Adequate intake of fluoride in childhood.
Unwaxed dental floss to remove plaque and calculus.
Regular dental checkups.
Proper alignment of occlusal forces.
Avoidance of refined sugar.

General Treatment Measures

General measures to control inflammatory diseases of the oral cavity include the following:

Avoidance of hot, acid, and irritating foods and fluids.
Frequent and gentle cleansing of inflamed tissues with saline mouthwashes (1 tsp of table salt to 8 oz of lukewarm water).
Avoidance of tobacco.
Adequate hydration.
Adequate rest.
Topical or systemic (or both) analgesics.

WHITE LESIONS OF THE ORAL CAVITY

White lesions of the oral mucosa are common. The whiteness may be due to hyperplasia of the epithelium or to a change in the nature of the keratin, allowing it to imbibe water and appear soggy. Various benign conditions may present as white lesions (Table 48–1).

1. LEUKOPLAKIA

Leukoplakia has been defined as a white patch or plaque on the oral mucosa that cannot be wiped off and which is not clearly recognized as a specific condition (Fig 48–1). A white plaque compels the observer to establish a diagnosis. If obvious measures such as correction of damage due to trauma or cessation of tobacco use do not lead to resolution of the leukoplakic lesion, a biopsy should be obtained. The pathologist will grade the changes as benign, dysplastic, or malignant, and treatment can then be planned accordingly.

Benign or mildly dysplastic leukoplakic lesions require frequent periodic examinations, biopsy of indurated areas, removal of offending factors, and good oral hygiene. Lesions of the tongue, soft palate, anterior pillar complex, and floor of the mouth should be treated early by surgery because the potential for malignant transformation is higher than that of buccal,

Table 48–1. White lesions of the oral cavity.

White Plaque	Characteristics	Comment
Linea alba	White ridge of buccal mucosa opposite occulsal plane of teeth	Recognition
Leukedema	Filmy white opalescent quality	Recognition
Traumatic keratosis	Results from chronic low-intensity trauma; thickened patches	Remove trauma
White sponge nevus	Spongy, thickened, chamoislike; may be folded	Biopsy to confirm
Smoker's keratosis	Leukoplakia with nicotine stains	Stop tobacco use
Stomatitis nicotina	Smoker's keratosis of hard palate	Stop tobacco use
Candidiasis	Acute and chronic forms	See text
Lichen planus	Erosive and plaque	See text
Lupus erythematosus	Discoid type	See text

labial, or palatal lesions. Lesions elsewhere with moderate or severe dysplasia also should be treated surgically.

2. ERYTHROPLASIA

Red plaques of the oral mucosa may be benign but must be sampled and studied histologically. These lesions are frequently asymptomatic and should be recognized by clinical examination. There are 2 types of erythroplasia suggestive of oral cancer. The first is a granular, velvety red patch that may be stippled with white areas. The second is a smooth macular plaque. Both types have an abraded appearance and indistinct borders, and induration is often absent. Persistence of an erythroplastic patch for 10–14 days requires biopsy to exclude the possibility of squamous cell carcinoma. Approximately 80% of these lesions show invasive carcinoma on histologic examination.

3. ORAL CANCER

Oral squamous cell carcinoma accounts for 5% of neoplasms in men and 2% in women. These tumors are usually firm patches that may be ulcerated. Risk factors include heavy tobacco and alcohol use in persons in the fifth decade and older. Unfortunately, 60% of oral cancers are in an advanced stage at the time of discovery, so that a 5-year survival rate of 30% prevails. This should be contrasted with a 5-year survival rate of 95% for patients with skin and lip cancers. Patient delay in reporting symptoms is an important variable, as is physician delay in obtaining biopsy specimens. Because many early oral cancers are asymptomatic, careful clinical examination, recognition of suspicious lesions, and frequent periodic examinations and tissue sampling of benign or mildly dysplastic leukoplakic lesions are necessary to improve the prognosis for these patients.

OTHER ORAL TUMORS

Virtually any benign or malignant tumor that can occur in other areas of the body can occur in the oral cavity. In addition, tumors can develop in structures unique to the oral cavity. Most of these lesions are properly managed by the dentist or oral surgeon. A biopsy can be done to confirm the clinical diagnosis or to rule out cancer.

1. MESENCHYMAL TUMORS

Various benign mesenchymal tumors occur in the oral cavity. **Fibromas** are firm, dome-shaped, smooth, slowly growing nodules covered by normal mucosa (Fig 48–2). **Lipomas** are softer and deeper. Benign tumors of the nerve sheath (neurofibromas and neurilemmomas) are also slowly growing, well-circumscribed mucosal nodules. All of these lesions should be conservatively excised.

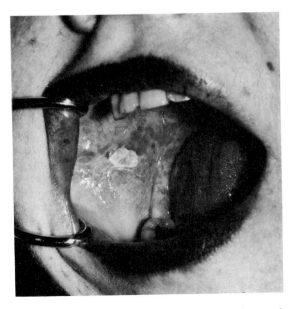

Figure 48–1. Leukoplakia is a white patch or plaque of the oral mucosa that cannot be wiped off. The term is descriptive, not diagnostic.

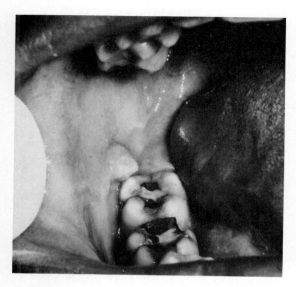

Figure 48–2. Oral fibromas are firm, dome-shaped nodules of the oral mucosa. They are benign, grow slowly, and are covered by normal mucosa.

Vascular tumors such as **lymphangiomas, hemangiomas**, and **pyogenic granulomas** can occur. Diagnosis is usually made on the basis of clinical findings. Management of each differs. Lymphangiomas should be conservatively excised if possible. Hemangiomas in infancy often regress spontaneously and should be managed conservatively. Pyogenic granulomas should be surgically excised or destroyed. They often are seen as bleeding sessile nodules. The gingival tumor of pregnancy is a pyogenic granuloma of the gums.

2. CYSTS

An **eruption cyst** is a bluish, dome-shaped nodule that overlies an erupting tooth. It may be treated simply by incising the overlying tissue.

A **mucocele** is a soft, well-demarcated nodule that occurs most often on the lower lip or floor of the mouth. It results from disruption of a salivary gland duct, allowing pooling of mucin or saliva in the lamina propria. Observation is a reasonable first approach, as the lesion may involute. If the mucocele persists, intralesional injection of triamcinolone acetonide (0.1–0.2 mL of 5 mg/mL solution) is reasonable treatment. Incision and drainage, surgical excision, or marsupialization may be necessary.

Dermoid and epidermoid cysts are trapped embryonic remnants. Rubbery, firm, slowly growing nodules may develop along the midline of the mouth. Surgical excision is the treatment of choice.

3. PIGMENTED LESIONS

The **amalgam tattoo** is an asymptomatic blue or black macule seen on the gingival, buccal, or sulcular mucosa. It results from the inadvertent introduction of silver amalgam into the tissue. No therapy is necessary unless the lesion is bothersome, in which case simple excision will suffice.

Lentigines are small, flat, hyperpigmented, single or multiple gray to brown macules. They may occur on the oral mucosa as well as the skin. If the macules are numerous and distributed on the lips, Peutz-Jeghers syndrome should be considered. Biopsy or simple excision can confirm the diagnosis.

Intraoral melanocytic nevi may occur, though they are far less common than cutaneous nevi. These lesions should be conservatively excised. Both lentigo maligna and malignant melanoma may arise on the oral mucosa.

CANDIDIASIS

Essentials of Diagnosis
- Opportunistic infection.
- White curdlike patches or red atrophic patches.
- Burning, painful symptoms.
- Hyphal elements in scrapings.
- Positive culture does not necessarily mean infection.

General Considerations

Candida albicans is an opportunistic pathogen that can adapt to various local and systemic conditions to cause active disease of the oral mucosa. The organism lives commensally in the mouths of 40% of the population without causing disease. Thus, culturing *Candida* organisms from the oral cavity does not necessarily implicate them as pathogens. Since *Candida* organisms must penetrate the outer layers of the mucosa in order to produce disease, the presence of hyphal forms in a scraping from the affected tissue is more diagnostic than is a positive culture. Situations in which *Candida* may become pathogenic include poorly controlled diabetes, endocrinopathies such as hypothyroidism, ecologic imbalances occurring with antibiotic therapy, local abrasions, surgical trauma, stomatitis from cancer chemotherapy, and any condition in which the host has been rendered immunoincompetent (corticosteroid administration, cancer chemotherapy, congenital or acquired immunodeficiency including AIDS).

A. Acute Candidiasis (Thrush): Acute pseudomembranous candidiasis (thrush) occurs in debilitated adults and children as well as newborns. Soft, almost fluffy, raised white patches are seen on the oral mucosa, with a predilection for the tongue, cheeks, and palate (Fig 48–3). When the plaque is scraped

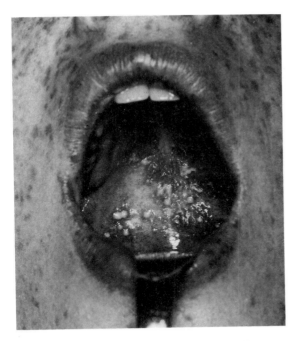

Figure 48–3. Thrush is an acute pseudomembranous candidiasis characterized by soft, almost fluffy raised white patches with a predilection for the buccal, tongue, and palatal mucosae.

away, a red, raw base is seen. The plaque contains matted organisms and desquamating epithelial cells.

B. Acute Atrophic Candidiasis: Acute atrophic candidiasis is a red, painful generalized inflammation of the oral mucosa that occurs in debilitated patients. This form of candidiasis occurs in patients who are receiving broad-spectrum antibiotics and in those undergoing therapy with cytotoxic and immunosuppressive drugs.

C. Chronic Atrophic Candidiasis: Chronic atrophic candidiasis is manifested by red, patchy, or confluent inflammation of the palatal mucosa of denture wearers. The patient often complains of a burning sensation or a sore mouth limited to the sites of the dentures, which are often worn 24 hours a day. Constant occlusion provides an ideal opportunity for *Candida* to invade the tissue. These patients often have angular cheilitis (perlèche).

D. Chronic Hyperplastic Candidiasis: Chronic hyperplastic candidiasis appears as a white, thickened plaque on the oral mucosa. These lesions are the result of systemic factors (eg, endocrinopathies) or local factors (eg, other lesions, trauma) that permit tissue invasion and a hyperplastic response. Median rhomboid glossitis probably represents a chronic hyperplastic form of candidiasis.

E. Chronic Mucocutaneous Candidiasis: Chronic mucocutaneous candidiasis is a complex group of diseases in which the invasion of *Candida* organisms produces mucosal, cutaneous, and occasionally paronychial lesions. The causes are multifactorial, but they are usually related to an underlying immunodeficiency state.

Differential Diagnosis

The differential diagnosis of candidiasis includes the white lesions of the oral cavity (Table 48–1).

Treatment

Treatment of the various forms of candidiasis is directed both at the infection and at the underlying causes. After gentle cleansing of the mouth, an antimycotic preparation such as nystatin solution should be applied. Clotrimazole or nystatin troches can be held in the mouth until they dissolve and are swallowed. The patient should use the antibiotic after meals and hold it on the mucosa long enough to allow the drug to act. To prevent relapse, treatment should be continued for 7 days after a clinical cure. Ingestion of ketoconazole, 200 mg/d, or application of a 0.5% solution of gentian violet judiciously and infrequently can be helpful in refractory disease. For *Candida* denture stomatitis, the dentures should be soaked in an antimycotic solution at night. During the day, they may be used as a fixed dressing to maintain an antimycotic cream in opposition to the inflamed mucosa. Early construction of properly fitting dentures is important.

Prognosis

Unless there is some profound underlying condition, the candidiasis should clear in 7–14 days with appropriate therapy. Recurrence or chronicity of candidiasis indicates the need for a careful medical evaluation of underlying factors.

VIRAL INFECTIONS OF THE MOUTH

The oral cavity is a common site of viral infections, whether localized or systemic (Table 48–2). Specific treatments, if available, are discussed in Chapter 14. The treatment for infection localized to the oral mucosa is supportive, as outlined in General Principles of Management, above.

BACTERIAL INFECTIONS OF THE MOUTH

Bacterial infections of the oral cavity are unusual. Certain organisms, however, can attack the debilitated host. Cases of diphtherial stomatitis, deep fascial plane infections with facultative anaerobes, and "thrush" from organisms other than *Candida* have been reported.

Table 48–2. Viral infections of the oral cavity.

Infection	Presentation	Site	Age	Comment
Herpes zoster	Painful grouped vesicles	Unilateral	Adults > children	Skin lesions
Herpetic gingivostomatitis	Painful grouped vesicles	Diffuse, lips	Children > adults	Fever, malaise
Recurrent herpes	Painful grouped	Single group, lips	Adults > children	Rare intraoral
Herpangina	Scattered tiny vesicles, petechiae	Posterior mucosa	Children > adults	Fever, pharyngitis
Infectious mononucleosis	Scattered tiny vesicles	Posterior mucosa	Adults > children	Fever, pharyngitis
Hand, foot, and mouth disease	Scattered tiny	Posterior mucosa	Children > adults	Hand, foot lesions
Varicella	Scattered tiny vesicles	Posterior mucosa	Children	Skin lesions
Measles	Bluish macules with red halo	Buccal mucosa	Children	Skin lesions
Rubella	Petechia	Posterior mucosa	Children	Skin lesions

Acute necrotizing ulcerative gingivitis (trench mouth, Vincent's infection) is an acute infectious disease of the gingiva caused by a fusiform bacterium and a commensal spirochete acting synergistically. Lesions are usually localized to the interdental papillae but may involve the buccal mucosa and pharynx. Clinically, the lesions are necrotic, punched-out ulcers with a yellowish exudate. Considerable discomfort attends the infection.

In the presence of fever or lymphadenopathy, systemic antibiotic therapy with penicillin or metronidazole is indicated and is usually followed by rapid improvement in 4 or 5 days. During the acute phase, a warm hydrogen peroxide mouth rinse should be used. After the acute phase has passed, cleaning the teeth and oral hygiene measures should be instituted. Occasionally, gingivectomy is necessary to recontour the remaining gingival tissue. Emotional stress, fatigue, and smoking are predisposing factors that should be controlled.

SEXUALLY TRANSMITTED DISEASES

Lesions of sexually transmitted diseases are becoming more common on the oral mucosa. Herpes simplex, gonorrheal stomatitis, pharyngitis, and syphilis can all cause mouth disease. These are discussed in detail in Chapter 13.

Oral lesions may be seen in all stages of syphilis. In congenital syphilis, abnormal central incisors (Hutchinson's teeth) and molars (mulberry molars) and scars radiating from the angles of the mouth (rhagades) may be seen. In primary syphilis, chancres may be noted on the lips or oral mucosa.

Pharyngitis or mucous patches can accompany secondary syphilis. The mucous patches may be subtle, or there may be an obvious white plaque. Scraping the surface leaves a raw, red, eroded, and highly contagious base. Gummas of tertiary syphilis classically involve the palate or tongue.

ORAL MUCOSAL MANIFESTATIONS OF SYSTEMIC DISEASES

1. SJÖGREN'S SYNDROME

Sjögren's syndrome is a chronic inflammatory disorder characterized by diminished function of the salivary and lacrimal glands. There are 3 forms: (1) a primary form, (2) a form associated with autoimmune diseases, and (3) a form associated with aggressive lymphocyte behavior. Two of the following 3 criteria are required for the diagnosis: (1) xerophthalmia (keratoconjunctivitis sicca), diagnosed by slit-lamp examination; (2) xerostomia, by biopsy of the labial minor salivary glands; and (3) an associated autoimmune or lymphoproliferative disorder.

Oral symptoms include painful tongue (glossodynia), altered taste (dysgeusia), dry mouth (xerostomia), angular cheilitis, and dental caries of the cervical portion of the teeth. Between one-third and one-half of patients have salivary gland enlargement. Other symptoms include xerophthalmia, photophobia, conjunctivitis, nasal or vaginal dryness, bronchitis, and pneumonia. Extraglandular symptoms include Raynaud's phenomenon, purpura, and symptoms associated with autoimmune disease.

The differential diagnosis of the sicca complex of

Table 48–3. Autoimmune disease associated with Sjögren's syndrome.

Systemic lupus erythematosus
Rheumatoid arthritis
System scleroderma
Mixed connective tissue disease
Dermatomyositis
Polymyositis
Graves' disease
Graft-versus-host disease
Celiac sprue
Dermatis herpetiformis
Chronic active hepatitis
Primary biliary cirrhosis

xerostomia (dry mouth) and xerophthalmia (dry eyes) includes sarcoidosis, amyloidosis, hyperlipoproteinemias, hemochromatosis, and the use of anticholinergic drugs. The primary form of Sjögren's syndrome is the sicca complex only. The sicca complex may be associated with an autoimmune disease (Table 48–3).

Patients with Sjögren's syndrome suffer an increased risk of developing lymphoproliferative disorders, such as B cell lymphoma, non-Hodgkin's lymphoma, and dysproteinemias. The risk is 43 times greater than normal. Indications that the immunologic disturbances attending Sjögren's syndrome are evolving toward a lymphoproliferative disorder include lymphadenopathy, splenomegaly, increased parotid gland swelling, and a decrease in the previous hyperglobulinemia.

Therapy for Sjögren's syndrome should be directed toward the autoimmune disease, if present. The xerostomia is treated palliatively with increased fluids, oral rinses with 2% methylcellulose, sugar-free sialagogues, and scrupulous oral hygiene and dental care. Xerophthalmia is treated palliatively by the use of artificial tears, prompt treatment of infections, and the wearing of diving goggles to maintain ocular humidity.

2. GRANULOMATOUS DISEASES

Wegener's granulomatosis is characterized by locally necrotizing granulomas of ear-nose-throat structures, the lungs, and the kidneys. Ragged, heaped-up ulcers of the oral mucosa, particularly posteriorly, may be seen.

Oral lesions are seen in one-fourth of patients with **sarcoidosis**. The most common lesion is a yellowish-red papule or nodule that has a predilection for the palate and tongue, though the lesions may be diffusely dispersed. Involvement of the salivary glands (Heerfordt's syndrome) is another characteristic form of sarcoidosis.

The **histiocytosis X syndromes** may involve the oral mucosa. Granulomatous gingivitis, granuloma-

tous nodules, and bony destructive lesions leading to tooth exfoliation are seen in histiocytosis X.

3. GASTROINTESTINAL DISEASES

The oral cavity may a be a reliable indicator of gastrointestinal disease. The oral manifestations are presented in Table 48–4.

4. HEMATOLOGIC DISEASES

Iron-deficiency anemia may provoke oral paresthesias and xerostomia before the pale, smooth, depapillated tongue is recognized. **Plummer-Vinson syndrome (sideropenic dysphagia)** affects middle-aged women, in whom the signs and symptoms of iron deficiency anemia plus leukoplakia and an atrophic oral mucosa are noted. Nail changes of koilonychia (spoon-shaped nails) and dysphagia secondary to esophageal webs or strictures—along with achlorhydria, angular cheilitis, and splenomegaly—complete the syndrome.

Pernicious anemia is classically associated with a smooth, red to magenta, beefy, painful tongue. Erythematous macules of the buccal mucosa and angular cheilitis may accompany this megaloblastic anemia. Interestingly, the nuclei of the oral mucosal epithelial cells show the typical megaloblastic

Table 48–4. Oral manifestations of gastrointestinal disease.

Disease	Manifestations
Crohn's disease	Aphthous stomatitis, oral Crohn's disease, cobblestone edema
Ulcerative colitis	Aphthous stomatitis, pyostomatitis vegetans
Peutz-Jeghers syndrome	Lentigines of lips, oral mucosa
Hemochromatosis	Blue-gray oral mucosal pigmentation
Blue rubber bleb nevus syndrome	Compressible blue, domed angiomas
Peptic ulcer disease	Cherry angiomas, venous lakes, and grouped capillaries of lips
Acrodermatitis enteropathica	Nonspecific stomatitis, cheilitis
Sprue	Glossodynia, aphthous stomatitis
Pernicious anemia	Glossodynia, fiery-red tongue, flabby tongue, aphthous stomatitis
Malabsorption	Sore mouth, glossitis, stomatitis, cheilitis
Gardner's syndrome	Supernumerary teeth, bone cysts
Plummer-Vinson syndrome	Glossodynia, pale smooth tongue, leukoplakia, oral cancer

changes of hyperchromatism, prominent nucleoli, nuclear enlargement, and serrated, marginated chromatin seen in peripheral leukocytes and bone marrow specimens.

The **leukemias** are associated with several changes of the oral mucosa. In acute leukemia, gingival swelling results from the accumulation of leukemic cells in the gingivae. Purpura and ulceration may attend the leukemic infiltration. Petechiae, purpura, ecchymoses, or spontaneous bleeding of the gingivae may at times be the presenting complaint. In chronic leukemia, ulcerative oral lesions are more common than gingival swelling.

Cyclic neutropenia is a periodic disease in which attacks occur at 3-week intervals. Fever, headache, malaise, and cervical lymphadenopathy accompany the gingival and oral necrotic ulcers. **Agranulocytosis** is often accompanied by gingivitis, superficial

erosions, or large, necrotic ulcers. With **polycythemia**, the mucosa is edematous, congested, and livid and bleeds easily. The **hypereosinophilic syndrome** may present with mucosal ulcers. Eosinophilic ulcer of the tongue is a benign and self-limited process characterized by infiltrating eosinophils in the lamina propria and mucosa.

ORAL MANIFESTATIONS OF GENODERMATOSES (Table 48–5)

The oral cavity is a rich site of manifestations of various genodermatoses. Many of these disorders are reflected in changes in the oral mucosa, while others are reflected in tooth or bony disturbances.

Some of these genodermatoses are associated with

Table 48–5. Oral manifestations of genodermatoses.

Disorder	Inheritance	Oral Lesions	Other Manifestations
Acrodermatitis enteropathica	Autosomal recessive	Erosive stomatitis, candidiasis	Alopecia, growth retardation, diarrhea (inherited zinc-deficiency state)
Multiple endocrine neoplasia, type 2b	Autosomal dominant	Papular and nodular neuroma tumors of lips and tongue	Corneal neuromas, pheochromocytoma, medullary carcinoma of thyroid
Darier's disease	Autosomal dominant	Cobblestone papules of oral mucosa	Hyperkeratotic, crusted plaques in intertriginous and seborrheic areas
Pachyonychia congenita, type 1	Autosomal dominant	Oral leukokeratosis	Palmoplantar hyperkeratosis, hyperhidrosis, keratosis pilaris, nail dystrophy
White sponge nevus	Autosomal dominant	Spongy, white oral plaques	May involve anus, vulva, vagina
Peutz-Jeghers syndrome	Autosomal dominant	Orificial and oral tiny pigmented macules	Hamartomatous gastrointestinal polyps
Hereditary hemorrhagic telangectasia	Autosomal dominant	Telangiectases of lips, tongue, and mucosa	Telangiectases of many visceral organs, skin, arteriovenous fistulas
Neurofibromatosis[1]	Autosomal dominant	Oral nodules, unilateral macroglossia	Neurofibromas in visceral organs, skin, café-au-lait spots, axillary freckles, central nervous system involvement (gliomas, epilepsy, oligophrenia), bony abnormalities
Tuberous sclerosis	Autosomal dominant	Oral fibromas	Adenoma sebaceum, periungual fibromas, shagreen patch, ash-leaf white macule, epilepsy, phakomas, renal tumors
Cowden's syndrome[1]	Autosomal recessive	Cobblestone papules of oral mucosa	Verrucous skin papules, punctate palmoplantar keratoderma, facial papillomas, soft tissue tumors, multiple visceral anomalies including malignancies
Nevoid basal cell carcinoma syndrome[1]	Autosomal dominant	Jaw cysts	Multiple basal cell carcinomas, bony abnormalities
Gardner's syndrome[1]	Autosomal dominant	Osteomas of facial bones, supernumerary teeth	Epidermoid cysts, osteomas, soft tissue tumors, polyposis of gastrointestinal tract
Papillon-Lefèvre syndrome	Autosomal recessive	Exfoliation of primary and permanent teeth	Palmoplantar hyperkeratosis and hyperhidrosis, psoriasiform rash of elbows and knees
Sturge-Weber syndrome	· · ·	Unilateral oral angiomas	Cutaneous, ocular, intracranial angiomas

[1]Associated with malignancies.

the development of cancer, which may be prevented by prophylactic surgery (as in Gardner's syndrome) or treated early if the association is recognized (as in Cowden's syndrome). In all, a proper diagnosis is important for prognostic reasons and for genetic counseling. Recognition of the oral manifestations, some of which are among the earliest signs or symptoms, is important to diagnosis. (See also Chapter 20.)

CONTACT STOMATITIS

All forms of contact stomatitis are uncommon because of the brief period of contact of irritants or allergens with mucosal surfaces while eating; because of neutralization, dilution, and buffering of irritating chemicals by saliva; and because of the rapid removal of the antigen by the vascularized mucosa and the paucity of keratin available to form a complete antigen. Irritant contact stomatitis is more common than allergic contact stomatitis. Contact stomatitis usually presents as a generalized inflammatory condition of the mucosa with edema, erythema, and occasionally erosions and ulcers. The patient may complain of paresthesias and taste disturbances, with few objective findings.

Allergic causes include flavorings, coloring agents, preservatives, benzocaine, detergents and abrasives found in dentifrices, mouthwashes, topical anesthetics, and oral medications. Dental metals and resins and denture materials are occasionally allergens.

Allergic gingivostomatitis is a characteristic fiery red, edematous, troublesome inflammation of the gingivae attached to underlying bony structures such as the alveolar ridges and palate (Fig 48–4). Occasionally, it can affect the soft tissues of the oral mucosa. It is most often caused by flavorings and

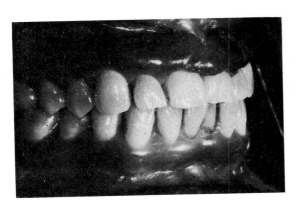

Figure 48–4. Allergic gingivostomatitis is a characteristic fiery red, edematous inflammatory reaction affecting the gingivae attached firmly to the underlying alveolar bone.

coloring agents included in dentifrices, mouthwashes, candies, mints, and chewing gum.

Treatment

Identification and removal of the offending agent allows for healing of the tissues. Gentle oral hygiene usually suffices, but topical corticosteroid preparations are occasionally necessary if the inflammation is severe.

STOMATITIS MEDICAMENTOSA

Adverse reactions to systemically administered medications can affect the oral mucosa only or the oral mucosa as a part of a more generalized adverse reaction. The former is exemplified by gingival hyperplasia caused by phenytoin and the latter by erythema multiforme with oral, ocular, genital, and cutaneous lesions. These adverse reactions are listed in Table 48–6.

Postantibiotic stomatitis is a diffuse erythematous stomatitis in which the tongue is red, smooth, and tender. Recovery is slow, even after use of the antibiotic is discontinued. Supportive measures and treatment of superimposed *Candida* infection may be necessary. The diffuse **toxic stomatitis** that attends cytotoxic anticancer therapy is also characterized by slow recovery. Management is the same as for postantibiotic stomatitis.

RECURRENT APHTHOUS STOMATITIS

Essentials of Diagnosis
- Recurrent oral ulcers.
- Three morphologic types: minor, major, and herpetiform.

Table 48–6. Stomatitis medicamentosa.

Reaction	Drug
Gingival hyperplasia	Phenytoin
Lichen planus-like eruption	Gold, penicillamine, oral antidiabetic agents
Black, hairy tongue	Antibiotics, griseofulvin
Glossodynia	Lithium, antibiotics, griseofulvin
Taste dysfunction	Lithium, antibiotics, griseofulvin, metronidazole
Gingivitis	Oral contraceptives
Candidiasis	Oral contraceptives, antibiotics, cytotoxic agents, corticosteroids
Diffuse stomatitis	Antibiotics, cytotoxic agents
Ulcerative stomatitis	Cytotoxic agents
Hyperpigmentation	Chloroquine, quinacrine, alkylating agents
Xerostomia	Antihistamines, anticholinergics, antihypertensives

- Few lesions at a time.
- Intense pain early, less intense later.
- Complete healing between episodes.
- Characteristically affects young people.

General Considerations

Recurrent aphthous stomatitis (canker sore) is the most common cause of recurrent oral ulcers, afflicting at least 20% of the general population at some time. Onset after age 30 is uncommon. It is not a distinct entity but the mucosal manifestation of several conditions. About 25% of cases can be related to some underlying cause; the remainder are classified as idiopathic.

Clinical Findings

Symptoms and Signs: There are 3 types of recurrent aphthous stomatitis: minor aphthous ulcers, major aphthous ulcers, and herpetiform ulcers. **Minor aphthous ulcers** are the most frequent (80%) type. Multiple small, shallow ulcers surrounded by an erythematous halo affect the anterior oral mucosa (Fig 48–5). The ulcers typically resolve in 7–14 days, without scarring. The average patient suffers 3–4 episodes per year.

Major aphthous ulcers are less common (10% of cases). Single or multiple large, deep ulcers surrounded by an erythematous halo affect the anterior or posterior oral mucosa (Fig 48–6). The ulcers may require 14–30 days to resolve and usually leave a scar.

The elemental lesion in **herpetiform ulcers** is a vesicle with a surrounding halo of erythema. The vesicles are grouped like the vesicles of herpes simplex (Fig 48–7). However, herpetiform ulcers are not caused by herpes simplex virus; canker sores are not a viral infection. Groups of vesicles may affect any oral mucosal surface, and the patient may have as many as 100 individual lesions. The vesicles usually coalesce

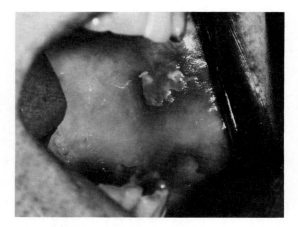

Figure 48–6. Major aphthous ulcers are another type of canker sore. These are single or multiple large, deep ulcers surrounded by an erythematous halo.

into plaques, then into large ulcers. Healing may require several weeks and leave scars.

The lesions of recurrent aphthous stomatitis are probably produced as an immunologic attack on some antigen. Some authors report that 15% of patients with recurrent aphthous stomatitis have deficiencies of vitamin B_{12}, folate, iron, or a combination of these substances. When the deficiency is identified, corrected, and replaced, most sufferers undergo a complete or marked remission. Other correctable causes include systemic diseases such as celiac sprue, Crohn's disease, ulcerative colitis, gluten sensitivity, and Behçet's syndrome.

Some women develop lesions in the latter half of the menstrual cycle, when serum estrogen levels are low. These patients give clear histories of association of their oral ulcers with their menstrual cycles, and they respond to the use of estrogens or estrogen-dominated oral contraceptives.

B. Laboratory Findings: Deficiencies of vitamin B_{12}, folic acid, or iron may be present even when the complete blood count and peripheral smear are normal. For this reason, specific assessments for deficiencies are indicated.

Differential Diagnosis

Lesions of oral lichen planus and the oral blistering diseases are continuous; they are neither recurrent nor characterized by complete healing between episodes. Cyclic neutropenia can cause mouth ulcer. Both the neutropenia and the ulcers have a regular 3-week periodicity.

Treatment

Individual episodes can be ameliorated by caustics such as silver nitrate, which convert an immunologic lesion to a more readily healing traumatic one, or by

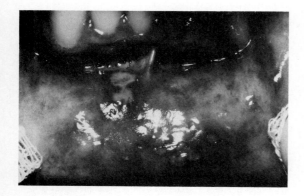

Figure 48–5. Minor aphthous ulcers are a type of canker sore. These are multiple, small, shallow ulcers surrounded by an erythematous halo.

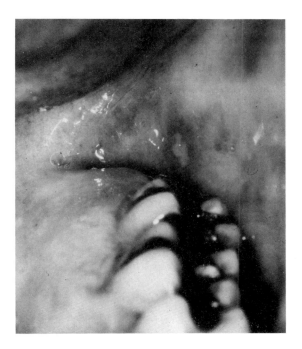

Figure 48–7. Herpetiform ulcers are a third type of canker sore. The elemental lesion is a tiny vesicle. These are often grouped (herpetiform) and become confluent into larger ulcers. They are not caused by herpesvirus.

the frequent application of topical fluorinated corticosteroids to early lesions. Once the lesion is fully developed, the above methods should be avoided, as they may delay healing. Supportive oral therapy as outlined at the beginning of this chapter is indicated to allow spontaneous healing. Pain may be temporarily relieved by the use of viscous lidocaine or dyclonine applied topically with a cotton-tipped swab.

Prognosis

Most patients with recurrent aphthous stomatitis undergo a spontaneous remission during the second or third decade of life.

ORAL LICHEN PLANUS

Lichen planus may affect the skin only, the skin and oral mucosa, or the oral mucosa only (see Chapter 41). Middle-aged and older persons are most commonly affected. As an oral ulcerative disease, it is differentiated from recurrent aphthous stomatitis by its persistence and morphologic appearance. A spontaneous remission of oral lichen planus occurs in 50% of patients by 12 months. Morphologically, the ulcers of lichen planus are usually set in an erythematous background, often overlaid with or adjacent to reticu-

lar, whitish, netlike striae. The tongue and the buccal and labial mucosae are favored sites, though any oral mucosal surface, including the gingivae, may be involved. Lichen planus may take 2 forms: nonerosive (linear, papular, plaques) or erosive (atrophic, erosive or bullous, ulcerative).

Oral lichen planus may be asymptomatic, particularly the thickened, raised plaques. If pain is present, the intensity remains relatively constant. Whitish plaques develop on the buccal mucosa or lateral borders of the tongue (Fig 48–8). Erosive lesions have lost the covering epithelium and are therefore sensitive to acidic, spicy, and thermal stimuli. Erosive lesions are surrounded by the hyperkeratotic whitish network that characterizes lichen planus. Complete healing does not occur.

A biopsy specimen from the border of a lesion (thickened white tissue) will confirm the diagnosis. Differentiation from recurrent aphthous stomatitis is not difficult (Figs 48–5 to 48–7).

The combination of red and white lesions should suggest the possibility of oral cancer. Malignant degeneration of oral lichen planus is quite unusual, though patients with chronic lichen planus should be followed closely.

Treatment of oral lichen planus is palliative. Suppression of inflammatory events with fluorinated topical corticosteroids applied 3–4 times daily is beneficial. If a drug is responsible, it should be discontinued if possible.

BULLOUS DISEASES

Blisters on mucosal surfaces break easily and leave erosions and ulcers. The history of a blister should stimulate the clinician to consider the differential diagnosis of oral blistering diseases (Table 48–7). The liberal use of routine histopathologic and immunofluorescent studies of tissue and serum is critical to the diagnosis of the oral blistering diseases. Early diagnosis is important to an early, aggressive treatment program, which can control the disease before it becomes generalized or advanced. (See Chapters 8 and 42.)

LESIONS OF THE TONGUE

Varicose veins are commonly seen on the undersurface of the tongue in patients in middle life and older and have no pathologic significance.

Black hairy tongue is caused by hyperplasia of the filiform papillae. Black pigment derived from the metabolic by-products of oral microflora also may be seen. This condition sometimes occurs after the administration of antibiotics. Simple tongue brushing with a dentifrice may suffice as treatment. If not, brushing for 3 minutes after the application of 40%

Table 48–7. Oral blistering diseases.

| Disease | Presentation | Histologic Features | Immunofluorescence | | Comment |
			Direct	Indirect	
Pemphigus vulgaris	Oral	Blister, acantholytic	Intercellular space	Intercellular space	Oral lesions in 50% ante-date skin lesions
Bullous pemphigoid	Oral and skin	Subepithelial blister	Basement membrane zone	Basement membrane zone	Skin lesions often first
Cicatricial pemphigoid	Oral and ocular	Subepithelial blister	Basement membrane zaone	Negative	Oral lesions first, may involve other mucosa, scarring
Erythema multiforme	Oral and skin	Subepithelial blister	Vessels	Negative	Target lesions, urticarial lesions simultaneous onset of skin and oral lesions

urea may be considered. The pigment can be bleached with 3% hydrogen peroxide.

Oral hairy leukoplakia causes subtle white striae on the sides of the tongue. It is a relatively specific oral manifestation of systemic infection with human immunodeficiency virus (HIV) and can be treated by applying tretinoin solution (Retin-A) 0.05% daily.

Furred tongue results from failure to properly desquamate or from hypertrophy of the filiform papillae. It is seen with febrile illnesses, smoking, and upper respiratory infections. Brushing the tongue with a dentifrice and a soft-bristled toothbrush usually suffices as treatment.

Smooth tongue results from the absence or atrophy of the filiform papillae. It is classically associated with nutritional deficiencies such as iron deficiency anemia, Plummer-Vinson syndrome, pernicious anemia, and malabsorption states (sprue and pellagra). Therapy is directed to the underlying condition.

Fissured tongue is a developmental defect seen with Down's syndrome. It may be acquired during the course of several diseases (Sjögren's syndrome, Melkersson-Rosenthal syndrome) or as an isolated defect associated with advancing age. No therapy is necessary.

Geographic tongue results from hyperplasia of patterned areas of the tongue. Other areas may be normal or atrophic, yielding the picture of a bas-relief map. This condition is more common among young patients and those with the atopic diathesis. Topical tretinoin or fluorinated corticosteroids may ameliorate the occasional symptomatic geographic tongue.

Median rhomboid glossitis has traditionally been attributed to a developmental defect presenting in later life, ie, the persistence of the embryonic tuberculum impar. The patient discovering the midline mass is often concerned about cancer. Median rhomboid glossitis is benign and may represent a form of chronic hyperplastic candidiasis. If the lesion does not respond to anticandidal therapy, biopsy examination should be done to confirm the diagnosis and allay anxiety.

GLOSSODYNIA

Glossodynia (idiopathic orolingual paresthesias, "burning tongue") is one of the more vexing causes of sore mouth. It has been described as a burning, itching, stinging, sandy sensation of the mouth, particularly the tongue. The typical patient is a postmenopausal woman with persistent distressing symptoms but no observable lesions. Table 48–8 lists the causes of glossodynia. Only after these have been excluded can the clinician attribute the symptoms to psychologic causes.

DENTURE SORE MOUTH

Denture sore mouth may be a cause of glossodynia. In a series from the UK, 5% of patients in a general dental practice, 10% of patients in a diabetic clinic, and 25% of patients in a menopause clinic complained of burning mouths. In most of these pa-

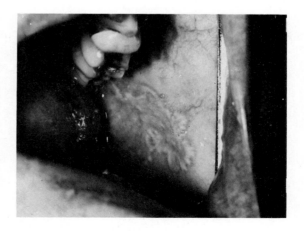

Figure 48–8. The plaque-like lesions of oral lichen planus are characterized by a central plaque with a surrounding zone of white, reticulated inflammatory activity.

Table 48–8. Causes of glossodynia.

Iron deficiency anemia
Folate deficiency
Pernicious anemia
Diabetes mellitus
Menopause (estrogen deficiency)
Dentures
Contact dermatitis
Candidiasis
Xerostomia
Oral habits
Coincidental dental disease
Depression
Anxiety or cancerophobia
Drug reactions

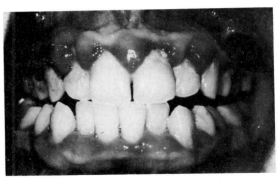

Figure 48–9. Periodontitis is the inflammatory response of the gingiva to the accumulation of plaque and calculus (note surfaces of teeth). The gingivae become swollen and inflamed, and pockets (pyorrhea) develop around the neck of the tooth.

tients, denture defects were part of the problem. However, other causes such as iron, folate, or vitamin B_{12} deficiency, diabetic medication, estrogen deficiency, dental abscess, and anxiety or cancerophobia also were important. In many cases there was more than one cause.

Patients suffering from denture sore mouth often have denture defects that cause chronic trauma, and most have associated candidiasis along with the other causes. If a patient wears dentures 24 hours a day, occluded tissues may not have an opportunity to recover from the chronic trauma. Removing the dentures for 1–2 weeks and treating for oral candidiasis frequently alleviate the symptoms. (See also Chronic Candidiasis, above.)

XEROSTOMIA

Dryness of the mouth is a relatively common complaint of patients aged 50 years or older. Drugs such as anticholinergics, antihypertensives, antipsychotics, and antidepressants may be responsible. In some patients, the symptom is a manifestation of aging and hypofunction of the salivary glands. In others, sicca symptoms may represent Sjögren's syndrome or other organic causes (postradiation therapy; replacement of glands by tumor or inflammatory tissue).

If the patient can masticate and swallow a saltine cracker without fluids, xerostomia is mild. In such instances, oral fluids (for lubrication of the oral mucosa) are all that is necessary; a glass of water for rinsing at the bedside is helpful for quenching nocturnal thirst. If the patient cannot masticate and swallow the saltine cracker, xerostomia is severe. Patients

with moderate or severe xerostomia are likely to have dental caries and candidiasis. Fluoride mouth rinses, scrupulous oral hygiene, regular dental prophylaxis, and anticandidal therapy are helpful adjuncts.

In all patients with xerostomia, a search should be made for organic causes.

GINGIVITIS & PERIODONTITIS

Gingivitis and periodontitis are the most common inflammatory reactions involving dental supporting structures. Gingivitis involves the interdental, marginal, or attached gingivae and is caused by the accumulation of plaque (mucinous and bacterial deposits) and calculus (hard deposits) at the interface of the tooth and gingival tissues. Thorough prophylaxis and scaling, coupled with meticulous oral hygiene and the use of nonwaxed dental floss, can usually control the gingivitis.

When the inflammatory process spreads to involve the supporting structures of the tooth (periodontal ligament and alveolar bone), periodontitis is present (Fig 48–9). Untreated periodontitis leads to extensive bone resorption, separation of the gingivae from the teeth (pocket formation), and eventual tooth loss or pyorrhea or both. If the periodontal pocket attains sufficient depth, surgical correction will be necessary to restore full dental health.

REFERENCES

Altman J, Perry HO: The variations and course of lichen planus. Arch Dermatol 1961;84:179.
Andreasen JO: Oral lichen planus. 1. A clinical evaluation of 115 cases. Oral Surg Oral Med Oral Pathol 1968;25:31.
Basker RM, Sturdee DW, Davenport JC: Patients with

burning mouths: A clinical investigation of causative factors, including the climacteric and diabetes. Br Dent J 1978;145:9.

Bean SF: Diagnosis and management of chronic oral mucosal bullous diseases. Dermatol Clin 1987;5:751.

Beitman RG, Frost SS, Roth JL: Oral manifestations of gastrointestinal disease. Dig Dis Sci 1981;26:741.

Conklin RJ, Blasberg B: Oral lichen planus. Dermatol Clin 1987;5:663.

Daniels TE et al: The oral component of Sjögren's syndrome. Oral Surg 1975;39:875.

Decker J, Goldstein JC: Risk factors in head and neck cancer. N Engl J Med 1982;306:1151.

Fisher AA: Contact stomatitis. Dermatol Clin 1987;5:709.

Gorlin RJ, Pindborg JJ (editors): Syndromes of the Head and Neck. McGraw-Hill, 1964.

Gorlin RJ: Genetic disorders affecting mucous membranes. Oral Surg Oral Med Oral Pathol 1969;28:512.

Hutton KP, Rogers RS III: Recurrent aphthous stomatitis. Dermatol Clin 1987;5:761.

McCarthy PL, Shklar G (editors): Diseases of the Oral Mucosa, 2nd ed. Lea & Febiger, 1980.

Nashberg A, Garfinkel L: Early Diagnosis of Oral Cancer. American Cancer Society, 1978.

Nuss DD et al: Multiple hamartoma syndrome (Cowden's disease). Arch Dermatol 1978;114:743.

Powell FC: Glossodynia and other disorders of the tongue. Dermatol Clin 1987;5:687.

Randle HW: White lesions of the mouth. Dermatol Clin 1987;5:641.

Ray TL: Oral candidiasis. Dermatol Clin 1987;5:651.

Reeve CM, Vanroekel NB: Denture sore mouth. Dermatol Clin 1987;5:681.

Rice DH: Advances in diagnosis and management of salivary gland diseases. West J Med 1984;140:238.

Rogers RS III (editor): Disorders of mucous membranes. (Symposium.) Dermatol Clin 1987;5:641. [Entire issue.]

Rogers RS III: Recurrent aphthous stomatitis: Clinical characteristics and evidence for an immunopathogenesis. J Invest Dermatol 1977;69:499.

Shklar G: Modern studies and concepts of leukoplakia in the mouth. J Dermatol Surg Oncol 1981;7:996.

Staffileno H Jr: Periodontal disease: Special emphasis, recognition diagnosis, and indications for dental and medical management. J Am Acad Dermatol 1980;3:95.

Strand V, Talal N: Advances in the diagnosis and concept of Sjögren's syndrome (autoimmune exocrinopathy). Bull Rheum Dis 1980;30:1046.

Zelickson BD, Rogers RS III: Oral drug reactions. Dermatol Clin 1987;5:695.

Mitchell H. Friedlaender, MD

The skin of the eyelids is susceptible to the same types of infections, hypersensitivity disorders, and tumors that involve the skin elsewhere. Eyelid skin is extremely thin, and the loose subcutaneous tissue allows fluid to accumulate and become walled-off by the orbital septum. The mucous membrane of the eye—the conjunctiva—is the target of many infections and immunologic processes, including the bullous dermatoses. The cornea, protected by the eyelids and by the conjunctiva, may be affected secondarily in skin and mucous membrane disorders. It may be the primary target of certain immunologic diseases.

ATOPIC (ALLERGIC) KERATOCONJUNCTIVITIS

Atopic keratoconjunctivitis, the ocular counterpart of atopic dermatitis, is seen in a small percentage of patients with atopic dermatitis—particularly those with severe involvement. Rarely, ocular symptoms may be the most prominent feature of the disease. Atopic dermatitis is discussed in Chapter 40.

Atopic keratoconjunctivitis can affect men or women at any age. Adolescents and young adult men are particularly susceptible, and in these patients the disease typically runs a course of 5–15 years.

Clinical Findings

The skin of the eyelids may show erythematous and exudative lesions. In later stages, scaling and crusting may occur. Infection of the lid margins with *Staphylococcus aureus* is common.

The conjunctiva may appear red and swollen. A watery discharge and photophobia are frequently noted. Less commonly, cobblestonelike elevations ("giant papillae") may be observed on the palpebral conjunctiva. These papillae consist of edematous tissue containing numerous eosinophils, plasma cells, lymphocytes, and mast cells. Examination of conjunctival scrapings nearly always reveals numerous eosinophils. In long-standing atopic disease, scarring of the palpebral conjunctiva may be observed.

Atopic cataracts (Fig 49–1) are seen in 8–10% of patients with atopic keratoconjunctivitis but usually not for at least 10 years after onset of the skin disease.

Atopic cataracts typically show a shieldlike opacification of the anterior lens cortex. Keratoconus, a form of corneal ectasia, is more common in atopic individuals than in the general population.

Differential Diagnosis

Vernal keratoconjunctivitis may be difficult to distinguish from atopic keratoconjunctivitis on ocular examination. It is rarely seen after age 20 years. This disorder is associated with warm climates and is worse in the spring and summer. Conjunctival scarring does not usually occur, and skin lesions expected with atopic dermatitis are generally not present.

Treatment

If symptoms are mild, cool compresses and vasoconstrictor antihistamine eye drops (eg, Albalon-A, Vasocon-A) may be sufficient. In more severe cases, topical corticosteroid eye drops may be needed to control the inflammation, but ocular corticosteroid therapy is best conducted by an ophthalmologist, because these medications may be associated with severe ocular complications such as glaucoma, cataract formation, and superinfection. They are particularly hazardous in patients with corneal herpes simplex infection, in whom their improper use may lead to irreversible corneal damage and blindness. Any patient receiving ocular steroid therapy should have slit-lamp

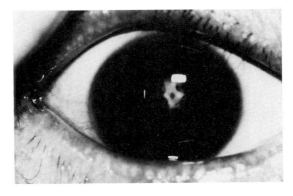

Figure 49–1. Atopic cataract in a patient with long-standing atopic keratoconjunctivitis.

examination and tonometric evaluation at regular intervals. Steroid therapy of the skin of the eyelids also has been associated with cataract formation. In some patients, this may be due to the dermatitis or atopic state. Because systemic steroids can cause cataracts and precipitate glaucoma, it is useful for patients receiving chronic systemic steroids to have a baseline eye examination with follow-up examination at 6- to 12-month intervals.

Cromolyn sodium (Opticrom) 4% eye drops 4 times a day provide marked relief of itching, redness, and photophobia in patients with atopic keratoconjunctivitis and other allergic ocular disorders.

If the lid margins are infected, a topical antibiotic may help.

CONTACT DERMATITIS

The skin of the eyelids is particularly susceptible to contact allergy (see also Chapter 33). Although almost any chemical can elicit dermatitis, several eye drops commonly used in ophthalmology are potent contact sensitizers. Neomycin, a frequently used topical antibiotic, produces contact dermatitis in some patients who chronically use it as drops. Atropine and its derivatives, used as mydriatics, are also contact sensitizers. Topical anesthetics, antihistamines, eyelid cosmetics, preservatives in eye drops, and even fingernail polish have also been implicated. Occasionally, glaucoma medications such as echothiophate iodide may produce contact sensitivity.

Clinical Findings

The eye is a frequent site of involvement in contact dermatitis. The lower eyelid is preferentially involved when exposure to eyedrops is responsible, whereas the upper eyelid is more dramatically involved in reactions to other contactants such as nail polish. Conjunctivitis may be present, characterized by a papillary response, pronounced vasodilatation, chemosis, and watery discharge. Erythematous blepharitis may also occur, as can keratitis in severe cases.

Treatment

The best treatment is to terminate exposure to the allergen. It is often possible to substitute other drugs when eye drops are involved. Cool, soothing compresses give relief. Weak topical corticosteroid creams or ointments can be used for a week or so if there is periorbital involvement.

CICATRICIAL PEMPHIGOID

Cicatricial pemphigoid can be a severe debilitating and blinding disease (see Chapter 42). It is a bullous dermatosis that affects mucous membranes much more severely than skin. Eye involvement occurs in 50–75% of cases as early as 10 years before or as late as 20 years after the onset of other mucosal or skin lesions.

Clinical Findings

A. Symptoms and Signs: The disease may begin as a nonspecific conjunctivitis involving one or both eyes. Early symptoms include burning, a foreign body sensation, excessive tearing, sticking together of the eyelids, and photophobia. Occasionally, blisters may be seen on the bulbar conjunctiva or lid margins. Hyperemia and thickening of the conjunctiva may be noted, and a ropy mucoid discharge may be present.

In later stages, symblepharon formation may occur (Fig 49–2). The inferior cul-de-sac is usually more involved than the superior. Symblepharon formation may progress relentlessly and lead to obliteration of the fornices, adhesions of the bulbar and palpebral conjunctiva, and restriction of eye movements. Frequently, the lacrimal puncta are also obliterated. In the later stages, cicatricial entropion may be seen.

The cornea may be severely affected in the later stages of the disease. This is due to lack of wetting by lid movement, partly from paucity of tears and entropion. The dryness results from progressive scarring of the conjunctiva, obstruction of the lacrimal ducts, and loss of goblet cells from the conjunctiva. About one-third of patients with the disease become blind, usually in both eyes.

B. Laboratory Studies: Direct immunofluorescence studies show linear deposits of IgG or IgA in the basement membrane zone in approximately 40% of cicatricial pemphigoid patients. In addition, one may find deposition of IgM, components of the complement system (C1q, C4, C3), properdin, and fibrin. A small percentage of cicatricial pemphigoid patients—mostly women with extensive disease—have circulating basement membrane zone antibodies of the IgG or IgA class. Antinuclear antibodies

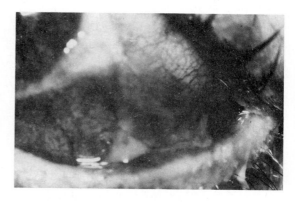

Figure 49–2. Symblepharon formation and shortening of lower conjunctival fornix in a patient with cicatricial pemphigoid.

(ANA) have been demonstrated in two-thirds of patients with ocular manifestations of cicatricial pemphigoid, but neither the ANA levels nor the titer of anti-basement membrane zone antibodies appears to correlate with the clinical course of the disease.

Differential Diagnosis

Ocular findings indistinguishable from cicatricial pemphigoid may be seen in Stevens-Johnson syndrome, pemphigus vulgaris, and toxic epidermal necrolysis. Alkali burns and drug-induced cicatrization of the conjunctiva may also be similar. The age of the patient, the history, involvement (or not) of other mucous membranes, and immunofluorescent studies usually help distinguish cicatricial pemphigoid from other ocular disease.

Treatment

The treatment for cicatricial pemphigoid is unsatisfactory. Topical corticosteroids have little or no effect on the disease. Systemic steroids may have no effect in preventing the relentless conjunctival cicatrization. Cytotoxic drugs such as cyclophosphamide and azathioprine have some effect, especially when used in combination with oral corticosteroids.

Extensive conjunctival scarring associated with cicatricial pemphigoid leads to inturning of the eyelashes and erosion of the cornea. Eyelashes should be removed when they abrade the cornea. This can be done by simple epilation with a cilia forceps, by electrolysis, or by cryotherapy of inturned lashes.

A major complication of cicatricial pemphigoid is a dry eye syndrome due to loss of goblet cells and stenosis of the lacrimal ducts. Artificial tears and mucus substitutes often help.

PEMPHIGUS

Pemphigus is a chronic, progressive autoimmune bullous disorder that occurs in several different forms (see Chapter 42).

Clinical Findings

A. Symptoms and Signs: Ocular involvement is rare in pemphigus. Catarrhal or purulent conjunctivitis is sometimes seen. Vesicles that rapidly rupture and erode may involve the inner canthus or palpebral conjunctiva. These are acutely painful but generally disappear in 7–10 days, leaving no scar. Repeated bulla formation may lead to conjunctival cicatrization with progressive contraction of the conjunctival sac, especially the lower fornix.

B. Laboratory Findings: Direct immunofluorescent studies demonstrate IgG and complement in the intercellular spaces of the epidermis and in the conjunctiva. Most patients also possess a circulating IgG antibody with affinity for the intercellular spaces of squamous epithelium.

Treatment

Corticosteroids have greatly improved the prognosis for this disease. Cytotoxic drugs such as azathioprine, cyclophosphamide, and methotrexate have been employed in conjunction with corticosteroids. Treatment is discussed in more detail in Chapters 42 and 53. In general, patients with pemphigus should be cared for by specialists, because the disorder is potentially fatal and very difficult to treat satisfactorily.

Topical combination antibiotic-corticosteroid eye drops can be used for the treatment of conjunctivitis accompanying pemphigus. The conjunctivitis often responds to systemic treatment at the same time the skin lesions improve. Removal of lashes when trichiasis is present may help reduce corneal complications. Artificial tears should be used for symptomatic relief.

STEVENS-JOHNSON SYNDROME

Stevens-Johnson syndrome is an acute bullous eruption involving the skin and mucous membranes (erythema multiforme major). The syndrome consists of fever; a variety of cutaneous lesions, including erythematous papules, "target" lesions, and bullae; and erosions or bullae on the mucous membranes. When the process affects only the skin, it is called erythema multiforme minor or simply erythema multiforme. The cause is unknown, but drug reactions and infections are often suspected. Stevens-Johnson syndrome frequently involves the conjunctiva.

The disease may occur at any age but is most common in children and young adults. Prodromal symptoms suggesting an upper respiratory tract infection such as fever and malaise may precede by several days the appearance of skin lesions. There may be extensive involvement of the skin, lips, oral mucosa, and other mucous membranes. Ocular involvement produces a clinical picture resembling cicatricial pemphigoid. Erythema multiforme is discussed further in Chapter 35.

Clinical Findings

Ocular involvement is common in the severe bullous form with mucous membrane involvement. The eyelids may show a generalized eruption with hemorrhagic crusting at the lid margins. There may be mild conjunctivitis that resolves without complications or severe conjunctival involvement with blisters, pseudomembranes, and symblepharon. Purulent conjunctivitis may result from secondary infection. The raw conjunctival surfaces can heal with formation of symblepharon or ankyloblepharon. Lid deformities and trichiasis result from cicatricial changes. Loss of goblet cells in the conjunctiva, tear deficiency, and dry eye syndrome may result. Corneal complications secondary to conjunctival and lid abnormalities are the most serious ocular complications of the disease. Corneal ulceration and even perforation can result. Ocular complications occur in about 50% of patients with Stevens-Johnson syndrome.

Treatment

Systemic treatment is discussed in Chapter 35. Topical corticosteroid eye drops may quiet the acute inflammation, but their efficacy is unproved. Topical antibiotics can be used to treat secondary infections. Good hygiene and lubrication of the eye with artificial tears and ointments may help. Consultation with an ophthalmologist is recommended.

In chronic cases, tear supplements are given frequently to prevent corneal epithelial breakdown. Treatment of trichiasis and lid deformities is similar to that used for cicatricial pemphigoid.

TOXIC EPIDERMAL NECROLYSIS

Mucopurulent or pseudomembranous conjunctivitis is the most common ocular finding in toxic epidermal necrolysis. Conjunctival scarring and corneal complications may develop in severe cases. This disorder may be a severe generalized form of the Stevens-Johnson syndrome and is often a manifestation of hypersensitivity or toxicity to a drug. It can also occur as a form of graft-versus-host reaction. (See also Chapter 35.)

Clinical Findings

The skin of the eyelids and periocular region may show changes similar to those observed elsewhere. Eyelashes may be lost. A mucopurulent conjunctivitis, usually mild, is the most common sign, but in severe cases symblepharon formation may occur. Immobility of the lids may lead to exposure keratitis. Corneal ulceration, scarring, and vascularization may develop. Perforation of the globe has occurred rarely.

Treatment

Ocular involvement may require nothing more than good lid hygiene and crust removal. Attention should be given to corneal exposure and trichiasis, because corneal ulceration may result. Topical lubricants and topical antibiotics help prevent corneal complications. As with treatment of the Stevens-Johnson syndrome, the use of systemic corticosteroids is controversial. Evaluation by an ophthalmologist is strongly advised.

Prognosis

Conjunctival scarring may lead to a dry eye, corneal exposure, and even corneal perforation. If the eye is kept well lubricated and the cornea well covered by the eyelids, ocular complications are unlikely.

PSORIASIS

Lid lesions, conjunctival changes, and corneal vascularization occur in 10% of patients with psoriasis. These complications are twice as frequent in males as in females. They may be the only manifestations of the disease.

Clinical Findings

Ocular symptoms may be minimal or pronounced. The lashes may be covered with scales and the lid margins erythematous and crusted. Squamous blepharitis may lead to inflammatory ectropion with trichiasis. Aside from the lid changes, a common ocular finding is nonspecific conjunctivitis, catarrhal or purulent. Symblepharon, xerosis, and trichiasis occasionally follow the healing phase.

Treatment

The ocular manifestations are managed symptomatically. Good hygiene should be practiced. Topical corticosteroids may be used when necessary. The uveitis accompanying psoriatic arthritis requires monitoring by an ophthalmologist for increase in intraocular pressure, cataract formation, and the development of synechiae. Short-acting mydriatics may be used if there is a tendency to synechia formation.

Prognosis

The ocular findings in psoriasis are usually mild, and the visual prognosis is excellent. In uveitis associated with psoriatic arthritis, there is potential for significant ocular morbidity. Fortunately, this condition is rare.

ROSACEA

The eye is affected in about 50% of patients with rosacea. Ocular involvement may be mild, associated with conjunctival irritation; or severe, complicated by corneal involvement (see Chapter 26).

Clinical Findings

Ocular findings may occur before skin manifestations are noted. A chronic, nonulcerative blepharitis may be seen. There may be conjunctival hyperemia and a mild papillary reaction on the palpebral surfaces. The hyperemia may come and go and may be exacerbated by hot or spicy foods. Nodular conjunctivitis is sometimes present.

The cornea can be extensively involved. Infiltrates near the limbus may be seen intermittently; these may scar and lead to peripheral corneal vascularization.

Treatment

Oral tetracycline (eg, 250 mg 4 times daily) leads to considerable improvement in virtually all cases of ocular rosacea. Relapse may occur, however, within a few days after stopping the drug.

The corneal lesions respond to topical steroids in low doses. However, steroids promote corneal thinning within these lesions, so that patients undergoing topical steroid treatment should be seen every few days and examined with the slit lamp.

HERPES SIMPLEX

Herpes simplex virus is one of the most important infectious agents producing ocular disease. Corneal scarring secondary to herpes simplex keratitis is one of the leading indications for corneal transplantation. For general discussion of infection with this virus, see Chapter 14.

Clinical Findings

A. Eyelids: Blepharoconjunctivitis with vesicular lesions on the lid margins can occur with initial or recurrent infection. This may be seen in the newborn if the mother has active genital herpes. Occasionally, a diffuse chorioretinitis and associated encephalitis can develop.

B. Conjunctiva: Primary herpes simplex infection often begins as conjunctivitis, sometimes associated with conjunctival membranes and a palpable pre-auricular node.

C. Cornea: Herpes simplex keratitis is currently the leading cause of corneal blindness in the USA. The classic corneal lesion is the dendritic ulcer (Fig 49–3), which is usually unilateral and multiple and involves the epithelium. This lesion is accompanied by complete or partial loss of corneal sensation. The dendritic lesions are associated with replicating virus, and the linear nature is probably due to a sliding in of the corneal epithelium to cover the defect created by proliferating virus. Most dendritic ulcers last 7–14 days, though they may persist for longer periods. Larger geographic ulcers may occur, especially in immunocompromised individuals. These take longer to heal.

The deeper layers of the cornea can be affected in herpes simplex infection, and this generally leads to severe and prolonged disease. Disciform keratitis appears as a round area of corneal stromal edema. It may represent a hypersensitivity reaction to herpetic antigen, because live virus cannot be isolated from the stroma in most cases. Variable amounts of corneal stromal infiltration can be seen in severe herpetic corneal lesions. These lesions have a protracted course and may lead to permanent corneal scarring. Occasionally, inflammation of the cornea extends to the anterior chamber, resulting in herpetic uveitis and sometimes glaucoma. With deeper lesions, the likelihood of visual morbidity is increased.

Prevention

Ultraviolet light, fever, and stress are recognized triggers of herpes simplex infections. Patients are cautioned to reduce fevers and to avoid direct sunlight.

Treatment

The aim of treatment in herpetic ocular disease is to preserve vision and reduce the morbidity caused by recurrent inflammation. Herpes simplex keratitis is a self-limited disease that usually resolves within a few months.

The disease is usually treated by ophthalmologists. Dendritic corneal ulcers can be treated effectively by epithelial debridement. Alternatively, antiviral agents such as idoxuridine, vidarabine, trifluridine, and acyclovir are effective. Topical corticosteroids enhance viral proliferation and are therefore contraindicated in the presence of active herpetic epithelial disease.

Course & Prognosis

Deep herpetic corneal infections may last for years and lead to severe visual loss. Epithelial disease is usually mild and short-lived.

HERPES ZOSTER

Herpes zoster is a problem for ophthalmologists when it affects the ophthalmic division of the fifth cranial nerve. In such cases, the skin on one side of the forehead and nose and the adjacent upper eyelid

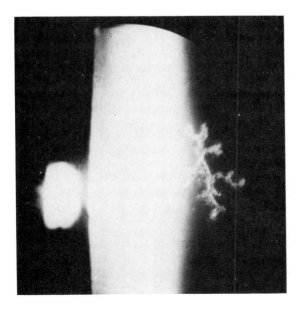

Figure 49–3. Dendritic corneal ulcer in herpes simplex keratitis. The ulcer is highlighted by retroillumination using a slit lamp photomicroscope.

develop vesicles on a red base. The conjunctiva, cornea, and uveal tract may be affected and lead to losss of vision.

Clinical Findings

A. Eyelids: The skin lesions (on lids and lid margins) of herpes zoster appear as grouped, red, painful macules that become papules, vesicles, pustules, and crusted ulcers. They usually heal within 2 weeks and only rarely lead to scarring.

B. Conjunctiva: The conjunctiva may be hyperemic and infiltrated by inflammatory cells. A papillary reaction is generally seen, but membranes, follicles, and transitory vesicles may be present. Permanent scarring may develop, leading to entropion and trichiasis.

C. Cornea: Small dendritic lesions of the corneal epithelium differ from herpes simplex dendrites in that those of zoster are elevated and do not have knoblike endings. A coarse punctate epithelial keratitis may be seen, almost always accompanied by corneal stromal lesions, which may be round or nummular. Corneal vascularization may develop.

D. Uvea: Iridocyclitis is a common ocular complication of herpes zoster. Inflammation may be mild or severe. The iris may be edematous and hyperemic. Later, sector atrophy and adhesions of the iris to the lens may be seen. Some color change of the iris may occur as a result of atrophy of the pigment layers. Secondary glaucoma is not uncommon in ophthalmic zoster. Occasionally, the posterior pole of the eye can be affected by focal choroiditis or hemorrhagic retinitis.

E. Other: Patients with zoster involving the fifth cranial nerve are among the most likely to develop postherpetic neuralgia. Age is a factor in the occurrence of this complication, because neuralgia is uncommon in patients under age 50 years.

Various neurologic disturbances are associated with herpes zoster, including pupillary abnormalities, ptosis, and other cranial nerve palsies.

Complications & Sequelae

Visual loss can occur as a result of corneal scarring and vascularization or because of glaucoma. Patients with fifth nerve involvement should be examined by an ophthalmologist so that a diagnosis of ophthalmic zoster can be made at an early stage.

Treatment

Usually the disorder is treated by ophthalmologists or after consultation with ophthalmologists. The skin lesions of ophthalmic herpes zoster should be treated with supportive therapy. If bacterial superinfection occurs, topical antibiotics are indicated.

Oral acyclovir appears to be effective in limiting the severity of herpes zoster ophthalmicus. Topical corticosteroids can suppress inflammation dramatically but may prolong the disease. If significant iritis is present, the pupil should be kept dilated with frequent instillation of a short-acting mydriatic.

Course & Prognosis

Zoster is generally self-limited.

LEPROSY

About 90% of patients with lepromatous leprosy have ocular manifestations; one-third show significant visual loss (see Chapter 12).

Clinical Findings

A. Lepromatous Leprosy: The supraciliary ridges are thickened, and there is loss of the eyebrows, beginning during the early stages of the disease. Nodules—histologically resembling xanthomas—appear on the face and lids. Lashes may show poliosis. In the later stages, there may be marked loss of cilia and eyebrows and disfigurement of the brows, nose, and lips. Hyperemic keratoconjunctivitis may occur, followed by symblepharon formation and lid deformities.

B. Tuberculoid Leprosy: Skin lesions may affect the lids and brows, leading to loss of eyebrows and cilia and to degenerative changes involving the brows and lid margins.

Treatment & Prognosis

Leprosy treatment is discussed in Chapter 12.

SARCOIDOSIS

Sarcoidosis is a multisystem disease of unknown cause characterized by a number of immunologic abnormalities (see also Chapter 47). The disease affects chiefly the lungs and lymph nodes, though almost any organ can be involved. Ocular findings are present in about 25% of cases. An ocular syndrome having the characteristic findings of sarcoidosis but lacking systemic disease may also be seen.

The immunologic abnormalities in sarcoidosis can be classified into 3 main areas: (1) depression of cellular immunity, (2) lymphoproliferation with increased serum gamma globulins, and (3) granulomatous reactions.

Clinical Findings

Small "millet-seed" nodules may be seen on the eyelids as on the skin elsewhere. Conjunctival nodules are frequently present on the palpebral conjunctiva and may be biopsied to confirm the diagnosis. Yellowish sarcoid nodules are sometimes seen on the episclera, especially over the insertion of the rectus muscles. The most common corneal manifestation of sarcoidosis is calcific band keratopathy. This usually develops after several episodes of uveitis.

Inflammation of the uveal tract is often characterized by the formation of "mutton fat" keratic precipitates. Nodules on the surface of the iris (Koeppe and Busacca nodules) are also typical features of sarcoidosis. A nonspecific chorioretinitis may develop, leading to scarring and pigment clumping in the retina. Scattered exudates on the retina that have been described as "candle wax drippings" may also be seen. Retinal vasculitis is not uncommon. Granulomas of the optic nerve have also been described. The lacrimal gland may also contain granulomatous inflammation.

Treatment

The mainstay of treatment in sarcoidosis is the use of systemic corticosteroids. Steroid therapy may be applied topically to the eye or injected subconjunctivally. Dilating drops may be necessary to prevent the iris from sticking to the lens (posterior synechiae). The prognosis is usually good; however, in certain cases, especially in blacks, the ocular disease may be severe and progressive and lead to significant visual loss.

REFERENCES

Bean SF, Halubar K, Gillett RB: Pemphigus involving the eyes. Arch Dermatol 1975;111:1484.

Friedlaender MH, Cyr R: Contact sensitivity in the guinea pig eye. Curr Eye Res 1981;1:403.

Friedlaender MH: *Allergy and Immunology of the Eye.* Harper & Row, 1979.

Jenkins MS et al: Ocular rosacea. Am J Ophthalmol 1979;88:618.

Person JR, Rogers RS III: Bullous and cicatricial pemphigoid: Clinical, histopathologic, and immunopathologic correlations. Mayo Clin Proc 1977;52:54.

50

Autoimmune Rheumatologic Skin Diseases

Denny L. Tuffanelli, MD

Scleroderma, dermatomyositis, and lupus erythematosus have in the past been collectively termed collagen diseases, connective tissue diseases, or collagen-vascular diseases. They are often grouped among the autoimmune rheumatologic skin disorders because they are systemic disorders of the dermis that are associated with various autoantibodies. Each of these disorders is usually regarded as a distinct clinical entity, though combinations of them can occur. The link between these multisystem diseases is evident from their many shared clinical and laboratory characteristics; cutaneous changes such as sclerosis, calcinosis, poikiloderma, periungual telangiectasia, and Raynaud's phenomenon are common to all. Likewise, systemic features such as myositis, arthralgias, and esophageal changes are seen in all 3 disorders. In scleroderma and lupus erythematosus in particular, levels of autoantibodies to cellular organelles and macromolecules are markedly increased.

A disease characterized by Raynaud's phenomenon and antibodies to extractable nuclear antigen (ENA) and ribonucleoprotein has been called "mixed connective tissue disease." The term "undifferentiated connective tissue disease" is preferred for that form of the disease in which patients lack ribonucleoprotein antibody. If monitoring is carried on long enough, the disease changes so that the physician can usually diagnose a more specific autoimmune rheumatologic skin disease. Although overlapping, undifferentiated autoimmune disease does occur and presents special problems in diagnosis and treatment, most patients with autoimmune rheumatologic skin diseases present with classic symptoms specific for one of the 3 major disorders.

SCLERODERMA

Scleroderma is a general term for several chronic autoimmune rheumatologic skin diseases of unknown but possibly immunologic cause, There are both localized cutaneous and systemic forms. The systemic form is called progressive systemic sclerosis. The localized cutaneous forms of scleroderma include morphea, generalized morphea, linear scleroderma, morphea profunda, eosinophilic fasciitis, and pansclerotic morphea.

Morphea usually occurs as discrete sclerotic plaques that slowly resolve over 3–5 years and leave areas of hyperpigmentation. In more extensive morphea, lesions may be generalized and involve deeper layers of tissues, eg, the panniculus (morphea profunda); lesions may also be mutilating (pansclerotic morphea). Patients with generalized morphea only rarely develop features of systemic scleroderma.

1. PROGRESSIVE SYSTEMIC SCLEROSIS

Essentials of Diagnosis
- Cutaneous sclerosis, usually acral in distribution but at times diffuse.
- Raynaud's phenomenon, cutaneous calcinosis, telangiectatic mats on face, lips, and hands.
- Dysphagia, arthralgias, myalgias, cardiopulmonary involvement.

General Considerations
Progressive systemic sclerosis (systemic scleroderma), a disease characterized by pathologic changes of the cutaneous, gastrointestinal, vascular, pulmonary, cardiac, and renal systems, is thought to be due to immunologic and vascular aberrations. The onset is insidious and the course unpredictable. Initial presenting symptoms usually include Raynaud's phenomenon, arthritis, or acrosclerosis. Raynaud's phenomenon and cutaneous sclerosis may be the only symptoms for long periods. Variants of systemic scleroderma with a different prognosis include the CREST syndrome (calcinosis, Raynaud's phenomenon, esophageal hypomotility, sclerodactyly, and telangiectasia), classic "diffuse" scleroderma, and inflammatory scleroderma. There is no standardized classification of systemic scleroderma.

The presence of numerous autoantibodies in the serum of patients with scleroderma (Table 50–1) suggests an immunologic pathogenesis. Antinuclear antibodies occur in 40–90% of patients with scleroderma, depending on the substrate used in immunologic studies. Immunofluorescent patterns include homogeneous, speckled, particulate, and so forth (Fig 50–1).

Table 50–1. Antibodies in scleroderma.

As defined by morphologic patterns on immunofluorescent staining:
"True" speckles
Large speckles
Particulate
Nucleolar
Homogeneous
Peripheral (rim)
As defined by the antigen reacting with the antinuclear antibodies:
4S-6S RNA
Scl-70
As defined by the antigen reacting with cellular organelles
Centromere
Centriole
Nucleolus
Mitochondrion
Lamins

Specific antibodies to nucleoli, centromeres, centrioles, and mitochondria have been demonstrated in scleroderma and account for many of the patterns. Patients with CREST syndrome often have anticentromere antibodies.

Clinical Findings

A. Symptoms and Signs: Cutaneous features include Raynaud's phenomenon, digital ulcers, cutaneous sclerosis (most commonly acral), calcinosis, telangiectases, and hyper- and hypopigmentation (Fig 50–2). Telangiectases may be periungual or matlike and involve the face, lips, and palms in particular. Cuticular thickening is common.

All organs may be involved; esophageal, articular, pulmonary, and renal involvement are the most sig-

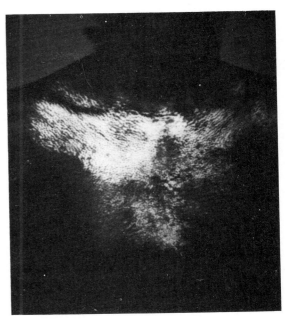

Figure 50–2. Extensive depigmentation of the chest in systemic scleroderma.

nificant. Gastrointestinal disturbances include dysphagia, regurgitation, weight loss, malabsorption, and constipation.

Arthralgias and myalgias predominate in the inflammatory form of systemic scleroderma. Biliary cirrhosis associated with mitochondrial antibodies occurs occasionally, as does thyroiditis associated with thyroid antibodies. Pulmonary symptoms include progressive exertional dyspnea and cough; recurrent pneumonia is not uncommon. Diffuse fibrosis in the lower two-thirds of the lung is typical. Only a few patients have clinical renal disease, which may cause renal failure, seizures, and death.

B. Laboratory and Other Diagnostic Studies: The diagnosis of systemic scleroderma is usually made clinically, though laboratory examinations may aid in evaluation of the activity and prognosis of the disease. The most helpful diagnostic laboratory findings include cutaneous sclerosis on skin biopsy, decreased esophageal motility on cine-esophagography or manometry, pulmonary fibrosis on x-ray, and tests reflecting diminished intestinal absorption. The blood count is rarely abnormal, but there may be eosinophilia or an elevated sedimentation rate. Cold agglutinins and rheumatoid factor may be present. Antinuclear antibodies are present in 40–90% of patients; the homogeneous (diffuse) pattern is seen most frequently on indirect immunofluorescent staining, but the nucleolar pattern is more specific and occurs more commonly in scleroderma than in any other disorder. Anticentromere and anticentriole antibodies

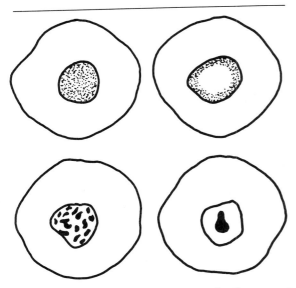

Figure 50–1. Patterns of antinuclear antibodies as seen by indirect immunofluorescence. (Clockwise from top left: homogeneous, peripheral, nucleolar, and particulate.)

also appear to be relatively specific for scleroderma. Antithyroid and antimitochondrial antibodies should also be sought during the evaluation. Anti-DNA, anti-ENA, and complement studies help to differentiate systemic scleroderma from other autoimmune disorders.

Differential Diagnosis

The differential diagnosis of systemic scleroderma includes other connective tissue diseases, overlapping connective tissue diseases, scleredema, scleromyxedema, eosinophilic fasciitis, porphyria cutanea tarda, bleomycin toxicity, amyloidosis, and chronic graft-versus-host disease.

Complications

The course of systemic scleroderma is variable; in some patients the course is rapidly progressive, but in most it is chronic and characterized by increasing morbidity. Cutaneous sclerosis may become extensive, and digital ulcers and gangrene may represent severe complications; amputation of digits is frequently necessary. Articular disability, marked ankylosis (Fig 50–3), and loss of function of digits are common. Cardiac, pulmonary, and renal lesions indicate a poor prognosis. Causes of death include renal, cardiac, or respiratory failure; perforation of the gastrointestinal tract; and intercurrent infection.

Treatment

There is no specific therapy for systemic scleroderma; treatment is supportive and directed toward the organ system involved. General measures include avoiding exposure to cold and refraining from smoking. Patients should avoid cold beverages, ice cubes, and occupational exposure to cold and should wear appropriate protective clothing (eg, gloves) in cold weather. Physiotherapy that includes whirlpool baths, casts, traction splints, paraffin casts, massage, and exercise may help prevent contractures. Application of topical antibiotics to digital injuries early in the course of the disease is helpful. The most common management problems are Raynaud's phenomenon and digital ulcers. A one-eighth-inch cylinder of nitroglycerin ointment may be applied topically. Biofeedback therapy is of limited use. Sympatholytics may be helpful early. Phenoxybenzamine (Dibenzyline) has been used, but nifedipine (Procardia), 10 mg 3 times daily, has proved most useful to prevent or lessen symptoms of Raynaud's phenomenon. Low-molecular-weight dextran and intra-arterial reserpine are used in patients with incipient gangrene. Cutaneous calcinosis is resistant to therapy.

There is no agent of proved efficacy for cutaneous sclerosis. Dimethyl sulfoxide (DMSO) is of no benefit. Corticosteroids may be useful in the acute inflammatory stage, and sulfasalazine (Azulfidine, others) has provided apparent benefit. Penicillamine is currently being used by some clinicians but is extremely toxic. Plasmapheresis is an expensive experimental approach. Gastrointestinal symptoms are often alleviated by cimetidine and esophageal dilation. Tetracycline is beneficial for malabsorption. Arthralgias and myalgias may be treated with nonsteroidal anti-inflammatory agents, systemic corticosteroids, or antimalarials. Prazosin, captopril, and dialysis have been lifesaving in patients with incipient renal failure. Many of these agents have serious side effects, and clinicians must be thoroughly familiar with each drug they prescribe.

Prognosis

The course of systemic scleroderma is fulminating in 10–30% of patients, who usually die within 5 years after diagnosis. In 70–90% of patients, the disease pursues a slow course, with increasing morbidity and disability. Rarely, the disease may become inactive.

2. LOCALIZED SCLERODERMA

Essentials of Diagnosis

- Morphea: hard, slightly yellow to white plaques with surrounding violaceous borders.
- Eosinophilic fasciitis: large, ill-defined areas of sclerosis of skin associated with limitation of movement.
- Linear scleroderma: hard, slightly yellow plaques, sometimes slightly depressed, occurring in a linear configuration, often on the scalp, face, or extremity.

General Considerations

These related disorders are characterized by sclerosis. Collagen fibers are thick and tightly packed,

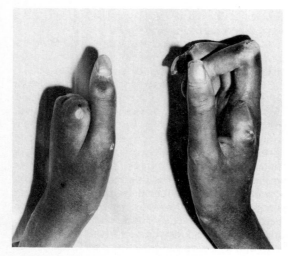

Figure 50–3. Ankylosis and loss of digits in systemic scleroderma.

and the zone of dermal connective tissue is wide. In morphea, most of the collagen is in the dermis. In morphea profunda, the collagen and inflammation are in the subcutaneous fat. In eosinophilic fasciitis, the fascia is the area of thick collagen. In disabling pansclerotic morphea, even the underlying muscle tissue may be inflamed and sclerosing. Linear scleroderma may affect all layers, including bone.

Clinical Findings

A. Symptoms and Signs: The lesions begin in indurated patches that are flesh-colored or faintly purplish, smooth, and shiny but feel firm. Pigmentation may occur. Guttate lesions and lesions that clinically resemble lichen sclerosus et atrophicus may occur.

In linear scleroderma, involvement of underlying bone and muscle leads to atrophy of the face or extremity and the resulting disturbing cosmetic appearance is a serious problem. If an extremity is affected, the disease is a major physical handicap as well.

B. Laboratory Findings: In localized scleroderma, particularly linear scleroderma, serologic abnormalities may be present, eg, antinuclear antibody, rheumatoid factor, antibody to single- and double-stranded DNA, and hypocomplementemia.

Differential Diagnosis

Localized scleroderma must be differentiated from such diseases as lichen sclerosus et atrophicus, the atrophodermas, lipoatrophy, lupus erythematosus, panniculitis, and other forms of panniculitis, scleredema, and Romberg's disease.

Complications

The major complications of localized scleroderma are severe cosmetic deformities when the scalp or face is involved and functional impairment when an extremity is involved.

Treatment

Plaquelike and guttate morphea lesions usually regress spontaneously. Topical and intralesional administration of corticosteroids is occasionally beneficial. Acute generalized morphea may respond to a brief course of systemic corticosteroids, eg, prednisone, 40 mg/d for 1 month, then tapered to complete withdrawal over the following 2 weeks. The management of morphea profunda, pansclerotic morphea, and linear scleroderma is difficult. Antimalarials and phenytoin are advocated by some.

Prognosis

Morphea often resolves spontaneously or with treatment. Linear scleroderma involving the scalp, face, or an extremity is often associated with progressive atrophy of underlying muscle and bone. Features of systemic autoimmune disease may develop.

LUPUS ERYTHEMATOSUS

Essentials of Diagnosis

- Photosensitivity, with skin lesions in areas exposed to sunlight.
- Specific and nonspecific cutaneous lesions; specific lesions include discoid lupus erythematosus, "butterfly" eruption, and annular lesions of subacute cutaneous lupus erythematosus.
- Discoid skin lesions: nummular scaling plaques with follicular plugs, atrophy, scarring, and telangiectases.
- Annular skin lesions: ringlike scaling plaques, usually with central hypopigmentation.
- Butterfly erythema: a fixed, sometimes sharply marginated red patch over the nose and cheeks.
- Joint symptoms in 90% of patients.
- Serologic abnormalities, including antinuclear antibodies, antibodies to double-stranded DNA, and hypocomplementemia.
- Involvement of internal organ systems (systemic form).

The American Rheumatism Association has proposed that a diagnosis of systemic lupus erythematosus can be made with reasonable probability if 4 of the following 11 criteria are present, serially or simultaneously, during any interval of observation:

Malar rash
Discoid rash
Photosensitivity
Oral ulcers
Nonerosive arthritis
Serositis
Renal disorder
Neurologic disorder
Hemolytic anemia, leukopenia, lymphopenia, or thrombocytopenia
Positive anti-DNA, anti-Sm, or false-positive serologic test for syphilis
Positive antinuclear antibody.

General Considerations

Lupus erythematosus is a connective tissue disorder of unknown cause with a broad spectrum of manifestations ranging from purely cutaneous involvement (discoid lupus erythematosus) through mild systemic illness to serious and potentially fatal disease. Systemic lupus erythematosus is probably not one but several conditions. Multisystem involvement occurs frequently, but the disease may affect only one organ, eg, skin or kidney. Although it is typically a disease of young women, it affects both sexes and all age groups, and there is no particular racial incidence. Remissions and exacerbations are common. Genetic predisposition, autoimmunity, certain drugs, sex hormones, ultraviolet light, viruses, and circulating antigen-antibody complexes play a role in etiology.

Clinical Findings

A. Symptoms and Signs: Cutaneous lupus erythematosus may be acute, subacute, or chronic, and lesions may be scarring or nonscarring. Patients with all forms of cutaneous lupus, including discoid lupus erythematosus, may develop systemic lupus erythematosus. There is a spectrum of disease between the purely cutaneous and systemic forms.

Classic lesions of discoid lupus erythematosus are well-defined plaques that are characterized by erythema, follicular plugging, telangiectasia, scarring, atrophy, hyperpigmentation, and hypopigmentation. Lesions are frequently limited to sun-exposed areas but may involve the ears, mucous membranes, and other areas not exposed to the sun. Subacute cutaneous lesions are most commonly annular or papulosquamous (Fig 50–4). Patients with subacute cutaneous lesions usually have mild systemic disease. Cutaneous lesions frequently noted in systemic lupus erythematosus include facial erythema in a butterfly distribution over the nose and cheeks, petechiae, purpura, leg ulcers, infarctive digital lesions, and digital

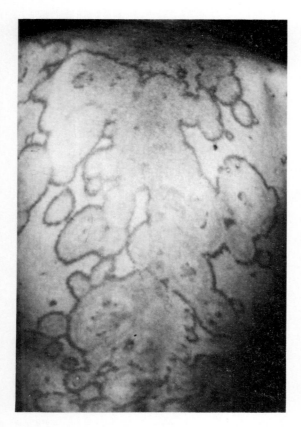

Figure 50–4. Subacute cutaneous annular lesions of lupus erythematosus.

gangrene. Raynaud's phenomenon occurs in about 20% of patients with systemic lupus erythematosus. Mucous membrane lesions occur in the purely cutaneous as well as the systemic forms. Bullous lesions may occur as part of lupus erythematosus; however, erythema multiforme, pemphigus, bullous pemphigoid, and dermatitis herpetiformis are also associated (rarely) with cutaneous lupus. Other unusual manifestations include erythromelalgia, multiple dermatofibromas, soft tissue calcification, and erythema annulare centrifugum.

Numerous variants of cutaneous lupus erythematosus are seen. In lupus panniculitis, panniculitis without vasculitis occurs deep in the subcutaneous fat. Firm, well-defined nodules up to 5 cm in diameter occur and leave an area of lipoatrophy upon resolution. The face, back, upper arms, and buttocks are most affected. The overlying skin may be normal, or cutaneous lupus erythematosus may be present. Therapy with antimalarial drugs (eg, hydroxychloroquine, 200 mg daily) or low doses of systemic corticosteroids (eg, prednisone, 15 mg each morning) is usually beneficial. The differential diagnosis includes Weber-Christian disease, pancreatic disease, traumatic or factitial panniculitis, and morphea profunda. (See Chapter 25.)

Lupus erythematosus and lichen planus coexist in an occasional patient. Chronic, painful, erythematous plaques on the extremities and palmar or plantar hyperkeratotic lesions usually occur, whereas pruritus and photosensitivity are rare. The lesions of lupus erythematosus and lichen planus cannot be easily differentiated clinically, histologically, or immunologically. Patients usually show a poor response to therapy.

A cutaneous lupuslike syndrome has been reported in patients with various complement deficiencies, most commonly in women with homozygous C2 deficiency. Most of these patients have photosensitivity and discoid lupus erythematosus. Rheumatoid arthritis occurs frequently. There is a low incidence of anti-DNA antibodies and renal disease. Complement-deficient patients with this syndrome present first to a dermatologist, and a very low total hemolytic complement (CH_{50}) determination (not C3 assay, which may be normal) suggests the diagnosis.

Fever is common. Musculoskeletal symptoms are present in most patients; persistent arthralgia and stiffness—with no permanent changes in the joints—are common. Myalgias are also common; muscle weakness due to myopathy associated with lupus erythematosus is seen less often. Patients with vacuolar myopathy associated with systemic lupus erythematosus have been described. Numerous cases of patients with systemic lupus erythematosus and concomitant avascular bone necrosis have been reported; the disease itself or systemic corticosteroids may cause the necrosis.

Renal disease is a feature of systemic lupus

erythematosus that has serious clinical implications; the finding of more than 5 red blood cells per high-power field in a clear urine specimen indicates active kidney disease. Proteinuria of over 1 g/24 h, red blood cell casts, oval fat bodies, and impaired renal function (elevated serum urea nitrogen or serum creatinine) indicate renal disease. The absence of renal involvement is best demonstrated by renal biopsy, because test results on urinalysis may be negative in active disease. Nephrotic syndrome is common in children with renal lupus erythematosus. In general, patients with decreased renal function and lupus nephritis have a poor prognosis, though exceptions occur.

Cardiac disease in lupus erythematosus may appear as pericarditis, myocarditis, or cardiomegaly and, later, heart failure. Pericarditis has been estimated to occur in 25% of cases.

Pleurisy with or without effusion is the most common clinical pulmonary finding mainly related to lupus erythematosus; true lupus pneumonitis is rare.

Esophageal involvement similar to that in scleroderma, with loss of peristalsis and dilatation of the esophagus and small intestine, may occur.

Jaundice is usually due to hemolytic anemia or hepatitis.

Central nervous system disease is the second most frequent cause of death in patients with lupus erythematosus. Kidney failure is first. Neurologic signs are usually mild and transitory. Symptoms of central nervous system disease are present in 25% of patients and peripheral neuritis in 12%. Convulsions, psychoses, and disturbances of mental function are common. Convulsions and coma are grave prognostic signs. Psychoses in systemic lupus erythematosus may occur as a result of treatment with systemic corticosteroids, may be intrinsically related to active systemic lupus erythematosus, or may represent psychiatric illness precipitated by systemic lupus erythematosus.

B. Laboratory Findings: When a diagnosis of cutaneous lupus erythematosus is first made, patients are concerned about the prognosis and confused about the possible systemic progression of disease. For this reason, a complete evaluation is performed when the patient first presents. If test results are normal, the patient is reassured that the disease is mainly cutaneous and likely to remain so and that it is chiefly a cosmetic problem. Tests performed at the first visit include a complete blood count, sedimentation rate, and urinalysis; antinuclear antibody, anti-DNA, CH_{50}, and C3 assays; and appropriate skin biopsies.

In patients with possible systemic lupus erythematosus, more extensive studies are performed to evaluate involvement of other organs. Laboratory studies in such patients may commonly demonstrate anemia, leukopenia, thrombocytopenia, or urinary tract abnormalities with systemic involvement. The sedimentation rate is often elevated.

The determination of antinuclear antibodies is the basic screening test for lupus erythematosus (Table 50–2). (The LE cell preparation is rarely used and is mostly of historical importance.) Serum from patients with systemic lupus erythematosus almost always demonstrates antinuclear antibodies, as does serum from many patients with discoid lupus erythematosus. Immunofluorescent staining techniques reveal that the homogeneous pattern is the most common;

Table 50–2. Antinuclear antibodies.

Antigens	Clinical Correlations
Deoxyribonucleic acid	
Double-stranded DNA (ds-DNA)	Systemic lupus erythematosus
Single-stranded DNA	Systemic lupus erythematosus, rheumatoid arthritis, Sjögren's syndrome
Single-stranded DNA (ss-DNA)	Rheumatic and nonrheumatic disease
Deoxyribonucleoprotein (DNP)	
Complex of DNA and histone	Systemic lupus erythematosus
Histone	Idiopathic systemic lupus erythematosus (60%) and drug-induced lupus erythematosus (95%)
Acidic nuclear proteins	
Extractable nuclear antigens (ENA)	
Sm	Systemic lupus erythematosus (30%)
RNP (ribonucleoprotein)	High in mixed connective tissue disease; lower titers in rheumatic diseases
SSA/Ro	Sjögren's syndrome, systemic lupus erythematosus with photosensitivity, subacute cutaneous lupus erythematosus, neonatal lupus erythematosus, C2-deficient lupus erythematosus
SSB/La/Ha	Sjögren's syndrome (60%), systemic lupus erythematosus (15%)
Scl-1, Scl-70	Scleroderma
Jo-1	Polymyositis
Pm-1	Polymyositis
Nucleolus	
Nucleolar 4S-6S RNA	Raynaud's disease, scleroderma
Centromere	Scleroderma, CREST syndrome
Centriole	Scleroderma
Lamins	Scleroderma

the nucleolar pattern is occasionally seen in lupus erythematosus but is more common in scleroderma. The outline (peripheral, ring) pattern usually reflects high titers of DNA antibodies and is seen in patients with active systemic lupus erythematosus. Speckled and particulate patterns are also noted. These morphologic patterns frequently correspond to specific nuclear antigens; these relationships are currently being studied. Dilution of serum and the substrates used may alter the patterns observed. Anti-double-stranded DNA antibodies are found in one-third to two-thirds of patients with lupus erythematosus and are specific for the disease. Patients with discoid lupus occasionally have DNA antibody, but such patients often develop systemic lupus erythematosus. High titers of DNA antibody correlate strongly with active disease. The *Crithidia luciliae* immunofluorescence assay is a test for double-stranded DNA.

Antibodies to extractable nuclear antigens (ENA) are often found and may provide a clue to the diagnosis and possibly the prognosis. Of the ENA antibodies, antibody to ribonucleoprotein is often associated with mixed connective tissue disease. Sm (Smith) antibody is associated with a relatively benign form of systemic lupus erythematosus, a higher incidence of Raynaud's phenomenon, and a lower incidence of central nervous system involvement and progressive nephritis than is DNA antibody alone. The cytoplasmic antigens Ro and La may be associated with a negative antinuclear antibody titer if certain substrates are used. Patients with antibodies to Ro or La usually have a positive antinuclear antibody titer if tissue culture or human tissue substrates are used to perform the test. Ro and La may be markers for a group of patients with cutaneous lupus erythematosus and photosensitivity who subsequently develop systemic lupus erythematosus.

Serum complement levels are often low in patients with active systemic lupus erythematosus. C3 and CH_{50} are the most commonly measured elements; C3 levels are used to follow disease activity. Assay of cryoglobulins and circulating immune complexes is useful. Falling levels of C3 and rising levels of anti-DNA antibodies and circulating immune complexes indicate increased disease activity.

C. Special Examinations: Study of cutaneous biopsy specimens by both light and immunofluorescence microscopy is useful in diagnosis. Pathologic changes in cutaneous lupus erythematosus usually correlate with the age of the lesion. Early skin lesions usually show only sparse and nonspecific changes, including atrophy of the epidermis, hydropic degeneration of the basal cell layer, and edema of the epidermis with vasodilatation and extravasation of red blood cells. In typical older discoid lesions, hyperkeratosis and follicular plugging may be seen in addition to lymphocytic infiltrates around hair follicles and sweat glands. In active systemic lupus erythematosus, fibrinoid changes are noted in the

ground substance. Arteries may show hyaline and fibrinoid necrosis of the media that is frequently associated with intimal and adventitial proliferation, lymphocytic infiltration, thrombi, and infarcts and may present as cutaneous vasculitis.

Direct immunofluorescence studies of skin biopsies are most useful in the diagnosis of lupus erythematosus. Immunoglobulins (predominantly IgG) and complement are bound to the region of the dermal-epidermal junction. Homogeneous, granular, and thready patterns have been described. In systemic lupus erythematosus, the band of immunofluorescent immunoglobulin may be seen in clinically uninvolved skin (Fig 50–5) as well as in involved areas, whereas in discoid lupus erythematosus only the lesions show deposition of immunoreactants. Antibodies to basement membrane or circulating antigen-antibody complexes due to exogenous or autologous antigens comprise these deposits.

Dermal-epidermal deposition of immunoglobulins is found in all forms of cutaneous lupus erythematosus and is useful in confirming the diagnosis of systemic lupus erythematosus in patients without typical skin lesions. The presence of the band of complement in clinically normal skin suggests increased disease activity.

Differential Diagnosis

The differential diagnosis of cutaneous lupus erythematosus commonly includes polymorphous light eruption, seborrheic dermatitis, rosacea, tinea barbae, erythema following treatment with cortico-

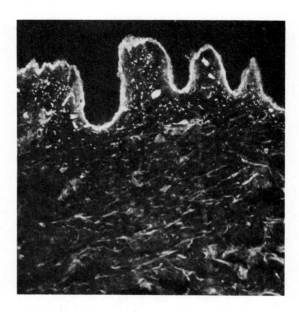

Figure 50–5. IgG deposited at the dermal-epidermal junction in normal-appearing skin in systemic lupus erythematosus.

steroids, lichen planus, psoriasis, and actinic keratoses. The cutaneous lesions of systemic lupus erythematosus vary widely and must often be distinguished from drug eruptions and other causes of vasculitis, bullae, mucous membrane lesions, etc. The differential diagnosis of various internal disorders is equally vast.

Pregnancy & Lupus Erythematosus

Birth control, pregnancy, and childbirth must be discussed with women patients who have lupus erythematosus. Birth control pills should be used with caution, if at all; other methods of contraception are preferable. Each patient must be individually counseled about the advisability of pregnancy. Fertility is not affected, but the abortion rate is about twice that of the normal population. Corticosteroid therapy is usually not harmful to the fetus. Maternal antinuclear antibodies can be transmitted placentally but disappears permanently by the time the infant is 4 months old.

Newborn infants of mothers with lupus erythematosus rarely demonstrate the features of discoid or systemic lupus erythematosus, but if newborns are affected, skin lesions of discoid lupus erythematosus, leukopenia, and thrombocytopenia are most frequently noted. The rash in neonatal lupus erythematosus is often periorbital in location and associated with prominent telangiectasia. The disease is usually self-limited but has persisted in several patients. Congenital heart block may occur in infants born of mothers who have Ro antibodies in their sera; the usual clinical presentation is bradycardia in utero or soon after birth.

Women should be reassured that they need not be overly concerned about passing the disease to their children, but the mother's disease may remain the same, worsen, or even go into remission during pregnancy. Although symptoms usually worsen with pregnancy, most women with systemic lupus erythematosus tolerate pregnancy well. Serious exacerbations occur occasionally. The outlook for women with mild systemic lupus erythematosus who contemplate pregnancy is usually good.

Treatment

A general medical examination and periodic blood counts, determination of the erythrocyte sedimentation rate, urinalysis, anti-DNA antibody and C3 levels are used to follow patients with active systemic disease. A common error in management is to generate undue alarm in patients with minimal cutaneous lupus erythematosus, eg, to create a phobia about sunlight. Patients with demonstrated photosensitivity should avoid exposure to the sun. Photosensitivity can usually be determined by the history, but testing is occasionally helpful (see Chapter 38). Plaques of discoid lupus erythematosus occur in traumatized areas, so that the patient should be advised to avoid picking and scratching. For patients with extensive, disfiguring scars from discoid lupus erythematosus, expert advice on the use of wigs and makeup by a cosmetologist is a positive approach. Sunscreens should be used when excessive exposure to sunlight is anticipated.

Use of local corticosteroid creams and ointments is the simplest, most effective therapy, particularly for early erythematous plaques; fluorinated preparations are particularly effective though more expensive. Application of topical corticosteroids followed by occlusion with pliable plastic film increases absorption and is often worthwhile. Intralesional injection of corticosteroids (eg, triamcinolone acetonide, 2–10 mg/ml) may be useful in refractory lesions, though the injected area may develop temporary or permanent subcutaneous atrophy. Surgical procedures are ineffective.

The decision to use antimalarial drugs in discoid lupus erythematosus is difficult. If lesions are refractory to treatment and cause excessive disfigurement, antimalarial drugs, including hydroxychloroquine (200–400 mg/d), chloroquine (250–500 mg/d), or quinacrine (100 mg/d), may be used, usually in that order of preference. Patients with photosensitivity or cutaneous lesions respond especially well to antimalarial therapy. Antimalarial drugs are recommended for some patients to reduce the dosage of corticosteroids required for concurrent therapy. Each has disadvantages. Some lesions will respond to one antimalarial but not to another. The dose is lowered when the patient responds. Side effects include gastrointestinal disturbances, itching, leukopenia, thrombocytopenia, myasthenia, and cycloplegia. Pigmentary changes of the skin, hair, nails, and hard palate are occasionally noted. Serious ocular changes include reversible keratopathy and irreversible retinopathy. Ophthalmologic consultation, including slit lamp and fundus examination, should be obtained before therapy is begun and every 3–6 months thereafter. A complete blood count and urinalysis are performed occasionally. Oral corticosteroids and cytotoxic agents may occasionally be of benefit for extensive cutaneous lesions but should be used only when the disease is not controlled; referral to a dermatologist is recommended.

In patients with systemic lupus erythematosus, a careful assessment of disease activity must be made, and any infections must be treated rapidly. Drug reactions are common, so drug therapy should be conservative. Blood transfusions should be given only in life-threatening situations.

A therapeutic trial of salicylate alone is often indicated. Aspirin or its equivalent, 4–6 g/d with milk, may be tried. The dosage may be increased until significant clinical improvement occurs or salicylism appears.

In some patients with the milder, chronic form of

lupus erythematosus, in whom rest, salicylates, and antimalarials may not adequately control signs and symptoms, corticosteroids—eg, prednisone, 2.5–10 mg/d orally—may be added to the aspirin-antimalarial regimen. Corticosteroids are always administered to patients who are febrile, toxic, and critically ill from systemic lupus erythematosus. Other indications include thrombocytopenia, hemolytic anemia, significant nephropathy, pericarditis, and central nervous system involvement. In severely ill patients, prednisone, 40–80 mg/d orally, is given to start, and the dosage is increased until symptoms are controlled; the dosage is then diminished as rapidly as possible. Side effects of corticosteroids are proportionate to the dosage. Frequent determinations (eg, once every 2–3 weeks) of blood pressure and weight, urinalysis, and blood counts should be obtained. In stressful situations such as operation or infection, the dosage must be significantly increased.

Immunosuppressive agents are used occasionally, particularly in the therapy of lupus nephropathy. Patients experiencing severe side effects from corticosteroid therapy or those who have failed to respond are candidates for immunosuppressive therapy. Immunosuppressive agents have both immunosuppressive and anti-inflammatory effects and should be used only by clinicians experienced in their use. Antimetabolites (eg, azathioprine), alkylating agents (eg, cyclophosphamide and mechlorethamine), and folic acid antagonists (eg, methotrexate) have been used.

Course & Prognosis

The relationship between pure discoid (cutaneous) lupus erythematosus and systemic lupus erythematosus has long been controversial. The incidence of patients who present with discoid lupus erythematosus that later progresses to systemic lupus erythematosus ranges from 2% to 20% and varies with the definitions used in classification and the patient populations studied.

It is not unusual for typical systemic lupus erythematosus to remit and leave lesions of chronic discoid lupus erythematosus. Discoid lupus erythematosus may spontaneously subside, remain at the same level of activity, worsen (with resultant scarring and disfigurement), or progress to active systemic lupus erythematosus, either slowly or acutely following some stress or insult.

Discoid lupus erythematosus per se can be localized (lesions only above the neck) or generalized (lesions on the trunk or extremities). Clinical and serologic abnormalities are greater in generalized discoid lupus erythematosus. Most observers agree that systemic lupus erythematosus with discoid lesions represents a more benign form of the disease, and survival time is longer than for patients with systemic lupus erythematosus without discoid lesions.

The prognosis for patients with systemic lupus erythematosus varies with the organs involved; renal or central nervous system involvement implies a poor prognosis. In most patients, the disease is chronic, with a 10-year survival rate over 90%.

POLYMYOSITIS-DERMATOMYOSITIS

Essentials of Diagnosis

- Periorbital edema and purplish (heliotrope) coloration over the upper eyelids.
- Gottron's sign: pink papules over the interphalangeal and metacarpal joints.
- Cuticular and periungual telangiectases.
- Proximal muscle weakness of the extremities.
- Elevated serum levels of muscle enzymes, eg, CK, AST (SGOT).

General Considerations

Polymyositis-dermatomyositis is a systemic connective tissue disorder of unknown cause; when skin lesions are present, the disease is termed dermatomyositis. Skin, connective tissue, and striated muscle are involved. Childhood cases usually occur before the age of 10 years. Most adult cases occur between the ages of 40 and 60 years. The reported incidence of associated cancer in adults varies from 10% to 40%. The primary tumor may occur in the lung, stomach, rectum, kidney, breast, uterus, or testis. Dermatomyositis may occur before the tumor is discovered.

Clinical Findings

A. Symptoms and Signs: Classic cutaneous signs include a violaceous (heliotrope) discoloration of the eyelids, a scaly malar erythema, and erythematous atrophic papules over the extensor surfaces of the interphalangeal and metacarpophalangeal joints (Gottron's papules; Fig 50–6). Cutaneous lesions may precede the onset of myositis by months or

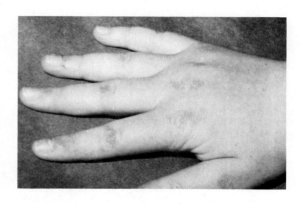

Figure 50–6. Papular erythema (Gottron's sign) over the joints in an 8-year-old child.

even years. Isolated dermatologic manifestations in the absence of systemic disease occur rarely. Cuticular thickening and cuticular and periungual telangiectases are common. Erythema over the upper cheeks and forehead and a dusky red rash of the arms and upper back are noted. Calcinosis, which appears most commonly in children, occurs in about 50% of patients as small nodules on the extremities, shoulder, and pelvic girdle that may ulcerate and extrude (Fig 50–7). Lesions of vasculitis with small cutaneous ulcerations of the trunk and arms occur occasionally.

Myopathy may occur before or after the appearance of cutaneous lesions. Typically, systemic proximal muscle weakness of the extremities and weakness of the anterior neck flexors and abdominal muscles occur. Subcutaneous edema may occur over the affected muscles. Flexural contractures of the elbows, hips, knees, and ankles are prominent. Hypopharyngeal involvement with diminished deglutition is a grave prognostic sign. Palatal, pharyngeal, and the upper third of the esophageal musculature are also affected, and aspiration pneumonia may be a serious associated problem. Respiratory difficulty due to intercostal and diaphragmatic weakness may require a respirator. Gastrointestinal ulceration secondary to vasculitis is seen in the childhood form of the disease.

B. Laboratory Findings: Serial studies of muscle enzyme levels (CK, AST [SGOT], aldolase, and LDH) are useful in evaluating disease activity. When enzyme levels are interpreted, hepatic and cardiac disease must be ruled out. In patients with chronic dermatomyositis, enzyme levels may be minimally elevated or normal. Electromyography may distinguish myopathy from neuropathy and is useful to help plan the site of muscle biopsy. Skin and muscle biopsies usually confirm the diagnosis; the latter demonstrates an inflammatory myositis. Elevated levels of gamma globulin and rheumatoid factor occur occasionally. Antinuclear antibodies are rarely present. Anemia is uncommon.

Differential Diagnosis

Differential diagnosis includes other connective tissue diseases, particularly scleroderma, lupus erythematosus, and mixed connective tissue diseases. Early cutaneous signs may resemble contact dermatitis or other inflammatory dermatoses.

Complications & Sequelae

Childhood dermatomyositis has a high incidence of complications, including contractures and generalized calcinosis. Soft tissue calcifications are not metabolically active, so they are difficult to treat. Gastrointestinal hemorrhage in children secondary to vasculitis is often fatal.

Because cancer and dermatomyositis are so often associated, studies must be performed to detect underlying cancer in all adults with dermatomyositis.

Treatment

Early diagnosis is essential. Laboratory tests of muscle enzyme levels are used to assess disease activity. In the early stages of active disease, corticosteroids, eg, prednisone, 25–100 mg orally each morning, are necessary; the dosage is thereafter tapered in accordance with the patient's response. The disease is often chronic, and therapy may be required for months or years. Most patients respond to corticosteroids. In patients who fail to respond to treatment, immunosuppressive agents—eg, methotrexate, cyclophosphamide, azathioprine, and chlorambucil—have yielded favorable results. Combination therapy with prednisone and methotrexate is probably most effective. Management of calcinosis is difficult and disappointing; nothing works. Physiotherapy can prevent contractures. Patients with an associated neoplasm have a poor prognosis, though remissions of dermatomyositis may occasionally follow removal of the tumor.

Course & Prognosis

The course of dermatomyositis is variable and unpredictable. The acute phase may become quiescent

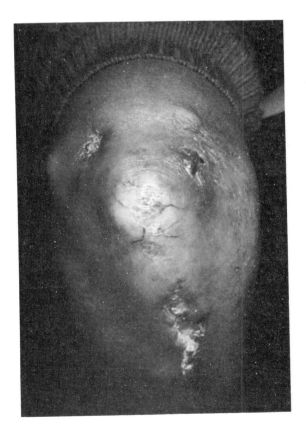

Figure 50–7. Cutaneous calcinosis.

and result in only minimal change, or the disease may become fulminant, with death ensuing within a year. Some patients develop severe contractures or exten-

sive calcinosis. Death is often due to hypopharyngeal paralysis and aspiration pneumonia.

REFERENCES

Crowe WE et al: Clinical and pathogenetic implications of histopathology in childhood polydermatomyositis. Arthritis Rheum 1982;25:126.

Nimelstein SH et al: Mixed connective tissue disease: A subsequent evaluation of the original 25 patients. Medicine 1980;59:239.

Rodnan GR: When is scleroderma not scleroderma? The differential diagnosis of progressive systemic sclerosis. Bull Rheum Dis 1981;31:7.

Rowland LP, Clark C, Olarte M: Therapy for dermatomyositis and polymyositis. Adv Neurol 1977;17:63.

Tanenbaum L, Tuffanelli DL: Antimalarial agents: Chloroquine, hydroxychloroquine, and quinacrine. Arch Dermatol 1980;116:587.

Section X:
Skin Disorders in Specific Populations

Skin Disease in Infants

51

Amy S. Paller, MD & Nancy B. Esterly, MD

The diagnosis and treatment of dermatologic disorders in neonates and young infants offer special challenges to the physician. Infants are not merely little adults. They may be affected by a wide range of problems peculiar to their age group or may display unusual manifestations of the more common skin disorders, making definitive diagnosis troublesome. Furthermore, examination of an infant is often made difficult by lack of cooperation, so that patience and playfulness on the part of the examining physician are critical for adequate assessment.

Many dermatologic disorders of infants are associated with systemic abnormalities; therefore, a complete physical examination is important for making the proper diagnosis or eliminating other possible diagnoses. Finally, therapy of dermatologic disorders in infants is complicated by the various effects and risks of systemic and topical medications in infants, eg, the risk of growth retardation must be considered when using systemically administered corticosteroids on a daily basis.

SPECIAL CHARACTERISTICS OF THE SKIN OF INFANTS

The skin of the neonate and young infant differs from that of the adult. Knowledge of these differences facilitates understanding of skin disorders in infants and especially the results of administration of topical agents. Differences in transepidermal water loss, vulnerability to physical and chemical insults, and percutaneous absorption of topically applied agents have been described.

Although transepidermal water loss is slightly decreased in healthy term infants in comparison with adults, it is greatly increased in preterm infants, probably because of the thinner stratum corneum, increased water content, and increased permeability of premature skin. Percutaneous absorption of drugs is increased in neonates, especially in premature infants younger than 32 weeks of gestational age. The skin barrier function of the preterm infant rapidly improves within the first 2 weeks of life to match that of the term infant, regardless of gestational age.

The anatomic and physiologic factors that account for the differences in percutaneous absorption between infants and adults are poorly understood. The stratum corneum, the major barrier to percutaneous absorption, is no thinner in infants younger than 3 months of age than in older children and adults. In addition, no biochemical differences in epidermal keratins have been found. The epidermis, however, does increase in thickness during the first few months of life, particularly owing to the development of the rete ridges. In addition, the ratio of surface area to body weight in the infant is 2.7 times that of the adult, so that treatment of an equivalent surface area would lead to greater systemic absorption. Other factors heighten the effects of percutaneously absorbed agents.

The metabolism, distribution, and excretion of drugs are altered in neonates and young infants. Organ systems in the neonate, such as the liver, kidneys, and brain, are neither structurally nor functionally fully developed. The immaturity of the kidneys and liver leads to altered urinary excretion and metabolism, and the brain and liver are proportionately larger in relation to the rest of the body. In addition, total body water and extra- or intracellular water are increased and adipose tissue is decreased.

These alterations in percutaneous absorption account for the increased toxicity of topically applied drugs and chemicals. The most notorious offenders are phenol, boric acid, salicylic acid, lindane, and hexachlorophene. Topical corticosteroids may also cause considerable toxicity, particularly fluorinated corticosteroids applied to the skin of preterm or low-birth-weight infants with cutaneous denudation or inflammation. Chronic suppression of the pituitary-adrenal axis with growth impairment is the greatest risk. Suppression of the pituitary-adrenal axis by topical hydrocortisone is minimal and rapidly reversible.

TRANSIENT LESIONS

Several benign and relatively transient skin lesions are frequently observed in the newborn infant. These conditions are important because they often cause anxiety in parents and require an explanation and reassurance. The most common of these disorders are discussed below.

MILIA

Epidermal cysts are found in about 40% of full-term infants and appear as multiple tiny, firm, yellow-white papules usually localized to the forehead, cheeks, and nose. Spontaneous exfoliation during the first weeks of life can be expected.

SALMON PATCH

These common macular vascular lesions are found in 30–50% of normal newborns. The salmon patch is pale pink with a diffuse border; however, the color intensifies with temperature changes and crying. Sites of predilection are the glabella, the eyelids, and the nape of the neck. Salmon patches tend to be smaller and less intense in color than nevus flammeus and usually resolve spontaneously. Eyelid lesions tend to fade by 1–2 years, while nuchal lesions are more persistent and may be found in 25–50% of school-age children.

ERYTHEMA TOXICUM

This self-limited eruption usually occurs within the first few days of life and tends to disappear by the end of the first week. The lesions are evanescent and consist of yellow-white papules or pustules on a broad erythematous base or splotches of erythema lacking a central papule. Lesions may be sparse or profuse and develop in all areas except for the palms and soles, where they occur only rarely. The infants are asymptomatic.

A monomorphous collection of eosinophils is evident on Wright-stained smears of pustular contents. This finding permits distinction from staphylococcal pustulosis, in which the smears contain leukocytes

and gram-positive cocci in clusters. Candidal pustules can be distinguished by demonstrating the pseudohyphae and spores on a KOH preparation. Pustules of transient neonatal pustular dermatosis contain only scattered neutrophils and cellular debris. Erythema toxicum requires no treatment and is of no significance in terms of future health.

TRANSIENT NEONATAL PUSTULAR MELANOSIS

This disorder occurs in about 5% of black infants and less than 1% of white infants. The lesions are usually detectable at birth as small superficial vesiculopustules that leave a fine collarette of scale on rupturing or hyperpigmented macules that fade during subsequent months. New lesions may continue to erupt over a period of several days. The cause of the disorder is unknown, and infants are otherwise well. Areas of predilection include the forehead, nape, anterior neck and submental area, lower legs, and back. When lesions are widespread, staphylococcal and candidal infections must be excluded. No treatment is necessary, as the disorder is self-limited and harmless.

MILIARIA

Obstruction of eccrine gland ducts may occur when the neonate is exposed to an excessively hot and humid environment. These lesions, called miliaria, occur in 2 forms. In miliaria crystallina, noninflamed superficial vesicles containing clear fluid result from retained sweat just beneath the stratum corneum. In miliaria rubra, the intraepidermal portion of the sweat duct has ruptured, causing an intraepidermal inflammatory vesicle; the lesions in this form of sweat retention are small grouped erythematous papules. Miliaria resolves quickly when the infant is transferred to a cooler environment. At times, these lesions may resemble other vesicular disorders, erythema toxicum, staphylococcal pustulosis, or candidiasis. Appropriate cultures and studies should be performed to distinguish these eruptions.

HARLEQUIN COLOR CHANGE

This phenomenon is most commonly seen in premature newborn infants during the first week of life and results from vascular autonomic imbalance. When the infant is lying on the side, the dependent half of the body becomes red and is sharply demarcated from the superior portion, which is pale by comparison. The phenomenon may be evanescent or last up to 20 minutes.

CUTIS MARMORATA

Cutis marmorata is a marbled appearance of the skin of infants when chilled. The mottling results from capillary and venular dilatation and usually disappears on rewarming. Persistent and prominent cutis marmorata is often associated with trisomies 18 and 21 and with the Cornelia de Lange syndrome. The mottling of cutis marmorata is generally not as vivid as that of cutis marmorata telangiectatica congenita, tends to be more evanescent, and is diffusely distributed.

NEONATAL ACNE

Acne may occasionally present during early infancy, presumably owing to hormonal stimulation of the sebaceous glands. This problem occurs more frequently in male infants. The eruption consists of comedonal plugs and erythematous papules and pustules; nodulocystic lesions are rare. The problem is self-limited, but therapy with mild topical agents such as benzoyl peroxide usually suffices.

HEMANGIOMAS

CAPILLARY & CAVERNOUS HEMANGIOMAS

Essentials of Diagnosis

- Often not present at birth; appear during first weeks.
- Grow, then recede.
- Superficial red lobulated or deeper blue-red masses.

General Considerations

Cutaneous hemangiomas are exceedingly common in neonates. Approximately two thirds of them are superficial, 15% are subcutaneous, and 20% are mixed. There appears to be no genetic predisposition to developing hemangiomas, but girls are affected more often than boys. Only 20–30% of hemangiomas are present at birth, but 90% are evident by 2 months of age. Almost all have developed by 9 months of age.

Differentiation between "capillary" and "cavernous" hemangiomas is based on histopathologic appearance. Capillary hemangiomas consist of masses of dilated capillaries with variable endothelial cell proliferation. Cavernous hemangiomas are composed of large dilated vessels filled with blood that compresses the thin endothelial lining. The term "straw-berry nevus" is a commonly used designation for a capillary hemangioma.

Clinical Findings

The classic strawberry hemangioma is a lobulated, bright red, well-circumscribed lesion that is elevated but compressible. A bluish-red or skin-colored mass with less distinct borders suggests a subcutaneous component. When the entire tumor is subcutaneous or deep in the dermis, the overlying skin may look normal or appear slightly blue in color. In the newborn, the precursor lesion may present as a sharply demarcated pale patch that subsequently develops telangiectases and finally evolves into a typical capillary hemangioma.

The most common areas of involvement are the face, back, scalp, and anterior chest. Hemangiomas are generally solitary, although some children have multiple lesions.

Differential Diagnosis

Hemangiomas may occur as a feature of other syndromes.

A. Diffuse Neonatal Hemangiomatosis: These infants have visceral hemangiomas most commonly involving the liver, gastrointestinal tract, lungs, or central nervous system. Virtually all have cutaneous hemangiomas as well that are usually multiple, widely disseminated, red-blue papular lesions present at birth or developing within the first few weeks of life. Neonates may suffer from gastrointestinal hemorrhage, central nervous system damage, respiratory tract obstruction, and high-output cardiac failure and may die despite supportive therapy, corticosteroid administration, operation, or radiation.

B. Blue Rubber Bleb Nevus Syndrome: Vascular lesions of the bowel are associated with characteristic deep blue, rubbery, compressible cutaneous nodules that are sometimes present at birth in infants with this syndrome. The cutaneous lesions vary in number, may be painful, and do not regress spontaneously. Severe anemia may result from recurrent gastrointestinal bleeding.

C. Rare Syndromes: These include Riley-Smith syndrome (macrocephaly, pseudopapilledema, and multiple cavernous hemangiomas), Bannayan's syndrome (macrocephaly, lipomas, and hemangiomas), Maffucci's syndrome (cavernous hemangiomas with dyschondroplasia), and Gorham's syndrome (cavernous hemangiomas and disappearing bones).

Complications

Ulceration is a complication that usually occurs during the early phase of rapid expansion of the hemangioma and may result in scarring, secondary infection, and disfigurement (Fig 51–1). Hemangiomas may bleed freely if traumatized, but the blood loss is rarely of great magnitude. An unusual but serious complication is Kasabach-Merritt syndrome,

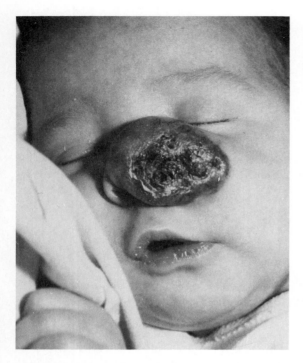

Figure 51–1. Ulcerated hemangioma on the nose of a young infant.

in which thrombocytopenia occurs owing to sequestration of platelets within the hemangiomatous mass. Associated coagulation defects occur, and severe bleeding results in anemia. Kasabach-Merritt syndrome usually occurs during the first few weeks of life and is heralded by rapid expansion of the hemangioma.

Treatment

For most hemangiomas, no treatment is indicated. Bleeding from trauma can usually be controlled by compression, and secondary infection is best treated by wet compresses and appropriate antibiotic therapy. When lesions interfere with essential functions such as respiration, feeding, or vision, prompt intervention is necessary. Acceptable treatment modalities include surgical excision, administration of oral prednisone, or intralesional injection of steroid. Kasabach-Merritt syndrome may require surgical therapy or a course of oral corticosteroid therapy. In addition, replacement transfusions of red cells, fresh-frozen plasma, and platelets and measures for control of high-output cardiac failure and bleeding may be necessary.

Course & Prognosis

Hemangiomas may enlarge rapidly during the first 6 months of life; involution may begin during the latter part of the first year or may occur much later. Approximately 50% of raised hemangiomas disap-

pear by 5 years of age; 98% have involuted by 9 years. The involution process occurs spontaneously and is reflected by flattening and softening of the mass and the appearance of pale gray areas on the surface indicating beginning fibrosis. The time and rate of involution cannot be predicted by the size or location of the lesion. Residual skin changes occur in about 10% of patients and usually consist of redundant skin, pallor, or telangiectases.

NEVUS FLAMMEUS
(Port Wine Stain)

Essentials of Diagnosis

- Sharply marginated.
- Pink, red, or port wine color.

General Considerations

Nevus flammeus represents a permanent congenital defect. Histopathologically, numerous dilated capillaries without endothelial proliferation are present in the dermis of these lesions.

Clinical Findings

Nevus flammeus is usually sharply demarcated and flat, though the surface may occasionally be slightly pebbly in texture. The color varies from pink to purple to almost black in deeply pigmented individuals. The most common location is the face in unilateral distribution. Mucous membranes may be involved. The size varies from a few millimeters to almost half the body surface.

Sturge-Weber syndrome and Klippel-Trenaunay syndrome are multisystem disorders that regularly include nevus flammeus as a feature. In Sturge-Weber syndrome, or trigeminal angiomatosis, a port wine nevus is associated with seizures, ipsilateral intracranial calcifications, contralateral hemiparesis, and ocular abnormalities. Nevus flammeus is usually unilateral and localized to the first trigeminal region of the face, though it may occur also at other sites. Intraoral involvement is common, but the palate and mandibular gingiva only rarely demonstrate vascular hyperplasia. Ocular abnormalities are frequent and include buphthalmos, glaucoma, choroidal angioma, optic atrophy, and hemianopic defects. Neurologic manifestations result from atrophy of the cerebral cortex or irritation from calcification related to the intracranial angiomas. While some patients are developmentally delayed or have behavioral disturbances, these defects do not predictably correlate with the severity of the vascular change. Skull x-rays often show pathognomonic "tram-line" calcification of the ipsilateral cerebral cortex, but these radiographic changes are absent in the neonatal period. Computed tomographic scans often show calcifications in early infancy, and both MRI and CT scans show the cortical atrophy.

Klippel-Trenaunay syndrome consists of venous varicosities and overgrowth of soft tissue and bone in association with the cutaneous vascular nevus. The defect is usually unilateral, with a lower extremity involved more frequently than an upper extremity. The vascular lesion varies from pink to deep purple and may be macular or show considerable thickening and surface irregularity. Arteriovenous shunts and lymphangiomatous abnormalities may be present.

Miscellaneous conditions occasionally associated with nevus flammeus include trisomy 13, Rubinstein-Taybi syndrome (broad thumbs and toes, slanted palpebral fissures, and hypoplastic maxilla), Beckwith-Wiedemann syndrome (macrosomia, macroglossia, and omphalocele), pseudothalidomide syndrome (facial nevus flammeus with phocomelia, flexion contractures, cloudy corneas, and growth retardation), and Wyburn-Mason syndrome (arteriovenous aneurysm of the midbrain with retinal vessel abnormalities ipsilateral to a facial nevus in a trigeminal distribution).

Differential Diagnosis

Port wine stain should be differentiated from salmon patch and from an early capillary hemangioma. An attempt should be made to distinguish those patients with a syndromal group of anomalies.

Complications

An isolated nevus flammeus can be regarded as mainly a cosmetic problem. The neurologic and ophthalmologic aspects of Sturge-Weber syndrome may cause major difficulties and require a multidisciplinary approach to management. Complications associated with Klippel-Trenaunay syndrome include edema, thrombophlebitis, and ulceration and infection of affected limbs.

Treatment

A. Port Wine Stain: Laser therapy is most effective in obliterating lesions and is currently the treatment of choice. Excision and grafting of smaller lesions and tattooing of larger lesions are alternative approaches. Cosmetics such as Covermark can be used to mask lesions on a daily basis.

B. Sturge-Weber Syndrome: Seizures can be controlled with anticonvulsant medications in over 50% of patients. Ophthalmologic consultation is necessary because treatment of glaucoma can avoid blindness. Gingival overgrowth can be ameliorated by scrupulous dental hygiene and, if necessary, surgical excision of the excess tissue.

C. Klippel-Trenaunay Syndrome: Venous varicosities can be prevented or slowed in progression by the use of elastic support stockings. Orthopedic procedures may be indicated for associated problems such as bone length discrepancies. Partial or total removal of the hypertrophic tissue has been helpful in some cases.

Course & Prognosis

The nevus flammeus is a fixed lesion and maintains its size relative to the growing child.

CUTIS MARMORATA TELANGIECTATICA CONGENITA

This lesion is presumably due to a developmental abnormality of the veins and capillaries, with resultant vascular ectasia. The histopathologic findings vary from dilated mature blood vessels in the dermis and subcutaneous tissues to a normal histologic appearance.

Clinical Findings

Reddish-blue vascular marbling of a portion of the skin is noted from birth. The reticulated bands are often restricted to a single extremity or portion of the trunk, frequently in segmental distribution. The demarcation between normal and abnormal skin is sharp and often is at the midline. The color of the reticulated pattern deepens with crying or fluctuations in temperature.

Differential Diagnosis

This disorder must be differentiated from cutis marmorata in the infant, a physiologic vascular response.

Complications

Telangiectatic capillary hemangiomas and areas of nevus flammeus may be associated with this disorder. Ulcers occasionally develop in the skin over the reticulated bands, especially when there is atrophy of the underlying subcutaneous tissue. Atrophy and hypertrophy of the soft tissues and bones of the affected part—as well as various other developmental anomalies—can occur in these patients.

Treatment

Only local treatment is indicated if complications such as ulcerations develop.

Course & Prognosis

Many lesions fade with increasing age, though the marbling persists into adulthood in some patients.

LYMPHATIC DISORDERS

LYMPHANGIOMAS

Lymphangiomas are hamartomatous malformations of dilated lymphatic channels lined by cuboidal or flat lymphatic endothelium. They are often associated with abnormalities of the regional lymphatic vessels. The hamartomas vary in location and pattern. Hemangiomas may be associated.

Clinical Findings

Lymphangioma circumscriptum may be present at birth or may develop later in childhood and is probably the most common of the lymphangiomas. The lesion consists of small clusters of vesicles filled with clear fluid and is usually skin-colored. If a hemangiomatous component is present, the blebs may be purple or blue-black. Lymphangioma circumscriptum is superficial in location but may be associated with abnormalities of the regional deep lymphatic vessels as well. The most common sites are the perineum, axillary folds, proximal limbs, and oral mucosa. Lesions may be linear in distribution and may become verrucous.

Cystic hygroma is a multiloculated hamartoma most commonly noted in the neck area but found also in the groin, axilla, or popliteal fossa. Cystic hygromas tend to enlarge rapidly.

Simple lymphangiomas are well-circumscribed, solitary, skin-colored subcutaneous or dermal tumors that may also involve the mucous membranes. Deep lymphatic involvement is occasionally associated. The simple lymphangioma either slowly enlarges or remains stable, but serous exudation from the surface is at times noted following trauma.

Cavernous lymphangiomas are more diffuse and consist of large cystic lymphatic dilatations that may also involve the intermuscular septa.

Differential Diagnosis

Lymphangioma circumscriptum may be confused with herpes simplex infection or clustered lesions of molluscum contagiosum. Those that appear verrucous or are arranged linearly may resemble a verrucous epidermal nevus, but the serous material within the lymphangioma serves to differentiate these 2 entities. Cystic hygromas must be distinguished from bronchogenic and thyroglossal duct cysts as well as from lipomas. Cavernous lymphangiomas may be confused with cavernous hemangiomas or lymphedema when large portions of the limbs, trunk, and face are involved, particularly with enlargement of the tongue and lips.

Treatment

Cystic hygromas and uncomplicated simple lymphangiomas can be excised. Large lymphangioma circumscriptum lesions are difficult to remove because of involvement of the deep lymphatic vessels and may require grafting after excision; carbon dioxide laser therapy results in temporary clearance, but the hamartoma may recur within the treated area. Partial removal of cavernous lymphangiomas is often all that is practical.

LYMPHEDEMA

Primary noninflammatory congenital lymphedema occurs more often in female patients and is usually present at birth. The most common site is the lower limbs, though the face, genitalia, or upper limbs may be affected. Rarely, abnormalities of the visceral and parietal lymphatics lead to chylothorax or chylous ascites.

The involved tissues are edematous and brawny, with fibrosis developing as lymphatic dysfunction progresses. Secondary infections are common and may be recurrent.

Lymphangiography demonstrates dilatation, tortuosity, and hypoplasia of the lymphatic vessels. Aplasia is unusual. The lymphedema may respond to treatment with diuretics or elevation and pressure bandaging or pump compression applied to the involved limb. Adjunctive surgery may also offer some palliation.

Lymphedema occurs in Milroy's disease, an autosomal dominant congenital disorder that usually involves the legs and feet; in lymphedema with obstructive jaundice, a familial entity consisting of chronic recurrent obstructive jaundice, progressive lymphedema of the lower extremities, and cutaneous hemangiomas; and in gonadal dysgenesis (Turner's syndrome), in which striking lymphedema of the hands and feet may be a prominent feature.

DEVELOPMENTAL ABNORMALITIES

AMNIOTIC BANDS

Ringlike constrictions particularly involving the limbs and digits are thought to result from encirclement by fibrous amniotic strands that are formed following rupture of the amnion in utero. When a limb is involved, these partial or complete constrictions may lead to amputation of a portion of the extremity.

APLASIA CUTIS
(Congenital Absence of Skin)

These localized defects are found most commonly on the posterior scalp near the midline but may occur elsewhere on the scalp or rarely on the face, trunk, or limbs. The lesions can be solitary or multiple but on the trunk and limbs are usually bilateral and symmetric. At birth, the defect may be covered by a tough smooth membrane or may be raw and ulcerated or crusted. On the scalp, these lesions tend to be circular, sharply marginated, and hairless. Denuded areas heal slowly, resulting in a flat or hypertrophic scar. Secondary infection and hemorrhage are uncommon complications. Biopsy demonstrates absence of the epidermis, a paucity of hair follicles, sweat glands, and sebaceous glands, and often a decrease in dermal elastic tissue. Deeper defects may extend through the subcuticular layer and periosteum. Occasionally, an underlying bony defect can be detected on skull films, but these defects heal spontaneously during the first year or 2 of life.

Although usually sporadic, familial cases have been documented with both autosomal recessive and autosomal dominant transmission. Congenital absence of skin has been associated with a variety of other malformations and is seen with increased frequency in some syndromes such as trisomy 13. Therapy should be conservative; however, surgical excision of poorly healing lesions and large or unsightly scars may ameliorate cosmetic problems.

ABNORMALITIES OF THE HAIR, SWEAT GLANDS, & NAILS

Ectodermal structures may be abnormal in a wide spectrum of multisystem disorders. In many of these conditions, recognition of the cutaneous manifestations facilitates diagnosis but the cutaneous markers are otherwise insignificant. A few of the disorders consist of cutaneous findings predominantly and will be discussed briefly. Additional syndromes associated with adnexal structural defects are listed in Tables 51–1 to 51–5.

Table 51–1. Disorders of hair with hypertrichosis.

Localized
  Turner's syndrome: low posterior hairline.
  Trisomy 18: back and forehead
  Ring chromosome E: low hairline
  Congenital hemihypertrophy with hypertrichosis
  Hairy nevi
  Hairy ears
  Hairy elbows syndrome
Generalized
  Mucopolysaccharidoses
  Cornelia de Lange syndrome
  Leprechaunism
  Congenital lipodystrophy
  Craniofacial dysostosis with dental, ocular, and cardiac abnormalities
  Hypertrichosis lanuginosa universalis
  Hypertrichosis with gingival fibromatosis

Table 51–2. Disorders associated with hypotrichosis.

Anhidrotic (hypohidrotic) ectodermal dysplasia
Atrichia with papular lesions
Congenital alopecia
Ectrodactyly, ectodermal dysplasia, and cleft lip and palate syndrome
Hidrotic ectodermal dysplasia
Hypotrichosis, syndactyly, and retinitis pigmentosa
Immunodeficiency with short-limbed dwarfism (cartilage-hair hypoplasia)
Incontinentia pigmenti
Keratosis follicularis spinulosa decalvans
Oculo-dento-digital syndrome
Oral-facial-digital syndrome
Progeria
Rothmund-Thomson syndrome
Seckel's dwarfism
Severe ichthyosis (various types)

PACHYONYCHIA CONGENITA

This disorder is inherited as an autosomal dominant condition with variable expressivity. Nail dystrophy generally appears at birth or shortly thereafter and involves both the fingers and the toes. The nails are thickened, hard, and elevated at the distal edge. Paronychia is common and at times results in shedding of the nail plate. Additional features include keratoderma of the palms and soles, hyperhidrosis, oral leukokeratosis, and keratosis pilaris. Less frequently, verrucous skin lesions, epidermal cysts, scrotal tongue, natal teeth, and corneal dystrophy may be associated. There is no effective treatment. Avulsion

Table 51–3. Morphologic disorders of hair.

Fine, light-colored	Phenylketonuria Pierre Robin syndrome Tyrosinemia
Fine, fragile	Hartnup disease Homocystinuria
Atrophic bulbs	Citrullinemia Trisomy 21
Fine, rough, brittle	Marinesco-Sjögren syndrome
Abnormal curliness	Woolly hair Hereditary enamel hypoplasia with kinky hair
Small caliber shafts	Cartilage-hair hypoplasia
Trichorrhexis invaginata	Netherton's syndrome
Trichorrhexis nodosa	Argininosuccinicaciduria
Pili torti	Menkes' syndrome Bjornstad's syndrome Marie-Unna hypotrichosis
Trichoschisis	Trichothiodystrophy
Monilethrix	
Pili annulati	
Pili triangulati et canaliculi	Uncombable hair syndrome

Table 51–4. Syndromes with abnormal nails: Nail aplasia, hypoplasia, or dysplasia.

Acrocephalosyndactyly (Apert's syndrome)
Acrodermatitis enteropathica
Anonychia and ectrodactyly
Basan skin hypoplasia with nail dystrophy
Cartilage-hair hypoplasia
Chromosomal abnormalities: trisomy 13, trisomy 18, Turner's syndrome, long-arm 21 deletion syndrome
Deafness with nail dystrophy
Dyskeratosis congenita
Ellis-van Creveld syndrome
Enamel hypoplasia with curly hair
Epidermolysis bullosa
Goltz's syndrome (focal dermal hypoplasia)
Gorlin-Pindborg syndrome (glossopalatine ankylosis, hypodontia, microglossia, and abnormalities of the extremities)
Incontinentia pigmenti
Lamy-Maroteaux syndrome (pyknodysostosis)
Larsen's syndrome
Nail-patella syndrome
Otopalatodigital syndrome
Popliteal web syndrome
Progeria
Rothmund-Thomson syndrome

of the troublesome nails and the use of keratolytic agents for skin lesions may be palliative.

NAIL-PATELLA SYNDROME

This autosomal dominant disorder is characterized by absent patellas, nail changes—especially of the thumbs and index fingers—and renal dysplasia. Hypoplasia of the humeral and radial heads, osseous horns on the iliac crests, and mental retardation may be associated as well. The prognosis is poor for infants with renal involvement, because glomerular and tubular lesions may progress to chronic renal failure.

PARONYCHIA

In infants, local injury in the paronychial region complicated by secondary infection is usually due to vigorous thumb sucking. The common pathogens implicated are *Staphylococcus aureus, Pseudomonas aeruginosa,* and *Candida albicans.* Bacterial and fungal cultures should be obtained and proper treatment instituted with soaks and antibacterial or anticandidal agents. Recurrent or persistent candidal infections

Table 51–5. Syndromes with hypertrophic nails.

Congenital hemihypertrophy
Familial hyperpigmentation with nail dystrophy (Touraine and Soulignac)
Pachyonychia congenita
Rubenstein-Taybi syndrome

may imply an underlying immunologic defect or chronic mucocutaneous candidiasis.

ECTODERMAL DYSPLASIAS

Ectodermal dysplasia is a descriptive term for disorders affecting appendages and skin. The 2 best defined entities are hidrotic and hypohidrotic (anhidrotic) ectodermal dysplasia. Ectodermal dysplasia is also associated with ectrodactyly and cleft lip and palate ("EEC syndrome").

Hidrotic ectodermal dysplasia is an autosomal dominant disorder characterized by variably absent, hypoplastic, or thickened nails; sparse hair; hyperkeratotic palms and soles with normal sweating; and carious but otherwise normal teeth.

Hypohidrotic (anhidrotic) ectodermal dysplasia, in contrast, includes absent or diminished sweating due to partial or complete absence of eccrine sweat glands that can result in episodic hyperthermia. Dentition may be incomplete, and the teeth are often discolored and conical. Caries are frequent. The hair is sparse, and the skin is dry, thick, and hypopigmented. Affected individuals have a characteristic facies with frontal bossing and hypoplasia of the central face, periorbital pigmentation, thick everted lips, and prominent chin and ears. Variable findings include stenotic lacrimal puncta, corneal dysplasia, hearing loss, hypoplasia of the mucous glands of the respiratory and gastrointestinal tracts, gonadal abnormalities, and hypoplasia of the nipples and breast tissue. Atopic disorders also occur with increased frequency in these children.

BLISTERING DISORDERS

EPIDERMOLYSIS BULLOSA

Essentials of Diagnosis
- Variable findings, depending on type.
- Inherited; family members often affected.
- Bullae at sites of trauma.

General Considerations
Epidermolysis bullosa is a group of rare hereditary mechanobullous disorders that differ in severity and prognosis. They may be divided into scarring and nonscarring types and are further subdivided by location of blister formation and the pattern of inheritance (Table 51–6). Most recently, electron microscopy and immunofluorescence mapping have facilitated classification. In all types of epidermolysis bullosa, lesions can be produced by heat and mechanical trau-

Table 51-6. Common forms of epidermolysis bullosa.

Type	Inheritance[1]	Skin	Oral	Nails	Teeth	Other	Histopathologic Changes
Epidermolysis bullosa simplex	AD	Nonscarring blisters; may be generalized	+	+		Worse in summer	Basal cell cytolysis
Weber-Cockayne syndrome	AD	Nonscarring blisters on hands and feet				Worse in summer	Cleavage through upper epidermis or basal cells
Epidermolysis bullosa letalis (Herlitz)	AR	Generalized blisters; heal with atrophy; vegetative growths in survivors	+++	+++	+++	Most die early; growth retardation; anemia in survivors	Cleavage through lamina lucida; decreased hemidesmosomes
Epidermolysis bullosa dominant dystrophic	AD	Generalized blisters; heal with milia and scarring	+	++			Cleavage below lamina densa; decreased anchoring fibrils
Epidermolysis bullosa recessive dystrophic	AR	Generalized blisters; heal with milia and scarring; flexion contractures and digital fusion	+++	+++	+++	Early demise common; esophageal strictures and ulceration; growth retardation; highest risk of cutaneous cancer; increased collagenase	Cleavage below lamina densa; decreased anchoring fibrils

[1]AD = autosomal dominant; AR = autosomal recessive.

ma. The pathogenesis of all forms of epidermolysis bullosa remains unclear.

Clinical Findings

The clinical presentation differs among the various types of epidermolysis bullosa. The most common forms that are nonscarring are epidermolysis bullosa simplex and junctional epidermolysis bullosa (lethalis). Epidermolysis bullosa simplex, which is autosomal dominant in inheritance, is present at birth or develops in early infancy. Bullae occur most frequently on the legs, feet, hands, and scalp (the most common sites of trauma) and heal without scarring. The nails are involved occasionally. Secondary infection of the skin is frequent, but the infant otherwise remains in good health. On biopsy of a blister, there is cytolysis of the basal cell layer of epidermis and intraepidermal cleavage at that site.

Junctional epidermolysis bullosa (Herlitz type, epidermolysis bullosa letalis) is inherited in an autosomal recessive manner and is almost always present at birth. The bullae are generalized but tend to spare the palms and soles. Lesions of the scalp and perioral area are characteristic. The nails may be involved, but digital fusion does not ensue. Mucosal surfaces are frequently affected, including the esophageal and anal mucosa. The dentition is also defective. Although the bullae are nonscarring, secondary infection and ulcerations are common and result in moist vegetative growths. Most infants are growth-retarded and at least moderately anemic. Early death from septicemia is not uncommon. Skin biopsy of an intact blister from affected infants demonstrates separation at the dermal-epidermal junction through the lamina lucida zone.

The most common scarring forms of epidermolysis bullosa include an autosomal dominant and a severe autosomal recessive form. The less severe dominant form may begin at birth, although it frequently appears later. The extent of involvement varies. The lesions are often restricted to the hands, feet, and sacral region. Mucous membrane lesions are mild, if present, and the nails are often dystrophic. Scarring of the hands and feet with milia formation may occur but is not nearly as severe as in the recessive form. The site of separation is beneath the basement membrane (subepidermal blister).

The recessive (polydysplastic) form is often observed at birth, with blisters or hemorrhagic erosions, especially on the feet. Blisters develop at sites of trauma, but they may also appear spontaneously. Scars and milia form at sites of blistering, and the digits gradually become fused within a mittenlike encasement of scar tissue. Oral and esophageal mucous membrane changes may be severe, the teeth are carious, and the nails are lost. These infants fail to thrive and experience retardation in growth and development, recurrent infections, and moderate to severe anemia. The cleavage plane of the blister is beneath the basement membrane (subepidermal), and anchoring fibrils are absent on electron microscopy. These patients tend to have elevated collagenase levels in the skin, but the role of this enzyme in the pathogenesis of the disease is unclear.

Differential Diagnosis

In occasional cases the lesions of epidermolysis bullosa resemble aplasia cutis or bullous impetigo. The lesions of herpes simplex, bullous mastocytosis, and immunologically mediated blistering disorders may rarely be considered.

Treatment

Care of an infant with epidermolysis bullosa is directed at minimizing trauma. Clothing, toys, and crib coverings should be soft and nonabrasive. Adhesive materials should not contact the skin. Special devices to diminish intraoral trauma from feeding, such as those used for infants with cleft palates, are helpful. Sponge baths with minimal handling of the baby may prevent separation and loss of large portions of the epidermis. When bullae arise, they should be punctured and the collapsed blister top left intact to serve as a protective covering. The use of topical antibiotics may decrease the frequency of bacterial infection in denuded areas. Mittenlike wound dressings may encourage healing and protect skin from further trauma.

Nutritional problems are common when oral and esophageal lesions are present. Thinned or puréed foods facilitate swallowing, and topical anesthetics such as viscous lidocaine or diphenhydramine may alleviate discomfort when administered before feeding. Because the anemia in babies with epidermolysis bullosa is due to iron deficiency, transcutaneous protein loss, and chronic inflammation and infection, supplemental iron and a high-protein diet are beneficial.

INCONTINENTIA PIGMENTI

Essentials of Diagnosis

- Female sex predilection.
- Grouped vesicles, often in linear configuration.
- Later, verrucous papules and bizarre pigmentation resembling marbled cake.
- Risk for seizures, dental and ocular abnormalities, mental retardation.

General Considerations

This congenital hereditary disorder may affect other organ systems as well as the skin. Most affected children are females, and there is a high abortion rate among female carriers, suggesting an X-linked dominant inheritance pattern with lethality for males.

Clinical Findings

The first cutaneous stage of the disease is often present at birth or during the first few weeks of life. It consists of grouped vesicles on an inflammatory base that erupt in crops and tend to be linear in distribution, affecting mainly the limbs and scalp. In the second stage, hyperpigmented verrucous papules and nodules are found on the limbs. These develop several weeks later when the vesicular phase is no longer evident. The third stage, from which the disorder derives its name, consists of flat hyperpigmented streaks and whorls that mainly involve the trunk. The hyperpigmentation often fades considerably by late childhood, and many patients subsequently have hypopigmented, atrophic streaks. Nail dystrophy and small areas of alopecia may occur as well. Infants occasionally present with the second or even third stage of incontinentia pigmenti, bypassing the previous stage.

Defective dentition, ocular abnormalities, and central nervous system defects—including developmental delay, seizures, microcephaly, and spasticity—may coexist or become apparent later in infancy.

Peripheral eosinophilia is often noted in infants concurrent with the blistering stage of the disease. On skin biopsy, the intraepidermal vesicles are characteristically filled with eosinophils.

Differential Diagnosis

Because of the configuration and distribution of the vesicular lesions, the major consideration in differential diagnosis is herpes simplex infection. A Tzanck smear for multinucleated giant cells and, if necessary, culture for herpes simplex virus will distinguish the 2 conditions. The presence of myriads of eosinophils on a smear of vesicle fluid will also help to differentiate incontinentia pigmenti from all other conditions except erythema toxicum, which differs in clinical presentation and course. Epidermolysis bullosa, epidermolytic hyperkeratosis, bullous mastocytosis, and other vesicular processes are blistering disorders that have no tendency for patterned distribution and have other distinguishing features. The hyperpigmented streaks and whorls must be distinguished from early epidermal nevi and linear and whorled nevoid hypermelanosis.

Treatment

The inflammatory vesicular lesions may become secondarily infected and can be treated with compresses, topical corticosteroids, and antibiotics as required. Periodic examinations are necessary throughout childhood to detect involvement of other systems. Associated defects such as anomalous dentition may necessitate participation of other specialists for optimal care. The parents should receive genetic counseling.

Course & Prognosis

The course is variable and depends on the severity of associated defects, especially those of the central nervous system. Some children with only cutaneous manifestations experience complete resolution without sequelae; however, as affected individuals they must receive appropriate genetic counseling.

SCALING DISORDERS

Shedding of skin is a normal, transient phenomenon in the newborn period. It is especially prominent in postmature or dysmature infants; however, when extensive scaling is present, one must consider the ichthyoses, a group of disorders that may cause considerable problems for the neonate. Some of these disorders are discussed again in Chapter 21.

ICHTHYOSIS

There are 4 major types of ichthyosis. Three types occur during the neonatal period: X-linked ichthyosis, lamellar ichthyosis, and epidermolytic hyperkeratosis. The fourth type, ichthyosis vulgaris, is the most common form in older children but rarely develops before 3 months of age. The terms "collodion baby" and "harlequin fetus" are used to describe the appearance of certain affected newborn infants but may not be specific types of ichthyosis.

Clinical Findings

A. X-linked Ichthyosis: Up to one-third of affected males are abnormally scaly at birth, and almost all have manifestations by 3 months of age. The scales are large and brown, so that the infant appears dirty. The entire body surface is usually affected with the exception of the central face, palms and soles, and most of the flexural areas. In addition to the cutaneous findings, deep corneal opacities visible by slit lamp examination often develop by adulthood but provide no impediment to vision. Female carriers may also have corneal opacities but demonstrate no cutaneous manifestations.

The cellular kinetics of the skin in X-linked ichthyosis are normal; however, the skin biopsy findings are similar to those of lamellar ichthyosis: hyperkeratosis, an increased granular layer, a thickened stratum spinosum, and dermal perivascular lymphocytic infiltrates. A deficiency of sterol sulfatase in several types of cells has been demonstrated as a consistent finding in patients with this disorder.

B. Lamellar Ichthyosis: Patients with "lamellar ichthyosis" have now been subclassified as having classic lamellar ichthyosis or nonbullous congenital ichthyosiform erythroderma. These infants are born with generalized erythroderma and desquamation or may have the phenotype of collodion baby. Palms, soles, and flexural surfaces are affected. With increasing age, the intense erythroderma fades and generalized scaling predominates, with accentuation in the flexural areas. The scales vary in color from yellow to dark brown, are large, and may be extremely thick. Although ectropion may be severe in later life, it is rarely a significant problem in the newborn infant. These infants can become sec-

ondarily infected because of the large areas of macerated skin. Patients in the classic lamellar ichthyosis subgroup have darker, larger scales and more extensive alopecia and ectropion, whereas patients with congenital ichthyosiform erythroderma have a more intense erythroderma and scales that are finer and white.

The turnover rate of the skin in congenital ichthyosiform erythroderma is markedly increased. On biopsy, hyperkeratosis, an increased granular layer, a thickened stratum spinosum, and mononuclear infiltrates around dermal blood vessels are seen. The disorder is usually inherited in an autosomal recessive manner, but the pathogenesis is unknown. Patients with the congenital ichthyosiform erythroderma form have elevated levels of hydrocarbons (*n*-alkanes) in their scale.

C. Epidermolytic Hyperkeratosis (Bullous Congenital Ichthyosiform Erythroderma): During the neonatal period, affected infants develop bullae over large areas, resulting in significant denudation in addition to dryness, desquamation, and erythema. The bullae tend to occur in crops and may be several centimeters in size. Secondary infection is a frequent complication, and sepsis may ensue, especially in young infants. The scales of epidermolytic hyperkeratosis are warty and easily shed in large amounts. Palms and soles are generally normal. Ectropion is not seen.

The epidermal cellular kinetics are altered as in nonbullous congenital ichthyosiform erythroderma. Skin biopsy is diagnostic, demonstrating large clumped keratohyaline granules in association with extensive vacuolization of the granular layer and midepidermal cells. Hyperkeratosis and thickening of the stratum spinosum are present to varying degrees. Epidermolytic hyperkeratosis is inherited in an autosomal dominant fashion.

D. Collodion Baby: At birth, these infants are enclosed in a taut yellow cellophane-like membrane that may result in temporary distortion of facial features, especially the ears, lips, and eyelids. The membrane may be perforated by lanugo and scalp hair. Soon after birth, cracking and peeling of the membrane begins, revealing an underlying erythema. Complete shedding of the membrane may take several weeks, and a new membrane may form in some areas before the process is complete. Affected children usually develop the lamellar ichthyoses, but, less commonly, collodion membranes have been reported in infants with certain other forms of ichthyosis as well. In a rare infant with collodion membrane, the skin remains normal after shedding.

Collodion babies are much less severely affected than are harlequin fetuses. Although they are frequently born prematurely, the neonatal course is otherwise uncomplicated. A more severely affected infant may have temporary difficulty with feeding and respiration. Secondary bacterial and candidal infections are another frequent problem, particularly if the skin becomes macerated from high humidity in the isolette.

E. Harlequin Fetus: These infants have the most severe form of ichthyosis and usually die within the first hours or days of life. The skin is yellow-gray, very thick and hard, with deep moist fissures. The fissuring occurs mostly over areas of movement, ie, the joints, neck, thorax, axillas, and groin.

Marked ectropion and eclabium are present; the ears are underdeveloped and flattened; and the hair and nails may be absent or hypoplastic. Flexion deformities of all joints result from the extreme cutaneous inelasticity, and the hands and feet may be ischemic.

Complications include hypothermia, inability to feed due to perioral inelasticity, hypoventilation with secondary pneumonia, and cutaneous infection with sepsis. The pathogenesis is unknown. X-ray diffraction analysis of the stratum corneum of one infant demonstrated an abnormal keratin as a major horny layer component; however, subsequent studies of 3 such infants failed to confirm this finding. A defect in epidermal lipid metabolism has also been identified in a single harlequin fetus. There are reports of affected siblings, suggesting an autosomal recessive form of inheritance.

F. Other Desquamative Processes:

1. Physiologic desquamation– Infants born between 40 and 42 weeks' gestation tend to have increased frequency and amount of scaling.

2. Dysmature infants– These neonates are stressed in utero and tend to have additional features that distinguish them from newborn infants with physiologic desquamation. Characteristic findings include decreased subcutaneous fat, absence of vernix caseosa, unusually long hair and nails, and, frequently, meconium staining of skin, umbilical cord, and nails.

3. Staphylococcal scalded skin syndrome– This bullous desquamative process results from a toxin produced by *S aureus,* especially phage group II strains, and can be confused with epidermolytic hyperkeratosis. In contrast to ichthyosis, generalized scaling is absent. The bullae are flaccid, Nikolsky's sign is positive, and the epidermis peels in large sheets, leaving a moist erythematous base. The cleavage plane of the blisters is intraepidermal at the level of the granular layer. (See Chapter 12.)

4. Psoriasis– Although very rare in infancy, psoriasis may appear as diffuse macerated scaly areas in the diaper area, as an erythroderma, or as localized plaques of scale. A positive family history and disease-specific skin biopsy findings will help to substantiate the diagnosis.

5. Keratoderma of the palms and soles– A number of rare hereditary disorders are manifested by hyperkeratosis localized to the hands and feet. These disorders include tylosis, mutilating keratoderma,

progressing keratoderma, mal de Meleda, and Papillon-Lefèvre syndrome.

G. Other Ichthyosis Syndromes:

1. Ichthyosis linearis circumflexa– This autosomal recessive condition is manifested by generalized polycyclic lesions bordered by white scale (often double-edged) and flexural hyperkeratosis.

2. Erythrokeratoderma variabilis– Geographic plaques of thick yellow-brown scales and discrete transient and migratory macular erythematous patches are characteristic of this autosomal dominant disorder. The face, buttocks, and extensor surfaces of the limbs are affected most frequently.

3. Netherton syndrome– This autosomal recessive disorder is characterized by hair shaft defects, especially trichorrhexis invaginata, an atopic diathesis; and ichthyosis, usually ichthyosis linearis circumflexa.

4. Sjögren-Larsson syndrome– Spastic paralysis, mental retardation, and nonbullous congenital ichthyosiform erythroderma are the triad of findings that comprise this syndrome. These patients have recently been found to have a defect of the fatty acid cycle.

5. Chondrodysplasia punctata– Inherited in an autosomal recessive, autosomal dominant, or X-linked dominant form, this disorder is manifested by stippled epiphyses, short dysplastic femora or humeri, cataracts, and a patterned ichthyosis (25%). Peroxisomal abnormalities are associated.

6. Rud's syndrome– Ichthyosis in association with mental retardation and other neurologic defects and infantilism occurs rarely; some of these patients are a subgroup with X-linked ichthyosis.

7. Refsum's syndrome– This autosomal recessive disorder, due to inability to metabolize phytanic acid, results in polyneuritis and atypical retinitis pigmentosa, with a variable ichthyosis that usually develops after the first decade of life.

8. Trichothiodystrophy– An autosomal recessive disorder, this syndrome includes delayed growth and development, hair defects (especially trichoschisis), ichthyosis, and nail dystrophy as well as other variable features. Low sulfur content of the hair and a banded appearance under polarizing microscopy are the markers for this disorder. Some of the infants have presented in the newborn period as collodion babies.

Treatment

Safe and relatively effective therapy for ichthyosis is limited to topical preparations. Liberal use of emollients may be all that is necessary to keep an infant relatively comfortable and well lubricated. Keratolytic agents such as lactic and citric acid, urea, and topical vitamin A acid preparations can be used as tolerated to minimize scaling but are rarely necessary in the newborn period. Oral retinoids, though promising, are not yet of proved safety for long-term therapy of these disorders. Systemic and topical antibacterial and antifungal agents may be required for secondary infections; antihistamines may help to control pruritus if present.

Prognosis

Other than the harlequin fetus, infants with ichthyosis tend to fare well. Apart from the risk of secondary infection and annoying pruritus in some infants, the major problems are cosmetic.

NEONATAL INFECTIONS

BACTERIAL INFECTIONS

1. BULLOUS IMPETIGO

These blisters, usually caused by a coagulase-positive *S aureus,* phage group II, tend to develop after a few days of life as opposed to those of congenital noninfectious blistering diseases. The bullae are flaccid and vary in size, number, and distribution (Fig 51–2). They are filled with straw-colored or turbid fluid and, upon rupture, leave a red denuded base with a varnishlike crust.

Gram staining of blister fluid will demonstrate clusters of gram-positive cocci, and culture can be performed to identify the causative organism. Often the peripheral white blood cell count is elevated, with a shift to the left. Any newborn suspected of having

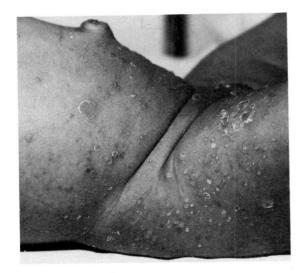

Figure 51–2. Multiple pustules and flaccid bullae of staphylococcal impetigo.

bullous impetigo should have blood cultures performed and should receive intravenous antistaphylococcal antibiotic therapy. Strict isolation procedures should be instituted to avoid spread of staphylococcal infection to other infants in the newborn nursery. Compresses of normal saline or aluminum acetate solution, applied intermittently, will facilitate rupture and drying of the bullae and decrease the spread of infection.

Bullous impetigo is most often confused with epidermolysis bullosa, but a number of other disorders such as epidermolytic hyperkeratosis, herpes simplex infection, and incontinentia pigmenti are also included in the differential diagnosis. The blisters in these disorders are usually present at birth and are free of bacterial organisms unless secondary infection supervenes. (See Chapter 12.)

2. STAPHYLOCOCCAL SCALDED SKIN SYNDROME

Staphylococcal scalded skin syndrome (formerly called Ritter's disease in infants) is caused by *S aureus,* usually of the group II phage type. This infection occurs primarily in infants and young children. The initial manifestation is a rapidly progressive intense erythroderma associated with cutaneous tenderness, and the infant resists being held or comforted. Flaccid bullae appear and become confluent, and large areas of epidermis may peel away in sheets. The perioral area, groin, neck folds, and axillae are frequently the initial sites of blistering. In less severely affected infants, frank blisters do not develop but the reddened skin acquires a sandpaper quality resembling that of streptococcal scarlet fever. Hyperemia of the oral mucous membranes and conjunctivitis are frequently present. With progression, the skin changes are accentuated around the mouth, producing a characteristic "sad man" facies.

The disorder is due to an erythrodermic toxin produced by the organism, and—although the infant may appear toxic—bacteremia is unusual. Nevertheless, as in bullous impetigo, blood cultures should be obtained and antistaphylococcal therapy should be initiated. (See Chapter 12.)

3. SYPHILIS

Syphilis is a transplacentally transmitted disease whose manifestations depend upon the duration of untreated maternal disease. Most babies born to untreated mothers with early syphilis will become infected before delivery. About 25% die in utero, and the majority of liveborn infants are born prematurely with evidence of syphilis noted during the first weeks or months of life. In general, syphilis cannot be detected in the fetus of affected mothers prior to the

18th week of gestation, probably because of an inadequate fetal immunologic response early in gestation.

The clinical manifestations are variable in early syphilis and are usually noted between 2 and 6 weeks of age. The most common cutaneous eruption consists of oral pink maculopapules that gradually become copper-colored and scaly. The anogenital and perioral areas as well as the palms and soles are sites of predilection. At times, annular lesions, ulcers, and hemorrhagic vesicles and bullae are present. Not uncommonly, the palms and soles are thickened, fissured, and erythematous; the nails may be deformed owing to paronychial involvement. Petechiae may be present if the infant has thrombocytopenia. Without treatment, the cutaneous lesions tend to clear spontaneously during the next few months, leaving variable pigmentary changes. Syphilitic chancres may occur with primary infections but are unusual. Mucous membrane lesions are frequently present, and rhinitis ("snuffles") is an early manifestation.

3. MISCELLANEOUS INFECTIONS

Group B streptococci are the most common bacterial organisms causing infection in the newborn. They tend to cause sepsis in the immediate neonatal period and meningitis as a late manifestation. Skin abscesses and omphalitis may be associated.

A small percentage of infants with *Listeria* sepsis have cutaneous lesions. They are generally widespread and can be papules, pustules, petechiae, or, rarely, vesicles. Conjunctival and oropharyngeal blisters are occasionally present. Omphalitis may be an additional feature. The organism can be cultured from the cutaneous lesions.

Although omphalitis may be an early manifestation of *Pseudomonas* infection, the cutaneous lesions can be recognized as characteristic of infection with this organism. The initial lesions are vesicles set in an erythematous base, but they rapidly become hemorrhagic pustules. The pustules rupture to form punched-out necrotic ulcers with surrounding violaceous cellulitis. Cultures and Gram-stained smears of material obtained from the intact vesicopustules permit identification of the infectious agent. Treatment should be initiated as early as possible, because sepsis is likely and the prognosis is poor if lesions are widespread.

CANDIDIASIS

The most common forms of candidiasis affecting infants are diaper dermatitis and thrush; however, a generalized cutaneous eruption may also be observed at birth or during the first week of life.

Candidal diaper dermatitis presents as sharply demarcated, erythematous, elevated, scaly plaques,

usually involving the intertriginous areas, and is often studded by pustules that may develop in the plaque and beyond the margins (satellite pustules) (Fig 51–3). Less often, dermatitis consisting of erythematous papules or pustules is the presenting feature. Because *Candida* is found in the stool of many of these infants, perianal accentuation or erythema is not unusual. However, no pattern is universal and the flexures and perianal areas may be spared.

The infection must be differentiated from other infectious and irritant eczematous reactions involving the diaper area. A potassium hydroxide preparation and culture of scales or pustule contents provide a definitive diagnosis. Other infectious agents causing diaper dermatitis include *S aureus* and gram-negative organisms, especially *Escherichia coli*. Erythematous pustules with weeping, crusting, and punched-out ulcers may be seen. Gram-stained smears of pustular material and cultures are helpful in determining the causative agent.

The choice of systemic or topical antibiotics depends upon the organism involved, the extent of the eruption, and the age of the infant. The dermatitis usually responds quickly to anticandidal topical agents such as nystatin, clotrimazole, or miconazole.

During the first week of life, congenital candidal infection may be manifested as a generalized eruption. In infants with skin lesions at birth, the infection is presumed to have occurred in utero as an ascending infection from a vaginal or cervical focus. The amniotic fluid may be culture-positive for organisms, and the cord and chorionic plate may have demonstrable lesions as well.

The eruption of congenital cutaneous candidiasis is characteristically erythematous and papulopustular. Pustules are often present on the palms and soles, and there is relative sparing of the diaper area as well as the oral mucosa. The nails may also be involved.

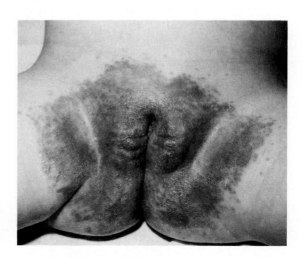

Figure 51–3. Candidal diaper dermatitis.

With progression, desquamation becomes a predominant feature. In the majority of infants, viscera are uninvolved, and these babies respond well to topical anticandidal agents. Disseminated infection involving viscera carries a grave prognosis even when the infant is treated systemically. Infants most at risk for visceral involvement are prematures under 1500 g and infants with respiratory distress.

Thrush (oral candidiasis) is seen in 5% of newborn infants, though it may occur at any age. It is most commonly acquired during passage through the vaginal canal and becomes apparent 1–2 weeks after birth. It is typically detectable as white adherent patches on an erythematous base on the buccal mucosa, tongue, gingivae, and occasionally the posterior pharynx. A 10- to 14-day course of oral nystatin suspension is usually curative.

Chronic mucocutaneous candidiasis is very unusual and is most commonly seen in infants who are immunocompromised or in association with the later development of endocrinopathies. Crusted, weeping erythematous plaques as well as dry scaly patches are found on the scalp and face, especially in the perioral area, on acral and paronychial skin, and on the oral and genital mucosa. In some children, the granulomatous lesions have a verrucous character, and hornlike projections develop in involved areas. A KOH preparation and culture of lesional material will verify the presence of *C albicans*. This form of candidiasis tends to be refractory to standard anticandidal therapy but is usually at least partially responsive to orally administered ketoconazole.

VIRAL INFECTIONS

Viral infections in the newborn tend to disseminate rapidly. Because the clinical manifestations can be similar, it is often difficult to distinguish the various congenital infections until cultures prove positive or serum titers are elevated.

1. HERPES SIMPLEX INFECTION

Herpes simplex virus causes considerable morbidity and mortality in the neonate. Cutaneous manifestations vary from a single plaque of grouped vesicles on an erythematous base to a diffuse vesiculobullous eruption. Visceral involvement is most commonly reflected by pneumonitis, hepatosplenomegaly, ocular abnormalities, and meningoencephalitis. A tentative diagnosis can be made if multinucleated giant cells are found on Tzanck smear of an intact vesicle, though the lesions of varicella-zoster virus will also yield giant cells, and the cutaneous features of disseminated herpes simplex infection and varicella may be identical. A culture for herpes simplex virus will be positive after 2–3 days and permits

definitive diagnosis. Serum antibody titers to herpes simplex virus may be elevated.

The introduction of intravenous vidarabine and acyclovir has improved the outlook associated with neonatal herpes simplex virus infection. Preventive measures—including careful observation and cultures for maternal genital herpes near term as well as cesarean section within 4 hours after amniotic membrane rupture for women with active infections—have decreased the risk of ascending infection. Transplacental intrauterine herpes infection has been reported but with a lower frequency. Any newborn suspected of having a herpes simplex infection as well as medical personnel or a mother with a mucocutaneous herpetic lesion should be protected from contact with healthy neonates.

Other congenital viral infections do not cause vesicles but do cause visceral abnormalities similar to those of disseminated herpes simplex infection and different cutaneous findings.

2. CYTOMEGALOVIRUS INFECTION

Infants with cytomegalovirus infection are often small for gestational age or born prematurely. Visceral changes include hepatosplenomegaly, respiratory distress, microcephaly, convulsions, chorioretinitis, and jaundice. Anemia and thrombocytopenia are common. The cutaneous manifestations are not specific but include petechiae, purpura, and dark blue to red papulonodules that represent islands of extramedullary dermal erythropoiesis (blueberry muffin lesions). Occasionally, a generalized papular eruption has been noted.

The diagnosis is suggested by the finding of intracytoplasmic and intranuclear inclusion bodies in the enlarged cells of the viscera or in fresh urine. Viral isolation may be accomplished from urine or tissue, and previously elevated or increasing serum titers provide further confirmation of infection. In severely affected infants, especially those with neurologic manifestations, the prognosis is poor. There is no available satisfactory therapy.

3. RUBELLA

The skin changes of congenital rubella are similar to those of cytomegalovirus infection. Petechiae and purpura are apparent at birth but usually clear by 6 weeks of age; extramedullary dermal erythropoiesis is also common. Occasionally, persistent cutis marmorata reflects ongoing vasomotor instability. Visceral manifestations include intrauterine growth retardation, microcephaly with central nervous system changes and psychomotor retardation, cataracts, deafness, cardiac lesions—especially patent ductus arteriosus and congestive heart failure—pneumonitis, and hepatosplenomegaly with hepatitis. The presence of congenital malformations indicates infection during the first trimester of pregnancy.

4. ACQUIRED IMMUNODEFICIENCY SYNDROME (AIDS)

AIDS has been reported in increasing numbers of children since 1983. Presently, most pediatric cases of AIDS are acquired perinatally by transplacental transmission of the human immunodeficiency virus (HIV). Transplacental transmission of AIDS is not inevitable but is estimated to occur in 50% of susceptible infants. Infants may acquire the virus from infected breast milk or from the administration of infected blood products (see also Chapter 15).

Clinical Findings

Clinical evidence of AIDS is usually detectable in infants by 3–6 months of age, though 28% of affected infants are small for gestational age at birth. Failure to thrive, recurrent fever, upper and lower respiratory tract infections, diffuse lymphadenopathy, hepatosplenomegaly, chronic diarrhea, and recurrent otitis media are the most common clinical signs. Mucocutaneous candidiasis occurs in 75% of infants, and an eczematous rash resembling that of atopic dermatitis has been noted in 19%. Kaposi's sarcoma may involve the skin or lymph nodes of infants with AIDS but is extremely rare.

Dysmorphology may be associated with intra-uterine HIV infection. The typical features include growth failure, microcephaly, ocular hypertelorism, a boxlike appearance of the forehead, flat nasal bridge, mild obliquity of the eyes, elongated palpebral fissures and blue sclerae, short nose with flattened columella, and triangular philtrum and patulous lips.

T cell immunodeficiency with a depressed T helper to T suppressor-cytotoxic cell ratio occurs in patients with clinical manifestations. Lymphopenia is rarely found in affected children despite its frequency in adults. Although total immunoglobulin levels are usually elevated, many children demonstrate absent or decreased levels of IgG$_2$. Anti-HIV antibodies are detectable in all patients with AIDS and are found also in infants without clinical and laboratory evidence of AIDS who are at risk. The most common infecting agents are *Candida*, cytomegalovirus, and *Pneumocystis carinii*. Epstein-Barr virus, herpes simplex, adenovirus, *Cryptococcus, Mycobacterium intracellulare, Toxoplasma, Cryptosporidium,* and *Entamoeba* infections are also described. These infants are susceptible to pyogenic pneumonia and bacterial sepsis, primarily from *Staphylococcus, Streptococcus,* pneumococcus, *E coli,* and *Salmonella*. Death in infancy is usually due to opportunistic infections.

Differential Diagnosis

AIDS should be suspected in any infant—particularly one born of a mother in a high-risk group—who develops an opportunistic infection or shows features characteristic of AIDS. Other immunodeficiency disorders, especially severe combined immune deficiency (SCID), should be considered but are differentiated by the absence of anti-HIV antibodies. Secondary immunosuppression from drugs must also be distinguished.

TOXOPLASMOSIS

Toxoplasmosis shares many of the features of the congenital viral infections but is caused by an intracellular protozoon, *Toxoplasma gondii*. Infected infants may be born prematurely or be stillborn, and manifestations may present at birth or during the first few days of life. Associated problems include microcephaly, hydrocephaly, chorioretinitis, pneumonitis, lymphadenopathy, vomiting and diarrhea, hepatosplenomegaly, jaundice, and anemia. A maculopapular rash occurs in 1–25% of patients with generalized disease. The eruption tends to be widespread but spares the scalp, palms, and soles and usually clears within 2 weeks. Serum titers of IgM type antibody against *T gondii* are elevated in the affected newborn, and the organism may be demonstrated by Giemsa staining of affected tissues or cerebrospinal fluid or by inoculation of a laboratory mouse with tissue suspensions or body fluid sediment. The treatment of choice is a combination of pyrimethamine and sulfadiazine, but this therapy is useful only in preventing further tissue damage. Morbidity and mortality rates are high, with nervous system and ocular abnormalities occurring as residua in over 50% of infants.

INFILTRATIVE PROCESSES

HISTIOCYTOSIS X (Langerhans Cell Histiocytosis)

Essentials of Diagnosis

- Erythema and scaling, especially at scalp, neck, axillae, and groin.
- Vesicles, ulcers; occasionally petechiae.
- Systemic signs (variable).
- Diagnostic skin biopsy.

General Considerations

This designation refers to a group of nonlipid reticuloendothelioses whose visceral and cutaneous manifestations vary. The skin lesions all show a similar histologic picture that permits diagnosis. Masses of pale-staining histiocytes invade the upper dermis and epidermis, often in association with abundant eosinophils. On electron microscopy, the abnormal histiocytes contain racket-shaped organelles called Birbeck granules that are normally present in epidermal Langerhans cells. The functional and etiologic significance of these granules has not been determined. The histiocytic cells usually stain with S100 and have CD1 on their surface.

Clinical Findings

A. Symptoms and Signs: Affected infants may be acutely ill or may be well except for the cutaneous lesions. Systemic signs and symptoms include fever and irritability, poor weight gain, pallor, bleeding, pain with movement, dyspnea, hepatosplenomegaly, lymphadenopathy, suppurative otitis, oral lesions, and bone tumors.

The most common cutaneous manifestation in older infants is an erythematous papular scaling eruption of the scalp, neck, axillae, and groin. Petechiae, vesicles, and ulcerations may be intermingled. Lesions present at birth or developing during the neonatal period are often vesiculopustular. Erythematous nodules have also been noted.

B. Laboratory Findings: Laboratory examinations should include a complete blood count with differential and platelet count, serum transaminase levels, immunoglobulin levels, and tests of T cell function (see Differential Diagnosis, below). A chest x-ray and skeletal survey as well as biopsies of cutaneous and mucous membrane lesions are indicated.

Differential Diagnosis

Histiocytosis has been associated with immunologic deficiency; rarely, siblings develop histiocytic infiltration of skin and viscera manifested variably by generalized skin rash, hepatosplenomegaly, lymphadenopathy, diarrhea, hypogammaglobulinemia, T cell dysfunction, and eosinophilia. The condition is rapidly fatal and appears to be inherited in an autosomal recessive pattern. A fetal thymus transplant resulted in normalization of T cell function and clearance of disease in a single patient.

Complications

Cutaneous bacterial or candidal infection may supervene and result in sepsis. Bone infiltration may be progressively destructive.

Treatment

Skin lesions may be treated locally with wet compresses and topical corticosteroids. Infections should be managed with appropriate systemic antibiotics or topical anticandidal agents. Unless there is evidence of extracutaneous dissemination or rapid progression of disease, treatment may not be indicated; histiocytosis X limited to the skin may resolve spontaneously without systemic treatment. Patients with systemic histiocytosis X diagnosed before 24 months of age tend to fare less well. Treatment includes systemic corticosteroids, antimetabolic agents, and radiation therapy (See Chapter 44).

JUVENILE XANTHOGRANULOMA

Essentials of Diagnosis

- Dome-shaped, yellow-orange papule.
- Does not urticate when stroked.
- Diagnostic skin biopsy.

General Considerations

This benign problem arises during the first 2 years of life with onset at birth in 20% of cases. There is no hereditary, racial, or sex predisposition. A skin biopsy of a mature lesion demonstrates Touton giant cells characterized by multiple nuclei surrounded by a rim of foamy cytoplasm. Lipid deposition is evident on fat stains. The histologic picture is diagnostic of juvenile xanthogranuloma.

Clinical Findings

Typical xanthogranulomas are sharply demarcated, firm, dome-shaped, yellow-orange papules that almost always occur on the head, neck, or upper trunk. They vary in size from a few millimeters to several centimeters and may enlarge rapidly. Both solitary and multiple lesions can occur. Affected infants are healthy, and the process generally remains confined to the skin. Serum cholesterol and triglyceride levels as well as other laboratory studies are always normal.

Differential Diagnosis

A solitary juvenile xanthogranuloma may resemble a mastocytoma but never urticates when stroked. Xanthomas due to hyperlipoproteinemia are not seen in the neonatal period. In the older infant, a Spitz nevus (spindle cell nevus) or pyogenic granuloma can also mimic a juvenile xanthogranuloma.

Complications

Whereas the lungs, pericardium, and testes have rarely been the site of juvenile xanthogranulomas, the majority of extracutaneous lesions arise in the ocular tissues. Eye lesions may predate the onset of skin changes or may occur in the absence of cutaneous manifestations. Ocular involvement may result in glaucoma, hyphema, uveitis, and severe acute proptosis.

Course & Prognosis

Ocular xanthomas require treatment to prevent ensuing damage from glaucoma. Skin lesions generally regress spontaneously within 6 months to 2 years after onset. Following involution, altered pigmentation or a flat atrophic area may remain (See Chapter 43).

3. MASTOCYTOSIS
(See Chapter 30.)

Cutaneous mast cell disease in infants presents in various forms ranging from solitary mastocytoma to diffuse infiltration of the skin. Diagnosis of all types of mast cell lesions can be confirmed by skin biopsy sections stained with Giemsa or toluidine blue stain that demonstrate the infiltrate of mast cells in the dermis.

Mastocytoma is a solitary lesion, present at birth or developing during the first few months of life. Ten to 15% of cases of mastocytosis are solitary tumors. Typical lesions appear as oval, pink-yellow to tan plaques that feel infiltrated or rubbery. They occur most commonly on the wrist but may be found anywhere, and the lesions are usually smaller than 6 cm in diameter. When traumatized, mastocytomas urticate and, during infancy, may develop vesicles or bullae (positive Darier's sign) on the surface.

Generalized maculopapular or nodular eruptions (urticaria pigmentosa) most commonly appear during infancy or early childhood but are occasionally present at birth. These lesions often spare the face, palms, and soles but may be scattered elsewhere. They range from yellow to brown, may be soft or firm, are sharply or poorly defined, and vary in size from a few millimeters to several centimeters. Darier's sign (urtication after stroking) is usually positive and supports the diagnosis. Dermographism may also be elicited on uninvolved skin. Rarely, visceral organs may be affected, most notably the gastrointestinal tract, bones, liver, spleen, lymph nodes, and bone marrow.

DISEASES OF SUBCUTANEOUS TISSUE

SUBCUTANEOUS FAT NECROSIS OF THE NEWBORN

This problem usually occurs in healthy newborn infants and generally begins within the first few days of life. On skin biopsy, the subcutis contains necrotic fat cells and the edematous, thickened fibrous septa are infiltrated with inflammatory cells. Calcium is frequently deposited in areas of necrosis.

The lesions of subcutaneous fat necrosis are sharply circumscribed, indurated, or nodular plaques with overlying red to violaceous skin. Sites of predilection include the thighs, buttocks, back, arms, and cheeks.

The lesions are frequently tender initially. The cause is unknown, though excessive chilling and obstetric trauma have been implicated in some instances. Rarely, the infant has associated pancreatitis or hypercalcemia.

Differential Diagnosis

Several entities can be confused with subcutaneous fat necrosis.

Sclerema neonatorum occurs during the first few days of life, more commonly in preterm or debilitated neonates, and is characterized by firm, taut, nonpitting skin over most of the body surface. The joints and face may be relatively immobile. These infants are frequently seriously ill, and some observers view sclerema as a poor prognostic sign because many infants subsequently die. In infants who survive, sclerema rarely persists for more than 2 weeks. Treatment is directed toward the underlying disease, because nothing can be done to alleviate the skin manifestations. The skin biopsy findings are similar to those of subcutaneous fat necrosis except that inflammation, fat necrosis, and calcification are usually absent.

Edema neonatorum can be distinguished by its propensity to pit easily and localization to dependent parts.

Cellulitis is often the most difficult problem to differentiate. Bacterial cultures of material obtained by careful needle aspiration should be obtained if infection is strongly suspected. Laboratory data supporting an infectious origin are critical to establishing this diagnosis.

Cold panniculitis has a similar clinical appearance and occurs most commonly on the cheeks in susceptible infants. Warm, erythematous, indurated plaques appear hours to days following exposure to cold, and the lesions may be reproduced by a application of ice for 2 minutes to the skin of affected infants. Laboratory studies, including measurement of plasma cryoglobulins, cryofibrinogen, cold agglutinins, and cold hemolysins, are normal. The inflammation resolves in 2–3 weeks, but postinflammatory hyperpigmentation may follow.

Weber-Christian panniculitis is rare but has been described in infants. Typically, erythematous nodules arise in the arms, thighs, and buttocks and may be associated with hepatomegaly, fever, and an elevated erythrocyte sedimentation rate.

Treatment

Most infants should be managed expectantly. In markedly fluctuant areas of fat necrosis, needle aspiration before rupture may decrease the incidence of subsequent scarring, but drainage of lesions is almost never required. Aspiration carries with it the risk of bacterial contamination. Infants with hypercalcemia may require restriction of calcium or administration of systemic steroids.

Course & Prognosis

Subcutaneous fat necrosis is self-limited, and lesions resolve spontaneously within weeks to months. Residual scarring or atrophy is unusual, but on occasion these changes follow extensive calcium deposition. In some patients, the contents of the necrotic nodules may liquefy and drain spontaneously, resulting in scarring.

PIGMENTARY ABNORMALITIES

Pigmentary changes may be visible at birth or may develop during the first few months of life as melanin production increases. Lesions with altered pigment may be localized, as in café au lait spots or white spots, or generalized, as in albinism.

HYPERPIGMENTED LESIONS

1. CAFÉ AU LAIT SPOTS

These macular lesions are occasionally evident in the newborn period but more commonly appear during the first year of life. Most are present by 5 years of age. Nineteen percent of normal children have a single café au lait spot. Multiple or large café au lait spots are associated with neurofibromatosis and McCune-Albright syndrome.

2. CONGENITAL MELANOCYTIC NEVI

Melanocytic nevi are occasionally present at birth and vary greatly in site, location, and appearance. The giant pigmented nevus (congenital hairy nevus; garment nevus) has a propensity to develop malignant melanoma at some time in life in approximately 10% of patients. These lesions may occupy up to 35% of the body surface. The color may range from light brown to black and is often uneven within a particular lesion (Fig 51–4). Localized thickening of the skin and growth of coarse hair from the surface are variable features. Leptomeningeal melanocytosis is an infrequent complication and may result in enlargement of the head, seizures, and other neurologic abnormalities.

It is the prevailing opinion that these nevi should be removed because of the relatively high risk of malignant transformation. Excision of giant congenital nevi is best accomplished during the early years of life,

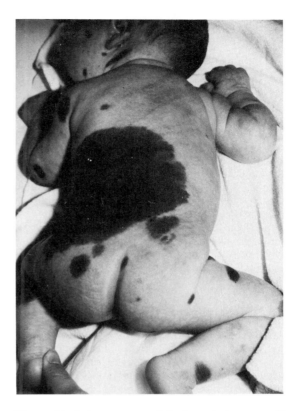

Figure 51–4. Large congenital pigmented nevus with satellite lesions.

because 60% of associated melanomas occur during the first decade. The procedure is usually done in stages and often requires extensive grafting or balloon expansion techniques. Smaller congenital nevi can usually be removed more easily. While some dermatologists feel that nevi smaller than 1.5 cm pose little risk of melanoma, others advocate removal of all congenital nevi. When lesions are located at sites where removal is difficult, such as the face or the tip of the penis, the risk of cosmetic or functional disturbance may be greater than that of malignant transformation. Observation rather than excision is probably best in those instances.

3. BLUE NEVUS

Blue nevi are raised and usually oval in shape, with a blue hue that results from the localization of spindle-shaped melanocytes within the dermis. The blue nevus must be differentiated from the Mongolian spot, which is always completely flat, gray-blue in color, and found most often over the buttocks and lower back in black, Indian, or Oriental babies. On occasion, a blue nevus may be confused with a hemangioma.

4. EPIDERMAL NEVUS

Epidermal nevi tend to resemble streaks or patches of dirt on the skin during the first weeks of life. They result from thickening of the epidermis and thus have an increased number of intraepidermal melanin granules. Several different clinical presentations include velvety plaques, linear lesions, grouped or linear papillomas, or warty hyperkeratotic lesions distributed in a localized or widespread fashion. Some patients with epidermal nevi have associated anomalies, mainly of the musculoskeletal and central nervous system (epidermal nevus syndrome). Treatment of the cutaneous abnormality is frequently not indicated. It can be treated with keratolytic agents or surgical removal by excision.

5. NEVUS SEBACEUS

This congenital nevus usually consists of a hairless, yellow-orange, well-defined plaque on the scalp. Less commonly, it is located on the face, ear, or neck. Occasionally, this lesion is mistaken for a melanocytic nevus or an area of aplasia cutis. Sebaceous nevi should be removed during childhood because of their predisposition to transform into basal cell carcinomas and other benign or malignant adnexal tumors during adulthood.

6. INCONTINENTIA PIGMENTI

Although whorls and streaks of macular hyperpigmentation represent the third stage of incontinentia pigmenti, occasionally the bullous and verrucous stages are bypassed. The pigmented lesions must be distinguished from an epidermal nevus or epidermolytic hyperkeratosis.

7. MASTOCYTOSIS

The yellow-brown lesions of urticaria pigmentosa are occasionally macular and may be mistaken for café au lait spots.

HYPOPIGMENTED LESIONS

1. GENERALIZED HYPOPIGMENTATION

Generalized hypopigmentation may result from a biochemical defect resulting in pigment dilution, as in

phenylketonuria, or from a nutritional deficiency, as in kwashiorkor. In albinism, the skin, eyes, and hair are devoid of pigmentation, and photophobia, nystagmus, and impaired visual acuity of variable degree are associated. Some patients have a deficiency of the enzyme tyrosinase required for melanin synthesis (tyrosinase-negative albinism). The underlying biochemical or cellular defect in the majority of cases is unclear.

These children must use protective sunscreens because of their increased risk of developing actinic keratoses, basal cell carcinomas, squamous cell carcinomas, and melanomas. Generalized reduction in pigmentation is also seen in Chédiak-Higashi, Cross-McKusick-Breen, and Hermansky-Pudlak syndromes.

2. LOCALIZED REDUCTION OF PIGMENTATION

Hypopigmented patches may be present at birth or may become noticeable for the first time as the infant develops additional pigment during the first year of life. White macules in a newborn infant may be the initial manifestation of tuberous sclerosis, with the associated seizures, mental retardation, adenoma sebaceum, shagreen patches, and periungual fibromas developing later. These hypopigmented macules are best detected with Wood's lamp, which accentuates the contrast between the normal skin and the area deficient in pigment. White leaf macules of tuberous sclerosis must be differentiated from nevus anemicus (a localized defect in vascular responsiveness), areas of postinflammatory hypopigmentation, and, later in infancy, pityriasis alba.

Piebaldism is a rare autosomal dominant disorder manifested by patches of amelanotic skin and hair, especially on the central forehead and anterior scalp, chin, thorax, back, mid arm, and mid leg. Islands of normal pigmentation may be found within amelanotic sites. The amelanotic areas are fixed; progression or repigmentation is not expected. Vitiligo can be distinguished by a later onset, positive family history, lack of lesions at birth, and changing pattern of the skin lesions. Differential diagnosis also includes Waardenburg's syndrome, an autosomal dominant condition of variable expressivity that includes lateral displacement of the ocular inner canthi, synophrys, heterochromia of the irides, deafness, white forelock, and sites of decreased cutaneous pigmentation.

Incontinentia pigmenti achromians (hypomelanosis of Ito) is a neurocutaneous syndrome with distinctive macular streaks and whorls of hypopigmentation that is present in the neonate or develops during infancy. Up to 50% of these children have seizures, developmental delay, or ocular or musculoskeletal abnormalities.

ECZEMATOUS DERMATITIS

SEBORRHEIC DERMATITIS OF INFANCY

Essentials of Diagnosis

- Eczematous dermatitis.
- Begins with cradle cap.
- Not present at birth.
- Favors scalp, face, and body folds.

General Considerations

This eczematous process frequently begins in the first weeks of life with scalp involvement (cradle cap). Its cause is unknown. While seborrheic dermatitis may resemble atopic eczema or occur in a child who later develops atopic dermatitis, these 2 disorders can be distinguished clinically most of the time.

Clinical Findings

Seborrheic dermatitis is characterized by nonpruritic plaques of scaling and erythema, especially on the scalp, face, retroauricular areas, neck folds, axillae, and groin (Fig 51–5).

Occasionally, the process becomes more generalized. The scales are usually yellow and greasy in character but may be white and dry. The child is otherwise healthy. Most commonly, the rash begins at 2–3 weeks of age but may have its onset at any time during the first year of life.

Differential Diagnosis

Atopic dermatitis is the most common eczematous disorder after the third month of life but rarely occurs during the first month. Often there is a positive family history of eczema, asthma, or allergic rhinitis. As opposed to seborrheic dermatitis, the entire skin surface is usually xerotic, and the child is bothered by intense pruritus. Areas of predilection in infants with atopic dermatitis are the face and extensor surfaces of the limbs. Acute lesions are moist and weeping—in contrast to those in seborrheic dermatitis, which are usually dry. Chronic lesions of atopic dermatitis are dry, but lichenification is a prominent feature.

Infants with Leiner's disease develop a generalized exfoliative dermatitis within weeks after birth in addition to diarrhea and failure to thrive. A variety of immune defects have been associated. This disorder is extremely rare.

In histiocytosis X, an erythematous scaling rash may be present, especially on the scalp, around the ears, and in flexural areas. Petechiae or ulcerations may be present in the neonate with histiocytosis X, and the rash may have a pustular morphology. Gingival lesions, hepatosplenomegaly, lymphadenopathy, and rales on chest auscultation are supportive evidence for histiocytosis; the skin biopsy is diagnostic.

Particularly in the diaper area, an eczematous process may be due to an irritant reaction to exogenous substances, candidal infection, or psoriasis, all of which can simulate seborrheic dermatitis.

Secondary infection with bacteria and *C albicans* can be detected by performing the appropriate smears and cultures.

Treatment

Seborrheic dermatitis usually responds to applications of a nonfluorinated topical corticosteroid such as 1% hydrocortisone. The scalp can be treated with an antiseborrheic shampoo followed by a topical sulfur or corticosteroid preparation if needed. Weeping lesions may require compressing with saline or Bur-

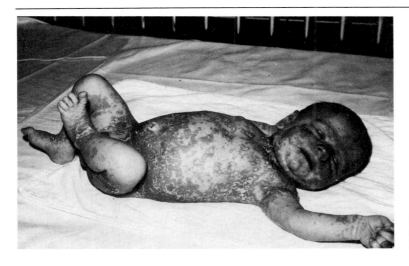

Figure 51–5. Extensive seborrheic dermatitis on the face, trunk, and limbs of a young infant.

ow's solution, followed by application of a protective ointment. Appropriate topical anticandidal agents and systemic or topical antibiotics are indicated for secondary infection.

Course & Prognosis

Seborrheic dermatitis responds rapidly to treatment but often recurs periodically during the first year of life. Remission beyond the first year is usual.

DIAPER DERMATITIS

Irritant diaper dermatitis is more common than infectious or allergic dermatitis. The most frequent causes are prolonged contact of diaper-area skin with urine or feces and improper cleansing. The skin initially appears reddened and, with chronicity, becomes dry and scaly. In chronic severe dermatitis, hypertrophic papules, blisters, and erosions develop—lesions that can be mistaken for bacterial infection and condylomata lata of syphilis. Meticulous hygiene, avoidance of irritants, and a brief course of therapy with a mild topical corticosteroid and a protective ointment will usually clear this type of dermatitis. If weeping lesions are present, compresses with saline or Burow's solution are indicated. Plastic or other occlusive pants should be avoided.

Allergic contact dermatitis represents a true delayed hypersensitivity reaction to a particular contactant. Although frequently suspected, these reactions are in fact quite rare in infants. Seborrheic and atopic dermatitis may involve the diaper area, as may the less common disorders such as psoriasis, histiocytosis X, Leiner's disease, and acrodermatitis enteropathica.

Infections in the diaper area are due most frequently to *C albicans*, *S aureus*, and gram-negative organisms (see section above on infections).

NEONATAL LUPUS ERYTHEMATOSUS

Neonatal lupus erythematosus is a rare disorder characterized by the cutaneous lesions of lupus erythematosus or congenital heart block. Cutaneous lesions may be present at birth or may develop during the first 3 months of life. They may be annular, scaly erythematous plaques or may resemble those of discoid lupus with central epidermal atrophy and dyspigmentation but without follicular plugging and residual scarring. The cutaneous lesions are most commonly located on the face and scalp but may occur elsewhere on the body. Although sunlight is not a prerequisite for development of these lesions, photosensitivity is suggested by their localization to the face and scalp and by the history of sun exposure prior to their development.

Mothers of affected infants have circulating SSA and, less commonly, SSB autoantibodies, and these antibodies are acquired transplacentally by the affected infants. Only 33% of infants are ANA-positive. Mothers may have a variety of autoimmune disorders, especially systemic or subacute cutaneous lupus erythematosus and Sjögren's syndrome, or may be asymptomatic. Not uncommonly, an asymptomatic mother may later develop clinical evidence of the disease.

Clinical Findings

Histopathologic examination of involved skin shows degeneration of basal cells of the epidermis, superficial infiltration of the dermis with mononuclear cells, and variable epidermal atrophy. Immunofluorescence analysis of lesional skin may demonstrate granular IgG at the dermal-epidermal junction.

Congenital heart block occurs in up to 50% of patients, and neonatal lupus erythematosus is now thought to be the most common cause of this problem. The block is usually complete, though 2:1 atrioventricular block has also been described. The atrioventricular system shows inflammation and fibrosis. Occasionally, coexistent myocarditis and congestive heart failure complicate the picture. Hepatomegaly and splenomegaly are found in 20% of patients, and hematologic abnormalities—including thrombocytopenia, hemolytic anemia, and leukopenia—affect 15% of infants. Lymphadenopathy and pneumonitis have also been reported.

Differential Diagnosis

The lesions of neonatal lupus erythematosus must be differentiated from those of other scaling conditions, including seborrheic dermatitis, superficial fungal infections, psoriasis, and atopic dermatitis.

Treatment

Bland lubricants and sun protection are the most important elements of therapy. Mild topical corticosteroids may be useful for patients with more severe cutaneous involvement. A pacemaker may be required for infants with complete heart block.

Course & Prognosis

The cutaneous and systematic abnormalities—other than the permanent cardiac block—resolve between 6 and 12 months of age, corresponding to the disappearance of the maternally transmitted autoantibodies. To date, 2 infants with cutaneous neonatal lupus erythematosus and 6 with cardiac block have subsequently developed autoimmune disorders.

REFERENCES

Alper J, Holmes LB: The incidence and significance of birthmarks in a cohort of 4,641 newborns. Pediatr Dermatol 1983;1:58.

Enjolras O, Riche MC, Merland JJ: Facial port-wine stains and Sturge-Weber syndrome. Pediatrics 1985;76:48.

Esterly NB: Cutaneous hemangiomas, vascular strains and associated syndromes. Curr Probl Pediatr 1987;17:1.

Esterly NB, Maurer HS, Gonzalez-Crussi F: Histiocytosis X: A seven-year experience at a children's hospital. J Am Acad Dermatol 1985;13:481.

Evans NJ, Rutter N: Development of the epidermis in the newborn. Biol Neonate 1986;49:74.

Haber RM et al: Hereditary epidermolysis bullosa. J Am Acad Dermatol 1985;13:252.

Hebert AA, Esterly NB: Bacterial and candidal cutaneous infections in the neonate. Dermatol Clin 1986;4:3.

Hurwitz S: *Clinical Pediatric Dermatology.* Saunders, 1981.

Solomon LM, Cook B, Klipfel W: The ectodermal dysplasias. In: *Dermatologic Clinics: The Genodermatoses.* Alper JC (editor). Saunders, 1987.

Solomon LM, Esterly NB: *Neonatal Dermatology.* Saunders, 1973.

Storer JS, Hawk RJ: Neonatal skin and skin disorders. In: *Pediatric Dermatology.* Schacher LA, Hansen RC (editors). Churchill-Livingstone, 1988.

Williams ML, Elias PM: Genetically transmitted generalized disorders of cornification: The ichthyoses. In: *Dermatologic Clinics: The Genodermatoses.* Alper JC (editor). Saunders, 1987.

52   Skin Disorders in Black Patients

Sandy Martin, MD & Theodore Rosen, MD

Diagnosis and treatment of cutaneous disorders of black patients require an understanding of significant differences from those of whites. There are differences not only in genetically determined pigmentation, anatomic characteristics, and reactivity of the skin and its appendages but also in the incidence of certain dermatologic conditions that may be influenced by these and other—chiefly cultural—factors.

While almost all skin disorders are common to every race, the presentation of skin disease in blacks might make recognition more difficult for physicians trained primarily to observe disorders of fair skin. Inflammatory and pigmentary changes in black skin, for example, may be obscured or take on a different coloration than might be expected. The texture and thickness of the skin may be different. Certain patterns of response are more common in black skin than in white skin. Exaggerated hyperpigmentation or hypopigmentation may follow injury to the skin. The active, dynamic pilosebaceous unit in blacks accounts for the prominent follicular involvement and annular configuration that are seen in black skin. There is a tendency in blacks toward excessive fibroblastic tissue response (eg, keloids) and granuloma formation.

Some cutaneous diseases are common in blacks, while others are rare. Acne keloidalis nuchae is rare in whites but a common disabling disorder in blacks. Disseminated and recurrent infundibulofolliculitis is described chiefly in black patients. On the other hand, photosensitivity reactions, acne rosacea, and cutaneous xanthomas occur far less frequently in black than in white patients.

This chapter will emphasize some variations of skin disorders seen in blacks.

ACNE KELOIDALIS NUCHAE

Essentials of Diagnosis
- Discrete and confluent hard hypertrophic papules and nodules on the back of the neck.
- Secondary infection and weeping are common.

General Considerations
Acne keloidalis nuchae is a disorder nearly unique to black patients. Its cause is unknown, but the disor-

der may involve a foreign body type of reaction to ingrown hairs or a bacterial folliculitis.

Clinical Findings
Early cases resemble folliculitis on the back of the neck. With time, globoid hypertrophic follicular and perifollicular papules and nodules develop. As keloidal scarring progresses, sinus tracts, pustules, abscesses, and drainage are seen (Fig 52–1).

Complications
Infection is the most common complication. Some patients may have limitation of range of neck movement due to scarring. Squamous cell carcinoma may rarely develop.

Treatment
Early aggressive therapy may limit morbidity. Topical and systemic antibiotics may reduce folliculitis and the tendency for keloid formation. Smoldering secondary infection is perhaps the most common source of chronic provocation. Topical and intralesional corticosteroids and medicated shampoos containing antimicrobial agents (eg, chloroxine [Capitrol], selenium sulfide [Selsun]) are helpful to debride crusts, reduce the numbers of microbes, and suppress inflammation. Once keloids have formed, treatment is difficult (see below).

INFANTILE ACROPUSTULOSIS

Essentials of Diagnosis
- Pruritic vesicopustules primarily on the hands and feet of infants.
- Little response to topical steroids or antibiotics.

General Considerations
This newly described eruptive disorder is severely pruritic and associated with restlessness and fretfulness. The cause is unknown. It begins between 2 and 10 months of age in children with no history of atopy. Black infants seem especially prone to its development.

Clinical Findings
A. Symptoms and Signs: Pinpoint erythematous macules evolve into papules, then discrete pustules on

626

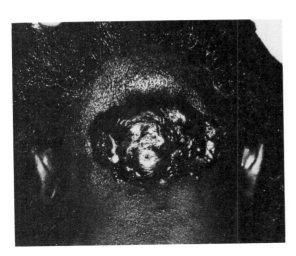

Figure 52–1. Acne keloidalis nuchae. Alopecia and hypertrophic scarring result from an active inflammatory process involving the follicles.

the hands and feet. Scattered lesions may be seen elsewhere. The disorder resolves by 2 or 3 years of age.

B. Laboratory Findings: Cultures and wet mounts are negative. Histologic examination shows intraepidermal pustules containing neutrophils.

Differential Diagnosis

Dyshidrosis, impetigo, scabies, transient neonatal pustular melanosis, tinea, and pustular psoriasis all must be considered.

Treatment

Soporific doses of diphenhydramine may help suppress itching. Dapsone has been helpful in some cases because of its effect on neutrophils, but it is infrequently indicated because the risk of side effects usually outweighs the need for treatment.

AINHUM

Ainhum is a disorder almost unique to blacks. There is no known cause. A fibrous constriction develops that ultimately—over a period of several years—leads to autoamputation of the affected digit. The disorder must be differentiated from "pseudoainhum," which is caused by trauma, scleroderma, congenital anomalies, leprosy, syringomyelia, or diabetes.

ATOPIC DERMATITIS

Atopic dermatitis is a common disease with no racial predilection. The disorder appears different in

blacks because it tends to affect hair follicles, leading to follicular prominence. Black children may show widespread follicular papules before developing eczematous morphology. Lichenification and hyperpigmentation are common.

DERMATITIS CRURIS PUSTULOSA ET ATROPHICANS ("Nigerian Skin Disease")

Dermatitis cruris pustulosa et atrophicans may represent a localized pyogenic infection from prolonged application of oils. It is reported mainly in blacks in Nigeria and Trinidad. Follicular pustules lead to shiny atrophic areas on the involved skin. Scaling may be prominent. The arms are occasionally involved, along with the legs. Affected patients should discontinue applications of topical oils. Benzoyl peroxide gels (5 or 10%) along with topical or systemic antibiotics such as tetracycline, 250 mg 3 times daily, may be helpful.

DERMATOSIS PAPULOSA NIGRA

Dermatosis papulosa nigra is a group of seborrheic keratoses that develop on the faces of black patients. It is a common cosmetic affliction and occurs earlier

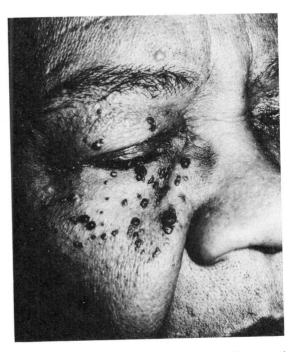

Figure 52–2. Dermatosis papulosa nigra. Clusters of dark verrucous papules and papulonodules appear on the right paranasal area. Histologically, these are pigmented seborrheic keratoses.

in life than the seborrheic keratoses in fair-skinned individuals.

The number of keratoses increases with time, but lesions show no malignant potential. They do not spontaneously subside. They are most common over the malar regions but may be seen on the neck, chest, and back (Fig 52–2).

Treatment is basically destructive and may be followed by pigmentary or keloidal changes. Cryosurgery can be used, but melanocytes are easily destroyed; hyperpigmentation often results. Cautery may be better tolerated but can cause scars to form. Sometimes it is worthwhile to treat only a lesion or 2 so the physician and patient can assess the cosmetic result before proceeding with wholesale removal.

DISSEMINATED & RECURRENT INFUNDIBULOFOLLICULITIS (Hitch & Lund Disease)

Disseminated and recurrent infundibulofolliculitis is a not uncommon pruritic papular eruption that does not respond well to therapy. It is almost unique to black skin. The discrete follicular papules wax and wane on the trunk and buttocks and show little tendency toward lichenification or confluence and resemble gooseflesh (Fig 52–3). Histologic examination shows a lymphocytic infiltrate surrounding the infundibulum (upper hair follicle) and follicular plugging.

The differential diagnosis includes atopic dermatitis, contact dermatitis, lichen nitidus, keratosis pilaris, phrynoderma, lichen planopilaris, secondary syphilis, Darier's disease, and Kyrle's disease.

Anti-inflammatory and antipruritic agents may occasionally be helpful, but treatment is often unsatisfactory.

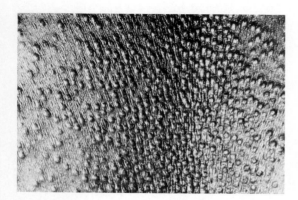

Figure 52–3. Disseminated and recurrent infundibulofolliculitis. Sharply defined follicular papules resemble those of cutis anserina. The tendency toward follicular prominence is marked in black skin.

FOX-FORDYCE DISEASE

Fox-Fordyce disease is a stubborn persistent pruritic dermatosis of the apocrine gland regions. The axillae, areolae, and pubic region are most commonly involved. Most patients are black. The disease has been known as "apocrine miliaria" because there is obstruction of the apocrine sweat duct and subsequent rupture of the duct, analogous to true miliaria of the eccrine glands. Complications include secondary infection and lichen simplex chronicus. The differential diagnosis includes folliculitis, follicular neurodermatitis, and candidiasis. Administration of oral contraceptive agents occasionally has been useful though not usually recommended specifically for Fox-Fordyce disease. Topical vitamin A (tretinoin) cream may help.

FUTCHER'S LINES

Futcher's lines (also known as Voigt's lines) are normal color patterns seen in pigmented individuals, especially blacks and darkly pigmented Japanese. The interface between the darker segment of skin (usually anterolaterally on the upper arms) and the lighter segment of skin (anteromedially) is marked by a discrete line. There are no complications. Eczematous processes such as contact dermatitis may be mistakenly diagnosed.

HAMARTOMA MONILIFORMIS

This is an asymptomatic disorder more common in institutionalized individuals, primarily blacks. The linear, beaded papules are flesh-colored and do not coalesce or scale. They are seen on the forehead, clavicle, and neck.

Histopathologic study reveals hyperplasia of sebaceous glands, nerves, and collagenous and elastic fibers but is not diagnostic.

HOT-COMB ALOPECIA

Young black females commonly use a combination of hot combs and petrolatum to straighten or curl their hair. Chronic use is associated with follicular inflammation and alopecia, followed by eventual scar formation and atrophy. Biopsy may be indicated to rule out other causes of scarring alopecia, such as lupus erythematosus, sarcoidosis, lichen planopilaris, or scleroderma. Inflammation will stop when the hot-comb treatments are stopped. Scarring alopecia may be permanent.

KELOIDS
(See also Chapter 24.)

Keloids are firm, raised, shiny exaggerated nodules devoid of hair. Most keloids form at sites of trauma, such as on the earlobes after ear piercing, but some appear to develop spontaneously. Keloids represent an exaggerated fibroblastic proliferation particularly common and annoying to blacks. This common tendency can complicate simple wounds, earring punctures, acne (Fig 52–4), and major surgery.

Although common in blacks, keloids occur in all races. The ratio of incidence in blacks to that in whites is variously given as 20:1 to 5:1. Trauma and inflammation or infection can lead to keloids. Complications include limitation of function or range of movement, cosmetic dysfunctions, pain, tenderness, or itching.

Intralesional corticosteroid injection (usually triamcinolone acetonide, 5–10 mg/mL) is the most common and effective therapy. Cryosurgery may be utilized with or without intralesional corticosteroid therapy. Occasionally, keloids must be removed surgically. The tendency for recurrence may be lessened by injecting triamcinolone acetonide, 5–10 mg/mL, into the wound site at the time of surgery and periodically thereafter.

LICHEN PLANUS

Lichen planus is not more common in blacks than in whites. However, lichen planus in blacks commonly is hypertrophic. In addition, both the erosive and the ulcerative plantar variants are more common.

Typically, lesions are a deep purple color in black patients with lichen planus. Oral lesions are relatively uncommon in blacks, compared to whites. Lesions

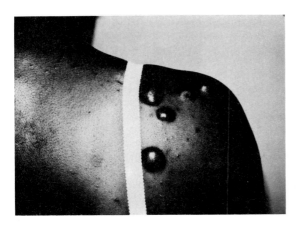

Figure 52–4. Keloids. Exaggerated scar tissue response can be a source of aggravation, both cosmetically and because of itching or tenderness.

often resolve to leave intense hyperpigmentation, which slowly fades (see Chapter 41).

MIDLINE HYPOPIGMENTATION

A midsagittal band of hypopigmentation is considered a variant of normal black skin. It may be prominent or barely visible. Its incidence may approach 30–40% of blacks. Midline hypopigmentation may be inherited as an autosomal dominant characteristic. One may also find hypopigmented macules beneath the clavicles or in the periareolar region.

MONGOLIAN SPOT

Mongolian spots represent areas of dermal melanocytosis. Approximately 40–90% of black neonates have them. It is thought the patches represent an arrest in migration of melanocytes from the neural crest to the epidermis. Mongolian spots may be solitary or multiple. They tend to fade in time. Occasionally they are mistaken for melanomas or hematomas. No treatment is required.

NAIL PIGMENTATION

Diffuse or longitudinal nail plate pigmentation is common in blacks. While absent at birth, this phenomenon appears in young adult life. The pigmented bands are asymptomatic. This pigmentation is the result of excessive melanin within the nail plate rather than in the underlying soft tissue (nail bed). This variation of normal must be differentiated from subungual nevus or melanoma, contact with silver- or mercury-containing topical agents, pigmentation due to ingestion of antimalarial drugs, Addison's disease, and postirradiation melanonychia. In white patients, a pigmented band in a nail is usually an indication for biopsy of the nail matrix. In most blacks this is not necessary—though it should always be considered—since the bands are common; ie, they are much less likely to be melanomas. Diffusion of pigment into the cuticular skin, however, should raise serious concern about subungual malignant melanoma. No treatment is indicated. The long-term prognosis is benign.

ORAL PIGMENTATION

Oral pigmentation is a frequent incidental finding in blacks. While absent at birth, this condition is fully manifested at age 20 years. Any portion of the oral mucosa may be affected, though the gingivae are affected most frequently. Colors may range from gray-blue to brown-black.

The differential diagnosis includes heavy metal exposure, antimalarial and phenothiazine therapy, to-bacco staining, Addison's disease, Peutz-Jeghers syndrome, and pigmentation associated with hemochromatosis.

There are no symptoms, and no therapy is indicated.

PAPULAR ERUPTION OF BLACKS

Essentials of Diagnosis
- Widespread symmetric papular eruption.
- Intense itching refractory to therapy.
- No evidence of systemic disease.

General Considerations
This recently described disorder of unknown cause occurs primarily in young adult black men. The incidence is unknown.

Clinical Findings
A. Symptoms and Signs: Firm, monomorphous, dermal flesh-colored papules arise in a symmetric fashion not necessarily associated with hair follicles. The epidermis is not affected. Sites of predilection include the upper arms, the postauricular region of the neck, and the upper trunk. The disorder is characterized by severe pruritus that fails to respond to most attempts at management.

B. Laboratory Findings: Biopsy reveals a dense perivascular infiltrate composed of mononuclear cells and eosinophils.

Differential Diagnosis
Sarcoidosis, lymphoma cutis, and papular granuloma annulare are considered in the differential diagnosis, but most of these do not itch.

Treatment
Most methods of treatment are ineffective. Short-term remission may be induced in some cases with systemic corticosteroids.

Prognosis
The long-term outlook for clearing is bleak. Lesions tend to multiply with time.

PITYRIASIS ROSEA

There are some unusual and important aspects of pityriasis rosea in blacks. Instead of being salmon-pink, lesions are reddish to dark brown. Papular and vesiculopapular presentations seem to be more frequent in blacks. There may be protracted hyperpigmentation following involution of the acute eruption; this is a rare sequela in other ethnic groups.

Because pityriasis rosea may lead to distressing cosmetic complications in blacks, therapy is advis-able in florid cases. Systemic corticosteroids (eg, intramuscular triamcinolone, 40–60 mg) may decrease inflammation or hasten resolution. Phototherapy, while sometimes useful in white patients, should be avoided in blacks as it may exacerbate postinflammatory pigmentary changes (see also Chapter 41).

POMADE ACNE

Pomade acne is a disorder of persons who use greasy ointments and oils on or near the affected skin. Because this practice is widespread in the black community, pomade acne is more common in this group. Women are affected more frequently than men.

Because pomade application is most common on the scalp, the resulting eruption frequently favors the forehead and temples. Open and closed comedones, pustules, and erythematous papules as well as postinflammatory pigmentation are found. Deep cystic lesions are uncommon.

Usual acne therapies are employed (see Chapter 26). Mild abrasives are particularly helpful (eg, use of a Buf-Puf to rub the area daily). The patient must discontinue pomade application if treatment is to be effective, in which case the outlook is good.

PSEUDOFOLLICULITIS BARBAE

Essentials of Diagnosis
- Numerous inflammatory papules in a hairy area, usually the beard.
- Pustules or hyperpigmentation may be present.
- Disease resolves if hair is allowed to grow.

General Considerations
This very common disorder of blacks is the result of reentry of coiled hairs into the skin. Shaving facilitates the process of ingrown hairs by "sharpening" the free hair end. Short curly hairs are also more prone to penetrate the skin than long ones.

Clinical Findings
Pseudofolliculitis may occur in any shaved location. Pseudofolliculitis barbae, axillaris, capitis, pubis, and corporis all have been reported—the beard area being most often affected.

Early lesions consist of erythematous papules intermixed with pustules. In long-standing disease, indolent firm papules (often hyperpigmented) predominate. Coiled hairs may sometimes be detected under the skin. Keloidal scars may result in patients so predisposed.

Differential Diagnosis
Acne vulgaris, tinea barbae, and sarcoidosis must be considered in the differential diagnosis.

Treatment

Discontinuance of shaving reduces the number of new lesions and ultimately allows some of the embedded hairs to "pop out." When this is impractical, prevention of a "close" shave will avoid immediate penetration by sharpened hairs. Chemical depilatories are useful but require careful patient instruction. A single-blade razor (rather than double-blade) should be employed, and shaving should be done in one direction only (with the grain) after thorough hydrating of the hair with compresses or by washing. Use of special razors that prevent close shaving may be of benefit, eg, "PFB, The Bump Fighter." Alternatively, electric shavers are available that allow hair to grow out longer, eg, "The Black Pro." A preshaving scrub with an abrasive sponge (Buf-Puf) helps loosen embedded hairs. In some patients, application of topical tretinoin (Retin-A) will help in the long term, though some increased irritation may be present when this therapy is initiated.

Prognosis

The condition can be improved considerably with modification of shaving habits and often clears completely if shaving is stopped. Otherwise, the condition is a chronic one and requires continued management.

PSORIASIS

Psoriasis is relatively uncommon in black patients, an incidence of 0.1–1.4% having been reported. The typical bright red plaques may be absent in black patients, the lesions assuming a blue, violaceous, brown, or even black hue. Postinflammatory changes (hypo- or hyperpigmentation) may follow resolution of lesions (see Chapter 41).

SARCOIDOSIS

Essentials of Diagnosis

- Variable morphology (a "great imitator" disease).
- Violaceous nodules or papules near facial orifices.
- Erythema nodosum.
- Systemic (ocular, pulmonary, osseous) manifestations.

General Considerations

Sarcoidosis is more common among blacks in the USA (up to 18:1 ratio compared to whites). Females outnumber males about 2 to one. Sarcoidosis tends to be more aggressive in blacks, with higher morbidity and mortality rates compared to whites. In some patients, disease is confined to the skin, while in others it affects internal organs as well.

Clinical Findings

A. Symptoms and Signs: A variety of unusual cutaneous manifestations may appear in blacks, including ichythyosis-like scaling, ulcerative deep subcutaneous nodules, verrucous plaques, and hypopigmented macules. The disease in blacks as well as whites is a great imitator and mimics many different disorders depending on morphologic features. Flesh-colored papules scattered over the chest or back are common. Papules along the corners of the nose or mouth suggest the disorder. Scarring scalp alopecia as a presentation of sarcoidosis is generally limited to blacks.

Systemic sarcoidosis is also a great imitator of other diseases. Systemic signs and symptoms include malaise, weight loss, fatigue, and lethargy. Cough, chest pain, and night sweats are common. Other signs and symptoms depend upon which organ systems are affected and where. Lung lesions are common and include hilar adenopathy, miliary lesions in the parenchyma, and fibrosis. Lymphadenopathy, hepatomegaly, and splenomegaly can occur. Sausage-shaped swelling of the finger joints, cardiac arrhythmias, odd neurologic abnormalities, uveitis, conjunctivitis, and swelling of the salivary glands may also develop.

1. Erythema nodosum– In sarcoidosis this usually is associated with hilar adenopathy. It occurs in about one-third of all patients with systemic sarcoidosis and resolves spontaneously, usually within months.

2. Papules– Widely disseminated dermal nonscaling papules are common. In blacks they are flesh-colored but may be yellow-orange, brown, or violaceous red. Sometimes papules form annular configurations.

3. Plaques and nodules– Variable morphology suggests many disorders. Flesh-colored or blue-red nodules occur symmetrically over the trunk, thighs, and shoulders. Confluence of lesions produces indurated plaques.

4. Lupus pernio– Nodules and plaques occur on the nose, cheeks, or ears to produce purple bulbous deformities. Lesions are typically indurated and blue-red to purple.

5. Scar sarcoid– For some reasons, granulomatous infiltrates like to form in scars and often give them a purple-red color and an indurated, inflamed appearance.

6. Angiolupoid sarcoid– Soft reddish swellings adjacent to the nose over the cheeks often have telangiectasia over the surface.

B. Laboratory and Other Diagnostic Studies: Laboratory findings also depend upon the type of sarcoidosis, the organs involved, and the extent of involvement. Typically, laboratory findings are unaffected by sarcoidosis limited to the skin. The histologic picture is characteristic in papular skin lesions and in many other forms as well. There is a "naked tubercle" of epithelioid cells in the dermis without the mantle of lymphocytes seen in many other granulomatous diseases.

Serum calcium levels may be elevated. Angiotensin-converting enzyme levels are elevated, especially when the lung is affected. Hypergammaglobulinemia is common, but measures of cell-mediated immunity are often depressed. Liver function tests such as the AST (SGOT), LDH, and alkaline phosphatase may be abnormal.

Chest x-ray may show diffuse infiltration, hilar adenopathy, or other disorder.

Differential Diagnosis

Sarcoidosis mimics many diseases and can often be considered in the differential diagnosis of various systemic and cutaneous problems. In the skin, the disease commonly suggests granuloma annulare, xanthomas, lichen planus, psoriasis, lupus erythematosus, necrobiosis lipoidica, rosacea, granuloma faciale, leprosy, syphilis, diseases causing scarring alopecias (see Chapter 28), or diseases causing pigmentary changes or ulcerations.

Treatment

If only the skin is involved, topical or intralesional corticosteroids are the treatment of choice, though they are relatively ineffective. Systemic corticosteroids work well but cause predictable side effects over the long periods of time usually required. There is no standard way to use systemic corticosteroids, because doses and regimens depend on the organs affected, the extent of disease, systemic signs, and duration of therapy as well as other factors.

Therapeutic maneuvers are essentially the same in blacks as in other groups. Antimalarial medications may be useful in some patients; quinacrine is more suitable for use in blacks than in whites, because the complication of yellow skin discoloration is often inapparent.

SICKLE CELL ULCERS

Essentials of Diagnosis

- Nonhealing ulcers, lower extremities.
- Recurrent attacks of fever; pain in the anus, legs, or abdomen.
- Associated with sickle cell anemia.

General Considerations

Sickle cell anemia is nearly unique to blacks. Skin ulcerations associated with this hemoglobinopathy usually begin between ages 10–20 years. The incidence of this phenomenon in homozygotes is about 50%. Partial vascular obstruction and a decreased local oxygen tension due to abnormal hemoglobin and erythrocyte morphology account for these lesions.

Clinical Findings

A. Symptoms and Signs: Sickle cell ulcers present as well-demarcated "punched-out" defects. Lesions usually appear close to the malleoli. Ulcers are painful and slow to heal and may be complicated by infection or joint deformity.

B. Laboratory Findings: Anemia, jaundice, or reticulocytosis may be present. Peripheral blood smear shows characteristic sickle-shaped erythrocytes. Hemoglobin electrophoresis demonstrates hemoglobin S. This is done last and is not generally available.

Treatment

Some principles for the treatment of leg ulcers of various causes are discussed in Chapter 23. The affected leg should be immobilized and elevated. The ulcers can be cleansed with hydrogen peroxide or antibacterial solutions such as chlorhexidine. Devitalized tissue should be debrided. Dextranomer (Debrisan) beads may prove useful in cleansing and debriding and have been effective in promoting healing. Blood transfusions are indicated when the hemoglobin count falls below 12 g/dL.

STEROID-INDUCED HYPOPIGMENTATION

Corticosteroids may induce hypopigmentation by damaging melanosomes. This phenomenon is more likely to be noted in dark-skinned persons. Both topical application and intralesional injection can produce hypopigmentation. Repigmentation is gradual but generally complete. There is no treatment that will hasten repigmentation.

Steroid treatment should be discontinued in affected areas if feasible.

TRANSIENT NEONATAL PUSTULAR MELANOSIS

This uncommon asymptomatic dermatitis occurs almost exclusively in black neonates. Vesicopustules and pigmented maculas develop on the trunk, palms, and soles. Biopsy reveals a subcorneal blister filled with leukocytes (polymorphonuclear and eosinophilic). Erythema toxicum neonatorum, congenital viral infections, and staphylococcal impetigo are major diagnostic considerations.

No therapy is indicated. The lesions resolve promptly and spontaneously.

VOLAR MELANOTIC MACULES

This condition is prevalent among black patients. The presence and severity of hyperpigmented macules correlate roughly with the degree of overall pigmentation. Volar macules are the result of local accumulations of melanin.

The hyperpigmented macules are usually small (< 1 cm in diameter), multiple, and haphazardly patchy in distribution. Asymptomatic lesions possess irregular outlines and variability in shape and size. Plantar macules are more often prominent on or near the ball and heel of the foot.

The major differentiation is from lesions of secondary syphilis. Malignant melanoma and acral-lentiginous melanoma must also be considered if there is only one lesion.

Lesions persist throughout life but do not require therapy.

MALIGNANT EPIDERMAL NEOPLASIA

Malignant epidermal neoplasms are much less common in black patients than in those with fair complexions. In all probability, this relates to the photoprotective benefits of increased melanin in the skin, thus decreasing the penetration of carcinogenic ultraviolet radiation. Cutaneous neoplasia accounts for only 1.5–7% of all cancers in blacks, in contrast to 20% (or more) in whites. Basal cell epitheliomas contribute about 20% of all such tumors, while in situ and invasive squamous cell carcinomas as well as melanoma make up the remainder.

When basal cell epitheliomas do occur in blacks, there is no significant epidemiologic difference from those in other ethnic groups. Most basal cell epitheliomas occur on the head and neck (exposed) region and demonstrate a clinically typical morphology. Lesions are relatively indolent and usually respond to standard methods of therapy (see Chapter 43).

In contrast, squamous cell carcinoma in blacks often occurs in nonexposed (covered) areas of the body and is frequently the result of an antecedent cutaneous condition. Any chronic scarring skin disease may give rise to squamous cell carcinoma in blacks, especially discoid lupus erythematosus, traumatic and burn scars, erythema ab igne, and hidradenitis suppurativa. Such secondary neoplasms often demonstrate rapid growth, local aggressiveness, and a substantial metastatic rate. Thus, the prognosis is less favorable when compared to similar tumors arising in sun-damaged skin of whites.

Squamous cell carcinoma in situ (Bowen's disease) seems uncommon in black patients. When it occurs, arsenic exposure (medicinal, occupational, environmental) should be suspected. Histologic and clinical features are the same in blacks as in other groups.

Malignant melanoma is an uncommon but not rare tumor in blacks. The relative incidence of this tumor in whites, however, is estimated to be 4 times that in blacks. About two-thirds of all melanomas in blacks arise on the lower extremities, particularly on the soles. Subungual melanomas may occur. In contrast to whites, the head, neck, and trunk are not common sites of melanoma in blacks. Reported poor survival rates suggest that this tumor behaves even more aggressively in blacks than in other groups, but this may be due to the time of diagnosis, because it is more commonly delayed in blacks. Clinical features are identical to those delineated elsewhere.

TINEA VERSICOLOR

While this disorder affects individuals of all races, it is often more florid in black patients (see Chapter 16). The exact incidence is unknown. Flare-ups are frequent in spring and summer. Several distinctive features are encountered in blacks. This fungal infection begins as multiple macules covered with dustlike white scale. Follicular accentuation is prominent among black patients and may remain the pattern throughout the disease course. Alternatively, perifollicular macules may coalesce to form widespread large patches. In either case, the lesions of tinea versicolor in blacks are hypo- or hyperpigmented rather than fawn-pink (as is typical in whites). Moreover, facial involvement is more common in blacks than in other races. The degree of itching varies from mild to severe.

In black patients, the differential diagnosis includes hypopigmented seborrheic dermatitis, pityriasis alba, leprosy, macular sarcoidosis, and postinflammatory hypopigmentation. Treatment is the same (see Chapter 16). The disorder can usually be brought under control, but relapses are frequent.

REFERENCES

Altman A et al: Basal cell epithelioma in black patients. J Am Acad Dermatol 1987;17:741.

Barr RJ, Globerman LM, Werber FA: Transient neonatal pustular melanosis. Int J Dermatol 1979;18:636.

Brauner GJ: Cutaneous disease in the black races. In: *Dermatology,* 2nd ed. Moschella SL, Hurley HJ (editors). Saunders, 1985.

Chapel TA, Taylor RM, Pinkus H: Volar melanotic macules. Int J Dermatol 1979;18:222.

Coleman WP III et al: Nevi, lentigines, and melanomas in blacks. Arch Dermatol 1980;116:548.

Conte MS, Lawrence JE: Pseudofolliculitis barbae: No "pseudoproblem." JAMA 1979;241:53.

Cosman B, Wolff M: Acne keloidalis. Plast Reconstr Surg 1972;50:25.

Gross MD et al: Nodular subcutaneous sarcoidosis. Arch Dermatol 1977;113:1442.

Hall JC et al: Pseudofolliculitis: Revised concepts of diagnosis and treatment. Report of three cases in women. Cutis 1979;23:798.

James WD, Carter JM, Rodman OG: Pigmentary demarcation lines: A population survey. J Am Acad Dermatol 1987;16:584.

Jarratt M, Ramsdell W: Infantile acropustulosis. Arch Dermatol 1979;115:834.

Kahn G, Rywlin AM: Acropustulosis of infancy. Arch Dermatol 1979;115:831.

Kauh YC, Goody HE, Luscombe HA: Ichthyosiform sarcoidosis. Arch Dermatol 1978;114:100.

Kenney JA: Management of dermatoses peculiar to Negroes. Int J Dermatol 1970;9:110.

Labow TA, Atwood W, Nelson CT: Sarcoidosis in the American Negro. Arch Dermatol 1964;89:682.

Leyden JJ, Spott DA, Goldschmidt H: Diffuse and banded melanin pigmentation in nails. Arch Dermatol 1972;105:548.

LoPresti P, Papa CM, Kligman AM: Hot comb alopecia. Arch Dermatol 1968;98:234.

Martin S, Rosen T, Locker E: Metastatic squamous cell carcinoma of the lip: Occurrence in blacks with discoid lupus erythematosus. Arch Dermatol 1979;115:1214.

Matsuoka LY, Schauer PK, Sordillo PP: Basal cell carcinoma in black patients. J Am Acad Dermatol 1981;4:670.

Mora RG, Burris R: Cancer of the skin in blacks: A review of 128 patients with basal cell carcinoma. Cancer 1981;47:1436.

Murray JC, Pollack SV, Pinnell SR: Keloids: A review. J Am Acad Dermatol 1981;4:461.

Owen WR, Wood C: Disseminate and recurrent infundibulofolliculitis. Arch Dermatol 1979:115:174.

Rosen T: Squamous cell carcinoma: Complication of chronic skin disorders in black patients. J Natl Med Assoc 1986;78:1203.

Rosen T, Algra RJ: Papular eruption in black men. Arch Dermatol 1980;116:416.

Rosen T, Martin S: *Atlas of Black Dermatology.* Little, Brown, 1981.

Rosen T, Stone MS: Acne rosacea in blacks. J Am Acad Dermatol 1987;17:70.

Rosen T, Tucker S, Tschen J: Bowen's disease in blacks. J Am Acad Dermatol 1982;7:364.

Serjeant GR: Leg ulceration in sickle cell anemia. Arch Intern Med 1974;133:690.

Wyre HW Jr, Murphy MO: Transient neonatal pustular melanosis. Arch Dermatol 1979;115:458.

Section XI:
Therapeutics & Surgery

Medical Dermatologic Therapy

53

Jo-David Fine, MD & Kenneth A. Arndt, MD

Most disorders affecting the skin can be ameliorated or cured with appropriate medical therapy. Although many conditions respond to purely topical treatment, some require concomitant or principal use of oral or parenteral systemic agents. Many of the systemic drugs discussed herein have potentially serious side effects. Referral to an appropriate specialist is often prudent.

GENERAL PRINCIPLES OF MEDICAL THERAPY OF CUTANEOUS DISEASE

PRETREATMENT CONSIDERATIONS

Before instituting definitive therapy, the diagnosis or a reasonably confident differential diagnosis must be determined. This may require one or more tests, including a potassium hydroxide preparation, a Tzanck preparation, examination of a Gram-stained smear, lesional cultures, and skin biopsy. Selected serum and urine tests may prove helpful. Unless the diagnosis is readily apparent, it is best to defer treatment until the results of such studies are known, so that morphologic alterations resulting from nonspecific treatment will not obscure the diagnosis. The patient with symptoms such as itching or pain can be treated symptomatically while tests are pending.

Unfortunately, many dermatologic conditions respond only gradually to treatment. Patients are sometimes seen in consultation complaining of previously

"incorrect" treatment when in fact treatment was appropriate but not continued long enough to yield a favorable response.

BARRIER FUNCTION & DRUG PENETRATION

In normal skin, the stratum corneum serves as a barrier against easy penetration into the body by external agents and against uncontrolled fluid loss from underlying tissues. When the stratum corneum is absent or damaged as a result of external insult (burns, chemicals, abrasions, fissures), cutaneous inflammation, or other abnormalities, there is increased percutaneous penetration from outside in and from inside out, resulting in increased risk of exudation and fluid loss and of cutaneous and systemic bacterial infection. Furthermore, topically applied agents may be more readily absorbed when the skin barrier is damaged.

Barrier function is also affected by the degree of skin hydration. A well-hydrated epidermis permits penetration of many topically applied drugs. Ointments generally provide a better vehicle for penetration of agents such as corticosteroids compared with creams, perhaps because they increase the hydration of the skin by occlusion. Similarly, occlusive airtight dressings or wraps promote increased percutaneous penetration or toxicity of most topically applied agents. Dermatologic vehicle formulations are complex and may contain one or more chemicals (ie, propylene glycol) meant to enhance cutaneous transport of the active drug.

Some cutaneous disorders are characterized by thick scale or crust that might hinder penetration of topically applied agents. In these situations, it is beneficial first to chemically disrupt or physically remove the scale or crust and then to apply agents helpful against that particular disease.

Other factors that may affect percutaneous absorption and efficacy of therapy are infection, frequency of drug application, and tachyphylaxis.

Coexisting Infection

Many patients with skin disorders have secondary bacterial skin infections. Extensive infection may obscure the signs of the underlying primary skin disease; after the infection is eliminated, specific treatment can be directed to the underlying disease. Simultaneous treatment of primary disease and secondary infection may be impractical. For example, the application of topical corticosteroids under occlusion to lichenified areas of eczema which are secondarily impetiginized will lead to worsening of the secondary infection.

Frequency of Application

There is little pharmacokinetic information pertaining to the optimal dose-response characteristics of topical medication; what information does exist pertains primarily to topical corticosteroids but may apply more generally. However, even the latter findings may pertain only to the specific strengths and types of corticosteroids employed. One study of patients with steroid-responsive dermatoses showed 6 treatments a day to be no more effective than 3 per day. Another study showed that once-daily application is as effective as applying the agent 3 times a day. Overnight application of medication to hydrated skin—with or without occlusion—also may be as effective as multiple daily applications. These findings may correlate with animal studies showing that percutaneous absorption of hydrocortisone was significantly increased when a large amount was applied as a single daily dose as compared to one-third of that dose applied once or 3 times daily.

Tachyphylaxis

Patients treated chronically with topical corticosteroid preparations may find after a short time that the medication no longer seems beneficial. Tachyphylaxis—the rapid decrease of response to the anti-inflammatory and antimitotic effects of topical corticosteroids—may occur after only 1–2 weeks use. After a 4- to 7-day rest period, however, responsiveness to the drug usually returns. Substitution with a different corticosteroid (similar potency but slightly different chemical structure) may result in continued therapeutic response. Even though the effectiveness of topical corticosteroids may decrease with continuous use, penetration through skin may actually increase, leading to unwanted systemic effects. These and other topical agents should not be used casually and chronically but with care and for as short a time as possible.

Regional Variation in Percutaneous Absorption

It is clear that stratum corneum and epidermal thickness vary markedly in different body sites (ie, palm versus genitalia versus eyelid). As such, it is reasonable to expect that percutaneous and systemic absorption of some topically applied agents would be enhanced in areas having less physical barrier. In addition, some adverse side effects, most notably steroid atrophy, are seen more readily in sensitive skin sites following prolonged treatment with potent topical agents.

ADVERSE SIDE EFFECTS

The use of any topical or systemic agent is accompanied by a risk of unwanted side effects. This is especially true when potent corticosteroids are applied topically. Atrophy, telangiectasia, and striae can appear within weeks, particularly in susceptible skin sites such as the face, genitalia, and intertriginous regions (inframammary, inguinal). In small children, the use of topical corticosteroids over widespread areas may lead to significant systemic absorption and, as a result, growth retardation or adrenal suppression. Adverse effects from systemic corticosteroids will be discussed in greater detail elsewhere. Knowledge of potential toxic or allergic adverse effects of drugs is as important as expertise in their therapeutic use.

Some skin conditions require potent systemic medications, such as the cytotoxic drugs cyclophosphamide and azathioprine; in such patients, bone marrow suppression may occur and is usually dose-related. Other adverse effects may occur that are specific for a particular drug (eg, hemorrhagic cystitis or painful oral erosions may develop during treatment with cyclophosphamide but not with azathioprine).

Surface Area-to-Volume Ratio

Increased systemic levels of a drug and systemic side effects or toxicity may result from the application of topical agents over wide areas of the body. It is essential to be cautious when treating large skin surface areas, especially with occlusion techniques; in particular, infants and children have a higher surface area-to-volume ratio than adults and are therefore at greater risk.

Similarly, a major consideration when using wet compresses is their effects on thermoregulation; when large areas are covered, patients may develop marked hypothermia with attendant discomfort, as well as the possible masking of fever and other signs of occult infection. Therefore, open wet dressings should be applied only to small areas at a time, especially in children.

OTHER CONSIDERATIONS

Fixed-Combination Preparations
Many commercial topical preparations contain more than one active agent; some may be beneficial and more economical than an identical mixture by the pharmacist. Often, however, addition of a second agent adds little benefit and may increase the risk of drug intolerance. For example, addition of neomycin to topical corticosteroid formulations adds little benefit in most clinical situations but may result in allergic contact sensitization and exacerbation of the underlying skin eruption. As in choosing appropriate combinations of oral drugs for systemic disease, in skin conditions it is often better to prescribe several topical medications used concurrently rather than relying on a single commercial combination. If it is deemed desirable to use several agents in a single preparation, many formulations are commercially available or can be prepared by the pharmacist.

Quantity of Medication
Topically applied medications are often expensive, especially when prescribed in small commercially prepared containers. For patients using large quantities, such as in generalized psoriasis or dermatitis treated with topical corticosteroids, there will be significant savings if these drugs are dispensed in large prepackaged amounts.

Awareness of the amount of topical material needed to cover a particular body area will prevent dispensing too little medication to the patient, who might otherwise run out of drug before an adequate course of treatment can be completed. In general, approximately 30–60 g of an ointment or cream is necessary to cover the entire adult body in a single application. Twice as much lotion is required to cover a similar area.

When using potentially hazardous topical (eg, fluorouracil) or systemic (eg, prednisone, methotrexate) agents, it is prudent to dispense only the amount of medication needed until the next appointment. Unmonitored or unnecessary drug use is more apt to be avoided if the amount of drug available to the patient is closely controlled.

Choice of Vehicles
Not only should the correct active agent be used when topical medications are chosen, but the agent should be incorporated into an appropriate vehicle. In acute inflammatory conditions characterized by vesiculation or exudation, aqueous preparations such as wet dressings, lotions, aerosols, and creams should be used. The specific choice of vehicle depends on the degree of drying effect required. In more chronic conditions characterized by thickened, lichenified skin, scale formation, and dryness, ointment-based preparations may be more advantageous in better hydrating skin and allowing enhanced penetration of active drug into the lesions.

TYPES OF TOPICAL PREPARATIONS

In general, topical medications may be classified as open wet dressings, powders, liquids, creams, ointments, and pastes. The specific choice depends on the characteristics of the eruption.

Open Wet Dressings
Open wet dressings are especially useful in conditions characterized by vesicles, pustules, exudates, and crusts.

Such dressings cool and dry the skin by evaporation. As wet dressings are removed, they help debride crusts and exudate from the surface. With appropriate use of open wet dressings, the exudative and acute inflammatory aspects of dermatoses can be decreased, allowing subsequent treatment with other topically applied agents and vehicles.

Powders
Powders are useful as drying and lubricating agents. They act by increasing the effective skin surface area. Powders may be inert and nonabsorbent (eg, talc) or absorbent and contain pharmacologically active ingredients. Powders are used primarily in intertriginous areas, where maceration may adversely affect primary skin disorders.

Liquid Preparations
Liquid preparations are commonly used as lotions or tinctures. A **lotion** is a suspension of powder in water. **Tinctures** are solutions containing alcohol. Both preparations induce coolness and dryness as they evaporate on the skin surface. In addition, powder is left on the skin following evaporation of a lotion. These preparations are most frequently used in acute skin eruptions or in hirsute body areas.

Shake Lotions
Shake lotions, which must be agitated to suspend the powder, contain zinc oxide, talc, glycerin, and water. Calamine lotion contains zinc oxide and ferric oxide and imparts a pink color to the skin. Other ingredients may be added to the basic lotion depending upon the effects desired. Additional drying may be achieved by adding small amounts of alcohol; an antipruritic effect may be imparted by the addition of menthol, phenol, or camphor; scaling dermatoses may benefit from the addition of salicylic acid or coal tar solution.

Creams

Creams are semisolid oil-in-water (o/w) emulsions. They are water-soluble, cosmetically elegant, and "vanish" after rubbing into the skin. They are useful in both acute and chronic skin disorders. Although not as occlusive as ointments, creams are more easily used and are usually more acceptable to patients.

Gels

A gel is a transparent, colorless, semisolid emulsion. Gels liquefy upon contact with the skin, leaving a nonocclusive, greaseless film on drying. Gels may contain water, alcohol, propylene glycol, or acetone. Gels containing large amounts of water and sometimes other solvents are called jellies.

Ointments

In an emulsion base, if the amount of oil exceeds the amount of water, the preparation is an ointment. Ointments are water-in-oil (w/o) preparations and are more lubricating and occlusive than creams. Ointments may be either soluble or insoluble in water. Water-soluble ointment bases tend to be greaseless and are especially useful when compounding water-soluble drugs. Ointment bases that are water- repellent are composed of hydrophobic hydrocarbons (eg, petrolatum), hydrogenated vegetable fats, or silicones. In general, ointments are not easily washed off of the skin.

Pastes

Pastes are combinations of finely ground powder and ointment and may be protective against exogenous irritants and sunlight. They are usually poor vehicles for delivering active agents and—except for zinc oxide paste—are infrequently used today. They are also difficult to remove from the skin.

SPECIFIC TOPICAL MEDICATIONS
(Alphabetical Order)*

ACNE PREPARATIONS

Benzoyl Peroxide

Topical benzoyl peroxide is useful in the treatment of acne vulgaris, reflecting its bacteriostatic activity against *Propionibacterium acnes*. It may also be comedolytic or have sebostatic effects. Benzoyl peroxide preparations, most often used in 2.5%, 5%, and

10% concentrations in creams, lotions or gels, may be irritating; the lowest concentrations should be used initially. They may induce allergic contact sensitization. For most patients with papulosquamous acne, benzoyl peroxides are initially the topical drug of choice.

Topical Antibiotics

Three antibiotics—clindamycin, erythromycin, and tetracycline—are commonly employed in mild to moderate acne vulgaris, frequently in conjunction with benzoyl peroxide or retinoic acid. They are routinely formulated in lotion form in alcohol or propylene glycol solutions, most often in 1–2% concentration. All are effective against *P acnes*. In terms of topical efficacy, clindamycin and erythromycin may be somewhat more beneficial than tetracycline, though all have been shown useful.

Topical tetracycline may impart a temporary yellowish discoloration to the skin; it may brightly fluoresce when such skin is subsequently exposed to long wave ultraviolet light such as "black" light. A few patients have developed diarrhea and pseudomembranous colitis following topical use of clindamycin; therefore, clindamycin is contraindicated in patients with an active or past history of inflammatory bowel disease or pseudomembranous colitis and should be discontinued in any patient developing persistent diarrhea.

Tretinoin

Tretinoin (retinoic acid; vitamin A acid) is particularly effective in comedonal and papular acne. Tretinoin increases epidermal cell turnover, inhibits tonofilament synthesis, and decreases attachment between keratinocytes. The same effect presumably occurs in the hair follicle and sebaceous duct; it prevents development of keratinaceous plugs and loosens cellular debris in those areas. Used nightly or every other night, this drug predictably produces a transient acne flare 3–6 weeks into treatment. However, continued use leads to clinical improvement. Use should be decreased during the summer because of problems with exaggerated sunburn and unresolved questions about photocarcinogenicity. Tretinoin is an irritant, especially when used in higher concentrations. Exposure to eyes, mouth, and nares should be avoided.

Tretinoin has been reported to be useful alone or in combination with other drugs in many disorders, such as oral lichen planus, ichthyosis, Darier's disease, melasma, nevus comedonicus, senile comedones, linear verrucous nevus, keratosis palmaris et plantaris, pseudofolliculitis, acanthosis nigricans, Fox-Fordyce disease, reactive perforating collagenosis, and geographic tongue. Most recently, it has been proposed for the treatment of photoaged skin.

Other Drying & Peeling Agents

Several preparations utilize sulfur in combination

---

*Scabicides and pediculocides are described in Chapter 18.

with salicylic acid, resorcinol, or alcohol; these have been recommended for use in acne because of their peeling effect. However, they may in fact produce much nonspecific irritation. Their overall effectiveness in acne is relatively minimal compared to other available agents.

Other Topical Agents Used in Acne

In patients with active severe cystic acne, some relief may be achieved with the use of hot sulfurated lime compresses (Vleminckx's solution).

ANESTHETICS

Topical anesthetics are most frequently used by the dermatologist in treating painful areas on mucosal or mucocutaneous sites, especially the oral or anogenital areas, because such tissues lack stratum corneum and the active agents are locally absorbed. They may be useful for patients with extensive aphthous stomatitis, recurrent oral or genital herpes simplex infection, severe oral erosions of pemphigus vulgaris or cicatricial pemphigoid, and venereal warts and condylomata acuminata being treated with chemical or physical destructive modalities. When used on intact skin, however, there is no significant beneficial effect, mostly due to lack of penetration through the stratum corneum. In addition, the use of benzocaine-containing preparations may produce allergic contact sensitization, further arguing against their use on nonmucosal surfaces.

Topical anesthetics may be divided into amides (eg, dibucaine, lidocaine), aminobenzoate esters (eg, benzocaine, tetracaine hydrochloride), and non-amide, nonaminobenzoate esters (including dimethisoquin, dyclonine hydrochloride, pramoxine hydrochloride). Benzocaine, a common topical anesthetic in sunburn preparations, is a p-aminobenzoic acid (PABA) derivative. Twenty-five percent of patients sensitive to benzocaine are also sensitive to paraphenylenediamine, hydrochlorothiazide, sulfonamides, and PABA ester-based sunscreens. There may be cross reactions with other local anesthetics including procaine and tetracaine. Lidocaine may be used safely in patients allergic to benzocaine. Of all topically applied anesthetics, those with the longest duration of action include dimethisoquin and pramoxine; anesthesia is noted within the first few minutes after application and lasts up to 2–4 hours.

ANTHRALIN

Anthralin, a derivative of anthracene, has been used in psoriasis treatment for over 60 years. It is effective when used alone or in combination with tars and ultraviolet B light. In vitro, this drug inhibits cell growth and thymidine incorporation in human cultured cells. It inhibits mitochondrial DNA replication and repair synthesis. In the past, anthralin was usually used in 0.1%, 0.25%, 0.5%, or 1% concentration in a base containing salicylic acid, the latter added to prevent oxidation of anthralin to an inactive form. Although many psoriasis patients were well controlled using anthralin applied to the skin for 4–12 hours, this regimen was not universally popular because it frequently proved to be too irritating and caused discoloration of skin and clothing. More recent studies have demonstrated that anthralin may be just as effective but less irritating if one of the higher concentrations (0.5–1%) is applied to psoriatic lesions for only 15–30 minutes ("short contact therapy") and then washed off.

ANTIBACTERIAL OINTMENTS

Several antibacterial ointments are commercially available; most contain combinations of the "nonabsorbable" antibiotics, bacitracin, neomycin, polymyxin B, or gramicidin. A topical preparation of gentamicin is also available. These preparations may be useful in the early treatment of superficial cutaneous wounds. In more extensive bacterial skin infections, they are ineffective, and appropriate systemic antibiotics must be administered.

Bacitracin, a polypeptide elaborated by *Bacillus subtilis,* is bactericidal against many gram-positive organisms, especially *Streptococcus, Staphylococcus,* and pneumococcus, but inactive against most gram-negative organisms. Anaerobic cocci and tetanus are also among the bacteria sensitive to this drug.

Neomycin is an aminoglycoside antibiotic effective against most gram-negative organisms. It is approximately 50 times more active against *Staphylococcus* than bacitracin (by weight), but bacitracin is 20 times more active against *Streptococcus.* Neomycin causes more allergic contact sensitivity than any other topical antibiotic.

Polymyxin B, a cyclic polypeptide elaborated by *Bacillus polymyxa,* is effective against gram-negative bacteria except *Proteus* and *Serratia.* It has little action against most gram-positive bacteria.

Gramicidin is bactericidal against many gram-positive bacteria.

Gentamicin is an aminoglycoside antibiotic used primarily by intravenous route for systemic gram-negative infections. It is also effective against *Staphylococcus aureus* and group A β-hemolytic streptococci. The drug may be used topically, although it may produce allergic contact sensitization; there is no advantage in its use compared to those previously mentioned. It is not recommended for routine wound management.

Mupiricin is a newly approved topical antibiotic

that has been shown to be highly effective in the treatment of cutaneous streptococcal infections. In many patients, mupiricin may used in lieu of systemic antibiotics for the treatment of primary and secondary forms of impetigos.

ANTIFUNGAL AGENTS

Several topical antifungal agents are effective in the treatment of both dermatophytosis and candidiasis. These include imidazole agents such as clotrimazole, miconazole, econazole, and ketoconazole and nonimidazole drugs such ciclopirox olamine, haloprogin, tolnaftate, and naftifine. However, dermatophyte infections of hair and nails require treatment with systemic griseofulvin or ketoconazole.

In those mucocutaneous infections caused by *Candida* albicans where broad spectrum antifungal agents are not desired, nystatin may be tried though systemic ketoconazole or amphotericin B may still be required. Nystatin, a polyene antibiotic that acts by affecting fungal cell membranes, is ineffective in dermatophytosis and is poorly absorbed after oral administration but is still effective when used orally to rid the gastrointestinal tract of excessive *Candida* organisms.

Amphotericin B is available for topical and parenteral use. Administered intravenously, this is a very effective drug for many systemic fungal infections. Topically, it is useful only for *C albicans* infections, and it may cause some staining of the skin. It has no advantage over the drugs previously described and is not recommended for routine use against cutaneous *Candida* infections.

Although broad spectrum topical antifungal agents are effective against tinea versicolor, as well as dermatophyte and *Candida* infections, the former may also be simply and less expensively treated with any of the following: 2.5% selenium sulfide suspension, zinc pyrithione solution, or 25% sodium thiosulfate solution. In patients with *C albicans* paronychia, good response may be seen when the nailfold areas are treated with 2–4% thymol in absolute alcohol.

Recent studies have also demonstrated the efficacy of topical ketoconazole in the treatment of seborrheic dermatitis, perhaps due to its effect on *Pityrosporum* colonization.

ANTIPRURITIC AGENTS

Generalized pruritus is difficult to alleviate unless the causative disease or mediator can be specifically treated. Oral antihistamines are often prescribed but are most effective in histamine-mediated conditions (eg, urticaria, mastocytosis). Some patients with localized pruritic disorders may derive transient benefit from one of several topical preparations usually containing menthol, phenol, or camphor. Menthol in 0.25–2% concentrations exerts its antipruritic effect mainly through the cooling sensation it induces. Phenol in 0.5–2% concentrations reduces pruritus through temporary anesthesia of cutaneous nerve endings. Camphor in 1–3% concentrations has a local anesthetic effect. Other agents less frequently used include dilute solutions of salicylic acid and coal tar. In addition, some reduction of pruritus may be achieved by the use of "shake" lotions such as calamine lotion with or without addition of one of the previously mentioned compounds. Commercial preparations containing benzocaine or diphenhydramine should be avoided, since both may produce allergic contact sensitization.

ANTISEPTIC CLEANSERS

Antiseptic agents may be bacteriostatic or bactericidal. They are used as local or generalized skin cleansers, may be used for wound irrigation, and are particularly useful in patients in whom reduced cutaneous bacterial counts are desired. Two commonly used agents are chlorhexidine and iodine compounds.

Chlorhexidine is a nonstaining antiseptic active against gram-positive and gram-negative bacteria as well as many fungi and yeasts. It has a rapid onset and long duration of effectiveness, is not inhibited in the presence of blood, and is well tolerated by most patients.

Antiseptic **iodinated compounds** are water-soluble and brownish-yellow. These materials slowly liberate iodine on contact with reducing substances and are effective against bacteria, fungi, yeasts, protozoa, and viruses. One of the most frequently used preparations is povidone-iodine. Such compounds may require minutes of contact on the skin before killing bacteria; they may become ineffective in the presence of blood or serum.

In the past, **hexachlorophene** was widely used as an antiseptic agent. Hexachlorophene is bacteriostatic against many gram-positive organisms including *Staphylococcus* and has a cumulative effect if used repeatedly. However, this agent cross-reacts with some halogenated phenol derivatives involved in primary photosensitivity reactions and, more importantly, has been associated with neurotoxicity when used in children or in burn patients. There is no advantage in using hexachlorophene instead of the safer and equally or more effective agents chlorhexidine and iodinated compounds.

ANTIVIRAL AGENTS

Acyclovir

Acyclovir is the generic name for the acyclic nucleoside of guanine. This drug has been shown to be effective against herpesviruses, including herpes simplex and zoster-varicella. The drug may be given by intravenous, oral, or topical routes. Following uptake into cells, it is phosphorylated to the monophosphate, which requires the phosphorylating enzyme thymidine kinase. This enzyme is present in cells infected by herpes simplex virus and absent in unaffected normal cells. Cellular kinases subsequently transform acyclovir monophosphate to the triphosphate, at which point the drug can inhibit herpesvirus DNA polymerase. Acyclovir appears to have little toxicity because of its selective effect against viral-induced DNA polymerase. Strains of herpes simplex virus resistant to acyclovir have been reported. This may result when the virus does not code for thymidine kinase or when the drug is no longer inhibitory against viral DNA polymerase.

When given by intravenous route, acyclovir achieves substantial blood levels quickly and is subsequently excreted through the kidneys. Although poorly absorbed orally, there are still sufficient peak serum concentrations to be inhibitory against the herpes simplex virus.

Topical application of acyclovir during the initial episode of genital herpes is associated with reduction in the duration of viral shedding, hastening of the resolution of lesions, and decreased symptomatology. Topical acyclovir does not prevent new lesion formation during the course of disease, nor does it prevent the development of latency. In patients with recurrent genital herpes, acyclovir therapy reduces the duration of viral shedding but does not enhance resolution or provide symptomatic relief. Similarly, topical acyclovir may promote healing in localized zoster. Topical use of acyclovir should be confined to patients with an initial episode of genital herpes or localized zoster.

Oral acyclovir has been successfully employed in the management of primary and recurrent herpes simplex infections (including eczema herpeticum) and localized zoster.

Acyclovir has been shown to be beneficial in patients receiving bone marrow transplants if given parenterally to prevent subsequent development of herpes simplex infection or shortly after confirmation by culture of active cutaneous herpes infection. Similarly, intravenous acyclovir is routinely given to patients with disseminated herpes simplex infections, immunocompromised patients with localized herpetic infections, and selected individuals with localized and disseminated herpes zoster infections.

ASTRINGENTS

Astringents are used to reduce weeping from the skin surface. They precipitate protein and therefore "seal" the affected skin surface. Commonly used astringents include aluminum acetate, aluminum chloride hexahydrate, potassium permanganate, and silver nitrate. One of the most commonly used astringents for wet dressings is **aluminum acetate (Burow's solution),** used in 1:40 to 1:10 dilutions; it is clear and colorless. Some astringents may also be germicidal, though in the concentrations used for aluminum acetate salts there is no added antimicrobial activity.

Potassium permanganate, thoroughly dissolved in water for baths (1:25,000) or compresses (1:4000–1:16,000), is astringent and germicidal and thought to be active because of its oxidizing ability. At one time very popular, it is no longer commonly used because it imparts a purple stain to skin, nails, and clothing. In addition, if the potassium permanganate crystals are not fully dissolved, they produce a chemical burn on contact with skin.

Silver nitrate (0.1–0.5%) serves as an astringent and germicidal agent, the latter presumably due to precipitation of bacterial protein by liberated silver ions. It is used principally in the topical care of thermal burns. This material will also cause skin staining and may be irritating if used in greater concentrations. Other astringents used on the skin include copper and zinc sulfate.

BURN PREPARATIONS

Two topical agents commonly used in burn therapy are silver sulfadiazine and mafenide. **Silver sulfadiazine (Silvadene)** is used in 1% cream form and is primarily indicated for the topical treatment of second- and third-degree burns. It is particularly useful in maintaining sterility of burn sites, thereby reducing the risk of secondary sepsis. This agent is bactericidal for many gram positive (*S aureus, S epidermidis,* β-hemolytic streptococci) and gram-negative organisms (the latter including *Pseudomonas, Enterobacter, Klebsiella, E coli, Serratia,* and *Proteus*). It exerts its bactericidal effect by acting on the cell membrane and cell wall of the organism. In addition, silver sulfadiazine is effective against *C albicans.*

Since silver sulfadiazine is a sulfonamide derivative and may be systemically absorbed in patients with burns, its use is contraindicated in patients hypersensitive to other sulfonamide drugs. It should not be used in newborns or premature infants because of increased risk of kernicterus associated with the use of sulfonamides. Silver sulfadiazine may lead to severe hemolytic anemia in patients deficient in the enzyme glucose-6-phosphate dehydrogenase. Occasional patients have developed hyperosmolarity as a result of absorption of propylene glycol from the cream base.

Mafenide acetate (Sulfamylon) is bacteriostatic against many gram-positive and gram-negative organisms including *Pseudomonas* and some anaerobes. It is systemically absorbed through burn sites, metabolized, and then excreted through the kidneys. Its activity is unaltered in the presence of serum or pus. It is unclear whether there is cross-reactivity with other sulfonamides. Fatal hemolytic anemia has been reported in association with the use of this drug in patients with glucose-6-phosphate dehydrogenase deficiency. Both the active drug and its metabolites inhibit carbonic anhydrase, and some patients—particularly burn victims with renal impairment—may develop metabolic acidosis.

CHEMOTHERAPEUTIC AGENTS

Mechlorethamine (Nitrogen Mustard)

Mechlorethamine is a nitrogen mustard frequently used topically in the treatment of the patch or thin-plaque stage of mycosis fungoides. Used properly, mechlorethamine may result in long-term remissions. It may be administered in either liquid or ointment form. When given topically (at a dilution of approximately 0.02%), the drug may be of benefit for considerable periods of time. The most common side effect is the development of contact hypersensitivity. Should this occur, mechlorethamine may be safely reapplied in much lower concentrations. The drug should be discontinued if diffuse hyperpigmentation occurs. Mechlorethamine is not effective in patients with tumor-stage mycosis fungoides. Chronic use may lead to the development of cutaneous squamous cell or basal cell carcinomas.

Fluorouracil

Fluorouracil is an antimetabolite that inhibits thymidylic synthetase and prevents the conversion of deoxyuridylic acid to thymidylic acid and inhibits DNA synthesis. It is used in 1–5% concentration and is recommended for the treatment of multiple actinic keratoses. It has also been used in the treatment of flat, genital, and intraurethral warts, Bowen's disease, and superficial basal cell carcinoma. This drug may also be used for treating keratoacanthomas (topical or intralesional use), porokeratosis of Mibelli, or psoriasis. Towards the end of the treatment course, patients develop intense inflammation exacerbated by exposure to ultraviolet light. Patients with extensive lesions are frequently not treated until wintertime. When treating superficial basal cell carcinoma or Bowen's disease, the more concentrated (5%) preparation should be utilized for at least 1 month. Development of an irritant reaction is not a contraindication to subsequent use.

TOPICAL CORTICOSTEROIDS

The most widely used agents for inflammatory skin diseases are topical corticosteroids. A myriad of different preparations are currently available that vary in relative potency depending on the concentration of corticosteroid as well as the chemical structure of the specific corticosteroid molecule employed. In addition, considerable variation in bioactivity may be seen in some generic topical glucocorticoids. Topical corticosteroids have a marked anti-inflammatory effects and inhibit epidermal cell division. They are useful in a variety of unrelated inflammatory conditions such as allergic contact dermatitis and atopic dermatitis and in some hyperproliferative diseases, most notably psoriasis.

One means of increasing the potency of a corticosteroid is to attach a halide moiety to the molecule; other methods include changing the vehicle or perhaps adding urea or some other keratolytic agent to the compound. Use of an ointment will increase the occlusiveness of the preparation, enhance hydration of the skin, and increase percutaneous absorption.

Topical corticosteroids, if applied over large surface areas for long periods, may result in some of the side effects that occur with chronic systemic corticosteroid use, especially if applied under occlusive dressings. It is possible to alter the normal hypothalamic-pituitary-adrenal gland axis if topical corticosteroids are used injudiciously. Local side effects from the chronic use of potent corticosteroid preparations include atrophy, stria formation, hyperpigmentation, telangiectasia, and hypertrichosis. Use of occlusive wraps or ointment vehicles may result in increased skin maceration, folliculitis, or acneiform eruptions. Some patients complain of burning, itching, or erythema secondary to topical corticosteroids, usually not due to sensitivity to the steroid but an irritant or allergic reaction to one or more of the vehicle constituents.

Because of potential irreversibility of some side effects such as cutaneous atrophy, those skin sites most susceptible, such as the face, genitalia, inguinal folds, and axillae, are best treated only briefly (days) with potent corticosteroids or, preferably, with medium- or low-potency corticosteroids. In particular, 1% hydrocortisone is best suited for use in these areas. Any corticosteroid preparation applied around the eyes may, in a susceptible patient, lead to increased intraocular pressure and acute glaucoma. In addition, it may be possible to produce cataracts in some patients if corticosteroids are applied chronically around the eyes.

In extensive and severe dermatoses, potent corticosteroids are usually chosen for initial treatment; later, the potency and frequency of application are decreased.

Table 53–1 lists the relative potencies of some topical corticosteroids.

DEPIGMENTING AGENTS

Hydroquinone (paradihydroxybenzene) is frequently used to reduce the intensity of pigmentation

Table 53–1. Comparison of relative potency of different topical corticosteroids.[1] (Listed in descending order of potency from most potent [1] to least potent [7].)

1 (most potent)

Betamethasone dipropionate cream or ointment, 0.05% (in optimized vehicle)

Clobetasol propionate cream or ointment, 0.05%

Diflorasone diacetate cream or ointment, 0.05% (in optimized vehicle)

2

Amcinonide ointment 0.1%

Betamethasone dipropionate ointment, 0.05% (regular vehicle)

Desoximetasone cream or ointment, 0.25%

Diflorasone diacetate ointment, 0.05% (regular vehicle)

Fluocinonide cream, ointment, or gel, 0.05%

Halcinonide cream and ointment, 0.1%

3

Betamethasone benzoate gel, 0.025%

Betamethasone dipropionate cream, 0.05%

Betamethasone diacetate cream, 0.05%

Diflorasone diacetate cream, 0.05%

Triamcinolone acetonide ointment, 0.1%, or cream, 0.5%

4

Amcinonide cream, 0.1%

Betamethasone benzoate ointment, 0.025%

Betamethasone valerate lotion, 0.1%

Desoximetasone cream, 0.05%

Flucinolone acetonide cream, 0.2%, or ointment, 0.025%

Flurandrenolide ointment, 0.05%

Hydrocortisone valerate ointment, 0.2%

Triamcinolone acetonide ointment, 0.1%

5

Betamethasone benzoate cream, 0.025%

Betamethasone dipropionate lotion, 0.05%

Betamethasone valerate cream or lotion, 0.1%

Clocortolone pivalate cream, 0.1%

Fluocinolone acetonide cream, 0.025%

Flurandrenolide cream, 0.05%

Hydrocortisone butyrate cream, 0.1%

Hydrocortisone valerate cream, 0.2%

Triamcinolone acetonide cream or lotion 0.1%; cream, 0.025%

6

Alclometasone dipropionate cream, 0.05%

Desonide cream, 0.05%

Fluocinolone acetonide solution, 0.01%

7 (least potent)

Dexamethasone sodium phosphate cream, 0.1%

Hydrocortisone cream, 0.5%, 1%, and 2.5%

Methylprednisolone acetate cream, 1%

[1]Adapted from Arndt KA: *Manual of Dermatologic Therapeutics,* 4th ed. Little, Brown, 1989—as modified from Cornell RC, Stoughton RB: Arch Dermatol 1985;121:63, and Stoughton RB, Cornell RC: Semin Dermatol 1987;6:72.

of melasma, freckles, and senile lentigines as well as the epidermal component of postinflammatory hyperpigmentation. When applied to skin over 6–8 weeks, these areas become somewhat lighter in color as a result of the inhibitory effect on the tyrosinase system. Hydroquinone also affects the formation, melaninization, and degradation of melanosomes and may cause necrosis of whole melanocytes. Application results in gradual and usually temporary skin lightening. It may be combined with other agents (eg, tretinoin) to further enhance skin hypopigmentation. Rarely, however, increased ("pseudo-ochronosis") rather than decreased pigmentation may result as an adverse reaction to treatment with hydroquinone. **Monobenzone,** the monobenzyl ether of hydroquinone, results in permanent skin bleaching and is used solely in severe cases of vitiligo to permanently remove residual areas of normal pigmentation.

Another novel depigmenting agent, **azelaic acid,** was originally identified as the etiologic factor in the hypopigmentation associated with tinea versicolor. Subsequently it has been shown to inhibit tyrosinase in vitro and to have a direct cytotoxic effect on melanocyte mitochondria. Studies are still ongoing to determine its role, if any, in the treatment not only of lentigo maligna but of malignant melanoma as well.

KERATOLYTICS

Keratolytic agents are used to soften keratin and remove scales. Salicylic acid, for example, produces desquamation by solubilizing the intracellular cement; it enhances shedding of stratum corneum cells by decreasing cell-to-cell adhesion. Application of high concentrations of these preparations may produce irritation. Keratolytics are frequently used in the management of psoriasis, ichthyosis, warts, calluses, corns, and other hyperkeratotic lesions.

LUBRICANTS

Lubricants are topical preparations containing fats or oils alone or in emulsions with water; they are used as vehicles as well as for hydrating and protecting the skin. They soften the skin by trapping water within the stratum corneum, thereby making the skin more pliable. Lubricants work much better if the skin is previously hydrated by first soaking for 5–10 minutes; otherwise, the only moisture trapped is that which is normally lost through transepidermal water loss. These preparations may contain combinations of vegetable oils (eg, olive and peanut oils), animal fats (especially lanolin), hydrocarbons (paraffin, petrolatum, mineral oil), and waxes. Lanolin is a yellowish material obtained from sheep wool; it rarely may produce an allergic contact dermatitis. Compounds such as paraffin and spermaceti are used to raise the melting point. Waxes are frequently added to harden ointment bases.

Lubricants may vary considerably in their consistency; some feel greasy, although they provide an excellent occlusive barrier. Choice of preparation will depend on the use intended (eg, as a cosmetically elegant vehicle versus one that provides maximal occlusiveness) and personal taste.

MINOXIDIL

Minoxidil is a potent vasodilator originally marketed for the treatment of severe refractory hypertension; one side effect of systemic administration was the induction of generalized terminal hair growth. Subsequent studies have been performed with topical preparations to determine the potential usefulness of this drug in the treatment of a variety of scalp disorders associated with hair loss. Evidence suggests that a minority of patients with male pattern (androgenic) alopecia—as well as some patients with less extensive alopecia areata—may benefit from its chronic use. At least 4 months of treatment may be required to determine its efficacy, and even longer time periods may be needed to ascertain the extent of regrowth of first vellus and then, later, terminal hairs. In androgenic alopecia, milder forms of vertex (but not frontal) hair loss respond best. In some patients, this drug may prove more useful in preventing additional hair loss than in regrowing hair. New hair growth is not permanent; hair loss recurs following cessation of treatment.

Side effects, most commonly irritant or allergic contact dermatitis, from the topical application of minoxidil are rare, though the risk is increased if the drug is applied to inflamed scalp. Although blood levels of minoxidil can be detected following topical application, there is no significant incidence of systemic side effects as a result of percutaneous absorption.

PIGMENTING AGENTS & PHOTOCHEMOTHERAPY (PUVA)

Psoralens are tricyclic furocoumarin-like chemicals that—when used along with UVA ultraviolet light (PUVA)—are helpful in the treatment of vitiligo, psoriasis, cutaneous T cell lymphoma (mycosis fungoides), and several other less common diseases. The 2 commonly used agents are trioxsalen and methoxsalen. These agents may be used orally or, in the case of trioxsalen, topically, with subsequent judicious exposure to natural or artificial ultraviolet light. They produce photoadducts with DNA following exposure to ultraviolet A radiation (320–400 nm) and produce gradual repigmentation in vitiliginous areas or diminution or clearing of areas of psoriasis or mycosis fungoides. Patients receiving excessive amounts of drug or ultraviolet light develop severe cutaneous burns. Chronic PUVA therapy may lead to an increased incidence of cutaneous squamous cell carcinoma.

SHAMPOOS

Shampoos are solutions used for local scalp hygiene and as vehicles for application of one or more compounds. Nonmedicated shampoos contain detergents and other chemicals added primarily for cosmetic reasons. Medicated shampoos are especially useful in treating localized seborrheic dermatitis or psoriasis of the scalp; commonly used preparations contain selenium sulfide, zinc pyrithione, tar, or salicylic acid and sulfur. Some of these agents may be effective by direct inhibition of epidermal cell mitosis; others may simply work by local debridement of scales.

SOAPS

Soaps work by removing foreign material and emulsifying fat from the skin surface. They may be of alkaline or neutral pH. Those preparations that are alkaline or coarsely made may prove irritating to sensitive skin. "Superfatted" soaps contain increased contents of fat or oil but are not necessarily milder. Many soaps contain chemicals added to provide fragrance or color; in some patients, exposure to such agents may result in allergic contact dermatitis.

SUNSCREENS

Sunscreens may be chemical or physical in nature. Chemical sunscreens contain one or more compounds that absorb ultraviolet light, thus acting as a radiation filter. These preparations are usually colorless, nonvolatile, and chemically stable. Chemical sunscreens include *p*-aminobenzoic acid (PABA), benzophenones, cinnamates, anthranilates, and salicylates. Physical sunscreens contain particulate materials that act by reflecting and scattering ultraviolet and visible radiation. Such preparations are cosmetically less acceptable than chemical sunscreens. Physical sunscreens include preparations containing zinc oxide, titanium dioxide, magnesium silicate, ferric chloride, kaolin, and ichthyol.

Chemical sunscreens may be compared by their sun protection factor (SPF) values. The SPF value is the ratio of the time required to produce erythema through a sunscreen to the time required to produce the same degree of erythema without the sunscreen. SPF values range from 2 (minimal) to 30 or more (maximal). The efficacy of a sunscreen is affected by the amount of ultraviolet radiation absorbed by the active compound or compounds as well as by the ability of the preparation to withstand excessive sweating or exposure to water. Choice of a sunscreen should take into consideration skin type (ie, relative sensitivity to ultraviolet light) and the particular wavelengths of ultraviolet light harmful to an underlying disease. Those patients having extreme sensitivity to ultraviolet and visible light may require physical sunscreens.

Effective sunscreens diminish but do not totally

prevent melanogenesis in the skin. Several adverse effects may occur from the use of topical sunscreens: (1) Contact and allergic photocontact dermatitis have been reported with several preparations. (2) Patients with allergy to benzocaine, procaine, sulfonamides, or paraphenylenediamine may develop allergic reactions when subsequently exposed to PABA or PABA esters. (3) Eczematous dermatitis occasionally occurs in patients exposed to topical PABA in conjunction with systemic administration of thiazide diuretics or sulfonamides.

TAR COMPOUNDS

Tars are obtained by the destructive distillation of various woods, coals, petroleum, and shale. These preparations contain numerous organic chemicals, including many aromatic compounds. The specific active ingredients in dermatologic tar formulations are unknown. Tars are black, viscous, and only slightly soluble in water. Several solvents enhance tar solubility. Tars have been used for many skin conditions but are now primarily used—alone or in combination with other drugs or modalities—for the treatment of psoriasis. Tars suppress DNA synthesis, and it is for this reason that they are felt to be efficacious in psoriasis. In one standard treatment for psoriasis, the Goeckerman regimen, patients are treated with topical tars and subsequently exposed to ultraviolet B radiation. One study has demonstrated that the addition of tar to aggressive ultraviolet light therapy has no more benefit than the combination of a simple emollient with subsequent exposure to UVA light. However, use of tars may have a "light-sparing" effect and allow clearing with less intensive UVL exposure.

WART REMOVAL PREPARATIONS

Common and flat warts may often be treated with keratolytic agents such as liquid preparations composed of 5–26% **salicylic acid** (some in combination with 5–20% lactic acid) and adhesive pads containing 40% salicylic acid. These medications work by local destruction of affected keratinocytes and may thus provide a stimulus to the immune system for subsequent rejection of the virus. Mosaic warts tend to be less responsive.

Another agent used for such lesions is **cantharidin**, a chemical which through its effect on cell membranes and mitochondria results in blister formation and subsequent elimination of infected skin. (Use caution.)

Acids such as **mono-, di-, and trichloroacetic acids** may also be effective when applied directly to warts. (Use caution.)

Fluorouracil in 1–5% concentration has been re-

ported useful in some otherwise recalcitrant urethral and rectal venereal warts.

The accepted topical agent for the treatment of moist warts, condyloma acuminata, is **podophyllum resin** (eg, 20–40% in tincture of benzoin, washed off well in 2–6 hours). This plant extract is cytotoxic, causing mitotic arrest in metaphase. Podophyllum resin may be extremely irritating, especially in higher concentrations, when left on the skin for excessive periods. When applied to extensive skin surfaces or mucous membranes, this drug may produce significant central nervous system side effects.

SYSTEMIC THERAPY FOR DERMATOLOGIC DISORDERS (Alphabetical Order)

ANTIBIOTICS

Antibiotics most commonly prescribed empirically by the dermatologist are erythromycin, tetracyclines, and penicillin and its derivatives.

Erythromycins

The erythromycins are bacteriostatic or bactericidal for gram-positive organisms. Of particular interest is the effectiveness of erythromycin against streptococci and staphylococci. Although some erythromycins are destroyed by gastric acid, acid-resistant preparations are available. These drugs are primarily excreted in bile.

Erythromycin is particularly useful for penicillin-allergic patients with streptococcal or staphylococcal disease and for acne vulgaris patients who are intolerant or unresponsive to oral tetracycline. Erythromycin (like high-dose tetracycline) may also be beneficial in pityriasis lichenoides.

The most common side effect from erythromycin is gastrointestinal distress (nausea, vomiting, diarrhea). Erythromycin estolate has been known to produce acute cholestatic hepatitis.

Tetracyclines

In moderate to severe acne vulgaris, tetracycline is usually the first systemic antibiotic chosen, since it is inexpensive, effective, and usually well-tolerated. This bacteriostatic drug achieves high concentrations within sebaceous follicles after oral administration and inhibits bacterial lipase. Tetracyclines have somewhat irregular absorption from the gastrointestinal tract. Absorption is adversely affected by the concurrent intake of cationic chelating materials (ie, calcium, aluminum, and iron, as found in dairy products, antacids, and vitamin preparations).

Tetracyclines bind to calcium; they are deposited in growing bones and teeth and as such are not routinely recommended for use in children under the age of 12. For similar reasons, tetracycline is not used during pregnancy.

Much of the orally administered tetracycline remains within the lumen of the gut and is subsequently excreted in the feces; that which is absorbed is excreted in bile and urine.

Side effects from tetracycline are uncommon but include recurrent candidal vaginitis and gastrointestinal symptoms (most notably nausea).

Minocycline, a member of the tetracycline group, is extremely effective in some patients with acne vulgaris unresponsive to other tetracyclines. As opposed to some other tetracylines, minocycline absorption is not substantially affected by concomitant intake of calcium-containing dairy products. Adverse reactions to minocycline include nausea, vomiting, and dizziness or vertigo. In addition, a small number of patients develop a bluish-gray discoloration within acne lesions, scars, or unaffected skin.

Penicillin & Derivatives

Penicillins comprise a group of antibiotics characterized by the presence of a β-lactam ring plus a common nucleus, 6-aminopenicillanic acid. These drugs have an inhibitory effect on microbial cell wall synthesis and are especially effective against gram-positive organisms. In dermatologic practice, penicillinase-resistant penicillins are usually used to treat those staphylococcal infections (eg, bullous impetigo) which are frequently unresponsive to erythromycin. These drugs, which may be administered orally or intravenously, cross react with other penicillins and therefore must not be used in patients with previous history of allergic reactions (including rashes or anaphylaxis) to penicillin.

ANTIFUNGAL AGENTS

Griseofulvin

There are presently 2 oral antifungal agents used in the United States. The older drug, griseofulvin, is an antibiotic derived from a species of *Penicillium* and is fungistatic and fungicidal against various species of *Microsporum, Epidermophyton,* and *Trichophyton* but ineffective against deep fungi, *Candida albicans,* and tinea versicolor. This water-soluble drug binds to cellular lipids and causes metaphase arrest in cells with rapid turnover. There is considerable variability in upper small intestinal absorption; most ingested griseofulvin is detected unchanged within the feces. Two approaches to increase absorption—and hence bioavailability—are to administer ultramicrosize formulations of the drug and to have each dose taken with a high-fat meal. Griseofulvin can be detected within the stratum corneum within 48–72 hours after beginning treatment.

Side effects include headache, other protean neurologic symptoms, nausea, vomiting, and diarrhea. Serum sickness, angioedema, and estrogen-like effects have been reported. The use of this drug in patients with several types of porphyria may result in acute crisis. Laboratory abnormalities may include leukopenia, monocytosis, proteinuria, and cylindruria. If given concurrently with anticoagulants, griseofulvin may reduce drug-induced hypoprothrombinemia.

Griseofulvin is used for superficial dermatophyte infections involving widespread skin areas, hair, and nails. Despite prolonged treatment, many nail infections do not respond entirely or subsequently relapse. Resistance may develop to this drug.

Ketoconazole

Ketoconazole is a water-soluble imidazole derivative effective in the treatment of dermatophytosis (including infections unresponsive to griseofulvin), candidiasis, chronic mucocutaneous candidiasis, tinea versicolor, coccidioidomycosis, paracoccidioidomycosis, histoplasmosis, and chromoblastomycosis. This drug interferes with the synthesis of the fungal sterol ergosterol, leading to subsequent lethal abnormalities within fungal plasma membranes. At the dosage administered to humans, ketoconazole appears to be fungistatic. In the treatment of dermatophytes, glabrous skin responds more rapidly than palmoplantar skin, hair, or nails. The most frequently observed side effects are nausea and pruritus, though other side effects seen with griseofulvin (headache, dizziness, gastrointestinal symptoms) may also occur. Ketoconazole is dissolved only at low pH; therefore, it is poorly absorbed in patients who are achlorhydric or who are taking concurrent cimetidine, anticholinergics, or antacids. Ketoconazole passes the blood-brain barrier poorly and is excreted in feces and urine.

The most notable adverse effects of ketoconazole to date are the development of elevated hepatic enzyme levels, acute toxic hepatitis, gynecomastia, decreased libido, or oligospermia in a small number of patients. A history of prior hepatitis should be a contraindication to the use of this drug; serum liver function tests should be followed closely in patients treated with ketoconazole. This drug may also potentiate the effects of warfarin. There is no information about its safety when administered during pregnancy.

ANTIHISTAMINES

Antihistamines act by competitive inhibition with histamine for receptor sites on various target cells. The classic antihistamines, H_1-blockers, are most useful in the treatment of acute urticaria. They have no effect on non-histamine-mediated pruritus. All antihistamines are well absorbed following oral administration, have an onset of action within 15–30 minutes, and last up to 6 or more hours.

Five major classes of H_1-antihistamines include the ethanolamines (eg, diphenhydramine), ethylenediamines (tripelennamine, hydroxyzine), alkylamines (eg, brompheniramine), propylamines (eg, cyproheptadine), and phenothiazines (eg, promethazine). Although all these drugs have similar actions, their efficacy may vary considerably from patient to patient. In some patients, it may be necessary to combine 2 or more different classes of antihistamines to achieve the appropriate effect.

Some patients may find that one or more of these groups produces more sedation than others. These drugs may, in addition, exert an atropine-like action manifested by dry mouth, blurred vision, and urinary retention. Some patients may note marked sedation or central nervous system excitation. Terfendine or astemizole are often tolerated well by these patients. Patients receiving antihistamines should be warned of these potential side effects and, in particular, should be urged to avoid operating motor vehicles or aircraft or dealing with other potentially dangerous machinery until it has been established that the patient does not experience sedation from the drug. In addition, the drug should not be used by older men with prostatic hypertrophy, to avoid the risk of urinary retention. When taken in extremely large amounts (eg, overdose), ataxia, incoordination, convulsions, and later coma, cardiorespiratory arrest, and death may occur.

Over-the-counter preparations are available that contain diphenhydramine for topical application. Topical antihistamines should be avoided because of lack of efficacy as well as risk of inducing allergic contact dermatitis. The use of diphenhydramine solution within the oral cavity, however, may be beneficial for temporary numbing of the oral mucosa in patients with severe aphthous stomatitis or other oral diseases characterized by blisters and erosions.

ANTIMALARIALS

The 2 most commonly used antimalarials in dermatology are hydroxychloroquine (Plaquenil) and quinacrine (Atabrine; mepacrine). These drugs have been beneficial in the treatment of cutaneous aspects of lupus erythematosus as well as in patients with polymorphous light eruption, solar urticaria, and cutaneous eruptions of dermatomyositis and in selected individuals with porphyria cutanea tarda. Although their mode of action is not known, a myriad of effects have been noted including drug binding of DNA, inhibition of the LE cell phenomenon, suppression of lymphocyte transformation, inhibition of in vitro complement-mediated hemolysis, cellular membrane

stabilization by calcium ion competition, and stabilization of lysosomes.

The antimalarials are almost completely absorbed in the gastrointestinal tract and reach maximum plasma concentrations within 8–12 hours. Subsequently, the drugs maintain high tissue levels and may be detectable up to years following use. Antimalarial excretion occurs mainly via the kidneys.

Hydroxychloroquine and chloroquine may produce an irreversible retinopathy that may progress even after cessation of drug treatment. This retinal damage appears dose-related; it occurs primarily in patients who have received a total cumulative dose of at least 200 g. The suggested safe daily dosage for hydroxychloroquine is 7 mg/kg body weight per day. As opposed to these 2 drugs, quinacrine does not produce retinopathy. In patients treated with hydroxychloroquine or the less frequently used drug chloroquine, patients require an initial baseline ophthalmologic examination and follow-up examinations every 4–6 months while on treatment.

The antimalarials may produce severe leukopenia, especially during the first 3 months of treatment. Even more frequently, aplastic anemia has been reported. These drugs are still distributed with a precaution against their use in patients who are deficient in glucose-6-phosphate dehydrogenase, though hemolytic reactions have been seen only with primaquine. A frequent side effect from the use of quinacrine is a reversible yellowish discoloration of the skin and sclera that may be mistaken for jaundice. Any antimalarial may result in a graying of hair. Some patients treated chronically with antimalarials develop a bluish-black discoloration of the palate, face, pretibial, and nailbed areas. This condition, referred to as pseudo-ochronosis, slowly improves following drug cessation. Other infrequent cutaneous side effects include lichenoid dermatitis, urticaria, exfoliative erythroderma, and exacerbation of psoriasis.

For most skin conditions requiring the use of antimalarials, hydroxychloroquine is used in dosages of 200–400 mg/d. The dosage of quinacrine is 100–300 mg/d. The amount of drug used is slowly reduced as disease manifestations resolve. Chloroquine may be useful in selected patients with porphyria cutanea tarda but is given in one of several low-dose regimens (eg, 125 mg once or twice weekly) to avoid severe reactions, including toxic hepatitis. Occasional patients with cutaneous lupus erythematosus may benefit from the combination of hydroxychloroquine and quinacrine when poorly responding to either agent alone.

BLEOMYCIN

Bleomycin, a cytotoxic polypeptide antibiotic mixture isolated from a soil fungus, has been shown to be effective as an intralesional agent in the treatment of recalcitrant warts. Side effects include pain at the time of injection, localized edema, and the development of a hemorrhagic eschar.

CORTICOSTEROIDS

Systemic corticosteroids are highly effective in the treatment of many cutaneous disorders, especially the autoimmune bullous dermatoses, including pemphigus, bullous pemphigoid, cicatricial pemphigoid, epidermolysis bullosa acquisita, and herpes gestationis. In some patients with pemphigus vulgaris, very high doses of prednisone, often exceeding 150 mg/d, may be either life-saving or necessary to achieve complete remission. Although usually given orally, rare patients with pyoderma gangrenosum and pemphigus vulgaris have benefited by treatment with brief courses (eg, 5 days) of very high doses of prednisone administered intravenously ("pulse therapy"), followed by lower doses given orally either alone or in conjunction with a second immunosuppressive drug. Other serious or even life-threatening cutaneous disorders that may benefit by systemic corticosteroids include pyoderma gangrenosum and toxic epidermal necrolysis. Abbreviated courses of systemic corticosteroids may be of benefit for severe allergic contact dermatitis (including poison ivy), generalized atopic dermatitis, other types of generalized eczematous dermatitis, acne fulminans, leukocytoclastic vasculitis, systemic lupus erythematosus, dermatomyositis, and Sweet's syndrome. Intralesional corticosteroids are helpful in a variety of conditions, including inflammatory epidermal or acne cysts, psoriasis, localized eczematous dermatitis, discoid lupus erythematosus, localized lichen planus, alopecia areata, and necrobiosis lipoidica diabeticorum.

In normal individuals, cortisol is normally produced every morning by the adrenal cortex in amounts equivalent to a daily morning dosage of 5–7.5 mg of prednisone. This production is under control of the hypothalamic-pituitary-adrenal axis. As serum cortisol levels decrease, the hypothalamus produces corticotropin-releasing factor, which then stimulates the production of adrenocorticotropic hormone (ACTH) by the anterior lobe of the pituitary gland. ACTH then stimulates the adrenal gland to produce more cortisol. When exogenous corticosteroids are necessary, most patients are given a single oral dose in the early morning to mimic the normal cyclic release of cortisol by the adrenal gland and thereby produce the least alteration in the normal hypothalamic-pituitary-adrenal gland axis. Some patients respond to the use of alternate-day steroid therapy, thus reducing the risk of developing almost all the common complications.

Chronic use of corticosteroids does result in suppression of normal adrenal gland production of cortisol. Therefore, abrupt discontinuation of such therapy may result in a hypoadrenal state. In addition, because of the lack of adrenal cortisol reserve, patients receiving chronic corticosteroid therapy require increased steroid supplementation during surgery or with other serious injury or illness. Tapering of corticosteroid dosage is necessary in all patients except those having received short (4-week) treatment courses. After achieving remission, the dosage of corticosteroid is slowly reduced in a way that will produce the least amount of side effects and still allow little or no disease activity. Many steroid-responsive skin diseases may be unpredictable in the dosage of corticosteroids required for remission, and individual patients often have marked temporal variations in dosage requirement.

Corticosteroids can be divided into 3 groups depending upon their duration of ACTH suppression: (1) Short-acting glucocorticoids act for approximately 24–36 hours and include cortisone, hydrocortisone, prednisone, prednisolone, and methylprednisolone. (2) Intermediate-acting glucocorticoid preparations, which act for approximately 48 hours, include triamcinolone and paramethasone. (3) Long-acting corticosteroids, including dexamethasone and betamethasone, have activity for at least 48 hours. Most physicians use prednisone, prednisolone, or methylprednisolone, since any of these may be suitable in alternate-day as well as in daily therapy. Prednisone becomes effective only after hepatic conversion to prednisolone. Patients with liver disease may not benefit as much from prednisone because of the difficulty in this metabolic conversion.

There are many possible complications to the chronic systemic use of corticosteroids. These include striae, easy bruisability, growth disturbances in children, obesity, hypertension, moon facies, increased appetite, increased susceptibility to infections, delayed wound healing, osteoporosis and bony fractures, myopathy, carbohydrate intolerance, personality or emotional disturbances, and the development of posterior subcapsular cataracts. Abnormal laboratory tests may include hyperglycemia, neutrophilia, lymphocytopenia, and monocytopenia. Patients receiving long-term corticosteroid therapy may have decreased cell-mediated immunity. Increased sodium and potassium excretion also occurs. On alternate-day regimens, all complications will be decreased except cataracts. Most studies suggest that systemic corticosteroids may be taken during pregnancy without risk to the fetus. There are still a few reports of slightly increased frequencies of spontaneous abortion and stillbirths or instances of cleft-palate after corticosteroid use. Patients with past histories of peptic ulcer disease or tuberculosis—or those having concurrent bacterial infections—are preferably not treated with systemic corticosteroids.

In some clinical situations, the use of intramuscular corticosteroids may be advantageous. Many are long-acting (some up to 3–4 weeks after injection). However, the slow and erratic absorption and metabolism of intramuscularly placed corticosteroids results in continued release of the drug in a nonphysiologic (nondiurnal) manner. In addition to the previously mentioned side effects of systemic corticosteroids, local cutaneous atrophy may result when intralesional or intramuscular injections are used.

CYCLOSPORINE

Cyclosporine, an 11-amino-acid polypeptide derived from a soil fungus, is used primarily for the prevention and treatment of organ transplant rejection. Recent studies have demonstrated its possible role in the treatment of several skin diseases, including recalcitrant psoriasis vulgaris, pemphigus vulgaris, graft-versus-host disease, bullous pemphigoid, and Behçet's disease. Isolated patients having severe atopic dermatitis, alopecia universalis, ichthyosis vulgaris, epidermolysis bullosa acquisita, pyoderma gangrenosum, systemic lupus erythematosus, cutaneous T cell lymphoma, and sarcoidosis have also been reported to benefit from cyclosporine treatment. Its use in autoimmune bullous disorders and systemic lupus may be primarily as a steroid-sparing immunosuppressive agent.

Following oral administration, cyclosporine is erratically absorbed from the gastrointestinal tract, necessitating careful monitoring of serial blood levels. The largest percentage of absorbed drug is bound to erythrocytes, but the drug is widely distributed throughout the body. Cyclosporine is metabolized primarily by the liver; toxicity may occur in the presence of hepatic dysfunction. One of the major adverse effects is nephrotoxicity, which occurs in most patients receiving chronic therapy. Although renal function usually returns to baseline following cessation of treatment, some patients have developed irreversible renal dysfunction as a result of interstitial fibrosis. Other side effects may include hypertension, hepatotoxicity, neurologic injury, gastrointestinal symptomatology, myalgias, arthralgias, fatigue, gingival hyperplasia, hypertrichosis, and the development of secondary cancers (mainly lymphomas) and infections.

CYTOTOXIC DRUGS

Azathioprine (Imuran)

Azathioprine is a chemical derivative of 6-mercaptopurine. It is well absorbed from the gastrointestinal tract, subsequently metabolized to 6-mercaptopurine, and eventually converted to 6-thiouric acid by the enzyme xanthine oxidase (therefore, the use of allopurinol in patients concurrently on azathioprine may result in toxic levels of mercaptopurine). Ap-

proximately 30% of azathioprine is bound to serum protein. Azathioprine and its metabolic product 6-mercaptopurine are undetectable in serum 8 hours after oral ingestion. This drug is primarily excreted by the kidney in the form of mercaptopurine; in the presence of renal insufficiency, normal oral dosage will result in excessively high levels of mercaptopurine.

There are relatively few side effects when this drug is given orally. Infrequently, patients may complain of nausea, vomiting, diarrhea, steatorrhea, fever, arthralgias, alopecia, and skin eruptions. Other potential adverse effects include hematopoietic suppression and, rarely, severe cholestatic hepatitis. In animals, azathioprine is teratogenic. Renal transplant patients treated with azathioprine develop increased number of cutaneous and systemic cancers. Temporary chromosomal abnormalities associated with azathioprine use have been reported.

The 2 diseases shown to benefit from the use of azathioprine—in which it is usually used initially in conjunction with corticosteroids—are bullous pemphigoid and pemphigus vulgaris. In addition, cicatricial pemphigoid, epidermolysis bullosa acquisita, and pityriasis rubra pilaris may also improve.

Cyclophosphamide (Cytoxan)

Cyclophosphamide is an alkylating agent structurally related to mechlorethamine. Although this drug is not commonly used in high doses and is usually used intravenously for various types of noncutaneous cancers, it has been used with some success in patients with pemphigus vulgaris and bullous pemphigoid unresponsive to other drugs. When used for selected dermatologic conditions, cyclophosphamide is usually administered in a dosage of 100–150 mg once daily.

Cyclophosphamide is an immunosuppressant, especially affecting cell-mediated immune response. It is well absorbed orally and is metabolically activated following absorption. Maximal plasma levels are detectable 1 hour after oral administration. The serum half-life is approximately $6\frac{1}{2}$ hours, with subsequent elimination through urine and stool.

When cyclophosphamide is given in the dosages normally used for dermatologic therapy, the 2 most common side effects are hematologic suppression and sterile hemorrhagic cystitis. Hematopoietic suppression is usually reversible with temporary cessation of the drug. Hemorrhagic cystitis may occur in up to 5–10% of patients as a result of direct irritation of the bladder mucosa by drug metabolites and may occur within the first few hours of its administration. This side effect may be avoided if the patient drinks large amounts of water shortly before and up to 2 hours after intake of the drug by mouth and then frequently voids so as to dilute the metabolites present within the urine as well as keep the bladder essentially empty.

Should severe hemorrhagic cystitis develop and persist, it may be necessary to treat the bladder with chemical instillation or even electrofulguration.

Less frequent side effects, primarily noted in patients given high intravenous dosages of cyclophosphamide, include oral ulcerations, increased coloration of the skin and nails, alopecia, jaundice, clotting abnormalities, renal tubular necrosis, enterocolitis, and azoospermia or anovulation. Cyclophosphamide is teratogenic. Patients with cancer or rheumatoid arthritis treated with cyclophosphamide appear to have an increased risk of later developing an initial or second cancer; however, this has not yet been reported in patients given low doses for skin disease. In addition to some severe bullous disorders (eg, pemphigus vulgaris, cicatricial and bullous pemphigoid, epidermolysis bullosa acquisita), other diseases with cutaneous manifestations that may benefit from treatment with cyclophosphamide include Wegener's granulomatosis, lupus erythematosus, cutaneous vasculitis, and pyoderma gangrenosum. Many patients with advanced forms of mycosis fungoides have been treated with multidrug chemotherapy, including cyclophosphamide.

Hydroxyurea (Hydrea)

Hydroxyurea is an anticancer agent that inhibits DNA synthesis. Although used primarily in the treatment of chronic myelocytic leukemia and some solid tumors, some patients with extensive psoriasis may also benefit from therapy with this drug. In psoriasis, hydroxyurea is utilized in 500–1500 mg/d dosage and is administered orally. The drug is well-absorbed in the gastrointestinal tract, has a peak serum concentration within the first 2 hours, and is almost completely excreted within 24 hours through the kidneys. Side effects include hematopoietic depression and megaloblastic erythropoiesis unassociated with vitamin B_{12} or folic acid deficiency. Patients who have received prior radiation therapy may experience exacerbation of postirradiation erythema following the administration of hydroxyurea. This drug may also be associated with gastrointestinal disturbances, skin eruptions, and, infrequently, various neurologic signs and symptoms. It is teratogenic in animals and is contraindicated in pregnancy. Hydroxyurea may also cause temporary renal impairment and therefore should not be given in patients with preexisting kidney disease.

Methotrexate

Methotrexate, a folic acid analogue, has as its site of action the enzyme dihydrofolate reductase. This drug is used by dermatologists primarily for extensive psoriasis uncontrollable by standard topical methods or photochemotherapy. Some special forms of psoriasis otherwise difficult to treat—including localized pustular psoriasis, acute pustular psoriasis of von Zumbusch, psoriatic erythroderma, and psoriatic arthritis—may also respond. Methotrexate has also been used successfully as a steroid-sparing drug in patients with some severe autoimmune bullous disorders (particularly pemphigus vulgaris and bullous pemphigoid) and some forms of vasculitis.

Methotrexate is fairly well absorbed by the gastrointestinal tract; about 50–90% of the drug is detectable unchanged in the urine within the first 8 hours. Some of the drug is retained within tissues, especially kidney and liver, for weeks to months. Approximately 50% of plasma methotrexate is protein-bound; this is important since several drugs, including salicylates and nonsteroidal anti-inflammatory agents, displace methotrexate from albumin, thereby increasing the potential for toxicity. Other drugs may similarly interact with methotrexate to increase toxicity by reducing renal elimination, enhancing toxic effects (eg, ethanol), reducing tubular secretion (eg, sulfonamides), or increasing intracellular accumulation of methotrexate (eg, probenecid, dipyridamole). Patients with renal impairment are particularly at risk for methotrexate toxicity because of the extent of kidney excretion of this drug.

Methotrexate interferes with normal embryogenesis and should not be given during pregnancy. Patients should be advised to use contraceptive measures during treatment and for at least 12 weeks afterward because of the long retention of the drug within tissues.

Some otherwise normal psoriatic patients may, with long-term methotrexate therapy, develop liver fibrosis or cirrhosis. Patients with a past history of hepatitis, cirrhosis, or alcoholism, or those shown to have histologic evidence of liver damage prior to therapy, are not treated with this drug except in the most urgent circumstances. Close monitoring of serum liver enzymes is performed in all patients receiving methotrexate, and the drug is discontinued if persistent liver abnormalities arise. Significant liver damage may occur prior to the development of serum enzyme abnormalities. Liver biopsy is obtained if enzyme levels become elevated or when a cumulative dose of 1.5 g has been given and after each additional 1–1.5 g has been taken; some authorities recommend baseline liver biopsies prior to initiation of therapy.

Methotrexate is usually given weekly by intramuscular or oral routes. The most common side effects are malaise, nausea, and leukopenia. The administration of methotrexate a few days following ultraviolet irradiation may reactivate an acute sunburn reaction.

RETINOIDS

One of the most exciting recent advances in dermatology has been the development and release of 2 oral retinoids for the treatment of several skin diseases. These drugs were initially examined because of clinical evidence that vitamin A given in high doses benefited several skin conditions, most notably cystic acne. The 2 synthetic oral retinoids currently available are isotretinoin (13-*cis*-retinoic acid) and etretinate; others with potentially equal clinical efficacy but reduced side effects (or shorter tissue half-lives) are now in clinical trials.

When given for approximately 4–5 months, isotretinoin results in an excellent response in most patients with previously recalcitrant nodulocystic acne. Patients continue to improve for many months following cessation of treatment. This drug is effective in clearing nodulocystic lesions as well as other inflammatory (papules, pustules) and to a lesser extent noninflammatory acne lesions (open and closed comedones). Isotretinoin is less effective when hidradenitis suppurativa or dissecting cellulitis of the scalp accompanies acne.

Acne patients receiving isotretinoin have rapid and marked inhibition of sebaceous gland secretion. Sebum levels on the skin are markedly reduced, and the skin surface lipids show a reversal of lipid pattern to that seen in children. Ultrastructural examination of skin from patients treated with isotretinoin confirms that the pilosebaceous units are reduced in size.

Retinoids have also been found beneficial in the treatment of several disorders of keratinization. Psoriatic patients, particularly with pustular psoriasis or psoriatic erythroderma, usually benefit significantly when treated with etretinate; as such, some authorities now recommend etretinate therapy over methotrexate in these specific psoriatic subsets. Unfortunately, the response to etretinate by patients with other more common forms of psoriasis is usually far less dramatic. In general, the response of psoriatics to etretinate is less striking than that seen with isotretinoin in acne; furthermore, when etretinate proves to be beneficial, the response lasts only during the actual course of treatment—in contrast to the sustained action seen by isotretinoin in acne. Isotretinoin is far less effective than etretinate in the treatment of psoriasis. Other diseases noted to be at least partially improved with etretinate include Darier's disease, pityriasis rubra pilaris, lamellar ichthyosis, harlequin fetus, epidermolytic hyperkeratosis, and hyperkeratosis palmaris et plantaris. Isotretinoin has been reported to be of benefit also in discoid lupus erythematosus and gram-negative folliculitis.

In patients with basal cell nevus syndrome, the use of isotretinoin may result in reduction of skin tumor size and lead to partial or complete regression of some tumors. As an experimental correlate, there is growing literature to support the concept that retinoids may be beneficial as tumor-preventive agents.

Side effects with oral retinoids are common and include cheilitis, pruritus, headaches, blepharoconjunctivitis, erythema, dryness or desquamation of the skin, myalgias, arthralgias, and, in some patients, temporary thinning of scalp hair or other hair-bearing areas. Some acne patients treated with isotretinoin may develop areas of exuberant granulation tissue; similar findings have been noted with etretinate. Other findings that may be seen are elevated liver enzyme tests and, in approximately 25% of patients, elevations of serum triglyceride levels, the latter rarely leading to eruptive xanthomas or acute pancreatitis. A substantial minority of patients have been noted to have asymptomatic calcification of ligaments, especially along the spine. Long-term use of etretinate may lead to premature closure of the epiphyses in children.

Isotretinoin and etretinate are highly teratogenic; fetuses exposed to these drugs may have major anomalies of multiple organs, including the central nervous system. Therefore, exposure during pregnancy must be avoided. Female patients must be counseled about the risks of the drug to the developing fetus during pregnancy and the need for adequate contraception during and after treatment. Whereas isotretinoin may exert a teratogenic effect up to 2 months after cessation of treatment, there is evidence that etretinate may exert a similar effect for an even longer time (up to 2 years). A reliable method of contraception must be continued at least during these intervals following completion of retinoid therapy.

SULFONES & SULFONAMIDES

The sulfones and sulfonamides most commonly used in dermatologic practice are dapsone and sulfapyridine. They are most often given in the treatment of dermatitis herpetiformis, a pruritic vesicular eruption characterized histologically by neutrophilic microabscesses in the papillary dermis and immunologically by the presence of IgA in granular or linear array along the dermal-epidermal junction. However, the most common use of dapsone in the world today is in the treatment of leprosy. Other diseases of dermatologic interest in which dapsone or sulfapyridine has been reported effective include subcorneal pustular dermatosis, acne conglobata, pyoderma gangrenosum, bullous pemphigoid, cicatricial pemphigoid, chronic bullous dermatosis of childhood, erythema elevatum diutinum, relapsing polychondritis, granuloma annulare, granuloma faciale, bullous eruption of systemic lupus erythematosus, leukocytoclastic vasculitis, actinomycotic mycetoma, alopecia mucinosa, pustular psoriasis, herpes gestationis, pemphigus, Weber-Christian panniculitis, brown recluse spider bites, and Hailey-Hailey disease. Some of these conditions have as a unifying feature the presence of granulocytes as the major infiltrating cell within the dermis.

These drugs exert a bacteriostatic effect as a result of interference with bacterial folate biosynthesis and inhibition of choline incorporation into the lecithin of cell membranes. These drugs are oxidants and therefore have an influence on glutathione. Dapsone inhibits lysosomal enzyme activity and interferes in the myeloperoxidase-hydrogen peroxide-halide-related system in neutrophils. In addition, dapsone may have an effect on neutrophil chemotaxis.

Approximately 80% of the oral dose of dapsone is absorbed from the gastrointestinal tract. Peak serum levels occur within 2–6 hours. The serum half-life ranges from 2–4 days. Following gastrointestinal absorption, dapsone is metabolized via acetylation and hydroxylation into several metabolites. Differences in acetylator phenotypes appear to have no correlation with drug efficacy or degree of side effects. Ninety percent of dapsone dosage is excreted by the kidneys, and 10% can be detected in bile. In patients receiving long-term treatment with dapsone, the drug may be found for long periods within the body as a result of both high protein binding and enterohepatic recirculation. As opposed to dapsone, sulfapyridine is less well absorbed by the intestinal tract. It is metabolized by the liver and excreted mainly via the kidneys.

An expected side effect in the use of dapsone therapy is the development of hemolysis and methemoglobinemia. The drug is contraindicated in patients deficient in the enzyme glucose-6-phosphate dehydrogenase, who will develop profound erythrocyte hemolysis following such exposure. Methemoglobinemia may be seen, especially in patients taking high doses; it may be partially corrected by the coadministration of methylene blue. Other side effects that appear to be dose-related include nausea, vomiting, headache, weakness, fatigue, dizziness, nervousness, and shortness of breath. Peripheral neuropathies may be noted in some patients treated with very high dosages. Infrequent findings have also included marked hypoalbuminemia, nephrotic syndrome, psychosis, and cholestasis. There are limited data suggesting that congenital malformations may occur if dapsone is administered during pregnancy. Rarely, patients have developed agranulocytosis following treatment with dapsone or sulfapyridine.

Patients require frequent laboratory evaluation, which includes a complete blood count with differential white count, a chemistry profile to include renal and liver tests, urinalysis, and methemoglobin level.

SELECTED OTHER SYSTEMIC DRUGS

Clofazimine

Clofazimine is a substituted iminophenazine dye used primarily in the treatment of leprosy. This drug is effective in selected patients with pyoderma gangrenosum, discoid lupus erythematosus, erythema nodosum leprosum, acne fulminans, pustulosis palmaris et plantaris, pustular psoriasis of von Zumbusch, and granuloma faciale.

Extensive animal studies have shown a remarkable lack of toxicity. Follow-up of a series of 51 patients treated for 8 years has confirmed this lack of toxicity. There is no evidence of mutagenic or teratogenic activity.

Clofazimine is highly lipophilic. Patients treated with clofazimine have drug deposits within subcutaneous fat, bone, skeletal muscle, liver, spleen, small intestine, gallbladder, adrenal glands, and mesenteric lymph nodes; it has been detected within lymph nodes as long as 4 months following cessation of therapy. Clofazimine crosses the human placental barrier, resulting in pigmentation of offspring.

Clofazimine is administered orally. Approximately 70% is absorbed within the small intestine and at least 35% is subsequently excreted within the feces, with less than 0.1% of the initial dosage detectable in urine. The half-life of this drug in humans is at least 70 days.

The most apparent side effect is pink, red, or brownish-black discoloration of the skin, especially over sunlight-exposed surfaces. Hair, sweat, sputum, urine, and feces may similarly become discolored. This side effect is dose-related and slowly reversible upon discontinuation of therapy. Other cutaneous side effects may include xeroderma, ichthyosis, pruritus, photosensitivity, and acneiform or nonspecific eruptions. Gastrointestinal side effects include nausea, vomiting, abdominal pain, and diarrhea.

Clofazimine is given in divided oral doses (usually 300 mg total daily dosage) with meals or milk. The total dosage is decreased or the time interval between doses increased should gastrointestinal symptoms develop. For most skin conditions, at least 2 months of treatment may be necessary before a beneficial effect is seen. Serial routine laboratory examination (blood, urine) is necessary for all patients being treated with this agent.

The drug is contraindicated during the first trimester of pregnancy, in patients prone to recurrent abdominal pain or diarrhea, and in those with preexisting liver or kidney disease.

Colchicine

Colchicine is an alkaloid used primarily for treatment of gout. Recently, there has been renewed interest in the use of colchicine for selected skin conditions. Laboratory studies with colchicine have shown it to be intimately involved in the inhibition of microtubule assembly. Colchicine also affects cAMP and the chemotaxis of polymorphonuclear leukocytes and monocytes.

Conditions that may benefit from colchicine include dermatitis herpetiformis, psoriasis, necrotizing vasculitis, Behçet's syndrome, familial Mediterranean fever, localized and systemic scleroderma, calcinosis universalis, sarcoid arthritis, relapsing polychondritis, rheumatoid arthritis, acute pseudogout, and Paget's disease of bone. Striking chromosomal abnormalities have been noted in gout patients receiving colchicine. Therefore, colchicine is contraindicated in pregnant women and should be used in nonpregnant women only if strict contraceptive measures are concurrently being used.

The limited dose factor for colchicine is usually the development of nausea, vomiting, diarrhea, and abdominal pain. Other side effects include hematopoietic suppression, alopecia, amenorrhea, myopathy, peripheral neuritis, and azoospermia.

Gold Therapy (Chrysotherapy)

Gold salts have been used for years in the treatment of rheumatoid arthritis. More recently, intramuscular gold has been found effective in the treatment of pemphigus vulgaris. As in the case of rheumatoid arthritis, patients with pemphigus vulgaris are given weekly intramuscular injections.

Two gold preparations are used in dermatology. **Gold sodium thiomalate** is water-soluble; **aurothioglucose** is oil-based. Recently, an oral gold preparation—auranofin—has been released for use in rheumatoid arthritis, but experience is limited in its use in dermatologic conditions.

The most common side effect of chrysotherapy is the development of a macular or papular eruption. Less frequently, lichen planus-like or pityriasis rosea-like eruptions may occur; very rarely, exfoliative dermatitis has been seen. Stomatitis, gingivitis, or glossitis may also develop. Following temporary discontinuation of chrysotherapy, skin eruptions resolve, although it may require 3–4 months. Following that time, most patients can be given further gold without recurrence of cutaneous side effects.

Some patients experience a vasomotor (nitritoid) reaction characterized by flushing, generalized erythema, weakness, vertigo, syncope, and hypotension within minutes after administration of the water-soluble gold preparation. Other reactions seen within 24 hours after gold sodium thiomalate injections include joint stiffness, arthralgias, myalgias, and malaise. Fewer than 1% of patients treated with gold develop hematologic side effects, but these may include leukopenia, agranulocytosis, thrombocytopenia, and, rarely, aplastic anemia. In approximately 2–10% of patients, proteinuria may occur, especially in those who receive large amounts. Gastrointestinal side effects are rare and may include intrahepatic or granulomatous bowel disease. Other side effects of gold therapy may include diffuse pulmonary infiltrates, pneumonic consolidation or diffuse interstitial fibrosis, corneal ulceration, or diffuse deposition of metallic gold within body tissues, including skin (chrysiasis).

Patients to be treated with intramuscular gold are generally given an initial test dose of 1 mg. If no untoward reactions occur, the patient may receive slowly increasing intramuscular dosages up to 50 mg/wk. In pemphigus vulgaris, there may be no significant improvement until 400–500 mg of cumulative dose has been received. If no response has been noted after a total of 1 g, the patient is usually considered refractory to this treatment and therapy is discontinued. In patients who receive significant benefit, the therapy may be decreased in frequency to every 2 and, later, every 4 weeks after receiving 1 g of gold. Because of the multiple potential side effects that may occur with chrysotherapy, it is necessary to monitor patients with serial complete blood counts, platelet counts, urinalysis, and liver function tests.

Pentoxifylline

Pentoxifylline, a derivative of methylxanthine, was originally marketed for the symptomatic treatment of intermittent claudication. This drug is incorporated into erythrocyte cell membranes and appears to have clinical utility by increasing erythrocyte deformability. As such, erythrocytes are better able to traverse tiny blood vessels within diseased skin, providing needed oxygen. Pentoxifylline also affects various in vitro functions of granulocytes and platelets. Several cutaneous disorders are said to be benefited by this drug, including Raynaud's phenomenon, vasculitis (including livedo variant), leg ulcers, atrophie blanche, cutaneous infarcts of systemic lupus erythematosus, necrobiosis lipoidica, granuloma annulare, and pityriasis lichenoides et varioliformis acuta. Other proposed uses, some based upon anecdotal experience, include enhancement of pedicle flap and skin graft survival and treatment of pyoderma gangrenosum, eosinophilic fasciitis, lymphedema, myxedema, keloids, and leg ulcers associated with cryoglobulinemia.

MISCELLANEOUS THERAPIES

In addition to the medical treatment methods previously discussed, a variety of others have been reported within the past few years for selected dermatologic conditions. Some await confirmation of efficacy in larger numbers of patients treated in a controlled double-blinded fashion; others are of proved efficacy but have only limited clinical utility either because of the rarity of diseases affected or the potential severity of side effects.

Among the most promising new therapies is parenteral **alpha interferon** for widespread condylomata acuminata; response has also been reported in cutaneous T cell lymphoma and in verrucous lesions of epidermodysplasia verruciformis. Others include **phenytoin** (for recessive and some junctional forms of epidermolysis bullosa), **nifedipine** (for Raynaud's phenomenon, and possibly urticaria pigmentosa and atrophie blanche), **thalidomide** (for severe discoid lupus erythematosus, reactional lepromatous leprosy, severe aphthosis, and recalcitrant prurigo nodularis), **disodium cromoglycate** (for urticaria pigmentosa), **papaverine** and **evening primrose oil** for atopic dermatitis, **saturated solution of potassium iodide** (for erythema nodosum), **topical testosterone and oral potassium para-aminobenzoate** (for lichen sclerosus et atrophicus), **cimetidine** (in combination with H$_1$

blockers) for chronic urticaria, topical **carmustine** (for lymphomatoid papulosis), topical **capsaicin** (for postherpetic neuralgia), topical or oral **metronidazole** (for rosacea), and topical **dinitrochlorobenzene immunotherapy** (for recalcitrant warts). Parenteral **zinc** remains the therapy of choice for acrodermatitis enteropathica, and oral supplementations with **vitamin D and fish oil** have been reported to be of clinical benefit in some patients with psoriasis.

REFERENCES

Ahmed AR, Hombal SM: Cyclophosphamide (Cytoxan). A review on relevant pharmacology and clinical uses. J Am Acad Dermatol 1984;11:1115.

Ahmed AR, Hombal SM: Use of cyclophosphamide in azathioprine failures in pemphigus. J Am Acad Dermatol 1987;17:437.

Allenby CF, Sparkes CG: Halogenation and topical corticosteroids: a comparison between the 17-butyrate esters of hydrocortisone and clobetasone in ointment bases. Br J Dermatol 1981;104:179.

Arndt KA: Manual of Dermatologic Therapeutics. With Essentials of Diagnosis, 4th edition. Little, Brown, 1989.

Aso M: Effects of potent topical corticosteroids on adrenocortical function. J Dermatol 1983;10:145.

Bagatell FK et al: Evaluation of a new antifungal cream, ciclopirox olamine 1% in the treatment of cutaneous candidiasis. Clin Ther 1985;8:41.

Balfour HH Jr et al: Acyclovir halts progression of herpes zoster in immunocompromised patients. N Engl J Med 1983;308:1448.

Barthelemy H et al: Treatment of nine cases of pemphigus vulgaris with cyclosporine. J Am Acad Dermatol 1988;18:1262.

Bickers DR, Hazen PG, Lynch WS: Clinical Pharmacology of Skin Disease. Churchill Livingstone, 1984.

Brown MD et al: Therapy of dermatologic disease with cyclosporin A. Adv Dermatol 1989;4:3.

Bryson VJ et al: Treatment of first episodes of genital herpes simplex virus infection with oral acyclovir: Randomized double-blind controlled trial in normal subjects. N Engl J Med 1983;308:916.

Bunney MH: Viral Warts: Their Biology and Treatment. Oxford University Press, 1982.

Buxman M et al: Therapeutic activity of lactate 12% lotion in the treatment of ichthyosis. J Am Acad Dermatol 1986;15:1253.

Chalker DK et al: Efficacy of topical isotretinoin 0.05% gel in acne vulgaris: Results of a multicenter, double-blind investigation. J Am Acad Dermatol 1987;17:251.

Corey L et al: A trial of topical acyclovir in genital herpes simplex virus infections. N Engl J Med 1982;306:1313.

Cornell RC, Stoughton RB: Correlation of vasoconstrictor assay and clinical activity in psoriasis. Arch Dermatol 1985;121:63.

Cornell RC, Stoughton RB: Use of topical steroids in psoriasis. Dermatol Clin 1984;2:397.

de Vivier A: Tachyphylaxis to topically applied steroids. Arch Dermatol 1976;112:1245.

Devillez RL: Topical minoxidil therapy in hereditary androgenic alopecia. Arch Dermatol 1985;121: 197.

Diette KM et al: Psoralen and UV-A and UV-B twice weekly for the treatment of psoriasis. Arch Dermatol 1984;120:1169.

DiGiovanni JJ et al: Extraspinal tendon and ligament calcification associated with long-term therapy with etretinate. N Engl J Med 1986;315:1177.

Eells LD et al: Topical antibiotic treatment of impetigo with mupiricin. Arch Dermatol 1986;122:1273.

Ellis CN et al: Cyclosporine improves psoriasis in a double-blind study. JAMA 1986;256:3110.

Ellis CN et al: Isotretinoin therapy is associated with early skeletal radiographic changes. J Am Acad Dermatol 1984;10:1024.

Ellis CN, Voorhees JJ: Etretinate therapy. J Am Acad Dermatol 1987;16:267.

Ely H: Pentoxifylline therapy in dermatology: A review of localized hyperviscosity and its effects on the skin. Dermatol Clin 1988;6:585.

Farber EM, Abel EA, Cox AJ: Long-term risks of psoralen and UV-A therapy for psoriasis. Arch Dermatol 1983;119:426.

Feingold DS, Wagner RF Jr: Antibacterial therapy. J Am Acad Dermatol 1986;14:535.

Gallant C, Kenny P: Oral glucocorticosteroids and their complications. A review. J Am Acad Dermatol 1986; 14:161.

Gammon WR et al: Comparative efficacy of oral erythromycin versus oral tetracycline in the treatment of acne vulgaris. A double-blind study. J Am Acad Dermatol 1986;14:183.

Gerber LH et al: Vertebral abnormalities associated with synthetic retinoid use. J Am Acad Dermatol 1984; 10:817.

Gibbons RB: Complications of chrysotherapy: A review of recent studies. Arch Int Med 1979;139:343.

Goette DR: Topical chemotherapy with 5-fluorouracil. J Amer Acad Dermatol 1981;4:633.

Goldberg LH et al: Oral acyclovir for episodic treatment of recurrent genital herpes. Efficacy and safety. J Am Acad Dermatol 1986;15:256.

Gollnick H et al: Acitretin versus etretinate in psoriasis. J Am Acad Dermatol 1988;19:458.

Grimes PE et al: Determination of optimal topical photochemotherapy for vitiligo. J Am Acad Dermatol 1982;7:771.

Haas AA, Arndt KA: Selected therapeutic applications of

topical tretinoin. J Am Acad Dermatol 1986;15:87.

Hay RJ et al: A comparative double blind study of ketoconazole and griseofulvin in dermatophytosis. Br J Dermatol 1985;112:691.

Hay RJ, Midgeley G: Short course ketoconazole therapy in pityriasis versicolor. Clin Exp Dermatol 1984;9:571.

Hayes ME, O'Keefe EJ: Reduced dose of bleomycin in the treatment of recalcitrant warts. J Am Acad Dermatol 1986;15:1002.

Hirschmann JV: Some principles of systemic glucocorticosteroid therapy. Clin Exp Dermatol 1986;11:27.

Jones HE: Ketoconazole. Arch Dermatol 1982;118:217.

Juhlin L, et al (symposium editors): Current concepts in the mode of action of anthralin in the treatment of psoriasis. Br J Dermatol 1981;105(Suppl 20):3.

Kaplan RP, Russell DH, Lowe NJ: Etretinate therapy for psoriasis: clinical responses, remission times, epidermal DNA, and polyamine responses. J Am Acad Dermatol 1983;8:95.

Katz SI: Commentary: Sulfoxone (Diasone) in the treatment of dermatitis herpetiformis. Arch Dermatol 1982;118:809.

Kligman AM et al: Evaluation of ciclopirox olamine for the treatment of tinea: multicenter, double-blind comparative study. Clin Ther 1985;7:409.

Kligman AM et al: Topical tretinoin for photoaged skin. J Am Acad Dermatol 1986;15:836.

Koranda FC: Antimalarials. J Am Acad Dermatol 1981;4:650.

Lang PG Jr: Sulfones and sulfonamides in dermatology today. J Amer Acad Dermatol 1979;1:479.

Levine MJ, White HAD, Parrish JA: Components of the Goeckerman regimen. J Invest Dermatol 1979;73:170.

Leyden JJ, Shalita AR: Rational therapy for acne vulgaris: an update on topical treatment. J Am Acad Dermatol 1986;15:907.

Lin AN, Reimer RJ, Carter DM: Sulfur revisited. J Am Acad Dermatol 1988;18:553.

Lowe NJ et al: Anthralin for psoriasis: short-contact anthralin compared with topical steroid and conventional anthralin. J Am Acad Dermatol 1984;10:69.

Lowe NJ, David M: New retinoids for dermatologic diseases: uses and toxicity. Dermatol Clin 1988;6:539.

Lowe NJ, Lazarus V, Matt L: Systemic retinoid therapy for psoriasis. J Am Acad Dermatol 1988;19:186.

Luby J: Therapy in genital herpes. N Engl J Med 1982;306:1356.

Maddox JS, Ware JC, Dillon HC Jr: The natural history of streptococcal skin infection: prevention with topical antibiotics. J Am Acad Dermatol 1985;13:207.

Malkinson FD: Colchicine: new uses of an old, old drug. Arch Dermatol 1982;118:453.

McKendrik MW, McGill JI, White JG: Oral acyclovir in acute herpes zoster. Br Med J 1986;293:1529.

Millikan LE et al: Naftifine cream 1% versus econazole cream 1% in the treatment of tinea cruris and tinea corporis. J Am Acad Dermatol 1988;18:52.

Monroe EW: Chronic urticaria: review of nonsedating H₁ antihistamines in treatment. J Am Acad Dermatol 1988;19:842.

Mosher DB, Parrish JA, Fitzpatrick TB: Monobenzylether of hydroquinone: a retrospective study of treatment of 18 vitiligo patients and a review of the literature. Br J Dermatol 1977;97:669.

Nazzaro-Porro M: Azelaic acid. J Am Acad Dermatol 1987;17:1033.

Olsen EA, DeLong ER, Weiner MS: Dose-response study of topical minoxidil in male pattern baldness. J Am Acad Dermatol 1986;15:30.

Page EH, Wexler DM, Guenther LC: Cyclosporin A. J Am Acad Dermatol 1986;14:785.

Parish LC, Witkowski JA, Muri JG: Topical corticosteroids. Int J Dermatol 1985;24:435.

Parrish JA et al: Photochemotherapy of psoriasis using methoxsalen and sunlight: A controlled study. Arch Dermatol 1977;113:1529.

Parrish JA et al: Photochemotherapy of vitiligo. Arch Dermatol 1976;112:1531.

Pathak MA: Sunscreens: topical and systemic approaches for protection of acute and chronic sun-induced skin reactions. Dermatologic Clin 1986;4:321.

Pearlman DL, Youngberg B, Engelhard C: Weekly pulse dosing schedule of fluorouracil: a new topical therapy for psoriasis. J Am Acad Dermatol 1986;15:1247.

Peck GL et al: Prolonged remissions of cystic and conglobate acne with 13-cis-retinoic acid. N Engl J Med 1979;300:329.

Peck GL et al: Treatment and prevention of basal cell carcinomas with oral isotretinoin. J Am Acad Dermatol 1988;19:176.

Penneys NS: Gold therapy: Dermatologic uses and toxicities. J Am Acad Dermatol 1979;1:315.

Pochi PE et al: Guidelines for prescribing isotretinoin (Accutane) in the treatment of female acne patients of childbearing potential. J Am Acad Dermatol 1988;19:920.

Pochi PE: Oral retinoids in dermatology. Arch Dermatol 1982;118:57.

Poulin Y, Perry HO, Muller SA: Pemphigus vulgaris: results of treatment with gold as a steroid-sparing agent in a series of thirteen patients. J Am Acad Dermatol 1984;11:851.

Price VH: Topical minoxidil in extensive alopecia areata, including 3-year follow-up. Dermatologica 1987;175(suppl. 2):36.

Provost TT, Farmer ER: Current Therapy in Dermatology 1985–1986. Mosby, 1985.

Reboli AC, Del Bene VE: Oral antibiotic therapy of dermatologic conditions. Dermatol Clin 1988;6:497.

Roenigk HH Jr et al: Methotrexate in psoriasis: revised guidelines. J Am Acad Dermatol 1988;19:145.

Rothman KF, Pochi P: Use of oral and topical agents for acne in pregnancy. J Am Acad Dermatol 1988;19:431.

Sanchez JL, Torres VM: Double-blind efficacy study of selenium sulfide in tinea versicolor. J Am Acad Dermatol 1984;11:235.

Savin RC: Double-blind comparison of 2% ketoconazole cream and placebo in the treatment of tinea versicolor. J Am Acad Dermatol 1986;15:500.

Skinner RB, Rosenberg EW: Double-blind treatment of seborrheic dermatitis with 2% ketoconazole cream. J Am Acad Dermatol 1985;12:852.

Stebben JE: Surgical antiseptics. J Am Acad Dermatol 1983;9:759.

Stern RS et al: Risk of cutaneous carcinoma in patients treated with oral methoxsalen photochemotherapy for psoriasis. N Engl J Med 1979;300:809.

Storrs FJ: Use and abuse of systemic corticosteroid therapy. J Am Acad Dermatol 1979;1:95.

Stoughton RB: Are generic formulations equivalent to trade name topical glucocorticoids? Arch Dermatol 1987; 123:1312.

Thiers BH, Ely H (editors): Dermatologic Therapy I. Dermatol Clin 1988;6(4):497

Thomas JR III, Doyle JA: The therapeutic uses of topical vitamin A acid. J Amer Acad Dermatol 1981;4:505.

Vonderheid EC et al: Long-term efficacy, curative potential, and carcinogenicity of topical mechlorethamine chemotherapy in cutaneous T cell lymphoma. J Am Acad Dermatol 1989;20:416.

Weiss JS et al: Topical tretinoin in the treatment of aging skin. J Am Acad Dermatol 1988;19:169.

Wheeler CE Jr (editor): Antiviral drugs and vaccines for herpes simplex and herpes zoster. Proceedings of a symposium held at the American Academy of Dermatology forty-fourth annual meeting. J Am Acad Dermatol 1988;18:161.

Yawalker SJ, Vischer W: Lamprene (clofazimine) in leprosy. Lepr Rev 1979;50:185.

Dermatologic Surgery

54

Henry H. Roenigk, Jr, MD

The treatment of many benign and malignant growths on the skin is surgical. Neoplasms are frequently biopsied or excised. Surgery is also used to remove unwanted skin, transplant hair, improve the cosmetic appearance of scars, and destroy unwanted pigment, growths, or blood vessels. Cosmetic procedures are becoming more common, and the dermatologist is often trained to perform these procedures. All physicians should be familiar with the advantages of the procedures available and the problems associated with them in order to better advise their patients.

HOW TO SET UP TO DO OFFICE SURGERY

The Room

Most dermatology offices can easily have one room set up for excisional surgery. The room should be larger than the standard examining room and should be used only for skin surgery. There should be adequate space, ventilation, and temperature control. Active perspiration during the procedure may lead to wound contamination and to discomfort for both patient and physician.

High-quality surgical lighting may be mounted on the ceiling or wall or can be achieved with various floor-stand models (eg, Burton lamp).

A high-quality power table is preferable. Separate controls for table height and head elevation should be included. It is helpful if the table can be placed in the Trendelenburg position. Some tables can be rotated 180 degrees on their base (eg, Ritter table). Several dental and podiatry chairs are comfortable.

Shelving and other surfaces should be stainless steel, facilitating cleaning and disinfection. A Mayo stand of adjustable height should be placed close to the operating area. A fully equipped updated emergency kit should be in the operating room whenever surgery is being performed (Table 54–1). Physicians should be familiar with the use of all drugs in emergency situations. Cardiopulmonary resuscitation (CPR) courses should be attended regularly by physicians and office staff.

Table 54–1. Essentials for emergency kit.

Oxygen supply system
"Ambu" resuscitating bag with adult and pediatric masks and tubing for connection to oxygen system
Intravenous equipment
Tourniquet
No. 18 needles and Angiocaths or Intracaths
Tape and arm board
Tubing and 500-mL bags of normal saline and D5W
Scalpel, hemostats, and suture for "cut-down" if needed (these may already be in excision kit)
Headboard to place under patient for cardiac massage
Medications
NaHCO$_3$, prepackaged 50-mL syringes (at least 2)
Epinephrine 1 : 1000 (1-mL ampule) for allergic reactions 1 : 10,000 (10-mL ampule with intracardiac needle)
50% dextrose (50-mL Ristojet ampules) for hypoglycemic reactions
Lidocaine 2% (5-mL syringe, 100 mg)
Aminophylline (10-mL, 250-mg ampules)
Naloxone (0.4 mg/mL), only if narcotics are used before or during surgery
Diazepam (10-mL ampule for intravenous use)
Diphenhydramine (50-mL ampule)

Sterilization & Skin Preparation

Surgical packs should be prepared and autoclaved with steam under pressure. It is best to obtain an autoclave with a separate door for dry heat sterilization (eg, Pelton-Crane). There is less damage to sharp instruments if they are wrapped in aluminum foil and dry-heat sterilized. These instruments may be placed on the open excision pack with a transfer forceps.

Prior to sterilization, all instruments should be scrubbed with ordinary detergent to remove visible debris. Further cleaning of cracks and crevices may be done with ultrasonic cleaners.

Mechanical scrubbing of the skin surface with chlorhexidine solutions or iodophors before surgery adequately decreases the surface bacteria count. Alternatively, 70% isopropyl alcohol may be used. A more effective solution may be obtained by adding 1% iodine to the isopropyl alcohol.

Because of the dangers of AIDS and hepatitis, the dermatologic surgeon and assisting personnel should protect themselves from contact with blood and body fluids. Wearing of proper gowns, masks, and gloves and meticulous attention to disposal and cleaning of instruments are essential.

The Surgical Pack

The surgical pack may be wrapped in suitable cloth material (eg, surgical towels) or in autoclave paper. If autoclave paper is used, the Mayo stand must be covered with a sterile impermeable sheet (eg, Barrier Field) to prevent contamination if the paper becomes moistened (eg, with lidocaine) during the procedure. Autoclave tape should be used to close the pack. This tape changes color when sterilization is complete. A typical surgical pack may contain the following items:

1. Several 4 × 4 gauze sponges.
2. A pointed wooden toothpick for drawing the line of excision.
3. A glass syringe, 5 mL (optional).
4. Towel drapes (disposable fenestrated drapes optional).
5. A No. 3 Bard-Parker handle with centimeter markings on one side.
6. A 4½-inch needle holder (Webster type—smooth jaws).
7. Two or 3 short, curved mosquito hemostats.
8. A small medicine cup (glass or metal, optional).
9. Small tissue forceps with medium teeth.
10. One forceps without teeth (Adson).
11. One short, curved, sharp iris scissors.
12. One or 2 skin hooks (optional).
13. One dissecting scissors (optional).

Disposable plastic syringes (5 mL) without needles attached and 18- and 30-gauge needles may be added to the excision set at the time of surgery. Disposable towel drapes are available with fenestrated holes of various sizes, or one can use a fenestrated drape with adhesive on one side (3M Steri-Drape). The Steri-Drape has the advantage of not allowing blood to run under the drape onto the patient. Draw lines of excision before placing the drape, because anatomic markings are lost at that time. Either gentian violet solution or methylene blue may be poured into a medicine cup for this purpose.

Instruments & Other Additions to Surgical Pack

The following may be added to a routine excisional pack:

1. One No. 15 and one No. 11 Bard-Parker blade.
2. A disposable hot cautery unit (eg, Concept unit) may be used directly. Coagulation of blood vessels can also be achieved by clamping vessels with mosquito hemostats and using an electrocoagulation unit, which should have a ground plate (eg, Bovie or Electricator).

3. Razor blade and razor blade breaker.
4. Suture material, including stapler and staples.

Absorbable sutures for subcutaneous suturing may be added. Synthetic absorbables such as Dexon (Davis & Geck), Vicryl (Ethicon), or chromic catgut may also be used. Nonabsorbable synthetics should be used for skin suturing (either subcuticular or interrupted). There is little reason to use silk suture in skin surgery.

The most commonly used suture materials are 5-0 and 6-0 Prolene or nylon. Prolene is perhaps slightly less reactive than nylon and seems somewhat more stretchable. Most sutures come prepackaged with appropriate-sized needles for the size of suture being used. Staple guns with metal staples are useful for scalp and other areas where sutures must be left in place for longer than 1 week.

EVALUATION OF & INSTRUCTIONS FOR THE SURGICAL PATIENT

A good history and physical examination are essential to preoperative evaluation. For office surgery, an extensive questionnaire is helpful. Blood pressure is especially important, because hypertensive patients frequently bleed profusely, especially when undergoing scalp surgery. Irregularities of pulse should be noted. A record of all allergies and present medications should be made.

Specifically ask if the patient is taking beta-blocking and monoamine oxidase inhibitor drugs. The patient also should be asked for a history of epilepsy, because larger doses of local anesthetic may induce convulsions. It may be prudent to learn if a patient has had hepatitis or falls in a high-risk category for infection with HIV. If the patient has a cardiac pacemaker, electrocoagulation should not be used. The entire skin surface can be examined to rule out bacterial or viral disease at distant locations.

For most dermatologic surgery performed on outpatients with local anesthesia, the patient should have a light breakfast with juice the morning of the procedure. This helps avoid syncope and vomiting. Ingestion of caffeinated beverages the day of the procedure may precipitate hypertension. Ingestion of aspirin or aspirin-containing products within 7–10 days before the procedure may prolong bleeding. Acetaminophen or codeine may be used as substitutes depending on the severity of pain (eg, in patients with severe arthritis).

ANESTHESIA

The selection of an appropriate anesthetic, its proper administration, and attention to preoperative anxiety and postoperative pain are essential to a successful surgical procedure.

Preoperative Medication

For most simple procedures (skin biopsy, excision, or short procedures), no preoperative medication is necessary. For long procedures (hair transplants and dermabrasions) in which much anxiety may be present, preoperative sedation is essential. Reassurance and explanation of the procedure are important. Intramuscular medications such as meperidine (Demerol), 50–100 mg, or diazepam (Valium), 5–10 mg, are useful.

Local Anesthetics

Anesthetics most commonly used in skin surgery are local anesthetics of the amide or ester linkage type. The amide linkage type (lidocaine is the most commonly used) has rapid onset and lasts 45 minutes to 2 hours. The incidence of allergic reactions is extremely low, and toxicity depends upon total accumulated dose over time. The main complications are central nervous system stimulation, convulsions, and cardiotoxicity. Epinephrine is frequently added to lidocaine to prolong local anesthesia. Lidocaine is available in 0.5%, 1%, and 2% solutions with or without epinephrine 1:200,000–1:100,000. Other local anesthetics include etidocaine (Duranest), bupivacaine (Marcaine), mepivacaine (Carbocaine), prilocaine (Citanest), procaine (Novocain), and chloroprocaine (Nesacaine). Etidocaine has a slower onset but more prolonged duration of action (3–5 hours). Epinephrine should not be given to patients receiving monoamine oxidase inhibitors because the interaction can result in extreme hypertension.

Luer-Lok disposable syringes and 30-gauge needles should be used to inject the local anesthetic very superficially (attempt to form a wheal in the tissue). Slow injection causes less pain from the injection. Field block anesthetics are sometimes helpful when treating the fingers, toes, or face.

OFFICE DERMATOLOGIC SURGICAL PROCEDURES

BIOPSIES

The cutaneous biopsy is often vital to the diagnosis of skin diseases such as vasculitis, bullous diseases, malignant tumors, lichen planus, granuloma annulare, adnexal tumors, and cutaneous granulomas.

Selection of the appropriate lesion and site for biopsy is essential. Biopsy of primary lesions is usually best. Biopsy of secondary lesions such as excoriations, fissures, or ulcerations usually is not helpful. A new and fully developed lesion is generally preferred over an old, healing one. When biopsying a blister, it is important to include a portion of the surrounding rim of normal tissue with the specimen. Once the site is selected, the area should be cleansed and locally anesthetized with lidocaine. Frigiderm spray applied to the blister will keep it intact during the biopsy.

Cutaneous Punch

The cutaneous punch (reusable or disposable, size 2–6 mm) should be directed through the skin with a rotary motion to a depth of approximately 4 mm—deep enough to include the entire dermis and some fat. When performing a punch biopsy, tension is held on the skin perpendicular to normal skin lines; when tension is released, the site of the biopsy will form an oval in the direction of the skin lines, giving wound closure a better cosmetic result. At the completion of the procedure, the skin can be closed with a suture that is removed in 5–10 days, depending on the location, or the wound can be left open to heal secondarily.

Excisional Biopsies

Excisional biopsies are useful for larger or deeper lesions not easily removed with a punch. Outline the lesion with gentian violet before anesthesia obscures normal markings. The excision is made along skin lines with a No. 15 scalpel blade. At completion of the procedure, the skin is closed with subcutaneous and skin sutures.

Shave Biopsies

Shave biopsies are usually performed on superficial lesions such as seborrheic keratoses, actinic keratosis, or nevi. The lesion is anesthetized and is raised by pressure between the thumb and the first finger. A single-edged razor blade or No. 11 blade can be used to shave off the lesion. Hemostasis is obtained by using a hot-tipped cautery, trichloroacetic acid, or other hematinic solutions such as solutions of ferric subsulfate or aluminum chloride.

Curettage

Curets come in various sizes with one sharp side used to "scoop" out tissue to be removed. Curettage is often followed by electrodesiccation. Curettage is frequently used for removal of warts, seborrheic keratoses, and basal cell carcinoma. Bleeding can be stopped with electrodesiccation or a topical hematinic agent. The use of curets to treat basal cell carcinoma allows the physician to "feel" the difference between tumor and normal skin. As in the other surgical techniques, tissue removed is always submitted for pathologic examination.

Incisional Biopsies

A dermatologist occasionally employs incisional biopsy for lesions such as keratoacanthoma or melanoma, which may be too large to excise. An elliptic incision is made into the lesion, including some normal adjacent tissue. In this way, an adequate biopsy specimen may be obtained without causing an extensive cosmetic defect.

EXCISIONS

The care given to planning a good surgical excision will be rewarded with a fine cosmetic result and a happy patient. The direction of the incision should correspond to Langer's skin tension lines or to natural wrinkle lines. Lesser scars are achieved by placing incision lines at right angles to the direction of muscle pull, thus helping to prevent hypertrophic scars. The use of various W- or Z-fashion wound closures allows a large scar more flexibility and minimizes stretching of scars. Proper hemostasis and prevention of infection by use of sterile technique are important. Damage to wound edges may occur if tissue is crushed with a forceps or allowed to dry out. Prophylactic antibiotics are seldom necessary except for extensive surgery (eg, scalp reductions). Avoid tension in wound closures by undermining subcutaneous tissue and using subcutaneous absorbable sutures. Large spaces in wounds can lead to hematoma formation and infection.

Excision of Benign Lesions

Excision of benign lesions such as nevi, fibromas, xanthelasmas, and epidermal cysts needs only a 0.5- to 1-mm border of normal skin. The use of a punch biopsy followed by closure often gives the best cosmetic result with the least amount of tissue removed. More often, elliptic excisions are preferred, especially for lesions larger than 5 mm.

Excision of Malignant Lesions

Malignant lesions of skin such as basal cell or squamous cell carcinoma need borders of 1–2 mm depending on clinical features. Microscopic control of borders (eg, Mohs' fresh tissue microscopically controlled chemosurgery) is very helpful in dealing with malignant tumors (see below). Location and histologic type of the tumor influence the choice of technique, as do the size of the border of tumor-free tissue and likelihood of recurrence. For example, carcinomas in the nasolabial fold and perioral area frequently penetrate deeper than is clinically evident, and the exact border of sclerosing basal cell carcinomas is difficult to determine clinically. These basal cell carcinomas are best treated with Mohs' chemosurgery rather than excision or curettage and

desiccation. Carcinomas arising de novo from burn scars, chronic draining sinuses, or ulcers are often more aggressive and require more extensive surgery and search for possible metastasis. The management of malignant melanoma is discussed elsewhere.

Microscopically Controlled Excisions (Mohs's Chemosurgery)

In the 1930s, Frederic Mohs developed a method for fixing tissue in situ without altering its architecture. Application of a paste containing 40% zinc chloride in stibnite was painful, but fixation in situ permitted scalpel excision of tissue in a bloodless field.

Subsequently, the same excellent results were obtained without the use of a chemical fixative. In the fresh-tissue technique, the layers are excised, followed by complete microscopic examination by a modified frozen-section technique repeated as often as necessary to remove the residual tumor in serial stages (Figs 54–1 and 54–2). The fresh-tissue method is quicker, and the patient experiences less pain.

Lesions to be treated by fresh-tissue Mohs surgery are ordinarily biopsied first for diagnosis. This biopsy should be processed by routine paraffin-embedded histologic methods and stained with hematoxylin and eosin stains. The Mohs technique traces that cancer through the skin until the tumor-free plane is reached. This is specialized surgery requiring a team of nurses, technicians, and a dermatologist with special training in the technique. In Mohs' micrographic surgery, the area is anesthetized by regional or local block and as

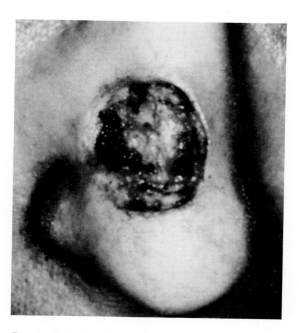

Figure 54–1. Basal cell carcinoma of nose after several stages of Mohs's chemosurgery.

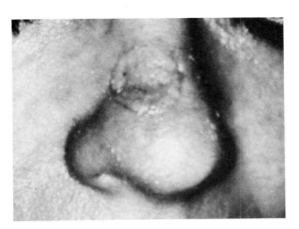

Figure 54–2. Skin graft used to repair defect created by Mohs's chemosurgery.

much of the clinically detectable cancer as possible is scraped away with a small curet. A tissue section of the remaining base is excised in a saucerlike manner, and hemostasis is obtained. The excised tissue is cut into 1-cm^2 pieces, marked, and mapped. Frozen sections are cut from each section. The histochemical staining process does not distort the dye markings. On microscopic examination of the undersurface of the tissue, the surgeon pinpoints the exact position on the tissue map of any remaining cancer and returns to the patient to excise additional tissue from that site.

Microscopic control allows the Mohs surgeon to formulate a 3-dimensional view of tumor extension, often extending a considerable distance beyond clinically apparent margins, yet the Mohs technique minimizes removal of normal tissue. Mohs surgery offers the highest cure rates with the most difficult tumors, especially recurrent tumors.

DERMABRASION

Dermabrasion consists of planing off the epidermis and a portion of the dermis using a motor- or pneumatic-driven metal brush or diamond fraise. Mild preoperative sedation is necessary, but anesthesia is obtained with ethyl chloride spray or 1% lidocaine by injection (local or field blocks). Postoperative care includes application of special hydrocolloid dressings (Vigilon). This dressing is replaced with a new Vigilon dressing each day. Erythema persists for about 30–60 days, and sunlight exposure is restricted for 2 months.

Indications for dermabrasion include acne scars, tattoos, multiple trichoepitheliomas, syringomas, traumatic scar revision, certain types of epidermal nevus, rhinophyma, multiple actinic keratoses, and many others.

Complications can include hyperpigmentation, hy-

popigmentation, keloid or hypertrophic scar formation, milia, persistent erythema, and secondary infection.

HAIR TRANSPLANTS & SCALP REDUCTIONS

Hair transplantation is possible because hair follicles from a hair-producing area (occipital scalp) will continue to grow when transplanted to a balding area (frontal scalp). After local anesthetic, recipient plugs prepared with 3.5- to 4-mm round punches are filled with donor plugs 0.5 mm larger, generally taken from the occipital or lateral scalp. After removal of the plugs, they are placed in sterile saline and all hair, foreign matter, and extraneous fragments of fat are removed before reimplanting in the recipient area. This is done in a carefully preplanned method to create a natural-appearing area of hair growth. Dressings are applied that can be removed in 24 hours. Small crusts that fall off in about 2 weeks form on each plug. The hairs in transplanted plugs fall out soon after the procedures; the follicular apparatus persists, so that new hair will reach the scalp surface in 2–3 months following surgery (Fig 54–3).

Scalp reduction is a procedure in which large areas of bald scalp (12 × 4 cm or greater) may be removed, thus reducing the need for hair transplantation. The procedure, in effect, stretches hair-bearing portions of scalp over an excised bald area. Scalp reduction can give a more natural and full appearance to scalp hair than transplanted hair alone. Scalp reduction requires special skills and assistance. Tissue expanders may be implanted under the scalp prior to surgery in order to facilitate closure.

SKIN GRAFTS

Skin grafts are defined by their thickness: full thickness, split thickness, epidermal pinch graft, or composite grafts of skin with muscle, cartilage, etc. Grafts are usually used in wounds that cannot be closed by first intention. The cosmetic results are always less satisfactory than with excisional surgery. Full- and split-thickness skin grafts can be performed as office procedures by dermatologic surgeons specially trained in the procedure.

Pinch grafts may be used in an attempt to re-epithelialize leg ulcers when there is good granulation tissue. Grafts 4–10 mm in diameter are taken from anesthetized skin (usually the upper thigh) by pinching up a small amount of skin with the tip of a small needle and slicing with a scalpel or razor blade. The grafts are placed in sterile saline and transferred to the ulcer bed with a 2-mm space between grafts. An adhesive spray and then a semipermeable dressing (OpSite) are applied with edges extending beyond the margin of the ulcer. Gauze and an elastic dressing

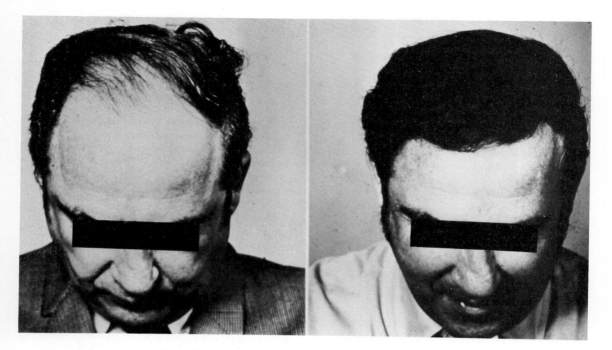

Figure 54–3. Male pattern alopecia before and after hair transplantation.

cover the wound, which is not disturbed for 3–4 days. Strict bed rest is necessary. Pinch grafts can be examined through the Op-Site, and fluid accumulating under the dressing can be drained. Infection can occur.

Dressings may be removed in 5–6 days or left in place if there is no infection. Careful cleansing with alcohol allows the wound to form a firm crust that will come off in 2–3 weeks. The grafts will extend to the skin of the adjacent graft and fill up the ulcer.

LIPOSUCTION

The removal of unwanted fat in such areas as the chin, abdomen, thighs, buttocks, handlebar areas, knees, etc, has become a popular technique in a society that values thin body contours as a beauty feature. Although some surgeons perform liposuction under general anesthesia, the procedure can be done safely under local anesthesia if only small areas are treated.

A patient with good skin turgor who is healthy and at near-normal weight is an ideal candidate for liposuction. Aspiration of fat is done with various-sized cannulas attached to a suction machine. To achieve a good result, the physician must know the proper amount of fat to remove. The fat removed can sometimes be injected into areas of fat atrophy as a method of soft tissue augmentation. Special training is necessary to perform this operation also.

REFERENCES

Epstein E Sr, Epstein E Jr: *Skin Surgery,* 6th ed. Saunders, 1988.
Roenigk RK, Roenigk HH Jr: *Dermatologic Surgery: Prin-* *ciples and Practice.* Marcel Dekker, 1988.
Stegman SJ, Tromovitch TA, Glogan RG: *Basis of Dermatologic Surgery.* Year Book, 1981.

Physical Methods of Therapy in Dermatology

55

Ervin Epstein, Sr, MD, Ervin Epstein, Jr, MD, & Mark V. Dahl, MD

By its location, the skin is accessible to various physical agents that can be used to treat skin disease. These include ultraviolet radiation, x-rays, other ionizing radiations, cryotherapy, electrosurgery, and lasers. This chapter presents background information. Indications for their use and specific treatment regimens are discussed under specific diseases. Referral to physicians with special training in many of these physical methods is prudent.

ULTRAVIOLET RADIATION

Ultraviolet radiation can be used to treat skin disorders such as psoriasis, atopic dermatitis, acne, and vitiligo. Ultraviolet radiation is electromagnetic radiation emitted by the sun and by various artificial light sources (Fig 55–1). Ultraviolet radiation penetrates and interacts with molecules in the skin such as DNA, RNA, and proteins. The radiation raises the molecule to a higher energy state and may cause a chemical change resulting in a photobiologic response. How ultraviolet radiation helps so many skin diseases is speculative. Different effects may help different diseases. There is no unifying reason why ultraviolet radiation should be considered good treatment for skin disease, but empirically the treatments often are very beneficial.

As discussed in Chapter 38 on photosensitivity disorders, the ultraviolet spectrum is divided into 3 parts. The UVC band consists of wavelengths between 200 and 290 nm. These wavelengths do not reach the earth's surface; they are absorbed instead by the ozone layer. The UVB band consists of wavelengths between 290 and 320 nm—the erythemogenic wavelengths that cause sunburn. The UVA band consists of wavelengths from 320 to 400 nm. These wavelengths easily pass through window glass. Both UVA and UVB radiation are used to treat skin disorders.

Sunlight can be used for treatment of skin disease, but it is difficult to control the dose delivered. Too little radiation may not be enough for effective treatment, and too much risks phototoxic reactions such as sunburn. Furthermore, relatively long exposures to sunlight are necessary to treat some diseases, and work or weather conditions may interfere with therapy. To obtain accurate graded doses, therefore, artificial sources of ultraviolet radiation often are used.

Sources emitting UVB include both mercury vapor lamps and fluorescent tube sunlamps. The gas molecules between the electrodes are ionized by electrons passing between them. The excited ions emit radiation. The exact spectrum of light emitted can be adjusted by the use of various phosphors in the source.

In practice, several fluorescent sunlamps are mounted parallel to one another on the walls of a cabinet. Patients needing treatment enter the cabinet,

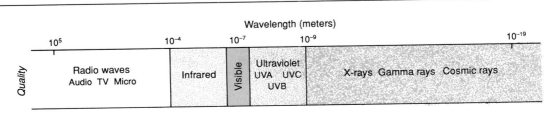

Figure 55–1. Electromagnetic spectrum.

and the lamps are turned on for varying periods of time depending upon skin type, the skin disease being treated, the number of previous treatments, the configuration of the booth, and the ultraviolet flux of the bulbs. The object is to use as high a dose of ultraviolet radiation as possible without producing erythema.

Daily exposure of the skin to increasing increments of UVB often induces complete remission of psoriasis after 3–4 weeks (see Chapter 41). Ointments or creams containing crude coal tar or its derivatives can be used to sensitize the skin and make it more permeable to radiation.

UVA is commonly produced by similar-appearing bulbs with different phosphors. These have peak emissions between 355 and 365 nm. UVA bulbs too are typically mounted in parallel in a cabinet phototherapy unit. Ordinarily, huge doses of UVA are required to produce discernible photobiologic reactions. For this reason, treatment with UVA is usually combined with administration of a psoralen drug. The drug is activated by photons in the UVA range to form photoadducts between DNA base pairs. This suppresses DNA synthesis and cell division. UVA also interacts with RNA, protein, and other cellular constituents.

Phototherapy is not without risk. Patients undergoing phototherapy with ultraviolet radiation may experience a painful sunburnlike reaction. Ultraviolet radiation damages the skin in the same ways as natural sunlight. Side effects of exposure to UVA and UVB include aging, wrinkling, pigmentary abnormalities, actinic keratoses, and skin cancers, particularly basal and squamous cell carcinomas. In general, the increased risks associated with phototherapy for skin disease have not been excessive, and the potential benefits often outweigh the risks.

Patients undergoing phototherapy should protect their eyes by wearing protective goggles opaque to UVA and UVB radiation while receiving treatment. Patients undergoing PUVA therapy must continue to protect their eyes from ambient UVA for at least 24 hours (preferably more) after each treatment. Because the psoralen can remain in the lens for long periods of time, it can interact with UVA there to cause cataracts.

IONIZING RADIATION

Superficial x-ray radiation, generated at 80–120 kV, is used chiefly to treat basal and squamous cell carcinomas of the face. The absorbed dose is measured in units called grays, an SI unit that has supplanted the older rad (radiation absorbed dose). One gray (Gy) is 1 joule (J) of absorbed energy per kilogram of tissue. One centigray (cGy) is equivalent to 1 rad. When total doses of 4000–5000 cGy are administered in approximately 10 treatments to a basal or squamous carcinoma and to a well-shielded surrounding area of clinically uninvolved skin, cure rates of about 95% are achieved. An acute radiodermatitis is produced by this dose, but characteristically it fades and leaves a scar with varying degrees of atrophy.

Most basal and squamous cell carcinomas are treated surgically by excision. However, in occasional patients x-ray radiation may be the treatment of choice. For example, elderly patients may prefer this treatment modality because it is nontraumatic and because it often better preserves the anatomic structures with a better cosmetic result, especially for cancers on the nose. X-ray radiation is also used to treat eyelid cancers.

Other cutaneous tumors may also be treated with superficial irradiation. These tumors include Kaposi's sarcoma and cutaneous T cell lymphomas (mycosis fungoides). Delivery of 3500–4000 cGy of electron beam irradiation to the whole skin surface may actually cure some patients with early cutaneous T cell lymphomas. Because the relatively heavy electrons penetrate tissue much less well than x-rays, these large doses do not damage extracutaneous tissues. Electron beam or deep orthovoltage irradiation may also be the most effective treatment for local palliation of tumors of cutaneous T cell lymphomas.

Various inflammatory cutaneous diseases also respond to superficial x-ray radiation, but the advent of effective drug therapy has markedly reduced the frequency with which it is used for inflammatory lesions. Grenz ray therapy consists of irradiation of 10–15 kV and is safer than therapy with deep x-rays. Grenz rays penetrate only the most superficial layers of the skin. Doses of 50–100 cGy are given each week for a total dose of approximately 1000 cGy to any one area during any one course of treatment.

CRYOTHERAPY

Skin cells can be destroyed by freezing. Liquid nitrogen is the cryogenic agent most frequently used for this purpose, though dry ice and other agents have occasionally been employed. Maximum tissue destruction occurs if the skin is frozen quickly but allowed to thaw slowly. Liquid nitrogen is typically delivered to a skin lesion by touching it with a cotton-tipped applicator soaked with the cryogen or by spraying liquid nitrogen from a special cryotherapy unit. The depth of freezing can often be judged by the diameter of the ice ball that forms in the treatment area. If more careful monitoring is necessary, thermocouple probes may be inserted under the skin to measure the depth of freezing more directly.

Tumors and skin lesions that can be destroyed using cryotherapy include warts, seborrheic keratoses, actinic keratoses, lentigos, skin tags, and basal cell carcinomas. Application of liquid nitrogen causes some pain, but it is usually well tolerated. Local anesthetics are not routinely necessary unless cryotherapy is extensive, such as that used to treat a basal cell carcinoma. Typically there is another burst of pain as the frozen tissue thaws. Treated lesions typically necrose. Bullae may occur on occasion and may be blood-filled. Treated sites typically heal within 2 weeks. The cosmetic scar is often quite acceptable and preferable to scars resulting from destruction using electrosurgery or other modalities.

Complications of cryotherapy include pain, infection, scarring, and damaged underlying nerves, especially on the fingers. Pigmentary disturbances are common, so cryotherapy should be used with caution in patients with dark skin. Because swelling occurs where cryotherapy is used, rings should be removed from fingers before treatment of lesions on the digits.

Cryotherapy may also be used to peel the skin. A "slush" consisting of acetone and dry ice can be applied to the skin for short periods of time as a poultice. Alternatively, the skin can be sprayed lightly with liquid nitrogen using special cryospray equipment.

ELECTROSURGERY

Electric currents can be used to "burn off" various skin lesions. Destruction can be by electrodesiccation, coagulation, electroexcision, cauterization, or electrolysis.

1. ELECTRODESICCATION

Electrodesiccation is performed with a monopolar current. A desiccating needle is inserted into the lesion or held a few millimeters above it. The current is activated and flows to and through the lesion. With many small tumors, this may be sufficient for cure. However, with larger growths, curettage is usually also employed. The bulk of the lesion is removed with a curet under local anesthesia to provide a specimen for histologic examination. The base can then be electrodesiccated. Because the electrodesiccating current does not penetrate deeply, prior curettage increases the efficiency of the procedure. For treating most basal and some squamous cell carcinomas, 3 "rounds" of curettage and electrodesiccation often are recommended. Bleeding may be controlled by simple electrodesiccation or the use of hemostatic chemicals. Electrodesiccation also can be used to remove warts, vascular tumors such as pyogenic granulomas, keratoses of all types, skin tags, and other benign lesions.

2. ELECTROCOAGULATION

In contrast to electrodesiccation, electrocoagulation uses a bipolar current. The current flows through the body from the lesion being treated to a grounding plate, usually inserted under the patient's back or thigh. Electrocoagulation achieves faster hemostasis than electrodesiccation.

3. ELECTROEXCISION

Bipolar current also can be used to cut tissue. Electroexcision is often preferred for vascular lesions because it cauterizes bleeding vessels as it cuts. A local anesthetic is typically injected beneath and around the periphery of the lesion. A starting incision is burned around the lesion at one end. The tissue is raised with a hook or a toothed forceps, and the block is separated from the underlying tissue by a horizontal burning cut. After the specimen has been completely removed, any residual bleeding can be controlled by electrodesiccation or by clamping and tying. The wound is allowed to heal by secondary intention. The epidermis and granulation tissue grow in from the sides and from the depths of the defect. In most locations, the wound heals with a linear scar despite the originally round excision, and grafting is usually unnecessary. Rates of healing vary but usually are complete within 1 month.

4. ELECTROCAUTERY

Electrocautery employs a heated electrical tip similar to that of a soldering iron. The heat chars the tumor or other tissue and cauterizes the lesion and weeping blood vessels at the same time. Electrocautery thus provides a way to destroy tissue with heat.

5. ELECTROLYSIS

Electrolysis is used to remove unwanted hair by destroying the bulb from which it grows. A fine needle is inserted along the shaft of the hair, and a direct current is passed through the needle. Properly performed, the treated follicle can be destroyed permanently with minimal scarring. Unfortunately, the large number of follicles makes electrolysis unsuitable for any but clearly delimited areas of the skin such as small areas of the face or breasts.

LASERS

When electrons in the laser medium excited by electrical current to higher orbits return to the ground state, photons of energy are released. These can start a chain reaction, and light can be emitted as a monochromatic (single wave length), coherent (in phase), highly collimated (nondivergent) beam. Upon reach-

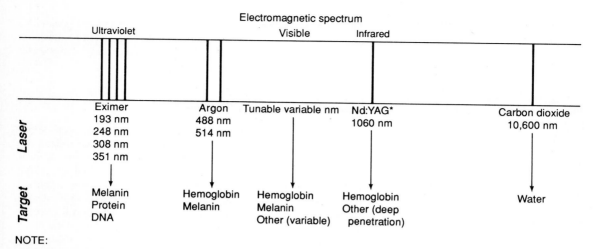

Figure 55–2. Emission spectra of lasers.

ing its target, the laser beam interacts with molecules in the tissue to cause tissue destruction.

The most common types of lasers in use are carbon dioxide lasers and argon lasers. There are also ruby lasers, helium-neon (HeNe) lasers, neodymium-yttrium-aluminum-garnet (Nd:YAG) lasers, and tunable dye lasers (Fig 55–2).

The most versatile laser system is the CO_2 laser. It can be operated in a focused or defocused mode. When defocused, the target area is approximately 2 mm and the beam causes surface vaporization and instantaneous cell destruction. The heating and destruction occur so quickly that very little heat is conducted to adjacent or deeper cells, and the zone of injury is small. The depth of penetration is only about 0.1 mm, and the zone of tissue destruction can therefore be carefully controlled.

In its focused mode, the beam diameter is only 0.1 mm and the power density approaches 50,000 W/cm². In this mode, the laser beam will cut tissue. The depth and precision of the incision depend upon the speed with which the laser beam is moved along the tissue. Because it generates heat, the laser actually sterilizes the cut as it goes and seals blood vessels so that the surgical field is bloodless unless a large blood vessel is encountered. Because the heat is conducted to only a slight extent, the tissue is preserved and can be subsequently examined histologically. Pain is minimal because nerve endings are sealed rather than frayed. Lymphatics are sealed, which limits postoperative swelling and theoretically may prevent dissemination of tumor excised by this technique.

The CO_2 laser can be used to remove tattoos. It

destroys tissue in a bloodless field, so that the pigment can be easily visualized as treatment proceeds. Warts can also be destroyed by this modality, but the plume of smoke generated may contain infectious particles.

The argon laser is used to treat vascular lesions because the red color of oxygenated hemoglobin selectively absorbs the blue-green color of the argon laser beam. Port wine stains may be treated in this way. It causes considerable lightening of dark port wine stains and flattens blebs and nodules. Telangiectases can also be treated with the argon laser, as can spider angiomas, venous lakes, and certain pigmented lesions such as lentigos.

Flashlamp-pulsed tunable dye lasers, as the name suggests, are tunable; ie, the wavelength of output can be adjusted to match the peak absorption wavelength of the target tissue. These lasers emit energy in short bursts that allow destruction of target tissue but minimize damage to surrounding tissues from heat diffusion. These lasers are especially useful for treatment of port wine stains.

Laser treatment is not without risk. The CO_2 laser beam is invisible, so the potential for damage to eyes is great. Typically, a small red helium-neon laser beam is associated with the CO_2 laser and coaxial with it, so that its red light marks the area being struck by the CO_2 laser beam. Even so, everyone in the room should wear full wraparound eye goggles. Because the beam generates heat, care must be taken to prevent fire, especially on surgical dressings. Wet dressings placed around the surgical site protect adjacent normal tissue and reduce the chances for ignition. Inflammatory solvents should not be used.

REFERENCES

Elton RF: Complications of cutaneous cryosurgery. J Am Acad Dermatol 1983;8:513.

Epstein E, Epstein E Jr: *Skin Surgery.* Saunders, 1987.

Goldschmidt H: *Physical Modalities in Dermatologic Therapy.* Springer-Verlag, 1978.

Roenigk RK, Roenigk HH Jr: *Dermatologic Surgery: Principles and Practice.* Marcel Dekker, 1988.

Tan OT, Morelli JG: Lasers in dermatology. Curr Probl Dermatol 1989;1:7.

Tan OT, Sherwood K, Gilchrest BA: Treatment of children with port-wine stains using the flashlamp-pulsed tunable dye laser. N Engl J Med 1989;320:416.

Wheeland RG, Bailin PL: Dermatologic applications of the argon and carbon dioxide lasers. Curr Concepts Skin Dis 1984;5:5.

Zacarian SA: *Cryosurgery for Skin Cancer and Cutaneous Disorders.* Mosby, 1984.

Glossary

Fredrick S. Fish, MD

Abrasion: The superficial loss of epithelium, usually by mechanical friction, that results in oozing and crusting.

Abscess: A well-demarcated inflammatory nodule, usually of infectious cause, containing polymorphonuclear leukocytes (pus).

Acantholysis: Loss of cohesion between epidermal cells or adnexal keratinocytes due to faulty formation of intercellular bridges or loss of intercellular binding substances.

Acanthosis: Increased thickness of the epidermis caused by hyperplasia of the spinous layer.

Acne: A chronic inflammation of the pilosebaceous units primarily of the face and trunk that occurs most frequently in adolescents and consists of comedones, papules, nodules, cysts, or pustules.

Acrochordon: A pedunculated fibrovascular papilloma or skin tag.

Actinic keratosis: Single or multiple discrete, rough keratotic macules or papules that occur on sun-damaged skin.

Adenoma: Hypertrophy or tumefaction of a gland.

Adnexa (of skin): The cutaneous structures that make up the hair, nails, and sebaceous, eccrine, and apocrine glands.

Albinism: The inherited inability to manufacture melanin. There are several types of albinism, each with different defects in melanin production.

Allergens: Antigens that induce allergic reactions.

Allergy: An altered state of immune reactivity, usually denoting hypersensitivity.

Alopecia: Loss of hair in any amount.

Alternative complement pathway: The system of activation of the complement pathway through involvement of properdin factor D, properdin factor B, and C3b, finally activating C3. Also called the properdin pathway.

Anaphylaxis: A reaction of immediate hypersensitivity that results from release of mediators from mast cells by cytotropic antibodies following exposure to antigen.

Anergy: Inability to react to common skin test antigens.

Angioedema: A large area of soft tissue swelling of skin from edema; usually related to vasodilatation.

Angioma: A tumor made up of blood vessels or lymph vessels.

Anhidrosis: Absence of ability to sweat.

Annular: Ring-shaped.

Antibody: An immunoglobulin molecule with a specific amino acid sequence that can combine with the antigen which stimulated its production.

Antifungal: An agent that is destructive to fungi or that suppresses the growth or reproduction of fungi.

Antigen: A substance capable of inducing a detectable immune response.

Antihistamine: A drug that counteracts the action of histamine.

Antinuclear antibodies (ANA): Antibodies directed against nuclear constituents; present in patients with various rheumatoid diseases, particularly systemic lupus erythematosus.

Aphthae: Inflammatory ulcers of the oral mucosa that usually appear on an erythematous base.

Aplasia: Lack of development of an organ or tissue.

Apocrine: A type of glandular secretion in which the apical portion of the secreting cell is cast off along with the secreted products.

Appendages: In dermatology, nail plates and hair shafts.

Arcuate: Curved.

Athlete's foot: A lay term for superficial fungal infections of the feet.

Atopy: A clinical hypersensitivity state with a hereditary predisposition.

Atrophy: A wasting away or diminution in size of a cell, tissue, or organ.

Auspitz's sign: Pinpoint bleeding observed when the scale of a lesion of psoriasis is forcibly removed.

Autoimmunity: Immunity to self-antigens.

B cell: A type of lymphocyte that can differentiate into plasma cells.

Balanitis: Inflammation of the glans penis.

Baldness: Absence of hair from the scalp.

Ballooning: Intracellular edema of keratinocytes leading to loss of stain affinity (pallor) and later cellular rupture with formation of multiloculated intraepidermal vesicles.

Bamboo hair: Abnormality of the hair shaft in Netherton's syndrome consisting of periodic invaginations.

Basal cells: Germinative cells of the epidermis found along the basal layer of the epidermis.

Beau's lines: Temporary transverse depressions of nail plates that move from the matrix to the free edge as the nail grows. They may develop during a serious illness.

Benign: Not malignant.

Blackhead: The darkened bit of sebum and keratin at the pilosebaceous ostium—a lay term for open comedo.

Blue nevus: A collection of intradermal melanocytes with a unique histopathologic appearance that produce a bluish or blue-black papule or nodule.

Bockhart's impetigo: A superficial form of folliculitis.

Boil: See Furuncle.

Bowen's disease: Intraepidermal squamous cell carcinoma.

Bromhidrosis: A condition caused by apocrine sweat that has become foul-smelling secondary to bacterial decomposition.

Bromoderma: A usually pustular skin eruption due to ingestion of bromides.

Bubo: An enlarged and inflamed lymph node, particularly in the axilla or groin, due to such infections as lymphogranuloma venereum, plague, tuberculosis, or syphilis.

Bulla: A fluid-filled blister, usually 2 cm or more in diameter.

Burrow: An excavation in the stratum corneum of variable size and shape that houses a parasite.

Café au lait spots: Pigmented brown patches seen in neurofibromatosis and other genodermatoses.

Calabar swelling: Posterior cervical adenopathy seen in association with loiasis.

Calcifying epithelioma of Malherbe: A neoplasm of the hair apparatus (now called pilomatrixoma).

Calcinosis cutis: The pathologic condition in which abnormal amounts of calcium are deposited in the skin.

Callus: Hypertrophy of the stratum corneum in localized areas, especially on the hands and feet.

Calor: Heat.

Candida: A genus of imperfect fungi characterized by yeast cells, mycelia, pseudomycelia, and blastospores.

Canker sore: Ulceration chiefly of the mouth and lips; also called aphthous ulcer.

Capillary hemangioma: A benign neoplasm made up primarily of capillary blood vessels.

Carbuncle: A necrotizing staphylococcal infection of skin and subcutaneous tissue composed of a cluster of furuncles.

Carcinoma: A malignant growth of epithelial cells that tends to invade surrounding tissues and give rise to metastases.

Carcinoma in situ: Limitation of a malignant process to the place of origin.

Carotenemia: Yellowing of the skin resembling jaundice caused by excess carotene in the skin.

Carpet tack scale: The spiked undersurface of the scale that can be removed from affected follicular orifices in well-developed lesions of discoid lupus erythematosus.

Catagen: The brief stage of the hair growth cycle in which growth stops.

Cauterization: Application of a caustic substance, electric current, or heat to destroy tissue.

Cavernous hemangioma: A neoplasm composed of large blood vessels that lies in the subcutaneous fat and deep dermis.

Cayenne pepper spots: Tiny red petechiae often associated with capillaritis.

Cellulitis: Purulent inflammation of the subcutaneous tissues, usually caused by bacteria.

Chancre: A papular lesion occurring at the site of entry of infection in the skin in diseases including syphilis and tuberculosis.

Cheilitis: Inflammation affecting the lips.

Chloasma: Hyperpigmentation, especially on the face, that can occur with pregnancy and increased estrogen states.

Chloracne: An acneiform eruption caused by exposure to chlorinated hydrocarbon products.

Chronic: Persisting over a long period of time.

Clavus: A corn.

Clubbing: A proliferative change of soft tissue near the terminal phalanges of the fingers or toes.

Cold cream: A pharmaceutical and cosmetic formulation of animal fat or mineral oil and a sodium salt. The vanishing quality is achieved by the addition of dispersing agents.

Cold sore: A lay term for herpes simplex infection, most often of the lips, which is often recurrent and which follows an upper respiratory infection.

Collagen: The main supportive protein of skin, tendon, bone, cartilage, and connective tissue.

Collodion baby: Infant with (usually) an ichthyotic condition that appears as if painted with collodion and distorted by the tight grip of the material.

Colloid milium: A papular dermatosis that usually occurs in sun-damaged skin on the face and consists of degenerated collagen.

Comedo: A plug in an excretory duct of the skin that often has a dark discoloration and is commonly referred to as a blackhead.

Compound nevus: A collection of benign melanocytes both at the dermal-epidermal junction and within the dermis.

Condyloma acuminatum (pl: condylomata acuminata): A soft papilloma commonly seen in the genital region caused by infection with human papilloma virus (genital wart).

Corn: A horny induration and thickening of the stratum corneum produced by friction and pressure that forms a conical mass pointing down into the dermis, producing pain and irritation.

Cream: A suspension of oil in water, usually with a thick consistency.

CREST phenomenon: Calcinosis, Raynaud's phenomenon, esophageal dysmotility, sclerodactyly, and telangiectasia—occurs in a subset of patients with progressive systemic sclerosis.

Crust: An outer layer of solid material formed by drying of a bodily exudate or secretion.

Cryoglobulin: An abnormal globulin that precipitates at low temperatures and redissolves upon warming to body temperature.

Cryotherapy: The therapeutic use of cold, such as freezing warts of actinic keratoses with liquid nitrogen.

Curet: An instrument with a spoon- or loop-shaped tip used to remove abnormal tissue growths.

Curettage: The removal of tissue with a curet.

Cutis: The skin.

Cyst: Any closed cavity or sac that contains a liquid or semisolid material.

Dandruff: A common term used for scaling of the scalp.

Darier's sign: Urtication and itching that occurs after stroking or rubbing lesions of urticaria pigmentosa.

Decubitus ulcer: Bedsore.

Degranulation: A process whereby cytoplasmic granules of cells discharge their contents.

Delayed hypersensitivity: A cell-mediated immune reaction that can be elicited by intradermal injection of antigen, with a subsequent cellular infiltrate and edema that are maximal between 24 and 48 hours after antigen challenge.

Delusions of parasitosis: An erroneous belief that skin is infested with parasites. Most patients are obsessional personalities with apparent monosymptomatic hypochondriasis.

Demodex folliculorum: A mite found in the hair follicles and in sebaceous secretions of humans, especially of the face and nose.

Depigmentation: The removal of pigment, generally melanin.

Depilatory: A chemical agent for removing or destroying hair.

Dermabrasion: Surgical removal of the epidermis and as much of the dermis as necessary by mechanical means using wire brushes or diamond fraises on a high- or low-speed hand-held power unit. This technique is used to remove scars, tattoos, pigmented nevi, or other irregularities of the skin.

Dermatitis: Inflammation of the skin.

Dermatofibroma: A dermal nodule occurring most frequently on the extremities and which is composed of fibroblasts, collagen, capillaries, and histiocytes.

Dermatoglyphics: Patterns of skin ridges on the fingers, palms, toes, and soles.

Dermatographia: Urtication induced by moderately firm stroking or scratching of the skin with a dull instrument.

Dermatome: 1. An instrument for cutting thin pieces of skin for skin grafting. 2. The area of skin supplied with afferent nerve fibers by a single posterior spinal root.

Dermatophytes: Superficial fungi that infect the skin; usually caused by the fungi *Microsporum, Epidermophyton,* and *Trichophyton.*

Dermatophytid: A secondary skin eruption that is an expression of hypersensitivity to a dermatophyte.

Dermoid: Resembling the skin.

Desmosome: A bipartite structure that forms the site of attachment between keratinocytes.

Diascope: A glass or clear plastic plate, usually a microscopic slide, that is pressed against the skin to observe the skin after the blood vessels are emptied.

Digitate: Having fingerlike processes.

Dolor: Pain.

Drug eruption: A skin rash caused by a pharmacologic agent.

Duct: A tube with well-defined walls, especially for the passage of secretions or excretions.

Dyskeratotic cells: Prematurely cornified keratinocytes that have eosinophilic cytoplasm and small dark-staining nuclei.

Ecchymosis: A blue or purple hemorrhagic patch in the skin or mucous membrane.

Eccrine: Pertaining to the common sweat gland and its related structures.

Ecthyma: A shallow ulcerative skin infection caused by bacteria that often results in scarring.

Ectoderm: The outermost of the 3 primary germ layers of the embryo. From it are developed the epidermis and epidermal tissues such as the nails, hair, and glands of the skin.

Ectothrix: A fungus that grows inside the hair shaft and produces a sheath of arthrospores on the outside of the hair shaft.

Eczema: A superficial inflammatory process involving the epidermis characterized by itching, redness, minute papules and vesicles, oozing, weeping, crusting, and later scaling, lichenification, and pigmentary changes.

Edema: The accumulation of excessive fluid in the skin.

Elastic fibers: Connective tissue fibers synthesized by fibroblasts that help the skin return to its normal position after stretching.

Elastosis: Degeneration of elastic tissue.

Electrocautery: 1. An apparatus for cauterizing tissue consisting of a platinum wire in a holder that is heated by an electric current. 2. The process of destruction of tissue by electrically produced heat.

Electrocoagulation: Coagulation of tissue produced by a biterminal high-frequency electric current.

Electrodesiccation: Dehydration and destruction of tissue by a high-frequency electric current.

Electrolysis: Use of galvanic electric current to remove excess body hair by destroying the follicle.

Embolus: Blood clot or other solid plug brought by the blood from a vessel and from a distant site forced into a smaller blood vessel and causing obstruction of the circulation.

Emollient: An agent that softens or smooths the skin.

Emulsion: A preparation of one liquid distributed in small globules throughout the body of a second liquid.

Endothelium: The layer of cells that lines the cavities of the blood and lymph vessels, the heart, and the serous cavities of the body.

Endothrix: A dermatophyte whose growth and spore production are confined chiefly within the shaft of the hair, without formation of conspicuous spores on the outside of the hair shaft.

Entoderm (also endoderm): The innermost of the 3 primary germ layers of the embryo. The epithelium of the pharynx, respiratory tract, digestive tract, bladder, and urethra are derived from this layer.

Eosinophilic: Readily stainable with eosin.

Ephelis (pl: ephelides): Freckle.

Epidermis: The layer of the skin that covers the dermis and contains the stratum basale, stratum spinosum, stratum granulosum, stratum lucidum, and stratum corneum.

Epidermolysis: A condition of the epidermis that allows easy separation of its various layers, so that blisters form either spontaneously or after trauma.

Epidermotropism: The presence of mononuclear cells

in the epidermis without spongiosis, as occurs in mycosis fungoides.

Epiloia: An acronym for tuberous sclerosis that designates epilepsy, low intelligence, and adenoma sebaceum.

Epithelioma: Any tumor derived from epithelium.

Eponychium: Commonly called the cuticle, it is a narrow band of epidermis that extends from the nail wall onto the nail surface.

Erosion: A shallow ulcer that involves only the epidermis and heals without scarring.

Eruption: Visible changes of the skin due to some abnormal state.

Erysipelas: Infection of the skin and subcutaneous tissue caused by *Streptococcus pyogenes* and marked by redness and swelling with rapid spread.

Erysipeloid: A skin infection caused by *Erysipelothrix rhusiopathiae* that usually begins in a wound and remains localized, rarely becoming generalized and systemic.

Erythema: Redness of the skin produced by congestion of capillaries, which may occur from a variety of causes.

Erythroderma: Redness over wide areas of the body.

Eschar: Necrotic crusted skin produced by thermal injury, corrosive agents, or gangrene.

Exfoliative: Characterized by diffuse scaling.

Factitial: Produced by artificial means.

Fibrillar: Pertaining to minute fibers or filaments that are often components of a compound fiber.

Fibroma: A tumor composed mainly of fibrous or mature connective tissue.

Figurate: Having a geometric, arcuate, annular, or circular pattern.

Filiform: Thread-shaped.

Fissure: A crack or split in the skin.

Fixed drug eruption: A localized drug eruption that recurs in the skin at the same anatomic site.

Flaccid: Lacking firmness; soft, lax.

Flap: A section of full-thickness skin with a blood supply that is surgically transferred to an adjacent or distant part of the body as a skin graft.

Flush: Transient redness and warmth primarily of the face and neck associated with certain medications and pathologic conditions.

Foam cell: A histiocyte that has imbibed lipids and appears to contain bubbles. Foam cells are seen in many xanthomatous conditions.

Follicle: A sac, cavity, or pouchlike depression.

Freckle: A brownish pigmented macule on the skin due to localized accumulation of melanin as a result of the stimulant effect of sunlight acting on clusters of melanocytes that have a higher than normal tyrosinase activity.

Fulguration: Destruction of tissue by electric sparks generated by a high-frequency current.

Fungus: A phylum of plants, including yeasts, rusts, molds, smuts, mushrooms, etc, characterized by the absence of chlorophyll and the presence of a rigid cell wall composed of chitin, mannans, and cellulose.

Furuncle: A skin infection caused by bacteria that enter through the hair follicles and form a painful pus-filled nodule.

Fusiform: Spindle-shaped (a pointed ellipse).

Gamma globulins: Serum proteins with slow mobility in electrophoresis that comprise the majority of immunoglobulins and antibodies.

Gammopathy: A lymphoproliferative disorder characterized by abnormal quantities or types of immunoglobulins.

Gangrene: Necrosis and death of tissue, usually considerable, generally associated with loss of vascular supply and followed by bacterial invasion and putrefaction.

Gel: A jellylike, clear vehicle that usually contains volatile solvents which evaporate quickly when applied to the skin.

Genodermatosis: A genetically determined disorder of the skin.

Geographic tongue: A disorder of the tongue that consists of white lines and plaques that move about and resemble the borders of political divisions on a map.

Glossitis: Inflammation of the tongue.

Glossodynia: Pain in the tongue.

Goeckerman regimen: An intensive treatment regimen for psoriasis using ultraviolet light and tar ointments.

Gooseflesh: Perifollicular papulation of the skin caused by cold or strong emotion.

Graft-versus-host reaction: The clinical and pathologic sequelae of immunocompetent lymphocytes from a donor reacting against cells of a recipient.

Granular: Consisting of or marked by the presence of granules or grains.

Granuloma: A chronic proliferative lesion containing lymphocytes, monocytes, macrophages, and either epithelioid cells or multinucleated giant cells or both.

Grenz rays: Very soft Roentgen rays having electromagnetic vibrations of wavelength about 0.2 nm, lying in the electromagnetic spectrum between Roentgen rays and ultraviolet rays.

Grenz zone: A border zone of uninvolved connective tissue separating the epidermis from a dermal cellular infiltrate.

Guttate: Drop-shaped.

Gyrate: Spiral-shaped.

Haloderma: Any skin eruption caused by ingestion of a halide.

Hamartoma: A benign tumor-like nodule composed of an overgrowth of normal mature cells and tissues.

Hangnail: A small torn piece of eponychium on the proximal or lateral nail fold.

Haplotype: The portion of the genotype determined by genes of a single chromosome inherited from one parent.

Hapten: A substance not itself immunogenic that can become an antigen by binding to a carrier protein.

Head louse: A wingless bloodsucking insect that is a human parasite of the head and scalp. This louse is responsible for pediculosis capitis.

Helper T cells: A subtype of T lymphocytes that induce B cells to differentiate.

Hemangioma: A benign tumor composed of blood vessels.

Hematoma: A localized accumulation of blood, usually clotted, in tissue, an organ, or a space, caused by a rupture in a blood vessel wall.

Hematoxylin: A crystalline stain obtained by extracting logwood with ether and used as a stain in microscopy.

Hemosiderin: An insoluble form of storage iron that is visible microscopically both with and without specific stains.

Herald patch: The initial erythematous scaling macule of pityriasis rosea. It may occur days before the eruption becomes generalized.

Herpes: Inflammatory skin diseases characterized by spreading or creeping small clustered vesicles.

Heterochromia: Diversity of color in a part or parts that should normally be of one color.

Hidradenitis: Inflammation of a (usually apocrine) sweat gland.

Histamine: A bioactive amine that causes smooth muscle contraction of human bronchioles and small blood vessels, increased permeability of capillaries, and increased secretion by nasal and bronchial mucous glands.

Histiocyte: Macrophage.

Hives: An eruption consisting of transient edematous papules and plaques. Same as urticaria.

HLA: The major histocompatibility genetic region in humans.

Hordeolum (sty): A localized, purulent, inflammatory staphylococcal infection of one or more sebaceous glands of the eyelids.

Horn: A pointed projection.

Humectant: A moistening substance.

Hutchinson's freckle: Lentigo maligna.

Hydropic degeneration: Damage to the cells of the basal layer, which produces tiny spaces or vacuoles in the cells.

Hypergranulosis: An increase in the number of keratinocytes in the granular layer, often associated with orthokeratosis.

Hyperhidrosis: Excessive sweating.

Hyperkeratosis: Hypertrophy of the stratum corneum.

Hyperpigmentation: Abnormally increased pigmentation.

Hyperplasia: An increase in the number of keratocytes that results in a thickened epidermis.

Hypersensitivity: A state of altered reactivity in which the body reacts with an exaggerated response to a foreign agent.

Hypertrichosis: Excessive growth of hair.

Hypertrophic scar: An enlarged or thickened scar.

Hypertrophy: An increase in size of keratinocytes that leads to a thickening of the epidermis.

Hypha: One of the filaments composing the mycelium of a fungus.

Hypogranulosis: A decrease in the number of keratinocytes in the granular layer.

Hyponychium: The thickened epidermis underneath the free distal end of the nail.

Hypoplasia: A decrease in the number of keratinocytes that results in a thinned epidermis.

Ichthyosis: Any of several generalized skin disorders characterized by dry, rough, scaling skin, which occurs as a result of excessive production or retention of keratinocytes or a molecular defect in keratinization.

Idiotype: A unique antigenic determinant of an immunoglobulin or antibody representing the antigen-binding site.

Immediate hypersensitivity: An immunologic reaction mediated by antibodies (especially IgE) and products released from mast cells minutes after the antigen combines with its appropriate antibody.

Immune complexes: Antigen-antibody complexes.

Impetigo: A superficial infection of the skin.

Indirect immunofluorescence: A technique for detecting antibodies in fluids. The fluid (usually serum) is incubated with a normal substrate and then overlaid with fluorescent conjugated anti-immunoglobulin. The substrate is then viewed microscopically under ultraviolet light.

Integument: The skin.

Interferon: A heterogeneous group of low-molecular-weight proteins elaborated by infected host cells that protect noninfected cells from viral infection.

Interleukin-1: A macrophage-derived factor that triggers proliferation of T cells.

Interleukin-2: A lymphocyte-derived factor that promotes long-term proliferation of T cells. Also called T cell growth factor.

Intertrigo: Skin inflammation occurring on apposed surfaces of skin such as the creases of the neck, the axillae, the folds of the groin, and beneath the breasts.

Iododerma: Any skin eruption resulting from iodine or iodide ingestion.

Irritant: An agent that produces irritation.

Isoantibody: An antibody capable of reacting with an antigen derived from a member of the same species as that in which it is raised.

Jarisch-Herxheimer reaction: A reaction following treatment of syphilis and other intracellular infections, caused by the release of large amounts of antigenic material into the circulation.

J chain: A glycopeptide chain that aids assembly of polymeric immunoglobulins, particularly IgA and IgM.

Jock itch: Tinea cruris.

Kappa chain: One of 2 types of light chains forming immunoglobulins.

Keloid: A sharply elevated, progressively enlarging scar composed of excessive amounts of collagen.

Keratin: A very insoluble protein that contains high amounts of sulfur. It is the principal constituent of epidermis, hair, nails, and horny tissues and forms the organic matrix of tooth enamel.

Keratoacanthoma: A rapidly growing papule with a central crater filled with keratinous material that is often difficult and sometimes impossible to distinguish from shallowly invasive squamous cell carcinomas.

Keratoderma: A skin disorder characterized by diffuse thickening of the stratum corneum on the palms and soles.

Keratohyaline granules: Deeply basophilic, irregularly shaped granules present in the granular layer of the epidermis.

Keratolysis: Dissolution of the stratum corneum.

Kerion: A nodular, boggy, exudative, circumscribed tumefaction covered with pustules and caused by a dermatophytic fungus.

Koebner's phenomenon: Lesions typical of skin disease induced by trauma eg, psoriasis.

Koilonychia: A dystrophy in which nails are thin and concave, with raised edges. Also called spoon nails.

Laceration: A torn, ragged wound.

Lamella: A thin plate.

Langerhans' cell: A dendritic cell present in the skin that plays an important role in antigen presentation.

Langer's lines: Lines of cleavage of the skin determined by the position and orientation of collagen bundles and elastic fibers.

Lanugo: The fine hair on the body of the fetus.

Laser: An acronym for light amplification by stimulated emission of radiation. An instrument that transforms light of various frequencies into a nondivergent beam of monochromatic radiation that can mobilize immense heat and power when focused at close range and can be used as a tool in diagnosis, physiologic studies, and surgical procedures.

Latrodectus mactans: Black widow spider.

Lentigo: A pigmented macule on the skin.

Leukemid: Any skin eruption associated with leukemia.

Leukonychia: Whitish discoloration of the nails.

Leukotriene: A vasodilatory lipoxygenase metabolite of arachidonic acid.

Levamisole: An anthelmintic drug with possible immunostimulatory capabilities.

Lichenification: Thickening of the epidermis with exaggeration of its normal markings.

Liniment: An oily liquid preparation.

Lipoma: A benign tumor composed of mature fat cells.

Livedo reticularis: A peripheral vascular condition characterized by a reddish blue netlike mottling of the skin, usually on the extremities.

Lotion: A liquid suspension or dispersion for external application to the body.

Loxosceles reclusa: The brown recluse spider.

Lues: An old term for syphilis.

Lunula: The visible portion of the nail matrix that forms a small whitish crescent.

Lymphokines: Soluble products of lymphocytes that act as mediators.

Lysosomes: Granules that contain hydrolytic enzymes and are present in the cytoplasm of many cells.

Macerate: To soften by wetting or soaking.

Macule: A nonpalpable flat area of skin that is different in color or texture from surrounding skin and less than 1–2 cm in diameter.

Malignant: Cancerous.

Mast cell: A tissue cell that can release mediators such as histamine.

Mastocytosis: An abnormal accumulation of mast cells.

Mees' lines: Single or multiple white transverse bands on the nails; a sign of inorganic arsenic poisoning, septicemia, or acute or chronic renal failure.

Melanocyte: A dendritic cell normally present in the basal cell layer of the epidermis and the hair matrix. Has the ability to form melanin through the enzymatic oxidation of tyrosine.

Melanonychia: Darkening of the nail by melanin pigmentation.

Mesoderm: The middle layer of the 3 primary germ layers of the embryo, lying between the ectoderm and the entoderm.

Milia: Small superficially located white cysts 1–2 mm in diameter.

Mites: A group of arthropods related to spiders, usually having transparent or semitransparent bodies.

Mole: A nevus composed of melanocytes.

Monilethrix: A disorder of hair shafts in which the hairs exhibit multiple constrictions so that the hair looks like a string of beads.

Morbilliform: Resembling the eruption of measles.

Morgan's line: A secondary crease commonly seen on the lower eyelids of patients with atopic dermatitis.

Mucin: A mucopolysaccharide or glycoprotein.

Munro's abscess: A microabscess composed of neutrophil fragments in the parakeratotic layer in psoriasis.

Mycosis: Any disease caused by a fungus.

Mycosis fungoides: A form of cutaneous T cell lymphoma, usually of malignant T helper cells. In its tumor stage, the lesions resemble mushrooms, a kind of fungus.

Myiasis: A condition caused by infestation by fly maggots.

Myxedema: A condition characterized by a dry, waxy type of swelling, with abnormal mucin deposits in the skin and other tissues, and frequently associated with thyroid disease.

Nail: The horny cutaneous plate on the dorsal surface of the distal end of a finger or toe.

Necrobiosis: Degeneration of collagen bundles within the dermis where there is loss of normal structure but not true necrosis. These changes are often seen in granuloma annulare and necrobiosis lipoidica diabeticorum.

Necrosis: Local death of cells.

Neurodermatitis: A general term for a dermatosis caused by scratching.

Neurofibroma: A tumor of Schwann cells.

Nevus: A circumscribed stable hamartomatous malformation of the skin with an excess or deficiency of normal epidermal, connective, adnexal, nervous, or vascular tissue.

Nevus pigmentosus: A benign tumor composed of melanocytes.

Nit: The egg of a louse.

Node: A small mass of tissue in the form of a swelling or protuberance.

Nodule: A deep solid mass usually 1–4 cm in diameter.

Nucha: The nape or back of the neck.

Oil: A greasy-feeling liquid usually composed of long-chain hydrocarbons.

Ointment: A greasy-feeling solid usually composed of long-chain hydrocarbons.

Onychauxis: Overgrowth or thickening of the nail.

Onychodystrophy: Malformation of a nail.

Onychogryphosis: A curved overgrowth of the nails.

Onycholysis: Loosening or separation of all or part of a nail from its bed.

Onychomalacia: Softening of the nails.

Onychomycosis: Fungal disease of the nails.

Onychorrhexis: Spontaneous splitting or breaking of the nails.

Orthokeratosis: Normal keratinization.

Pachyonychia: Thickened nails.

Paint: A pharmaceutical preparation in which evaporation of the vehicle leaves a hard film containing the active ingredient.

Panniculitis: Inflammation of the subcutaneous layer of fat tissue.

Papilla: A small elevation in the shape of a nipple.

Papilloma: A benign tumor of the epithelium with a nipple shape on a broad base.

Papule: A raised skin lesion less than 1–2 cm in diameter.

Parakeratosis: Abnormal cornification marked by keratinocyte nuclei in the stratum corneum.

Paronychia: Inflammation of the tissues around the nails.

Paste: A mixture of a powder and an ointment.

Patch: A flat area of skin that is different in color and texture from the surrounding skin and is larger than 3–4 cm in diameter.

Patch test: A means of reproducing allergic contact dermatitis by placing a suspected allergen in contact with unbroken skin for 48 hours. Positive reactions show redness and vesicles.

Pathergy: 1. Abnormal reactivity. 2. Multiple allergies.

Pautrier's abscesses: Small collections of leukocytes, or microabscesses, found in the epidermis of mycosis fungoides.

Pediculosis: Louse infestation.

Pemphigoid: A subepidermal bullous eruption resembling but distinct from pemphigus.

Pemphigus: A chronic intraepidermal bullous eruption.

Periderm: The outer of the 2 layers of fetal epithelium that generally disappears before birth and persists only as the cuticle.

Periodic acid-Schiff (PAS) stain: A stain consisting of periodic acid, which oxidizes hydroxyl groups to aldehydes, and Schiff's reagent, which reacts with aldehydes, giving a red product. Used to test for fungi.

Perlèche: Inflammation of the angles of the mouth.

Petechia: A minute spot resulting from intradermal or submucous capillary hemorrhage.

Phagedenic ulcer: An ulcer that spreads rapidly, consuming tissues and sloughing particles in the discharge.

Phakomatoses: Genetic conditions with both cutaneous and neuroectodermal anomalies, eg, neurofibromatosis, tuberous sclerosis, encephalo-trigeminal angiomatosis, and cerebroretinal angiomatosis.

Phlebectasia: Abnormal venous dilatation.

Phlegmon: Intense inflammation of connective tissue, often causing ulceration or abscess formation.

Photoallergy: Reaction to substances rendered allergenic by exposure to light or ultraviolet radiation.

Photodermatitis: Skin inflammation caused by light or ultraviolet radiation.

Photophytodermatitis: Skin inflammation caused by plant products on the skin activated by light or ultraviolet radiation.

Photosensitivity: An abnormal sensitivity of the skin to light or ultraviolet radiation.

Phototoxic: Pertaining to injury by ultraviolet radiation or light.

Phrynoderma: A papular eruption with perifollicular hyperkeratosis seen in severe vitamin A deficiency. Also called toad skin.

Piebaldism: A condition of 2-toned skin, white and black or brown.

Pilar: Pertaining to the hair.

Pitted nails: Small depressions of the nail plates, as seen in psoriasis.

Plasma cells: Cells derived from B lymphocytes that synthesize immunoglobulins and have an ellipsoid shape with one eccentrically placed nucleus.

Poikiloderma: Pigmentary and atrophic changes of skin causing a dappled or mottled appearance.

Poliosis: Gray hair.

Polymorphous: Having many forms.

Pompholyx: A vesicular eruption of the hands or feet of uncertain cause.

Pore: The opening of a sweat duct.

Porokeratosis: Hypertrophy of the stratum corneum around the ducts of the sweat glands or circumscribing small areas of skin.

Porphyria: A group of diseases resulting from abnormalities in porphyrin metabolism and marked by increased formation and excretion of porphyrins or their precursors.

Poultice: A moist mass applied to an area of skin to give moist heat.

Powder: A fine particulate material.

Prickly heat: A common term for miliaria rubra, a pruritic eruption resulting from obstruction of the sweat gland ducts.

Properdin pathway: See Alternative complement pathway.

Prurigo: Several itchy skin eruptions consisting of dome-shaped papules, vesicles, and crusts.

Pruritus: Itching.

Pseudopelade: An inflammatory condition of the scalp resulting in loss of hair and scarring. Distinct from alopecia areata, in which there is no scarring.

Psoriasiform: Like psoriasis. Clinically, a sharply marginated plaque with thick scales; histologically, a pattern characterized by hyperkeratosis, acanthosis, elongation of the rete pegs, and an inflammatory filtrate.

Pulex irritans: The common flea that attacks humans.

Purpura: A purple papule resulting from hemorrhage into tissues.

Pus: A liquid consisting of leukocytes, necrotic tissue, and edema fluid, the product of inflammation.

Pustule: An elevated skin lesion (typically < 1 cm) containing pus.

Pyoderma: A purulent condition of the skin.

Quartz lamp: A vacuum lamp of melted quartz glass used as a source of ultraviolet radiation.

Radiodermatitis: Inflammation resulting from exposure to ionizing radiation.

Rash: Skin eruption.

RAST: Radioallergosorbent test. A radioimmunoassay for detecting IgE antibody directed against specific allergens.

Raynaud's phenomenon: Intermittent attacks of severe blanching of the digits brought on by exposure to cold.

Rete ridges: Downward projection of epidermis at the dermal-epidermal junction, resembling a network of ridges.

Rheumatoid factor: An anti-IgG antibody present in the serum of patients with rheumatoid diseases.

Rhinophyma: Redness, sebaceous hyperplasia, and nodular swelling of the skin of the nose. A form of rosacea.

Rhus: Botanical genus including species commonly termed poison ivy, poison oak, and poison sumac.

Ringworm: A group of fungal skin diseases caused by dermatophytes and resulting in ring-shaped pigmented patches.

Rodent ulcer: A basal cell epithelioma that has become large and eroded.

Rosacea: A chronic inflammatory condition of the face marked by redness, telangiectasia, and acnelike pustules.

Rubor: Redness.

Sarcoma: A malignant neoplasm of mesodermal origin.

Scab: A crust that forms on superficial wounds of the skin.

Scabies: Infestation with *Sarcoptes scabiei*.

Scar: A lesion of fibrous tissue covered by atrophic epidermis remaining after healing of a wound.

Scarlatiniform: Resembling scarlatina, the delicate red exanthem of scarlet fever.

Scleroderma: An indurated condition of the skin. Caused by a thickened tissue layer as seen in systemic sclerosis and morphea.

Sclerosis: Induration or hardening.

Scratch: A mark resulting from the linear stroking of the skin with fingernails or a sharp instrument.

Seborrhea: Excessive secretion of sebum.

Sebum: The product of the sebaceous gland, a mixture of fatty acids, glycerides, phosphatides, and epithelial debris.

Serpiginous: Having a wavy or snakelike margin.

Serum sickness: A hypersensitivity reaction mediated by antigen-antibody complexes, consisting of fever, adenopathy, and vasculitis.

Shake lotion: A suspension of powder in a liquid, such as water or oil.

Shingles: Herpes zoster.

Shwartzman phenomenon: A severe reaction with tissue necrosis resulting from injection of killed microorganisms or toxins into the skin, followed by intravenous injection of filtrates of that or a different microorganism or toxin.

Sinus: A cavity or channel.

Skin: The outer covering of the body, consisting of dermis, epidermis, subcutaneous fat, and appendages.

Solution: A liquid containing ionized particles.

Sore: A common term for a lesion of the skin or mucous membranes.

Spirochete: A spiral-shaped microorganism of the order Spirochaetales.

Spongiosis: Intercellular edema of the epidermis, giving the area a spongy appearance.

Squamous cell: A flat cell lying between the basal and granular cell layers of the epidermis.

Sting: An injury caused by a plant or animal toxin introduced into the skin by mechanical trauma.

Stratum corneum: The most superficial layer of the epidermis, consisting of dead cells.

Stratum germinativum: The bottom layer of the epidermis, consisting of a single layer of dividing cells.

Stratum granulosum: The epidermal cell layer just below the stratum lucidum, consisting of 2 or 3 rows of cells containing keratohyaline granules.

Stratum lucidum: The epidermal cell layer between the stratum corneum and the stratum granulosum.

Stratum malpighii: The major layer of the epidermis, consisting of 6–10 rows of keratinocytes.

Stria: A streak or line.

Sty: See Hordeolum.

Subacute: Between acute and chronic.

Subcorneal: Just under the stratum corneum.

Subepidermal: Just under the epidermis.

Subungual: Just under the nail plate.

Sunburn: Skin injury with redness, tenderness, and sometimes blistering after excessive exposure to sunlight, produced by ultraviolet rays in the range of 280–320 nm.

Suppressor T cells: A subset of T lymphocytes that suppress antibody synthesis by B cells or inhibit other immunologic effects of T cells.

Sweat gland: The glands that secrete sweat, both eccrine and apocrine.

Swimmer's itch: An itching dermatitis caused by schistosome bites.

Syngeneic: Having identical genotypes.

Systematized: Referring to diseases or lesions that are widespread and arranged in an orderly fashion.

Tattoo: The deposition of exogenous pigments into the skin or mucous membranes, either intentionally or accidentally.

Telangiectasia: Dilatation of a small group of blood vessels.

Telogen: The resting or quiescent stage of the hair cycle.

Thèque: An island of melanin-producing cells situated at the dermal-epidermal junction or within the dermis.

Thrush: A superficial fungal infection of the mucous membranes of the mouth.

Tincture: A pharmaceutical preparation consisting of an alcohol solution.

Tinea: Superficial fungal infection of the skin.

Trichauxis: An increase in the size and number of hairs.

Trichiasis: Ingrown eyelashes.

Trichotillomania: A habit or compulsion to pull out one's own hair.

Trombicula: A genus of mites that can infest humans.

Tumefaction: A swelling.

Tumor: A swelling.

Tunga penetrans: A species of fleas found in tropical and subtropical America, commonly referred to as jiggers, sand flies, or chigoes.

Turban tumor: Multiple benign cylindromas covering the scalp.

Tylosis: Callus formation.

Tyndall light phenomenon: The reflection of light by particles suspended in a gas or liquid that imparts a blue tinge to objects in the dermis seen through the epidermis.

Tzanck test: Examination of cells from the floor of a vesicle.

Ulcer: A local defect on the surface of tissue caused by sloughing of necrotic material.

Ulerythema: An erythematous skin disease resulting in atrophy and scarring.

Ungual: Relating to the nail.

Unna's boot: An occlusive dressing of gelatin and zinc oxide paste applied to the foot and leg.

Urticaria: A skin condition characterized by wheals and itching.

Urticaria pigmentosa: Conglomerates of mast cells forming brown macules or plaques that become pruritic and urticated when irritated.

Vaccinia: A viral disease of cattle (cowpox) inoculated in humans to produce an antibody against smallpox.

Vacuolization: The formation of small spaces or vacuoles.

Variola: Smallpox.

Vasculitis: Necrotizing inflammation of blood vessels.

Vegetans: Growing lushly profusely (said of lesions).

Vellus: Fine hairs.

Venereal: Transmitted by sexual contact.

Verruca: An epidermal proliferation of viral cause.

Versicolor: Of many colors.

Vitiligo: Destruction of melanocytes in circumscribed areas of skin, resulting in depigmented patches.

Wart: An epidermal excrescence of viral or nonviral origin.

Weeping: Exudation of clear serum from a superficial inflammation of the epidermis.

Wheal: A smooth, elevated area of urticaria (hives) that is usually evanescent and pruritic.

Whitehead: A superficial pustule or milium.

Whitlow: A felon or abscess on the terminal phalanx of a finger.

Wickham's striae: A pale network of lines on the surface of the papules of lichen planus.

Winter itch: Xerosis and pruritus related to the winter season.

Wood's light: An ultraviolet lamp that emits long-wave ultraviolet radiation causing fluorescence in certain conditions, eg, fungal infections.

Wrinkle: A crease or furrow.

Xanthelasma: A cholesterol-containing yellow plaque on the eyelid.

Xanthoderma: Yellow discoloration of the skin.

Xanthoma: A yellow papule, nodule, or plaque of the skin.

Xerosis: Abnormal dryness of the skin.

Zoonosis: A disease communicated to humans by an animal.

Zosteriform: Following the distribution of a peripheral sensory nerve.

Index

Note: Page numbers in bold face type indicate a major discussion. A *t* following a page number indicates tabular material and an *f* following a page number indicates an illustration. Insofar as possible, drugs and chemical agents are listed under their generic or common names, and a cross reference is provided for the trade name.